NEONATOLOGY

Pathophysiology and
Management of the Newborn

NEONATOLOGY
Second Edition

Pathophysiology and Management of the Newborn

Edited by

GORDON B. AVERY, M.D., Ph.D.

Professor of Child Health and Development
George Washington University School of Medicine
Director, Division of Neonatology
Children's Hospital National Medical Center
Washington, DC

with 71 Contributors

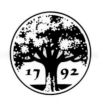

J. B. Lippincott Company
PHILADELPHIA   TORONTO

Second Edition

Copyright © 1981, by J. B. Lippincott Company. All rights reserved. No part of this book may be used or reproduced in any manner whatsoever without written permission except in the case of brief quotations embodied in critical articles and reviews. Printed in the United States of America. For information address J. B. Lippincott Company, East Washington Square, Philadelphia, Pennsylvania 19105

3   5   6   4

Library of Congress Cataloging in Publication Data

Main entry under title:

Neonatology: Pathophysiology and Management of the Newborn.

Bibliography
Includes index.
1. Infants (Newborn)—Diseases.   2.   Neonatology.
1.   Avery, Gordon B. [DNLM: 1.   Infant, Newborn, Diseases—Physiopathology.   2.   Infant, Newborn, Diseases—Therapy.   WS420 N441]
RJ254.N46   1981   618.92′01   80-21992
ISBN 0-397-50429-2

The authors and publisher have exerted every effort to ensure that drug selection and dosage set forth in this text are in accord with current recommendations and practice at the time of publication. However, in view of ongoing research, changes in government regulations, and the constant flow of information relating to drug therapy and drug reactions, the reader is urged to check the package insert for each drug for any change in indications and dosage and for added warnings and precautions. This is particularly important when the recommended agent is a new or infrequently employed drug.

To
HOWARD HOLTZER, who taught me science
    and
THOMAS E. CONE, JR., who taught me pediatrics

Contents

II   THE FETAL PATIENT

III   TRANSITION AND STABILIZATION

IV   THE NEWBORN INFANT

Contributors

R. Peter Altman, M.D.
Professor of Surgery
Columbia Presbyterian College of Physicians and
  Surgeons; and
Chief, Division of Pediatric Surgery
Babies' Hospital
Columbia Presbyterian Medical Center
New York, New York

Charles A. Alford, Jr., M.D.
Meyer Professor of Pediatric Research
Department of Pediatrics
University of Alabama in Birmingham
School of Medicine
Birmingham, Alabama

Kathryn D. Anderson, M.D.
Associate Professor of Surgery and of Child Health and
  Development
George Washington University School of Medicine; and
Senior Attending Surgeon
Children's Hospital National Medical Center
Washington, DC

Gordon B. Avery, M.D., Ph.D.
Professor of Child Health and Development
George Washington University School of Medicine; and
Director, Division of Neonatology
Children's Hospital National Medical Center
Washington, DC

Joseph A. Bellanti, M.D.
Professor of Pediatrics and Microbiology and
Director, International Center for Interdisciplinary
  Studies of Immunology
Georgetown University School of Medicine
Washington, DC

A. Barry Belman, M.D.
Professor of Urology and Child Health and Development
George Washington University School of Medicine; and
Chairman, Department of Urology
Children's Hospital National Medical Center
Washington, DC

Diane V. Bernstein, R.N.
Associate Clinical Unit Coordinator
Children's Hospital National Medical Center
Washington, DC

Attilio L. Boner, M.D.
Associate Professor of Pediatrics
University of Verona
Verona, Italy

Alfred M. Bongiovanni, B.S., M.D.
Professor of Pediatrics and of Pediatrics in Obstetrics
University of Pennsylvania School of Medicine; and
Director of Perinatal Endocrinology
Pennsylvania Hospital
Philadelphia, Pennsylvania

T. Berry Brazelton, M.D.
Chief, Child Development Unit
Children's Hospital Medical Center; and
Associate Professor of Pediatrics
Harvard Medical School
Boston, Massachusetts

Judyth Todd Brown, R.N., B.S.N.
Neonatal Nurse Clinician
Children's Hospital National Medical Center
Washington, DC

Philip L. Calcagno, M.D.
Professor and Chairman, Department of Pediatrics
Georgetown University School of Medicine
Washington, DC

Judith A. Cannon, R.N.
Transport Coordinator
Children's Hospital National Medical Center
Washington, DC

George Cassady, M.D.
Professor of Pediatrics and
Associate Professor of Obstetrics and Gynecology
University of Alabama in Birmingham
School of Medicine
Birmingham, Alabama

Richard M. Cowett, M.D.
Assistant Professor of Pediatrics
Brown University; and
Neonatologist
Women and Infants Hospital of Rhode Island
Providence, Rhode Island

Joseph Dancis, M.D.
Professor and Chairman, Department of Pediatrics
New York University School of Medicine
New York, New York

Michele M. Dombkiewicz, R.N.
Associate Clinical Unit Coordinator
Children's Hospital National Medical Center
Washington, DC

Mitzi L. Duxbury, F.A.A.N., B.S., M.A., Ph.D.
Professor of Nursing
University of Minnesota School of Nursing;
Assistant Dean for Graduate Studies and
Professor, Center for Health Services Division
Minneapolis, Minnesota

Gloria D. Eng, M.D.
Professor of Child Health and Development
George Washington University School of Medicine;
Chairman, Department of Physical Medicine and
    Rehabilitation
Children's Hospital National Medical Center
Washington, DC; and
Medical Director
Center for the Handicapped
Montgomery County, Maryland

Audrey E. Evans, M.D.
Director, Division of Oncology
Children's Hospital; and
Professor of Pediatrics
The University of Pennsylvania School of Medicine
Philadelphia, Pennsylvania

Murray Feingold, M.D.
Director, Center for Genetic Counseling and Birth
    Defect Evaluation
Tufts University School of Medicine and
Boston Floating Hospital for Infants and Children
Boston, Massachusetts

Pamela M. Fitzhardinge, M.D., F.R.C.P.(C)
Professor of Pediatrics
University of Toronto;
Associate Director of Pediatrics and
Director of the Neonatal Follow-up Program
Hospital for Sick Children
Toronto, Ontario, Canada

Anne B. Fletcher, M.D.
Director of the Nursery and
Associate Professor of Child Health and Development
George Washington University School of Medicine
Washington, DC

Roger K. Freeman, M.D.
Medical Director, Women's Hospital
Memorial Hospital Medical Center
Long Beach; and
Professor-in-Residence, Department of Obstetrics and
    Gynecology
University of California School of Medicine
Irvine, California

David S. Friendly, M.D.
Associate Professor of Ophthalmology and of Child
    Health and Development
George Washington University School of Medicine; and
Chairman, Department of Ophthalmology
Children's Hospital National Medical Center
Washington, DC

Donald C. Fyler, M.D.
Associate Professor of Pediatrics
Harvard Medical School; and
Associate Chief, Department of Cardiology
Children's Hospital Medical Center
Boston, Massachusetts

George P. Giacoia, M.D.
Associate Professor of Pediatrics;
Head, Division of Neonatology
University of Oklahoma
Tulsa Medical College; and
Director, Eastern Oklahoma Perinatal Center
Tulsa, Oklahoma

Harry H. Gordon, M.D.
Director Emeritus, Rose F. Kennedy Center for
    Research in Mental Retardation and Human
    Development; and
NARC–Grover F. Powers Professor Emeritus of
    Pediatrics
Albert Einstein College of Medicine
Yeshiva University
New York, New York

Paul P. Griffin, M.D.
Professor and Chairman, Department of Orthopedics
    and Rehabilitation
Vanderbilt University School of Medicine
Nashville, Tennessee

Joan E. Hodgman, M.D.
Professor of Pediatrics
University of Southern California School of Medicine;
    and
Director of the Newborn Division
Los Angeles County–University of Southern California
    Medical Center
Los Angeles, California

W. Alan Hodson, M.D.
Professor and Head, Division of Neonatal Biology
Department of Pediatrics
University of Washington School of Medicine
Seattle, Washington

Edward H. Hon, M.D.
Doré Professor of Obstetrics and Gynecology
Los Angeles County–University of Southern California
    Medical Center
Los Angeles, California

Mary Elizabeth L. House, R.N., B.S.N.
Neonatal Outreach Coordinator
Children's Hospital National Medical Center
Washington, DC

Y. Edward Hsia, B.M., M.R.C.P., D.C.H.
Professor of Genetics and Pediatrics
University of Hawaii School of Medicine
Honolulu, Hawaii

Pedro A. José, M.D., Ph.D.
Associate Professor and Chief, Pediatric Nephrology
Georgetown University School of Medicine
Washington, DC

Richard Koenigsberger, M.D.
Associate Professor of Neurology and Pediatrics and
Director, Division of Pediatric Neurology
College of Medicine and Dentistry of New Jersey
Newark, New Jersey

Kee S. Koh, M.D.
Assistant Clinical Professor
Los Angeles County–University of Southern California
    Medical Center
Los Angeles, California

Ernest N. Kraybill, M.D.
Associate Professor of Pediatrics and
Chief, Division of Neonatology
University of North Carolina School of Medicine
Chapel Hill, North Carolina

Peter Lang, M.D.
Instructor in Pediatrics
Harvard Medical School; and
Associate in Cardiology
Children's Hospital Medical Center
Boston, Massachusetts

Lula O. Lubchenco, M.D.
Professor Emerita, Department of Pediatrics
University of Colorado School of Medicine
University of Colorado Health Sciences Center
Denver, Colorado

M. Jeffrey Maisels, M.B., B.Ch.
Professor of Pediatrics and of Obstetrics and
    Gynecology
The Pennsylvania State University College of Medicine;
    and
Chief, Division of Newborn Medicine
The Milton S. Hershey Medical Center
Hershey, Pennsylvania

Andrew M. Marglleth, M.D.
Professor and Associate Chairman, Department of
    Pediatrics
Uniformed Services University School of Medicine; and
Attending Physician
National Naval Medical Center
Bethesda, Maryland and
Walter Reed Army Medical Center
Washington, DC

George H. McCracken, Jr., M.D.
Professor of Pediatrics
University of Texas Health Sciences Center
Southwestern Medical School; and
Attending Physician
Children's Medical Center and
Parkland Memorial Hospital
Dallas, Texas

Thomas H. Milhorat, M.D.
Professor of Surgical Neurology and of Child Health
    and Development
George Washington University School of Medicine; and
Chairman of Neurosurgery
Children's Hospital National Medical Center
Washington, DC

Thomas Moshang, Jr., M.D.
Associate Professor of Pediatrics
Hahnemann Medical College
Philadelphia, Pennsylvania

John Stephen Naulty, M.D.
Instructor in Anesthesia
Harvard Medical School; and
Senior Associate in Anesthesia
Brigham and Women's Hospitals
Boston, Massachusetts

Nicholas M. Nelson, M.D.
Professor and Chairman, Department of Pediatrics
The Pennsylvania State University College of Medicine
Milton S. Hershey Medical Center
Hershey, Pennsylvania

David J. Nochimson, M.D.
Associate Professor of Obstetrics and Gynecology and
Director, Maternal–Fetal Medicine
University of Connecticut School of Medicine
Farmington, Connecticut

William Oh, M.D.
Professor of Pediatrics and Obstetrics
Brown University Program in Medicine; and
Pediatrician-in-Chief
Women and Infants Hospital of Rhode Island
Providence, Rhode Island

Frank A. Oski, M.D.
Professor and Chairman, Department of Pediatrics
State University of New York
Upstate Medical Center
Syracuse, New York

Zoe L. Papadopoulou, M.D.
Assistant Professor and Chief, Pediatric Dialysis and
    Transplantation
Georgetown University School of Medicine
Washington, DC

Karen E. Pape, M.D., F.R.C.P.(C)
Assistant Professor of Pediatrics
University of Toronto; and
Assistant Director of the Neonatal Follow-Up Program
Hospital for Sick Children
Toronto, Ontario, Canada

Roderic H. Phibbs, M.D.
Professor of Pediatrics and
Associate, Cardiovascular Research Institute
University of California in San Francisco
San Francisco, California

Edward J. Quilligan, M.D.
Professor and Director, Division of Maternal–Fetal
    Medicine
Department of Obstetrics and Gynecology
University of California School of Medicine
Irvine, California

Judson G. Randolph, M.D.
Professor of Surgery
George Washington University School of Medicine; and
Surgeon-in-Chief
Children's Hospital National Medical Center
Washington, DC

David W. Reynolds, M.D.
Assistant Professor of Pediatrics
University of Alabama in Birmingham
School of Medicine
Birmingham, Alabama

Jeffrey G. Rosenstock, M.D.
Assistant Professor of Pediatrics
University of Pennsylvania School of Medicine; and
Director, Oncology Ambulatory Services
Children's Hospital
Philadelphia, Pennsylvania

Arnold J. Sameroff, Ph.D.
Professor of Psychology and
Associate Director of the Institute for the Study of
    Developmental Disabilities
University of Illinois at Chicago Circle
Chicago, Illinois

Jon W. Scopes, M.B., Ph.D., F.R.C.P.
Professor of Pediatrics
St. Thomas's Hospital Medical School
University of London
London, England

Sergio Stagno, M.D.
Associate Professor of Pediatrics
University of Alabama in Birmingham
School of Medicine
Birmingham, Alabama

Mildred T. Stahlman, M.D.
Professor of Pediatrics
Division of Neonatology
Vanderbilt University School of Medicine
Nashville, Tennessee

Jean J. Steichen, M.D.
Assistant Professor of Pediatrics and of Obstetrics and
    Gynecology
University of Cincinnati College of Medicine and
Children's Hospital Research Foundation
Cincinnati, Ohio

Leo Stern, M.D.
Professor and Chairman, Department of Pediatrics
Brown University; and
Pediatrician-in-Chief
Rhode Island Hospital
Providence, Rhode Island

**Paul R. Swyer, M.A., M.B. (Cantab), F.R.C.P.(C),
F.R.C.P.(Lond), D.C.H.**
Director, Division of Perinatal Medicine and
Senior Scientist, Research Institute
The Hospital for Sick Children; and
Professor, Department of Pediatrics
University of Toronto
Toronto, Ontario, Canada

Leticia U. Tina, M.D.
Associate Professor and Chief, Renal Clinic
Georgetown University School of Medicine
Washington, DC

William E. Truog, III, M.D.
Department of Pediatrics
Division of Neonatal Biology
University of Washington School of Medicine
Seattle, Washington

Reginald C. Tsang, M.B.B.S.
Professor of Pediatrics and of Obstetrics and
    Gynecology, and
Director, Diabetes in Pregnancy Program
University of Cincinnati College of Medicine and
Children's Hospital Research Foundation
Cincinnati, Ohio

Robert Usher, M.D.
Director of Neonatology
Royal Victoria Hospital
Montreal, Quebec, Canada

Joseph J. Volpe, M.D.
Professor of Pediatrics, Neurology, and Biological
    Chemistry
Washington University School of Medicine; and
Pediatric Neurologist and Neonatologist
St. Louis Children's Hospital
St. Louis, Missouri

Ruth D. Weise, R.N., M.A.
Assistant Professor of Nursing
University of Minnesota School of Nursing
Minneapolis, Minnesota

Barry Wolf, M.D., Ph.D.
Assistant Professor of Human Genetics and Pediatrics
Medical College of Virginia
Richmond, Virginia

Sumner J. Yaffe, M.D.
Professor of Pediatrics and Pharmacology
University of Pennsylvania School of Medicine; and
Director, Division of Clinical Pharmacology
Children's Hospital
Philadelphia, Pennsylvania

Preface

Neonatology, an "infant" field at the time the first edition of this book was published, has grown and developed considerably in the ensuing interval. An explosion of publications about the newborn has occupied perhaps a third of the space in pediatric journals and has left the clinician scrambling to keep up with modifications of care. The number of neonatologists has surged, as almost 200 training programs in the United States have graduated fellows who have moved into full-time positions in secondary and tertiary centers. Concern has begun to arise as to when the discipline will be saturated and graduates will no longer readily find jobs, although this time has not yet arrived. However, it has become obvious that the number of pediatric and neonatology trainees will not be sufficient to meet the need for around-the-clock bedside neonatal care supervision. Full-time physician groups, working in shifts, and neonatal nurse practitioners are among the arrangements with which institutions are experimenting to meet this need. It seems clear, however, that even small and frail infants will henceforth command the same diligent and intensive care as is afforded older children who are critically ill.

This book, in its second edition, has required extensive revision to take into account the developments of the past 5 years. Its general format and goals are nevertheless the same: to serve both as a guide to therapy and an aid to understanding the pathophysiology of diseases affecting the newborn. Six new chapters have been added. The first, on obstetric anesthesiology, reflects the increasing concern of neonatologists for the critical delivery room transition period. The second, on the behavioral characteristics of the newborn, is in keeping with a new awareness of the sensitivity of the newborn as a responsive individual. Indeed, it has recently been the lay public that has pressured the profession to provide more adequately for the humanistic aspects of childbirth. A third new chapter is written by a group of nurses and describes nursing care organization and practices in the intensive care nursery. Another new chapter details present knowledge of the outcome of follow-up of high-risk newborns, with concern for both major handicaps and for subtle perceptual and learning difficulties. The remaining two new chapters are devoted to mineral metabolism and to neonatal urology.

The neonatologist ideal for today's situation is a multitalented superman or superwoman who never sleeps. Both the scientific and intensely personal aspects of neonatal intensive care must be responded to on a case-by-case basis. But in addition, the neonatologist must coordinate a complex interdisciplinary team including nursing, social work, laboratory, respiratory therapy, pharmacy, and consulting medical and surgical specialties. Budgeting involves not only negotiations with hospital administration, but with state and federal agencies, third party payers, and fund raising through public and private grant mechanisms. Making all of these responsive to the unique needs of newborns is akin to administration of a small hospital within a hospital. With regionalization of care, these negotiation and coordination roles are further multiplied. An active interface is vital with both obstetrics and obstetric anesthesiology. Teaching, outcome feedback, and statistics-keeping must reach out to numerous referring hospitals. A transport mechanism must be created and continuously supervised and monitored. Public legislation must be followed and active participation given in the seemingly endless committees responsible for regional planning. Yet, at the same time, new techniques must be evaluated by controlled clinical trials, pathophysiology elucidated through laboratory research, publications scrutinized for new developments, and new equipment evaluated and budgeted.

Needless to say, few individuals can fill all these roles, and specialization within neonatology is beginning to occur both in areas of specific medical expertise and in administrative responsibility. However, our traditional training is biased strongly toward medical care of individual patients and is weak in many of the other areas vital to success of a program. In the future, it would be prudent for increased emphasis to be placed on administration, personnel policies, public health and epidemiology, statistics, teaching techniques, and the special skills of counseling and negotiation. Although there are aspects of these activities in other pediatric specialties, neonatology is, and will be for the forseeable future, a uniquely team-oriented discipline. It is permanently embedded in the matrix of total reproductive care, from personal hygiene and sex education, to general health and perinatal care, to high-risk obstetric clinics and delivery management, through neonatal intensive care, to follow-up and rehabilitative care of high-risk infants.

Looking to the future, certain areas of development seem likely. First, the regional perinatal care systems currently being planned and assembled will become more uniform and efficient. Persons with particular training and skills in health care systems management will be responsible for their coordination. Within individual perinatal systems, risk identification and preventive measures, including maternal transfer, will assume increasing importance. Our preoccupation will be more and more with the quality of survivors. To this end, new techniques of monitoring and management will allow care of the brain with sophistication and precision similar to that now possible with care of the lung. There are some interesting years ahead.

Gordon B. Avery, M.D., Ph.D.

Preface to the First Edition

Neonatology means knowledge of the human newborn. The term was coined by Alexander Schaffer, whose book on the subject, *Diseases of the Newborn,* was first published in 1960. This book, together with Clement Smith's *Physiology of the Newborn Infant,* formed cornerstones of the developing field. In the past 15 years, neonatology has grown from the preoccupation of a handful of pioneers to a major subspecialty of pediatrics. Knowledge in this area has so expanded that it now seems important to collect this material into a multiauthor reference work.

Although the perinatal mortality rate has declined over the past 50 years, the best presently attainable survival rates have not been achieved throughout the world, and indeed the United States lags behind 15 other countries, despite its vast resources. New knowledge and improvement in the coordination of services for mother and child are needed to drive down perinatal mortality further. And finally, far greater emphasis must be placed on morbidity, so that surviving infants can lead full and productive lives. One hopes that in the future the yardstick of success will be the quality of life and not the mere fact of life itself.

In this past decade, neonatology, as a rec-ognized subspecialty of pediatrics, has come into being around the intensive care–premature nursery. Needless to say, the problems of prematurity are far from solved. But neonatology is ripe for a broadening-out from its prematurity-hyaline membrane disease beginnings. The newborn is heir to so many problems and his physiology is so unique and rapidly changing that all conditions of the newborn should come within the concern of the new and expanding discipline of neonatology. It has long since become standard practice to admit to premature nurseries other high-risk infants such as those of diabetic or toxemic mothers. Here the criterion is the need for intensive care. However, the neonatologist's specialized knowledge should give him a significant role in the care of other infants in the first 2 to 3 months of life, whether or not they require intensive care, and whether or not they are readmitted for problems unrelated to prematurity and birth itself. Detailed knowledge of newborn physiology can assist in the management of congenital anomalies, surgical conditions of the neonate, failure to thrive, nutritional problems, genetic, neurologic and biochemical diseases, and a host of conditions involving delayed maturation. Thus one can conceive of a subspecialty sharply limited in age to early infancy, but broad in its study of the interaction of normal physiology and disease processes.

Neonatology must also grow in its relationship to obstetrics and fetal biology. In the best centers, an active partnership has developed between obstetrics and pediatrics around the management of high-risk pregnancies and newborns. Sometimes training has been cooperative, but in only a few instances have basic scientists concerned with fetal biology been brought into this effort. Important beginnings have been made in studying the fetomaternal unit, such as the endocrine studies of Egon Diczfalusy, the cardiopulmonary studies of Geoffrey Dawes, and the immunologic studies of Arthur Silverstein. But fundamental processes such as the controls of fetal growth and the onset of labor are not understood at this time. Centers or institutes bringing together workers of diverse points of view are needed to wrestle with the profound problems of fetal biology. At the clinical level, the interdependence of obstetrics and neonatology is obvious. As an ultimate development, these two specialties may one day be joined as a new entity, perinatology, at least at the level of training and certification. In the meantime, far greater mutual understanding and daily interaction are needed for the optimal care of mothers and their infants.

This book is organized around problems as they occur, as well as by organ systems. It hopes to achieve a balance between presentation of the basic science on which rational management must rest, and the advice concerning patient care which experts in each subarea are qualified to give. Individual chapter authors have approached their subjects in varying ways, and no attempt has been made to achieve a completely uniform format. In some instances, there is overlap of subject material, but the somewhat different viewpoints presented, and the desire to spare the reader hopscotching through the book after cross references, have persuaded me to leave small overlaps undisturbed.

It is appreciated that no volume such as this can have more than a finite useful lifetime. Yet while its currency lasts, I hope it will serve as a practical guide to therapy and an aid in the understanding of pathophysiology for those active in the care of newborns.

Gordon B. Avery, M.D., PH.D.

NEONATOLOGY

Pathophysiology and
Management of the Newborn

I

General
Considerations

1

Perspectives on Neonatology—1980

Harry H. Gordon

"The matter does not appear to me now as it appears to have appeared to me then."
Baron Bramwell, quoted by Supreme Court
Justice Robert Jackson

Modern practice is based on old and new, empirical and scientific observations. Experience with change over the past 50 years makes the author certain that the conventional wisdom of today will change even more rapidly, as new techniques and scientific concepts yield new "facts," and as new social forces impinge on their use. Changing sexual mores, the large number of pregnancies in adolescents, the legalization of abortions, the increasing number of mothers working outside the home, and the rise in consumerism are examples of such forces.

HISTORICAL BACKGROUND

A historical review is not the purpose of this chapter. However, the names of several giants on whose shoulders we stand have been chosen for mention: Pierre Budin, Arvo Ylppö, Albrecht Peiper, Julius Hess, Ethel Dunham, and Sir Dugald Baird.

Budin, a French obstetrician, extended his concerns beyond the delivery room to the infants whom he helped deliver. He established his first Consultation for Nurslings (the counterpart of our well-baby clinics) at the Charité Hospital in Paris in 1892, and later supervised a "special department for weaklings" estab-

lished at the Maternité by Madame Henry, the former chief midwife. His book, *The Nursling,* was translated into English by Maloney in 1907 with a stirring introduction by Sir Alexander Simpson, Emeritus Professor of Midwifery and Diseases of Women and Children, University of Edinburgh.[1] The book consists of ten lectures given to students in addition to the usual lectures in "Practical Obstetrics." He said, "I propose to study with you, successively,

1. infants born before term (*i.e.,* congenitally feeble infants).
2. infants born at term and their care in the Maternité.
3. infants after they leave the hospital."[1]

The first four chapters are devoted to the study of infants with congenital feebleness, usually, but not always, the product of premature labor. He distinguishes between those infants large- and small-for-gestational ages. He alludes to the former as doing poorly: were they born prematurely to mothers with chemical diabetes? He alludes to the latter as tiny, puny infants with great vitality who seemed never to rest: were they born to hyperthyroid mothers or were they ateliotic dwarfs, hyperactive in comparison with other babies of the same weight? Standards of intrauterine growth were not available for the clinical judgments which we now base on both birth weight and gestational age.[2,3]

In the fourth chapter, there is a plan of the Department for Weaklings at the Maternité. Couney, one of Budin's students, recognized the morbid public interest in prematurely born infants and established exhibits to which admission was charged. One of these was a Chicago exposition in 1914, and it may be no coincidence that a premature infant center was established soon thereafter by Julius Hess at the Michael Reese Hospital in Chicago.

Numerous centers were subsequently established throughout the United States by personnel who journeyed to Dr. Hess and Miss Evelyn Lundeen for instruction.[4] These centers embodied the principles of Budin, an obstetrician, and Hess, a pediatrician: segregating premature infants to assure that there would be nurses with unique temperaments and specialized training; adding facilities including incubators; and instituting strict procedures for prevention of infections. The center, established in 1947 at the University of Colorado with the aid of the U.S. Children's Bureau, was a joint project of the Departments of Obstetrics and Gynecology and Pediatrics at the University, and of the Colorado State Department of Health.[5] In addition to facilities for premature infants, beds were supplied for mothers with complications of pregnancy which might lead to premature birth, and training programs were developed jointly to be given in various parts of Colorado. Regional centers for both high-risk mothers and infants are now being established in many countries.

Budin described newborn infant feeding practices and presented numerous weight curves as criteria for adequacy of breast and supplementary feeding. Currently, short hospitalizations of newborn infants, desirable for many reasons, make such graphs rarer than the charts of typhoid fever. Budin was concerned with the maintenance of breast feeding and with detailed advice about artificial feeding when this became necessary. He recommended as a rule of thumb that infants who could not be breast fed be given cow's milk daily, amounting to 10% of their body weight. Because cow's milk contains, on the average, 3.5% protein, Budin's rule of thumb was in time converted into the protein allowance stipulated by the National Research Council Food and Nutrition Board as recently as 1953. Circularly, this became a recommendation in preparation of feeding mixtures for young infants of 100 ml cow's milk per kg/day in order to meet the protein requirements of young infants.[6]

Arvo Ylppö, leader of Finnish pediatrics for many decades, had an early interest in premature infants. Working in Charlottenburg, Germany, more than 60 years ago, he published classic monographs on the pathology, physiology, clinical findings, and growth and fate of premature infants, all subjects of continuing interest. These comprehensive reports once served as a knowledge base for pediatric practitioners, teachers, and investigators. His simple observation that the stools of prematurely born infants fed human milk were greasier than those of full-term infants was confirmed by numerous laboratory observations of decreased fat absorption. His findings have become part of conventional wisdom; some continue to be rediscovered in small and large costly studies. Many subjects of current investigation are listed in the indices to his monographs.[7,8,9] His recognition of the impact of social factors on the development of infants after leaving the nursery undoubtedly led to his emergence as the leader of social pediatrics in Finland.[10]

Albrecht Peiper, working first in Berlin and later as professor of pediatrics at the University of Leipzig, was interested in neurophysiologic maturation of prematurely born infants as early as 1924.[11] His monographs gave more emphasis to this phase of maturation than did most other publications.[12,13] In the preface to the first edition of his book, he wrote,

Ever since pediatrics first emerged as a specialty, it has particularly concerned itself with the role of diet of infancy. It has given comparatively minimal attention to the characteristics of cerebral function in infancy. . . . With few exceptions, even the neurologists have not paid heed to the emergence of brain function, since they usually deal with adults, seldom with children, only under exceptional circumstances with infants.[14]

One of the brightest features of the current scene is the great expansion of interest in developmental neurobiology, mostly, it must be admitted, outside departments of pediatrics.

Peiper's monograph on disorders of respiration in premature infants addressed itself particularly to the relation of the clinical manifestations to the function of the nervous system. He described respiratory distress syndrome (RDS) and noted that he had seen it in prematurely born infants without pneumonia.

Ethel C. Dunham made her major contributions to neonatology during the years 1919 to 1949, which she spent in the Department of Pediatrics at Yale and as director of the Division of Research in Child Development of the U.S. Children's Bureau in Washington. These contributions were recognized in her receipt of the John Howland Medal of the American Pediatric Society in 1957.[15] Her book, *Premature Infants, A Manual for Physicians,* subsequently revised by Silverman, has been an invaluable asset for all who wish to learn about the newborn.[16] On the flyleaf, she used an inscription from Ballantyne:

In writing this book, I have honestly tried to avoid the four grounds of human ignorance set forth so long ago by Roger Bacon: trust in inadequate authority, the force of custom, the opinion of the inexperienced crowd, and hiding of one's own ignorance with the parading of a superficial wisdom.[17]

It was particularly appropriate that Silverman, who succeeded Dunham as author of the book, was a leader in establishing the use of the carefully controlled trial in the premature nursery.[18]

Mimeographed sheets, prepared with colleagues at the Children's Bureau, became the basis of one of the best-known publications of the American Academy of Pediatrics: *Standards and Recommendations for Hospital Care of Newborn Infants, Full Term and Preterm.* Her good-humored tolerance of the foibles of colleagues from different disciplines made her an effective advocate of increased teamwork among obstetrician, pediatrician, biostatistician, pathologist, nurse, social worker, and public health administrator, all for the sake of mothers and newborn infants. She lifted this author's sights far above narrow interest in the metabolism of prematurely born infants to include, on the one hand, Needham's interest in chemical embryology and Barcroft's interest in fetal circulation and respiration, and on the other, concern with their social and public health problems.

The original legislative charge to the Children's Bureau was to "study and report" on matters pertaining to children. Dr. Dunham's early interest in clinical problems of the newborn led her to emphasize the importance of a continuing federal monitor of data on mortality of newborn infants. This served as a base for federal policy, reflected in later legislation, which increased support of maternal and infant care services, as well as support of perinatal and neonatal research. The disparities she noted in different socioeconomic strata of the country continue to spur those concerned with the fate of children.

Sir Dugald Baird, currently Professor Emeritus of Obstetrics and Gynecology at the University of Aberdeen, established the Obstetric Medicine Research Unit and its successor, the Medical Social Research Unit, with the support of the British Research Council. The relative uniformity of obstetrical services supplied by the University department to women in all social strata, the good records, the welcomed participation of members of disciplines other than medicine (*e.g.,* sociology, behavioral science, education, and biostatistics), and the relative stability of the population permitted long-term follow-up and more precise isolation of the impact of socioeconomic factors on outcome. Using maternal height within social class as an index of previous health, he stressed the importance of considering reproduction in the context of the whole life cycle (*i.e.,* of health and nutrition during early childhood and adolescence as well as during pregnancy).[19,20,21] He saw children who became parents and their children who became parents as continuous developmental units, a broad point of view neglected by most obstetricians and pediatricians.

Improved collaboration of obstetrician and pediatrician is apparently possible, as exemplified in the growth of the subspecialty of perinatology. Alfred Beck's simple maxim that "the purpose of pregnancy is a happy, healthy baby" is not reflected, however, in widespread mutually respectful relations between practicing obstetricians and pediatricians, perhaps as a reflection of the differences in personality which lead physicians to their choice of specialty.[22] *The American Journal of Obstetrics and Gynecology* was known, as late as 1920, as *The American Journal of Diseases of Women and Children,* but it is now impossible to interest directors of training programs in assigning obstetric house officers to nurseries to follow the course of newborn infants, or pediatric house officers to the antenatal clinic to learn of mothers' anxieties.

THE DEVELOPMENT OF PERINATAL MEDICINE

The rapid rate of development of the prematurely born infant and his diminished "factor of safety" in the function of various organs and systems have always made study of the premature infant a treasure trove for new information in human biology.[23] Clement Smith's book, *The Physiology of the Newborn Infant,* helped to delineate the neonate's ability to maintain extrauterine homeostasis and supplied guidelines for practical application.[24]

In this country, during the third and fourth decades of the century, limited support for research came from the Children's Bureau and private foundations. This was increased in the 1950s by the National Institutes of Health which instituted a study section on human embryology and development, a developmental biology training grants committee, and a large collaborative study of perinatal morbidity. In 1962, the National Institute of Child Health and Human Development was created to foster, *inter alia,* specific research programs in the fields of maternal health, perinatal biology, and mental retardation. Furthermore, the report of President Kennedy's Panel on Mental Retardation resulted in increased funds, not only for research, but also for establishment of centers for high-risk infants and for maternal and infant care. In other countries, national health and other social welfare plans had earlier permitted the establishment of centers for high-risk mothers and infants, and these were used for productive clinical studies without the benefit of the extensive research funds available in the United States. Subsequent chapters in this book will detail the great advances in care resulting from basic and applied research in many countries. The remainder of this chapter will touch on some of the changes in care, and on some old and new problems.

Neonatal Intensive Care. The most striking change has been the conversion of the relatively quiet centers for prematurely born infants into bustling intensive care units for high-risk infants, regardless of gestational age or birth weight. The earlier premature-infant cen-

ter supplied specialized but essentially domiciliary care. Its provisions met the peculiar needs of tenants who had been forced to vacate prematurely their warm, dark, and watery premises in which the maternal organism maintained body temperature, supplied nutrition, excreted wastes, and protected against infection and psychological trauma. In the premature center, body temperature was maintained by swaddling, hot water bottles, or heat lamps and then by incubators, the latter ultimately so refined as to respond automatically to changes in the infant's skin temperature. The importance of maintenance of body temperature was generally accepted on empirical grounds, although the possibility of individual levels of control had been discussed. The introduction of hypothermia into cardiac surgery raised some questions about possible benefits of hypothermia for the hypoxia of premature infants. The question was decisively answered in the negative by the exemplary clinical trials of Silverman, Day, and their colleagues.

In former nursery practice, the clinical problems of respiration—spontaneous attacks of apnea, irregular respiration, cyanosis, and respiratory distress—were attributed to defects in "neurohumoral control of respiration," insufficient development of capillaries in the lung and cerebral medulla, circulatory failure, cerebral anoxia or hemorrhage, and aspiration of amniotic contents, gastric mucus, meconium, or milk.[25] Feedings were delayed for from 12 to 48 and 72 hours, unnecessary handling of infants was interdicted, stimulant drugs were given, and oxygen was administered, not only for cyanosis but also to prevent irregular respiration. Only a flowmeter attached to the tank of oxygen guided the amount administered. With leaky incubators, the effects of oxygen in raising the blood oxygen levels were, of course, variable and not measured; with better incubators, oxygen poisoning produced retrolental fibroplasia.[26]

Feeding practice was determined first by a judgment of the infant's ability to suck and swallow, and second by the qualifications of available nursing personnel. Human milk was the food of choice for all feeble or sick infants. Medicine droppers with rubber tips were widely used, and infants were fed every 1 or 2 hours by patient nurses who could be expected to place in the infant's mouth a human milk or a cow's milk mixture at a rate not exceeding his ability to swallow. Because the consequences of exceeding this limit were immediate and severe—aspiration and apnea, respiratory distress, pneumonia, or death—the directions for feeding were rigidly followed. Several consequences followed this limitation in the method of feeding. Although infants gained slowly, because of inadequate caloric intake, longer periods of hospitalization were accepted by Hess as not altogether undesirable because early discharge to poverty-stricken homes was harmful. The long hospital stays increased the risk of exposure to hospital infections, and strict preantibiotic isolation measures (*e.g.*, handwashing, individual sterile gowns, caps, and masks) were instituted. Mothers and personnel from other parts of the hospital were excluded. The use of intermittent gavage, and then of the indwelling nasogastric tube,[27] was a big step forward.

The composition of the feeding mixture is still a subject for studies and refinement. Human milk had been the food of choice for all feeble or sick infants from time immemorial, and wet nurses were present in Budin's and other units when natural mothers were unavailable because of ill health, or they were made unavailable by nursery routines. Metabolic data supported previous clinical judgments that lower fat and higher protein intakes than those of human milk would be associated with more rapid weight gain.[28] New data on amino acid concentrations in the blood, particularly of phenylalanine and taurine suggest that rate of weight gain is in itself an inadequate criterion even or particularly in low-birth-weight infants. Interpretation of the significance of these and new data has seemed to depend in part on the interest of the interpreter in amino acids, acid-base balance, water and electrolytes, calcium and phosphorus, macrophages, intellectual development, kidney function, osteoporosis or rate of weight gain, or, in the case of commercial formulas, on the enlightened self-interest of the manufacturer. A recent study showed that supplementary phosphate cured florid rickets in a very small infant fed only human milk.[29]

Needless to say, only nurses of certain temperaments were willing to serve in premature nurseries, and most house officers and pediatricians found working under the constraints of the nursery uninteresting; they missed the presence of individual variability—there if one but looked and listened.[30]

Advances in obstetrical practice have included improved methods of monitoring and intervening in high-risk pregnancies: third trimester glucose tolerance tests; determination of maternal titers of Rh antibodies; amniotic sampling for heme derivatives; fetal cell cultures for biochemical or chromosomal studies; lecithin–sphingomyelin determinations; fetal electronic and biochemical monitoring; intrauterine fetal transfusions; establishment of regional centers for women with complications of pregnancy; and establishment of productive research centers in perinatal biology that combine the efforts of neurologists, obstetricians, pathologists, physiologists, psychologists, and pediatricians.

CONTINUING PROBLEMS AND CONCERNS

Electronic monitoring of the fetus, even in uncomplicated labor, has led to more diagnoses of intrapartum anoxia. This has been associated with a tripling of the rate of cesarian sections. A causal significance of the association has been questioned, but it has been the subject of a task-force report for the National Institute of Child Health and Human Development,[31] and has been discussed even at a senatorial investigation of obstetrical practices in the United States.[32]

A persisting problem is our lack of understanding of the causes and mechanisms underlying the reproductive disability called premature birth. The greatest clinical application, to date, of research on the physiology of reproduction has been the development of hormonal methods for prevention of pregnancy.

We do not seem to be able to convert our recognition of the association of poverty with increased incidence of high-risk pregnancies and births into knowledge of whether and how, specific components of poverty, such as poor nutrition, poor personal hygiene, infections, drug addiction, poor education, mores, and despair, disturb pregnancy. A report on the number of infants with birth weights less than 2500 g among 140,000 infants born alive, in New York City during 1968, documented again that a higher rate is associated with medical and social risks in the mother and inadequate antenatal care. Low-birth-weight infants accounted for 5.8% of live births to mothers at "no" risk with adequate antenatal care; the comparable rate was 19.6% for women at risk who received inadequate care.[33]

The benefits of the modern nursery for high-risk infants are being extended by regionalization.[34] Helicopters are being used for transport, a long step from the selected taxicabs whose owners were persuaded by Hess to put electrical outlets for incubators on their dashboards. New indications for, and dimensions of, vigorous intervention immediately after birth have been introduced. They include continuous monitoring of clinical signs and repeated monitoring of biochemical findings as guides to therapy for acidosis, hypoxia, hypercapnia, respiratory distress, circulatory failure, hyperbilirubinemia, and hypoglycemia. The interventions consist of early intravascular administration of glucose, amino acids, lipids, water, sodium bicarbonate, or other buffer solutions; exchange transfusions; phototherapy; almost-routine use of antibiotics; steroid therapy; ventilatory assistance; and drug therapy based on new knowledge of pharmacology, and respiratory and circulatory physiology. Advances in anesthesia and surgical skills and in postoperative parenteral alimentation have permitted successful surgical intervention in small infants with cardiac, pulmonary, gastrointestinal, and neural tube defects.

Although the interventions are still being refined, this activism has been associated with increased survival rates particularly of those infants weighing less than 1500 g at birth,[35] and with a decreased incidence of spastic diplegia;[36] however, this conclusion is not universally accepted.[37,38] Increase in survival is bringing increase in some forms of morbidity (e.g., chronic oxygen dependence, clotting disorders, and necrotizing enterocolitis). Other problems (e.g., hyperosmolality and hyperammonemia), are more easily recognized to be partly iatrogenic. Some practices are of too short duration to have been standardized.

Psychological considerations are also squeezing their way into the neonatal intensive care unit.[30,39,40,41] The opening of the nurseries to the traffic required by intensive care has, under the flawed shield of antibiotics, permitted mothers and fathers to come into closer contact with infants, in the hope of minimizing the disruption of mother-infant "bonding."[42] The term **early intervention** may mean something wholly different to the psychologist and the neonatologist; one may be concerned with later psychomotor development, while the other's struggle for the immediate survival of the infant leaves time and interest for too little else. In some regional centers the separation of mother and infant has been decreased by returning the infant to the referring nursery for intermediate care. The increased incidence of battered children among former low-birth-weight infants is gross evidence that perinatologists need to be actively concerned with parents and their lifestyles, particularly those who are unwed or have marginal incomes. The data with which to judge with assurance the long-term benefits of some specific medical or psychological interventions may not be available for a long time, if ever. Prolonged follow-up is particularly difficult among the indigent in a society as heterogeneous and mobile as that of the United States.

ETHICAL DILEMMAS

Certain ethical dilemmas arise acutely because we live in a society now more aware of civil rights, more informed (sometimes misinformed) and more suspicious of physicians and hospitals because of the publicity given to malpractice litigation.

One issue concerns the clinical research necessary to improve the fate of the high-risk fetus or neonate. The horns of the dilemma are the conflict between the Kantian stance of never using a person solely as a means and John Stuart Mills' choice of the greatest good for the greatest number—the latter a form of statistical morality. The problem is even more difficult when one questions the validity of proxy consent in clinical trials on the infants who are chosen for studies in which they may be put at risk by a therapeutic measure of possible harm, or by omission of a therapeutic measure of possible benefit in an appropriately randomized clinical trial.

The National Commission for the Protection of Human Subjects in Biomedical and Behavioral Research has wrestled with the problems in a praiseworthy, thorough, scholarly way. After hearing much testimony and studying carefully reasoned position papers on the proven values of clinical research, on the limits of animal research, and on the legal and ethical issues, they developed rules and regulations which apply specifically to research on the pregnant woman, the fetus, the infant and child.[43,44]

Institutional review boards, mandated by previous regulations, must satisfy themselves in the case of the infant that (1) the contemplated research is sound and significant; (2) it has already been performed in animals, adults and older children before infants, if this is possible and appropriate; (3) the permission of parents is obtained; (4) subjects are selected in an equitable manner; and (5) privacy and confidentiality are protected.

Furthermore, the risk must be *minimal,* that is, not greater than the risk infants run in the course of their daily lives. Obviously the high-risk neonate already runs a large risk, but the intervention studied must hold out the prospect for *direct* benefit to the patient with an anticipated benefit-risk ratio at least as favorable as other treatment alternatives.

In the case of the pregnant woman, no activity may be undertaken unless

1. appropriate studies have been completed on animals and non-pregnant individuals.
2. the risk to the fetus is minimized, and in all cases is the least possible risk for achieving the objectives of the activity, except where the purpose of the activity is to meet the health needs of the particular fetus.
3. individuals engaged in the activity will have no part in any decisions as to the timing, method, and procedures used to terminate a pregnancy; and in determining the viability of the fetus at the termination of the pregnancy.
4. any procedural changes which may cause greater than minimal risk are not introduced into the procedure for terminating the pregnancy solely in the interest of the activity.
5. no inducements, monetary or otherwise, are offered to terminate pregnancy for purposes of the activity.

Differences of opinion will of course arise in the mandated institutional review boards, in their judgments of benefit-risk ratios and validity of informed proxy consent. The writer believes the HEW recommendations (above) are fair and justified even though we will be forced to make bedside decisions with fewer clinical trials for support. The major cause for this decrease is the decline in the number of qualified people choosing careers in clinical science because of the constriction of federal funds for research training and research grants. At the same time, there has been a rise in funds supporting alternative, socially useful, satisfying professional opportunities.

The number of clinical investigations will decline, also, because of the restrictions imposed by the Commission's guidelines, no matter how much we need the studies as scientific guides to improvements in care. This decrease may come in one of two ways. The investigator may submit a protocol developed from justified curiosity, honed to be "scientifically sound and significant" and acceptable, by thinking that emphasizes the "greatest good for the greatest number." The Institutional Review Board, however, with less curiosity, may decline approval because it is not satisfied with the minimal risk or proxy consent. Alternatively, the restriction may come because the investigator himself subscribes to the ethic of "never using a person solely as a means," curbs his curiosity, and declines to even plan a clinical investigation.

What shall we do in the face of decreased prospects for carefully randomized clinical trials even though we need the information? Above all, we must maintain curiosity and skepticism. Astute clinical and laboratory observations of what McQuarrie once termed "experiments in nature" continue to be fruitful. An example is the recent report of transient hyperammonemia.[45] Furthermore, we will have to rely more on animal studies to give leads for cautious interpretation of their clinical counterparts. An example is in the production by excessive oxygen of lesions in the retina of newborn mice and rats similar to those of retrolental fibroplasia in the infant. We shall also have to use epidemiologic analyses of the natural course of physiologic disorders and disease states, even though the associations, found or not found, leave gaps in judgment of causality. Procedures for judging associations without direct experimental intervention are discussed in detail by Susser.[46] He points out that complexity in causation may leave residual uncertainty, which, in fact, has to be tolerated not only in epidemiology but in other sciences as well. The physician is asked to allow neither the commendable quest for certainty nor residual uncertainty to "sap the will for action."

We shall have to rely more on "disciplined intuition." Discipline comes from an understanding of biostatistical methods and values, knowledge of the scientific literature, and skepticism nurtured *inter alia* by the reading of letters to the editor and commentaries on original reports. Intuition comes from extensive personal experience and recollection of accurate clinical observations. The latter supplement, but do not replace, those that can be analyzed statistically. Some belong in the category described by Margaret Mead:

. . . our knowledge of ourselves and of the universe comes . . . from two sources . . . from our capacity to explore human responses to events . . . through introspection and empathy, as well as from our capacity to make objective observations in physical and animate nature.[47]

A classic example of the "capacity to explore human responses . . . through introspection and empathy . . ." is in the loving transaction between mother and infant caught by Picasso in his famous 1905 painting of a nursing mother. Such an observation, as well as the others we make in clinical practice, is simply not food for a computer.

We continue to make decisions under uncertainty. With the advances in technology, some of these have become life and death matters, posing ethical dilemmas with intense emotional overtones. The physician can be helped by the logic of the moral philosopher to sort out those parts of the decision process which are based on *medical facts,* and those based on *moral values,* even though, by virtue of his technical skills and professional training, he makes and should continue to make the final decisions about continuation of life supports. This is a common source of tension in the neonatal ICU as in other intensive care units.[48] The medical judgments of prognosis of the infant for survival and for future development are not always made with certainty. The physician is then asked to make a value judgment of the quality of the life he may save. Needless to say, in a profession in which the primary ethical imperative will always be to

save lives, inclusion of the need to consider the quality of those lives may become a source of conflict.

Considerable literature is now available to help physicians make decisions based on both medical judgments and moral values. McCormick has described the varied conclusions of moral philosophers.[49] His own conclusion is that quality-of-life judgments can be considered as extensions of, and not as conflicts with, reverence for the sanctity of life. Saving lives is not the only aim of medicine; the question of future suffering needs also to be considered if the neonatologist is to be more than an intensive care technologist. Jonsen and Garland have edited a comprehensive discussion by members of different disciplines and developed nine ethical propositions as guidelines for physicians.[50] Their sixth proposition states that life-preserving intervention should be considered as doing harm to an infant who cannot survive infancy, or who will live in intractable pain or cannot participate even minimally in human experience. The latter is, of course, most difficult to judge and requires that the physician take account of the values and feelings of the parents without sacrificing his own judgment.[51] The physician with ultimate responsibility for the patient is asked to function not only as a professional technician, but also as a fellow human being respecting the autonomy of the patient and family, and listening to the opinions of others concerned: nurse, social worker, religious counselor, and hospital administrator, as well as the physicians who supply specialized technical skills. On a *case-by-case* basis, one must then decide *what one should do of what one can do.*

RELATION TO NORMAL DELIVERY

Finally, it should not be, but is, necessary to point out that the overwhelming majority of pregnant women and newborn infants are not high-risk. A cesarian section rate of 15% to 20% is hard to justify; it represents the result of "high-risk thinking" and an excessive fear of litigation. When perinatologists narrow their interests to the high-risk mother and her infant, productive and exciting though this may be, the subspecialty separates itself, in a counterproductive way, from obstetrics and pediatrics and the reasons for its existence: promotion of the health and development of infants and their mothers. The prenatal clinic, the nursery for normal infants, the well-baby clinic, and the neighborhood family health center are proper responsibilities of the well-rounded perinatologist, as are the delivery room, the high-risk nursery, the perinatal biology research laboratory and the special high-risk clinics. It may be that the role of the obstetrician and the neonatologist will become a supervisory one for allied health personnel in normal pregnancies and deliveries, but they cannot become supervisors or team leaders without developing a deeper understanding of mothers and fathers and families. It is a challenge to our elitism to find time to listen with a "third ear" to parents from different cultural backgrounds and with varying amounts of information, education, understanding, and anxiety. A lack of such understanding has led to institutional practices that have been stridently termed a cultural warping of childbirth.

In perinatology, as in all of medicine, clinical and laboratory sciences and technology are necessary but not sufficient for our tasks as physicians. Consumers are demanding that respect be mutual, a relationship that should exist without their having to demand it, in what has been described as a covenant based on mutual trust between doctor and patient.[52-54]

REFERENCES

1. **Budin P:** The Nursling: The Feeding and Hygiene of Premature and Full Term Infants. Maloney WJ (trans). London, The Caxton Publishing Co., 1907
2. **Lubchenco LO, Hansman C, Dressler M, Boyd E:** Intrauterine growth as estimated from liveborn birth weight data at 24 to 42 weeks of gestation. Pediatrics 32:793, 1963
3. **Battaglia FC, Lubchenco LO:** A practical classification of newborn infants by weight and gestational age. J Pediatr 71:159, 1967
4. **Hess JH, Lundeen EC:** The Premature Infant: It's Medical and Nursing Care. Philadelphia, JB Lippincott, 1941
5. **Taylor ES, Gordon HH:** The premature infant program in Colorado. The Mother (Quarterly Bulletin of the American Committee on Maternal Welfare) 10:1, 1948
6. **Gordon HH, Ganzon AF:** On the protein allowances of young infants. J Pediatr 54:503, 1959
7. **Ylppö A:** Pathologische Anatomische Studien bei Frühgeborenen. Z Kinderheilkd 20:212, 1919
8. **Ylppö A:** Zur Physiologie, Klinik und zum Schicksal der Frühgeborenen. Z Kinderheilkd 24:1, 1919
9. **Ylppö A:** Das Wachstum der Frühgeborenen von der Geburt bis zum Schulalter. Z Kinderheilkd 24:111, 1919
10. **Raiha CE:** Professor Arvo Ylppö. Ann Med Int Fenn 36:351, 1947
11. **Peiper A:** Beiträge zur Sinnesphysiologie der Frühgeburt. J Kinderheilkd 104:195, 1924
12. **Peiper, A:** Unreife und Lebensschwäche. Leipzig, Georg Thiem Verlag. 1937
13. **Peiper A:** Die Atemstörungen der Frühgeburten. Ergeb Inn Med Kinderheilkd 40:1, 1931
14. **Peiper, A:** Cerebral Function in Infancy and Childhood, 3rd rev ed. Nagler B, Nagler H (trans). New York, Consultant's Bureau, 1963
15. **Gordon HH:** Presentation of the John Howland Medal and Award of the American Pediatric Society to Dr. Ethel C. Dunham. Am J Dis Child 94:367, 1957
16. **Dunham EC:** Premature Infants: A Manual for Physicians, Publication No. 325 of the US Children's Bureau. Washington, DC, US Government Printing Office, 1948
17. **Ballantyne JW:** Manual of Antenatal Pathology and Hygiene, Vol 1, The Fetus. Edinburgh, William Green & Sons, 1902
18. **Silverman WG:** The physical environment and the premature infant. Pediatrics 23:166, 1959
19. **Baird D:** Social factors in obstetrics. Lancet 1:1079, 1949
20. **Baird D:** Social factors in obstetrics. In Greenhill JP (ed): Year Book of Obstetrics and Gynecology. Chicago, Year Book Medical Publishers, 1969
21. **Birch H, Richardson S, Illsley R, Horobin G, Baird D:** Mental Subnormality in the Community: A Clinical and Epidemiological Study. Baltimore, Williams & Wilkins, 1970
22. **Kubie LS:** Some unsolved problems of the scientific career. Am Sci 41:596, 1953; 42:104, 1954
23. **Gordon HH:** Some biological aspects of premature birth. In Askin JA, Cooke RE, and Haller JA Jr (eds): A Symposium on the Child. Baltimore, The Johns Hopkins Press, 1967
24. **Smith CW:** Physiology of the Newborn Infant, Springfield, ILL, Charles C Thomas, 1945
25. **Levine, SZ, Gordon HH:** Physiologic handicaps of the premature infant, I. Their pathogenesis; II. Clinical applications. Am J Dis Child 64:274, 1942

26. **James LS, Lanman JT (eds):** History of oxygen therapy and retrolental fibroplasia: Report of the Committee on Fetus and Newborn of the American Academy of Pediatrics. Pediatrics 57:591, 1976

27. **Royce S, Tepper C, Watson W, Day R:** Indwelling polyethylene nasogastric tube for feeding premature infants. Pediatrics 8:79, 1951

28. **Gordon HH, Levine SZ:** The metabolic basis for the individualized feeding of infants, premature and full term. J Pediatr 25:464, 1944

29. **Rowe JC, Wood DH, Rowe DW, Raisz LG:** Nutritional hypophosphatemic rickets in a premature infant fed breast milk. N Engl J Med 300:293, 1979

30. **Horton FH, Lubchenco LO, Gordon HH:** Self-regulatory feeding in a premature nursery. Yale J Biol Med 24:263, 1952

31. Predictors of Intrapartum Fetal Distress: Report of Task Force to NICHD Consensus Development Conference on Antenatal Diagnosis, NIH Publication 79-1973. Bethesda, US Department of Health, Education and Welfare, Public Health Service, National Institutes of Health, April 1979

32. Obstetrical Practices in the United States, 1978. Hearing before the Subcommittee on Health and Scientific Research of the Committee on Human Resources, U.S. Senate. April 17, 1978. Washington, US Government Printing Office, 1978

33. Infant Death: An Analysis by Maternal Risk and Health Care: Contrasts in Health Status. Washington, DC, National Academy of Sciences, 1973

34. **Gluck L (ed):** Symposium on organization for perinatal care. Clin Perinatol, 3:265, 1976

35. **Lee K, Paneth N, Gartner LM, Pearlman MA, Gruss L:** Neonatal mortality rate: An analysis of the recent improvement in the United States. AM J Public Health 70:15, 1980

36. **Fitzhardinge PM:** Follow-up studies on the low birth weight infant. Clin Perinatol, 3:503, 1976

37. **Jones RAK, Cummins M, Davis PA:** Infants of very low birthweight: A 15 year analysis. Lancet 1:1332, 1979

38. **Jones RAK, Cummins M, Davis PA:** Letter to the editor. Lancet 2:523, 1979

39. **Hasselmeyer EG:** Behavior patterns of premature infants. Public Health Service Publ #840, Washington, D.C., 1961

40. **Caplan G:** Patterns of parental response to the crisis of premature birth. Psychiatry 23:365, 1960

41. **Barnett CR, Leiderman PH, Grobstein R, Klaus MH:** Neonatal separation: the maternal side of interactional deprivation. Pediatrics 45:197, 1970

42. **Klaus MH, Kennell JH:** Maternal–Infant Bonding. St. Louis. CV Mosby, 1976

43. **Jonsen AR:** Research involving children: Recommendations of the National Commission for the Protection of Human Subjects of Biomedical and Behavioral Research. Pediatrics 62:131, 1978

44. Task Force on Pediatric Research, Informed Consent and Medical Ethics: AAP Code of Ethics for the Use of Fetuses and Fetal Material for Research. Pediatrics 56:304, 1975

45. **Ballard RA, Vincur B, Reynolds JW et al:** Transient hyperammonemia of the preterm infant. New Engl J Med 299:920–925, 1978

46. **Susser M:** Causal Thinking in the Health Sciences: Concepts and Strategies of Epidemiology. New York. Oxford University Press, 1973

47. **Mead M:** Towards a human science. Science 191:903, 1976

48. **Frader JE:** Difficulties in providing intensive care. Pediatrics 64:10, 1979

49. **McCormick RA:** The quality of life, the sanctity of life: A theological perspective. Hastings Cent Rep 8:30, 1978

50. **Jonsen AR, Garland MJ (eds):** Ethics of Newborn Intensive Care. San Francisco, The Health Policy Program, School of Medicine, University of California; and Berkeley, Institute of Governmental Studies, University of California, 1976

51. Decision Making and the Defective Newborn. In Swinyard CA (ed): Proceedings of a Conference on Spina Bifida and Ethics. Charles C Thomas, Springfield, ILL, 1978

52. **Ramsey P:** The Patient as Person: Explorations in medical ethics. New Haven, Yale University Press, 1970

53. **Dyck AJ:** On human care: An introduction to ethics. Nashville, Abingdon, 1977

54. **May WF:** Code and covenant or contract and philanthropy. In Reiser SJ, Dyck AJ, Curran W (eds): Ethics in Medicine: Historic Perspectives and Contemporary Concerns. Cambridge, MA, MIT Press, 1977

2

The Morality of Drastic Intervention

Gordon B. Avery

STATEMENT OF THE PROBLEM

Should a severely malformed infant be resuscitated in the delivery room? An obvious trisomy 13? An intended abortion weighing 560 grams? Should a "no code" order be written on a severely asphyxiated infant with seizures, depressed tone and reflexes, and unstable vital signs? Should a baby with meningomyelocele and hydrocephalus have aggressive surgical intervention? If leg paralysis is total? If hydrocephalus is advanced? If the spinal defect is extensive and scoliosis is present? Should an infant with trisomy 18 have surgery for intestinal obstruction? Cardiac surgery? Should the respirator be turned off when a small premature with hyaline membrane disease is discovered to have a moderate intraventricular hemorrhage? A massive hemorrhage with dilated, fixed pupils and decerebrate posturing?

Such situations occur regularly in every intensive care nursery. They raise the question of whether therapy should be withheld or withdrawn in the face of a seemingly hopeless outlook for meaningful recovery. Duff and Campbell reported in 1973 that 14% of 299 consecutive deaths in a major tertiary nursery were the result of withdrawal or withholding of treatment.[1] An even higher percentage would characterize the policy of many nurseries in more recent years; yet, there are some centers in which life is almost always sustained regardless of the prognosis. The need to decide places a severe burden on nursery staffs already subjected to the battlefield pressures of intensive care.

A major problem is our uncertainty about the prognosis. There are no clinical or laboratory means to assess neurologic potential with precision in the young infant. In extreme cases, there is little doubt that brain damage is catastrophic and recovery is impossible, but individual babies come with every shade of ambiguity as to their prognoses. Thus, we must decide what is appropriate therapy for each individual infant in the context of his family.

THE LAW AND THE COURTS

Although each nursery has had to evolve a philosophy for dealing with these issues, there is little legal guidance in either specific laws or in judicial precedents. Many states have laws defining brain death, usually with very strict criteria implying total cerebral necrosis, supported by absent reflexes and a flat electroencephalogram.[2,3] The precedents concerning "no code" orders are few and somewhat contradictory. Thus, one decision requires prior judicial review, while another appears to place such matters within the scope of medical practice—in consultation with the responsible family.[4,5] Furthermore, decisions arising from adult medical situations apply poorly to neonates, with their long years of helpless dependence, severe congenital malformations, and lack of self-awareness or established relationships with the family. This chapter advisedly bears the word *morality* in its title, rather than *legality,* because, at this time and for the foreseeable future, our basic beliefs about the meaning and purpose of life will provide the principal coordinates by which we steer.

The law does specifically forbid any active measures to terminate life. Although some may think it a fine distinction between *allowing* a baby to die and *causing* a baby to die, this distinction is well established in law and tradition. Thus, when we discontinue a respirator, we must either be withdrawing an extraordinary therapy no longer justified by the child's condition, or have judged the child already to be dead.

PRIMUM NON NOCERE— FIRST, DO NO HARM

Neonatologists must take the long view in assessing the consequences of their decisions. It has been estimated that custodial care, over a lifetime, of a single defective child will cost about $400,000.[6] The cost in terms of human suffering is incalculable. In one series, 62% of families of children with meningomyelocele and hydrocephalus were judged to have made poor adjustments, and 43% of the parents were divorced or separated.[7] There is a dignity in the natural order—birth, illness, care within the family, and death—that should not be capriciously interfered with. The treatment we choose for our patients may have grave and long-lasting effects upon the quality of life of both the child and his family. We must be certain that the goals to be achieved are sufficient to justify the suffering that may ensue.

Many feel that judgment can come into play when extraordinary measures are required to preserve and extend life. The Roman Catholic Church takes this view, contending that ordinary care must always be given, but that other considerations may enter in when extraordi-

nary means are being contemplated.[8] In general, Protestant and Jewish theologians concur.[9,10] The problem lies in drawing the distinction between the ordinary and extraordinary. The use of respirators has become common in large medical centers, but may be judged as extraordinary means of prolonging partial life after severe brain damage has occurred.[11]

We sometimes unnecessarily prolong the misery of both baby and family when a hopeless situation could be terminated by withdrawing extraordinary therapy. We operate, ill-advisedly at times, on babies whose prognoses for meaningful life is nil. In my opinion, we would serve our patients better if we stopped to consider the consequences more carefully before using our new techniques.

INTERESTED PARTIES TO THE DECISION

The decision for or against intervention in a critically ill baby is made on behalf of a number of interested parties. Most obvious is the child himself. Few would question that, under most circumstances, the child's right to life is the preeminent consideration. But the child's right to life of reasonable quality must also be considered. The parents and siblings have a stake in the decision; their family life may be profoundly affected by what is decided. The specific medical institution caring for the baby may be involved, as overcommitted resources and uncollectable bills may make it impossible to render satisfactory care to other children with a much better prognosis. Finally, society at large may be responsible for the expenses of catastrophic illness and sustained custodial care. Obviously, these various considerations have different weights in making complex decisions. But automatic, unthinking, minute-by-minute prolongation of life can no longer be considered the only valid choice.

WHO DECIDES

The responsible physician must make a decision about what should be done, availing himself of consultation if necessary, and discussing the problem with the entire medical team. He must report the situation to the family, and be responsive to their wishes. But, as the individual with knowledge of the medical realities of the case, with some degree of objectivity, and with close contact with the family, the physician is in the best position to make a sound recommendation.

The family is always ambivalent. They want their baby to live, not to die. Yet the prospect of purposeless suffering and lifelong responsibility for a retarded child is frightening. The parents understand the medical alternatives largely as they are explained by the doctor; hence, he can profoundly bias their choice by how he feels and how he slants his presentation. Ultimately, the family has the authority to accept or reject the recommendation of the physician, but it is unfair to place the whole burden of decision on them. Regardless of the outcome, most parents will feel guilty and will need compassionate support.

Some have proposed that committees with medical and, perhaps, legal, theological, and lay members review cases involving the limitation of intervention. However, committees are clumsy instruments for decisions on individual cases; they are difficult to convene in the middle of the night and difficult to inform about the complexities of a clinical situation.

THE HANDLING OF FEELINGS

In caring for critically ill babies, the first feelings we must deal with are our own. We must master our anxiety, frustration, and discouragement, if we are to be of help to our patients and their families. Yet, at the same time, we cannot defend ourselves by completely hardening our hearts. The price of empathy with the family is a partial sharing of their pain. A physician caring for the dying must work through his own feelings about death. The various stages of dying have been sensitively described by Dr. Elisabeth Kübler–Ross: shock, denial, anger, depression, bargaining, acceptance, and separation.[12] In neonatology, we encounter these feelings most strikingly in the parents, but we should be aware of them when they occur in ourselves and in other members of the medical team.

Nurses caring for sick newborns become, to some degree, surrogate mothers. They feel love and pride for their babies, and experience grief and depression at their death. The "burn out" phenomenon in ICN nurses, discussed in Chapter 4, is partially the result of the many babies each has loved and lost. Because these feelings are very real, physicians must be careful to share the reasons for their decisions, and to show consideration and understanding.

The feelings of parents will be influenced by what we tell them and by the degree of respect we show to their babies. They should understand, if the baby dies, that every effort that had any reasonable hope of success was made. If the condition was in no way their fault and will not recur in subsequent pregnancies, these points should be emphasized. Though damaged or malformed, if we call the infant by his first name and refer to and touch and handle him as befits an individual having some dignity and value, the impact on the parents may be profound. Young nurses just coming on the unit are often worried that they do not know what to say to desperate, grieving, anxious parents. Yet little gifts of love given to the baby are perceived and appreciated far beyond the parents' ability to put their feelings into words, and soften the grieving process.

When we conclude that it is time to turn off a respirator, we first search for any signs of hope that would call for continued efforts, always giving the baby the benefit of any reasonable doubt. Then we discuss the situation within the medical team, especially including the nurses most closely involved with the baby. Ordinarily, the family has been in close communication, and appreciates that all reasonable hope has been exhausted. If they cannot accept the recommendation to terminate therapy, we wait and continue to discuss the worsening picture, until a time comes when we and they are jointly resolved that it is time to stop. We offer the opportunity for the parents to come into the nursery and see their baby for the last time, and, if they choose, to hold the baby while he dies. If not, we assure them that somebody from our team will stay with the infant constantly, and will hold and comfort him during his last minutes. The person taking responsibility for the decision must stay and not leave the nurse alone with a dying baby whose respirator has been turned off. Though death cannot be avoided, and, in such a case, may be unopposed, it must be respected.

Aftercare of the family is important and is often neglected. In the weeks after a baby's death, questions will arise in the parents' minds which they were initially too shocked to formulate. Guilt and self-blame are almost universal. A return visit to interpret autopsy results and give genetic counseling is often helpful. For those left with a handicapped child, continuing care must be arranged so that they do not feel abandoned with an unmanageable problem. At present, our facilities for residential care of defective children in their first year or two of life are very inadequate, and these must be improved as part of our collective responsibility for tragedies that should not fall solely on individual families.

SUMMARY

In the years ahead, I have no doubt that new science will help us judge more accurately the prognoses of critically ill newborns. Increased public awareness should spare the physician from some of his present isolation in making decisions on the use of drastic intervention. One would hope that the community will develop new resources for assisting families left with the responsibility for a defective child. Yet there still will remain gray areas in which judgments must be made without help from firm scientific standards and without established social and ethical guidelines, by the responsible physician working with the family and drawing on whatever resources he has of common sense, sensitivity, and concern.

REFERENCES

1. **Duff RS, Campbell AGM:** Moral and ethical dilemmas in the special care nursery. New Eng J Med 289:890–894, 1973
2. **Black P McL:** Brain death. New Eng J Med 299:338–344; 393–400, 1978
3. **Sweet WH:** Brain death. New Eng J Med 299: 410–412, 1978
4. **Schram RB, Kane JC Jr, Roble DT:** "No code" orders: Clarification in the aftermath of Saikewicz. New Eng J Med 299:875–878, 1978
5. **Smith BT:** "Code" or "no code": A nonlegal opinion. New Eng J Med 300:138–140, 1979
6. **Jonsen AR, Garland MJ:** Ethics of Newborn Intensive Care, p. 84. San Francisco, Health Policy Program and Institute of Governmental Studies, University of California, 1976
7. **Kohn JS, Scherzer AL, New B, Garfield M:** Studies of the school-age child with meningomyelocele: social and emotional adaptation. J Pediatr 78:1015, 1971
8. **Paton A:** Life and death: Moral and ethical aspects of transplantation. Seminars in Psychiatry 3:162, 1971
9. **Bentley CGB:** Decisions about life and death. Church Information Office, London, 1965. In Wolstenholme, GEW and O'Connor, M (eds): Ethics in Medical Progress with Special Reference to Transplantation, p. 72. London, Churchill, 1966
10. **Ramsey R:** The Patient as a Person, p. 98. New Haven, Yale University Press, 1970
11. **Smith HL:** Ethics and the New Medicine, p. 144. Nashville, Abingdon Press, 1970
12. **Kübler–Ross E:** On Death and Dying. New York, MacMillan, 1971

3

The Organization of Perinatal Care with Particular Reference to the Newborn

Paul R. Swyer

INTRODUCTION

The Spectrum of Care in Reproductive Medicine

The discipline of neonatology cannot be considered in isolation from the continuum represented by the reproductive cycle and the multiplicity of genetic, environmental, and social factors which influence reproductive success. Horizons have been widened. The obstetrician becomes a fetal physiologist and continues his interest to include the postnatal state of the baby, while the neonatologist becomes the prenatal advocate and diagnostician of the fetus and watches over his postnatal growth and development. The anesthesiologist is increasingly recognized as a valuable member of the team with his dual responsibility to ensure the comfort and safety of the mother, while safeguarding the integrity of the fetus and helping in management of the newborn. These three primary disciplines are supported by other medical and pediatric disciplines and subspecialties in the care of the mother and infant. In many areas, the nurse-midwife plays the major role in managing normal pregnancy with satisfactory results. The clinical nurse specialist in obstetrics and neonatology is playing an increasingly impor-

tant part in the clinical care of mother and infant.

Many factors, psychologic, economic, social, geographic, and organizational, are involved in successful reproduction beyond these medical influences. It is the purpose of this chapter to suggest how a systematic organization for the delivery of reproductive medical care can contribute to reproductive success and to suggest further that the narrow view in terms of neonatology or even perinatology should be replaced by the wider concept of reproductive medicine.

As a consequence of the greatly increased body of knowledge in reproductive medicine and, hence, possibilities for effective intervention, specific medical subspecialties of perinatology have formed within Obstetrics and Pediatrics, and, in the United States, subspe-

The author acknowledges his debt to the members of the Fetus and Newborn Committee of the Canadian Paediatric Society, the parallel committee of the Society of Obstetricians and Gynaecologists of Canada, the members of the Advisory Committee to the Minister of Health for Ontario, and the members of the Fetus and Newborn Committee of the American Academy of Pediatrics, from whom ideas and information presented in this chapter have been derived.

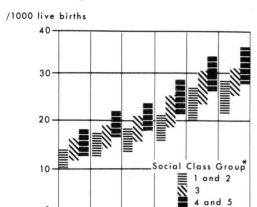

Fig. 3-1. Calculated perinatal mortality rate in mothers of different age groups, parity, social class (husband's occupation), according to smoking habits in pregnancy. Based on singleton births to mothers of 157.5 cm height or over, without severe toxemia. The top of each bar represents the risk in smokers, and the bottom the risk in nonsmokers. For the British Perinatal Mortality Survey social class was grouped on the paternal occupation according to the Registrar General's Classification of Occupations published in 1952, as shown below:

1. Professional or managerial
2. Supervisory
3. Skilled workers
4. Semi-skilled workers
5. Unskilled workers

(Adapted from Butler NR, and Alberman, ED: Perinatal Problems. E & S Livingstone. Ltd, 1969)[1]

cialty Board certifications in these disciplines are now extant. It is hoped that these new departures will not lead to undue isolation from the respective parent disciplines of obstetrics and gynecology and pediatrics.

The New Strategy of Disease Prevention in Reproductive Medicine

During recent years, emphasis has been placed on the development of a regionalized system of reproductive medical care. This system has hitherto been, to a large extent, disease oriented. With increased knowledge, the possibilities of prevention are becoming recognized. A regional organization, by reason of its multidisciplinary and comprehensive approach, is capable of furthering this goal. Two-thirds of infant mortality and morbidity occurs in infants of low birth weight (< 2500 g), either

because of prematurity or of growth retardation *in utero*. Most of the remainder is related to congenital defects. Thus, strategies must be aimed at reduction of the incidence of low birth weight, at prenatal diagnosis of congenital defects, and at genetic counseling.

For these strategies to be successful, a major effort in public and professional education will be needed. Recent consumer interest in the environmental setting of childbirth is a positive indication that a receptive attitude could be developed, aimed at increasing public awareness of and responsibility for health during pregnancy and childbirth. Figure 3-1 shows the estimated increase in risk from social and environmental factors,[1] and Figure 3-2 shows the perinatal mortality ratio according to previous obstetric history.[2] Delineation of the influence of risk factors is rendered more difficult by the coexistence of several in the same pregnancy. Poor social circumstances are, for example, often accompanied by several other adverse factors, such as small stature, more than the average number of previous pregnancies, heavy smoking, and advanced age. Multivariate analysis has been applied in the British Perinatal Mortality Survey to show that these factors are truly independent of each other in their effect on perinatal mortality, although associated and cumulative.[1,3] Thus, lack of prenatal care, poor nutrition, low socioeconomic and educational status, teen-age pregnancy, and the deleterious effects of alcohol,[4] smoking,[5] and drug usage[6] in pregnancy are all highly relevant to the prevention of low birth weight. Most of these are amenable to influence by education and specific intervention. The recently (1979) issued U.S. Surgeon General's Report on Health Promotion and Disease Prevention, *Healthy People,* emphasizes the element of personal responsibility for health.[7] Thus, a regional organization for reproductive medical care should develop public and professional educational programs and intervention strategies, (*e.g.,* school educational programs, early pregnancy registration and antenatal care, risk assessment, nutritional support programs, and genetic counseling) which reinforce and support this personal responsibility for health care and eugenics in and out of pregnancy. These and associated services should be regarded as an integral and extremely important part of a regionalized system for reproductive medical care, and

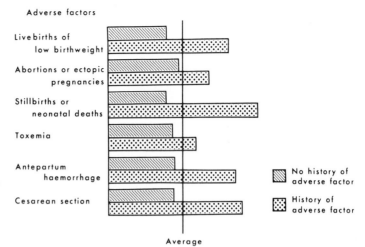

Adverse factors

Live births of
low birthweight

Abortions or ectopic
pregnancies

Stillbirths or
neonatal deaths

Toxemia

Antepartum
haemorrhage

Cesarean section

No history of
adverse factor

History of
adverse factor

Average

Fig. 3-2. Perinatal mortality ratio in multiparae according to previous obstetric history. Impact of each factor is indicated by the length of the bar for mortality *with* a history of that factor, versus the adjacent bar for mortality *without* that history. (Adapted from Butler NR: The Glaxo Volume 37:24. 1972)[2]

though the remainder of this chapter will be dealing with the more conventional aspects of regional organization, these preventive services must be recognized to be of paramount importance. Suitable resources and budgeting should be included in the regional plan.

Changing Social Attitudes Toward the Newborn

Historically there has been a marked change in attitude toward the newborn. Resigned acceptance of neonatal mortality rates of the order of 100 to 200 per thousand births or even condoned infanticide in earlier times has given way to intense concern for survival, which is now being tempered to a more balanced concern for quality of survival. Fortunately, with modern techniques of care, evidence is accumulating that the achievement of the first entails the second. Concern for quality of survival is receiving powerful impetus from the planned nature of pregnancies, following the wider availability of effective contraception, eugenic advice, and therapeutic abortion. This increasingly implies that every pregnancy is planned and wanted, although this desirable state of affairs is not yet universal. Scott, for example, reported that 50% of pregnancies in a recent hospital survey were unwanted before delivery; 20% remained unwanted after delivery.[8]

Influence of Abortion Laws

Liberalized abortions, many of which are authorized for medicosocial reasons (*e.g.*,

poor health, extremes of age, unmarried mother, poor socioeconomic circumstances), have the immediate effect of eliminating fetuses who, because of unfavorable social or medical conditions, would be subsequently at high risk of perinatal death. This fact is reflected in the low perinatal mortality rates for such countries as Bulgaria and Rumania, which on the other hand have relatively high post-neonatal mortality rates. However, these countries tend to have a high incidence of low-birth-weight delivery (up to 25%), which may be related to cervical incompetence from repeated nonparturitional cervical dilatation.[9]

Improvements in socioeconomic conditions and a new understanding of the causes and control of infection, in the more developed parts of the world, have resulted in major reductions in maternal, infant and perinatal mortality from the late 19th Century to the 1940s.[10] Maternal mortality and morbidity in particular were largely controlled, but fetal and neonatal mortality and morbidity, though reduced, remain a substantial problem.

The Modern Revolution in Reproductive Medical Care

Fundamental advances in knowledge concerning growth and development *in utero,* fetal physiology, pathology, and the mechanisms of the birth process have gone far to transform obstetrics from an art to a science, an adjustment which is still in the process of achieving the right balance.

With the post World War II era, important

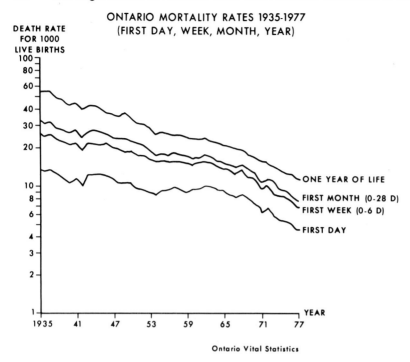

Fig. 3-3. Ontario mortality rate, 1935–1977.

technologic advances opened the way for research into the pathophysiologic mechanisms of disease in the newborn infant. Therapeutic advances followed, sometimes without critical and controlled appraisal. The epidemic of retrolental fibroplasia in the 1950s, causing blindness in newborns from excess oxygen usage, brought the recognition of the necessity for a more scientific and, hence, ultimately a more humane approach.[11]

Subsequently, increased knowledge of the pathophysiology of the neonatal period has produced spectacular advances in therapy, reflected by a continuing decline in perinatal mortality and morbidity (Figs. 3-3, 3-4). However, with this improvement has come the realization that the stage is often set, prior to birth and even prior to conception, for the remaining mortality and morbidity by a complex of factors: cultural, socio-economic, genetic, toxicologic, environmental, psychologic, as well as purely medical. Advances in knowledge surrounding the reproductive process have not always necessarily been matched by organizational changes designed to make available the benefits of this increased knowl-

edge to each and every pregnant woman and her fetus. For this new knowledge to benefit the woman carrying a risk pregnancy, an organization is required to identify the risk and to provide the service necessary to deal with the risk, preferably by prevention.

These facts provide the background and justification for the modern thrust to re-organize the delivery of health care services to pregnant women and their offspring and thus to safeguard the right of the child to be well born, while ensuring the psychological and physical health of the mother and family.

The Need for Specialized Facilities

Baird has shown that marked reductions in mortality can be achieved by coordinating rural and urban maternity services and by providing special hospital facilities for identified risk pregnancies.[12,13] In fact, those countries presenting the better perinatal statistics are generally characterized by integrated systems of delivery of reproductive medical care on a regional basis, often, as in several European countries, relying on allied health professionals and midwives to provide most normal care. Until fairly recently, relatively undifferentiated hospital facilities for the mother and newborn were adequate because of the limited possibilities for correctly oriented intervention. This is no longer the case, and the instant availability of skilled treatment and complex facilities may be crucial to survival and, even more importantly, to the subsequent integrity of the newborn.

Perinatal Statistics as an Aid to Planning

In the present era, maternal mortality and residual morbidity in the mother have been reduced to very low levels by skilled obstetrics (*e.g.*, 5.7 maternal deaths/100,000 live births in Ontario in 1977) and the control of infection (Table 3-1).[14] Risk situations in pregnancy are reflected more in poor fetal and newborn outcome with relatively minor mortality and morbidity for the mother. The perinatal mortality rate is therefore a sensitive index of the health care of both mother and newborn.

Perinatal and neonatal mortality rates have been falling steadily in most developed countries since the turn of the century (Figs. 3-3, 3-4). Improving socioeconomic circumstances makes a major contribution to the reduction in mortality rates, but advances in the medical care of the fetus and newborn over the last two decades have also been highly influential. Table 19-1, Chapter 19, demonstrates the fall in mortality experienced in The Hospital for Sick Children, Toronto, since 1960, for infants weighing less than 1500 g at birth, a reduction in mortality from 85% to 32% (see Chap. 19).

There are wide variations in perinatal mortality in many countries at a comparable level of general development. The information in Table 3-2 implies that a significant proportion of perinatal deaths is preventable if the standards of the better countries could be achieved by all. The Quebec Perinatal Mortality Committee has estimated an irreducible minimum perinatal mortality rate of 8.5 per 1000 live births.[15,16] It is significant that the province of Uusimaa in Finland, with a population of 1 million, has a perinatal mortality rate of 9.5 per 1000 live births, counting all newborn deaths weighing more than 600 g.[17,18]

Usher has suggested that, as a result of recent reductions in the population at risk (*i.e.*, predominantly infants of low birth weight), the minimum possible perinatal mortality rate (fe-

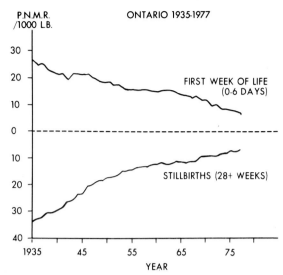

Fig. 3-4. Ontario stillbirths and perinatal mortality rate, 1935–1977.

tal and neonatal deaths up to 7 days, both weighing more than 1000 g) is 5.5/1000 live births made up of a stillbirth rate of 3.7 and a neonatal mortality rate of 1.8.[19]

Causes of Perinatal Mortality

Precise Pathological Information. Full postmortem information is essential to an understanding of the causes of perinatal deaths. Figure 3-5 categorizes the main pathologic lesions. Many of these conditions may be influenced by modern methods of perinatal

Table 3-1. Live Births and Maternal Mortality in Ontario from 1921 to 1977

Year	Live Births	Maternal Deaths	
		Number	*Rate**
1921	74,152	387	522
1931	69,209	372	538
1941	72,262	219	303
1951	114,287	97	84
1961	157,663	67	42
1971	130,395	25	19
1976	122,700	10	8
1977	122,757	7	5.7

* Rate per 100,000 live births (Ontario Vital Statistics 1977; Reports to Council, Ontario Medical Association)

Table 3-2. Perinatal Deaths—International Comparison

Country	Late Fetal Mortality	Neonatal Mortality	Perinatal Mortality
Canada	7.9	10.0	16.6 (1974)
Sweden			
1974	6.7	7.5	13.3
1975	5.8	6.4	11.3
1976	5.5	6.3	10.7
1977	5.1	5.8	10.2
Denmark	6.6	7.3	12.7 (1976)
Switzerland	7.2	7.4	13.5 (1975)
Finland	6.6	8.6	13.9 (1974)
Netherlands	7.7	7.6	14.0 (1975)
Norway	8.1	7.3	14.2 (1975)
New Zealand	8.3	9.6	16.5 (1975)
Japan	8.3	9.6	16.5 (1975)
German Dem. Rep.	7.9	11.7	17.6 (1975)
England and Wales	9.8	9.7	17.9 (1976)
Australia	10.4	10.0	19.2 (1975)
Germany, Fed. Rep. of	7.7	13.8	19.4 (1975)
France	11.7	9.9	19.5 (1977)
Poland	7.6	12.0	19.6 (1975)
Belgium	9.5	11.8	19.7 (1975)
USA	10.7	11.6	20.7 (1975)
Yugoslavia	7.6	19.4	21.9 (1975)
Italy	11.0	16.0	24.1 (1975)
Hungary	8.3	26.7	31.6 (1975)

(World Health Statistics Annual, 1:1978, WHO Geneva 1978)

management. Congenital malformations, both anatomic and biochemical (*e.g.,* enzymatic defects), are assuming increased importance as a cause of death as modern treatment reduces the more amenable diseases. Even in these cases, genetic counseling and prenatal diagnosis offer hope in avoiding certain lethal genetic conditions, while other malformations, such as diaphragmatic hernias, may in the future be diagnosed by fetography, and preparations made for immediate operation shortly after birth to improve the infant's chance of survival.

Similarly, new techniques of monitoring fetal growth by ultrasonography[20] and fetoscopy;[21] and fetal maturity by amniotic fluid analysis;[22] fetal condition by continuous fetal heart,[23-25] respiration rate monitoring,[26,27] fetal acid base and blood gas status,[28,29] and maternal urinary estriol[30] and/or placental lactogen excretion[31]

all have given a new precision to the management of risk pregnancy and labor, and have reduced the incidence of asphyxial and traumatic birth and unnecessary premature delivery.

Statistical Evaluation as an Aid to Improving Reproductive Medical Care. Standardization of definitions and perinatal mortality recording practices would provide a firmer basis for national and international comparisons and would help in determining the social, medical, and maternal characteristics which influence perinatal mortality. The greater the precision with which these factors can be delineated, the greater the possibilities for deployment of the appropriate corrective measures. Linkage of birth and death certificates would be important for extracting the relevant information.

There is, then, need for standardization of definitions of perinatal statistics which should conform to World Health Organization Standards as follows:*

Birth is the complete expulsion or extraction from its mother of a fetus weighing 500 g or more, irrespective of the gestational age.

Live Birth is the complete expulsion or extraction from the mother of an infant weighing 500 g or more who breathes, shows beating of the heart, pulsation of the umbilical cord, or definite movement of the voluntary muscles.

Stillbirth is the complete expulsion or extraction from the mother of a fetus weighing 500 g or more who shows no sign of life at or after birth.

Abortion is the complete expulsion or extraction from the mother of a fetus or embryo weighing less than 500 g.

First Week Death is the death of a live-born infant weighing 500 g or more at birth who dies during the first 7 completed days of life up to, but not including, the moment he becomes 168 hours of age.

Low Birth Weight refers to fetuses or infants less than 2500 g at birth.

Full Size refers to fetuses or infants weighing 2500 g or more at birth.

Gestational Age refers to the number of completed weeks/days which have elapsed between the first day of the last normal menstrual period to delivery of the fetus or infant.

Neonatal Period refers to the interval from the time of birth to the first 28 completed days of life.

Regarding fetal deaths, classification on the basis of gestational age is probably impractical, particularly for those deaths occurring between 20 and 30 weeks. The WHO Committee has suggested the definitions shown in Table 3-3.

For statistical analysis of neonatal deaths, it is suggested, however, that cohorts at 250-g intervals should be used.

Finally, the distinctions between perinatal death rate and ratio and total perinatal

---

* Based on World Health Organization (WHO) recommendations as interpreted by the Committee on the Fetus and Newborn of the Canadian Paediatric Society and the Society of Obstetricians and Gynaecologists of Canada.

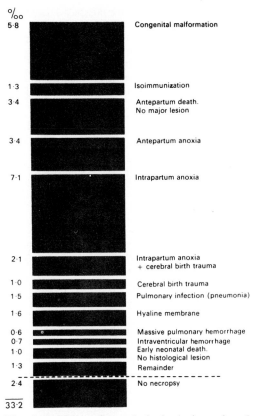

‰	
5·8	Congenital malformation
1·3	Isoimmunization
3·4	Antepartum death. No major lesion
3·4	Antepartum anoxia
7·1	Intrapartum anoxia
2·1	Intrapartum anoxia + cerebral birth trauma
1·0	Cerebral birth trauma
1·5	Pulmonary infection (pneumonia)
1·6	Hyaline membrane
0·6	Massive pulmonary hemorrhage
0·7	Intraventricular hemorrhage
1·0	Early neonatal death. No histological lesion
1·3	Remainder
2·4	No necropsy
33·2	

Fig. 3-5. The main pathologic lesions found at necropsy for a perinatal mortality rate of 33.2/1000 births. (Butler NR: Perinatal Mortality. E & S Livingstone Ltd, 1972)[2]

loss rate and ratios should be appreciated in Table 3-4.

There should be a continuing system for the statistical surveillance of the total system of reproductive medical care, with particular reference to morbidity and mortality statistics and the costs of services. Thus, the data to be gleaned from scrutiny of antenatal, natal, and postmortem records, linked with statistics on morbidity and costing, should be surveyed in order to monitor the effectiveness of the program in relation to cost, in order to provide for necessary modification of practice. In this connection, the U.S. Department of Health, Education, and Welfare required, as of January 1, 1979, the use of a new system called the International Classification of Diseases (Ninth Revision, Clinical Modification [ICD-9-CM]) to co-ordinate statistics on health problems

Table 3-3. Suggested Classifications of Live Births and Fetal Deaths by an Expert Committee of the World Health Organization. (The weight divisions at 500 g and 1000 g correspond approximately to gestational ages of 20 and 28 weeks.)

Group	Live Birth	Fetal Death
I	≤ 500 g	≤ 500 g (early)
II	501–1000 g	501–1000 g (intermediate)
III	> 1000 g	> 1000 g (late)

and care in hospitals. Universal use of such a system should ensure comparability of data in perinatal morbidity statistics.

Reasons have been cited for regarding poor perinatal statistics as "isolated specific phenomena which almost certainly represent a peculiar social and medical attitude to the particular area of human reproduction . . . the required medical care and facilities being so different from those needed for general illness that such care can only be given with concentrated facilities by people with special training".[32] This statement remains broadly true.

However, to be effective, such facilities must not only be available, they must be used by both the public and the primary providers of care. This requires education of the public and the medical profession. In France, financial incentives for the family (family allowance) linked to adequate medical control, pre- and post-natally, seem to be efficacious in improving use of the system.[18,33–36]

The Required Reorganization of Reproductive Medical Care

International comparisions show the United States and Canada to have somewhat worse statistical indicators of the status of perinatal care than many, though not by any means all, of the comparably developed countries (Table 3-2). In the 1950s, some countries, notably Great Britain and Sweden, began to evolve a system for the delivery of health care with geographic regional organization. This system has become highly developed in Scandinavian countries such as Sweden and Finland, where maternity services of all levels of sophistication tend to be concentrated in large county hospitals.[17] Many factors other than the operation of a regional medical system have contributed to these countries' preeminent positions with regard to reproductive health

Table 3-4. Definitions of Death Rates and Ratios.

Perinatal Death Rate	$\dfrac{\text{Fetal deaths + First-week deaths* (both 1,000 g or more in weight)}}{\text{Live births + Fetal deaths (both 1,000 g or more in weight)}}$	× 1,000
Perinatal Death Ratio	$\dfrac{\text{Fetal deaths + First-week deaths* (both 1,000 g or more in weight)}}{\text{Live births (1,000 g or more in weight)}}$	× 1,000
Rate for Total Perinatal Loss	$\dfrac{\text{Fetal deaths + First-week deaths* (both 500 g or more in weight)}}{\text{Live births + Fetal deaths (both 500 g or more in weight)}}$	× 1,000
Ratio for Total Perinatal Loss	$\dfrac{\text{Fetal deaths + First-week deaths* (both 500 g or more in weight)}}{\text{Live births (500 g or more in weight)}}$	× 1,000
Fetal Death Rate	$\dfrac{\text{Fetal deaths (1,000 g or more in weight)}}{\text{Live births + Fetal deaths (both 1,000 g or more in weight)}}$	× 1,000
First-week Death Rate	$\dfrac{\text{First-week deaths* (1,000 g or more in weight)}}{\text{Live births (1,000 g or more in weight)}}$	× 1,000

* 7 days are estimated as seven periods of 24 hours.

care indicators, particularly improvement in socioeconomic circumstances. However, those countries with better statistics generally have created a regionalized system of reproductive medical care, usually hospital based. Holland is a major exception, in that home delivery hitherto has been emphasized. Holland is amongst those countries with marginally better perinatal statistics than those in North America (Table 3-2). In 1977, 44.4% of deliveries were in the home,[37] the proportion falling steadily over recent years in favor of hospital delivery.[37] However, all pregnancies are carefully screened for actual or potential problems and only those devoid of ascertainable risk go forward to home delivery, which is itself supported by a highly organized emergency service in a small country with excellent internal communications. Despite these measures, the mortality for "low-risk" delivery in the home approaches that for hospital deliveries at all levels of risk. The level of training and skill of the individual selecting mothers for home delivery is crucial. Thus, GJ Kloosterman, a specialist obstetrician, reported a perinatal mortality rate of 2.5 per 1000 live births in women selected by him as expecting a normal delivery.[38] By contrast, Eskes reported rates of 14.0 per 1000 live births (28 weeks to plus 7 days) in deliveries selected for home birth by general practitioners and midwives.[39] These figures compare with an overall rate for the Netherlands of 16.9 per 1000 live births comprising all degrees of risk in 1974. Thus, selection for home delivery appears less than optimal unless carried out by a highly skilled individual.

While the concerned professions remain generally opposed to home delivery for reasons of safety, few in the medical professions or in the public would deny that a reappraisal and restructuring of hospital practices surrounding maternity is necessary to make the birth process more humane and psychologically acceptable in a family setting, promoting parental-infant attachment. This restructuring is in fact taking place in many centers. A useful guide to aid this process has recently been published.[40]

Alternatives to the conventional type of hospital delivery are under trial, such as the use of "alternative birthing centers" and so-called "in-and-out" delivery when the mother and infant remain in the hospital for only 24 hours or less. Little data currently exist regarding the former, though one approach that seems to work reasonably well[41]* is to situate such units within hospitals, adjacent to the regular obstetric department.[41] In-and-out delivery deserves further controlled evaluation. The economic advantages, however, are less than might at first appear, because of the highly organized follow-up services which are necessary for both mother and infant.

There is room for innovation and change in the delivery setting and practice, particularly with regard to the low-risk pregnancy. There seems to be no reason to situate "alternate birthing centers" outside hospitals, particularly in view of the relatively frequent recourse which may have to be made to conventional facilities, even for selected low-risk pregnancies. In one recent experience of an alternative birthing center, 23% of the first 500 births to low-risk mothers required such referrals. These included 44 caesarean sections, 13 electing anaesthesia, 25 for failure to progress, and 32 for augmentation of labor.†

The success of the French economic incentive system, whereby antenatal care is linked to maternity and child allowances, is noteworthy, and is associated with a modern system of reproductive medical care with significant effects on perinatal statistics,[18,42] the perinatal mortality rate having fallen from 24 per 1000 in 1968 to 14.7 per 1000 in 1977.[34]

Regional Reproductive Medical Services. A feature common to most countries with better reproductive medical statistics is the existence of a regional system of reproductive medical services. This has to provide for 24 hours a day, 7 days a week availability of consultants and junior staff, laboratory and investigational facilities, and special, professionally staffed transport for mother, infant, or both. Statistics indicative of the effectiveness of reproductive medical care often do not follow other indicators of community health care; they are extremely sensitive to the conditions under which specific medical reproductive care is delivered. The exact form that such a system takes depends a great deal on local circumstances, including social and professional attitudes, economic resources, available medical manpower, local geography, and climate.

---

* Ballard R: personal communication, 1979
† Ballard R: personal communication, 1979

There is no single solution to suit all circumstances, and operational flexibility is extremely important, particularly in view of the rapidly advancing areas of knowledge within the field.

The Effect of Regionalization in Improving the Outcome of Reproductive Medical Care

Prior to the introduction of regionalized programs, reproductive medical care had been rendered by physicians and hospitals of all degrees of expertise and facility, without a defined system for the identification of risk pregnancies or for matching the degree of risk to the expertise and level of equipment in the institution selected for delivery. Until recently, very few institutions existed in which integrated facilities for high-risk obstetric/fetal intensive care and neonatal intensive care were available for the approximately 15% of all pregnancies defined as "at risk."

The reproductive process is influenced by a multiplicity of psychologic, genetic, environmental, socioeconomic, cultural, and medical factors which control reproductive success. The influence of some of these factors is shown in Figure 3-1. No doubt variability in these and related factors partly explains the wide variations in health indicators in reproductive medicine among different countries and among different census tracts of the same city,[43] even when, as in the latter case, there is no financial or geographic barrier to obtaining medical care under the Ontario Provincial insurance scheme. In the United States, states with the highest mortality have rates that are about double those with the lowest. Since 1975, the Robert Wood Johnson Foundation has partly funded regionalized programs for Reproductive Medical Care in eight major areas of differing demographic and geographic characteristics.[44] Evaluation of the full impact of these programs on perinatal health indicators is in progress and the results are awaited.

There is, however, an extensive and increasingly convincing literature tending to show that it is the availability and the appropriate utilization of special medical facilities unique to reproductive medical care which have the major bearing on successful reproductive outcome.[45-48] There are now numerous reports showing that the introduction of successive modalities of special care is associated with successive improvements in mortality.[16,19,44-56]

Some of the Canadian evidence is documented in Table 3-5.

Improved mortality after introduction of special care in a regionalized system is exemplified by the findings of the Quebec Perinatal Committee, which, on the basis of mortality statistics reported by certain regionalized Quebec hospitals, has extrapolated its experience to the approximately 100,000 births for the whole Province (Tables 3-6, 3-7).[16] These numbers demonstrate the savings in lives to be anticipated following the universal application of each level of care as needed in a regionalized system. Savings of more than 1000 lives annually are projected, with reduction in provincial deaths from about 1900 infants per year to 850, and concomitant reductions in asphyxial morbidity if the performances of the worst units can be brought up to that of the best (Table 3-7).

Certain hospitals have mortality figures comparable to, or better than, the best quoted in Tables 3-5, 3-6, and 3-7, as have certain European countries, notably Sweden, Denmark, and Holland, with France improving rapidly. Sweden, for example, had a perinatal mortality rate of 10.2 in 1977 (Table 3-2).[58] The Finnish province of Uusimaa, including Helsinki and all social classes, has a perinatal mortality rate of 9.5 per 1000 live births, counting all fetuses weighing more than 600 g at birth.[17] These figures approach the "irreducible minimum" (with present knowledge) of 8.5 per 1000 live births (Table 3-7), in which the mortality is due solely to lethal congenital malformations and currently unpredictable accidents of labor. If the figures for the more successful hospitals (usually teaching hospitals which tend to attract risk pregnancies but which nevertheless have perinatal mortality rates of approximately 11 per 1000 live births)[59] could be matched by all hospitals, the national rate would fall by up to 50% for a saving of up to 30,000 lives annually in the United States.

In contemporary times, pregnancies are increasingly planned, wanted, and limited in number so that each becomes more precious both to the parents and to the community. This may partially explain the special care and attention given to the area of reproductive medicine by countries such as Sweden, Finland, France, and Switzerland, all of which have low birth rates (less than 15 per 1000 population).

Table 3-5. Impact of Intensive Care (IC)[8,32,49-53]

Hospital	Before IC	After IC	Year	
Stillbirth Rate (SB/1000 births)				
St. Boniface, Winnipeg	8.8	3.5	1973	
St. Joseph's, London	10.4	7.3	1969	
Women's College, Toronto	–	8.3	1978	
Royal Victoria, Montreal	–	6.9	1970–72	Fetal and neonatal IC
Queen's, Halifax	20.8	12.0	1965–68	
Neonatal Mortality Rate (0–6 days; rate per 1000 live births)				
St. Boniface, Winnipeg	5.0	3.5	1973	> 1000 g
Women's College, Toronto	10.6	6.2	1971	
Women's College, Toronto	–	5.6	1978	
Jewish General, Montreal	7.6	6.4	1973	
Jewish General, Montreal	–	3.7	1974	
Jewish General, Montreal	–	3.4	1975	
Queen's, Halifax	17.0	9.9	1965–68	> 500 g
Perinatal Mortality Rate (per 1000 live births)				
St. Boniface, Winnipeg	13.9	7.0	1973	> 1000 g
St. Joseph's, London	21.6	19.0	1969	> 500 g + SB
Women's College, Toronto	20.5	14.8	1971	Neonatal IC
Women's College, Toronto	–	13.9	1978	Fetal and neonatal IC
Royal Victoria, Montreal	19.1	15.2	1970–72	Neonatal IC
Royal Victoria, Montreal	–	11.6	1970–72	Fetal and neonatal IC
Jewish General, Montreal	20.9	14.9	1973	
Jewish General, Montreal	–	9.0	1974	
Queen's Halifax	–	8.9	1975	
Grace, Halifax	12.5	7.7		Before and after fetal IC

Table 3-6. Perinatal Mortality and Utilization of Neonatal Intensive Care Services, Quebec 1967–1969.

	Intramural Neonatal IC	Referral Neonatal IC	Neither Intramural nor Referral Neonatal IC
Number of births	20,176	35,289	105,467
Neonatal mortality per 1000 live births			
1001–2500 g	64	74	81
Over 2500 g	2.0	2.1	3.4
Total	6.3	7.4	9.4
Stillbirth rate per 1000 total births	8.5	9.5	9.9
Perinatal mortality per 1000 total births	14.7	16.9	19.1

(Data obtained from obstetric services in Montreal and Quebec City delivering more than 1000 infants per year, considering births over 1000 g birth weight and deaths up to 7 days; By permission of the Quebec Perinatal Committee, 1973)

Quality of Survivors

Perhaps an even more important consequence than the reduction in perinatal mortality by such an organization combining obstetric and pediatric neonatal expertise, is the avoidance of perinatally-determined morbidity as exemplified by Table 3-8 (See also Chap. 19). A recent survey has revealed variation in the incidence of severe asphyctic birth from 2.6 to 16.5 per 1000 live births in different hospitals in the province of Ontario, though they may serve similar populations.* CNS complications varied from 1.6 to 9.4 per 1000 live births. If the worst could attain the record of the best, there would be a very substantial reduction in the estimated 300 to 400 new patients with perinatally-determined cerebral palsy added to the provincial population each year,[60] as well as reduction in certain other types of perinatally determined handicaps. An analysis of the obstetric histories of a sample of patients presenting for treatment of cerebral palsy was

* Chance GW: personal communication, 1978

able to identify avoidable factors in 84% of patients.[61]

In Arizona, a review of the patients in a long-stay institution suggested that in 43% there was causative factors which are currently avoidable by the full application of knowledge of all facets of reproductive medicine, including genetic counseling and prenatal as well as perinatal care.[54] French estimates suggested that up to 65% of handicap was perinatally determined and potentially avoidable.[18] The financial implications of these estimates for long-term care are obvious and will be discussed further. Moreover, such figures represent only the "tip of the iceberg" of perinatally-determined morbidity.

The Commission on Emotional and Learning Disorders in Children (CELDIC) Report in Canada states: "The quality of health care at the time of birth and immediately postnatal is of critical importance in the prevention of neurological conditions or brain damage that may lead to learning disorders or mental retardation."[62] Beyond this, the quality of health care prior to conception and during pregnancy is also of critical importance in prevention.

It has been estimated that, in the United States there are 440,000 cerebrally palsied persons, 430,000 epileptics (many related to perinatal damage) and 2,620,000 persons with mental retardation.[63] In addition, there are an estimated one million in Canada,[62] and therefore probably at least ten million in the United States, who have so-called minimal brain damage, as manifested by poor school performance, delinquency, retardation of speech development, and reading skills. The incidence of handicap depends on definition, but recent estimates report 12% to 16% of all children have exceptional needs.[63–66]

The British Columbia Central Registry of Handicapped Children and Adults (0–20 years) defines a handicapped child as one "who has a disability severe enough to interfere with normal living, obtaining an education, and later earning a livelihood." Such persons are therefore severely affected long-term. Of the childhood population of British Columbia, 2.75% are registered: 70% for physical, organic, or sensory disabilities; 22% for mental retardation; and less than 8% for psychoneurosis or personality disorders (Annual Reports from the Registry).[65]

The United Kingdom survey entitled *11,000*

Table 3-7. Predicted Perinatal Mortality after Integration of Obstetrical Services into Larger Units

	Predicted Perinatal Mortality over 1000 g (per 1000 total births)	Approximate Number of Deaths per 100,000 births per year in Quebec
Conventional Care*	19.1	1910
Referral neonatal intensive care*	16.9	1690
Intramural neonatal intensive care*	14.7	1470
Intramural fetal and neonatal intensive care	11.6	1160
Irreducible minimum	8.5	850

* From Table 3-6
(Reproduced with modifications by permission of the Quebec Perinatal Committee, 1973)

Table 3-8. Reduction in Perinatal Asphyxia with Perinatal Intensive Care (Royal Victoria Hospital, Montreal)

	1965–1969 prior to perinatal unit	1970–1972 with peri-natal unit in operation	1970 Province of Quebec
Number of births	14,619	5,784	
Severe birth asphyxia/1000	11.7	5.9	
Postasphytic convulsions/1000	1.2	.2	
Postasphytic cerebral depression/1000	2.8	1.7	
Asphyxic Fetal deaths during labour/1000	3.6	1.2	2.8

(Adapted from Gosselin P, Roy A, Desjardins P, DeLeon A, Usher R; By permission of the Quebec Perinatal Committee, 1973)

Seven Year Olds reported that 14% of children born in 1958 had special needs.[64] In Canada, according to the 1966 census, 22% of the total population, or 8.4 million children, were 19 years of age and under. If we accept the incidence figures of 10% to 15%, this means that between 840,000 and 1,260,000 children and youths in Canada have emotional and learning disorders.[62] For the United States, this would translate into 8.4 to 12.6 million similarly afflicted.

It is uncertain how much of this formidable burden of handicap is determined by conditions which are amenable to prevention by optimal reproductive medical care. The evidence suggests that it may be of great, if not

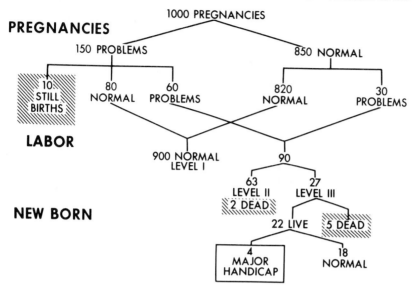

Fig. 3-6. Schematic pregnancy outcome.

paramount, importance if the whole gamut of reproductive medical care is considered, including health education of parents; adequate nutrition; genetic counselling; and prenatal, natal, and postnatal care. The potential economic savings to be realized are obviously very great if a substantial proportion of handicap could be eliminated, quite apart from the humanitarian aspect.

Severe handicap was expected in 40%–70% of infants weighing less than 1500 g in the 1950s, while recent figures emanating from special centers integrating both obstetric and pediatric neonatal care show a handicap incidence rate of less than 15%.*[65–67] Purely neonatal referral centers (*e.g.,* Toronto's Hospital for Sick Children) have a somewhat worse experience (19%), which is thought to be due to the impossibility of remedying prenatal, intranatal, and/or peripartum injury by postpartum transfer and treatment.[70] Such data are now sufficient to assure that the introduction of perinatal intensive care has not increased the incidence of damaged survivors.*

In 1968, it was estimated in France that there were 40,000 handicapped survivors annually from 833,000 live births (4.8%).[18] Various estimates quoted by Wynn and Wynn suggest that about 1% of all live births will be severely handicapped.[18] It has been conservatively estimated from improved experience in The Hospital for Sick Children in Toronto that a more recent (1976) figure for the severest handicap might be about 0.4% of all live births (Fig. 3-6).†

Table 3-9 shows the high incidence of antecedent obstetrical problems in the mothers of newborns admitted to an ICN. This represents an argument for fully integrated obstetric and neonatal services and the antenatal referral of risk pregnancies (15% of all pregnancies) which are predictable by current methods to Level II (12%) or Level III (3%) facilities. Tables 3-9, 3-12, 3-13, and 3-14, emphasize the prenatal, intranatal, and immediate postnatal origin of many problems which can only be palliated by neonatal intensive care as opposed to prevention or cure by total integrated reproductive medical care.

The schematic (Figure 3-6) demonstrates the outcome of 1000 unselected pregnancies, according to the broadly averaged current experience in developed countries. This outcome includes ten stillbirths, seven neonatal deaths, and four infants surviving with a major handicap, a conservative figure.[71]

Financial Implications. The humanitarian and financial implications for avoidance of

Table 3-9. Antecedent Obsteric Features.*

	Number	Percent†
Small for gestational age	132	10.9%
Multiple pregnancy		
Twin	102	(51 sets)
Triplet	3	(1 set)
Complicated pregnancy	439	36.2%
Membranes ruptured over 24 hours.	150	12.4%
Complicated delivery	937	77.25%

* In 1213 admissions, Neonatal Intensive Care Unit, The Hospital for Sick Children 1976.

† Percentage figures do not add to 100% because many patients have more than one condition cited.

reproductive casualty are very substantial indeed. With annual births of 3.3 million in the United States and a conservative estimate of incidence of severe brain damage of 0.5% to 1%, between 16,500 and 33,000 severely handicapped persons are added to the population annually, each entailing an average overall lifetime cost estimate at about $100,000 (1971 prices).[18] Data from North America suggest that this cost is over $0.5 million at current prices.[72] Comparison of the general average of mortality and morbidity with data from specific hospitals having the better perinatal statistics suggests that the full application of current knowledge in a reproductive medical care system would result in an approximately 50% reduction in the incidence of severe handicap and a saving of up to 5000 neonatal lives annually in the United States. The proportion of <1500 g survivors achieving normality has tripled from 30% to more than 85% in institutions combining intensive care during and after labor for the mother, fetus, and newborn;[70] while the absolute number of surviving undamaged has quadrupled because of reductions in mortality. These results however are only achieved if the appropriate care facilities are available and are appropriately used, as data from the Quebec Perinatal Committee and from other centers make clear.

Disparities in Regionalization. What are the reasons for these disparities? Geographic factors of remoteness and climate are obviously important but can be overcome with modern transport and communication technology although at some expense. However, geography cannot be blamed for the variations within metropolitan districts or cities. Here, variances more often seem based on socioeconomic, cultural, and educational differences in attitudes toward pregnancy and medical care because medical facilities are frequently locally available and financially accessible with the advent of universal, often state-supported, medical insurance plans.[43] Economic factors are not necessarily paramount. The United States, one of the richer countries in the world, has higher mortality rates than some less prosperous countries.

Nor is this mainly a rural community problem. Comparisons of rural and urban statistics in regions with and without high-risk obstetric-neonatal facilities show that domicile is of no importance, providing that optimal reproductive care facilities are both available and used.[73] Furthermore, maternal mortality and perinatal mortality statistics are closely linked but do not necessarily parallel infant mortality or older population mortality. This suggests that facilities for reproductive care are different from those needed for general health care, and that it can be given adequately only by people with special training using specific facilities. As a result, many jurisdictions, notably France[18,34,42,74] and 90% of the states in the United States,[56] have been rapidly developing and establishing regionalization plans.

The Costs and Potential Financial Benefits of a Regional System

The costs of operating a regionalized system have to be set against the savings achieved by reduction in damaged survivors needing long-term support. To be deducted from the costs of a new system would be those of the obstetric/pediatric reproductive medical service system currently in place, which would be absorbed and superseded by a regionalized program.

Also to be considered is the contribution in costs of genetic and chromosomally determined problems to perinatal morbidity and mortality, conservatively estimated at 2% of live births.[75] The genetic component is formidable, as indicated by the demonstration that approximately 30% of admissions to a pediatric hospital have some genetic involvement.[76] Some of these problems are avoidable by genetic counseling or therapeutic abortion, where acceptable.[75]

It is questionable whether it is possible or valid strictly to use cost/benefit analysis in the health field in relation to avoidance of mortality. This is because, in computing costs of early death in terms of lifetime earnings, productive capacity, and taxes as lost contributions to the community, one must take into account the fact that each individual is also a consumer of goods and services that missed consumption, which may largely cancel out contribution.[77] Benefits may have to be assessed on other grounds entirely: humanitarian and social. However, there does seem to be considerable potential for reduction in long-term morbidity (about 50%) by the proper application of present-day knowledge in reproductive medicine, and, here, cost/benefit analysis is much more convincing.

A detailed examination in France of the cost of perinatally determined handicaps, and the economic benefits of prevention, was initiated on the highest level in 1966 by Georges Pompidou, then Prime Minister of France. This initiative resulted from studies in the Fifth French Plan, which had shown the great cost and numbers of handicapped children. A series of studies culminated in designation of the reduction of "the damaging consequence in human, economic and financial terms of death and handicap attributable to pregnancy and childbirth" as the "Priority of Priorities."[18] Action was subsequently taken as part of the French Sixth Plan (1971–1975) and continued in the Seventh Plan, starting in January 1976.

The French have therefore produced, and partly implemented, a national perinatal policy with the objective of reducing perinatal handicap. Previously, this had been estimated as

an annual flow of 40,000 handicapped individuals eventuating from 833,000 live births in 1968. Of these, 8330, or one-fifth, were severely handicapped in the sense that the consequences were exceedingly costly, a figure corroborated by several other studies.[18,62,78,79]

There has been concern that programs aimed at reducing perinatal handicap might, by improving the chances of survival of handicapped individuals, paradoxically increase the total burden of handicapped. For example, over 70% of mongoloid infants now survive to school age, as compared to 10% 50 years ago.[18] Similar improvements in survival could be cited for hydrocephalus and spina bifida. On the other hand, advances in detection and prevention of such conditions as rhesus isoimmunization and phenylketonuria have markedly reduced or eliminated consequential handicap conditions. The French have stated that any program which resulted in a reduction in mortality but an increase in morbidity should be reconsidered. It is too early to obtain information on the overall impact of their program on morbidity, although a significant reduction in the incidence of prematurity has been registered between 1973 (8.2%, <36 weeks) and 1975–6 (6.8%, <36 weeks, p <0.001).[35]

While the objective has primarily been reduced perinatal morbidity rather than mortality, there has been a spectacular reduction in mortality. The French figure for 1970 was 23.4 per 1000 live births and a target of 18 per 1000 live births was set for 1980. in fact, the figure for 1977 is 14.8 per 1000 live births.*[34]

The French estimate was that each of their most seriously affected children (8300 in total, or 1% of annual live births) would cost about $300,000 at 1976 prices. While the most severely handicapped present the most visible problem, it may well be that the cost of the reduced employability of the much larger numbers of lesser handicapped[18] [estimated in the CELDIC Report to be one million individuals in Canada (extrapolated) to 10 million in the United States] is much greater.[62]

French data suggest that it is worth spending at least $60,000 in France (1970 prices or about $108,000 in 1978) to prevent one child from becoming handicapped.[18] Current estimates of the average cost of caring for one high-risk

* Salle B: personal communication, 1978

pregnancy and one problem newborn are of the order of $8,000* and $6,600[80] (1978 prices) respectively, not taking into account the cost of those in whom care is unsuccessful or which results in death or handicap. The approximate cost then of caring for and delivering one high-risk pregnancy is about $15,000.

Pomerance and associates, in the United States, have recently estimated the cost per "normal" survivor <1000 g to be $88,058, including an allowance for cases resulting in death or handicap.[81] Other United States estimates set the cost of lifetime support for a seriously handicapped person at about $750,-000 in 1978 prices. The French estimated that the total cost of reproductive casualty in France in 1976 amounted to $4,000 million annually, or $4,800 million, scaled to 1978 dollars.[18]

While society must be the final arbiter, the economics of preventive perinatal care appear compelling, to say nothing of the intangible humanitarian value.

Planning Regionalization

There has been an authoritative publication under the auspices of the American Academy of Family Physicians, the American Academy of Pediatrics, the American College of Obstetricians and Gynecologists, and the American Medical Association, assisted by the National Foundation–March of Dimes, entitled *Toward Improving the Outcome of Pregnancy, 1976.*[82] The principles of regionalization have most recently been described and further endorsed by the American Academy of Pediatrics in its publication *Standards and Recommendations for Hospital Care of Newborn Infants, 1977.*[83]

Such plans aim at providing a standard of care according to need, in conformity with the distribution of risk and morbidity in pregnancy and childbirth as set out in Fig. 3-6. It is recommended that three levels of reproductive medical care be made available on a regionalized basis as follows:

Level I (for 85% of pregnancies). Equipped and staffed to look after normal, low-risk pregnancies, deliveries, and newborns only, but with a capability to deal with emergencies aided by a predetermined contingency plan for support from the nearest level II or level III center.

* Effer SB: personal communication, 1979

Level II (for 12% of pregnancies). Equipped and staffed as in level I above, but, in addition, capable of providing services for pregnancies, deliveries, and newborns at moderate to high risk.

Level III (for 3% of pregnancies). Containing level I and level II services, but, in addition, capable of managing ultra-high risk pregnancies, deliveries, and newborns.

Eventually, level I services in hospitals or nursing stations should be free standing only in rural or isolated areas to provide for normal pregnancies. Elsewhere, level I services would gradually be integrated into institutions containing level II services, and, in the case of major referral centers, both level II and level III services. When the system is fully developed with time, most deliveries would take place in hospitals with both level I and level II facilities.

The exact nomenclature used for describing facilities in order of capability (*e.g.,* levels I, II, and III) is unimportant. It is essential, however, that there should be triage of pregnant and laboring women into low- (level I), moderate- (level II), and high- (level III) risk categories, and that facilities should be available in proportion to the estimated numbers in each category.

Each region would contain institutions offering all levels of care, but the levels and institutions would be organized in a collaborative system such that mutual consultation, support, and referral would be available to each level of care, appropriate to the needs of the individual patient. Such support would be supplied through the specialized services of level II and level III facilities, with the objectives of reducing perinatal mortality and morbidity.

The U.S. National Health Planning and Resources Development Act (PL 93-641) of 1974 requires that guidelines be prepared by the Department of Health, Education, and Welfare to include standards on the appropriate supply, distribution, and organization of health services. In 1977, proposed guidelines for Health Systems Agencies were published and there has since been an intense dialogue between Health, Education, and Welfare and professional and public organizations, resulting in increased flexibility and modification of the guidelines as originally published. Specifically, the guidelines were changed to provide for the

Table 3-10. Level II Numerical Considerations.

Population base						
(millions)	0.25	0.5	0.75	1	1.5	2
Live births (lb)	3,750	7,500	11,250	15,000	22,500	30,000
Incidence low birth weight						
/1000 lb	70	70	70	70	70	70
Needing Level II						
care/1000 lb	70	70	70	70	70	70
Patients/year						
level II	262	525	787	1,050	1,575	2,100
from level III*	93	187	282	375	562	750
	355	712	1,069	1,425	2,137	2,850
Length of stay						
(average)	7	7	7	7	7	7
Patient/days/year	2,485	4,984	7,483	9,975	14,959	19,950
Occupancy rate						
(%)	85	85	85	85	85	85
No. beds						
level II	6	12	18	24	36	48
from level III*	2	4.3	6.5	8.6	13.2	17
	8	16	24	33	49	65
Neonatologists						
(equivalents)	1†	1.5†	2	3	4	5

* Convalescent patients from level III
† Single-handed operation not possible.

integration of obstetric and pediatric neonatal services and to provide for four neonatal special care beds for intensive (level III) and intermediate (level II) care for 1000 live births/year, while allowing proportional adjustments in accordance with local geographic and demographic conditions such as an unusually high incidence of low-birth-weight deliveries in the community. It is advised that the four special care beds be divided into one for intensive care and three for intermediate care. In addition, there will need to be provision for 2 beds/1000 live births for continuing convalescent care for low-birth-weight infants. A recent survey[84] has identified 210 tertiary care units in the United States, integrated with varying degrees of regional organization.[56] The average bed number/unit was 31, 13.5 of which were at the intensive care level.

There has been discussion concerning the desirable size for tertiary and secondary care units. Generally, a compromise has to be reached between the distributional needs of the population in regard to accessibility and a unit large enough to provide a volume of patients sufficient to maintain the expertise of personnel and to afford economical use of expensive equipment and resources. It is obviously impossible to equip and staff every delivering hospital to the capability of a tertiary care unit. It should, however, be possible to equip and staff most hospitals in urban areas at least to the standards of a secondary care institution capable of managing all except the most complicated obstetric and neonatal problems. However, this may call for some consolidation of beds to achieve a reasonable patient volume. At least 1500 deliveries/year are required by the National Guidelines for Health Planning. However to maintain utilization of the mandated minimum of 15 beds (3 beds/1000 live births, intermediate [level II] and 2 beds/1000 live births continuing convalescent care [level I]), 3000 deliveries/year would be the required volume unless there was an active policy of referral to level II of patients from surrounding level I units. Health-planning agencies are therefore urged to consider merger and consolidation of maternity facilities to achieve this volume. It can even

Table 3-11. Level III: Numerical Considerations.

Population base					
(millions)	0.25	0.5	0.75	1	1.5
No. live births (lb)					
(15/1000 population)	3,750	7,500	11,250	15,000	22,500
Incidence low birth weight					
/1000 lb	70	70	70	70	70
Needing level III					
/1000 lb	30	30	30	30	30
Patients/year	112	225	338	450	675
Length of stay					
(average) days	10	10	10	10	10
Patient/days/					
year	1,125	2,250	3,375	4,500	6,750
Occupancy rate					
(%)	85	85	85	85	85
No. of beds	4	8	11	15	22
Neonatologists					
(equivalents)	1.5*	1	2	3	4

* Single handed operation not possible unless parttime comparably skilled help available or level II neonatologist associated.

be argued that facilities supplying all three levels of care would be the most effective because all facilities for any perinatal eventuality are on site and the necessity for either maternal or infant transfer is eliminated. Such a system is exemplified by the large county hospitals of Sweden and Finland, as well as by most of the functioning level III units in North America, which have been incorporated into regional plans.

Specialized publications should be consulted for information regarding equipment scales and staffing levels for each level of care.[32,56,57,71,85,87,88] Tables 3-10 and 3-11 give an idea of the numbers of beds and neonatal pediatric specialists needed for population bases varying from 0.25 million to 2 million.[71,91]

THE REGIONAL ORGANIZATION FOR REPRODUCTIVE MEDICAL CARE

A. The Problems to be Addressed

A coordinated system for the delivery of reproductive medical care is required to address the following problems and considerations:

1. The identification of the risk pregnancy and newborn and their referral to the appropriate level of care for the identified problem.
2. The high cost of perinatal intensive care and the limited availability of suitably trained personnel, equipment, and plant.
3. Not all hospitals with obstetric and neonatal services are capable of supplying high-risk care, with the result that some high-risk patients may not receive necessary care.
4. Developments in knowledge and the technology of care for the pregnant woman and newborn infant may not be applied systematically according to need.
5. In some areas, improved care may not be available.
6. Avoidance of duplication of personnel and facilities

In order to deal with these problems and considerations, it is necessary to develop a plan providing for the identification of risk at the primary care level, by means of an antenatal risk scoring system,[93-95] and to provide facilities in three levels of increasing capability according to identified risk level:

Level I   Normal pregnancy, delivery, and newborn care

Level II Care appropriate to moderate risk in the mother, fetus, and newborn

Level III Care appropriate to high risk in the mother, fetus, and newborn

The guiding principles for this organization are

1. That risk patients be identified early in pregnancy and appropriately referred.
2. That infants be born in facilities best adapted to care for expected problems within a regional organization.
3. That high-risk perinatal care (level III) be concentrated, usually in regional centers, for reproductive medical care, situated in major hospitals, often, but not necessarily, university affiliated.
4. That such centers should contain all three levels of care.
5. That level II centers should contain both level II and level I facilities.
6. That small hospitals in urban areas amalgamate and consolidate obstetric and neonatal services so that they can provide for all but the highest level of risk (*i.e.*, consolidate level II and level I services).
7. That the system provide for linkage between the different components to ensure optimal prenatal, natal, and postnatal care; professional and public education; data retrieval; and follow-up of outcome. All centers, regardless of level, should be able to provide immediate management of unpredictable problems and emergencies.
8. That patients be free to move between different levels of care within a hospital or between hospitals in the region, based on need.
9. That the level III institution—the regional center for reproductive medical care—be responsible for coordinating the operations within the region, providing for education and outreach programs, and conducting research in reproductive medicine.
10. That the system take account of the culture, demography, geography, climate, and the resource strengths of a region and be suitably flexible.

The specifications for, and the detailed implementation of, such a system have been accumulated in an extensive literature, from Canada,[71,85−87,90] the United States,[54,57,82,83,88−91] and other countries.[17,18,92]

It is more difficult to be precise about the specifications for a level II facility than for a level III. This is because the type and severity of diseased patients admitted, both maternal and infant, are less clearly defined and indeed should be flexible. Essentially similar basic staff and services will be required at both levels except that the range of highly specialized life support, and consultative and laboratory services will be curtailed for the level II facility. It is, for example, obviously impracticable and unnecessary to mandate genetic tissue culture laboratories in each level II facility. However, local conditions of geography, climate, expertise, and staffing level may well determine, for example, whether an infant is mechanically ventilated beyond about 1 hour in a given level II facility or whether the infant is transferred to a level III unit for this purpose, with corresponding variations in personnel and equipment scales.

As far as the mother is concerned, an identified moderate pregnancy risk score from the antenatal record will suggest consultation with a view to delivery in a level II facility, while a score in the high range will have similar implications for level III.

Regarding the infant, the following conditions would suggest consideration for consultation or transfer from Level I to Level II:

Gestation of less then 35 weeks or weight less than 2.5 kg
Neonatal sepsis or infection
Respiratory distress persisting beyond two hours of age
Evidence of neonatal blood loss, pallor, low blood pressure, or low hemoglobin
Hypoglycemia
Hemolytic disease
Infants of mothers taking hazardous drugs
Infants needing more than routine observation.

At level I the most pressing need is for the updating of personnel skills and equipment for neonatal resuscitation.

B. Risk Factors Associated with Pregnancy and Delivery

Risk factors prior to and during pregnancy include preexisting maternal disease, low socioeconomic level, vaginal bleeding, infection, hydramnios, and heavy smoking. Obstetric factors include mechanical complications and uterine inertia, toxemia, and isoimmunization.

Table 3-12. Risk Factors—Preconception.

Factor	Risk
Social	Poor antenatal care
Low-income level	Multiparity
	Eclampsia
Heavy work during pregnancy	Placental insufficiency
	Antepartum hemorrhage
Poor diet	Fetal malnutrition
	Prematurity
Lack of cooperation	Undetected hypertension
with physician	Anemia
	Albuminuria
Illegitimacy	Poor antenatal care
	Increased birth risks
Medical	Prematurity
Anemia due to iron or	
vitamin B_{12} deficiency	Malnourished babies
Diabetes mellitus	Hypertension
	Preeclampsia
	Toxemia
	Large-for-dates babies
	Congenital abnormalities
	Increased cesarian section rate
Hereditary disease	Cystic fibrosis
	Meconium ileus
Renal and cardiac disease	Toxemia
	Maternal cardiac decompensation
	Increased maternal death rate and
	perinatal mortality
Obesity	Hypertension
	Pelvic disproportion
Living at high altitude	Low birth weight
Obstetric	
<16 or >40 years	Abortion
	Toxemia
	Congenital abnormalities
Older primipara	Increased risks to baby
Multiparity >3	Ante- and postpartum hemorrhage
Previous history of fetal loss	Fetal risk
Low-birth-weight infant	
Multiple pregnancy	

(Based on details by Segal S: Personal communications, 1973)

These factors are explained more fully in Tables 3-12, 3-13, and 3-14.

In 1967, the Ontario Perinatal Mortality Committee showed that broadly identifiable risk factors could be determined in 32% of pregnancies, generating approximately 60% of neonatal problems.[96] Since that time, refinements have narrowed the definition to 15% of all pregnancies carrying significant risk (*i.e.,* 150 per 1000 live births).[97] Ideally, prenatally defined risk pregnancies should be selected for delivery in level II and III centers, according to the level of risk.

The delineation of all risk factors associated

Table 3-13. Risk Factors—Pregnancy.

Factor	Risk
Medical	
Infective	
VIRAL	
Rubella in 1st trimester	Congenital heart disease
	Cataracts
	Nerve deafness
	Bone lesions
	Prolonged virus shedding
Rubella, 2nd and 3rd trimesters	Hepatitis
	Thrombocytopenia
Herpes simplex	Neonatal hepatitis
Cytomegalovirus	Neonatal hepatitis
	Encephalopathy
Vaccinia (especially 1st trimester)	Congenital vaccinia
Maternal varicella	Congenital varicella
BACTERIAL	
Syphilis	Abortion
Tuberculosis	Congenital syphilis
Coliform urinary tract infection	Neonatal transplacental transmission
	Premature delivery
	Neonatal infection
PROTOZOAL	
Toxoplasma	Retinal, CNS lesions
	Hepatitis
	Microcephaly
	Thrombocytopenia
Malaria	Transplacental spread
Noninfective	
Hypertension and other	Premature birth
cardiovascular disease	Fetal embarrassment
Hyperthyroidism	Neonatal goiter from antithyroid drugs
	Neonatal thyrotoxicosis (LATS)
Myasthenia gravis	Exacerbation and resistance to drug
	therapy
Preeclampsia, nephritis,	Premature births
hypertension, excessive	Intrauterine growth retardation with
smoking by mother	small-for-dates babies
Unusual maternal medication	Congenital abnormalities
or addictive drug abuse	Neonatal withdrawal symptoms
Falling urinary estriol levels	Failing placental (placental insufficiency)
	function, fetal risk

(Based on details by Segal S: Personal communications, 1973)

with a given pregnancy requires not only a definite strategy on the part of the primary physician but also a system of consultants, professional and nonprofessional aides, as well as laboratory and hospital facilities. Identification of a risk pregnancy is aided by the use of prognostic scoring systems.[71,93–95,98] It is suggested that the center be notified of each

Table 3-14. Risk Factors-Labor.

Factor	Risk
OBSTETRICAL	Prematurity
Abnormal presentation	Malformation
	Cesarean section
Abruptio placentae	Fetal asphyxia
	Fetal exsanguination
	Perinatal mortality
Eclampsia, preeclampsia	Fetal morbidity, mortality
Fetal heart aberrations	Fetal distress
	Paroxysmal tachycardia, heart block
Multiple births	Small-for-dates babies
	Prematurity
	Feto-fetal transfusion
	Failure to recognize
	Increased perinatal mortality
Oligohydramnios	Postmaturity
	Congenital malformation
	Renal lesions
Hydramnios	Esophageal or other high alimentary tract atresias
	CNS anomalies
	Myelocele
	Hydrops
Precipitate delivery	Tentorial tears
	Neonatal asphyxia
Prolonged labor	Fetal asphyxia
	Intracranial birth injury
Rhesus or blood group sensitization	Hydrops
	Icterus gravis
	Neonatal anemia
	Kernicterus
	Hypoglycemia
Uterine rupture	Fetal asphyxia
Early rupture of the membranes >48 hours before delivery	Infection
Postcontraction fetal bradycardia	Fetal asphyxia
Fever	Premature delivery
	Neonatal infection
Meconium staining of liquor	Fetal asphyxia indicated by fetal scalp sample of blood pH <7.2

(Based on details by Segal S: Personal communications, 1973)

pregnancy on a standardized form to allow access to the system of pregnancy health care.[71] This form can serve to initiate a dialogue between primary physician and the consultant in case of need. Delivery can then be planned to take place in a facility at the appropriate level of complexity, whether for a normal delivery or for a pregnancy carrying a high risk, demanding all the resources of a major perinatal center. It should also be made possible for the primary physician to continue to take appropriate responsibility for his patients at all levels, with consulting help from the specialist team if necessary.

Such a scheme seems to be straightforward, but the element of unpredictable risk has to be allowed for in the system: (*i.e.*, a sudden accidental antepartum hemorrhage in a level I unit). Thus, facilities at all levels should be equipped to deal with emergency situations and to initiate, with support from the organization, a contingency plan to deal with the emergency.

C. Referral and Transport

A recognized need in a regionalized system is the ability to transport the risk mother before delivery from a level I to a level II or III facility. Increasing *in utero* referral can be expected to reduce the need for difficult neonatal transport.[99,100]

There is a definite necessity for personnel especially trained in the transport of mothers (prior to labor) and of sick infants.[99-104] There will be a limited requirement for skilled medical coverage of both types of medical personnel who will also need special background knowledge of transportation procedures.

The regional hospital center is the logical place to locate the majority of the transport services for the region. These services might include cars to bring patients to and from clinics, ambulances, and flying squad units— specialized vehicles with head room and services for monitoring and life-support, including skilled professional personnel for the transport of the seriously ill patient (mother and/or baby). Mobile units can be provided for the transport of public health personnel going into the community to carry out maternal and child health care, preventive medicine, and educational programs. Transport may also be needed to enable attendance at special facilities which cannot be duplicated locally such as genetic counseling, family planning, and premarital or marital counseling.

D. Evaluation and Data Collection

Continuous improvement in the delivery of perinatal care necessitates the availability of certain statistical data. It is necessary to have accurate figures on the distribution of perinatal deaths by hospital, by clinical referral area,

and by region. As well, these data must be available in such a way that they can be linked to the many known causes of perinatal morbidity and mortality for the following reasons:

1. To ensure the availability of accurate perinatal mortality rates (including stillbirth and early neonatal death rates)
2. To provide educational feedback to health care professionals
3. To monitor changes in perinatal mortality rates as a consequence of the way the delivery of reproductive care is organized
   a. to monitor variations among hospitals
   b. to monitor regional referral patterns and the efficiency of identification of high-risk pregnancies.
   c. to monitor the relationship between perinatal morbidity and mortality and the numbers of deliveries at levels I, II or III
4. To identify areas of need or deficiency due to regional variations, to social or eugenic factors, or to changes in mortality over time
   a. to monitor the incidence of prematurity and small-for-gestational-age infants
   b. to monitor survival rates among birth weight and gestational age categories
   c. to monitor survival rates related to mothers' age and parity
   d. to monitor variations in causes of stillbirth and neonatal death
5. To identify relationships between perinatal mortality and morbidity, and maternal morbidity
6. To provide planners and researchers with a useful data base
7. To facilitate planning activities leading to policy recommendations
   a. concerning regional referral patterns
   b. concerning special assistance for areas of need
   c. concerning minimum case load standards
   d. concerning specialized services and technologies
8. To assist the surveillance of congenital anomalies

With this information, it should be possible to analyze the various risk factors which have contributed to perinatal death or morbidity. With further analysis of these data with respect to regions, clinical referral areas, and hospitals, it should be possible to determine whether services in antenatal, intrapartum, or postnatal care need to be modified. Furthermore, such analysis should have educational value for the attending staff, to indicate the relevance and importance of these factors in patient management. Feedback of such data will enable perinatal review committees in hospitals and regions to monitor comparative data from their own and others' areas.

E. Communication

Free flow of data, information, and consultation among individuals and levels of care is very important to the operation of a regional reproductive care system, especially so in the identification of risk by means of the antenatal risk score form. Confidentiality should be maintained. It is unnecessary that the patient's name be revealed when statistical information only is being sought.

The level III facility should comprise an information and data retrieval center for the region with access to computer facilities. This center should coordinate and collect data from each institution and level of care within the region, with regard to incidence of risk pregnancy; numbers of admissions and births at each level; outcome, including incidence of handicap; and cost accounting. It should maintain a pregnancy risk register and a register of handicaps originating at birth. Central linkage of birth data (birth certificate), mortality data, and morbidity data from follow-up programs is strongly advised.

Telephone Facilities. Special telephone arrangements, such as a non-dial, "hotline" linkage between referring and referral institutions, results in a significant reduction in mortality.[105] Radio-telephone links are especially helpful during air transfer and have been found most useful during road transport in terms of logistics, scheduling of transport, and consultation concerned with the clinical management of the patient before and in transit. Information from a tape library can be relayed on a subject in which up-to-date knowledge is required. Transmission of educational video tapes on closed circuit TV can also be encouraged. No-toll telephone line service for these video and other tapes is advantageous. Arrangements could even be made to tape the conversations

and, after review, forward further relevant information including reprints of pertinent articles.

F. Responsibilities of the Regional Center

Level III units in health sciences centers should have responsibilities beyond patient care in teaching, research, and regional administration.

Professional Education. As part of medical school training, there will be responsibility for the undergraduate teaching of the obstetric and pediatric components of reproductive medicine. Post-graduate instruction of interns, residents, and fellows (subspecialists in training) should also be undertaken. Similarly, the counterparts of this teaching are necessary for professional nursing as well as for the paramedical disciplines. The tertiary center should also have a responsibility for outreach programs at all levels to the hospitals in the region.

Despite these teaching requirements, it is likely that the service load will be more than that required to provide adequate teaching material for these programs. This should be recognized in developing a global budget, taking into account both the teaching and service needs of the institution.

There is also a responsibility to educate the public regarding the facts surrounding successful reproduction and family life. In this connection, the contribution of other groups, medical (*e.g.*, public health) and lay, should be recognized and their help and cooperation sought.

Education of the Public. The provision of exemplary reproductive care is of no avail if it is not used; for example, 20% of women presenting for delivery on the nonreferred ward service of the Winnipeg General Hospital had received no prenatal care, according to a recent survey.* There is an inverse relationship between the number of prenatal examinations and perinatal mortality[63] and morbidity.[74]

There needs to be a sustained effort to instruct the public in sex education, family planning, genetics, and the antenatal, natal, and postnatal care required for optimal reproductive performance. The logical place for this

* Roulston M: Personal communication, 1970

education to commence is in the schools, where virtually 100% of the prospective re-producing population can be reached at a receptive age. Instruction in the school can be reinforced by a continuing campaign in the press, radio, or television, as well as on a personal basis through physicians, public health nurses, and allied health workers.

Research

The tertiary care center should be involved in basic, developmental, and operational re-search in reproductive medicine in the region. Research is essential not only to develop new knowledge, but also as a means of maintaining a critical attitude toward standards of care and of developing a cadre of knowledgeable indi-viduals able critically to evaluate recent ad-vances in the field from other jurisdictions, and to abstract them for current application locally when indicated.

Monitoring and Operational Research

The tertiary center should be responsible for monitoring the functioning of the regional system by evaluation of health indicators, both numerical and qualitative, providing feedback on performance to the component units in the region.

Regional Administration

While each component at the primary, sec-ondary, or tertiary level should be largely autonomous, the level III center should facil-itate the system for referral, consultation, and emergency support inherent to the regional system, including coordination of the transport network. It is also possible that there might be economies of scale in central purchasing of certain items in use throughout the region.

Staffing at all levels should take account of responsibilities beyond direct service to pa-tients. The administrative and monitoring func-tions suggest the need of a data and commu-nications facility at the regional center. The overall functioning of the system should be monitored by a committee representing the regional health authority, medical profession-als, and the public, with suitable statistical and secretarial resources.

The regional responsibilities of the regional center transcend the local responsibilities of the institution within which the facility hap-pens to be situated. The level III facility should

therefore have an administrative structure and budget separate from, though cooperative with, the institution in which it is situated.

Personnel

The personnel involved in the care of the mother and her infant may range from unskilled labor (home-helpers, baby-sitters, and so on) to highly skilled professionals specializing in obstetric and neonatal care. It is essential that some organization of personnel resources exist so that the services may be used in an eco-nomical and efficient manner. An estimate must be made of the numbers of highly skilled and less skilled personnel required to provide the necessary services, and this information should be distributed to medical schools, pub-lic health services, nursing schools, health science centers, and interested professional societies and licensing bodies. This informa-tion assists those desirous of further training in specialized fields to enter appropriate train-ing programs to meet the needs of the country.

The optimal care of both mother and child requires the services of a number of medical and paramedical personnel working as a team to care for the patient throughout her preg-nancy, delivery, and postnatal period. Appro-priate deployment of personnel is facilitated if established lines of communication and pat-terns of referral are developed. Ideally, medical personnel working in close liaison with par-amedical personnel can provide both impatient and outpatient care. Group practice facilitates this type of service.

The specialist medical staff in regional cen-ters can be responsible for the supervision of the nonspecialist staff within the regional hos-pital center itself and in community or periph-eral hospital centers. The provision of a ro-tating visiting service by specialized personnel for community hospital centers can be estab-lished and a two-way traffic encouraged (i.e., medical staff from the community center can also be encouraged to visit the regional center for postgraduate courses and meetings).

The regional center can be responsible for the provision and maintenance of maternal, fetal, and neonatal life-support equipment from a central pool. There can be a regional approach to purchasing and services such as pharmacy and medical supplies, laundry, and long-term storage of relatively inactive records.

Consulting and Support Services in a Regional System

The requirements for consulting and support services for level III are stringent because serious, difficult, and relatively rare disease is being treated in both mother and infant. For level II, the usual resources of a large general hospital with a pediatric component are adequate. More specialized consulting services should be made available by the level III center to levels II and I on request. A detailed listing of consulting and support services for reproductive medicine is available in several recent publications.[56,57,71,83,86-88]

Laboratory Services. These should be organized within the regional center to provide specialized tests not only for patients within the center, but also for the community, district hospitals, and clinics in the region. Examples are the genetic, cytologic, chemical, and spectrophotometric analysis of amniotic fluid and estriol determination.

Blood Bank. The regional center can provide a typing laboratory and depot for the storage of donor blood. Delivery of mothers in hospitals that do not carry donor blood is not advised. At least one unit of group O Rh-negative blood can be kept on hand and arrangements made for cycling replacement within 72 hours of blood required both for the obstetric and neonatal patients.

Risk Registers. Prenatal risk registers for the mother and postnatal risk registers for the infant can be maintained at the regional center. These registers can be used as tools to ensure that risk patients are identified and provided with care appropriate to their needs.

Special Outpatient Facilities. Provision can be made for those specialized services needed by the community such as premarital counseling, family planning, genetic counseling, and marriage counseling. These should be coordinated from, and may be situated in, the regional center, although it may be necessary for personnel to take their facilities to more remote areas within the region.

Outpatient services can usually be based in the hospital which provides inpatient services, thus establishing both a human and a documentary link. In some circumstances, however, considerations of geography, transportation, or personal choice may make it necessary for the outpatient and community services for prenatal and postnatal care of mother and infant to be rendered in a hospital, clinic or doctor's office, closer to the patient's residence. In these instances, the patient can still travel to the more distant obstetric unit for delivery.

G. Implementation

The intention would be to develop a regionalized system of primary, secondary, and tertiary care, integrating preventative, public health, obstetric and pediatric services by a phased reorganization of existing institutions and personnel. Because the institutional and staffing structure is largely in place, though poorly integrated, the costs of reorganization into a regional system should be relatively small and could be offset by rationalization and elimination of duplications, the changes necessary being gradually implemented over a number of years. Furthermore, informed estimates indicate that significant savings in health care costs can be realized by application of current knowledge.[18,54,71,89,90,92]

The location and distribution of level I and II units will largely be determined by the existing situation. The designation of existing facilities into levels I and II should be decided by consultation among the local professional and lay organizations, the responsible level II center, and the local health authority, having regard for local conditions and requirements. In urban centers, level I units should progressively be incorporated into level II units. There are two guiding principles which are, to a varying degree, antithetical and require compromise:

1. To achieve, where possible in relation to population density, an efficient and economic size (1,000–3,000 live births/year)
2. To preserve accessibility by population and staff

In this connection a travel time of not more than 30 minutes is suggested. In non-urban areas, this standard may need to be modified. Free-standing level I units might be retained or even newly created where travel times would be excessive.

Implementation should be time-phased, with goals to be achieved within a finite time period. Hospitals to be approved as Level II and Level III centers should provide documentation to ensure the availability of resources, both physical and personal, and identify the goals to be achieved. The centers should be required to self-evaluate their activities and results as related to defined goals.

Geographic remoteness and severe climatic conditions in some areas may justify the development of a degree of capability for level III care, as well as the full range of special secondary and primary care, despite a relatively small patient volume. The difficulty in the development of such limited tertiary care facilities resides in the relative failure to achieve the necessary critical numbers of patients needed to maintain expertise in staff and economical use of expensive resources. It has been suggested that 15 to 20 intensive care beds represent the minimum size of a tertiary newborn intensive care unit for economic staffing, equipping, and efficient operation.[18,71,83,85,88,90,91]

It is inherently unlikely that the full range of services of a tertiary care center could be provided without the resources of a health sciences center. Lack of residents and fellows in training, a legitimate service component in health sciences centers, would enjoin a relatively larger establishment of senior staff with a full-time or major part-time geographic commitment to perinatal medicine. It would also be very difficult to maintain the wide range of laboratory and special services essential to the operation of a complete tertiary care center.

CONCLUSION

The needs of the patient must always be the guiding principle in the whole organization of regional care. Factional local and jurisdictional conflicts must all be solved with the patient's prime interest in mind. Resolution of problems is usually signally aided by this approach.

REFERENCES

1. **Butler NR, Alberman ED:** Perinatal Problems: The Second Report of the 1958 British Perinatal Mortality Survey, p 44. Edinburgh and London, E & S Livingstone, 1969
2. **Butler NR:** Perinatal mortality: A world problem. The Glaxo Volume 37:24, 1972
3. **Butler NR, Bonham DG:** Perinatal Mortality: The First Report of the 1958 British Perinatal Mortality Survey (under the auspices of the National Birthday Trust Fund). Edinburgh, E & S Livingstone, 1963
4. **Morrison AB, Maykut MO:** Potential adverse effects of maternal alcohol ingestion on the developing fetus and their sequelae in the infant and child. Can Med Assoc J 120: 826–828,1979
5. **Miller HC, Merritt TA:** Fetal Growth in Humans p 103. Chicago and London, Year Book Medical Publishers, 1979
6. **Blinick G, Wallach R, Jereg E, Ackermann BD:** Drug addiction in pregnancy and the neonate. Am J Obstet Gynecol 125:135, 1976
7. U.S. Surgeon General's Report on Health Promotion and Disease Prevention: Healthy People. 1979
8. **Scott KE, Stone SH:** The unwanted pregnancy: Inevitable, burdensome, the cause of overpopulation (abstr). Ann. R. Coll. of Physicians Surg. of Canada, 6:51, 1973
9. **Wynn M, Wynn A:** Some consequences of induced abortion to children born subsequently. London, Foundation of Education and Research in Childbearing, 1972. See also editorial, Br Med J 1:506, 1973
10. **Swyer PR:** New trends in maternal, fetal, and neonatal medicine. Dimens Health Serv 56: 5 48–50, 1979
11. **James LS, Jonathan TL:** History of oxygen therapy and retrolental fibroplasia. Pediatrics [Suppl] 57:4 (Part 2) 591–642, 1976
12. **Baird D:** Perinatal mortality. Lancet I:515, 1969
13. **Baird D:** An area maternity service. Lancet I:515, 1969.
14. Reports to Council. Ontario Medical Association, 1977
15. **Usher RH:** Clinical implications of perinatal mortality statistics. Clin Obstet Gynecol 14: 885, 1971
16. Quebec Perinatal Committee: Perinatal Intensive Care After Integration of Obstetrical Services in Quebec: A Policy Statement of the Quebec Perinatal Committee. Quebec City, Ministry of Social Affairs, 1973
17. **Wynn M, Wynn A:** The Protection of Maternity and Infancy: A Study of the Services for Pregnant Women and Young Children in Finland with Some Comparisons with Britain. London, Council for Children's Welfare, 1974
18. **Wynn M, Wynn A:** Prevention of Handicap of Perinatal Origin: An Introduction to French Policy and Legislation. London, Foundation for Education and Research in Child-Bearing, 1976
19. **Usher RH:** Changing mortality rates with perinatal intensive care and regionalization. Semin Perinatol 1:309, 1977

20. **Miller HC, Merritt TA:** Fetal Growth in Humans p 155. Chicago, Year Book Medical Publishers, 1979

21. **Benzie RJ, Mahony MJ:** Fetoscopy and fetal tissue sampling. Report of international workshop on perinatal diagnosis: past, present, and future. Can Med Assoc J in press

22. **Doran TA, Benzie RJ, Harkin JL, Jones-Owen VM, Potter CJ, Thompson DW, Liedgren SI:** Amniotic fluid tests for fetal maturity. Am J Obstet Gynecol 119:829–837, 1974

23. **Hon EH, Hellegher A (ed):** Conference on Perinatal Research: Status of Fetus. Report of the 64th Ross Conference on Pediatric Research, Columbus, Ross Laboratories, 1971

24. **Caldeyro-Barcia R, Mendez-Bauer C, Poseiro JJ, Escarcena LA et al:** Control of human fetal heart rate during labour. In Cassels DE (ed): The Heart and Circulation in the Newborn Infant, pp 7–36. New York, Grune & Stratton, 1966

25. **Effer SB:** Intensive care: Obstetrical considerations. In Goodwin JW, Godden JO, Chance GW (eds): Perinatal Medicine, p 578. 1976

26. **Dawes GS:** Prenatal life: Fetal respiratory movements rediscovered. Pediatrics 51:965, 1973

27. **Reid L:** The lung: Its growth and remodeling in health and disease. Am J Roentgenol 129: 777–788, 1979

28. **Saling E:** Amnioscopy and foetal blood sampling: Observations on foetal acidosis. Arch Dis Child 41:472, 1966

29. **Low JA, Boston RW, Pancham SR:** The role of fetal heart rate patterns in the recognition of fetal asphyxia with metabolic acidosis. Am J Obstet Gynecol 109:922, 1971

30. **Cohen SL:** Estrogens and pregnancy. In Goodwin JW, Godden JO, Chance GW (eds): Perinatal Medicine, p 363. 1976

31. **Friesen HG, Singer W:** Human placental lactogen and chorionic thyrotropin. In Goodwin JW, Godden JO, Chance GW (eds): Perinatal Medicine, p. 347. 1976

32. **Swyer PR, Goodwin JW (eds):** Regional Services in Reproductive Medicine, p 7. Toronto, The Joint Committee of the Society of Obstetricians and Gynecologists of Canada and the Canadian Pediatric Society, 1973

33. **Flusin MF, Fournel M, Raddi A:** Resultats statistiques de l'exploitation des certificats de sante du 8e jour et du 9e mois dans le departement du Doubs. La Revue de Pediatrie XIV:276–280, 1978

34. **Beaufils F, Bouet A:** France. Lancet II:1352, 1979

35. **Revellin R, Salle B, Magnin P:** Evolution de la frequence et du pronostic de la prematurité a l'hôpital Edouard Herriot au cours des dernières annés (1970–1976). Rev Franc Gynec 73:319–322, 1978

36. **Rumeau-Rouquette C:** Evaluation epidemiologique du Programme de Perinatologie, Enquêtes Nationales 1972 et 1975–1976. Rapport de l'unité 149 de L'INSERM, 1978

37. **Netherlands Pocket Year Book, 1977:** Netherlands Central Bureau of Statistics. S'Gravenhage Staatsuitgeverij, 1977

38. **Kloosterman GJ:** De Voortplanting van de Mens (Human Reproduction). Centen, Bussum, 1973

39. **Eskes TKAB:** Lecture: Department of Obstetrics and Gynecology and Physiology. Denver, University of Colorado Medical Centre, April 5, 1976

40. Interprofessional Task Force on Health Care Family Centered Maternity/Newborn Care in Hospitals. Chicago, American College of Obstetrics and Gynecology. 1978

41. **Ferris C, Read F, Clyman R, Leonard C, Irwin N:** Safety of a hospital base antenatal birthing center. Clin Res 26:197, 1978

42. Editorial La Perinatalité. Nouvelle Presse Medicale, 7:3684, 1978

43. **Anderson UM:** Infant survival differential in the city of Toronto: A challenge to health planning and research. Can Fam Phys 16: 945–50, 1970

44. **Karel F (ed):** The Robert Wood Johnson Foundation. Special Report No 2, 1978

45. **McCarthy JT, Butterfield LJ:** Newborn country U.S.A. revisited. Rocky Mt Med J 135, 1978

46. **Williams RL:** Measuring the effectiveness of perinatal medical care. Med Care 17:95, 1979

47. **Williams RL, Hawes WE:** Caesarean section, fetal monitoring and perinatal mortality in California. Am J Public Health 69:864, 1979

48. **Kwang-Sun L, Paneth N, Gartner LM, Pearlman MA, Gruss L:** Neonatal mortality: An analysis of the recent improvement in the United States. Am J Public Health 70:15, 1980

49. **Effer SB:** Management of high-risk pregnancy: Report of a combined obstetrical and neonatal intensive care unit. Can Med Assoc J 101:389–397, 1969

50. **Shennan AT, Milligan JE:** Role of prematurity in perinatal mortality. Ontario Med Rev 47: 105, 1979

51. **Gosselin P, Roy A, Desjardins P, DeLeon A, Usher R:** Perinatal Intensive Care after Integration of Obstetrical Services in Quebec (Quoted in Quebec Perinatal Committee); Quebec City, Quebec Ministry of Social Affairs, 1973

52. **Koh KS, Greves D, Yung S, Peddle LJ:** Experience with fetal monitoring in a university teaching hospital. Can Med Assoc J 112:455, 1975

53. **Papageorgiou A, Masson M, Shatz R, Gelfand M:** The development of intramural neonatal and perinatal intensive care units and their impact on perinatal mortality (Abstr). Ann R Coll Phys Surg Can 9:82, 1976

54. **Baum FK, Daily WJR, Harris TR, Hart MC, Meyer HPB, Sells E:** The Arizona State newborn transport and intensive care programs. In Report of the Task Force of the National Foundation–March of Dimes, White Plains, New York, 1973

55. **Gluck L:** Foreword. Clin Perinatol 3:265, 1976

56. **Butterfield LJ:** Organization of regional perinatal programs. Semin Perinatol 1:217, 1977

57. Ross Laboratories: Planning and Design for Perinatal and Pediatric Facilities. Columbus, Ross Laboratories, Division of Abbott Laboratories, 1977

58. **Karlberg P, Ericson A:** Perinatal mortality in Sweden. Acta Paediatr Scand (Suppl) 275: 28, 1979

59. Vital Statistics, Ontario, 1977

60. **Whittaker JS, Chance GW:** The need for improved perinatal care in prevention of cerebral palsy. Can Fam Phys 25:732–736, 1979

61. **McManus F, Rang M, Chance GW, Whittaker J:** Is cerebral palsy a preventable disease? Obstet Gynecol 50:71, 1977

62. **Crainford L (ed):** CELDIC Report—One Million Children: A National Study of Canadian Children with Emotional and Learning Disorders. Ottawa, Commission on Emotional and Learning Disorders in Children, 1970

63. **Kohl SG:** Quoted in Wallace HM: Factors associated with perinatal mortality and morbidity. Clin Obstet Gynaecol 13:13, 1970

64. **Kellmer-Pringle ML, Butler NR, Davie R:** 11,000 Seven-Year-Olds: Studies in Child Development, pp 36–40. London, Longman, 1966

65. Department of Health Services and Hospital Insurance: Annual Reports from the Registry for Handicapped Children and Adults. Division of Vital Statistics, Health Branch, Department of Health Services and Hospital Insurance, Victoria, British Columbia

66. **Brimblecombe FSW:** A new approach to care of handicapped children. J R Coll Physicians Lond 13:4, 231–236, 1979

67. **Rawlings G, Stewart A, Reynolds EOR, Strang LB:** Changing prognosis for infants of very low birth weight. Lancet 1:516–519, 1971

68. **Calame A, Prod'hom LS:** Prognosis and quality of survival in prematures weighing 1500 g or less at birth, seen from 1966–1968. Schweiz Med Wochenschr 102:65–70, 1972

69. **Saigal S:** Low birthweight infants. CMA Affiliates News, Can Med Assoc J 119:385, 1978

70. **Fitzhardinge PM:** Follow-up studies on the low birth-weight infant. Clin Perinatol, 3:503, 1976

71. **Swyer PR (compiler):** A Regionalized System for Reproductive Medical Care in Ontario. Queens Park, Ontario, Information Service, Ontario Ministry of Health, 1979

72. **Quilligan EJ:** A study on custodial care from Connecticut state hospitals. Quoted in Swyer PR, Goodwin JW: Regional Services in Reproductive Medicine p 13. Toronto, The Joint Committee of the Society of Obstetricians and Gynaecologists of Canada and the Canadian Pediatric Society, 1973

73. **Scott KE:** Report of the committee on maternal and perinatal health of the province of Nova Scotia. NS Med Bull 49:81, 1970

74. **Manciaux M:** Organization of perinatal care in Europe: methodology of evaluation. In Bossart H, Cruz JM, Huber A, Prod'hom LS, Sistek J (eds): Perinatal Medicine pp 13–28. Bern, Hans Huber, 1973

75. **Lubs HA:** Quoted in Ontario Council of Health, Genetic Services, 1975

76. **Scriver CR, Neal JL, Saginur R, Clow A:** The frequency of genetic disease and congenital malformation among patients in a pediatric hospital. Can Med Assoc J 108:1111, 1973

77. **Hachette Fernand:** Benefit–Cost Analysis, Cost Effectiveness Analysis: A Brief Introduction. Unpublished paper, Ontario Ministry of Health, 1978

78. **Lewin D, Raiman J, Schroeder A:** La morbidité néonatale: facteurs medicaux et medico–sociaux. J Gynecol Obstet Biol Reprod (Paris) 1:731–743, 1972

79. **Niswander KR, Gordon M:** The Women and Their Pregnancies. Washington, DC Department of Health, Education and Welfare, 1972

80. **Swyer PR, Chalmers KM:** Unpublished data, 1978

81. **Pomerance JJ, Ukrainski CT, Ukra T, Henderson DH, Nash AH, Meredith JL:** Cost of living for infants weighing 1000 grams or less at birth. Pediatrics 61:908, 1978

82. Committee on Perinatal Health: Toward Improving the Outcome of Pregnancy: Recommendations For the Regional Development of Maternal and Perinatal Health Services. White Plains, The National Foundation–March of Dimes, New York, 1976

83. Committee on the Fetus and Newborn:

Standards and Recommendations for Hospital Care of Newborn Infants. Evanston, American Academy of Pediatrics, 1977

84. Ross Planning Associates: The Guide to Referral Centers Providing Perinatal and Neonatal Care. Columbus, Ross Laboratories, Division of Abbott Laboratories, 1978

85. Health and Welfare Canada: Special Care Units in Hospitals: Guidelines for Minimum Standards in the Planning, Organization and Operation of Special Care Units in Hospitals. Ottawa, 1975

86. Recommended Standards for Maternity and Newborn Care. Department of National Health and Welfare, Ottawa, 1968

87. Recommended Standards for Maternity and Newborn Care. Department of National Health and Welfare, Ottawa 1975

88. Callon, HF: Regionalization of Perinatal Care. Report of the 66th Ross Conference on Pediatric Research. Columbus, Ross Laboratories, 1974

89. Ryan, GM: Regional planning for maternal and perinatal health services. Semin Perinatol 1:255–265, 1977

90. Swyer PR: The regional organization of special care in the neonate. Pediatr Clin North Am 17:761, 1970

91. Swyer PR: Background paper: Special Care Units for Newborns: A Review Planning Method and Criteria for Neonatal Intensive Care Units. Boston, Boston University Centre for Health Planning, 1979

92. BPA/RCOG Liaison Committee: Recommendations for the Improvement of Infant Care during the Perinatal Period in the United Kingdom. London, The British Paediatric Association and The Royal College of Obstetricians and Gynaecologists Liaison Committee, 1978

93. Goodwin JW, Chance GW: New system for managing high-risk pregnancies. Ont Med Rev 46:563, 1979

94. Goodwin JW, Dunne JT, Thomas BW: Antepartum identification of the fetus at risk. Can Med Assoc J 101:458, 1969

95. Aubry RH, Nesbitt REL: High-risk obstetrics, Part 1. Perinatal outcome in relation to a broadened approach to obstetric care for patients at special risk. Am J Obstet Gynecol 105:241, 1969

96. Ontario Perinatal Mortality Study Committee: Second Report of Perinatal Mortality Study in Ten University Teaching Hospitals in Ontario Canada. Ontario Department of Health, 1967

97. Hebb M (Project Co-Ordinator): Report of the Nova Scotia Fetal Risk Project. 1969–1976

98. Ontario Council of Health: Perinatal Problems, Monograph No 2. Toronto, Ontario Department of Health, 1971

99. Harris TR, Isaman G, Giles HR: Improved neonatal survival through maternal transport: Outcome data from the Arizona high-risk maternal transport system. In Press, 1979

100. Merenstein GB, Pettett G, Woodall J, Hill JM: An analysis of air transport results in the sick newborn, Part II. Antenatal and neonatal referrals. Am J Obstet Gynecol 117: 1081, 1977

101. Chance GW, O'Brien MJ, Swyer PR: Transportation of sick neonates, 1972: An unsatisfactory aspect of medical care. Can Med Assoc J 109:847, 1973

102. Chance GW, Mathews JD, Gash J, Williams G, Cunningham K: Neonatal transport: A controlled study of skilled assistance. Mortality and morbidity of neonates less than 1.5 kg birthweight. J Pediatr 93:662–666, 1978

103. Gunn T, Outerbridge EW: Effectiveness of neonatal transport. Can Med Ascoc J 118: 646, 1978

104. Ministry of Health, Ontario: Report of the Project Team on Neonatal Transportation. Toronto, 1978

105. Perlstein PH: Neonatal hotline telephone work. Pediatrics 64, No 4:419–424, 1979

4

The Role of the Nurse in Neonatology

Theoretical and Administrative Considerations

Mitzi L. Duxbury

The growth of independent functions and responsibilities in perinatal nursing has considerably enriched and improved the quality of care rendered to the high-risk neonate and his/her family. Nurses are increasingly functioning in a collegial relationship with physicians. The central focus in this approach is the patient and the family. In order for the nurse to assume these increased responsibilities, the knowledge base of nursing science must be expanded, disseminated, implemented, and evaluated.

One of the measures of a professional is the use of a well-defined and well-organized body of knowledge to provide a service vital to human and social welfare.[1] Another criterion for professional practice implies autonomy. The profession of nursing depends on the discipline of nursing for its body of knowledge, although it has freely borrowed from other disciplines.

The Need for Rest. For example, Nightengale identified factors (propositions) related to placing the patient in "the best conditions for nature to act" (*i.e.,* heal). These include warmth, rest, diet, quiet, sanitation, space, and others.[2] These interconnected propositions hold true today, but we must ask ourselves the following questions. Are we indeed applying this theoretical model, or any other, in our daily care of the high-risk newborn and his/her family? Are we adding the uniqueness of nursing to the total care rendered or are we functioning as technical handmaidens? Do we apply a still-valid theory that is over 100 years old and at least "do no harm"? How do we ensure adequate rest for the sick neonate? How effectively can the body grow and heal when little or no rest is permitted?

Sleep is necessary for optimal growth because high levels of growth hormones are secreted during sleep.[3-6] Korones,[7] in a study of disturbance of infants' rest, identified the mean number of contacts per infant to be 132 in 24 hours, with a mean total duration of all contacts of 3.96 hours. This indicates that, on the average, each baby was disturbed 5.5 times every hour for an average of 9.6 minutes!

Can we not organize our care and that of others in a manner to better insure some periods of uninterrupted sleep? Should we not be planning and implementing our care based on the needs of this vulnerable neonate rather than those of the personnel? Who is responsible for ensuring rest if not the nurse? One might ask the same questions regarding noise and space; nursing often does not apply its all-too-limited scientific theory.

Holistic Approach To Patient Care

In the past three decades, several researchers have contributed to the discipline of nursing and its body of knowledge.[8-14] All theorists propose holistic approaches to nursing care that, when applied, articulate the uniqueness, or define the discipline of nursing. Riehl and Roy describe nursing as maintaining a person's life processes for the purpose of realizing his/her maximum potential, including health and harmonious interaction with his/her environment.[10] This definition of course includes the illness state but is not exclusive to it. It encompasses the maximum functioning of the total person.

Awrey discussed the medical–nursing collaboration as having three components: nursing, borderline, and medicine.[13] Olson's formulation of this approach provides a model for delivering care to the high-risk families in an ICN setting.[14] This model was developed specifically for preterm infants and their families.

Need for Critical Evaluation

It is imperative that nursing base its practices on knowledge rather than contemporary beliefs. Many so-called "theories" have been found completely invalid. Much of our practice today, I believe, is without a factual basis. We must continually test, retest, and redefine our practice. Failure to do so only perpetuates the "that's the way we do it here" system, and leads to an uncreative, bureaucratic nursing system.

NURSING ADMINISTRATION OF THE UNIT

The administrator of the unit should ideally hold a master's degree in nursing and have both knowledge and skill in the principles of administration. An adequate knowledge of perinatal nursing is also essential in order to articulate the needs of the unit in budget preparation, staffing, evaluating personnel, and other administrative tasks necessary for the operation of a large unit.

At the simplest level, the organizational ends defined by Hage should be adhered to.[15] These "ends" are efficiency, effectiveness, flexibility, and morale. The idea of "functional strains" means that all of these organizational ends or outcomes are related, and that an increase or maximization of one may result in the decrease or minimization of another. For example, an increase in efficiency (more babies in the unit with the same number of staff) would reduce the actual cost per baby but will probably result in a decrease in at least two of the other three outcomes: effectiveness (lowered quality of care per baby) and morale (the satisfaction nurses receive from their work). The nurse administrator must continually assess not only unit inputs but also outcomes.

Staffing the Unit

The approaches to nurse staffing of the ICN should be based largely on the functions or purposes of the unit.[16] If the unit is viewed as a tertiary care center and assumes some of the responsibilities of service and education for a defined geographic area, staffing patterns must support those needs. If, however, the unit is designated primarily to receive and/or transport sick infants, the staffing methodologies can be much more traditional. (See Chap. 3).

The goal of all health care institutions should be provision of high-quality patient and family care, and this primary goal must not be compromised by the educational or research goals of the unit. High-quality patient care must include preventive as well as episodic crisis care. It is difficult to incorporate any preventive modalities into a working model unless a regionalized systems approach is used, which includes the primary care providers in the geographically defined region. Prevention begins where the patient lives, and coordinated supportive working relationships must be effectively worked out.[16] Nursing coordination should emanate from the tertiary care center and the responsibilities for service and continued education must also be assumed there. This tertiary care center should maintain an affiliation with a graduate program in nursing.

Primary Nurse. Nursing history reveals many approaches to staffing. One approach, highly popular today, is **primary nursing.**

"Primary nursing is delivery of comprehensive, continuous, coordinated and individualized patient care through the primary nurse who has autonomy, accountability and authority to act as the chief nurse for her patients."[17] This approach to staffing assures total individualized care for the patient and his/her family on a continuous basis.

Concepts of primary nursing as identified by Ciske include[18]

1. Assignment of each patient to a specific (primary) nurse, who usually provides his care each day she is on duty until the patient's discharge or transfer.
2. Patient assignment by the primary nurse, who plans the care to be given when she is not on duty, when secondary or associate nurses care for her patients. Thus, 24-hour responsibility for care is actualized through the primary nurse's written directives on kardex and other communication tools.
3. Patient involvement in the care provided and identification of his goals relating to how the medical condition affects his life style.
4. Care giver to care giver communication—both in the nursing staff's daily reporting methods and between disciplines.
5. Discharge planning—including patient teaching, family involvement, and appropriate referrals.

An advantage of this approach to staffing is accountability; one person is accountable for the quality of nursing care and its continuity, and for ensuring that patient and family needs are fully comprehended and met.

Marram's study of primary care versus the team approach found that patients view the nurse in the primary care units as[19]

"1. Giving emotional support frequently, and
2. Treating them like special human beings;"

while the team patients' frequent responses were:

"1. Too much concerned with others' perceptions and not with what patients thought they needed, and
2. More concerned with finishing on time than giving good care."

Many more patients on the primary unit stated they were "extremely" satisfied with their care and the staff were more often satisfied with their work.

The level of nurse preparation appears to be an important variable in the quality of care delivered. Most primary care nurses should be prepared at the baccalaureate level in order to carry out the responsibilities necessary for this approach. The author observed several outstanding nurses without B.S. degrees who managed patients with a high degree of success. Generally, however, a B.S. degree should be the minimal requirement for these responsibilities. Ideally, masters' degree-prepared clinical nurse specialists should be available for consultation for all patients and should assume primary nurse responsibilities for those with unusually complex nursing problems.

Cost of Primary Nursing versus Traditional Approaches

Much additional study is required before definitive answers on cost will be obtained. Preliminary data suggests that a staffing pattern of primary care costs less than traditional approaches to care. A cost comparison study by Williams and Felton defined a cost savings of $4.35 per patient per day for primary care staffing over a team approach to staffing.[20] A more extensive study of cost effectiveness by Marram, Flynn, Abaravich, and Carey also supported cost savings and greater patient satisfaction than with team nursing.[17]

Long-term patient outcomes and cost studies must be undertaken to further assess implications for neonatal/perinatal care. Primary nurse staffing in institutions, coupled with assumption of their regionalized responsibilities, shows much promise for quality and cost-effective care.

BURN-OUT AND TURN-OVER

Burn-out and turn-over of staff have become a grievous, unmanageable problem in many ICNs. Some units studied have experienced a crude turnover rate of 70% per year.[21] Others have identified a crude turn-over rate of over 150% per year.

Veninga defined **burn-out** as ". . . a debilitating psychological condition resulting from work-related frustrations, which results in lower productivity and role."[22] **Tedium** is a term used by Pines and Kafry to describe a similar condition. The definition of tedium used by Pines and associates is "A general experience of physical, emotional and attitudinal exhaustion." This experience is characterized by feelings of strain and "burnout", by emotional as well as physical depletion and by negation of oneself and one's environment.

Turn-over has been associated with many variables, and burn-out is one of these. Many burned-out nurses probably resign, but others remain on the unit. The impact on both the person and the unit can be grievous when burned-out nurses remain.

In addition to burn-out as a variable associated with turn-over, many others have been identified. These include, but are not limited to, age, family income, size of the work unit, pay, hygiene factors, organizational climate, leadership in the unit, professional or bureaucratic orientation of the nurse, role deprivation, perceived pay equity, integration, communication, centralization of authority and decision making, commitment to career, routinization, and perceived administrative insensitivity.

Signs and Symptoms of Turn-over and Burn-out

The impact of burn-out and turn-over can affect a person in many ways, including the following:

1. Feeling helpless, impotent and unable to cope
2. Suffering from exhaustion, fatigue, and becoming physically run-down
3. Manifesting frequent physical symptoms, such as headaches, gastrointestinal upsets, weight loss, sleeplessness, depression, and shortness of breath
4. Becoming silent; a noncontributor at staff meetings; this applies especially to someone who is ordinarily talkative.
5. Exhibiting a quick temper, instant irritation, and frustration
6. Demonstrating suspicious attitudes from which paranoia may evolve
7. Becoming rigid and closed; the nurses's thinking is inflexible and change becomes impossible.
8. Exhibiting a decrease in risk-taking behavior or exhibiting an increase in risk-taking; (S)he may act without regarding the consequences.
9. Developing a negative attitude; (S)he becomes the staff cynic.
10. Becoming disagreeable; someone who "bad-mouths" any creative ideas
11. Becoming cynical regarding her/his own work and the organization
12. Fighting the system in an unproductive manner
13. Manifesting an increase in personal problems including alcoholism, mental illness, family conflict, and suicide
14. Unable to relax
15. Moving away from others and problems in the following ways: moving away from clinical practice into an administrative or teaching position; reducing personal involvement with clients and others; diminishing socialization with other staff members; and minimizing physical contact
16. Manifesting reduction in initiative so that her work becomes less efficient, particularly in times of stress

The unit, as well, is affected by burn-out and turn-over.

1. Adverse effects on the quality of care rendered
2. Other personnel and units affected
3. Creates difficulty with parents
4. More errors in judgment
5. Higher incidence of accidents
6. Increase in staff friction
7. Increase in sick time and disability
8. The leadership group, which is also the most committed, may be lost.
9. Increased bureaucratization

Assessing Turnover

Many methods for assessing turn-over in the unit are in use. Three rather simple techniques will enable the unit administrator to assess this movement in his/her unit.

Crude or Simple Turnover. The crude turnover (CTO) rate is compiled by dividing the number of nurses terminated in a given period by the average number of employees during that period, multiplied by 100.

$$CTO = \frac{\text{Number of leavers in a period}}{\text{Average employment in the same period}} \times 100$$

Survival-of-Leavers Curve. The survival-of-leavers curve is a graphic plot of the percentage of nurses leaving against the length of service of each. The survival-of-leavers curve for a given period is computed by the number of nurses terminated, plotted against the number of months each had been employed (Fig. 4-1).

Median Length-of-Service. The median length-of-service (stay) is computed from the survival-of-leavers curve, by identifying a point on the graph where 50% of those employed have left. In Figure 4-1, the median length of stay is 6 months.

It is important to go beyond assessment of CTO. A CTO rate of 100% can be read as

1. the entire labor force had turned over once during the year; or
2. half the labor force had turned over twice, the other half remaining stable; or
3. a quarter had turned over four times, and so on.

Thus, a CTO rate may not reflect a stable core of employees. In order to assess turnover in any individual unit, the CTO rate must therefore be viewed together with the survival-of-leavers curve.

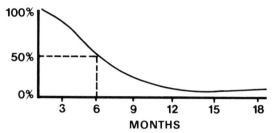

Fig. 4-1. Representative survival-of-leavers curve. Number of months of service is plotted against percentage of group leaving with that degree of longevity.

Strategies To Reduce Burn-out and Turn-over

Many strategies for reducing nurse burn-out and turn-over have been suggested. Some are directed toward the individual nurse and some to the organization or administrator. The gravity of this problem in many units mandates thoughtful attention and vigorous intervention.

Following is a list of ways in which an organization can decrease burn-out and turn-over:

1. Reduce the patient/staff ratio when it is higher than desirable.
2. Shorten staff work hours and provide more breaks and more part-time positions.
3. Allow for more opportunities for "time-outs" during the work day. Provide sanctioned time-outs.
4. Share the patient load through work sharing and rotation.*
5. Develop staff support systems.
6. Establish clear lines of communication.

7. Evaluate what are viewed as stress-producing hospital policies.
8. Discuss and resolve ethical dilemmas.
9. Clarify responsibilities and accountability.
10. Encourage both responsibility and accountability decision-making for all employees to increase their sense of success and control.
11. Provide for adequate job preparation.
12. Teach all the staff members to be aware of psychological and sociological components of neonatal care.
13. Provide critical care conferences as needed by any staff member.
14. Support occasional retreats to allow the staff members to get away together.
15. Develop a family committee composed of parents and staff members from all departments to view ICU functions and dysfunctions and to propose and implement solutions.
16. Encourage the development of a parent-to-parent program to supplement staff attention to family needs.
17. Provide opportunities for staff members to learn to deal with the emotional tensions of their work.
18. Establish and support mental health days for personnel in high-stress areas.
19. Do not recommend that a burned-out person be sent to encounter group sessions.
20. Teach personnel to deal with stress.

* Rotation: There is no agreement in the literature. Some feel rotation reduces stress, others say it does not and may even increase stress. It may depend, in part, on the individual nurse, the situation into which one is rotated, and so on.

Moral or Ethical Concerns for Nurses in Neonatal Intensive Care Units

Ruth D. Weise

Decision-making involves not only expertise in reasoning but also willingness to take risks. Nurses in neonatal intensive care units are constantly faced with circumstances that require deliberative action and that involve ethical issues, which require a rational framework within which to arrive at moral decisions.

Jacques Thiroux has developed a system of "humanitarian ethics" that identifies five major principles that might serve to guide nurses in neonatal units as they are faced with the many dilemmas that occur.[24]

1. The **value of life principle** propounds a

reverence for life and an acceptance of death.

2. **Principle of goodness or rightness**
   a. To promote goodness over badness
   b. To cause no harm or badness
   c. To prevent badness or harm
3. **Principle of justice or fairness** (in distributing goodness and badness)
4. **Principle of truth-telling or honesty**
5. The **principle of individual freedom** (encompasses the ways and means of being moral within the framework of the first four principles.

The nurse in a neonatal intensive care unit often deals with newborns who have severe malformations and/or genetic anomalies not presently responsive to medical prescription. Substantive ethical issues in these instances include passive euthansia, the "rightness" of medical research, financial stress for the parents of the infant, *complete* informed consent, maximum use of scarce or limited resources, patient and parent advocacy, colleagueal relationship with physicians. These are but a few of the infinite number of real or potential dilemmas for the nurse. To deal effectively with such problems requires that the nurse establish workable principles for responsible ethical behavior which provide some consistency in response. Chinn outlines an approach

(developed by Kinlein) for a nursing framework that emphasizes nursing rather than medical care, in defining "duty."[25]

For the nurse to carry out those responsibilities associated with professionalism, serious formulation of an ethical base is imperative. Murphy and Murphy[26] and Sigman [27] provide helpful guidelines to the development of a personal ethical system that has a rational base. With such a framework to assist in decision-making, collaborative rather than responsive relationships with the neonatologist become more available to the nurse practitioner.[28]

Physicians often see nurses as surrogate mothers who weep and wail at the loss of an infant for whom they have cared. If, however, the nurse has a well-defined ethical system and can share in the ultimate decision about management of the sick infant, the physician may well utilize the special "caring" capabilities of the nurse in assisting the parents of the sick infant. When the ICN nurse, as family advocate, addresses the five principles established by Thiroux, she enters the sphere of ethical practice in a highly stressful clinical area; care is given to patients rather than physicians, because a professional nurse is an extension of the patient, not the physician.

Neonatal Transport

Judith A. Cannon

HISTORY

Sophisticated infant transport systems are a creation of the last decade.[29] The need for these systems developed as the science of neonatology evolved. An improved outlook for small and seriously ill infants at regional neonatal centers made transfer of patients to these centers a practical and realistic expectation.

As early as 1948, the New York City Departments of Health and Hospitals realized that transporting sick infants from their place of birth, whether home or hospital, to "premature centers" decreased the deaths associated with prematurity.[30] An ambulance serv-

ice staffed by five transport nurses transported 1209 infants between 1948 and 1950; 85% of these weighed less than 2000 g. They had primative equipment by today's standards: an incubator heated by four hot water bottles, a gown and cap to dress the baby in, sterile supplies (including a DeLee mucus trap), bulb syringe, tuberculin syringe and 26-gauge needles, umbilical tape, hemostats, and scissors. The only other supplies carried were a rectal thermometer, a flashlight, and a bottle of water for baptism. The only medications used were aromatic spirits of ammonia, caffeine benzoate, and adrenalin. Yet, these nurses knew the basic principles of infant transport still important today. They realized the importance of keeping the infant warm and safe during transport and they always showed the baby, in his portable incubator, to the mother before leaving in the ambulance. Interestingly, the salary paid the ambulance drivers was $2800 per year; the nurse's salary was $2400 per year.[30,31]

Today, with the rapid advances and sophistication in neonatal care, the sick infant can best be managed in regional centers where resources, experts, and equipment can be localized. This avoids costly duplication of equipment and personnel and allows the best care possible for the infant.

METHODS OF TRANSPORT

In order for the infant to arrive at such a center, several modes of transport may be used.

Types of Transport

1. Maternal
2. Intrahospital
3. Ground: ambulance, van
4. Helicopter
5. Fixed-wing aircraft

Probably the safest and least costly is for the infant to be transported *in utero*. Identification of high-risk mothers and their referral to regional perinatal centers capable of caring for both mother and infant seems to be gaining in popularity. This method also seems to decrease infant mortality even more significantly than neonatal transfers.[32,33] However, not all sick infants can be identified prenatally. Therefore, an effective system of neonatal transport will always remain necessary.

Even if the distance to be transported is very short, such as from the delivery room to the nursery in the same hospital, the fundamental principles of transport must still apply. These fundamentals include warmth, stabilization by personnel with appropriate training and experience, and transport to the nursery under controlled conditions. Therefore, a neonatal resuscitation station should be established in each delivery room and be equipped with an overhead warmer or alternate heating device and other equipment necessary to stabilize and treat the distressed newborn.[34] Once safely moved to the nursery, the decision of whether to transfer the infant to a center for more specialized care can be made.

The method of transportation chosen for each region will depend on several factors. The time involved and the distance to be traveled are prime considerations. Centers in highly urbanized areas, such as the East Coast, rely primarily on ground transportation when serving areas in a 50 to 60 mile radius, with good roads. Where terrain is more hazardous or when speed is of critical importance, helicopters have also been used successfully. Disadvantages to this method are noise, vibration and difficulty of performing procedures en route. In many parts of the Western United States, where distances of over 150 miles must be covered, fixed-wing aircraft are the only practical alternative.

PERSONNEL

The expertise and competence of the personnel involved are the most important elements in the transport. Each member of the team must know his specific duties well and must be able to work independently and interdependently with all other members of the team in order to ensure smooth operation. Traditionally, the team has consisted of a physician and an assistant, usually a nurse. Many times, the physician was an intern or resident rotating through the nursery, with little or no experience in transporting sick newborns. The nurse chosen was often the one who could most easily be spared from a busy unit, not necessarily the one most qualified. The physician was responsible for medical evaluation, procedures, and management decisions, while the nurse cared for the patient and prepared the equipment. While a system such as this may be workable in some situations, it is not ideal, and because the trend is now toward limiting the ICN experience of house staff, the feasibility of providing a physician for every transport is disappearing.

Some centers have trained neonatal nurse specialists. These nurses are taught assessment skills, resuscitation skills, and technical skills such as intubation, umbilical vessel catheterization, measures to relieve pneumothorax, and IV insertion, in addition to advanced nursing management. They operate under standard protocols for care of the infant. They receive backup and advice from the neonatologists at the referral center and may request a physician to accompany transport when necessary.[35]

Thus, specially trained nurses may be the primary members of the transport team. They

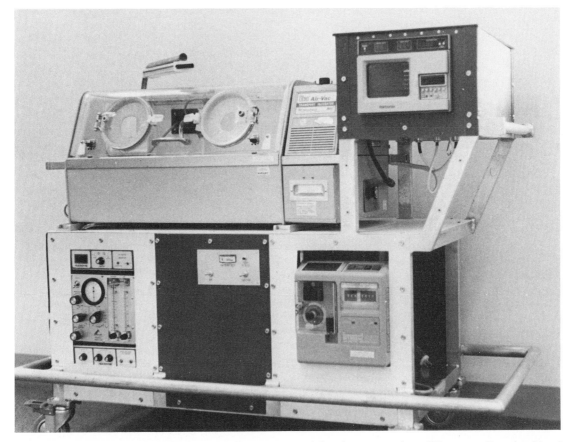

Fig. 4-2. Simple transport system with battery-operated incubator, monitor, IV pump, Doppler blood pressure apparatus, and tackle box with small supplies and equipment.

are aided by specially trained respiratory therapists, paramedics, or emergency medical technologists (EMTs) in various systems.[35,36,37,38] In addition, pilots and ambulance drivers who complete the team will function most effectively when they are taught basic principles of safe infant transport and are included in team decisions and problem solving.

EQUIPMENT

The equipment used for infant transport varies widely from system to system. It may be very complex, including a specially outfitted neonatal transport ambulance with built in radiant warmers, x-ray equipment, blood gas determination apparatus and myriads of other technical marvels. It can also be as simple as a portable incubator which will fit into any standard ambulance. The needs of the service area and the funds available for equipment purchase will determine what each system uses.

Equipment for Transport

1. Transport incubator
2. Cardiorespiratory monitor
3. Blood pressure device (doppler)
4. Oxygen mixing and measuring system
5. Portable ventilator and/or bagging set up
6. IV fluid pump
7. Equipment box with drugs and supplies

However, the basic components of most neonatal transport units include a portable battery-powered incubator which will allow visability and accessibility to the infant while maintaining a neutral thermal environment (Fig. 4-2). A monitoring device is needed for most transports because auscultation by stethoscope is difficult in transit. The monitor

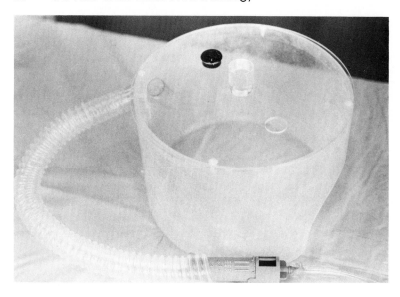

Fig. 4-3. Venturi device with oxygen hood for giving graduated oxygen concentrations in transit.

ideally should be compact and battery powered, and should have the capability to monitor temperature, heart rate, respiratory rate, and arterial blood pressure. We are currently using a Tektronix model 413 which has all of these capabilities. It has proved accurate and reliable. A Doppler device is also helpful to obtain peripheral blood pressures and to use as a backup pulse monitor. An oxygen source must also be provided with the ability to accurately control and analyze the concentration delivered to the infant. This can easily be accomplished by using a Venturi device with an oxygen hood. This device allows oxygen to mix with room air and can accurately vary $F_{I_{O_2}}$ concentration from 22% to 30% by 2% increments, and from 30% to 50% by 5% increments (Fig. 4-3). A more sophisticated system uses an oxygen blender with compressed air to achieve the desired concentration. In addition, a resuscitation bag with the ability to deliver positive end-expiratory pressure (PEEP) is needed. Appropriate size infant masks are also required. In systems which require traveling long distances, or which transport a high percentage of intubated infants, a portable infant ventilator is desirable. It should be able to deliver both ventilation with PEEP and continuous positive airway pressure (CPAP) during spontaneous breathing.

An intravenous infusion pump is also desirable. It, too, should be battery powered and portable. It must be capable of accurately and continuously infusing small volumes of fluid.

We have favored using the same pump for transport as is used in the neonatal intensive care unit. This allows less interruption when the infant is admitted to the unit and assures a backup pump if needed.

Other equipment needed for transport is listed in Table 4-1. The amount of supplies required may vary depending on the ability of the hospitals served to provide these materials. In addition to the above equipment, several forms must also accompany the transport personnel. These include a data sheet, permission forms, and a letter or booklet for parents, explaining transport and stating how they can remain in touch with the staff caring for their infant.

PROCEDURE FOR TRANSPORT

When an infant is born at a hospital that is not able to handle his problems, a well-organized referral system is vital to insure prompt and appropriate measures to meet his needs. Many areas have established regional referral centers with a "hot-line" toll-free number, or a direct-call number to handle such situations.

At the time of initial contact, basic data must be collected in order to handle the referral quickly and appropriately. The patient's name, referring hospital, and physician, and specific information about the patient's condition must be readily available. A telephone log is useful in collecting data and assures a permanent record. The person receiving the call must be able to evaluate the situation, advise the caller

Table 4-1. Transport Equipment

Equipment Box Drugs*	Equipment Box	Airway Supplies	Miscellaneous Supplies
1—50 ml vial 50% glucose	1—small catheter insertion tray	1—laryngoscope handle	1 each—size 5, 8 Fr. feeding tubes
1—50 ml vial sodium bicarbonate	1—umbilical tape	1—0 blade	1—bottle Dextrostix
1—amp. epinepherine 1:1000	1—scapel	1—1 blade	1—infant blood pressure cuff
1—amp. calcium gluconate 10%	1 each—size 3.5, 5, 8 Fr. umbilical catheters	2 each—extra batteries, light bulbs	Assorted needles, syringes, alcohol swabs
1—vial heparin 1000 units/ml	1 each—luer stub adaptors—size 16, 18, 20, 22	1—stylet	Tape
1—vial atropine	3—stopcocks	2 each—size 2.5, 3.0, 3.5, 4.0 Portex endotrachial tubes	Rubber bands
1—amp. Lasix (furosemide)	1—transducer dome	1—package infant airways	Safety pins
1—vial phenobarbital	1—pressure monitoring kit	1—DeLee mucus trap	Lubricant
2—vials 25% albumin	1—250 ml bottle 10% glucose	1—size 6.5 Fr. suction catheter	4 × 4 gauze pads
1—vial normal saline	1—Soluset, cassette, filter	1—size 8 Fr. suction catheter	
1—vial sterile water for injection	1—armboard	1—Laerdal bag, assorted masks, tubing	
1—heparin flushing solution 2 units/ml	2 each—size 25 short, 23 butterflies	1—O₂ analyzer	
1—60 ml bottle betadine solution	2 each—size 22, 20 Medicuts		
1—60 ml tincture of benzoin	2—T-connectors		

*As employed at Children's Hospital National Medical Center, Washington, D.C.

about methods of stabilization, and dispatch the transport team rapidly, or be able to promptly connect the caller with someone who can.

Hospitals using a referral service should be aware of what information and specimens will be required to accompany the patient. These usually include copies of the infant's and mother's charts, signed permission forms, x-ray films, laboratory data, a tube of the mother's blood, and may also include the placenta and a vaginal culture. In order to avoid delays, these should be available by the time the transport team arrives.

Preparations for Transport

1. Copy of infant's and mother's charts
2. Signed permits for transport
3. Copy of significant x-ray films and lab data
4. Tube of mother's blood
5. Mother's vaginal culture
6. Placenta (if available)

Once on the scene, transport team members must communicate with the referring staff to obtain pertinent history and information about the infant's condition. Next, they must evaluate and stabilize the infant, paying close attention to thermoregulation and airway management. Time spent stabilizing the infant is extremely valuable. Attempts to rush in and rush out should be avoided unless the only hope for the infant's survival is rapid transport to the referral center for surgery.

Once the infant is stabilized, an equally important part of the transport procedure is effective communication with the family. They are facing a very stressful situation. Many mothers fear that they will never see their newborns alive again. An honest appraisal of the infant's condition along with an explanation of where he is going, who will be caring for him, and how the parents can keep informed of his condition is greatly appreciated. Every effort should be made to allow the parents to see and touch their infant before transport. This may be accomplished by having

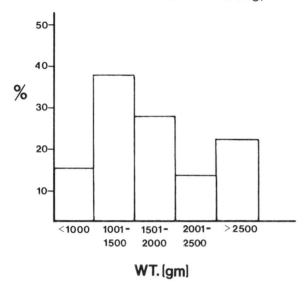

WT. (gm)

Fig. 4-4. Histograms showing frequency of transport by birth weight. Children's Hospital National Medical Center, Washington, D.C., July 1977–June, 1978.[39]

Table 4-2. Transports By Diagnosis, July 1977–June 1978*

Diagnosis	Number	Percent
Hyaline membrane disease	126	32.9
Asphxia	101	26.4
Transient tachypnea	37	10.3
Congenital pneumonia	4	1.0
Surgical	32	8.3
Multiple anomalies	28	7.3
Cardiac	27	7.0
Neurology/neurosurgery	16	4.1

*Children's Hospital National Medical Center[39]

the parents come to the nursery or the infant can be taken to the mother's room in the transport incubator when leaving the hospital. Parents should be prepared in advance for the appearance of the infant; explanation of tubes, wires, beeps, and equipment is vital. This contact is important in establishing parent–infant bonding.

Also important before departure is a quick call back to the referral center to inform them of the infant's current condition, equipment needed, and expected time of arrival. During the return transport, the infant is continuously observed and monitored. If stabilization has been effective, often little else is needed during the trip.

On arrival at the referral center, the transport nurse helps to admit and stabilize the infant, gives a report of history and transport activities to the staff assuming care, and calls the family to assure them that the infant arrived safely. Once this is done, the equipment is cleaned, restocked, and prepared for the next trip.

BABIES WITH SPECIAL NEEDS

A review of recent statistics at our institution revealed that many of the infants requiring transport were very small prematures. Almost one-half weighed less than 2000 g (Fig. 4-4).

The very small "premie" presents a great challenge to the transport team. He is often very difficult to keep warm; yet this is vital to his survival. Prewarmed blankets in the incubator and surgical gloves filled with warm water and covered with warm diapers placed next to his sides may help. A heat shield or plastic covering inside the incubator is also useful, as are plastic wrap and aluminized drapes.

The next largest group of infants in our series were those requiring transport for surgery (Tables 4-2, and 4-3). The infant with a diaphragmatic hernia is usually best transported by elevating his head, placing his affected side down, inserting a nasogastric tube, and avoiding bag and mask ventilation. If respiratory compromise is severe, he should be intubated prior to transfer.

Infants with tracheoesophageal fistula should be transported with their heads elevated and a Replogle tube or feeding tube in the esophageal pouch, which is gently suctioned frequently.

Omphalocele or gastroschisis requires close attention to thermoregulation because a large surface area of bowel is exposed. The defect should be covered with sterile, warm, isotonic saline dressing, wrapped with gauze, and covered with sterile plastic. Placing the infant in an adult bowel bag has been used successfully by some centers. Care must be taken not to kink or compromise the exposed bowel. A nastrogastric tube and IV line are also important. The infant with any type of gastrointestinal obstruction should have a nasogastric tube inserted and suctioned intermittently, and be transported with his head elevated to lessen respiratory compromise caused by abdominal distension.

Finally, infants with meningomyelocele require transport in a prone position, the defect being covered with a sterile dressing and every attempt made to prevent contamination of the defect with urine or stool.

REGULAR EVALUATIONS

Vital to the smooth functioning and improvement of the team is a periodic review of all transports. This should include an objective look at the data collected, the condition of the infant upon arrival of the team, measures undertaken to stabilize the infant, condition after intervention, and condition on arrival at the referral center. Data such as temperature, blood pressure, and blood gases can be reviewed and evaluated.

Also necessary is an evaluation of the function of the system as a whole. Were there any unduly long delays? What caused them: personnel delay, equipment malfunction, simultaneous calls, weather, uncertainty about bed

Table 4-3. Transports By Service, July 1977–June 1978*

	Number	Percent
Neonatal	301	78.8
Surgical	32	8.3
Cardiac	27	7.0
Neurology/neurosurgery	16	4.1
Endocrine	2	0.5
Other	3	0.7

*Children's Hospital National Medical Center[39]

availability? Only by such review meetings can the system be evaluated and improved. Ideally, such meetings should be attended by all team members and the medical director responsible for the transport service. Equally important to the evaluation of the team is continuing education for team members. They must keep up to date on new modes of therapy as well as periodically review all procedures, protocols, and equipment.

Patient Care in the ICN

Mary Beth L. House and Michele M. Dombkiewicz

STAFFING REQUIREMENTS

It is important that staffing patterns be based upon patient care requirements. Staffing assignment requires a tool by which one can objectively assess the level of care on a daily basis, in order to use the nursing staff more effectively. Documentation of the need for budgeted nursing positions should then be based upon the average census and average patient activity found in each individual patient unit. This should be reviewed and adjusted yearly.

For example, a classification system was developed by the Nursing Department at Children's Hospital National Medical Center under the leadership of Mrs. Lillian B. Williams, Director of Nursing, in conjunction with MacLeod Associates, Health Care Consultants. The classification tool uses a 1 to 10 coding system which takes into account the

needs of all ages of children including the neonate. Codes used to classify infants in the ICN range from special care, code 6 (one nurse to four patients), to code 10 (two nurses to one patient). All intermediate nursery care is code 7 (1:3). Codes 8 (1:2), 9 (1:1), and 10 classify all intensive patients.

Each code includes activity criteria, along with a table that shows the frequency of each activity by shift (Table 4-4). Each code indicates the level of care of a particular patient. The classifying is done by the clinical unit coordinator or her designee (usually the charge nurse) for a 24-hour period, including evenings, nights, and the following day. The evening shift then updates the classification sheet for the night shift, and the night shift does the same for the day shift. Carbon copies are sent each shift to the nursing office where the staffing coordinator determines the number of staff needed on all units for the following shift.

Table 4-4. Patient Activity Classification*

Code 6: under 2 years
A code 6 patient can have *up to* the following care needs per day:

Activity	Frequency By Shift			
	Day	*Eve*	*Night*	*Total*
Feed (parents/students do not assist)	2	2	2	6
Bed change	1	1	1	3
Diaper change	4	4	4	12
Complete bath		Day or Night		1
Rounds to patient	8	8	8	24
Rounds with physician	2	1	–	3
Take vital signs	2	2	2	6
Give meds (Oral and Injected)	3	3	2	8
Intake and output	6	5	3	14
Weigh patient	1	1	1	3
Instruct parents or play games	12 min	12 min	–	24 min
IVs (start, maintain, d/c)	8	8	8	24
Specimen collection (inc. S.G.)	1	1	1	3
Assist. Physician with procedure	½	½	–	\ 1

*As used by the Nursing Department of the Children's Hospital National Medical Center, Washington. The above example is only a guide to selecting a code 6 patient. Some patients may require other types of care activity not listed, but at the same time not require some of the activities listed above. Also, a patient may require a higher frequency of some activity and a lower frequency of another activity. If these types of *trade-offs* appear about equal, the patient is in Code 6.

Systems such as this allow for more objective and flexible staffing.

Staffing needs do not change through the 24-hour period. Therefore, the same number of nurses are required on each shift. The situation is more comparable to an ICU than to a general care unit.

ADMISSION

Admission is one of the most crucial time periods for the patient, the family, and the neonatal team. Most parents are overwhelmed at the sight of their infant and the ICN environment. From the beginning, a team effort should be made in establishing a relationship with the family. In this way, all members of the team approach the family with the same orientation. The primary nurse caring for the infant is usually the team member who spends the most hours with the family. She makes a nursing care plan and is in a good position to reinforce and explain information, support the medical plan of care, assess the family's needs, and coordinate the neonatal team efforts.

Stabilization

Upon arrival at the nursery from the delivery room or outside transport, the infant must be placed in a prepared environment. This includes a heat source for temperature stabilization; cardiopulmonary monitoring, oxygen and suction availability, manual resuscitator and appropriate size masks, emergency drugs, neonatal endotracheal tray, and blood pressure monitoring equipment (transducer or Doppler).

Nursing Care

Upon admission, the nurse obtains a weight and vital signs, including a blood pressure, Dextrostix, and abdominal girth. A nasogastric tube is inserted to expel air forced into the stomach from manual ventilation and to prevent aspiration of abdominal contents. Gestational age is assessed by the physician or nurse. A physical assessment is then performed.

The nursing admission note is quite detailed. Data includes the name, age, sex, admitting diagnosis, mode of admission, and any pertinent findings from the physical assessment.

Also included is any significant perinatal history. If the neonate had been home, the nurse records the time frame and progression of the illness, and what the baby's regimen was like (*e.g.,* bottle or breast fed, what type of formula, and so on). All of the data will go into preparing a nursing plan of care for the neonate.

GENERAL CARE

The art of nursing must always be present amidst the machinery, alarms, and monitoring necessary to deliver the best care to our patients. Providing for warmth, rest, and nutrition as well as observing, listening, and caring, remain the foundation for good nursing care.

Infection Control

A sick infant is at high risk for nosocomial infections. Infection control policies and procedures may vary depending on the type of nursery. The most important and recurrent directive that is found from nursery to nursery is strict handwashing. Medical and nursing personnel begin the day with a three-minute scrub to the elbow with an antimicrobial skin cleanser such as an iodophor preparation. Remove watches and jewelry before the scrub. After this, a good 15-second handwashing between babies is the most important thing we can do to prevent the spread of harmful organisms.

A cover gown must be worn over the uniform, scrub gown, or street clothes when the infant is being held against the body, such as during feedings or procedures. People with upper respiratory infections, diarrhea, herpes simplex lesions, sore throats, or other contagious illnesses should not be directly handling the infants.

An isolation area within the nursery may be needed for infants with suspected infection. In general, it is feasible, with good technique, to carry out wound, skin, and enteric isolation, but respiratory isolation is ineffective when common airspace is involved.

Visitation

Over the last 10 years, several studies have brought to light the extreme importance of maternal–child interaction and the effect this has on the progress and emotional well-being of the sick infant. Whereas visiting was once prohibited, most nurseries now encourage parents to visit as often as possible and to assist in their infant's care. Because many infants in an ICN are hospitalized for a month or more, 24-hour visitation gives parents flexibility. The standard hospital visiting hours are not helpful to parents who have home and work responsibilities.

A few nurseries are allowing grandparent visitation as support for the parents. In some instances, the grandparent may become the secondary caregiver, as the parents return to work. However, caution must be used in visitation policies. The numerous people entering the nursery and handling the baby may increase the risk of infection and cause increased congestion and noise which may be disturbing.

The period of the infant's illness can be very difficult on siblings. The household routine is changed and parents are away from home more frequently. Sibling visitation *within* the nursery room is discouraged. However, if there is a way for the brother or sister to see the baby from outside the nursery for short periods of time, it can be very helpful. Drawings made by the sibling can be placed at the baby's bedside. When the situation permits, an infant with a long-term illness may be taken to a separate room for the brother or sister to visit. It is important that the "wholeness" of the family not be completely lost during the infant's illness.

Identification

Every infant should have an identification band on at all times. It is also helpful to have a bed identification as well. A 3 × 5 card can be taped to the bed with the infant's name and the name of the primary nurse and the primary physician.

Bedside Check

The nurse should take time to see that the patient's environment is secure at the beginning of each shift. Warmers and isolettes must be plugged in and operating. When oxygen is required, humidity and temperature should be checked, as well as the percentage of administered oxygen. Ventilator settings and oxygen therapy should be checked against the last order. Appropriate limits must be set on all monitors and the alarms must be on and working. Upon request, the biomedical department may be able to adjust some of the monitors so that the alarms cannot be turned off.

Suction apparatus must be set up with suction catheters handy. The nurse should see that the correct IV solutions are hanging and infusing at the ordered rate. We recommend that the limit volume on the infusion pump be set at no more than three times the ordered hourly amount (3 hours worth of fluid). This is a safety precaution against the pump malfunctioning. Also, the alarm on the infusion pump must be set.

Many steps can be saved if supplies are gathered at the bedside of each patient at the beginning of the shift. It will also alert the charge nurse or unit clerk early on as to what supplies may need to be reordered.

Daily Care

Bath care is usually done on the evening shift. For one thing, it is the shift when infants on a 3-hour schedule are fed twice rather than three times. Most importantly, however, it is the shift the majority of parents are able to visit. After a demonstration by the nurse, parents are encouraged to take on the task of bathing their baby. Bath time is then adjusted to the time the parents are able to visit.

The infants should be bathed before a feeding, with warm water and a mild soap without hexachlorophene. The choice of sponge bath or tub bath depends on how critically ill the infant is. At this time, the infant's environment is cleaned. The warmer, bassinette, or crib, should be wiped down with a disinfectant and clean linen applied. Isolettes should be exchanged every three to four days to be thoroughly disinfected.

Skin Care

A mild lotion may be used to help prevent drying or breakdown of skin. However, lotions and creams are contraindicated on babies under phototherapy or heat lamps. Powder is not used because it can be irritating to the respiratory tract.

Paper tape is preferred to cloth tape when next to the infant's skin, particularly for the premature. Delicate tissue can be pulled off, leaving the infant more susceptible to infec-

tion. However, gauze pads can sometimes be placed between cloth tape and skin.

Cord Care

If the infant no longer needs an umbilical catheter, the cord should be cleaned daily with alcohol. Sponge baths are recommended initially to keep the area dry and free from infection.

Mouth Care

Mouth care should be given at least every 3 hours on infants who are taking nothing by mouth. Sterile water on a cotton swab is sufficient. Glycerin swabs are not recommended because salivary secretions seem to increase. This may put the infant at risk for aspiration. Also, excess secretions are contraindicated in many surgical conditions.

Diaper Care

The perineum must be cleansed with each diaper change. Air and cornstarch are two excellent methods of treatment for diaper rash. A heat lamp can be used two or three times a shift for about 10 minutes. Raised whitish pimples and satellite lesions may mean a *Monilia* infection, which will require a fungicide ointment.

Weights

The infants should be weighed at the same time each day, before a feeding. The night shift is preferred, so the new weight is ready for morning rounds. Never leave the infant alone on a scale. The same scale should be used each time to insure accuracy. Metric scales are preferred because nutritional and medicinal calculations are figured in metric units. The primary nurse must assess the infant's daily weight. Unusual losses or gains may indicate a change in the infant's condition or perhaps nutritional needs which are not being met. Be sure to note the addition or deletion of appliances from each day's weight (*e.g.,* IV boards, gastrostomy tubes, and so on).

Temperature

Axillary temperatures are taken to avoid injury to the rectal mucosa. A glass thermometer can be used, however, it must be left in place for 5 minutes for axillary temperatures. Electronic thermometers are safe, fast, and sanitary. Before the infant's discharge, parents should be encouraged to bring in a thermometer from home. The primary nurse can then teach the parents how to read and use their own thermometer.

FEEDINGS

Feedings require more caregiving time per shift than almost any other single nursing task. Infants are held for feedings whenever possible; they need to feel the warmth and security conveyed at feeding time (Fig. 4-5). The infant who must remain in the isolette or warmer needs to be gently stroked and talked to as if being held in the caregivers arms.

Feedings should be begun within one-half hour of the scheduled time. A feeding should take 15 to 30 minutes. Past this time, the infant may tire and use calories needed for growth. A propped bottle or unattended gavage tube feeding should be grounds for serious disciplinary action.

Breast Milk (See also Chap. 42)

Breast milk is used whenever possible. The nursing mother of a sick infant needs encouragement, support, and teaching to carry out this maternal task so important for her and the baby. A breast pump should be made available to the mother who is interested in nursing. By pumping her breasts, the mother can leave breast milk at the hospital to be used when she is unable to be there at the feeding time. The breast milk should be stored in the refrigerator at 4°C in sterile, disposable, plastic nurser bags or plastic baby bottles. The mother can purchase the bags or bottles at a grocery or drug store. They must be labeled with the infant's name, the time, and the date. Breast milk can be stored for up to 48 hours in the refrigerator. Do not use glass containers to store breast milk because white cells in the milk tend to cling to the glass. Breast milk is sometimes frozen; however, freezing destroys the cells.

If the infant is unable to suckle or needs a higher calorie/protein source for growth, the mother who wishes to nurse should be encouraged to continue pumping her breasts until the infant is able to suckle. Lloyd-B pumps are especially effective. A hand-bulb pump can be used; however, it is usually more successful after the milk supply is established.

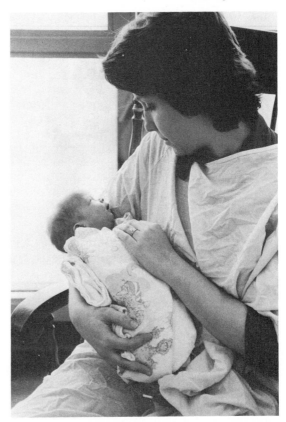

Fig. 4-5. Mother holding her baby in the ICN.

Nipple Feedings

The nurse must evaluate the suck/swallow coordination of the infant, which usually matures at about 34-weeks' gestation. Neurologic insults such as birth asphyxia and intraventricular bleeding, sepsis, and prematurity, may have an effect on the infants ability to nipple feed. Observe the infant for signs of respiratory distress, bradycardia, and cyanosis during feedings. Any untoward signs present at more than two feedings may indicate a need for an alternative feeding method. For an infant who has been tolerating feedings well, a change in feeding pattern is usually one of the first signs of illness.

Gavage Feedings

Intermittent oral or nasal gavage feedings are often used when an infant is unable to nipple feed. Gavage feedings are also used as a supplement to nipple feedings if the infant tires easily. The oral tube is inserted at the beginning of each feeding with care to avoid aspiration.

Up to about three months of age, infants are nose breathers. For a nasal gavage feeding, a number 5 French feeding tube is used for infants under 1600 g and a number 8 French feeding tube is used for most infants over 1600 g. The feeding tube is inserted according to the measurement taken from the bridge of the nose to the xiphoid. Choking or cyanosis may mean the tube is in the trachea.

After the tube is passed and secured, placement must be checked. This is done in two steps.

1. One cc of air is injected into the feeding tube. The air should be clearly heard entering the stomach by auscultation over the abdomen.
2. Stomach contents are aspirated into the feeding tube and then replaced.

Placing the end of the feeding tube into water to check for air bubbles from the lungs is not accurate because air may also be present in the stomach.

After the tube is passed and secured, the infant is checked for residuals. Residuals should be refed or the infant's buffer system and electrolyte balance may be altered. The decision of whether to subtract the residual from the feeding volume depends on the amount of the residual in relation to the amount of formula the infant has been taking.

A gavage feeding is a gravity feeding. The formula or breast milk should be no higher than 3 to 4 inches above the infant's abdomen. The infant should be placed on his right side during the feeding if he cannot be held. The baby should be burped with the gavage tube open to air. When removing the tube, it should be pinched and withdrawn smoothly so that milk does not enter the pharynx.

Normally the gavage tube is removed after the feeding. Infants on feedings every 2 hours can routinely have their gavage tube left in place to be changed once a shift. However, occasionally an infant may have episodes of apnea and bradycardia due to vagal stimulation as the tube is being passed. In this instance, the tube can be left in to be changed every 24 hours. However, the placement of the tube must still be checked before each feeding. An oral tube, in particular, is easily dislodged by the infant sucking on the tube.

Transpyloric Feedings (See Chap. 42)

Once the transpyloric (nasoduodenal, nasojejunal) tube is in place and feedings are begun, the infant should be watched for signs of necrotizing enterocolitis. The abdominal girth should be checked every two hours and recorded. All stools should be hematested. An oral gastric tube should be inserted along with the transpyloric feeding tube and the tube aspirated every 2 to 3 hours to check for gastric residual indicating paralytic ileus or overload. The gastric tube is left in place. Removal may dislodge the transpyloric feeding tube.

The osmolarity of the formula should be questioned if the infant has diarrhea. The feedings are given by constant infusion with a suitable pump. The pump setting for total volume should show no more than 3 hours worth of feeding in case of pump malfunction.

Gastrostomy Feedings

The gastrostomy tube is lowered to straight drainage about 15 minutes before the feeding, to check for residuals.

The height above the abdomen of the syringe barrel holding the formula should be adjusted within a 4-inch range so that the feeding takes approximately the same time as an oral feeding. The feeding should flow in by gravity: a plunger should never be used. If the baby has to vomit, the gastrostomy becomes a safety valve where the stomach contents can safely back up. The tube can then be lowered to straight drainage. If the feeding tube is too high above the abdomen or the plunger is left in the syringe, the stomach contents may regurgitate through the esophagus, putting the infant at risk for aspiration. The gastrostomy should not be clamped without a specific order.

Total Parenteral Nutrition

In some instances, it is not possible to feed an infant through the gastrointestinal tract. Contraindications include surgical lesions, necrotizing enterocolitis, intractable nonspecific diarrhea, and extreme prematurity. Parenteral nutrition is used to give these infants the proper nutrients. Total parenteral nutrition provides the infant with calories, protein, and essential fatty acids as well as vitamins and minerals. It is often overlapped with gastrointestinal feedings.

Parenteral alimentation includes amino acids to promote growth, glucose and lipid to meet caloric expenditures, and added vitamins and minerals. The infant is given approximately 100 to 110 calories/kg/day, beginning with a reduced dose and increasing slowly to full strength to prevent glycosuria leading to osmotic overload and dehydration. A 10% solution of Intralipid is the essential fatty acid infusate (See Chap. 42).

Infusion may be by either a central or peripheral venous line. When using a peripheral line, care must be given to prevent infiltration and damage to the infant's tissue. A dextrose solution of no greater than 10% should be infused in a peripheral line. To prevent blood stream contamination, the cutdown for a central venous line should be performed under strict asepsis. Usually the internal jugular vein is chosen, with tunneling under the skin to a remote skin exit behind the ear.

An antibacterial ointment is used before the sterile dressing is applied. The dressing should be changed every 48 hours. When changing the dressing, two nurses perform the procedure to maintain sterile technique and to prevent dislodging of the catheter. Preventing contamination of the line is a major consideration when caring for infants with total parenteral nutrition infusing through a central venous line.

Problems may occur during infusion of total parenteral nutrition. The nurse must monitor the infant carefully, noting any change in his status.

Nursing Intervention

1. A Dextrostix must be monitored every 4 hours initially, and at least once a shift when the infant is stable, during long-term total parenteral nutrition. Values between 45 and 130 mg/dl are considered safe.
2. Urine protein, sugar, and specific gravity are checked each voiding.
3. A constant IV flow rate should always be maintained. The nurse should never try to catch-up. This may lead to glucose overload and eventually cause dehydration through osmotic diuresis. An infusion running slower than the ordered rate will reduce caloric intake and may cause hypoglycemia.
4. The infant should be monitored for signs of sepsis.
5. Oral hygiene is important for any infant not taking fluids by mouth.
6. If the hyperalimentation is interrupted for any reason, a comparable dextrose solution must be hung in the interim.

Special Considerations for Intralipid

1. If the Intralipid is "piggybacked" with the hyperalimentation solution, it must be done close to the patient and below the filter. A filter may cause the fat emulsion to clump, putting the patient at risk for emboli.
2. During the test dose, the infant should be observed for adverse reactions. Dyspnea, cyanosis, flushing, vomiting, and elevation of temperature are signs of an untoward reaction. The Intralipid must be stopped immediately if any of these signs occur.
3. A serum lipemia check should be drawn every morning. It is necessary to stop the infusion 4 hours before the lipemia check for accurate results.

Most of the infants that receive total parenteral nutrition remain hospitalized for long periods of time. Parents must be encouraged to care for and handle their infant in order to foster development and bonding.

THE PREMATURE

Gestational Age (See also Chap. 12)

Tools for gestational age and growth assessment include the Dubowitz (Appendix D-1) and the Colorado Intrauterine Growth Chart (Appendix D-2). Problems of prematurity are a direct result of reduced gestational age.[36] The infant who is small for gestational age is undergrown for gestational age. The assessment is important in order to identify problems specific to premature and small-for-gestational-age infants and to develop a relevant plan of care.

The nurse must understand the fears and concerns of the parents whose infant is small for gestational age. Their infant may be doing well with adequate nutritional support. However, the parents may relate size to illness and be equating the critically ill premature's problems to those of their infant.[40]

Thermoregulation (See also Chap. 10)

An important responsibility of the nurse is to maintain a neutral thermal environment for the infant. Cold stress in a premature may cause acidosis, increased oxygen needs, apnea, poor perfusion, hypoglycemia, pulmonary hemorrhage, and without proper intervention, long-term complications or death. The infant's temperature should be maintained between 36.5°C and 37°C axillary. If an infant's temperature falls below 36.5°C, the temperature should be taken every 15 minutes to one-half hour until the baby is warmed and restabilized. The infant must be watched carefully; warming after cold stress may induce apnea.

In the delivery room, the infant should be dried and warmed as soon as possible. A free-standing warmer can be used to warm both mother and baby after delivery. Some institutions place a stockinette cap on all infants' heads immediately after delivery while the mother is holding the baby. The large, vascular surface over the cranium is an area of great heat loss. This method can also be used when taking the premature out of the isolette for feedings or treatment.

A radiant warmer allows the team access to the infant. However, attention must be paid to insensible water loss. Be sure the servocontrol is on and functioning. Hyperthermia will cause apnea and increased oxygen consumption, again pointing out the importance of a neutral thermal environment. A radiant warmer also leaves the infant an open target. The nurse must be sure infection control is maintained and stimulation is kept at therapeutic level.

An isolette provides warmth, humidity, and cleanliness. Once an optimum temperature is set, the isolette heat can be regulated by the infant's body temperature through the servocontrol thermistor. When an infant is septic, temperature instability (often hypothermia) is an early sign. The nurse must be aware of the normal isolette temperature settings according to the infant's weight and age (see Chap. 10). As the infant's temperature becomes unstable, the isolette temperature begins to rise or fall excessively as it tries to maintain a neutral

thermal environment. The nurse must be aware that a problem may be developing.

The isolette door should not be left open for any length of time because heat loss will occur. If a procedure cannot be done in the isolette, place the infant on a padded table and use a heat lamp or free-standing warmer. If the infant cannot be taken from the isolette and the door must be open for a significant amount of time, set the isolette heat control on manual rather than servocontrol and use a heat lamp.

Keep the isolette or warmer away from drafts or air conditioners. Be sure all alarms are on and functioning. Be aware of objects blocking the radiant heat source, such as phototherapy lights. Record the temperature of the isolette or warmer with other vital signs.

Nursing judgment must be used in bathing the premature. Any infant with temperature instability or a temperature under 36.5°C axillary should be cleansed in the isolette to prevent cold stress. Infants under 1500 g should always be bathed in their isolette, to avoid loss of heat through evaporation.

Very immature newborns may have excessive radiant heat loss even with these measures. If in an isolette, a heat shield of plastic, foil, or even Saran Wrap may aid temperature stability.

Apnea (See also Chaps. 14 and 39)

The premature is at high risk for apnea. Causes include failure to maintain a neutral thermal environment; metabolic disorders such as hypoglycemia and hypocalcemia; sepsis; hypoxia; anemia; hemorrhage; and immaturity of the respiratory center. Apnea is a pathologic condition accompanied by a change in color and bradycardia. Periodic breathing is the normal respiratory pattern of the premature and no significant hypoxia occurs.

There are several nursing measures to follow in caring for the infant with apnea:

1. The respirations *and* heart rate of the premature infant must be monitored.
2. Each episode must be assessed to determine true apnea.
3. An apnea flow sheet should be kept at the bedside to record the length of the episode, color change, bradycardia, stimulation required and any factors that may have precipitated the incident.
4. A Dextrostix should be done at least once per shift to monitor blood glucose.

5. An accurate record of blood output should be kept at the infant's bedside. Hemoglobin and hematocrit should be checked periodically.
6. The infant's temperature must be monitored closely.
7. If hypoxia occurs, blood gases will determine the need for oxygen therapy.
8. The nurse must be alert for signs of sepsis such as temperature instability, lethargy, and poor feeding.

In many instances, tactile stimulation such as rubbing the rib cage, gently tugging the leg, or flicking the bottoms of the feet will help the infant to breathe again. The nurse must always be gentle. Waterbeds can also be a source of stimulation.

Occasionally the infant will need more than tactile stimulation. There must be an oxygen setup with bag and appropriate size mask available for resuscitation. When apneic episodes become severe, mechanical ventilation may be required.

Aminophyllin and caffeine are sometimes used to stimulate the central nervous system where there seems to be no pathologic cause of apnea. Side effects of this therapy include tachycardia (a significant increase in heart rate, usually above 180), abdominal distention, and vomiting.

Growth and Development of the Premature

The nurse can foster development of the premature by providing visual, auditory, and tactile stimulation balanced with appropriate rest periods. Some programs have attempted to simulate an intrauterine environment through the use of voices, music, or a heartbeat, piped into the isolette.[41] Premature infants need to be held and rocked and to develop eye contact with their mothers. Waterbeds can also be used for vestibular stimulation. If a waterbed is used, there should be a "no-pins" warning on the isolette. Use body temperature water when filling the waterbed and add about 20 ml of chlorine bleach to prevent the growth of organisms. A waterbed will help avoid molding of the head and prevent pressure sores from developing. Place a roll under the infant's neck to maintain the airway of the small premature. The waterbed can be oscillated by a ventilator or other device to give gentle rocking.

THE NURSE'S ROLE IN GROWTH AND DEVELOPMENT

An important part of a nurse's daily plan of care is fostering the growth and development of the sick infant.[42-44] This is an ongoing process throughout the hospitalization and is individualized depending on the infant's age, condition, and length of stay. Continuity of care, through an implemented system of primary nursing, allows for this individualization and limits the number of caregivers.

Fostering growth and development begins with the comfort and warmth conveyed by the nurse at the bedside while carrying out tasks. The infant absorbs the nurse's feeling through her touch and tone of voice. Meeting basic daily needs such as hunger or diaper changing, and responding to crying within a reasonable length of time, help to make the infant's environment more secure.

The nurse, whenever possible, should plan physical care needs to avoid overstimulation and allow for adequate periods of rest. Planning vital signs before suctioning or feedings, and planning baths with procedures or blood drawing times, allow for longer uninterrupted sleep times. If intensive and intermediate infants are in different modules, intermediate care nurses can assess their patient's condition and appropriately dim a block of lights, creating a more home-like and restful environment during sleeping hours.

Mirrors and toys appropriate for the age, as well as singing, rocking, and talking, provide the infant with a variety of stimulation. Playpens can be used, particularly for the chronically ill infant, as a change of environment and a new source of visual stimulation. This change has soothed many infants with long-term illnesses who have become just plain tired of their bed and its surroundings.

Often a referral to occupational or physical therapy is appropriate for infants with extended stays to facilitate the continued development of muscular and motor coordination. The primary nurse and parents should be incorporated into the plan of therapy. The nurse can assume responsibility for the plan with further supervision as necessary. Parents can then continue this therapy after discharge.

Infant development is an ongoing process. It should be incorporated into the daily plan of care as naturally as the physical care given by the nurse.

SPECIAL CARE

For the pathophysiology of various diseases in infants, please refer to the individual chapters in this book. We have attempted to give nursing care guidelines for some of the special problems of the sick neonate.

Nursing Care of the Infant under Phototherapy

Phototherapy is usually begun when the indirect bilirubin is about one-half the exchange index. It is used to reduce tissue and serum bilirubin by direct exposure of the infant's skin to light, which breaks down the bilirubin to water-soluble, excretable products.

The infant should be undressed in order to expose the most skin surface. The baby should not be diapered. For female infants, a disposable diaper can be spread on the bed under the buttocks or perineum. For male infants, we have found that a paper mask can be tied at the hip. This allows maximum exposure while covering the genital area.

To prevent possible retinal injury, the infant's eyes must be protected from the phototherapy. There are several kinds of bilirubin masks available. Most require oval or gauze pads to be placed under the mask. The infant's eyelids must be closed before the pads are applied. The pads should be moistened with sterile water to prevent corneal abrasion. Eye infections caused by moistened eyepads have not been a problem at this institution.

When securing the bilirubin mask, the nurse must be sure it is snug but not so tight as to cause moulding. For the small premature, a stockinette or "ski cap" can be used over the eye pads instead of a bilirubin mask. This avoids pressure on the premature's head. The infant should be checked periodically to ensure the mask and pads have not slipped, exposing the infant's eyes to the light.

It is improtant to maintain temperature control. Most full-term infants with no other complications do well in a bassinette with warmth from the phototherapy lights. Occasionally an extra heat source may be needed. It is important that the genital area of a male infant be covered if the light bulb on the heat source is unprotected. These lights can be dangerous: a stream of urine on a hot light bulb may cause the bulb to break.

If a premature infant is in an isolette when phototherapy is necessary, be sure that the phototherapy light is not close to the thermometer in the isolette or over the thermistor on the infant's skin. A false high reading will keep the isolette from heating. Phototherapy lights do not emit enough heat to keep a premature warm.

Some radiant warmers have built-in phototherapy lights. Warmers without built-in lights may need two angled phototherapy units, placed at either side of the warmer. This gives enough energy for therapy and still allows heat to radiate to the infant.

A spectroradiometer is the best way to determine when the phototherapy lights should be changed. Use the meter daily and record the measurements in the nurse's notes. A normal reading is 4.0 to 6.0 μw/cm^2/nm. If there is no meter available, a card should be kept for each phototherapy unit. The nurse should mark the date and time the therapy was begun and discontinued. The total number of hours should then be tallied. Up to 400 hours usage is considered safe, although there is evidence that the radiant flux is good for as long as 1000 hours.

A bilirubin level should be checked every 6 to 12 hours, depending on the condition of the infant. Phototherapy lights should be turned off when drawing blood for bilirubin to prevent falsely low values. The nurse should be watchful for decreased urine output, increased specific gravity, and absence of stools. Infants under phototherapy should be well hydrated. Most full-term infants can tolerate a forced fluids diet. Feed formula or breast milk (measured into a bottle for accurate intake) every 4 hours. One or two ounces of sterile water can be fed 2 hours later and thereafter every 4 hours. The infant is then receiving fluids every 2 hours.

Side effects of phototherapy include lethargy, temperature change, and skin rash. Loose green stools usually occur and do not represent infectious diarrhea. The infant's perineum must be kept clean to prevent skin breakdown. No ointments should be used when the infant is under phototherapy; burns may occur.

It is important for parents to have contact with their baby. When the bilirubin level is not too near the exchange index, the infant is taken from phototherapy during feedings and the eye patches are removed for the parents to interact with their baby. If the bilirubin is high, sometime during the parent's visit turn the lights off and remove the eye patches for just a few minutes. Encourage the parents to feed and give as much care as possible during their infant's phototherapy.

Exchange Transfusion. Indications for exchange transfusion are given in Chapter 24. The infant is placed on a warmer with all extremities restrained and a cardiac/apnea monitor with oscilloscope and alarm is attached. To prevent vomiting and aspiration, the stomach contents should be emptied through a nasogastric tube, if the infant was recently fed. The baby should be diapered or should have a urine bag applied to protect the sterile field. The nurse should check the abdominal girth and a Dextrostix prior to exchange, which is usually done through an umbilical catheter. A preexchange bilirubin is drawn. The exchange blood and laboratory slip should be double-checked by a nurse and a physician for correct type and laboratory number. The blood must be run through a sterile coil tubing which is set in a blood warmer. No connections should be under water. The water in the blood warmer should be maintained at 37°C.

The patient should be observed and monitored closely throughout the exchange; any arrhythmias, cyanosis, seizures, rash, or change in vital signs should be noted. All blood output/input should be recorded with the time, and then the amount totalled to be sure it is the same. Periodically, the heart and respiratory rate should be recorded on the flowsheet. The nurse should be aware of the total volume to be exchanged. Postexchange blood must be sent to the laboratory for appropriate studies.

After the exchange, vital signs are taken every 15 minutes, twice and then every half-hour four times. Blood used in transfusions has a high glucose level and hypoglycemic rebound may occur. A Dextrostix should be checked every half hour four times and then every hour two times. If the catheter is removed after the exchange, the nurse should watch for bleeding at the umbilical site. Another rare side effect of exchange transfusion is necrotizing enterocolitis. The infant should be observed for signs of abdominal distention, increased girth, apnea, Hematest positive stools, and gastric residual. Phototherapy is often continued after the exchange.

Respiratory Care

Two-thirds of the infants in ICNs have serious respiratory problems. Much of the needed respiratory care is provided by the nurse at the bedside. Nursing assessment of respiratory and circulatory status is ongoing and includes physical assessment, laboratory analysis, and knowledge of bioinstrumentation.

The nurse must be able to operate and interpret a cardiopulmonary monitor with invasive pressure monitoring capabilities. This must be included in ongoing inservice education for the neonatal intensive care nurse, along with knowledge of ventilator care, use of the transcutaneous oxygen monitor, trend recorder, and other types of instrumentation.

Physical assessment includes both visual inspection and auscultation. The nurse should watch for nasal flaring and tachypnea (respirations above 60) and note intercostal, substernal and suprasternal retractions. She should check for circumoral cyanosis and cyanosis of mucous membranes and nail beds, and record all apneic spells, including duration, accompanying bradycardia, and other significant observations.

Grunting is another sign of respiratory difficulty. It may be audible or heard on auscultation. The stethoscope must also be used to evaluate breath sounds. Is air being moved? Are the breath sounds equal or diminished on one side? Are crepitant rales or rhonchi present? With experience, the nurse can pick up subtle changes in the respiratory function of the infant.

Oxygen is a drug that must be used with precision in infants with respiratory distress. The oxygen must be warmed and humidified. It is important for the nurse to check the temperature and humidity of the delivered oxygen. Humidity prevents the mucosa from drying. Over-humidification may obstruct the tubing with condensation, promote the growth of certain bacteria, as well as "drown" the infant who is intubated. The air-oxygen mixture should be warmed to slightly below body temperature. A stable oxygen temperature will prevent increased oxygen consumption from chilling.

There are essentially four ways of delivering oxygen to the neonate: oxygen hood, resuscitation bags, CPAP, and mechanical ventilation. An oxygen hood is used for infants breathing spontaneously who have less severe disease. The hood can be used in the isolette, basinette, or radiant warmer. Oxygen should not be piped freely into an isolette as the required percentage cannot be maintained steadily.

An interim measure of oxygenation is with resuscitation bag and mask. This increases the infant's P_{O_2} during manual ventilation. A bag and appropriate size mask should be at the bedside of all infants at risk. The oxygen blender should have enough outlets so that warmed, humidified oxygen through the bag and mask can be immediately available. The nurse should watch for chest movement and check breath sounds continuously during bagging. Over-ventilation may blow off too much CO_2 and cause apnea. Pressure from poor mask placement may cause corneal abrasion. During or after bagging, a gastric tube should be inserted to remove air in the stomach.

CPAP or PEEP (Positive End Expiratory Pressure) provide the infant with oxygen and positive pressure to help prevent alveolar collapse at end expiration. Positive pressure can be delivered through an endotracheal tube, or through nasal prongs, when assisted ventilation is not anticipated. The prongs are placed in the infant's nose and secured to prevent dislodging. Before inserting the prongs, apply a small amount of hydrocortisone cream, 0.125%, to the outside of the prongs and around the infant's nares. This helps to prevent breakdown and inflammation of the skin. Clean the prongs each shift to insure patency. An oral-gastric tube is inserted for stomach decompression.

Care of the Infant on a Ventilator. The criteria for mechanical ventilation are found in Chapter 22. As soon as the infant is intubated, breath sounds are checked for bilateral aeration. The endotracheal tube is then secured. An x-ray film is taken to confirm placement of the tube. The infant is attached to the ventilator and the ventilator tubing secured to a restraining device to prevent drag on the endotracheal tube. Place rolls on both sides of the infant's head to prevent movement and possible extubation. A small roll is placed under the shoulders to straighten the airway. Arterial blood gas values of infants receiving mechanical ventilation should be checked at least every 2 hours during the acute phase. This should be repeated 20 minutes after any ventilator settings (including

delivered oxygen) are changed. The nurse should record the amount of blood drawn for gases (and other tests) on a flow sheet. This, and blood pressure monitoring, will help alert one to hypovolemia and anemia. Also recorded is the amount of heparin flush used in a 24-hour period. Heparin flush can be prepared on the unit or in the pharmacy. As a precaution, even with a preservative added, heparin flush should be refrigerated. After 24 hours in room air, it should be discarded.

An infant receiving respiratory assistance requires close nursing observation. Hourly vital signs include an axillary temperature (36.5–37.0°C), apical pulse (120–180), respiration count (30–60), and blood pressure check. Normal mean central arterial blood pressure is 40 to 60 torr and normal central venous pressure is 2 to 8 torr. Be sure all alarms are set and functioning. The nurse should monitor the concentration, humidity, and temperature of inspired oxygen, and the temperature of the heating element.

Ventilator settings such as the rate, volume, PEEP, and peak inspiratory pressure (PIP), must be monitored by the nurse and recorded on the nursing or respiratory flow sheet between the respiratory therapists' rounds.

The positive pressure delivered through PEEP can reduce venous return. As PEEP is decreased, venous return to the heart increases. The nurse must closely watch the infant at risk for heart failure. As PEEP is increased and venous return decreases, the infant must be watched for signs of poor peripheral perfusion.

If peak inspiratory pressure begins to rise when the ventilator is volume- or time-cycled, check for an airway obstruction, pneumothorax or block in the tubing such as water or a kink.[45]

In order to ventilate certain agitated infants, drugs such as curare or pancuronium bromide (Pavulon) are sometimes used. By causing paralysis of the skeletal muscles, these medications prevent the infant from fighting the ventilator and may allow lower pressures to be used. The initial onset is within 5 minutes. Curare has a longer time duration than pancuronium bromide, lasting up to 20 minutes. Gastrointestinal bleeding and hypotension are side effects of curare. Tachycardia may occur with pancuronium bromide usage.

Frequent turning and range-of-motion exercises should be done while the infant is paralyzed. The infant's mouth may need frequent suctioning to remove collected secretions. A label should be placed at the infant's bedside to alert all staff that muscle paralysis is being used. It is extremely important that the physicians and nurses be aware that the infant is totally dependent on the ventilator; he will quickly die if any malfunctioning occurs and bagging is not immediately substituted. It may be necessary to Credé the bladder to avoid urinary retention. Artificial tears are used to prevent corneal drying.

Sudden deterioration in the infant's condition requires immediate action. The nurse must

1. call for assistance. Do not leave the infant unattended.
2. quickly scan the ventilator for mechanical failure. Too much pressure may indicate a blocked tracheal tube, too little may indicate a disconnection or extubation.
3. remove the infant from the ventilator and ventilate with a bag.
4. check the oxygen level and source.
5. listen to breath sounds. If breath sounds are totally absent with manual bagging, one must remove the endotracheal tube and ventilate with bag and mask.
6. begin full resuscitative efforts.

An emergency cart should always be available with equipment, as should drugs appropriate for neonatal resuscitation. An organized team approach to resuscitation should be implemented on the unit.

Postural Drainage and Suctioning should be performed every 2 to 3 hours on the infant receiving ventilatory assistance. Mucus adhering to the larger respiratory passages may cause obstruction of the airway and block the endotracheal tube or nasal prongs. The infant should be monitored and observed closely during the procedure. Vigorous postural drainage and prolonged suctioning can result in severe hypoxia and reflex bradycardia.

Percussion is done with a medicine cup wrapped with gauze or a padded nipple, followed by vibration with an electric toothbrush or similar device. Drainage is accomplished by positioning the infant and/or the warmer platform. A recent nursing study has shown the electric toothbrush alone provides the best results when compared with the padded nipple and appears to be least stressful to the infant.[46] The study itself makes nurses more aware of how the well-being of the compromised infant is affected by chest physical therapy and suctioning. Transcutaneous monitoring may heighten this awareness.

Endotracheal suctioning is done as a sterile procedure with sterile gloves and suction catheter. It is more easily performed by two people. (If this is not feasible a "one-glove" method can be used.) One person provides ventilation while the other does the suctioning. A brief period of 10 to 15 seconds of hyperventilation with bag and mask is done before, between, and after the suctioning to reexpand alveoli that may have collapsed. The nurse should monitor the infant and allow for periods of rest during the procedure.

In our unit, sterile normal saline (0.3 to 0.5 ml) is alternated every 2 to 3 hours with polymixin B solution (0.3 to 0.5 ml) and instilled into the endotracheal tube before suctioning. This helps liquefy and mobilize secretions. The nurse should turn the infant's head to both the right and left in order to suction both major bronchi. Suction should not be applied during insertion of the catheter. Sterile water is used to clean the catheter. Unless care is taken in passing the catheter, perforation of lung tissue can occur. A chart developed by Anderson and associates is used to measure the length which can safely be inserted (Fig. 4-6).[47] After the procedure, the nurse should check breath sounds for clarity and quality and record any pertinent information.

Pneumothorax. Too much pressure delivered to an infant being mechanically ventilated (manually or bagged) may cause rupture of alveoli, or pneumothorax. The signs of pneumothorax include respiratory distress, diminished breath sounds on the affected side, asymmetry of chest movement, deterioration in blood gases, and a shift in heart sounds to one side. Any infant at risk for a pneumothorax should have a #19 or #23 butterfly needle connected to a three-way stopcock and large syringe at the bedside. This is used as an emergency measure to tap the pleural space for air until a chest tube can be inserted.

Care of Chest Tubes. Once the chest tube is inserted the nurse should do the following.

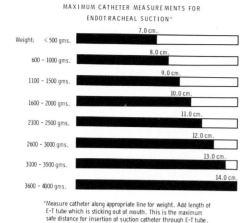

MAXIMUM CATHETER MEASUREMENTS FOR
ENDOTRACHEAL SUCTION*

Weight:	
< 500 gms.	7.0 cm.
600 - 1000 gms.	8.0 cm.
1100 - 1500 gms.	9.0 cm.
1600 - 2000 gms.	10.0 cm.
2100 - 2500 gms.	11.0 cm.
2600 - 3000 gms.	12.0 cm.
3100 - 3500 gms.	13.0 cm.
3600 - 4000 gms.	14.0 cm.

*Measure catheter along appropriate line for weight. Add length of
E-T tube which is sticking out of mouth. This is the maximum
safe distance for insertion of suction catheter through E-T tube.

Fig. 4-6. Chart showing safe length at which a catheter can be inserted for endotracheal suctioning. (Anderson K, Chandra R: J Pediatr Surg 11: 687, 1976)[43]

1. Make all connections firm.
2. Make sure the tubing is patent and not kinked or curled.
3. Mark and record the drainage level at the end of each shift.
4. *Not* clamp chest tubes if suction is interrupted. As long as the water seal remains intact, air cannot get into the pleural space. A clamped tube, however, allows pressure to build up in the pleural space, particularly if the infant is on a ventilator, creating a tension pneumothorax.
5. Usually there is little serous drainage from a chest tube inserted for a pneumothorax. ''Milk'' the tubing once per shift starting near the infant and working down. A wet wash cloth usually works very well.
6. Initially, there may be some bubbling in the water seal as air escapes from the pleural cavity. However, after that, bubbling in the water seal may mean an air leakage. The nurse should pinch the chest tube below its insertion. If the bubbling continues, the leak is somewhere in the system. All connections should be checked. If the bubbling stops when the chest tube is pinched, the air is coming from the pleural space. The pneumothorax may have recurred. The nurse should notify the physician and obtain a roentgenograph.
7. In a closed drainage system, the suction is controlled by the difference in the height of the water column between the suction control and water seal compartments. If 2 cm are used in the water seal, the column in the suction control section should equal the ordered cm of water suction + 2 cm.

Care of the Cardiac Infant (See also Chap. 23)

Recognition. Many of the individual signs and symptoms associated with heart disease are also indicative of other kinds of illness in the neonate. It is important, therefore, that the nurse look at the composite picture in order to recognize cardiac distress. Signs and symptoms include

1. Tachypnea: respirations over 60, particularly when the infant is at rest
2. Cyanosis: may be mild or severe, generalized or intermittent, such as during feedings or when crying; the nurse should check mucous membranes and nailbeds.
3. Dyspnea: this occurs particularly during feeding time.
4. Irritability: may be indicative of uncomfortableness due to oxygen hunger; the infant may be restless when sleeping.
5. Fatigue: tires easily during feedings or procedures
6. Retractions: sometimes accompanied by nasal flaring or grunting; if the heart is enlarged, the retractions may be seen laterally rather than substernally.[48]
7. Tachycardia: apical pulse above 170 even when at rest
8. Weight fluctuation: Poor weight gain may be seen soon after birth because of feeding problems and energy expenditure. Abnormal weight gain accompanied by edema is indicative of congestive heart failure.
9. Flaccid muscle tone
10. Vomiting
11. Weak cry
12. Hepatomegaly: caused by congestion of the liver
13. Diaphoresis: accompanies severe tachypnea

Often, the parents, upon bringing the child home, first notice problems and alert the medical team.[48] Therefore, it is important for nurses to closely assess the infant who is showing any signs of difficulty during the first days of life.

Diagnostic Procedures. Noninvasive diagnosis of the cardiac infant includes ECG, x-ray film, and an echocardiogram. Often, definitive diagnosis will require cardiac catheterization. The procedure is explained to the parents before the permit is signed. Be sure blood for emergency transfusion is made available for this procedure. The baby must have an empty stomach.

Postcatheterization, the extremity used may be cyanotic and cold, as the catheterization partially occludes a major vessel supplying blood to the limb. Observe the extremity for warmth, pulse, and color, and check the cutdown site for bleeding. Monitor vital signs. Keep the dressing dry and clean. Watch for signs of infection. Monitor the infant's output. Urine specific gravity may transiently be high (above 1.030) because of the dye used during catheterization. Barring any complications, the infant usually resumes feeding soon after the catheterization. Transfusion to replace sampling and blood loss may be needed.

Nursing Intervention. The cardiac infant requires careful monitoring and assessment of vital signs, weight, intake and output, and blood pressure. Chest sounds should be evaluated daily for increased congestion. Good pulmonary care is important in the prevention of pneumonia and atelectasis. The nurse should be sure the proper size cuff is used in monitoring the blood pressure or the reading will not be accurate. The width of the cuff should cover about ⅔ of the upper arm. The same cuff should be used each time for better accuracy.

Because of weakness from poor oxygenation, the infant's feedings may take a long time. It must be determined whether the baby can tolerate the stress of oral feedings. Sometimes a combined oral and gavage or total gavage feeding is in order. The cardiac infant is usually more comfortable in a partially upright position. When resting, a prone or side position also seems to help.[49]

Cardiac Drug Therapy Most frequently, medical stabilization of cardiac disease includes a diuretic such as furosemide (Lasix) or spironolactone (Aldactazide), and a cardiotonic preparation such as digoxin (Lanoxin).

Furosemide is a potent diuretic with a peak effect about ½ hour after the intravenous dose. It inhibits reabsorption of electrolytes. When used with digoxin, the nurse must keep in mind that excessive loss of potassium may increase digoxin toxicity.

Spironolactone is an oral preparation. The diuretic effects occur more slowly and are more prolonged. Although sodium and chloride are excreted with the water loss, there is a decreased excretion of potassium. Hyperkalemia can be a side effect, and is significant in infants with impaired renal function.

Strict intake and output must be measured on all infants under diuretic therapy. Diapers can be weighed to estimate output. Urine specific gravity and serum electrolytes must be closely monitored.

Digoxin allows the heart to pump with greater force but in a slower, more normal rhythm. Although digoxin is a lifesaver, it is also a potentially lethal medication. All dosages, particularly intravenous doses, must be calculated with extreme caution. In our institution, after the physician has written the order, a second physician must cosign the prescribed dosage. The nurse must also calculate the prescribed amount and dosage before transcribing the order onto the medication kardex. A decimal point in the wrong place can be fatal for the infant.

After digitalization, a digoxin level is obtained. The nurse must be aware of the signs of digitalis toxicity, such as irregularities in apical rhythm, bradycardia, vomiting, and poor feeding.

After stabilization, the infant may be sent home on oral digoxin. Good support, teaching, and guidelines must be provided for the parents. The infant may stay on digoxin therapy until the heart no longer needs the assistance or until corrective surgery can be done.

Cardiac Surgery. A highly skilled nursing team, with 24-hour, experienced medical backup, is essential for both closed- and open-heart cases. During open-heart surgery, infants may be on cardiopulmonary bypass or hypothermia. Postoperatively, cardiac infants require extensive arterial and venous monitoring. Along with normal postoperative care, these infants require assessment for dysrhythmias, cardiogenic shock, and emboli.

Parent Support. The road seems sometimes unending for the parents of a cardiac infant. The initial surgery may be many months away or repeated surgery may be necessary. An ongoing support group for parents whose children have cardiac problems may be useful, with leadership from professionals such as a clinical nurse specialist and/or cardiac social worker. Such groups allow parents to talk, share experiences, and comfort one another in a very special way.

Care of the Infant Who Requires Surgery (See also Chap. 34)

There are some fundamentals of nursing practice involved in the care of any infant requiring surgery. These include

1. safeguarding proper nutrition, including strict intake and output.
2. observing for localized and generalized infection.
3. maintaining a neutral thermal environment.
4. observing the incision area for bleeding and drainage and recording the amount.
5. observing for signs of shock from fluid or blood loss.
6. monitoring vital signs, abdominal girth, fullness of fontanel, and skin turgor.
7. observing for distress when gastric feeds are resumed.
8. monitoring electrolyte balance.

Keeping in mind the preceding nursing care requirements for all surgical infants, we have highlighted several of the conditions requiring special nursing intervention.

Gastrostomy Care. A gastrostomy tube is surgically placed in the stomach for decompression, removal of gastric juices, or for gastric feedings. The gastrostomy is initially placed for straight drainage. Sometimes 2 to 5 ml of a normal saline irrigation is necessary to keep the tube patent. After intestinal motility has resumed and drainage is minimal, the gastrostomy tube is elevated no more than four inches above the infant's abdomen. If this is tolerated, feedings are begun (see above). Should the infant vomit, the nurse should lower the gastrostomy tube. As gastrostomy feedings are tolerated, the tube will be clamped between feedings. This simulates normal feedings but removes the "blow-off" function of the gastrostomy. When oral feedings are tolerated, the tube will remain clamped until it is eventually removed.

The area at the entry site of the gastrostomy tube must be kept clean. Occasional leakage may occur. After surgery, the site must be checked and the dressing changed regularly. Half-strength peroxide may be used to cleanse the area. A cut is then made halfway down one side of a four by four and the dressing is slipped around the gastrostomy tube and taped. As the infant grows, a larger gastrostomy tube may be necessary.

If the infant goes home with the gastrostomy tube, the parents must be secure in feeding their infant and changing the dressing.

Peristomal Care. In babies with enterostomies, the peristomal skin is prepared by washing with warm water, rinsing well and patting dry. Using a stoma guide, a circle is drawn on the skin shield, the size of the stoma, and cut out. An opening is then made in the adhesive plate of the pouch about ⅛ inch bigger. The paper is peeled off the skin shield and placed sticky-side down with the stoma centered. The adhesive plate of the pouch is applied over the skin shield, centering it around the stoma. Tape is applied around the edges of the pouch, and the bottom of the pouch is folded and fastened with a rubber band or tape. The pouch should be emptied of feces frequently and wiped clean. This will help it to remain intact for a longer period of time. Warm water can be used to cleanse the pouch of thick or sticky feces. When it is clean, it is wiped dry and fastened again.

To keep the skin clean and help the pouch to adhere, creamy soap, oils, or lotions are not used around the stoma. If the adhesive tape becomes wet, new tape is applied. If the pouch leaks under the face plate, it is removed at once and a new one applied. The skin shield should be changed only when it comes loose, to minimize irritation to peristomal skin. Caution should be used in applying anything but warm water to cleanse and deodorize the inside of the pouch. The stoma tissue is living and will absorb chemical substances into the body.

Pyloric stenosis is the congenital hypertrophy of the muscle of the pylorus. The infant initially has intermittent vomiting which increases to persistent projectile vomiting. Because of the vomiting, these infants require assessment of hydration and electrolyte status upon admission. When the infant is calm and the stomach emptied, the hardened mass or "olive" can be felt in the right-upper quadrant. Postoperatively, a nasogastric tube may temporarily be inserted. Feedings usually begin 12 to 24 hours postoperatively, and progress gradually from clear liquids to full strength formula.

Necrotizing enterocolitis has numerous causes but occurs most frequently in asphyxiated premature infants. The signs include abdominal distention, gastric residual, the inability to tolerate feedings, apnea, and symptoms of sepsis. X-ray findings help to confirm the diagnosis.

Once necrotizing enterocolitis is suspected, the infant is given nothing by mouth. A nasogastric tube is inserted and all drainage and stool is measured and tested for blood. An abdominal girth is obtained every 2 hours. A girth increase greater than 1 cm in 4 hours is significant. The infant is started on antibiotics both intravenously and intragastrically. Gentamicin, diluted in 1 ml of sterile water, is inserted into the nasogastric tube which is clamped for ½ hour. Afterward, the tube is unclamped for drainage.

If the bowel becomes perforated, surgical intervention is necessary. Besides routine postoperative care, the infant may require gastrostomy and/or enterostomy care. The infant should be allowed nothing by mouth for up to several weeks to allow the bowel to rest and heal. Feedings are begun slowly, with residuals and abdominal girths checked prior to each feeding. Reducing substances are checked for in stools or ostomy drainage to determine whether the infant is tolerating feedings. If an extensive amount of bowel has been removed, the baby may be on long-term parenteral nutrition therapy. Throughout the recuperation period, the infant is observed for a recurrence of symptoms.

Omphalocele and Gastroschisis. An omphalocele is a herniation of abdominal viscera into the base of the umbilical cord. The sac, which may rupture, is thin and translucent, exposing the intestine and liver. Associated defects of the intestine, heart, and great vessels are common. Gastroschisis is not usually associated with other anamolies. This defect has no sac covering the evisceration. Most of the abdominal contents protrude from around the side of the umbilicus.

Preoperative care of both defects is similar. A nasogastric tube is inserted to prevent vomiting, aspiration, and intestinal distention caused by swallowed air. If the size of the defect is small, all of the contents may be completely reduced at surgery. If several reductions are necessary, a silon pouch is used to cover the evisceration. Special care is used to prevent infection. An antibacterial agent, such as povidone-iodine (Betadine), may be applied to the sac every few hours, using sterile technique.

The infant must receive good skin care. Immobility may cause skin breakdown. Strict intake and output is measured and fluid replacement may be necessary. The infant often has respiratory distress postoperatively because of pressure on the diaphragm. Heel sticks should be avoided, if possible, because circulation in the legs may be reduced by pressure on the inferior vena cava. The patient receives nothing by mouth for several weeks and hence is usually on total parenteral nutrition. When nasogastric drainage decreases and the patient begins to stool, feedings are begun slowly.

Tracheoesophageal Fistula (TEF) with Esophageal Atresia. Tracheoesophageal anomalies fall into several categories. Distal TEF with esophageal atresia is by far the most common, occurring in 85% to 90% of the cases. It is often accompanied by other midline anomalies such as imperforate anus, intestinal atresia, cardiac, and genitourinary anomalies. The mothers of these infants often have polyhydramnios. The upper esophagus does not connect with the stomach but rather ends in a blind pouch. The fistula is usually formed in the distal part of the trachea with the lower part of the esophagus connecting the trachea to the stomach.

Frequent choking, excess salivation, coughing, cyanosis, and the inability to pass a nasogastric tube are all signs of the anomaly. Because the stomach and upper esophagus are not connected, vomiting is not usually seen. If the infant is fed, he will cough or gag, and aspirate. The stomach may be distended with air passing from the trachea into the stomach.

Preoperative care is very important. The nurse must keep the oral pharynx clear of secretions. A Replogle tube may be passed into the esophageal pouch and placed on continuous suction. The infant is propped in an upright position to prevent reflux of gastric secretions. He is kept hydrated with an intravenous solution, and given nothing by mouth.

After the repair, a ventilator is usually required. Chest physical therapy is contraindicated postoperatively to avoid disturbing the repair. The infant remains in semi-Fowler's position. Gentle suctioning is often done and routine gastrostomy care is given. If primary repair is impossible, the upper esophagus may be brought out to the neck as a "spit fistula," requiring dressing and careful skin care.

Complications after repair include a leak at the site of the esophageal anastamosis, esophageal or tracheal stenosis, and pneumonia.

Diaphragmatic Hernia. If the pleuroperitoneal canal fails to close, a diaphragmatic hernia results, pushing intestinal contents into the chest cavity. Signs include severe respiratory distress, cyanosis, and shock. Nine out of ten defects occur on the left side. Heart sounds are heard on the opposite side because of mediastinal shift. Breath sounds are decreased or absent on the affected side and bowel sounds may be heard instead. The abdomen is scaphoid shaped (*i.e.,* empty or depressed).

Preoperatively, a nasogastric tube is inserted to prevent further abdominal distention. The head of the bed is elevated and the infant is positioned with the affected side down to minimize compression of the heart and facilitate expansion of the unaffected lung prior to surgery.

Postoperatively, chest drainage will be necessary. Extreme caution should be taken in milking the chest tubing and it should not be done without an order. The infant's position is changed frequently. If ordered, chest postural drainage is done very gently. Suctioning requires a measured catheter. If chest drainage is significant, fluid replacement may be necessary. Pneumothorax on the unaffected side may be rapidly fatal.

Even with quick intervention, the mortality rate is high. Pulmonary hypoplasia, hypoxia, cardiac tamponade, and pulmonary hypertension often result in fatality during the acute phase.

Care of the Infant with Hydrocephalus

Signs of hydrocephalus do not always appear at birth. Early on, a head circumference increasing too rapidly may be noted. As the head enlarges, the fontanel may become tense and begin to bulge. As pressure increases, there may be an increase in blood pressure, dilated scalp veins, vomiting, apnea, bradycardia, and "sunset eyes," caused by downward pressure on the orbit. The infant needs to be turned frequently to prevent pressure areas from developing. An infant water bed is excellent for relieving pressure and discomfort.

Ventricular Drain. A ventricular drain may be inserted for various conditions including ventriculitis, hemorrhage, and acute hydrocephalus. Care must be taken not to disturb the catheter entering the scalp into the ventricle, which otherwise may cause tissue damage and bleeding. The drain should be attached to sterile tubing which empties into a sterile collection bottle with an air vent. Be sure the air vent is functional. This setup should be changed every 24 hours by sterile procedure. Observe the infant for signs of shock caused by rapidly draining fluid. This may happen if the collection bottle is placed more than 10 cm lower than the level of the infant. If it is placed too high, no fluid will drain and intracranial pressure will rise. The level of the collection bottle must not be disturbed after it is placed and secured on the bed according to the appropriate level for drainage.

If the infant's level must change for a procedure such as weighing, the nurse should clamp the tubing. It is unclamped after the infant is returned to bed. The amount and color of the drainage is noted and the drainage bottle is marked with tape to indicate the level of fluid in the bottle at the end of each shift. When the infant cries, the fluid in the tubing should fluctuate. If the tubing is not patent, pressure will build. Also, if the drainage is bloody and is left in the tubing, the infant is at greater risk for infection.

The infant needs to be stroked and talked to. In most cases, the tube can be clamped for short periods during feedings or when parents are visiting, so that the baby is held several times a day.

Care of Ventriculoperitoneal Shunt. The infant should receive routine postoperative care. Check the incision sites for bleeding or drainage. It is more comfortable for the infant to be kept off the surgical site. This will also help prevent skin breakdown. The neurosurgeon should order the angle at which the baby's bed is to be elevated (usually about 30°).

Shunt failure may occur at any time. The nurse should watch the infant for signs of increased intracranial pressure. Throughout the hospital stay, as part of discharge preparation, the parents must be made aware of the signs of shunt failure. They must know what to do and who to contact should they fear something is wrong. They will need much support and encouragement before and after discharge.

DISCHARGE PLANNING

Discharge planning begins upon admission. Encouraging parents to participate actively in the daily care of their infant fosters infant development and helps the mother and father learn how to parent. We have identified nine basic elements of discharge planning:

1. *Routine Care.* Well baby care teaching, such as bathing, temperature taking, formula preparation, and breast feeding, can be introduced after the crisis period and becomes an ongoing process. The parents then have time to begin some of these tasks with the primary nurse available for questions.
2. *Special Procedures.* The parents will need to be taught care specific to their baby, such as medications, gastrostomy feedings, tracheostomy and enterostomy care. The primary nurse should allow sufficient time for optimal practice and support. The parents should be as comfortable as possible and demonstrate independence in these tasks before the infant is discharged.
3. *Infant's Personality.* It is helpful if parents understand certain patterns or traits unique to their baby. This will help the mother continue working through the identification process interrupted at birth.[50]
4. *Parent Readiness.* The primary nurse needs to assess the interaction between the parents and their infant. Is the visiting pattern consistent? When visiting, do the parents hold and cuddle their baby? Do they fondle and talk to their baby? Is there good eye contact established? Do the parents use pronouns and the baby's name when speaking to or about their infant? Are they making home preparations for their baby? The primary nurse must also be alert for signs of hesitancy and increasing concern in parents before discharge. Some fears can be worked through if they are identitifed. In our hospital, we have facilities for parents to room in with their infant for a few days before discharge. The parents can maintain a degree of independence, with the security of medical help nearby. This is particularly helpful for the extremely anxious parent or for parents who will be giving a high level of physical care at home, such as tracheostomy care.
5. *Referrals.* Community health agencies such as the Visiting Nurse Association, the Public Health Department, or Social Services, may be necessary for home teaching and support. They can assist the family in adapting emotionally, physically, and financially to the chronically ill infant.
6. *Growth and Development.* The development needs of the infant who has been hospitalized for a period of time must be assessed before discharge. A development program begun in the hospital can be continued at home. Or, the parents may be referred to an infant development program in the community.
7. *Medical Follow-up.* The infant must have medical follow-up with a pediatrician or well baby clinic. The primary nurse file should include a list of pediatricians and well baby clinics in the area, in case a family needs a referral. If an infant requires follow-up at a speciality (neonatology, neurology or cardiology) clinic, the appointment should be made before the infant is discharged.
8. *Medical Tests.* All infants must have a test for PKU and thyroid before discharge. Eye examinations should be done routinely on all premature infants and on infants who have had oxygen therapy. Sometime within a week before discharge, the eyes should be reexamined. At that time, if follow-up is necessary, an appointment can be made.
9. *Coordination.* During hospitalization, weekly multidisciplinary rounds are helpful to keep the team informed of the progress of the baby as well as the needs of the family as a whole. The rounds should include the primary nurse and physician, the attending, the social worker and the public health nurse.

Family-centered Nursing Care

Judyth Todd Brown and Diane V. Bernstein

HISTORICAL PERSPECTIVES

Extensive research and observation during the last decades have given us a wealth of information about the effects of illness and separation not only on the infant but on his family as well. As early as 1907, in his book, *The Nursling,* Pierre Budin, the father of neonatology, made the very cogent observation that "mothers separated from their young soon lost all interest in those whom they were unable to nurse or cherish."[51] Budin encouraged mothers to participate in care and breastfeed their infants. Unfortunately, this important aspect of premature care did not find its way into nurseries being established in the United States. With rare exceptions, most hospitals, concerned with preventing infection, excluded parents completely. This exclusion lasted in most hospitals well into the 1960s. By then it was becoming apparent that infants who had been separated from their parents for an extended period after birth were far more likely to return to the hospital later as ill-thriving or battered children.

Fortunately, ICNs now encourage parents to visit with no concomitant increase in infection. But even with open visiting policies, the birth and prolonged hospitalization of a premature or otherwise ill newborn is frightening and disruptive of the natural course of events surrounding birth. Before we can look at the effects of this disruption, we need to understand the formation of the normal mother-infant bond. Klaus and Kennell have described this bond as "the well spring for all the infant's subsequent attachments. Throughout his lifetime the strength and character of this attachment will influence the quality of all future bonds to other individuals."[50]

At one point, the dynamics of prematurity, neonatal illness and death, and the impact on parents and the family unit was neglected, with parents left out of close contact with their infant during hospitalization, and no one except their own families and friends to provide supportive care. In the not too distant past, the area of parental support seemed primarily to be the domain of the physician providing care for the baby, or the social worker. It was generally the physician who communicated to the family information about the infant and his illness, plans of therapy and prognosis, and shared with the family their fears, concerns, and disappointments. The nurse often performed the technical tasks of caring for the baby on a daily basis, giving supportive care to the family somewhat sporadically, often only in an acute crisis situation.

With changing perspectives in the delivery of health care on both medical and nursing levels, nurses are finding their roles expanded to include caring for and supporting the family unit during the illness and hospitalization of the neonate. Extensive research and observations over the last several decades have given us a wealth of information about the effects of illness and separation not only on the infant but on his family as well.

BONDING AND ATTACHMENT

Only within the past few years have the dynamics of maternal infant bonding been more fully explored, and the impact of that bonding been realized. We are now more aware that a mother brings to her pregnancy a total of many years accumulated experiences that will help her shape her perception of that pregnancy and her infant. Marshall Klaus and John Kennell have identified several key areas in a mother's own life that will help determine how she will be able to bond to and care for her infant.[50] These factors go back to the care that she received from her own mother, the very foundation for all subsequent nurturing experiences. Her attitudes are further shaped by lifelong experiences of caring, and are influenced by cultural and social values to some extent. The relationship that the mother shares with her family and the baby's father, as well as her experiences with previous pregnancies and childbirth, will impact on the bonding relationship that she will have with her infant. One might well add that many of these same factors will influence the father's ability to bond and care for the infant.

Many important steps towards attachment happen from the time of conception through delivery and after birth. Whether the pregnancy has been long planned for, or the parents find themselves surprised and caught unaware by the pregnancy, a certain period of time usually lapses until the mother finally accepts the pregnancy. The mother must adjust to her new role as mother, a role which may dramatically change her entire life-style.

As the baby develops and grows within her, the mother becomes more acutely aware of the baby as a separate individual. With fetal movement the "new person" within her attests to its own individuality, constantly reminding her of the impending advent and the new responsibilities that she will have to undertake. Real acceptance of the baby and pregnancy manifests itself as the mother starts to make physical preparations for the new baby.

With all conditions being optimal, a mother goes to delivery anxious to have her infant but awesomely aware of the responsibility of this new person she is about to bring into the world. There exists a time after delivery identified by Klaus and Kennell as the **maternal sensitive period.** It is during this time that "complex interactions between mother and infant help to lock them together."[50] It is felt that any circumstances which disrupt this period, such as premature birth, birth of an ill or malformed infant, and even deep maternal anesthesia, will detrimentally affect the bonding process between the mother and infant.

In order to minimize the effects of the disruption of bonding, nursing and medical personnel are encouraged to let the parents see, touch, and hold their infant, even if momentarily. Encourage parents to speak to their baby and to try to elicit eye-to-eye contact.

TRANSFER

When it is necessary to transfer an infant, the nurse plays a vital role not only in the stabilization and transport of the baby from an outlying hospital to a tertiary care center, but also in providing the parents with some baseline information about their newborn child. Through a comprehensive interview with the parents about the history of pregnancy, the astute nurse can start to gain a sense of the parents' attitudes about the pregnancy itself, and will be able to pass on information relevant to parental adjustment to the health care team. In most instances, the parents have been told that there is something wrong with their baby by the physician and have had at least some advance notice that the child is to be transferred. Because many physicians are hesitant to offer diagnosis or prognosis when unsure of what they are dealing with, this is often all the information that the parents have. Most parents are in a state of shock and disbelief and may be experiencing anticipatory grief. They are hesitant to see their infant, as a means of preparing themselves for the loss.

An important role of the nurse is to ensure that parents see and touch, and whenever possible, hold their infant prior to transfer to another health care setting. The ultimate goal should be to minimize the disruption of bonding. Taking the time to ask the parents if they have named their baby, and thereafter referring to him by name helps to reinforce the identity of the baby. Encouraging parents to look at, touch, and hold the infant, stressing the baby rather than the equipment helps the parents deal with the infant in a more realistic sense; he becomes a real person, no longer a fetus inside the mother's womb or a small, helpless "thing" attached to numerous wires and tubing. Encouraging the mother to place her finger in the infants hand, and assuring her that the infants reflex clasping signifies that he needs her, helps to make the experience of being a mother more real, especially when she may be hospitalized for a few days and unable to be near her baby. Pointing out the various physical characteristics of the baby that are similar to the parents, such as the color of hair or facial similarities, will help to reinforce the baby's uniqueness to the parents and facilitate attachment.

ADMISSION TO THE NEONATAL INTENSIVE CARE UNIT

Introduction to the Unit

There is much anxiety surrounding the illness of a newborn and the separation it necessitates. Added to this shock is the adjustment to the complex and often frightening ICN. Obviously, it is the staff's responsibility to reach out to these new parents with information and reassurance. Many nurseries accomplish this formally with an introductory letter or booklet designed to orient parents to this busy new place. Our booklet contains a statement of the staff's philosophy and concern. Other information includes maps of the physical layout of the hospital and intensive care unit, chapel, and cafeteria. Also included are names and phone numbers for social workers and chaplains. Visiting policies are explained and strict infection control measures outlined. The roles of the physicians, nurses, and other medical personnel are explained and telephone contact is strongly encouraged. There is also a valuable section containing a description, with pictures, of the specialized equipment which will be used with many of the infants.

The Personal Touch

Equally important is the informal, personal orientation parents receive when they first visit the nursery. Who does the orientation often depends on when the parents appear and who is available to speak with them. Ideally, the parents can speak with their infant's primary physician and nurse and identify them as the best sources of ongoing, comprehensive information. Regardless of who speaks with the parents, it is essential that parents' reactions and concerns be recorded and communicated.

The Role of the Father

In most cases, the father will be the first visitor. His normal, daily pattern of activities severely disrupted, he typically will be visiting the baby, reporting the infant's condition back to his convalescing wife, and working an 8-hour day. He may also have concerns about the care of other children. Fathers frequently report frustrations with limited visiting and telephone policies at hospitals of birth. The father often shares his wife's dismay that she cannot visit her child with him.[52] This is the time when problems can arise with fathers trying to shield their wives from what may seem to be the too harsh reality of their child's condition. Most nurseries make it clear from the outset that they withhold no information from either parent. Parents report over and over that knowing the facts, no matter how difficult, is better than "not knowing what is really going on."

The Mother's Role

Meanwhile, the mother, in another part of the hospital or in another hospital perhaps hundreds of miles away, has her own special problems. Along with her husband, she is experiencing anticipatory grief, but if she cannot see and touch her child, her fear and fantasies only intensify her grief. Many mothers desire to be moved from the postpartum unit to convalesce. Others prefer to stay, and postpartum nurses need to be sensitive to what a particular mother would rather do. But regardless of where she is, she needs frequent information about the baby. Ideally she will feel comfortable calling several times a day, but if she does not call the staff must pick up on this and call her. It must be determined why she has not called. Is she just afraid to "bother the staff" or is she overwhelmed and detaching herself from the infant? She may be compromised by other emotional or physical problems. Simple shyness can be overcome, but more serious problems will need counseling with a social worker.

Ideally, most phone conversations will be with a consistent nurse who knows what the mother has been told and her reactions to it. This one nurse cannot always be there. In a busy unit, especially if a nurse is speaking to a mother for the first time, there is a tendency to forge ahead with a barrage of facts and figures. Most phone conversations will be more beneficial if the nurse starts out by asking what the parent understands about the baby or what his condition was the last time the parent called. This encourages two-way conversation and helps bring misunderstandings to light. We need to remember that our tone of voice is just as important as the facts we give parents. Little things mean a lot. The nurse should call the baby by name and stress his individuality, and along with his ventilator settings, mention his temper or dimples or blond hair. She should ask how the parent is feeling, eating, and sleeping. Probably the most important, and often the most difficult: don't sound rushed.

The Mother's First Visit. Regardless of their obstetricians' recommendations, most mothers will immediately visit their child upon discharge. Through phone conversations, husband's reports, and pictures, a mother is somewhat prepared. Although many mothers are physically uncomfortable and emotionally overwrought during their first visit, most report that only after an introduction to the nursery and their baby can they begin to cope with baby's illness.[52] The staff needs to think of the mother's physical well-being because she is preoccupied with her infant. Provision of a wheel chair to get to the nursery and a seat at the bedside are helpful. Simple explanations of equipment will be needed initially but the nurse should be sensitive to what is preoccuping her. The mother should be allowed silence to look and touch and think. The simple question "Well, what do you think of your daughter?" can yield much information. The nurse should promise to repeat information and reanswer questions as often as necessary, and, again, stress the son or daughter lying there, not the equipment or disease.

CARE OF THE PARENTS OF THE CRITICALLY ILL CHILD

The birth of a premature or critically ill child immediately engulfs his parents in feelings of anxiety and guilt. The perfect, smiling, "Gerber baby" they expected is not the baby they have. Their child is ill, needs intensive care, may be damaged, and may even die. Parents of a premature have difficulty accepting that their child is actually born. The grieving process begins as shock and denial set in. Later parents can recall little of what was told to them during the first hours and days after their child's birth. They do, however, remember the gentle, patient willingness of the staff to repeat information over and over to them.

The first step in acceptance of this unexpected stranger comes as parents see and touch their child. At this time the mother in particular will begin to experience feelings of guilt and inadequacy, fearing something she did or did not do produced the prematurity or illness. If she cannot verbalize this fear, a staff person can help by asking her what she understands about why her child is premature or ill. Her answer can give the opportunity to correct misconceptions and to reassure her.[53]

Anxiety is the most obvious and intense emotion experienced by parents during this time. During the uncertain days when even survival is in question, parents will experience anticipatory grief. This is a reaction felt before the actual loss of a loved object. It is characterized by sadness, loss of appetite, inability to sleep, increased irritability, preoccupation with thinking about the baby, and feelings of guilt and anger. Episodes of crying, praying for the baby, depression, disbelief, thinking that the baby might die, and wanting to be left

alone are all perfectly normal. Parents are enormously relieved when assured that all of these painful emotions are to be expected.[54] Staff must allow parents to cry and be angry at what has happened to them. The expression of their emotions may even mean angry criticism and distrust of the staff. Tolerance and understanding of this behavior is difficult but productive, and gratitude will certainly be expressed later.[54]

While each infant's course and his parent's reactions to it differ somewhat, all families are placed in a crisis situation when their newborn is critically ill. Caplan defines crises as time-limited periods of disequilibrium, or behavioral and subjective upset, which are precipitated by an inescapable demand or burden to which the person is temporarily unable to respond adequately. During this period of tension, the person grapples with the problem and develops novel resources, by calling upon internal reserves and making use of the help of others. Those resources are then used to handle the precipitating factor and the person once more achieves a steady state. Unlike developmental crisis such as changing homes or jobs, the birth of a premature or ill child is an acute, unpredictable, unavoidable crisis which involves the pain and possible death of a loved one.[55]

Caplan, Mason, and Kaplan have identified three very useful catagories of grappling behavior which parents will employ as they struggle to achieve a steady state. After studying the responses and outcomes of 86 families to the births of premature, ill infants, they have further broken down these categories to identify behavior which portends a healthy or unhealthy outcome.[55]

1. Cognitive grasp of the crisis situation:
   Healthy Outcome. Parents continually survey the situation and gather as much information as possible about the baby and the causes and manifestations of the prematurity or illness. Their perceptions of the child are reality based and minimally distorted by irrational fantasies.
   Unhealthy Outcome. Parents do little active searching for evidence upon which a current assessment of the situation and a judgment about outcome or plans for handling it can be made. They suppress thoughts about danger or burden. Outcome is considered in terms of a global belief:

"All will be well" or "Luck will be bad." These beliefs, however, are more dependent on inner fantasies than on appraisal of external realities.

2. Handling of feelings:

Healthy Outcome. Parents show continual awareness of negative feelings throughout the crisis with free verbal and nonverbal expression of these feelings in interaction with others. Occasionally, at peak periods of stress, there will be temporary utilization of the defenses of denial, suppression, and avoidance, but anxiety, depression, and frustration soon give way to awareness, and a conscious attempt is made to master these feelings alone and with the help of others.

Unhealthy Outcome. Parents make little or no verbal admission of negative feelings and pretend to be cheerful, denying discomfort. Often the only negative feeling permitted open and continual expression is blaming others.

3. Obtaining help

Healthy Outcome. Parents actively seek help within the family or community in relation to tasks associated with care of their child. They also seek support and special attention to reassure, share anxieties and relieve guilt.

Unhealthy Outcome. Parents are reluctant, unable to see or accept help. They do not help each other in any consistent way, and when they do it is maladaptive grappling (*i.e.,* urging denial, stimulating blaming oneself or others, bickering).

These grappling behaviors are employed by parents as they move through what Caplan and associates call the four major psychological tasks necessary to master this painful situation and provide a healthy mother–infant relationship in the future.

1. Anticipatory grief involves withdrawing from the idea of the expected child. While the parents hope for survival, they prepare emotionally for death. Emotions must be expressed, and attachment to the real infant begun.
2. The mother must face her feelings of failure. She will struggle with these feelings until the chances for survival seem secure.
3. Characteristically there is a point at which the mother really begins to believe the baby

will survive. It may be an increase in weight, a change in feeding, a change in activity or appearance, or a change in the nurse's behavior.

4. The final task is learning how to care for her particular infant with his unique needs and personality. This comes with time, supervised experience participating in his care, and lots of encouragement. Home discharge has been identified as a time almost as stressful as the delivery itself. Discharge jitters can be minimized for parents and staff if assessment and teaching are started as soon as survival seems certain.

CARE OF PARENTS OF THE INFANT WITH A DEFECT.

Perhaps one of the most difficult tasks for medical personnel is helping parents of an infant with a congenital defect deal with the reality and acceptance of their infant.

It is generally accepted that parents must be told there is something wrong with their child as soon as a reliable diagnosis is made. Parents can easily sense a problem by the attitude and actions of the staff; they will lose trust in the staff if they are told that there is nothing wrong with their child because nonverbal communication negates this.

The task of telling parents about a baby with a congenital anomaly is, by its nature, very difficult and unpleasant. D'Arcy interviewed a large group of mothers about how, when, and from whom they first learned of their babys' defects and found that

mothers attached great importance to the approach and general attitude of the medical and nursing staff who told them about their babies, particularly if they learned soon after the baby's birth. Very often [the mother] could not remember exactly what had been said, but she could always recall whether the informant had an understanding approach and seemed aware of her suffering. Mothers who were hurt by seeming lack of sympathy towards them tended to attribute the abruptness to lack of feeling of the informant rather than to the likely cause— that is, the difficulty of imparting such information. Most mothers were impressed by the kindness and sympathy extended to them by medical and nursing staff. Small acts of kindness were clearly remembered years after the event.[56]

It is equally important that parents be given truthful information even if the truth regarding the diagnosis and prognosis is uncertain; it is always better to be honest than to tell the parents "not to worry, everything will be fine."

The medical staff must be aware of and sensitive to the multiple factors that make up the crisis of the birth of a child with a congenital defect. The emotional responses that parents exhibit may be prolonged. Shock and disbelief are followed by anger directed toward self, family members, and friends, and even the medical and nursing staff. Fear of the unknown, of complicated and extended medical health care, and of financial burden often compounds the anger. Parents experience a sense of guilt and personal responsibility at having produced a less than perfect child, and mourn the loss of the imagined normal infant. It is not uncommon for parents to experience depression characterized by a physical and emotional retreat and withdrawal. Patience, kindness, and understanding is the best medicine that staff can offer.

As parents are encouraged to ask questions, they will move into a state of data collecting. Many parents will visit the hospital library to gather as much information as they can about the defect. They search for a cause, a reason. They feel guilty and have a sense of personal responsibility. The parents may ask the same question of a multitude of staff, searching for an answer which may ease their feeling of guilt. These parents need consistent information to avoid misunderstandings and should be encouraged to communicate with their infant's primary physician and nurse. Most importantly, these parents need reassurance that they are normal and capable people; they need their fragile self-esteem bolstered.

The stigma that society places on a child with a congenital defect is another crisis that parents must face. Parents of an infant with an external or obviously visible defect may find this more difficult than parents of a child with an internal defect, as may parents with a child for whom there is no correctable surgery. Parents need to know that there are parent groups where they can find help from others facing the same problem.

After dealing with all of these conflicts the parents are confronted with the task of reorganization and attachment. If the attitude of the medical personnel has been reassuring and accepting, the parents will find it easier to believe in their self-worth and ability, and the worth of their infant. In helping parents to accept their infant, it is important that the medical personnel themselves foster a sense of worth and dignity of the infant. By encouraging the parents to recognize the human qualities of their infant, the responsive behavior the infant exhibits, and the positive physical characteristics that the infant has, the staff can help the parents towards accepting their baby as a unique individual with worth and ability to grow and develop in its own special way rather than as a damaged infant, a freak, or an accident of nature.[57]

CARE OF PARENTS OF THE CHRONICALLY ILL CHILD

Parents of infants who are chronically ill may be the most demanding and frustrating. Their infant has usually survived an acute crisis and the parents have faced shock, disbelief, and anger, and are trying to resolve and reorganize their lives in relation to their child. These parents are left in somewhat of a limbo, not knowing for certain whether their child will improve significantly and be able to grow and develop, or whether he will continue to maintain a state of chronic illness for an indeterminate period of time or die.

These parents may exhibit anger and hostility towards the staff as they see other infants admitted and discharged repeatedly while their child remains behind. Feelings that the staff is not doing enough to help their infant recover may be manifested by direct accusations of poor medical or nursing care or, conversely, by "bribing" staff members with praise and gifts in an effort to get what they believe will be better care. Playing staff against one another by requesting the same nurse to care for their child because "she gives such excellent nursing care," although flattering, can be an example of parents' manipulative behavior.

Parents of a chronically ill child need consistent caretakers and communicators. They need calm, patient, understanding personnel to quietly listen to their fears and anxieties without responding personally to accusations. These parents need to be guided to evaluate their infant's progress over a span of time (perhaps weekly, perhaps longer) rather than daily, to help relieve their feelings of frustration.

Parents may go through a period of time when they visit continually, and then suddenly not visit at all for awhile. This seemingly erratic visiting pattern is typical of parents who are saturated and overwhelmed with frustration and need a break to refresh and reorganize themselves. The staff should be understanding and supportive of the parents' behavior, and consistent staff members such as the primary physician and nurse should call the parents to touch base with them and let them know of any changes.

When parents do visit, they need to be encouraged to hold, cuddle, and provide tender loving care for their infant. They should be allowed to diaper and feed their baby if possible and to participate in as much care as they can. Reinforcing to parents their ability to love and care for their baby enables them to gain some sense of control and purpose during this long ordeal.

The Nurse's Role in Discharge Teaching. Early in the sick infant's course, it is not at all unusual for a mother to feel puzzling feelings of suspicion, resentment and jealousy towards the nurses who care for her child. The nurses are doing what she expected to be doing, caring for her child, and for the time being they are doing a more competent job than she can. Successful discharge teaching will facilitate the transition from these feelings of inadequacy and competition to feelings of self-assurance and attachment. Discharge teaching is most satisfying and successful if done by one nurse who knows the infant and his family well over some time. A comfortable relationship must be established between mother and nurse in order to foster the learning experience. Written tools and instructions are useful only when accompanied by a personal relationship, enabling appreciation of the uniqueness of each mother and infant.[53]

Readiness to Learn. As described earlier (components of maternal-infant bonding), there is a definite progression in the nature and amount of physical contact a mother has with a newborn and the extent of the self-involvement she feels in his care. This progression is interrupted when he is premature or ill. By encouraging gradual participation in his care as appropriate, the nurse helps reestablish this progression. Mothers have been known to call and interrupt their husbands at work to announce they have changed the diaper under their ventilator-bound son. It is essential that a mother understands that her presence and participation in care is very important to her ill infant's well-being. Furthermore, she needs to be assured that, with a little practice, she will get to know her baby better than anyone else and do the best job of all.

What a Mother Needs to Know. As nursery nurses, we have all known the frustration and confusion of discharging an infant we do not know well to a poorly prepared mother in a flurry of last minute instructions. We all realize that if discharge teaching is everybody's responsibility, it is nobody's responsibility. Early on in the hospitalization, and once survival is certain, one nurse, either a staff nurse in intermediate care or primary nurse, should assume responsibility for planning teaching. She should determine what this specific mother needs to know and do before she can successfully take her infant home. Every mother needs to learn how to bathe, feed, handle and dress her child. There are often additional specific teaching needs such as gastrostomy care or administration of medications. Appropriate medical follow-up must also be arranged with the parents' input. It is useful for the nurse to begin explaining these tasks to the mother in simple terms long before discharge. The mother needs gentle assurance that she will be comfortable with all tasks before discharge. Finally, the nurse should work out a timetable for learning with the mother. In this way, even the mother of a small, sick child, weeks from discharge, can set goals for herself and begin to feel that her ordeal will have an endpoint.

Teaching will be most successful if two principles are remembered. First, a mother will learn best from one sympathetic, supportive nurse with whom she has a continuous relationship. Second, an anxious mother can misunderstand the clearest and simplest instructions. She needs the opportunity to ask questions freely and digest material gradually over time.[53]

It is useful to have a written plan to document discharge teaching and to enable associate nurses to participate in teaching an an organized manner. This plan may be written in the patient's care plan or a specific discharge tool may be used.[58]

Finally, many mothers benefit from a day or two of "rooming in" with their infant in a private hospital room. Only the experience of total responsibility for her infant's care will dissolve those discharge jitters and make her finally feel like a mother.

Caring for the Parents of the Dying Infant

Despite our growing medical knowledge and aggressive sophisticated care, death does come to our nurseries. Engel states,

Death is an intensely poignant event which touches the deepest sources of human anguish, one which each of us yearns to be spared. Yet, as nurses and doctors, it is our constant companion. How can we protect ourselves from such repeated, personal suffering? One way and the easiest way, is to develop a shell, to insulate ourselves, to avoid engagement, to make out it does not occur or it is not our concern.[54]

Another more difficult way is to become "engaged," empathize and stick with a family through the illness, the dying, and the aftermath. Only in this way can we bring tenderness and meaning to death amidst machines.

As has been stated, from the time the infant becomes ill, parents will experience anticipatory grief, with sadness, loss of appetite, inability to sleep, increasing irritability and feelings of grief and anger. They are withdrawing from the expected child, and getting to know the actual child while anticipating his possible death.

Death may come within hours of birth, following several long nightmarish days, or after months of rollercoaster vigil. Each child, family, and story is different. Often survival is uncertain and even the staff cannot predict among themselves when or if an infant will die. The importance of staff support during this time of uncertainty has been discussed in previous sections.

As Death Approaches. It is not often that staff and family recognize the inevitability of death at the same time. The staff has had the experience of previous deaths and can recognize the clinical changes that mean death is likely. Although parents may see the changes and hear the prognosis, real acceptance on their part can take a long time. It is difficult to find anything positive or reassuring to tell parents who are desperately grasping at straws, and staff may try to avoid anything but superficial conversation with them. Understandably, parents can perceive this change in staff's attitude as rejection or abandonment. At this critical time, they need to feel the support of those whom they have come to identify as primary care givers and emotional supports. Frequent communication of information, concern for parent's well-being, and gentle repetition of the medical situation must continue. Parents need to be allowed to hope and to ventilate feelings of anger, bewilderment, and sadness. Often they hesitate to share feelings with busy staff. Understandably, they fear that showing anger could alienate staff and affect their infant's care. For these reasons and many others, a social worker needs to be involved in helping the parents of a critically ill and dying child, whenever possible.

Once staff feels an infant will die, it is only natural that we may find ourselves giving less vigorous care or "pulling away." Our attempts to detatch from the infant can be manifested by not wanting to care for the baby or "needing a break." Staff may also be angry about the situation. Anger and guilt may come as we face our inability to cure. We as staff need opportunities to ventilate these feelings. If left unrecognized, they burn us out. We must be especially mindful that these feelings can be misdirected toward parents when they do not behave as we feel they should. Sometimes we feel angry if they do not call or visit "enough," and we fancy ourselves more caring than they. Other times, we may criticize their denial and "blind hope" when they will not "listen" to our dismal predictions.

The Actual Death. Whenever possible, parents must be notified when death seems imminent. Some parents will very much want to be at their child's bedside. While their grief is painful, "being there" is all they feel they can do. Sensitivity on the staff's part is essential in helping these parents relate to their infant at this time. Every effort should be made to facilitate parent caretaking activities, such as holding, diapering, or just stroking and talking, if parents so desire. Obviously, no parent should be made to feel guilty if these activities are too difficult to face. Some parents' intense grief makes it impossible for them to even come to the hospital at the time of death.

In still other cases, mothers, particularly those with older infants, are placed in the difficult competitive position of giving up to nurses the caretaking they gave in the past. Engle stresses the need for staff to recognize and respect the mother's need to minister to her own child, yet be sensitive when she needs relief. In these cases, mothers' attempts to cope will swing from tender bedside care to frantic, inappropriate bedside activity, from exaggerated praise and gratitude of doctors and nurses to harsh criticism and complaints, from tearful sentimentality to philosophic resignation. The mother who cannot bear to leave her child as well as the mother who cannot bear to enter her child's room, are both suffering and need opportunities to share feelings and thoughts.[54]

Taking Leave. Around the time of death and certainly afterward, parents need a private area to confer with staff, meet with other family members or be alone. News of the death is best given in a private area where parents can behave naturally, and if possible, with other support people present. Numb shock may last minutes or hours before it gives way to tears and overwhelming sadness. Parents may not even remember what is said to them. Anyone who has sat with parents at this difficult time knows the gnawing feeling of "not knowing what to say." Actually, once the simple facts have been gently given, it is best to allow parents time to react and think. Silences which feel uncomfortable to us are not so to parents. Their minds and emotions are racing and, if we sit quietly, time will bring questions and reactions from them which we would not have anticipated.

Parents should be given the opportunity to take leave of their son or daughter as they wish. Often they will want to hold and be alone with their infant after death. They may ask to take pictures, particularly if this is the first time they have seen the infant or if it is the first time the infant has been clothed and disconnected from wires and tubes.

Various alternatives for burial arrangements need to be simply explained. At this time, permission for autopsy is usually requested. Once these details have been dealt with, parents are often eager to leave. This is only the beginning of their grief and should never be their last contact with the hospital. Each nursery has different arrangements for who will stay in touch with parents. Someone should call them within several days to see how they are doing. Often after the funeral is over and family and friends are gone, the parents' thoughts begin to clear. Questions can be answered and misconceptions clarified. Well-meaning relatives and friends will often begin

to try to erase the memory of the baby by dismantling the nursery, by not talking about the baby, or by reassuring the parents that "they can always have another baby." Parents are invariably relieved to hear you as a professional and a friend confirm their own feelings that while they may have other children, no one will ever take this child's place. Also, if their child was hospitalized his entire life, other family members did not have the same opportunity to watch the parents interact with their child that the staff did. We are in a unique position to commend the parents on their obvious love for their child and their faithfulness in calling and visiting even when it was frightening and painful. Finally, we as professionals can reassure them that the somatic upheavals of sleeplessness, loss of appetite, crying, bizarre dreams, and so on are entirely normal and will subside with time. Follow-up conferences need to be routinely scheduled to continue to help parents and detect any pathological problems. Parents should always feel free to call nursery staff if only just to be able to talk about the baby with someone who knew him. Beware of arbitrarily assigning a specific period of time as a "normal" period of grieving. Mourning may last a year or more. For years to come, painful memories will return unexpectedly. The parents may go on to have other children, but no child will truly ever take the place of the child they lost.

REFERENCES

1. **Kelly LY:** Dimensions of Professional Nursing, 3rd ed. New York, Macmillan, 1975
2. **Nightingale F:** Notes on Nursing: What It Is, and What It Is Not. (A facsimile of the first edition printed in London, 1859, with a foreword by Annie W. Goodrich). Philadelphia, Lippincott, 1966
3. **Chihara K, Kato Y, Maeda K, Matsukura S, Imura H:** Suppression by cyproheptadine of human growth hormone and cortisol secretion during sleep. J Clin Invest 57:1393, 1976
4. **Beck U, Brezinova V, Hunter WM, Oswald I:** Plasma growth hormone and slow wave sleep increase after interruption of sleep. J Clin Endocrinol Metab, 40(5):812, 1975
5. **Mendelson WB, Sitaram N, Wyatt RJ, Gillin JC, Jacobs LS:** Methscopolamine inhibition of sleep-related growth hormone secretion: Evidence for a cholinergic secretory mechanism. J Clin Invest 61:1683, 1978

6. **Mendelson WB, Jacobs LS, Reichman JD, Othmer E, Cryer PE, Trivedi B, Daughaday WH:** Suppression of sleep-related prolactin secretion and enhancement of sleep-related growth hormone secretion. J Clin Invest 56:690, 1975

7. **Korones SB:** Disturbance and infant's rest. Iatrogenic Problems in Neonatal Intensive Care. Columbus, OH, Ross Laboratories, 1976

8. **Peplau H:** Professional closeness. Nurs Forum 8:342, 1969

9. **King IM:** Toward a Theory for Nursing: General Concepts of Human Behavior. New York, Wiley, 1971

10. **Riehl P, Roy Sr C:** Conceptual Models for Nursing Practice. New York, Appleton-Century-Crofts, 1974

11. **Donaldson SK, Crowley D:** Discipline of nursing: Structure and relationship in practice. Communicating Nursing Research *10,* Western Interstate Commission on Higher Education, 1977

12. **Neal MV:** A conceptual framework for practice. In Neal MV (ed): A Conceptual Basis for MCH Nursing Practice: A Construct, Proceedings of a Perinatal Conference held by the School of Nursing, pp. 24–28. University of Maryland, March 10–12, 1976

13. **Awrey, JM:** Collaboration. In Neal MV, ed: A Conceptual Basis for MCH Nursing Practice: A Construct, pp. 162–175. Proceedings of a Perinatal Conference held by the School of Nursing, University of Maryland, March 10–12, 1976

14. **Olson VT:** A conceptual framework for mother-nurse interaction in an NICU. Univ. of Minn. School of Nursing, (unpublished paper), 1979

15. **Hage, J:** An axiomatic theory of organizations. Administrative Science Quarterly 10:289, 1965.

16. **Duxbury ML:** Personnel and staffing needs for perinatal programs. Seminars in Perinatology 1(3):267, 1977

17. **Marram G, Flynn K, Abaravich W., Carey S:** Cost-Effectiveness of Primary and Team Nursing. Wakefield (MA), Contemporary Publishers, 1976

18. **Ciske K:** Primary nursing: An organization that promotes professional practice. J Nurs Admin 4(2):28, 1974

19. **Marram G.:** Innovation on four tower west: What happened? Am J Nurs 73(5):356,1973

20. **Felton G:** Increasing the quality of nursing care by introducing the concept of primary nursing: A model project. Nurs Res 24(1):27, 1975

21. **Duxbury ML, Thiessen V:** Staff nurse turnover in neonatal intensive care units. J Adv Nurs 6:593, 1979

22. **Veninga R:** Quoted in Living, St. Paul MN Dispatch. August 23, 1978

23. **Pines A, Aronson E, with Kafry D:** Burnout: From Tedium to Personal Growth. New York, Free Press, In press

24. **Thiroux Jacques P:** Ethics: Theory and Practice, Encino, California, Glencoe Press, 1977

25. **Chinn Peggy L:** Issues in lowering infant mortality: A call for ethical action. Advances in Nursing Science 1:3, 63–78

26. **Murphy M, J Murphy:** Making ethical decisions systematically. Nursing '76, (May, 1976), 31–45

27. **Sigman Paula:** Ethical Choice in Nursing. Advances in Nursing Science 1:3, 37–52

28. **Grissum N:** How you can become a risk-taker and a role-breaker, Nursing '76, (November, 1976), 89–98

29. **Segal S (ed):** Transport of high risk newborn infants. Canadian Paediatric Soc, 1972

30. **Wallace HM, Losty MA, Baumgarten L:** Report of two years' experience in the transportation of premature infants in New York city. Pediatrics 9:439, 1952

31. **Losty MA, Orlofsky I, Wallace HM:** A transport service for premature babies. Am J Nursing 50:10, 1950.

32. **Merenstein GB, Petlett G, Woodall J, Hill JH:** An analysis of air transport results in the sick newborn II. Antenatal and neonatal referrals. Am J Obstet Gynecol 128:520, 1977

33. **Neil R, Ray D:** Neonatal transport. Med J Aust 2:862-4, 1977

34. **Hein H, Enenberg A, Lane N, Lundvall J:** Transport of the high risk neonate: Who, when, and how. J Iowa Med Soc 68(10): 348–57, 1978

35. **Honeyfield PR:** Staffing for Newborn Transport: Team Composition. In Newborn Air Transport, report of a conference held Feb. 9–10, 1978, Evansville, Mead Johnson Laboratories, 1978

36. **Mazzi E, Guterlet R, Phillips J:** The Maryland State Intensive Care Neonatal Program (MSICNP), Part 2: Role of the Maryland State Police aviation. Maryland State Medical J 26(12):48–50, 1977

37. **Guy M:** Neonatal transport. Nurse Clin North Am 13(1):3-11.

38. **McCaffree M:** Neonatal transport, 1976. J Okla State Med Assoc 71(1):10–4, 1978

39. **Short BL, Cannon J, Dombkiewicz M:** The infant transport system: review, evaluation and future plans. Clinical Proceedings, CHNMC, Washington, D.C., 36:194,1980

40. **Minor Holly:** Problems and prognosis for the small for gestational age and the premature infant. MCN 3:221, 1978

41. **Kramer L, Pierpont ME:** Rocking waterbeds

and auditory stimulation to enhance growth of preterm infants. Pediatrics 55:517, 1975

42. **Kaplan F:** The First Twelve Months of Life. New York, Grosset and Dunlap, 1977

43. **Schaffer HR, Callender WM:** Psychological effects of hospitalization in infancy. Pediatrics 24:538, 1959

44. **Salapatek S, Williams M:** A stimulation program for low birth weight infants. Am J Public Health 62:662–667, 1972

45. **Fuchs PL:** Continuous mechanical ventilation. Nursing 79 9:26–33, 1979

46. **Curran C, Kachoyeanos M:** The effects on neonates of two methods of chest physical therapy. MCN 4:309–313, 1979

47. **Anderson K, Chandra R:** Pneumothorax secondary to perforation of sequential bronchi by suction catheter. J Pediatr Surg 11:687, 1976

48. **Moreau Smith K:** Recognizing cardiac failure in neonates. MCN 4:98–100, 1979

49. **Gillon Janet E:** Behavior of newborns with cardiac distress. Am J Nurs 73:254, 1973

50. **Klaus MH, Kennell JN:** Maternal Infant Bonding. St. Louis, The CV Mosby Co., 1976

51. **Budin P:** The Nursling. London, Caxton Publishing Co., 1907

52. **Benfield DG, Leib SA, Rector J:** Grief response of parents following referral of the critically ill newborn. N Engl J Med 294:975–978, 1976

53. **Prugh DG:** Emotional problems of the premature infant's parents. Nurs Outlook 1: 461–463, 1953

54. **Engel G:** Grief and grieving. Am Nurs 64: 93–98, 1964

55. **Caplan G, Mason EA, Kaplan DW:** Four studies of crisis in parents of prematures. Community Ment Health J 1:149–161, 1965

56. **D'Arcy E:** Congenital defects: Mother's reactions to first information. Br Med J 3: 796–798, 1968

57. **Carr EF, Oppe JE:** The birth of an abnormal child: Telling the parents. Lancet 2:1075–1077, 1971

58. **Cagen J, Meier P:** A discharge planning tool for use with families of high-risk infants, Obstet Gynecol Nursing 8:146–148, 1979

II

The Fetal
Patient

5

Fetomaternal Interaction

Joseph Dancis

Reproduction, in the lower forms of life, is generally an inefficient process, requiring the production of large numbers of eggs to ensure the survival of relatively few offspring. Efficiencies were introduced by the development of internal fertilization, and by retention of the developing fetus within the mother. Placentation first appears among some fish and reptiles, reaching its most sophisticated form in the mammal. The mammalian fetus draws sustenance from the mother while protected from the hazards of an inclement and often threatening environment. The maternal organism, with her elaborate homeostatic mechanisms, becomes the external environment for the fetus (Fig. 5-1). To permit this arrangement, intimate anatomic and metabolic adjustments are necessary. Some of the more prominent interactions between mother and fetus are described in this chapter.

THE FETAL MEMBRANES

Membranes are an essential feature of life. Even a unicellular organism requires delimitation from its environment, and this is accomplished by a cell membrane. However, it is also necessary, even for a unicellular organism, to draw sustenance from its environment

through the same barrier. To accomplish both missions, a rather elaborate structure evolved.

The basic design of membranes is believed to be a double layer of lipids overlaid and invested by proteins.[1] The possible variations among membranes are almost limitless, introduced by differences in the composition of the lipids and of the proteins and their resultant interactions. Such modifications are necessary to permit the membranes to fulfill the varied functions demanded of them. To take two extreme examples, the need for insulation of nervous fibers is satisfied by one type of membrane, myelin, whereas capillaries have endothelial membranes that permit rapid exchange between circulating blood and interstitial fluid.

The fetal membranes are designed to facilitate the efficient transfer of nutrients to the rapidly growing fetus and for the excretion of fetal waste products. In the egg-laying species, the conceptus is deposited in a nutritive medium from which the fetal membranes extract the elements required for growth and development prior to hatching. In mammalian pregnancy, the fertilized ovum, surrounded by only a small amount of nutrient material which is quickly exhausted, must derive its nourishment from the mother. A new organ must be developed in which the maternal and fetal

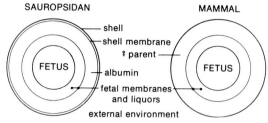

Fig. 5-1. The oviparous fetus derives its nourishment through fetal membranes from the albumin deposited in the egg, and is separated from its environment by the shell. In the mammal, the mother constitutes the external environment of the fetus, providing insulation and nourishment (Mossman HW: In Fetal Homeostasis, vol II. New York, New York Academy of Sciences, 1967)

circulations come into close juxtaposition over a very extensive area. This is accomplished in the human by modifying the chorionic and allantoic membranes to form the placenta.

COMPARATIVE PLACENTOLOGY

Although our emphasis will be on human pregnancy, it will be necessary at times to refer to observations in animals when suitable data are not available for the human. It is important to recognize the great variation in placentation among mammalian species as a precaution against assuming too simply that data collected in the animal is necessarily applicable to the human.

There is no completely satisfactory way to classify placentas. There are obvious differences in size, shape, number of cotyledons, and even number of placentas to a fetus (the rhesus monkey has two placentas). However, the most significant feature is probably the nature of the barrier between the maternal and fetal circulations. The most durable of the classifications, that of Grosser, emphasizes the number of tissue layers interposed between the maternal and fetal circulations from the "thick placenta" of the horse to that of the human, where the fetal villi dip directly into the maternal blood stream (Table 5-1).

This classification is necessarily an oversimplification ignoring the variability in membrane thickness existing in different areas of the same placenta, as well as the variations in one species of placenta at different stages of preg-

nancy.* However, it has served as a useful basis for discussion and also seems to have some correlation with function. The rate of diffusion of sodium across the placenta does correlate with the thickness of the placenta in several species. In the human, as pregnancy progresses, the placental membrane thins and the rate of sodium diffusion also increases.

A similar attempt to correlate antibody transfer with placental structure proved erroneous. It was noted that ungulates were born without maternal antibody, whereas the rodent and the primate were supplied with antibodies prior to birth. This was attributed to the "thinness" of the latter placentas. A fascinating series of studies by Brambell's group[2] demonstrated that, in the rodent, antibody transfer does not occur across the "thin placenta" at all, but across a specialized membrane derived from the yolk sac. Simple correlation proved misleading. The primate does not have a corresponding membrane, and antibody is transferred by the chorioallantoic placenta (*see* Immunological Interactions below).

IMMUNOLOGIC INTERACTIONS
The Fetal "Homograft"

The fetus, bearing paternal genes, elaborates proteins that are foreign to the mother and should, theoretically, fall victim to attack by maternal immunologic defenses. The success of the fetal "homograft" has elicited the interest of investigators in many disciplines because of its broad implications.

The placenta, interposed between mother and fetus, undoubtedly reduces the opportunity for immunologic reactions. However, although free intermingling of the maternal and fetal circulations is prevented, the barrier is considerably less than perfect. It has been known for many years that fetal erythrocytes may traverse the placenta and sensitize the mother, causing isoimmune disease. Histochemical methods for identifying fetal hemoglobin have demonstrated that such transfer is not a rare event but that fetal erythrocytes are regularly found during pregnancy in small numbers in maternal blood. Maternal antibodies against fetal white cells are also found,

* For a critical discussion, see Flexner LB (ed): Gestation, Transaction of First Conference. New York, Corlies, Macy & Company, Inc., 1955

Table 5-1. Classification of Placentation According to Number of Tissues Interposed Between Maternal and Fetal Circulations. (There is a progressive erosion of maternal tissue.)

Classification	Placental barrier						Species
	Maternal tissues			*Fetal tissues*			
	ENDOTHELIUM	CONNECTIVE TISSUE	EPITHELIUM	EPITHELIUM	CONNECTIVE TISSUE	ENDOTHELIUM	
Epitheliochorial	+	+	+	+	+	+	Pig horse
Syndesmochorial	+	+	–	+	+	+	Ruminants
Endotheliochorial	+	–	–	+	+	+	Carnivora
Hemochorial	–	–	–	+	+	+	Rodents Apes Man

(Adapted from Amorosa EC: In Gestation, Transactions of the First Conference. New York, Corlies, Macy & Co, Inc, 1954. As taken from Grosser A: Fruhentwicklung, Eihantbildung, und Placentation des Menschen und der Saugetiere, vol. 5. Munich, JF Bergman, 1927) suggesting that fetal leukocytes may also traverse the barrier.[3] Cells with male karyotype may be demonstrated in the blood of mothers bearing sons.[4]

It is possible that cells are transferred from the fetal to the maternal circulations through the intact placenta by diapedesis. The chorionic villi hang freely in the maternal blood stream. An increase in intracapillary pressure within the villus, possibly as a result of transient interference with venous return, could produce vasodilatation with enlargement of intercellular spaces in the endothelium, permitting leakage. This mechanism has been demonstrated experimentally in the guinea pig.[5] The leak disappeared immediately on lowering the pressure in the umbilical vein. Consistent with the above speculation, traffic in the reverse direction appears to be considerably less frequent. Clinically, there are relatively few reports of cancer cells in the offspring, although mothers with cancer are not rare. Either such cells are prevented from invading the fetus, or the fetus effectively rejects them. The transfer of any significant number of maternal lymphocytes would be expected to produce immunologic disease in the relatively defenseless fetus, and that is certainly not a common experience. However, it has been possible to experimentally produce runt or graft-versus-host disease in the fetal rat and rabbit by appropriately immunizing the mother, providing circumstantial evidence of transfer of maternal leukocytes.[6] A clinical example has also been described.[7]

Accepting the existence of an imperfect but effective cellular barrier, the question remains as to how the placenta, also of fetal origin, is tolerated even though intimately exposed to the maternal circulation. Evidence has been submitted that a homogenous, fibrinoid, noncellular layer covering the trophoblast may protect it immunologically.[8] However, the barrier appears to be discontinuous on electron-microscopy, so that protection would be incomplete.

Immunologic tolerance may provide a mechanism for protection. Invasion by a foreign agent induces a series of defensive responses in the host, among them the formation of circulating antibodies as well as the cellular response that is the primary instrument for transplantation rejection. Under certain circumstances, the antibodies may coat the invading cells and block cellular rejection, leading to tolerance. Hellström and coworkers demonstrated a serum factor, presumably antibody, in pregnant mice that protected fetal cells against rejection by sensitized lymphocytes.[9] In the human, fetal trophoblastic cells are regularly shed into the maternal blood stream, possibly playing a role in initiating and maintaining tolerance.[10]

Other factors, such as the endocrinologic changes associated with pregnancy, seem to modify the maternal immune response. It is indeed likely that multiple factors contribute to the success of the placental homograft, and it is possible that different factors are operative at different periods of gestation.[11]

Clinical examples of disruption of these normal processes have been rarely described. However, the diagnostic techniques are still difficult and not generally applied. It must be considered probable that at least some cases of abortion and immunologic disease in the newborn, possibly with subtle symptomatology such as "failure to thrive," will eventually be attributed to maternal sensitization.[7]

Immunological Status of Fetus and Newborn

The intimate association of mammalian pregnancy also affects the immunologic status of the fetus. The human fetus is capable of humoral and cellular immune responses long before birth, although not as efficiently as later in development. However, the circulating antibodies in the newborn are almost entirely maternal in origin. The absence of fetal antibodies is primarily the result of lack of exposure to foreign antigens during intrauterine life. On those occasions when the fetus is adequately exposed to a foreign antigen, it responds with IgM antibodies. Among other explanations that have been offered, is that maternal IgG circulating in the fetus suppresses that type of response.

The delivery of maternal antibody to the offspring, before or shortly after birth, is characteristic of mammalian pregnancy. It is evidently imperative for survival that the newborn have passive immunologic protection while developing its own immune defenses. The method by which maternal antibody is delivered to the fetus varies greatly among the species, and the variability of the mechanisms testifies to the importance of the goal.

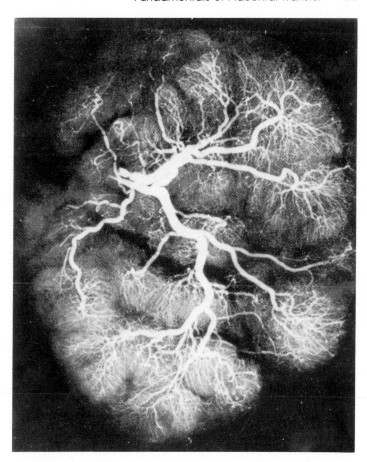

Fig. 5-2. A roentgenogram of the placenta following injection of the umbilical arteries with chromopaque (150 mm C-R length fetus). The cotyledonary structure is well demonstrated with rich fetal vasculature entering the villi. The maternal blood enters the placenta through spiral arterioles from the opposite surface, the basal plate, passing through the intervillous space and is collected into uterine veins. (Boyd JD, Hamilton WJ: The Human Placenta. Cambridge, W. Heffer & Sons, Ltd, 1970)

In the ungulate, such as the sheep, the lamb is born agammaglobulinemic, deriving its antibodies from the mother in colostrum. Proteins are efficiently absorbed through the intestine during the first days of life. The mouse and rat obtain some maternal antibody before birth and some after birth. The intestine in these species will absorb antibody for about 3 weeks postpartum, the duration of nursing. The rabbit and guinea pig get their quotas of maternal antibody before birth, but not through the allantoic placenta. The antibody is secreted into the uterine lumen where it is picked up by a fetal membrane, the splanchnopleure that is derived from the yolk sac.[3] In contrast, the human infant obtains most of his antibody directly through the chorioallantoic placenta.[13]

FUNDAMENTALS OF PLACENTAL TRANSFER

The placenta constitutes the main conduit through which pass the nutrients for the fetus as well as its excretory products. To maintain the extensive exchange needed by the rapidly growing fetus, the placenta increases in diameter and weight as pregnancy proceeds. Villous processes increase in number and fetal vasculature is progressively enriched so that toward term a very large surface area is available to the maternal and fetal circulations. The villi, with surface microvilli, are directly exposed to maternal blood spurting into the intervillous space from the spiral arterioles (Fig. 5-2). Nutrients circulating in maternal blood must cross the placental membrane (Fig. 5-3) to reach the fetal circulation.*

Circulatory Factors

In reviewing the principal factors affecting the amount of a nutrient delivered to the fetus

* For a discussion of this important subject, see Utero placental circulatory system. In Boyd JD, Hamilton WJ: The Human Placenta. Cambridge, W. Heffer & Sons, Ltd., 1970

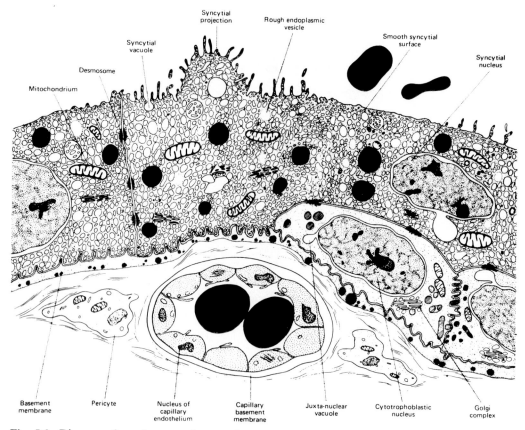

Fig. 5-3. Diagram of an electron-microscopic structure of a placental membrane.

The syncytial trophoblast **(upper portion of figure)** is exposed to maternal blood. Microvilli increase the area for transfer. Syncytial vacuoles may be part of the pinocytotic process for protein transfer. The rich mitochondrial and endoplasmic systems provide the machinery for intense synthetic activity. The syncytiotrophoblast, which is incapable of cell division, derives from the cytotrophoblast. Boyd JD, Hamilton WJ: The Human Placenta. Cambridge, W. Heffer & Sons, Ltd, 1970)

(Table 5-2), one must start with the maternal supply to the placenta. This may be expressed mathematically as the blood level in the maternal artery times the blood flow rate. Each of these factors depends on a series of others. The maternal blood level is affected by exogenous supply (generally nutritional) endogenous reserves, and the homeostatic mechanisms that normally stabilize the blood concentration. Disturbances in any of these features may influence the supply to the fetus. Similarly, reduction in blood flow through the intervillous space, such as may follow cardiac decompensation, a fall in blood pressure, or vascular pathology, will reduce the maternal supply to the placenta. The efficiency with which materials are removed from the placenta into the fetal circulation is affected by factors similar to those that control maternal supply.

The flow relations of the maternal to fetal circulation, whether concurrent, crosscurrent, countercurrent, or pool, probably play a less significant role. The human placenta does not seem to have an organized pattern of flow in the intervillous space and does not fit any simple classification. The anatomy of the intervillous spaces raises the possibility of arteriovenous mixing: oxygenated blood emerging from the spiral arteriole and mingling with venous blood receding from the villus towards the uterine veins. There may also be **shunting,** that is, arterial blood that completely fails to

Table 5-2. Major Factors Affecting the Placental Transfer of a Diffusible Substance

Maternal	Placental	Fetal

Amount delivered to the placenta
1. Blood concentration
    Exogenous and endogenous
      supplies
    Homeostatic mechanisms
2. Flow-rate in intervillous space
    Hemodynamic factors in
      mother
    Local circulatory factors
3. "Shunting" and arteriovenous
    mixing in intervillous space
	1. Area of diffusing membrane
	2. Diffusion pressure:
	    difference in concentration in
	    intervillous space and in villous
	    capillary
	3. Diffusion resistance
	    Characteristics of transferred
	      material-size, charge,
	      polarity, etc.
	    Characteristics of membrane
	      Physiochemical composition
	      Thickness
		1. Blood concentration
		2. Hemodynamic factors
		    Systemic
		    Local
		3. Flow characteristics
		    (Pool, crosscurrent,
		    and so on)

reach the villus resulting in a decrease in the efficiency of extraction. Indications of shunting are also evident in the fetal circulation.

What emerges from these considerations is that the circulation to the human placenta is not totally efficient for the transfer of materials. On the other hand, it is clearly adequate for the task. Babies are born alive and sufficiently developed to cope with the external environment. Compromises in the efficiency of transfer may serve other functions of the placenta.

Transfer by Diffusion

The driving force in transfer by diffusion is the concentration gradient across the placenta, defined by the difference in concentrations in maternal and fetal blood. The resistance to diffusion is dictated by the nature of the molecule (its size, water solubility, and electrical charge) and the nature of the membrane (its thickness and physiochemical structure; see also Chap. 46). The latter may also be altered pathologically, for example, by edema or by thickening of the basement membrane.

The principles determining molecular diffusion are generally applicable to biologic membranes, but the specifics have never been defined for the human placenta. There is similar uncertainty as to which nutrients are transferred solely by diffusion and which are assisted by active transport. Many judgments derive from studies with animal placentas or with nonplacental membranes. Among the materials that appear to be transferred by diffusion are water, sodium, urea, gases, and most lipid-soluble materials.

Protein Binding

Materials with very low water solubility are commonly bound to proteins for transport in blood. About 98% of oxygen is bound to hemoglobin. However, it is the small amount of physically dissolved oxygen that is responsible for creating the diffusion pressure. From this standpoint, binding to circulating proteins increases the amount delivered to the placenta but may reduce the rate of transfer. Counterbalancing this restraint on transfer from the maternal circulation is the availability for binding in the fetal circulation of the more avid fetal hemoglobin which, in high concentrations, facilitates transfer.

The same general principles apply to many lipid-soluble materials, such as steroids, bilirubin, and fatty acids. Protein binding increases the potential for transfer of these materials across the placenta. Placental transfer of iron is specifically enhanced by the transferrin-iron complex, probably through receptors, similar to the mechanism for transfer from plasma to reticulocyte.

Placental Metabolism

In the present discussion, we have referred to the placenta as a membrane although it is, in fact, an active metabolic organ with its own nutritive requirements. Perfusion experiments of human placenta indicate that oxygen is consumed at a rate of 10 ml/min/kg, and that this amount of maternal oxygen is diverted to placental use in the course of transfer to the fetus. This would amount to approximately

20% of the oxygen supplied to the conceptus.[14] Other nutrients are probably treated similarly.

Metabolic conversion within the placenta may be of such magnitude as to constitute a barrier to transfer. Over 50% of perfused adrenocorticosteroids are converted to more polar metabolites in the course of a single circulatory cycle.[15] Relatively little maternal glutamic acid reaches the fetus because of a slow transfer rate and rapid metabolism.[16]

Active Transport

The lipid nature of the placental membrane impedes the diffusion of most water-soluble molecules. Mechanisms within the placenta are needed to facilitate transport of those materials that must be supplied in large amounts to the fetus. The details of active transport systems are currently under intensive investigation, but certain operational characteristics have been known for many years. For example, the transfer of amino acids is stereospecific, the transfer rate of the natural L-form being more rapid than for the D-isomer.[17] Transfer requires energy and a gradient is established with levels about 30% higher in the fetal circulation.[18,19] Glucose also has a stereospecific transport system, but it does not require energy and the level is higher in the maternal circulation. The mechanism for glucose transfer is probably facilitated diffusion. Facilitated diffusion does not maintain a gradient across membranes, suggesting that the lower glucose concentration in the fetal circulation is a consequence of placental and fetal metabolism. The fetal level of several constituents (calcium, magnesium, water-soluble vitamins) is higher than that in the maternal circulation, an observation which is generally accepted as presumptive evidence of active transport. The transfer of iron in the rabbit appears to be directed only towards the fetus.[20]

Some proteins are transferred across the placenta in the human, but not in all mammals (see Immunologic Interactions). The rate of transfer is far slower than that of amino acids, the latter being the primary nitrogen source for fetal proteins. However, protein transfer is very significant to the immunologic defenses of the newborn infant. It is believed that proteins do not penetrate the membrane because of the large size of the molecules, but are engulfed by a process of pinocytosis and pass through the membrane in vacuoles. The process has a specificity unrelated to molecular size. IgG is transferred far more rapidly than IgA (about the same molecular weight) and twice as fast as albumin (less than half the molecular weight).

ANTEPARTUM NUTRITION

A logical discussion of antenatal nutrition might develop from a consideration of the nutritional requirements of the fetus *in utero*, and the ability of the mother to satisfy those requirements with the aid of the placenta. Unfortunately, the necessary information is very limited.

Flexner attempted to attack this problem by measuring the exchange rates of radioactive sodium across the placenta.[21] He concluded that the capacity for transfer of sodium to the fetus far exceeded its needs, as measured by the accumulation of sodium during growth. At that time it was not known that sodium transport may be intimately associated with the transfer of other substances such as amino acids, so that the apparently excessive exchange rate may be related to functions other than sodium deposition. The transfer of phosphorus in the guinea pig is approximately equivalent to fetal needs.[22] Flexner proposed that a reserve or "safety factor" existed for the transfer of certain nutrients, but transfer was marginal with others. The observations can be explained differently but the concept remains an interesting one.

There is little information derived from the human relating placental transfer rates to fetal metabolic requirements. Estimates of urea synthesis in the human fetus suggest significant amino acid catabolism, indicating amino acid transfer in excess of requirements for fetal growth.[23] In contrast, the transfer of free fatty acids, as measured in a perfusion system, is considerably less than that required for the deposition of fat in the last trimester, suggesting that the fetus synthesizes much of its fat from small fragments derived from glucose or amino acids.[24] Studies on the composition of fetal and newborn adipose tissue support this interpretation.

Clinical observations have provided some indirect information concerning antenatal nutrition. Although the primary source of fetal nutrients must eventually be the food consumed by the mother, a reasonably healthy baby may issue from a mother who is clearly malnourished. This has given rise to the notion that the fetus draws freely on maternal tissue reserves for its own welfare, existing as a ''parasite.''

Experimentalists have challenged this conclusion as being too simplistic. If a pregnant rat is placed on a diet deficient in protein and calories, her offspring will be small. Specific deficiencies are also readily induced. Placing a pregnant rat on a sodium-poor diet will rapidly reduce the serum sodium levels in both mother and fetus, indicating that the limited supplies of sodium are shared. However, potassium deprivation does not alter the fetal serum potassium level, even though the maternal level may fall to half the normal level.[25] A magnesium-deficient diet produces a rapid fall in both maternal and fetal serum levels; the mothers tolerate this without evident ill effect, but the fetuses are runted and desperately sick with severe hemolytic anemia.[26] The mother retains her tissue magnesium levels in spite of fetal needs. However, maternal iron (in the rabbit) is directed preferentially to the fetus where it is used in the synthesis of hemoglobin.[27] The nutritional arrangements between mother and fetus are evidently complex.

Interesting as these experiments are, their application to the human is uncertain. The rat produces a litter with a cumulative weight equivalent to 20% of the mother's after a 3-week gestation period. The human takes 9 months to produce an infant equivalent to about 5% of the mother's weight. During World War II, a reduction in birth weight was noted in Holland and particularly in Russia during periods of seige; however, starvation was severe. Low-birth-weight babies are common in underveloped countries where malnutrition is common, but the correlation may be spurious or only partially explanatory. A recent study in Guatemala has shown that the placentas are abnormal, with an increased incidence of infection and a reduction in the area of villous surface available for the transfer of nutrients.[28] Further data are needed on this important subject.

The possibility that fetal malnutrition may result from placental insufficiency is attractive. Experimentally, it has been produced in the rat and subhuman primate by reducing placen-tal blood flow by ligating some of the maternal vessels to the placenta. Undoubtedly, analogous situations occur in the human, though it is common clinical experience to observe multiple placental infarcts without visible effect on the fetus, indicating a reserve capacity in the placenta.

Clinical application of the concept of fetal growth retardation as a result of placental insufficiency was first made in the **postmaturity syndrome.** Flexner found a reduction in the transfer of sodium in the last weeks of human pregnancy in a limited number of cases, providing some support for the hypothesis.[21] With the development of tables describing the rate of growth of the human fetus, it has been recognized that a significant proportion of low-birth-weight newborns have suffered from intrauterine growth retardation. Attributing the growth retardation to antepartum malnutrition and specifically to placental insufficiency is usually presumptive. A variety of fetal factors, such as chromosomal anomalies and infection, may also cause growth retardation.

Toxemia is one clinical entity in which converging lines of evidence indicate that placental insufficiency contributes to the incidence of low-birth-weight infants. Placental clearance of radioactive sodium is reduced,[29] the amino acid gradient across the placenta is lower[30] and histologic studies reveal vascular involvement and a thickening of the placental basement membrane.[31] (For further details, see Chap. 15.)

ANTEPARTUM EXCRETION OF BILIRUBIN

The excretion of bilirubin provides an example of the interaction of fetus and mother to accomplish a given objective.[32] Bilirubin is a metabolite of hemoglobin which is not re-utilized and must be excreted. Newborn infants are rarely born icteric, but bilirubin rapidly accumulates in the blood after birth. Before birth, elimination of bilirubin from the fetus must take place across the placenta.

Bilirubin has limited solubility in water. Transport of bilirubin within the body is facilitated by binding to serum albumin, thus increasing its water solubility. To permit excretion into protein-poor aqueous media, such as bile or urine, water solubility must be increased. This is accomplished in the liver by conjugation, primarily to glucuronic acid.

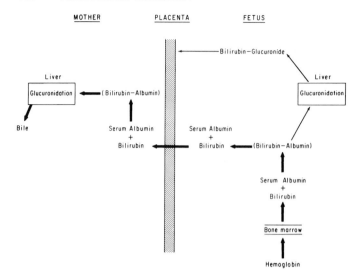

MOTHER   PLACENTA   FETUS

Fig. 5-4. Antepartum excretion of bilirubin. Fetal bilirubin is transferred from fetal serum albumin through the placenta to maternal serum, and then is conjugated by the maternal liver with glucuronic acid and excreted into the bile. Fetal glucuronidation is suppressed. The placenta is relatively impermeable to the glucuronide.

Before birth, excretion is across the placenta into protein-rich maternal plasma, permitting transfer of unconjugated bilirubin. In fact, the placenta is considerably more permeable to unconjugated bilirubin that to the glucuronide. Perhaps for this reason, conjugation of bilirubin in the fetus is suppressed. Following transfer of fetal bilirubin to the mother, it is efficiently conjugated and excreted (Fig. 5-4).

After birth, activation of the bilirubin glucuronidation mechanism is usually sufficiently rapid to keep the plasma bilirubin from reaching dangerous levels. Hyperbilirubinemia of the newborn must be viewed as a persistence of a physiologic adaptation to antepartum requirements.

THE PLACENTA AS AN ENDOCRINE ORGAN

Major differences in the endocrinologic control of pregnancy exist among the mammalian species.[33] The synthesis of large amounts of steroid hormones is required to induce and maintain the uterine changes associated with pregnancy, and this, in turn, involves the elaboration of trophic hormones (Table 5-3). Throughout pregnancy, in some species, and early in pregnancy in the human, the joint efforts of pituitary and ovaries are necessary. Characteristic of the human is the assignment to the placenta of roles ordinarily filled by the pituitary and ovary. In fact, after the first trimester, when the placenta is well estab-

lished, pregnancy will continue in the absence of the maternal pituitary and ovaries.

Human Chorionic Gonadotropin (HCG). Sensitive techniques have demonstrated that the secretion of HCG begins shortly after conception. The amount excreted into the urine reaches a peak during the first trimester and then falls to a relatively low level that is maintained throughout pregnancy.

The hormone is synthesized by the syncytiotrophoblast.[34] It had been long considered that HCG was synthesized by the inner layer of cells, the cytotrophoblast. There is now general agreement that the syncytial cells are equipped with the appropriate intracellular organelles (see Fig. 5-3) and constitute the endocrine factory. The syncytiotrophoblast, being incapable of cell division, arises from the cytotrophoblast. HCG cross-reacts immunologically with pituitary luteotrophic hormone which it resembles chemically and functionally.[35] Apparently, HCG replaces the pituitary hormone toward the end of the first trimester in maintaining the corpus luteum. It is not known whether it also exerts a trophic function on steroid synthesis by the placenta.

Human Placental Lactogen (HPL; chorionic somatomammotropin) is also synthesized by the syncytiotrophoblast. The amount synthesized increases throughout pregnancy reaching the amazing amount of 1.0 g daily.

HPL resembles pituitary growth hormone immunologically and in its biological actions, although its activity in the usual assay systems

Table 5-3. Hormone Levels During Pregnancy

Hormone	Serum level	Urine/24 hr
Chorionic gonadotrophin	40–100,000 IU/liter* 4–11,000 IU/liter	40–100,000 IU/liter* 4–11,000 IU/liter
Human placental lactogen	5.6 μg/ml	1 g
Estrone	10.0 μg/100 ml	2 mg
Estradiol	3.0 μg/100 ml	1.0 mg
Estriol	20.0 μg/100 ml	30 mg
Progesterone	15.0 μg/100 ml	

* Levels in first trimester. Remaining levels are typical of the third trimester. There is a wide normal range. Serial determinations are more informative in evaluating pregnancy. (Adapted from Ryan KJ: Amer J Obstet Gynec, 84:1695, 1962)[33]

is considerably lower.[36,37] Like HCG, it is secreted into the maternal circulation. The serum level in the mother approximates 5 to 10 μg/ml and only .02 μg/ml in the fetus. It is therefore assumed that HPL exerts its action through modifying maternal metabolism, possibly by increasing maternal dependence on lipids for energy, thereby releasing glucose for the fetus. In contrast, growth hormone elaborated by the pituitary circulates in the mother at a level approximating 5 ng/ml and in the fetus at 35 ng/ml. The fetal pituitary is evidently active during pregnancy and the placenta is relatively impermeable to these protein hormones.

A protein with thyrotropin-like activity has been extracted from human placenta. It cross-reacts immunologically with bovine thyroid stimulating hormone.[38] The concentration is extremely variable in different placentas, and the observation requires further study and confirmation.

Progesterone and Estrogens.[39,40,41] Both classes of steroids appear in the urine in progressive increasing amounts during preg-nancy. Progesterone is synthesized by placenta from cholesterol derived from the mother (Table 5-4). Some of the progesterone is used by the fetus to synthesize adrenal hormones, and the rest is excreted through the mother. The synthesis of estrogens requires an elaborate concerted effort on the part of the mother, placenta, and fetus (Table 5-5). Precursors for final conversion to estrogens are supplied to a limited extent by the mother, while considerably more originates from the large cortex of the fetal adrenal gland. Because of the dependence of these pathways on the fetoplacental unit, estrogen assays provide an index of fetal and placental function.

Recent Studies

The past few years have witnessed a renewed interest in the endocrinology of the placenta. *In vitro* studies have demonstrated luteinizing hormone-releasing factor in the placenta.[42] It has also been reported that ACTH is synthesized in placenta.[43] Further studies are awaited with interest.

Table 5-4. Major Pathways of Progesterone Synthesis

Mother	Placenta	Fetus
Acetate ↓ Cholesterol ——— Cholesterol ↓ ←———————— Progesterone ————→ Progesterone ↓ Aldosterone Hydrocortisone		

Table 5-5. Estrogen Synthesis

Mother	Placenta	Fetus

Cholesterol

DHA—SO$_4$ $\longrightarrow$ Dehydroepiandrosterone sulfate $\longleftarrow$ DHA—SO$_4$
(DHA—SO$_4$)

E$_1$—E$_2$ Estrone $\rightleftharpoons$ Estradiol
                (E$_1$)   (E$_2$)

Estriol

conjugation

Cholesterol

DHA—SO$_4$

16 α-hydroxydehydroepiandrosterone $\longleftarrow$ 16 α-OH-DHA-SO$_4$
(16 α-OH-DHA-SO$_4$) Sulfate

E$_3$ $\longleftarrow$ Estriol
              (E$_3$)

THE AMNIOTIC FLUID

A close interplay of mother and fetus is also evident in the formation and circulation of the amniotic fluid. Important gaps in our information remain but many significant details are already known.

The physiologic role of amniotic fluid is assumed to be mechanical, nutritive, and excretory.[44] The primary source of the fluid must, of course, be the mother, and experiments with isotopic water have demonstrated a rapid exchange rate (500 ml/hr) with maternal body water.[45] Early in pregnancy, the amniotic fluid resembles a transudate of maternal plasma. It is isotonic with a reduced protein concentration. Plasma proteins with molecular weights of up to 170,000 diffuse into the amniotic fluid.[46]

Later in pregnancy, the fetal contribution becomes more evident.[47] The tonicity of the fluid falls and urea and creatinine concentration rise, reflecting the contribution of hypotonic fetal urine. A circulation of amniotic fluid through the fetus is established with the fetus swallowing an estimated 500 ml daily.[48] Renal agenesis is commonly associated with oligohydramnios and esophogeal atresia with polyhydramnios.[49]

In recent years, investigations of the amniotic fluid have become very important clinically. The increased bilirubin concentration associated with isoimmune disease must be fetal in origin and is probably contributed by the stool or urine, though that has not been established. Similarly, abnormal metabolites associated with inborn errors of metabolism, such as the adrenogenital syndrome and methylmalonic aciduria, may be found in increased concentration in amniotic fluid. However, enzyme activities may originate from mother, fetus, or both.[50] Some of the enzymes are clearly fetal in origin permitting their use for antepartum diagnosis of such inherited diseases as Tay-Sachs. The usefulness of the lecithin:sphinogomyelin (LS) ratio in predicting maturity of the lung must have its basis in contributions from pulmonary fluids. In the fetal sheep, there is a constant outpouring of pulmonary fluid into the trachea.[51] There must be sufficient exchange with the amniotic fluid to influence the lipid content.

The desquamated cells floating in the amniotic fluid have proved most useful in the antepartum diagnosis of chromosomal and genetic diseases. The cells are presumed to arise in variable amounts from all the epithelia with which the amniotic fluid comes into contact: fetal membranes, fetal skin, genitourinary tract, and so on. Regardless of origin, the cells reliably reflect the chromosomal and genetic composition of the fetus. When grown in tissue culture, the karyotype is readily determined and an extensive list of enzyme assays can be performed.[52]

The central theme of the preceding chapter

is illustrated very simply in Figure 5-1. The mother and fetus must be viewed as a closely integrated unit, exposed to environmental influences. The intimacy of fetomaternal interactions require that the obstetrician and the pediatrician also interact. A variety of forces is driving the medical profession toward increasing specialization, and there are many benefits to be derived from this trend. However, unless a broad perspective of pregnancy is maintained, many problems will resist explanation and solution, thus bringing adverse effects on mother and child.

REFERENCES

1. **Hendler RW:** Biological membrane ultrastructure. Physiol Rev 51:66, 1971
2. **Brambell FWR, Hemmings WA, Henderson M:** Antibodies and Embryos. London, Athalone Press, 1951
3. **Payne R, Rolfs MR:** Fetomaternal leukocyte incompatibility. J Clin Invest 37:1756, 1958
4. **Walknowska J, Conte FA, Grumbach MM:** Practical and theoretical implications of fetal/maternal lymphocyte transfer. Lancet 1:1119, 1969.
5. **Dancis J, Brenner M, Money WL:** Some factors affecting the permeability of guinea pig placenta. Amer J Obstet Gynecol 48:570, 1962
6. **Beer AE, Billingham RE:** Maternally acquired runt disease. Science 179:240, 1973
7. **Kadowaki J, Thompson RI, Zuelzer WW et al:** XX-XY lymphoid chimaerism in congenital immunological deficiency syndrome with thymic alymphoplasia. Lancet 11:1152, 1965
8. **Currie GA, VanDoorninck W, Bagshawe KD:** Effect of neuraminidase on the immunogenicity of early mouse trophoblast. Nature 219: 191, 1968
9. **Hellström KE, Hellström I, and Brawn J:** Abrogation of cellular immunity to antigenically foreign mouse embryonic cells by a serum factor. Nature 224:914, 1969
10. **Thomas L, Douglas GW, Carr MC:** The continual migration of syncytial trophoblasts from the fetal placenta into the maternal circulation. Trans Assoc Amer Phys 72:140, 1959
11. **Anderson JM:** Transplantation—Nature's success. Lancet 11:1077, 1971
12. **Dancis J, Lind J, Oratz M, Smolens J, Vara P:** Placental transfer of proteins in human gestation. Amer J Obstet Gynecol 82:167, 1961
13. **Campbell AGM, Dawes GS, Fishman AP, Hyman AI, James GB:** The oxygen consumption of the placenta and fetal membranes in the sheep. J Physiol 182:439, 1966
14. **Challier J–C, Schneider H, Dancis J:** *In vitro* perfusion of human placenta, V. Oxygen consumption. Am J Obstet Gynecol 126:261, 1976
15. **Levitz M, Jansen V, Dancis J:** The transfer and metabolism of corticosteroids in the perfused human placenta. Am J Obstet Gynecol 132: 363, 1978
16. **Schneider H, Challier J–C, Mohlen KH, Dancis J:** Transfer of glutamic acid and glutamine across the *in vitro* perfused human placenta. Br J Obstet Gynecol in press
17. **Page EW, Glendening MB, Margolis A, Harper HA:** Transfer of D- and L-histidine across the human placenta. Amer J Obstet Gynecol 73: 589, 1957
18. **Crumpler HR, Dent CE, Lindan, O:** The amino acid pattern in human foetal and maternal plasma at delivery. Biochem J 47:223, 1950
19. **Schneider H, Panigel M, Dancis J:** Transfer across the perfused human placenta of antipyrine, sodium and leucine. Amer J Obstet Gynecol 114:822, 1972
20. **Dancis J:** The placenta in fetal nutrition and excretion. Amer J Obstet Gynecol 84:1749, 1962
21. **Flexner LB, Cowie DB, Hellman LM, Wilde WS, Vosburgh GJ:** Permeability of human placenta to sodium in normal and abnormal pregnancies and supply of sodium to human fetus as determined with radioactive sodium. Amer J Obstet Gynecol 55:469, 1948
22. **Fuchs F, Fuchs AR:** Studies on the placental transfer of phosphate in the guinea pig. I. The transfer from mother to fetus. Acta Physiol Scand 38:379, 1957
23. **Gresham EL, Simons PS, Battaglia FC:** Maternal-fetal urea concentration difference in man: Metabolic significance. J Pediatr 79:809, 1971
24. **Dancis J, Jansen V, Kayden HJ, Schneider H, Levitz M:** Transfer across perfused human placenta: II Free fatty acids. Pediatr Res 7: 192, 1973
25. **Dancis J, Springer D:** Fetal homeostasis in maternal malnutrition. I. Potassium and sodium deficiency. Pediatr Res 4:345, 1970
26. **Dancis J, Springer D, Cohlan SQ:** Fetal homeostasis in maternal malnutrition. II. Magnesium deprivation. Pediatr Res 5:131, 1971
27. **Bothwell TH, Pribella WF, Finch CA, Mebost W:** Iron metabolism in the pregnant rabbit. Iron transport across the placenta. Amer J Physiol 193:615, 1958
28. **Laga EM, Driscoll SG, Munro HN:** Comparison of placentas from two socioeconomic groups. I. Morphometry. Pediatrics 50:24, 1972
29. **Browne JC, Veall N:** The maternal placental blood flow in normotensive and hypertensive women. J Obstet Gynaecol Br Commonw 60: 141, 1953

30. **Butterfield LJ, O'Brien D:** The effect of maternal toxaemia and diabetes on transplacental gradients of free amino acids. Arch Dis Child 38:326, 1963

31. **Aherne W, Dunnill MS:** Morphometry of the human placenta. Br Med Bull 22:5, 1966

32. **Dancis J:** Aspects of bilirubin metabolism before and after birth. Pediatrics 24:980, 1959

33. **Ryan KJ:** Hormones of the placenta. Amer J Obstet Gynec 84:1695, 1962

34. **Thiede HA, Choate JW:** Chorionic gonadotrophin localization in the human placenta by immunofluorescent staining. II. Demonstration of HCG in the trophoblast and amnion epithelium of immature and mature placentas. Obstet Gynecol 22:433, 1963

35. **Friesen H, Astwood EB:** Hormones of the anterior pituitary. New Eng J Med 272:1328, 1965

36. **Josimovich JB, Atwood BL:** Human placental lactogen (HPL) a trophoblastic hormone synergizing with chorionic gonadotrophin and potentiating the anabolic effects of pituitary growth hormone. Amer J Obstet Gynecol 88:867, 1964

37. **Kaplan SL, Grumbach MM:** Serum chorionic "growth-hormone prolactin" and serum pituitary growth hormone in mother and fetus. J Clin Endocrinol Metab 25:1370, 1965

38. **Hershman JW, Starnes WR:** Placental content and characterization of human chorionic thyrotropin. J Clin Endocrinol Metab 32:52, 1971

39. **Solomon S, Bird CE, Ling W, Iwamiza M, Young PCM:** Formation and metabolism of steroids in the fetus and placenta. Recent Progr Horm Res 23:297, 1967

40. **Diczfalusy E:** Endocrinology of the fetoplacental unit. In Fetal Homeostatis, vol II. New York, New York Academy of Sciences, 1967

41. **Siiteri PK, MacDonald PC:** Placental estrogen biosynthesis during human pregnancy. J Clin Endocrinol Metab 26:751, 1966

42. **Siler-Khodr TM, Khodr GS:** Content of luteinizing hormone releasing factor in the human placenta. Am J Obstet Gynecol 130:216, 1978

43. **Liotta A, Osathanondh R, Ryan KJ, Krieger DT:** Presence of corticotrophin in human placenta: Demonstration of *in vitro* synthesis. Endocrinol 101:1552, 1977

44. **Ostergard DR:** The physiology and clinical importance of amniotic fluid. A review. Obstet Gynecol Survey 25:297, 1970.

45. **Plentl AA:** Formation and circulation of amniotic fluid. Clin Obstet Gynecol 9:427, 1966

46. **Usategui-Gomeg M, Morgan DF, Toolan HW:** A comparative study of amniotic fluid, maternal sera and cord sera by disc electrophoresis. Proc Soc Exp Biol Med 123:547, 1966

47. **Bonsnes RW:** Composition of amniotic fluid. Clin Obstet Gynecol 9:440, 1966

48. **Pritchard JA:** Fetal swallowing and amniotic fluid volume. Obstet Gynecol 28:606, 1966

49. **Wagner ML, Rudolph AJ, Singleton EB:** Neonatal defects associated with abnormalities of the amnion and amniotic fluid. Radiolog Clin North Amer 6:279, 1968

50. **Sutcliffe RG, Brock DJH:** Observations on the origin of amniotic fluid enzymes. J Obstet Gynaecol Br Commonw 79:902, 1972

51. **Adams FH, Fujiwara T:** Surfactant in fetal lamb tracheal fluid. J Pediatr 63:537, 1963

52. **Milunsky A, Littlefield JW, Kaufer JN, Kolodny EH, Shih VE, Atkins L:** Prenatal genetic diagnosis. New Eng J Med 283:1370, 1441, 1498, 1970

6

Management of the High-risk Pregnancy

Edward J. Quilligan,
David J. Nochimson,
and Roger K. Freeman

The past 20 years have witnessed a major step forward in obstetrics. This change has been both philosophic and technologic: philosophic in that the obstetrician has directed more of his attention toward the fetus, and technologic in that instrumentation has been developed (continuous fetal heart rate monitors and ultrasound) which allows evaluation of the fetus in the antepartum and intrapartum period. These two changes have been associated with a significant decline in perinatal mortality (Fig. 6-1). However, cause and effect cannot be proved, and there are those who feel that decreases in parity due to liberalized abortion and more effective birth control, increases in prenatal care, and dietary changes are more important in the decline of perinatal mortality. The probability exists that all of the above, including enhanced technology, have played a role in this decline, and that the attempt to attribute the decline to any single factor is naive.

One of the major tasks of the physician is to recognize the patient who is developing a problem. Because the obstetrician has two patients during pregnancy, the mother and fetus, he must be able to diagnose a problem developing in either one. The fetus, being totally dependent on the mother for its growth and maintenance, will naturally reflect problems occurring in the mother. It is well recognized, for example, that the fetus of a diabetic mother is subject to certain problems (*e.g.*, macrosomia, see also Chap. 16), as the fetus of a hypertensive mother is subject to others (*e.g.*, intrauterine growth retardation; IUGR), but both fetuses have one thing in common: a higher perinatal mortality. There are many other situations in obstetrics that are associated with an increased perinatal mortality. These conditions can develop in the antepartum or intrapartum period or they can be present in both time frames. The recognition of these situations of increased perinatal mortality are collectively referred to as high-risk pregnancy, high-risk infants or both. Several scoring systems using facts gained from the patient's history and from her present antepartum and intrapartum periods have been developed. The one most frequently used today is that of Hobel which encompasses all three periods.[1] In his system, problems are given risk scores, the more serious problem having a higher weighting (Table 6-1). Recently, he has modified this system and integrated it with a statistical approach to further assess probabilities of risk.[2] While these risk numbers may not be absolute, and although they do, indeed, change with changes in therapy, they alert the health care team to a

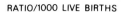

RATIO/1000 LIVE BIRTHS

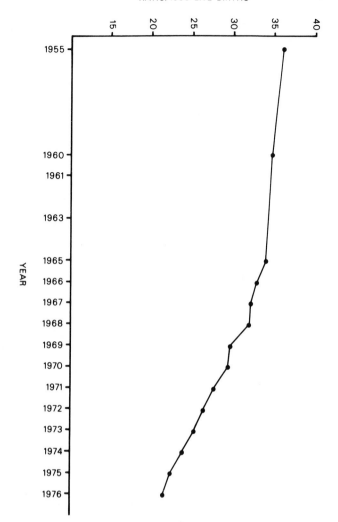

Fig. 6-1. Perinatal mortality (1955–1976). (Calculated from Facts of Life and Death, pp. 8–9. Washington, Department of Health Education and Welfare, Publication No. 79-1222, Nov. 1978)

problem and permit deployment of scarce resources to solving that problem. In this chapter, we shall attempt to describe, first, some of the resources now available to solve obstetric problems and, later in the chapter, some problem pregnancies and the way in which these resources are used to assist in good obstetric care.

FETAL MATURITY

It has been obvious for many years that the traditional antepartum evaluation of fetal maturity is subjective and imprecise. The idea of equating fetal size with fetal maturity has contributed to a significant perinatal mortality in both diabetic and IUGR pregnancy.[3] Also, inconsistencies in accurate dating of a pregnancy have caused the obstetrician to make erroneous estimates of gestational age and fetal maturity with subsequent increase in neonatal mortality.[4] Recently, progress has been made in organ system maturity evaluation, specifically of the fetal lung. All other methods of estimation of fetal age, size, and maturity are only indirect measurements.

Menstrual History

Although the last menstrual period (LMP) provides a time by which to date a pregnancy and determine gestational age and maturity, its shortcomings must be recognized. If a woman has had regular periods (*i.e.,* every 28 days), has kept a careful, written record of them, and was not on oral contraceptives prior to conception, the last menstrual period may be considered reliable.

Because the most constant time interval relating ovulation to menses is that from ovulation to the onset of menses rather than that from menses to ovulation, one can never be sure of the exact time of conception, even with an accurate LMP, unless ovulation is documented. Therefore, we make certain assumptions in dating ovulation 14 days before menstrual onset.

If a woman's cycle is 35 days rather than the usual 28, it can be assumed that she will ovulate on day 21 and not on day 14. Her expected date of confinement (EDC) will actually be 7 days past the 280 days usually calculated from her LMP. Oral contraceptives can also frequently delay ovulation after the last withdrawal period, a phenomenon seen in many pregnancies that go beyond 42 weeks.

If the LMP is delayed or is not normal, one should suspect early pregnancy bleeding that will make the EDC earlier. Therefore, it is obvious that careful history taking is the first important step in evaluating gestational age and fetal maturity.

Physical Examination

Another important method in providing close dating of the pregnancy is an early pelvic examination. If a patient is examined before the 10th week of gestation; if the uterine size is compatible with her last menstrual period; and if there are no uterine fibroids, uterine retroversion, or excessive obesity present; one can assume clinically that the pregnancy is firmly dated. Frequently, a pregnancy test is substituted for an early pelvic exam in a patient who presents herself very early in gestation. Valuable information is thereby lost.

Measurement of uterine fundal height serially with a tape measure is a much less accurate way to assess gestational age. By measuring the uterus abdominally from the symphysis pubis to the top of the uterine fundus, one may usually guess gestational age within ± a 4-week period. Roughly, in normal pregnancy, the uterine height measures 20 centimeters at 20 weeks' gestation, and 28 centimeters at 28 weeks' gestation in the absence of obesity, hydramnios, fibroids, or multiple gestation.

Table 6-1. Pregnancy Risk Factors

A. **Prenatal factors**	Score
1. Moderate to severe toxemia	10
2. Chronic hypertension	10
3. Moderate to severe renal disease	10
4. Severe heart disease, Class II–IV	10
5. History of eclampsia	5
6. History of pyelitis	5
7. Class I heart disease	5
8. Milk toxemia	5
9. Acute pyelonephritis	5
10. History of cystitis	1
11. Acute cystitis	1
12. History of toxemia	1

B. **Intrapartum factors**	Score
1. Moderate to severe toxemia	10
2. Hydramnios or oligohydramnios	10
3. Amnionitis	10
4. Uterine rupture	10
5. Mild toxemia	5
6. Premature rupture of membrane > 12 hr	5
7. Primary dysfunctional labor	5
8. Secondary arrest of dilation	5
9. Demerol > 300 mg	5
10. $MgSO_4$ > 25 g	5
11. Labor > 20 hr	5
12. Second stage > 2½ hr	5
13. Clinical small pelvis	5
14. Medical induction	5
15. Precipitous labor < 3 hours	5
16. Primary cesarean section	5
17. Repeat cesarean section	5
18. Elective induction	1
19. Prolonged latent phase	1
20. Uterine tetany	1
21. Pitocin augmentation	1

C. **Neonatal factors**	Score
1. Prematurity < 2,000 g	10
2. Apgar at 5 min < 5	10
3. Resuscitation at birth	10
4. Fetal anomalies	10
5. Dysmaturity	5
6. Prematurity 2,000–2,500 grams	5
7. Apgar at 1 min < 5	5
8. Feeding problem	1
9. Multiple birth	1

(Adapted from Hobel DH, Hyvarinen M, Okada D, Oh W: Amer J Obstet Gynecol 117:1, 1973)

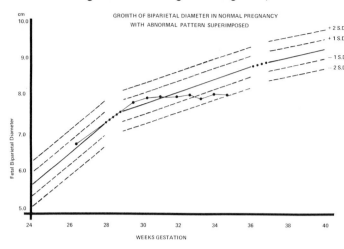

Fig. 6-2. Increase in fetal biparietal diameter from the 24th to the 40th week of normal pregnancy with one and two standard deviations from the mean is shown. The superimposed curve shows a flattened growth pattern over several weeks of gestation. (Martin CB et al: Obstet Gynecol 41:379, 1973)

Serial tape measurement of fundal height is useful in following uterine growth. The accuracy for dating pregnancy after 28 weeks, however, diminishes because of divergent fetal growth patterns in the third trimester.

Fetal heart tones are usually auscultated with a conventional fetoscope between 16 and 20 weeks' gestation. It is unlikely to hear fetal heart tones earlier than 16 weeks, except by newer ultrasonic methods. If dates are unsure and heart tones are not yet present, it is helpful in dating a pregnancy to see the patient on a weekly basis until fetal heart tones are heard.

Pregnancy Tests

New immunologic methods of pregnancy testing are now employed. The hemaglutination inhibition pregnancy tests have a sensitivity of about 1,000 IU of HCG per liter of urine. These tests are positive by 7 days after the first missed menstrual period. They are useful tools in helping to date pregnancy only if obtained early. A gradual fall in HCG makes the test unreliable after 12 to 14 weeks' gestation.[5]

Radiologic Methods

X-rays have been used for years to correlate the appearance of fetal epiphyseal centers and gestational age. Distal femoral epiphyses usually appear by 36 weeks, but this varies widely with the race and sex of the fetus. For instance, 50% of female infants weighing less than 2000 g have distal femoral epiphyses present. Proximal tibial epiphyses appear much later and are present in only about 50% of full-term Caucasian male infants.[6] Therefore, it is evident that the presence of epiphyseal centers is of little value in predicting fetal maturity.

Because fetal radiation is considered hazardous and because there are better methods available for estimating fetal maturity, it is no longer appropriate to employ x-rays for this purpose.

Ultrasound

Dating a pregnancy using ultrasound can be quite accurate. The measurement obtained with real-time or B-mode ultrasound depends on the gestational age of the fetus. During the first weeks of pregnancy, measurement of the crown-rump (C-R) length will date the pregnancy within one day. After this period, the measurement of the fetal biparietal diameter is accurate to within ±3 days, up to the 20th week of pregnancy.[7] Thereafter, dating a pregnancy using the biparietal diameter is hazardous because of the rather slow growth of the fetal biparietal diameter and the wide standard deviations in measurements (Fig. 6-2). Additional discussion is found under IUGR, below.

Amniotic Fluid

The amniotic fluid creatinine concentration and **lecithin-sphingomyelin ratio (L/S) ratio** is the most frequently used and most informative amniotic fluid study for evaluation of fetal maturity. At present, the most critical factor for neonatal survival is the maturity of the fetal lungs. Gluck suggested that amniotic fluid surface-active phospholipid levels reflect fetal pulmonary surfactant production.[8] He later related two phospholipids, lecithin and sphingomyelin, to the incidence of RDS.

Sphingomyelin levels in amniotic fluid remain rather constant with advancing gestational age (Fig. 6-3). Lecithin levels, however, surge abruptly at approximately 34 weeks, reflecting maturation of a more stable metabolic pathway for surface-active lecithin production in the fetus. It is when this stable lecithin pathway is established that the incidence of RDS begins to decrease markedly. The ratio of these two phospholipids has become the most useful and most reliable clinical tool for estimation of fetal pulmonary maturity.

When the L/S ratio is 2.0 or greater, there are essentially no deaths from hyaline membrane disease and a low morbidity from idiopathic RDS may be expected. When the L/S ratio is less than 2.0, a neonate may or may not develop RDS or hyaline membrane disease (HMD; Table 6-2). If the Apgar score is low, if the birth weight is low, or if gestational age is early, the likelihood of increased morbidity and mortality from these respiratory conditions is definitely increased.

Therefore, when a premature delivery is expected and the L/S ratio is less than 2.0, one should avoid any unnecessary stress during labor and delivery and prepare adequate resuscitation measures. Even with an L/S greater than 2.0, low Apgar scores contribute to an increased morbidity from RDS. It has been shown that the route of delivery (cesarean section versus vaginal) *per se* does not influence the incidence of RDS.[9]

Recently Hallman, Kulovich, and Gluck have demonstrated that a lung profile may be developed using the L/S ratio, plus the acetone precipitate fraction, and the amount of phosphatidylinositol and phosphatidylglycerol in amniotic fluid.[10] Phosphatidylinositol reaches a peak at 35 to 36 weeks and then starts to decline, whereas phosphatidylglycerol is present only after 35 weeks and is always associated with pulmonary maturity. The development of the lung profile has reduced some of the problems found in diabetic pregnancies, namely that an L/S greater than 2.0 was not adequate to predict the absence of RDS in the infant. If phosphatidylglycerol is present, RDS has not been found. The presence of phosphatidylglycerol assures pulmonary maturity when the L/S ratio is less than 2.0.

Other methods which will give a more rapid

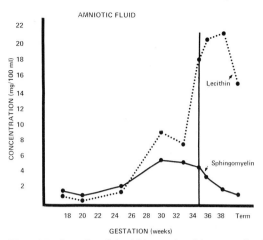

Fig. 6-3. Levels of lecithin and sphingomyelin in amniotic fluid at increasing gestational ages. (Gluck L et al: Am J Obstet Gynecol 109:441, 1971)

estimation of pulmonary maturity include the shake test, the microviscosimeter, and the optical density of amniotic fluid. The shake test, developed by Clements and his coworkers, is based on the ability of amniotic fluid with adequate surface-active material to maintain a stable foam when the fluid is mixed with alcohol.[11] The test has few false positives but many false negatives. The microviscosimeter test is a determination of the fluorescence polarization of amniotic fluid when mixed with the dye 1,6 diphenyl–1,3,5 hexatriene and incubated for 30 minutes. This test, like the shake test, has few false positives and a false-negative rate similar to the L/S ratio. Perhaps the simplest test is the determination of the optical density at 650 nm. An optical density of 0.15 or greater correlates well with a mature L/S ratio. In some studies, the false negative

Table 6-2. Deaths from HMD in Newborn Infants with Various Ranges of L/S Ratios

No.	L/S Ratio	Deaths from HMD (%)
3	≤1.0	100.0
6	1.1–1.3	33.0
16	1.4–1.6	25.0
23	1.7–1.9	8.7
347	≥2.0	0.3

(From Donald IR et al: Amer J Obstet Gynecol 115:547, 1973)

rate is as high as 30%. However, if the test is positive, HMD is rarely encountered.

CLINICAL ASSESSMENT OF PLACENTAL FUNCTION

Only recently has it been possible to assess placental function in the antepartum period with new biochemical and biophysical monitoring methods. When poor function is detected, it is termed **clinical uteroplacental insufficiency.** Clinical uteroplacental insufficiency is ill-defined and, in most instances, is believed to be secondary to a maternal condition rather than a primary disease entity.

The maternal conditions are usually related to chronic vascular disease syndromes, such as diabetes, hypertension, and renal vascular disease. In these conditions, a decreased intervillous space blood flow limits respiratory and metabolic exchange across the placenta.

This placental function impairment or chronic uteroplacental insufficiency can be associated with many clinical findings, including

1. failure of uterine growth in the third trimester.
2. meconium in the amniotic fluid prior to or during labor.
3. abnormal fetal heart tones during labor.
4. asphyxia neonatorum.
5. a small, infarcted placenta.
6. intrauterine fetal growth retardation.
7. neonatal meconium aspiration.
8. intrauterine fetal death.

Changes in uterine growth patterns with chronic placental insufficiency are not usually seen until the third trimester, but they should be suspected in the following situations: toxemia, diabetes, postdatism, oligohydramnios, elderly primigravida, third trimester bleeding, history of previous stillbirth, and cyanotic maternal heart disease.

Unfortunately, when chronic uteroplacental insufficiency and fetal jeopardy are recognized, the only treatment at present is delivery. This makes the concomitant assessment of fetal maturity of vital importance.

The methods currently employed in our institution for assessment of uteroplacental function are estriol, nonstressed monitoring, and the oxytocin challenge test (OCT). Many other substances have been linked to placental

function, including diamine oxidase, heat-stable alkaline phosphatase, leukocyte alkaline phosphatase, urinary pregnanediol, and human placental lactogen (HPL)

HPL has been employed more widely than the others. HPL has growth hormone-like activity, and is produced by the placenta in increasing amounts as pregnancy progresses. It is easily measured in maternal serum by radioimmunoassay or hemagglutination inhibition methods.

The amount of HPL in maternal serum increases gradually as pregnancy progresses to term. Spellacy has defined a fetal danger zone as being a value of less than 4 μg/ml after 30 weeks of gestation.[12] There seems to be a reasonable correlation between fetal distress in the patient with hypertensive vascular disease in pregnancy and low HPL values. The correlation is not good in the patient with diabetes or an erythroblastotic infant.

Estriol

Fluctuations in 24-hour urinary estriol determinations during pregnancy were first related to fetal jeopardy some 15 years ago.[13] The metabolism of steroids in the fetal and maternal tissues has been explored extensively since that time.[14]

It is known that estriol production during pregnancy exceeds that of the nonpregnant state and increases with gestational age, especially during the third trimester. The increased estriol production results from conversion of fetal adrenal androgen precursors to estriol by the placenta.

Estriol can be measured either in maternal plasma or in maternal urine. Both measurements have advantages and disadvantages. The urine measurements are simpler and one gets an integrated value over 24 hours; however, accurate collection is difficult and many drugs, such as ampicillin, alter the urinary values by disturbing the enterohepatic circulation of estriol. The plasma values are done by radioimmunoassay, and thus are more expensive. They are also subject to more diurnal variation. However, they are easy to collect and are not altered by renal disease in the mother or by drugs which influence estriol enterohepatic circulation. For the latter reasons, we have chosen to utilize plasma estriols to monitor our high-risk patients. Katagiri, Distler, and their coworkers have shown that

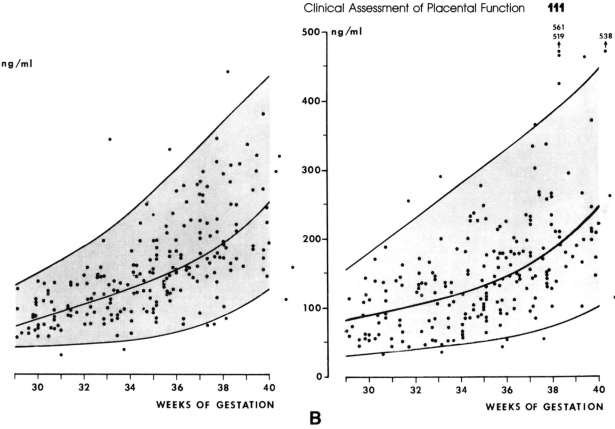

Fig. 6-4. A. Unconjugated plasma estriol. **B.** Total plasma estriol.

the best results are obtained when one uses the unconjugated plasma estriol fraction, the best results being the lowest diurnal variation, the best correlation with urinary estriol values, and the most accurate prediction of fetal distress.[15]

The mean unconjugated plasma estriol increases from 6 ng/ml at 28 weeks to 18 ng/ml at term. There are, as can be seen in Figure 6-4, rather wide variations which are within normal limits. Thus, the best indication of fetal distress is a decrease in estriol greater than the day-to-day variation. Buster and colleagues have shown a wide fluctuation in several values obtained over a 1 to 2 hour period and suggest multiple sampling to minimize this error. In our laboratory, we attempt to compensate for this by using as a standard the mean value of the three previous determinations. We then look for a decrease of 35% as indicative of fetal distress. In the diabetic, this can occur quite rapidly, so values must be obtained daily. On the other hand, the values

in patients with post datism, IUGR, and hypertension decrease more gradually; therefore, twice weekly values are adequate.

Interpretation of the chronically low estriol is the most difficult. Several causes for a diminished estriol excretion include

1. chronic uteroplacental insufficiency.
2. fetal growth retardation from causes other than chronic uteroplacental insufficiency (congenital anomalies, chronic fetal infections).
3. anencephaly.
4. congenital fetal adrenal insufficiency.
5. placental sulfatase deficiency.
6. error in dates.

The only category in the above list in which premature intervention may be indicated for fetal benefit is in chronic uteroplacental insufficiency. Thus, a low estriol excretion pattern is not specific, and further evaluation of uteroplacental function is required.

Although estriol excretion patterns are cur-

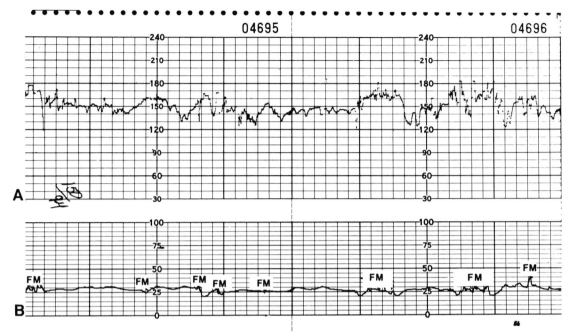

Fig. 6-5. Reactive nonstress test. **A.** Fetal heart rate. **B.** Simultaneous uterine tone. **FM.** Fetal movement.

rently in use clinically in the management of high-risk pregnancy, it remains to be proven that intervention on the basis of low or falling estriol actually improves perinatal mortality in the high-risk group.

Nonstress Monitoring

The use of fetal heart rate monitoring to evaluate fetal condition during the antepartum period received strong impetus from the development of the oxytocin challenge test (OCT) by Pose[17] and Ray[18]. However, the OCT had some disadvantages as a screening procedure: (1) it required 1 to 2 hours per test; and (2) it was contraindicated in any patient in whom one did not wish to see labor (*i.e.,* prior uterine scar, multiple pregnancies, and so on).

Hammacher[19] and Kubli[20] suggested using heart rate variability as an antepartum test of fetal well-being. However, some variability could be artificially induced by the equipment. Rochard and coworkers pointed out that the presence of fetal tachycardia (> 6 beats/min), occuring in conjunction with fetal movements, was associated with normal fetuses.[21] Evertson[22] and his colleagues defined a normal (reactive) fetus as one who demonstrated five

cardiac accelerations of 15 beats/minute, lasting 15 seconds, in association with fetal movement, during a 20-minute period (Fig. 6-5). They also found that only those fetuses with no or one cardiac acceleration, in a 20-minute period, had a suspicious or positive OCT.[23] We have modified our criteria for a nonreactive fetus to conform to this finding; that is, a reactive fetus is one who accelerates its fetal heart 15 beats or more for 15 seconds in association with fetal movement twice in a 20-minute period. If the fetus is initially nonreactive, it should be stimulated by moving it because about 25% of fetuses become reactive only after stimulation. If the fetus remains nonreactive after stimulation, then an OCT should be performed.

Oxytocin Challenge Test

This method of evaluating antepartum uteroplacental function is based on electronic fetal heart rate monitoring, advanced by Hon,[24] Quilligan,[25] Caldeyro-Barcia,[26] and others (see Chap. 7). Uniform fetal heart rate slowing following the peak of a uterine contraction during labor has been associated with fetal hypoxia measured by a decreased fetal P_{O_2}, fetal metabolic acidosis, low Apgar score, and intrauterine death. This fetal heart rate pattern is known as **late deceleration,** as described by Hon, or as a **Type II dip,** as described by Caldeyro-Barcia, and is considered to be ominous.

Kubli, Pose, and others have suggested observing the fetal heart rate responses to oxytocin-induced uterine contractions prior to labor as a measure of uteroplacental function.[20,17] The appearance of late deceleration is suggestive of a decreased uteroplacental respiratory reserve, similar to ECG changes on treadmill studies in patients with suspected coronary disease.

The test method currently used involves

1. semi-Fowler position for the patient in order to avoid supine hypotension syndrome.
2. blood pressure recording every 5 minutes.
3. external monitoring of uterine contractions and fetal heart rate.
4. oxytocin delivered intravenously by infusion pump with a usual starting dose of 0.5 mU/minute.
5. serial increase in oxytocin infusion every 20 minutes to obtain 3 uterine contractions in a 10-minute period.
6. repetition of the test weekly.

A definite negative or reassuring test requires adequate uterine activity, and three contractions every 10 minutes has been the arbitrary endpoint selected. Any persistent recurring late deceleration determines a positive test and the procedure should be terminated without further oxytocin stimulation.

Correlating this test with estriol and fetal outcome in a recent blind study from our institution, the OCT was found to become positive before any fall in the 24-hour urinary estriol.[18] Thus, the OCT has been found useful in helping to interpret a chronically low or confusing estriol pattern, and it is our initial means of quick evaluation for patients with suspected uteroplacental insufficiency because results can be obtained within 2 hours, compared to 24-hour urinary estriol collections.

While the OCT usually indicates fetal jeopardy when positive, we have had false-positive tests in a few patients who tolerated monitored labor and delivery without late deceleration, even though they had positive oxytocin challenge tests obtained at various times prior to labor. In over 600 OCTs in high-risk patients, there has been only one intrauterine fetal death within 1 week of a negative test. This death was probably caused by a cord accident rather than by uteroplacental insufficiency.

Therefore, we have been able to prevent premature intervention in patients who have had chronically low or confusing estriol patterns when the OCT has remained negative. The negative OCT reassures that the fetus is not in jeopardy, while a positive OCT is a warning sign of decreased placental respiratory reserve.

When the OCT is positive and fetal maturity has not been achieved, a 24-hour urinary estriol pattern in the normal range has allowed the pregnancy to continue without any fetal problems until the point at which the estriol begins to fall. However, if both tests have been abnormal, with the OCT positive and the estriol more than 2 standard deviations below the mean or falling more than 35% the intrauterine fetal prognosis is poor and intervention is recommended even with fetal immaturity. In the situation where fetal maturity has been achieved, we usually deliver the patient when either the OCT has become positive or the estriol has fallen significantly.

MANAGEMENT OF SPECIFIC HIGH-RISK SITUATIONS

Several maternal conditions, all hazardous to the fetus, are discussed below considering their management in the light of these new techniques.

Intrauterine Fetal Growth Retardation

The clinical suspicion of IUGR from failure of uterine enlargement is quite unreliable, but when suspected, we are faced with a long differential diagnosis including hypertension disorders, renal disease, diabetes, fetal viral infections, anomalies, maternal malnutrition, and cyanotic heart disease.[27] A clinical suspicion of IUGR may be confirmed by serial ultrasound scans detecting a decreased rate of growth of the fetal biparietal diameter.

The biparietal diameter of the fetal head is measured *in utero* on a serial basis. This diameter grows at a rate of about 1.8 mm/week during the last 10 weeks of pregnancy.[28,29,30] The absolute mean difference between the ultrasonic biparietal diameter and the neonatal caliper measurement ranges from 0.8 mm to 2.5 mm. Thus, serial determinations of fetal head growth can be accomplished quite accurately[31] (Fig. 6-2). Although fetal growth is the least affected dimension of an IUGR fetus, one may see a decreased rate of fetal head growth on serial measurements in this condition. Even with severe growth retardation, it is unusual to see the relatively declining biparietal values fall below 2 standard deviations from the mean for gestational age.[32]

In a patient with suspected IUGR, fetal well-being must be rapidly insured. An immediate OCT may allow one to avoid intervention and follow the patient on a longer term basis with twice weekly estriol collections and serial ultrasound A-scans.

Delivery is indicated with a positive OCT and reasonable assurance of fetal maturity. Again, IUGR itself is no cause for delivery until uteroplacental insufficiency appears.

Postmaturity

Perinatal mortality rises after 42-weeks' gestation, so that a high-risk group is identified by prolonged gestational age alone. The majority of patients with gestational ages past 42 weeks have erroneous dates, and indeed, even those with accurate dates generally have fetuses with no sign of postmaturity. The true syndrome includes oligohydramnios, meconium-stained amniotic fluid, loss of fetal subcutaneous fat, the "golden" vernix, long fingernails, and meconium staining of membranes and cord. This condition is indeed rare and it does not warrant a routine induction of all patients at 42 weeks or more.[33] Our approach then is to avoid intervention as often as possible.

When a patient is seen past 42 weeks' gestation, the following scheme is adhered to:

1. Plasma unconjugated estriols twice weekly
2. Once-weekly nonstress fetal monitoring
3. If the estriols decrease by more than 40% or if they are less than 2 standard deviations from the mean, or if the fetus is nonreactive, labor should be induced, assuming, of course, that there is no question about fetal age. If a question exists, pulmonary maturity should be checked with an L/S ratio.

Hypertensive Disorders

Hypertensive vascular disease in pregnancy exists when the blood pressure exceeds a systolic of 140, a diastolic of 90, or when there is a 30-point increase in systolic or a 15-point increase in diastolic pressure. Frequently accompanying the hypertension, there is evidence of proteinuria and water retention. The disease entities responsible include preeclampsia-eclampsia, essential hypertension, and chronic renal disease.

Preeclampsia-eclampsia is usually seen in the late second or in the third trimesters of pregnancy. It is most frequently present in a primigravid patient and is associated with an increase in mortality, directly proportional to the severity of the disease. In general, severe preeclampsia or eclampsia can be prevented by good prenatal care with early recognition and treatment of the disease. In its mildest form, it may be managed simply by an increase in bedrest at home. However, it is important that the physician see the patient frequently (every 3–4 days), and that he give her the warning signs of impending eclampsia; blurred vision, severe headaches, or severe epigastric pain. It is important during the course of even early therapy, to evaluate the fetus in addition to the mother. This can be done using nonstress fetal monitoring once each week and plasma estriols twice each week. If the disease seems to progress at all under conservative therapy, immediate hospital admission is mandatory. Immediate hospital admission is also mandatory if, on initial contact, the disease is more advanced (*i.e.,* a blood pressure over a 150 systolic or over 100 diastolic).

The treatment in the hospital consists initially of strict bedrest. The patient should be in the lateral recumbent position when in bed, and she should be evaluated thoroughly for daily weight changes; daily urinary output and urinary protein; blood pressures, at least four times each day; and hematocrits once or twice every week. If the disease is severe, a platlet count and fibrinogen evaluation should also be done. The fetus should be evaluated, as in the milder form of disease, with nonstress monitoring and plasma estriols. If the fetus is mature, as determined by L/S ratio or by any of the previously mentioned tests, delivery should be accomplished.

During the process of labor, convulsions are

more likely to occur; therefore, preventive therapy is frequently employed. This therapy consists of $MgSO_4$ given in adequate doses to prevent the majority of convulsive states. Magnesium sulfate may be given either intramuscularly or intravenously. Intravenously (IV), one should give a 3 g loading dose and then 1 to 2 g/hour. Intramuscularly (IM), the initial IV loading dose is given and followed immediately by 10 g deep into the muscle of the buttocks. This is followed every 4 hours by 5 g deep into the muscle. It is possible to achieve a toxic level of Mg in the blood. Fortunately, however, this can be anticipated by the loss of deep tendon reflexes. Therefore, the patient should be monitored when receiving $MgSO_4$ therapy with deep tendon reflexes and the dose should be adjusted downward if the reflexes are completely absent. One should also monitor urinary output and respiratory rate of these patients. Urinary output should be about 25 ml or more/hour and the respiratory rate should be above 12/minute. Magnesium sulfate should also be used in the more severe forms of preeclampsia, even when the patient is not in labor. When the patient is delivered, therapy should be continued for at least another 12 to 24 hours, depending upon the condition. In general, patients with this disease will start to respond immediately following delivery with a decrease in blood pressure and an increase in urinary output. If the patient is eclamptic when initially seen, immediate $MgSO_4$ is given IV to control the convulsions.

In some instances, the blood pressure reaches levels which are threatening to the mother from a standpoint of a cerebral vascular accident. At the same time it is perferable to keep perfusion pressure reasonably high to insure adequate oxygenation of the uterus. When one is faced with the dilemma of (a) attempting to prevent maternal stroke and (b) knowing that if the blood pressure is lowered too much, the fetus may suffer from hypoxia due to decreased uterine profusion, an arbitrary decision must be made. We have chosen a cut off diastolic blood pressure for treatment of 110 torr when the patient is pregnant. If it exceeds this value, the patient should receive treatment with hypotensive agents, the preferred agent being hydralizine, given in boluses of 2 mg every 5 minutes until the patient's blood pressure has dropped to about 100 dia-

stolic. If the patient is in a postpartum state, uterine perfusion does not pose a serious problem. In this instance, a cut-off blood pressure of 100 torr diastolic is used for treatment with hypotensive agents. Occasionally, patients will develop anuria, associated with preeclampsia. In this instance, treatment should be conservative, replacing only the fluids lost by the patient until she starts to mobilize her own fluid following delivery. If, inadvertently, the patient has received an excessive water load and develops pulmonary edema, diuretics should be used. This is the only situation in which diuretics should be used in preeclampsia. The preferred agent is furosemide, 40 mg.

If the patient has shown essential hypertension, she should be maintained on whatever drug regimen she had been taking prior to pregnancy. If the essential hypertension is discovered in the first trimester of pregnancy, we choose to start the patient on α-methyldopa, 250 to 500 mg qid, increasing to a total dose of 4 g/day, if necessary, to maintain the blood pressure at levels of about 90 diastolic and 140 systolic. These patients with chronic hypertensive vascular disease are much more liable to develop IUGR, so, in addition to the usual monitoring of the fetus with nonstress and stress monitoring and plasma estriols, ultrasound should be used to watch fetal growth. Like the chronic hypertensive patient, patients with chronic renal disease are also more prone to have an IUGR fetus, and the fetus should be monitored with the usual techniques plus serial biparietal diameters. These should be started sometime around the 24th to the 28th week of gestation, and should be done on a 2- to 4-week basis. Earlier measurements of biparietal diameter are helpful primarily for dating the pregnancy.

Diabetes Mellitus (See also Chap. 16)

About 1.5% of all pregnant women will have an abnormal glucose tolerance test. Because an abnormal glucose tolerance test in pregnancy is associated with a significantly higher fetal morbidity and potential maternal morbidity and mortality, it is imperative that the obstetrician recognize that patient who will be a diabetic during her pregnancy. The patient that has been diagnosed prior to pregnancy is

Table 6-3. Classification of Diabetes in Pregnancy. (A modification of White's classification)

Class A	1.	Abnormal glucose tolerance test with normal fasting blood sugar
	2.	Controlled with diet alone
Class B	1.	Insulin-treated diabetic
	2.	Onset over age 20
	3.	Duration under 10 years
	4.	No vascular disease or retinopathy
Class C	1.	Insulin-treated diabetic
	2.	Onset between age 10 and 20
	3.	Duration between 10 and 20 years
	4.	No vascular disease or retinopathy
Class D	1.	Insulin-treated diabetic
	2.	Onset under age 10
	3.	Duration over 20 years
	4.	Retinopathy
Class E	1.	Any pregnant diabetic with calcification of the pelvic vasculature
Class F	1.	Any pregnant diabetic with diabetic nephropathy

(Freeman RK, Mestman J: In Contemporary Obstetrics and Gynecology, Vol I. New York, McGraw-Hill, 1973)

relatively easy to recognize. However, about 40% of the patients who have an abnormal glucose tolerance test during pregnancy do so only during pregnancy.

Ideally, every patient who is pregnant should be screened for abnormal glucose metabolism. Because this is frequently a practical impossibility, criteria have been developed which will increase the yield of patients who have altered glucose metabolism. The criteria include patients with a previous macrosomic child (greater than 4,000 g); patients with a previous unexplained stillbirth; patients with a history of diabetes in the family; patients with unexplained congenital malformations in previous children; and patients who have glycosuria during the present pregnancy. Screening consists initially in making sure that the patient has had a reasonable carboyhdrate intake (300 g/day) for 3 days prior to seeing her. One then does a fasting blood sugar, gives the patient 100 g of carbohydrate (Glucola) to drink, and then takes a 2-hour postingestion blood sugar. The determinations are done on plasma; using a glucose oxidase method, the fasting blood sugar should not be greater than 100 and the 2-hour post glucose blood sugar

should not be greater than 140 mg/dl. If the patient has an abnormal 2-hour postprandial blood sugar, then a formal 3-hour oral glucose tolerance test should be performed. If the patients 2-hour postprandial glucose is normal, it should be repeated again in subsequent trimesters of pregnancy. If the patient has an abnormal glucose tolerance test, she is classified as a Class A or gestational diabetic (Table 6-3).

Class A diabetics should be observed carefully throughout their pregnancies.[34] They should be given a reasonable diet, consisting of 60 to 90g of protein each day, 250 g of carbohydrate, and, the remainder, of up to about 2000 to 2400 calories in fat. The patient should be seen on a biweekly basis until the last month of pregnancy when she should be seen every week. During each prenatal visit, it is important that, in addition to the routine measures, a fasting blood sugar be done to make sure the patient has not become an overt diabetic. As long at the fasting blood sugars remain normal, no special measures need be taken except to deliver the patient around the 40th week of gestation. These patients frequently have macrosomic infants (20–30%). Because a difficult delivery with shoulder dystocia and subsequent infant damage are not infrequent in these very macrosomic infants, we recommend cesarean section as a method of delivery. In order to accomplish this, of course, macrosomia must be diagnosed. Formerly, fetal weight was diagnosed primarily using abdominal palpation. More recently, the advent of real-time ultrasound, with the measurement of biparietal diameter trends, abdominal diameter, and intraamniotic fluid volume, as proposed by Hobbins, has allowed much more accurate weight estimations of the fetus.[35] The infants of Class A diabetics are also subject, after birth, to a higher incidence of hypoglycemia, hypocalcemia, and hyperbilirubinemia. The pediatrician should be aware of these complications so that they can be adequately managed in the nursery.

The Classes B through F diabetics are insulin dependent and are classified, according to the White classification, based on the duration of disease and the presence or absence of vascular complications (Table 6-3).[36] These patients require much more frequent observation and more rigid control. Control is established initially by admitting the patient to the hospital early in pregnancy for instruction in the care of the diabetes during the pregnancy, and by making certain that the blood sugars are reasonable. It has been demonstrated that the more nearly normal the blood sugar, both fasting and 2-hour postprandial, the lower the incidence of fetal macrosomia. One should attempt to keep the fasting blood sugars somewhere in the neighborhood of 80 to 90 mg/dl and the 2-hour postprandial blood sugars at less than 140. After control is established, the patient is discharged from the hospital to be followed in the ambulatory clinic. She should be seen on a weekly basis. At each visit, the fasting blood sugar and 2-hour postprandial blood sugar should be checked. The values mentioned above should be achieved if at all possible. If the patient's diabetes does not remain in control, she should be admitted to the hospital for control. She should also be admitted to the hospital if there is any question of infection because this will make diabetic control more difficult. Control is achieved through a combination of diet and insulin dosage. The diet prescribed should be 30 to 35 calories/kg of body weight, broken down into protein, 1 to 1.5 g/kg; carbohydrate, about 250 g; and the remainder in fat. Insulin control is usually achieved through a combination of the use of NPH or Lente insulin, plus regular insulin. The insulin is given twice each day, morning and afternoon; in general, two-thirds of the dose of long-acting insulin is given in the morning and one-third in the afternoon. The long-acting insulin is usually supplemented both morning and afternoon with regular insulin, given as a dose of regular insulin which is roughly one-fourth of the dose of the long-acting insulin, equally divided between morning and afternoon. Obviously, the combination of long-acting and regular-acting insulin, given above, are only guidelines and each individual patient must be tailored for optimal blood sugars.

When the patient has reached about 30 to 32 weeks of gestation, fetal nonstress testing should be begun on a once-a-week basis; plasma unconjugated estriols are also taken once a week. At approximately 34 weeks of gestation, we advise admitting the patient to the hospital for the remainder of the pregnancy. The diabetes is closely controlled. The patients have daily plasma estriols assayed and are given a weekly nonstress test for fetal well-being. The delivery date ideally should be after 38 weeks. The closer the patient is brought to term, the lower the infant morbidity. The delivery is chosen on the basis of (1) maternal indication for delivery; (2) fetal indications for delivery; or (3) elective delivery. Maternal indications for delivery include superimposed preeclampsia and diabetes that cannot be controlled.

Fetal indications for delivery include a decreasing plasma estriol (a drop greater than 40% of the previous 3 days' mean) and abnormal nonstress and stress monitoring of the fetus. The regimen that we use is as follows. If the fetus demonstrates pulmonary maturity, that is, an L/S ratio greater than 2.0 or the presence of phosphatidyl glycerol in the amniotic fluid, delivery is performed if either the plasma estriols or the fetal stress and nonstress tests are abnormal. If the fetus demonstrates pulmonary immaturity, fetal indications for delivery are present only when both tests (plasma estriols and nonstress tests) are abnormal. Elective delivery of the fetus should be performed during the 38th week, assuming fetal pulmonary maturity. This is because one can have false-negative, normal plasma estriols and stress and nonstress tests.

The route of delivery depends upon the ripeness of the cervix and the size of the fetus. If the fetus weighs less than 4000 g and the cervix is ripe, induction may be attempted using continuous fetal heart rate monitoring during the induction. On the day of induction, the patient's food should be withheld and her insulin dosage should be cut to one-third of its previous value; but some prefer to start the patient on a continuous insulin infusion, using roughly 1 unit of insulin per hour. The infant who is estimated to weigh over 4000 g or the mother who has an unripe cervix should be delivered by cesarean section. Following delivery, in the immediate postpartum period, the insulin dosage is cut to one-third of pre-pregnancy requirements.

Using the regimen outlined above, extremely satisfactory results in terms of perinatal mortality have been obtained. Overall perinatal mortalities of 3.5 to 4% have been reported by several groups. However, in the diabetic there still remains a sizeable problem of perinatal morbidity. The infant of the diabetic mother has a high rate of hypoglycemia, hyperbilirubinemia in the nursery (40%), increased incidence of hypocalcemia (20–25%), increased incidence of hypomagnesemia (20%) and increased incidence of congenital malformations (10%). With the exception of the congenital malformations, if these complications are recognized by the pediatrician and treated vigorously, no untoward effects should accrue to the newborn.

SUMMARY

By way of summary, then, a new era in obstetrics and pediatrics is emerging in which focus is on the quality of intrauterine life, in order to push back the resistant frontiers of perinatal mortality and morbidity.

Statistical methods and computer sciences are selecting high-risk factors as indices for precise identification of the high-risk pregnancy.

A centralization of obstetric care is creating high-risk centers and expanding departments of perinatal medicine.

The fetal surveillance methods discussed here will certainly attain wide usage in the near future and no doubt give way to even more exacting methods of study of the intrauterine passenger.

REFERENCES

1. **Hobel DH, Hyvarinen M, Okada D, Oh W:** Prenatal and intrapartum high risk screening. Prediction of the high risk neonate. Am J Obstet Gynecol 117:1, 1973

2. **Hobel C, Youkeles L, Forsythe A:** Prenatal and intrapartum high risk screening. II. Risk factors reassessed. Am J Obstet Gynecol (in press)

3. **Lubchenco LO, Hansman C, Dressler M, Goyd E:** Intrauterine Growth as estimated from liveborn birth weight data at 24 to 42 weeks of gestation Pediatrics 32:793, 1963

4. **Usher R, Allen A, McLean H:** Risk of respiratory distress syndrome related to gestational age route of delivery, and maternal diabetes. Am J Obstet Gynecol 111:826, 1971

5. **Mishell D, Vide L, Gemzell C:** Immunologic determination of human chorionic gonodotropin in serum. J Clin Endocrinol Metab 23:123, 1963

6. **Christie, A:** Prevalence and distribution of ossification centers in the newborn infant. Am J Dis Child 77:355, 1949

7. **Robinson JP:** Sonar measurement of fetal crown-rump length as a means of assessing maturity in the first trimester of pregnancy. Br Med J 4:28, 1973

8. **Gluck L, Kulovich M, Borer R, Brenner P et al:** Diagnosis of the respiratory distress syndrome by amniocentesis. Am J Obstet Gynecol 109:440, 1971

9. **Donald IR, Freeman R.K., Goebelsmann U, Chan WH, Nakamura RM:** Clinical experience with the amniotic fluid lecithin/sphingomyelin ratio. Am J Obstet Gynecol 115:547, 1973

10. **Hallman M, Kulovich M, Kirkpatrick E, Sugarman R, Gluck L:** Phosphatidylinositol and phosphatidylglycerol in anmniotic fluid: Indices of lung maturity. Am J Obstet Gynecol 125:613, 1976

11. **Platzker A, Tooley W et al:** Prediction of the idiopathic respiratory distress syndrome by a rapid new test for pulmonary surfactant in amniotic fluid. Clin Res 20:283, 1972

12. **Spellacy WN:** Monitoring of high risk pregnancies with Human Placental Lactogen. In Spellacy WN (ed): Management of the High-Risk Pregnancy, University Park Press, 1976

13. **Greene JW Jr, Touchstone JC:** Urinary estriol as an index of placental function. A study of 279 cases. Am J Obstet Gynecol 85:1, 1963

14. **Diczfalusy E:** Fetal viability and steariodogenesis in the human fetoplacental unit. Int J Gynaecol Obstet 8:770, 1970

15. **Katagiri H, Distler W, Freeman RK, Goebelsmann U:** Estriol in pregnancy. IV. Normal concentrations, diurnal and/or episodic variations, and day-to-day changes of unconjugated and total estriol in late pregnancy plasma. Am J Obstet Gynecol 124:272, 1976

16. **Buster JE, Meis PJ, Hobel CJ, Marshall JR:** Subhourly variability of circulating third trimester maternal steriod concentrations as a source of sampling error. J Clin Endocrin Metab 46:907, 1978.

17. **Pose SV, Costello JB et al:** Test of fetal tolerance to induced uterine contractions for the diagnosis of chronic distress. In Perinatal Factors Affecting Human Development. pp. 96–104. Washington, Pan American Health Organization, 1969

18. **Ray M, Freeman RK, Pine S, Hesselgesser R:** Clinical experience with the oxytocin challenge test. Am J Obstet Gynecol 114:1, 1972

19. **Hammacher K:** The clinical significance of cardiotocography. In Huntingford PJ, Juter KA Saling E (eds): Perinatal Medicine, pp. 80–93. Stuttgart Georg Thieme, 1969

20. **Kubli FW, Kaeser O et al:** Diagnostic management of chronic placental insufficiency. In Pecile A, Finzi C (eds): The Feto-Placental Unit. Amsterdam Excerpta Medica Foundation, 1969

21. **Rochard F, Schifrin BS, Sureau C:** Non-stressed

fetal heart rate monitoring in the antipartum period. Am J Obstet Gynecol 126–699, 1976

22. **Evertson L, Paul RH:** Antepartum fetal heart rate testing: The nonstress test. Am J Obstet Gynecol 132:895, 1978

23. **Evertson L, Gauthier R et al:** Antepartum fetal heart rate testing I. Evolution of the non-stress test. Am J Obstet 133:29, 1979

24. **Hon EH:** The fetal heart rate patterns preceeding death in utero. Am J Obstet Gynecol 78:47, 1959

25. **Hon EH, Quilligan EJ:** Classification of fetal heart rate, II. A revised working classification. Conn Med 33:779, 1967

26. **Caldeyro-Barcia R, Mendez-Bauer C et al:** Control of the human fetal heart rate during labor. In Cassels DE (ed): The Heat and Circulation in the Newborn and infant. New York, Grune and Stratton, 1966

27. **Bowes, W:** Personal communication.

28. **Willocks J, Donald I, Campbell S, Dunsmore IR:** Intrauterine growth assessed by ultrasonic fetal cephalometry. Br J Obstet. Gynaecol 74:639, 1967

29. **Kohorn EI:** An evaluation of ultrasonic fetal cephalometry. Am J. Obstet Gynecol 97:553, 1967

30. **Thompson HE:** The clinical use of pulsed echo ultrasound in obstetrics and gynecology. Obstet Gynecol Surv 23:903, 1969

31. **Campbell O:** An improved method of fetal cephalometry by ultrasound. Br J Obstet Gynaecol 75:568, 1968

32. **Ianniruberto A, Gibbons JM:** Predicting by ultrasonic B-scan cephalometry an improved technique with disappointing results. Obstet Gynecol 37:689, 1971

33. **Anderson GC:** Postmaturity: A review. Obstet Gynecol Survey 27:71, 1966

34. **Gabbe SG, Mestman JH et al:** Management and outcome of Class A diabetes mellitus. Am J Obstet Gynecol 127:465, 1977

35. **Gohari P, Berkowitz RL, Hobbins JC:** Prediction of intrauterine growth retardation by determination of total intrauterine volume. Am J Obstet Gynecol 127:255, 1977

36. **Gabbe SG, Mestman JH et al:** Management and outcome of pregnancy in diabetes mellitus, Classes B to R. Am J Obstet Gynecol 129:723, 1977

7

Management of Labor and Delivery

Edward H. Hon and
Kee S. Koh

For many years, the major concern of obstetricians has been the reduction of the maternal mortality and morbidity associated with the birth process. With the use of antibiotics, blood transfusions, better surgical techniques, and improved anesthesia, great progress has been made in these areas. Unfortunately, this progress in maternal care has not been matched by similar results in perinatal mortality and morbidity.

In recent years, there has been a reexamination of the factors that may play a part not only in survival of the infant but also in the quality of that survival. The importance of looking at the total picture of gestation is being emphasized. The general condition of the patient, together with the antepartum and intrapartum course, is being considered in conjunction with factors that may affect the neonate during its hospital stay and its growth and development. The fetal hazards of labor and delivery have received new attention, and techniques for management of labor and delivery are being carefully scrutinized.

Benson and coworkers have shown that stethoscopic sampling of the fetal heart rate (FHR) in the interval between contractions is inadequate for the early detection of fetal distress.[1] It is pertinent, therefore, to examine the more recent techniques of continuous electronic monitoring of the FHR[2–5] and fetal scalp blood sampling for its biochemical assessment.[6–9] Even though there have been few controlled studies using these techniques for fetal monitoring, on the basis of our understanding of their physiologic significance they appear to be reasonable approaches to the problem.[2,10–12] The preliminary clinical results are promising.[13–27] An important side effect is a new awareness of the fetus and the potentially damaging effects of labor and drugs upon it.

Effects of Labor on the Fetus

Traditionally, labor has been evaluated in terms of duration. Normal durations have been set up for primigravid and multiparous patients. Durations which exceed these norms are classified as prolonged labors. From the fetal standpoint, this method of defining normal labor is unacceptable. If the fetus is already compromised as the result of a maternal medical complication of pregnancy (*e.g.*, diabetes mellitus, chronic hypertension, Rh isoimmunization), it may not be able to tolerate the stress of even a few minutes of labor.[28,29] Normal labor, therefore, is better defined as that degree of labor that does not encroach

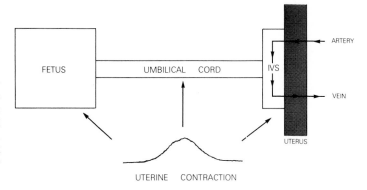

Fig. 7-1. Schematic diagram indicating that the mechanical effects of each uterine contraction may be seen on the fetal presenting part, umbilical cord, and intervillous space (IVS). (Hon, EH: An Atlas of Fetal Heart Rate Patterns. New Haven, Harty Press, 1968)

significantly on the fetal margin of reserve.[28] The acceptance of this concept is important if the fetal hazards of labor are to be minimized.

Each uterine contraction is a repetitive mechanical stress to the fetus and may affect it in a number of ways. Figure 7-1 indicates that the mechanical energy of the contracting uterus may be applied directly to the fetal body. This is usually the fetal vertex, where it may cause molding of the head, caput succedaneum, and even intracranial hemorrhage.

Because the umbilical cord is found around some portion of the fetal body about 25% of the time, it is not surprising that uterine contractions are associated with varying degrees of umbilical cord compression. A more subtle effect of uterine contractions is the impedance of intervillous space blood flow by each contraction.[2] As intramyometrial pressure rises, the venous outflow from the intervillous space is first shut off, producing congestion and a decrease in maternal-fetal transfer. As the intramyometrial pressure rises higher, the arterial inflow is also shut off so that the intervillous space is physiologically isolated from the mother. The net result is a transitory decrease in maternal-fetal transfer of which oxygen transfer is a significant part. It is clear then, that labor is made up of a series of repetitive stresses to the fetus that may be of sufficient magnitude to threaten its integrity and perhaps even life itself.

Fetal Heart Rate

Before the advent of continuous electronic monitoring of the FHR, FHR data was intermittently collected with a stethoscope in the interval between contractions. Furthermore, because it was difficult to hear the fetal heart beat during contractions, the little information available previously about FHR changes with contractions was inadequate and inaccurate. With the assessment of electronically acquired FHR data and new knowledge about FHR and the changes associated with uterine contractions, a new FHR classification became necessary.[30]

At present, it is customary to distinguish contraction-related changes in FHR from changes in FHR which are not contraction related. One such classification can be summarized as[30]

Periodic FHR—Changes in FHR associated with uterine contractions.
Baseline FHR—FHR changes in the absence of, or between periodic FHR changes.

Figure 7-2 illustrates the use of an FHR classification of this type.

Periodic FHR. Periodic FHR may be subdivided into the two major categories:

Acceleration —Uniform
　　　　　　 —Variable
Decelerations—Uniform (early, late)
　　　　　　 —Variable

Uniform FHR accelerations occur with each uterine contraction, and their onsets bear a consistent timing relationship to the beginning of associated contractions. While these FHR patterns have not been studied extensively, they seem to be the earliest sign of fetal stress and may be associated with the presence of increased fetal catecholamine levels. Not infrequently, they precede the development of late deceleration[28] which is associated with fetal hypoxia.[12]

Variable accelerations are those accelera-

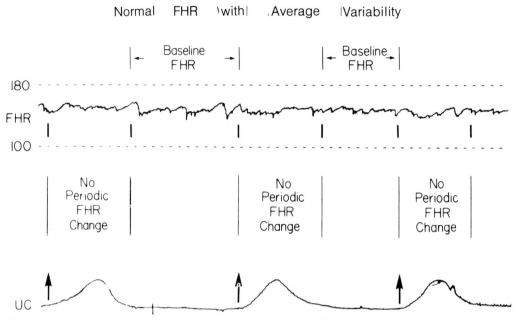

Fig. 7-2. Record of normal FHR showing division into baseline and periodic FHR. UC = uterine contraction. (Hon EH: An Atlas of Fetal Heart Rate Patterns. New Haven, Harty Press, 1968)

tions that do not possess a consistent timing relationship to uterine contractions. They are more angular in shape than uniform accelerations and are probably associated with fetal movement.

Baseline FHR. Research and clinical experience with electronic monitoring of FHR indicates that changes in the level of the baseline FHR provide less information about fetal well-being than do the periodic FHR changes. However, fetal tachycardia greater than 160 beats per minute should be viewed with caution. If the level of baseline FHR is rising during the course of labor, possible underlying factors such as excessive uterine activity, maternal hypotension, or fever should be carefully investigated. Likewise, fetuses in which the baseline FHR levels are less than 120 beats per minute should be carefully observed. The variability of the baseline FHR is of major importance also.[31-35] These fluctuations in baseline FHR appear to reflect the integrity of the nervous mechanisms controlling the fetal heart. If they are markedly diminished or absent, so that the FHR is smooth or fixed, this may indicate interference with FHR control by maternally administered drugs, fetal

asphyxia or immaturity of the fetal nervous system.

FHR Decelerations. The FHR deceleration patterns appear to be the most important for management of labor and delivery. Figures 7-3A, B, and C illustrate the three basic types. There are two uniform types (early and late deceleration), and one variable type (variable deceleration). The uniform and variable types are distinguished from each other by their shape and the timing relationship between the onset of the deceleration and the beginning of the associated uterine contraction.[28,30]

Figure 7-3A is an illustration of early deceleration in which each episode of FHR deceleration reflects the shape of the associated uterine contraction curve and the onset of the deceleration begins early in the contracting phase of the uterus. This particular pattern is thought to be caused by fetal head compression. From a clinical standpoint, it is considered to be innocuous because it has not been associated with depressed or acidotic fetuses or newborns. The middle trace (Fig. 7-3B) shows another uniform FHR deceleration in which the shape of each deceleration reflects the shape of the associated uterine contraction

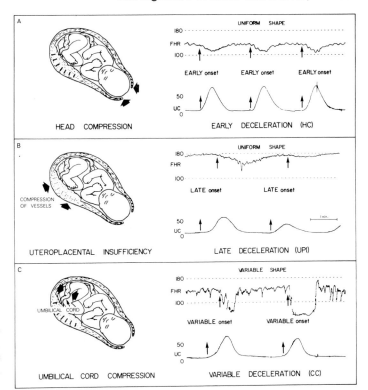

Fig. 7-3. Three FHR deceleration patterns of clinical significance. (Hon, EH: An Atlas of Fetal Heart Rate Patterns. New Haven, Harty Press, 1968)

curve. Here, however, the onset of the deceleration is late in the contracting phase of the uterus. This particular FHR deceleration is thought to be caused by uteroplacental insufficiency. From a clinical standpoint it is considered ominous insofar as it is associated with high-risk fetuses in which depression, acidosis, and fetal death have occurred.

Figure 7-3C is an example of variable deceleration in which the shape of the deceleration varies from contraction to contraction, as does the onset of the deceleration in relation to the beginning of the uterine contraction. This FHR deceleration is caused by umbilical cord compression and is therefore considered ominous because it can result in fetal asphyxia and death, if umbilical cord compression is severe and prolonged.

Fetal Scalp Blood Sampling

Over a decade ago Saling introduced the technique of fetal scalp blood sampling for the diagnosis of fetal distress.[6] The physiologic basis for the use of fetal scalp blood pH for the assessment of fetal hypoxia is illustrated in Figure 7-4.[7] In the breakdown of glucose to carbon dioxide and water, the initial anaerobic phase releases eight high-energy phosphate bonds. If adequate supplies of oxygen are present, an additional 30 high-energy phosphate bonds are generated during the aerobic phase of catabolism, thus making the total energy available 38 high-energy phosphate bonds.

In the absence of oxygen, the breakdown of glucose stops at the pyruvic acid level where it may be anaerobically metabolized to lactic acid at the cost of six high-energy phosphate bonds, thereby making available a net gain of only two high-energy phosphate bonds. In addition to the limited amounts of energy available from the anaerobic breakdown of glucose, there is an accumulation of pyruvic and lactic acid, thereby causing a metabolic acidosis in the fetus. Biochemical evaluation of a blood sample from the fetal scalp therefore has value for the detection of fetal hypoxia.

In practice, a number of modifying factors

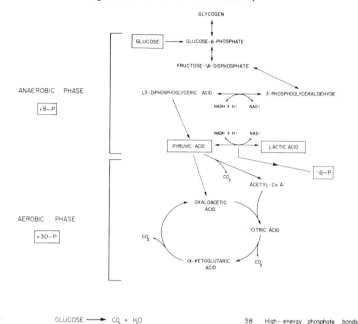

GLUCOSE $\longrightarrow$ CO₂ + H₂O   38 High - energy phosphate bonds

GLUCOSE $\longrightarrow$ PYRUVIC ACID $\longrightarrow$ LACTIC ACID   2 High - energy phosphate bonds

Fig. 7-4. Diagram illustrating anaerobic and aerobic phases of glucose catabolism. (Hon EH: Obstet Gynecol 33:219, 1969)

have to be taken into consideration when evaluating fetal hypoxia with fetal pH obtained from fetal scalp blood samples.[7] Because the maternal compartment is in intimate contact with the fetal compartment, the acid-base state of the mother has a marked effect on the fetal scalp blood pH. In all cases, a maternal blood sample should be obtained concurrently with the fetal sample. Edema, caput formation, and local vasoconstriction of the skin overlying the scalp may also produce spuriously low fetal pHs. In clinical use, these modifying factors must be taken into consideration when using fetal scalp sampling.

From a clinical standpoint, one of the major problems with fetal scalp blood sampling for fetal monitoring is the intermittency of the procedure and the need for repeated samples. The technique for obtaining the fetal scalp blood sample is more involved than that necessary for FHR monitoring. Additionally, it is necessary to have a biochemical technician available to do the determinations. Fortunately, a correlation exists between fetal scalp blood pH and FHR patterns. Kubli and coworkers demonstrated this correlation by comparing fetal scalp blood samples with FHR patterns that were present in the 20 minutes preceding the sampling time.[36]

Figure 7-5 is a graph reproduced from their studies. On statistical analysis of their data the various FHR patterns fell into four groups.

Group I: None (no deceleration); HC (head compression, *i.e.,* early deceleration); CC mild (cord compression mild, *i.e.,* variable deceleration, mild)

Group II: CC moderate (*i.e.,* variable deceleration, moderate)

Group III: UPI, mild (uteroplacental insufficiency, mild, *i.e.,* late deceleration, mild) UPI, moderate (*i.e.,* late deceleration, moderate)

Group IV: CC severe (*i.e.,* variable deceleration, severe) UPI severe (*i.e.,* late deceleration, severe)

It is obvious that, as the FHR patterns become more "ominous," there is an increasing fetal acidosis.

Management of Labor and Delivery

While electronic FHR monitoring and fetal scalp blood sampling are important adjuncts to the management of labor and delivery,

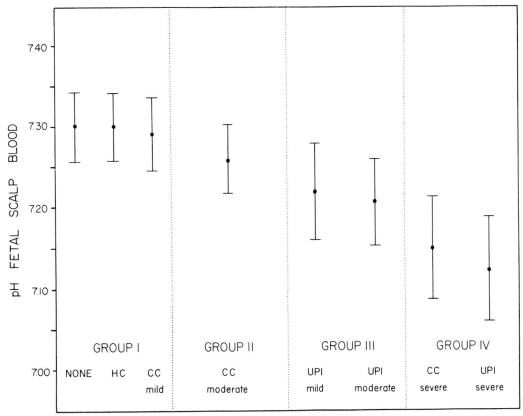

Fig. 7-5. Diagram correlating groups of FHR deceleration patterns and fetal scalp blood pH. See text for details. (Kubli F: Am J Obstet Gynecol, 104:1190, 1969)

careful observance of a number of other simple clinical procedures diminish the fetal hazards of labor.

1. Maintain the patient in as good a condition as possible.
2. Hydrate the patient sufficiently.
3. Choose with care the drugs used for analgesia and anesthesia so as to minimize fetal depression.
4. Keep the patient in a lateral position to avoid supine hypotension and exercise great care when using conduction anesthesia to keep maternal hypotension at a minimum.
·5. Monitor uterine hyperactivity with care, especially when inducing labor.
6. Exercise gentleness during delivery so as to minimize trauma to the fetus.

FHR Monitoring Equipment. At the present time, labor is managed with electronic monitoring of the FHR as a primary method of fetal surveillance. Fetal biochemical determinations are used as a complementary technique if unusual or confusing FHR patterns are detected. The aim of managing labor is to keep the FHR patterns normal. If this can be achieved, the probability of obtaining a good Apgar score at 5 minutes is about 99%.[37,38]

Two techniques are currently available for FHR monitoring: external (indirect) techniques and the internal (direct) techniques.

External techniques record FHR and uterine activity data from the abdominal wall of the mother and are used in situations in which the membranes have not been ruptured and/or in which the cervix is not dilated.

Two major methods are used to record the FHR from the maternal abdominal wall. The most popular is the Doppler ultrasonic technique which detects the changes in velocity of fetal blood or heart valve action associated

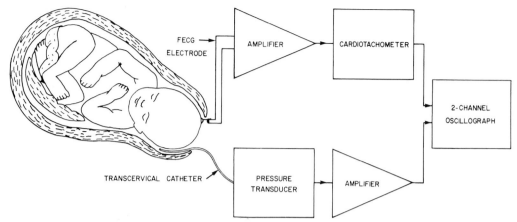

Fig. 7-6. Schematic diagram of techniques used for direct fetal monitoring. (Hon EH: An Atlas of Fetal Heart Patterns. New Haven, Harty Press, 1968)

with the fetal heart beat. The other method is the detection of the fetal heart sounds with a microphone. With both techniques the transducers are coupled to the maternal abdominal wall with a belt which encircles the maternal abdomen. The uterine contractions are detected with a tocodynamometer which gives the frequency of the uterine contractions, some indication of their duration but no quantitation of their amplitude. This latter measurement is modified to a large extent by the obesity and position of the patient and the tension of the encircling belt. The use of the fetal electrocardiogram from the maternal abdominal wall has also been used for this purpose, but it is not as useful as the above techniques.

The internal (direct) technique is the most efficient method of obtaining FHR and uterine contraction data. Figure 7-6 indicates that the FHR is calculated from the fetal electrocardiograms (FECGs) recorded from the fetal presenting part with a directly attached electrode. Two widely used electrodes are a clip[39] or a spiral type.[40] The intrauterine pressure is obtained with a polyethylene catheter which has been introduced into the uterus by the transcervical route. The data thus obtained are suitably amplified, processed and recorded on a two-channel oscillograph in such a manner that the FHR pattern and uterine pressure can be readily correlated. The internal technique gives the most precise measurement of FHR and uterine pressure currently available, and is used where the membranes have been rup-

tured and there is at least 1 cm of cervical dilatation.

Fetal Distress

In the evaluation of suspected fetal distress, consideration should be given to the degree of clinical risk present. FHR deceleration patterns of equal degree may have more significance in the high-risk fetus than they do in the normal fetus[41] because the former has been subjected to a compromised environment for an extended period of time; whereas the latter may be merely suffering a transitory stress.

To date, no real quantitation of fetal distress in terms of FHR and fetal pH have been developed so that considerable uncertainty exists when a diagnosis of fetal distress is made. Nevertheless, clinical decisions have to be made, so that guidelines must be used even though they may not be totally adequate.

Diagnosis. The diagnosis of fetal distress depends upon the ability to recognize ominous FHR patterns. If this is not possible, complementary use of fetal scalp blood sampling is a valuable adjunct. Extensive discussion of FHR patterns in fetal distress is beyond the scope of this report. However, 2 examples are given.

Figures 7-7A and **B** are examples of variable deceleration caused by umbilical cord compression. Note the increasing degrees of variable deceleration in both tracings.

Figures 7-8A, **B**, and **C** are examples of increasing late deceleration in the same pa-

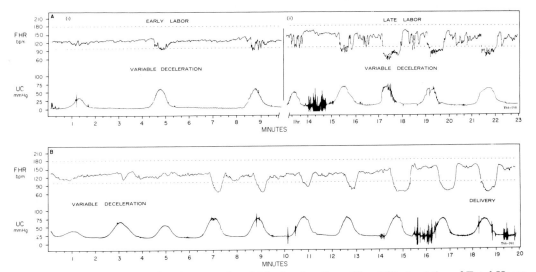

Fig. 7-7. Records of increasing degrees of variable deceleration. (Hon EH: An Atlas of Fetal Heart Rate Patterns. New Haven, Harty Press, 1968)

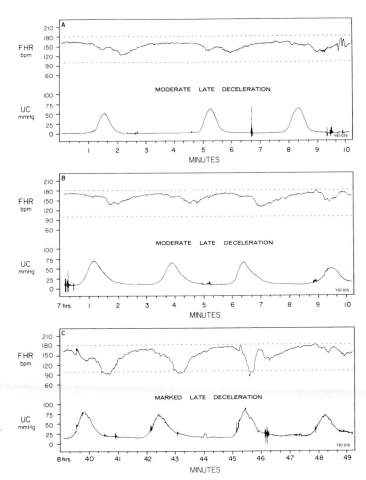

Fig. 7-8. Examples of increasing degrees of late deceleration. (Hon EH: An Atlas of Fetal Heart Rate Patterns. New Haven, Harty Press, 1968)

tient. The second to last episode of FHR deceleration in Figure 7-8C is a "mixed" FHR deceleration pattern in which the abrupt initial deceleration is that of variable deceleration and that immediately following it, is late deceleration.

General guidelines for the diagnosis of fetal distress are

Warning Signals

1. diminishing baseline FHR variability.
2. mild variable deceleration.
3. tachycardia of 160 beats per minute or greater.

Ominous Signs

1. variable deceleration lasting more than 1 minute and dropping to 60 beats per minute or less and getting progressively worse.
2. late deceleration of any magnitude, with or without tachycardia. If it is associated with a smooth baseline FHR the situation is more serious.

Treatment. Rational treatment of fetal distress is based on an understanding of the underlying mechanisms. Corrective measures should be directed at their alleviation. If these fail, labor must be terminated.

Corrective Measures

1. Change the position of the patient. This may remove pressure from the umbilical cord by changing the physical relations between it, the fetus, and the pelvis. If late deceleration is present because of supine hypotension, turning the mother to either lateral position will correct it.
2. Correct maternal hypotension. If this is due to the supine position Step 1 will suffice. Elevate the patient's legs; see that she is well hydrated and if conduction anesthesia is used, take precautions to avoid hypotension.
3. Decrease uterine activity. If oxytocin is being used for induction of labor, discontinue the infusion. Uterine relaxing drugs may also be used.
4. Administer oxygen at the rate of 6 to 7 liters per minute with a tight face mask. This measure may permit a slight increase in the oxygen delivered to the fetus and in some instances will alleviate or modify mild late deceleration.

5. Prepare for operative delivery.
6. If there is a question as to the clinical significance of any persisting FHR patterns after the above measures have been instituted, obtain a fetal scalp blood sample; if this is less than pH 7.20 on 3 serial samples, terminate labor.
7. In the case of severe variable deceleration, the situation may deteriorate so rapidly that it is not feasible to wait for fetal scalp blood sampling before operatively terminating labor.

Comments

The use of FHR patterns as a basis for the management of labor and delivery finds support in the fetal animal studies of Barcroft, Reynolds, and Paul; Myers and coworkers; and James and coworkers.[10-12,42,43] These studies indicate that the pattern of variable deceleration is associated with umbilical cord compression and that late deceleration is associated with fetal hypoxia and fetal hypotension, and, if permitted to persist for an extended period of time, the fetal animal develops brain damage similar to that found in the human.[12,42]

While the clinical studies to date are not extensive, Paul found a lower than expected intrapartum fetal mortality in a monitored high-risk group of patients than he found in a group of unmonitored lowrisk patients.[15] When FHR deceleration patterns were present with the low-birth weight baby, Hobel found an increased incidence of respiratory distress and death in the newborn infant.[41] Martin, in a similar study, confirmed these findings.* Gabert and coworkers, in a recent report, felt that FHR monitoring was instrumental in lowering infant mortality.[16]

A study of 483 patients by Haverkamp and coworkers indicated that there was no difference in clinical outcome between the electronically monitored group and the auscultated group.[44] However, with the former, the cesarean section rate was 16.5% as compared to 6.6% with the auscultated group.

Renou and coworkers reported that, in their experience with 350 patients, the umbilical artery blood of the electronically monitored fetuses was less acidotic than that of the

---

* Martin CB: Personal communication

unmonitored group. Furthermore, there was a significantly higher incidence of twitching, apnea, and convulsions in the unmonitored group. Additionally, four of this group were diagnosed as having brain damage. The authors felt the study should be discontinued because of the detrimental findings in the unmonitored patients.

In another small study of 504 patients, Kelso indicated that there was no difference in the clinical outcome between unmonitored and monitored fetuses, although there was one term intrapartum death in the unmonitored group and none in the monitored group.[20] Based on the sample size, the incidence may not be statistically significant, but one cannot ignore the implications of this observation.

In addition to these "controlled" studies, there have been a number of "uncontrolled" studies which appear to demonstrate that there is a marked decrease in intrapartum stillbirths with electronic fetal monitoring.[15-17,21] These studies, as well as the controlled studies, are compromised by the relatively small sample sizes and the formidable task of matching controls.

It is difficult to see how an adequately large controlled study of monitored and unmonitored patients could be attempted in the United States at the present time, given the mounting evidence that monitoring appears to be beneficial to the fetus and newborn.

A major criticism of electronic fetal monitoring is that it is a direct cause of the increasing cesarean section rate. While this may be so in many hospitals, it need not be, for a number of reports indicate that with fetal monitoring the section rate for fetal distress did not increase[13,26] and, in some instances, actually decreased.[22,45]

There is little doubt that much of the increase in the cesarean section rate for 'fetal distress' is not related to fetal compromise, but to anxiety and insecurity engendered in obstetricians by the lack of understanding of fetal heart rate patterns.

An estimation of the frequency of actual fetal distress can be approximated by adding the expected number of term intrapartum deaths (2/1000) to those of the high-risk fetus (4/1000) thus making a total of 6/1000. If one assumes an equal number of fetuses who may suffer nonlethal irreversible damage, this would make a total of 12/1000 or an incidence of 1.2%. Although these figures are admittedly imprecise, they do give a reasonable estimate of the incidence of fetal distress. Hence, if a hospital has a cesarean section rate of 10% for fetal distress, the major difficulty lies not with the fetus but with the obstetrician.

While the use of fetal minitoring is not supported by a conclusive controlled study, it now appears that if the FHR pattern is normal, both from the standpoint of baseline variability and absence of ominous decelerations, the probability of delivering a baby without low Apgar score is over 99%.[37,38] If abnormal or ominous FHR patterns are present, the accuracy in predicting a low Apgar score baby is between 60% and 20%.[37,38] Some of the difficulties are related to the relatively crude methods of visually assessing FHR patterns and the need for extensive education in FHR pattern recognition. Hopefully some of these problems will be reduced with the use of objective FHR evaluation techniques and increased educational programs.

Of prime importance in the evaluation of any technique for fetal monitoring is the need for a realistic reference point for performance. Unfortunately, there is not yet an adequate neonatal and infant follow-up program of fetuses who have been intensively monitored during labor and delivery. Until such a study is done, it will be difficult to evaluate the true significance of any fetal monitoring technique. In the interim, the present direction of fetal monitoring seems not unreasonable.

REFERENCES

1. **Benson RC, Shubeck F, Deutschberger J, Weiss W, Berendes H:** Fetal heart rate as a predictor of fetal distress. Obstet Gynecol, 32:259, 1968
2. **Hon EH:** Observations on "pathologic" fetal bradycardia. Am J Obstet Gynecol 77:1084, 1959
3. **Caldeyro–Barcia R, Mendez-Bauer C, Bieniarz J:** The Heart and Circulation in the Newborn and Infant. New York, Grune & Stratton, 1966
4. **Hammacher K, Huter KA, Bokelmann J, Werners PH:** Foetal heart frequency and perinatal condition of the foetus and newborn. Gynaecologia 166:349, 1968
5. **Maeda K:** Pathophysiology of Fetus. The 21st Annual Meeting of Japanese Obstetrical and Gynecological Society, 1969
6. **Saling E:** Die blutgasverhaeltnisse und der

saeurbasenhaushalt des fetus bei ungestoertem geburtsverlauf. Z Geburtsch Gynak 161:262, 1963

7. **Hon EH, Khazin AF:** Biochemical studies of the fetus. I. The fetal pH-measuring system. Obstet Gynecol 33:219, 1969

8. **Bowe ET:** Fetal blood sampling: Maternal-fetal relationships. In Bowe ET (ed): Fetal Growth and Development. New York, McGraw-Hill, 1968

9. **Beard RW, Morris ED, Clayton SG:** pH of fetal capilliary blood as an indicator of the condition of the fetus. J Obstet Gynaecol Br Commonw 74:812, 1967

10. **Barcroft J:** Researches on Prenatal Life. Springfield, (Ill.) Charles C Thomas, 1947

11. **Reynolds SRM, Paul WM:** Relation of brady-cardia and blood pressure of the fetal lamb in utero to mild and severe hypoxia. Am J Physiol 193:249, 1958

12. **Myers RE:** Two patterns of perinatal brain damage and their conditions of occurrence. Am J Obstet Gynecol 112:246, 1972

13. **Paul RH, Hon EH:** A clinical fetal monitor. Obstet Gynecol 35:161, 1970

14. **Tipton R, Shelley T:** An index of fetal welfare in labour. J Obstet Gynaecol Br Commonw 78:702, 1971

15. **Paul RH:** Clinical fetal monitoring. Experience on a large clinical service. Am J Obstet Gynecol 113:573, 1972

16. **Gabert HA, Stenchever MA:** Continuous electronic monitoring of fetal heart rate during labor. Am J Obstet Gynecol 115:919, 1973

17. **Paul RH, Hon EH:** Clinical fetal monitoring: V. Effect on perinatal outcome. Am J Obstet Gynecol 118:529, 1974

18. **Quilligan EJ, Paul RH:** Fetal monitoring: Is it worth it? Obstet Gynecol 45:96, 1975

19. **Renou P, Chang A, Anderson I et al:** Controlled trial of fetal intensive care. Am J Obstet Gynecol 126:470, 1976

20. **Kelso IM, Parsons RJ, Lawrence GF, et al:** An assessment of continuous fetal heart rate monitoring in labor. A randomized trial. Am J Obstet Gynecol 131:526, 1978

21. **Amato JC:** Fetal monitoring in a community hospital. A statistical analysis. Obstet Gynecol 50:269, 1977

22. **Edington PT, Sibanda J, Beard RW:** Influence on clinical practise of routine intrapartum fetal monitoring. Br Med J 3:341, 1975

23. **Johnstone FD, Campbell DM, Hughes GT:** Has continuous intrapartum monitoring made any impact on fetal outcome. Lancet, 1298, 1978

24. **Koh KS, Greves D, Young S et al:** Experience with fetal monitoring in a university teaching hospital. Can Med Assoc J 112:455, 1975

25. **Lee WK, Baggish MS:** The effect of unselected intrapartum fetal monitoring. Obstet Gynecol 47:516, 1976

26. **Shenker L, Post RC, Seiler JS:** Routine electronic monitoring of fetal heart rate and uterine activity during labor. Obstet Gynecol 46:185, 1975

27. **Tutera G, Newman RL:** Fetal monitoring: Its effect on the perinatal mortality and cesarean section rates and its complications. Am J Obstet Gynecol 122:750, 1975

28. **Hon EH:** An Atlas of Fetal Heart Rate Patterns. New Haven, Harty Press, 1968

29. **Ray M, Freeman R, Pine S, Hesselgesser R:** Clinical experience with the oxytocin challenge test. Am J Obstet Gynecol 114:1, 1972

30. **Hon EH, Quilligan EJ:** The classification of fetal heart rate. II. A revised working classification. Conn Med 31:779, 1967

31. **Hon EH, Lee ST:** The electronic evaluation of the fetal heart rate. VIII. Patterns preceding fetal death; further observations. Am J Obstet Gynecol 87:814, 1963

32. **McCrady JD, Vallbona C, Hoff HE:** Neuro-origin of respiratory heart response. Am J Physiol 211:323, 1966

33. **DeHaan J:** The short term irregularity in the foetal heart rate pattern. Drukkerij van Denderen, Gronigen, 1971

34. **Bemmel JH van:** Proefschrift. Nijmegen, 1969

35. **Yeh Sze-ya, Forsythe A, Hon EH:** Quantification of fetal heart beat-to-beat interval differences, a numerical approach. Obstet Gynecol 41:355, 1973

36. **Kubli FW, Hon EH, Khazin AF, Takemura H:** Observations on heart rate and pH in the human fetus during labor. Am J Obstet Gynecol 104:1190, 1969

37. **Hon EH:** The detection of fetal distress. p. 58. Fifth World Congress of Gynaecology and Obstetrics, Australia, Butterworth & Co., 1967

38. **Schifrin BS, Dame L:** Fetal heart rate patterns. Prediction of Apgar score. JAMA, 219:322, 1972

39. **Hon EH:** Instrumentation of fetal heart rate and fetal electrocardiography. III. Fetal ECG electrodes: further observations. Obstet Gynecol 30:281, 1967

40. **Hon EH, Paul RH, Hon RW:** Electronic evaluation of fetal heart rate. XI. The description of a spiral electrode. Obstet Gynecol 40:362, 1972

41. **Hobel CJ, Hyvarinen MA, Oh W:** Abnormal fetal heart rate patterns and fetal acid-base balance in low birth weight infants in relation to respiratory distress syndrome. Obstet Gynecol 39:83, 1972

42. **Myers RE, Mueller–Heubach E, Adamsons K:** Predictability of the state of fetal oxygenation from a quantitative analysis of the components

of late deceleration. Am J Obstet Gynecol 115: 1083, 1973

43. **James LS, Morishima HO, Daniel SS et al:** Mechanism of late deceleration of the fetal heart rate. Am J Obstet Gynecol 113:578, 1972

44. **Haverkamp AD, Thompson HE, McFee JG et al:** The evaluation of continuous fetal heart rate monitoring in high-risk pregnancy. Am J Obstet Gynecol 125:310, 1976

45. **Beard RW, Edington PT, Sibanda J:** Effects of routine intrapartum monitoring on clinical practice. Contrib Gynecol Obstet 3:14, 1977

8

Obstetric Anesthesia

John Stephen Naulty

Obstetric anesthesia has, since its inception in the 19th century, been a controversial practice. This controversy has arisen from the very nature of obstetric anesthesia: the administration of powerful and potentially dangerous drugs to the parturient. These interventions may be beneficial (as in cesarian section), are usually benign, but are occasionally deleterious to the fetus. Thus, when considering the administration of an anesthetic during the puerperium, the risk/benefit ratio to both mother *and* fetus must be assessed. Not infrequently, techniques that benefit the mother by relieving her pain have been shown to be excessively hazardous to the fetus (*e.g.,* "twilight sleep," paracervical block) and have been largely abandoned. It is the goal of the practitioner of obstetric anesthesia to devise and employ techniques which maximize the pleasurable aspects of parturition while minimizing the risks to both mother and fetus. This chapter is designed to introduce the neonatal practitioner to the scientific background and techniques of modern obstetric anesthesia, and to discuss the effects of these techniques on the fetus and neonate.

THE PAIN OF PARTURITION

Childbirth is described by most women as a painful process. Labor pain is a subjective sensory experience initiated by stretching of the cervix, distention of the lower uterine segment, and ischemia of uterine muscle fibers with accumulation of metabolites.[1] Nerve impulses stimulated by these factors travel from the uterus and birth canal via two major pathways.

Uterine and Cervical Pain

The afferent nerve fibers from the uterus and cervix are somatic sensory fibers which travel with the sympathetic nervous supply to the uterus. These fibers pass through the paracervical tissue along the uterine artery, and then through the inferior, middle, and superior hypogastric plexuses to the sympathetic chain. These impulses then enter the spinal cord through the 10th, 11th, and 12th thoracic nerves.

Perineal Pain

Impulses arising from the vagina, vulva, and perineum, however, travel a different pathway. Sensory innervation of this area is through the pudendal nerve, which enters the central nervous system at the second, third, and fourth sacral nerves.

Central Nervous System

Upon entering the central nervous system, these impulses undergo modulation in the posterior horn of the spinal cord, decussate, and ascend to the brain stem through the lateral spinothalamic tract. In the brain stem, these impulses stimulate the reticular formation and tegmental tract, and then continue upward to the ventral posterolateral nucleus of the thalamus. From there, fibers project to the sensory cortex for **localization** and **discrimination** of pain.

There are also projections to the prefrontal cortex and the limbic system, which stimulates the **motivational** and **affective** components of pain. It is this **motivational-affective** component that can be modulated by psychological factors such as attention, suggestion, anxiety, expectations, and prior conditioning.[2]

LABOR PAIN

The normal pattern of the pain of parturition, then, can be predicted from the above information. During the first stage of labor, increasing uterine contractions lead to progressive uterine muscle ischemia, cervical dilation, and distention of the lower uterine segment. This leads to a progressive increase in painful sensation, which is felt mainly in the distribution of the 10th, 11th, and 12th thoracic dermatomes. The most severe labor pains usually occur during the late acceleration phase of labor, when cervical dilation and the strength of uterine contractions reach their maximum.

In the second stage of labor and during delivery, stretching of the tissues of the vagina and perineum are added to the pain of uterine contractions. These sensations are mainly felt and referred to the distribution of the second, third, and fourth sacral dermatomes.

Reflex Effects of Labor Pain

In addition to the subjective sensation of pain, these impulses lead to stimulation of the autonomic nervous system, and reflex cardiovascular, respiratory, and musculoskeletal effects.

Cardiovascular

Cardiovascular sympathetic nervous system stimulation may cause an increase in cardiac output by as much as 60% during labor.[3] Tachycardia, hypertension, and arrhythmias may occur. Uterine blood vessels have been shown to be particularly sensitive to sympathetic tone. Shnider has demonstrated that experimentally produced pain can reduce uterine blood flow in pregnant ewes by release of endogenous catecholamines.[4,5]

Respiratory

Hyperventilation is a common response to painful stimulation. Arterial carbon dioxide is severely reduced in some patients during labor. The resulting respiratory alkalosis may produce fetal hypoxia by shifting the maternal oxyhemoglobin dissociation curve to the left,[6] leading to decreased oxygen release at the placenta.[7]

Musculoskeletal

Maternal skeletal muscle expulsive efforts ("bearing down") may become an uncontrollable urge as a result of labor pain. Obstetric anesthesia has been shown to control these reflexes, and decrease the metabolic acidosis which may result from excessive musuclar efforts.[8]

ADMINISTRATION OF OBSTETRIC ANESTHESIA

Benefits

Properly performed obstetric analgesia not only reduces the psychological or subjective component of pain but may also be beneficial in preventing undesirable reflex effects in some patients. For example, patients with severe mitral regurgitation may undergo cardiac decompensation and congestive heart failure as a result of sympathetic stimulation. Decreasing this stimulation with obstetric anesthesia may prevent these adverse effects.

Methods

The impulses arising from labor pain may be blocked in many ways, and numerous methods of pain relief have been developed. Selection of any given technique depends on the stage of labor, maternal condition, fetal condition, and experience of the anesthesiologist and obstetric team.

The pain of the first stage of labor may be relieved in many ways. Paracervical, paravertebral, epidural, and spinal anesthetics may be used to prevent noxious impulses from either entering or ascending the spinal cord. The sensation of pain may be also blocked by systemic analgesia with narcotics or by inhalational analgesia with N_2O, trichloroethylene, or methoxyflurane. Finally, the motivational-affective component of pain may be blocked with psychological methods, hypnosis, or acupuncture.

These techniques may be continued in the second stage of labor. In addition, the pudendal nerve may be blocked to relieve perineal pain. All of these techniques are currently used in obstetric anesthesia practice and will be discussed at greater length in the following section.

CURRENT OBSTETRIC ANESTHETIC PRACTICE

Obstetric anesthesia has traditionally been a stepchild in many anesthesia departments. Because of unpredictable and widely fluctuating manpower requirements, many anesthesia departments have declined to provide 24-hour obstetric anesthesia coverage. The American Society of Anesthesiologists (ASA) viewed this as an undesirable development and, in 1978, a position paper was published by the ASA which stated that parturients were entitled to the same level of anesthetic care as elective surgical patients.[9] This should ideally include the availability of a full-time anesthesiologist with modern equipment for administering anesthetics and monitoring the parturient. This ideal situation is far from reality today. In 1970, the American College of Obstetricians and Gynecologists performed a survey which revealed that in only 37% of hospitals were personnel specifically trained in anesthesia administering obstetric anesthetics. It is to be hoped that the growing interest in perinatal medicine will spill over into obstetric anesthesia and cause an improvement in this chronic staffing problem.

In another survey, anesthesia was directly responsible for 8% of 950 maternal deaths in the United States.[11] More than two-thirds of these deaths were judged to have been preventable. John Bonica in 1969 stated, "In case there is a choice between poorly administered anesthesia and no anesthesia, the latter should be selected."[12]

OBSTETRIC ANESTHESIA WITHOUT DRUGS

Psychoanalgesia

Psychoanalgesia is the term used to describe a number of techniques designed to minimize the noxious effects of the pain of parturition, such as the natural childbirth described by

Read in 1944,[13] Jacobsens' physiologic relaxation technique, and the Lamaze[15] and Bradley[16] techniques. Modern psychoanalgesic techniques combine a number of these approaches. They emphasize antenatal preparation and education to allay many of the anxieties associated with parturition; relaxation techniques to minimize the contribution of skeletal muscle spasm to labor pain; and the development of conditioned responses to uterine contractions which are designed to distract the parturient from the sensation of pain. These techniques do not make childbirth painless but rather are designed to convert the painful experience to a controllable positive experience. Psychoanalgesic techniques have proven to be very useful and generally adequate for delivery in about 20% to 30% of parturients.[17] When combined with other analgesic methods, psychoanalgesia may be effective in a larger percentage of the population.[18]

Psychoanalgesia, however, is not without risk. The breathing techniques of psychoanalgesia are designed to minimize hyperventilation, but some parturients develop severe hyperventilation, which shifts the maternal oxyhemoglobin dissociation curve to the left. This may interfere with placental oxygen exchange, and Saling and Ligidas in 1969 reported that neonates of hyperventilating parturients were more acidotic than a control group who did not hyperventilate.[19] Zador and Nillson in 1974 found that fetal acid-base balance during prolonged labor was better maintained during epidural anesthesia than in control patients who received no anesthesia.[20]

In addition, psychoanalgesic technique requires a high level of personal concentration and is not entirely reliable. Some enthusiasts of psychoanalgesic technique promote them as being applicable to all deliveries. Therefore, a woman who experiences severe pain during parturition and who wishes further anesthesia may feel as if she has failed. It is important to stress to the parturient that not all patients will find the technique adequate and further anesthetic intervention may be desirable or necessary.

A technique which is frequently associated today with psychoanalgesia is the so-called LeBoyer delivery. This method consists of birth in a semi-darkened, quiet, warm room; the neonate is placed immediately on the mother's abdomen; and the cord cut only after pulsations cease. The neonate is then immersed in a tub of warm water. The benefits of this method of delivery are debatable,[22] and one must be aware of the difficulty experienced in recognizing and treating the unexpectedly depressed neonate in such a situation. There is no justification for performing emergency neonatal resuscitation in semi-darkness with the neonate either on the mother's abdomen or in warm water. A physician called upon to resuscitate a neonate during a Leboyer delivery should first obtain adequate lighting and positioning of the neonate.

Hypnosis

Another method of disrupting the motivational affective element of the pain of parturition is hypnotic suggestion. One can provide adequate maternal analgesia with hypnosis in patients with high suggestibility. There appears to be no interference with normal reflexes and no depression of the infant.[23] Preparation of the patient for hypnosis requires a series of conditioning sessions prior to delivery. During these sessions, the parturient is taught to produce analgesia on some part of the body and is then conditioned to transfer this analgesia to the abdomen and perineum to provide pain relief for labor and delivery. A successful series of conditioning sessions allows the parturient to perform this maneuver during labor without the hypnotist actually being present. The hypnotic state may shorten labor,[24] and the acid-base status of neonates is apparently improved at birth and in the hour following, compared with other methods of analgesia.[23]

Notwithstanding these advantages, hypnoanalgesia is only rarely employed in obstetric practice today. Its lack of usage probably arises from relative paucity of skilled practitioners and from the staffing problems in obstetric units in general. In addition, Wahl reported a high incidence of psychological complications ranging from frank anxiety to psychosis following hypnosis for obstetric anesthesia.[25] Certainly, further investigations of the use of hypnosis in obstetric anesthesia should be carried out.

Acupuncture

Since acupuncture would seem to be completely safe for mother and newborn, its use for the relief of labor pain has been investi-gated. Wallis, *et. al.,*[26] reported that 19 of his 21 patients had analgesia using the traditional acupuncture points for vaginal hysterectomy and dysmemorrhea. None of the 21 subjects was judged by the investigator to have adequate analgesia. Acupuncture is useful in many pain states, but its role in obstetrical analgesia at this time remains unclear.

OBSTETRIC ANESTHESIA USING DRUGS

Labor pain that cannot be controlled with the above techniques may require additional anesthetic intervention. These techniques employ either intramuscular (IM), intravenous (IV), or inhalational administration of sedative or analgesic drugs, or the perineural application of local anesthetic drugs. These drugs and the techniques currently used will first be presented, and then their effects on the maternal-fetal unit will be discussed.

Techniques of IV or IM Medication

The systemic administration of sedatives, tranquilizers, and narcotics to the parturient is probably the most popular method of obstetric analgesia today. In the past, large doses of the drugs were employed to create the state of "twilight sleep." Increasing realization of the adverse affects of excessive medication on both mother and fetus has led to a reduction in dosage of these drugs. In addition, as discussed in Chapter 46, better understanding of maternal uptake, distribution, and placental transfer has led to a more rational and safer selection of methods of administration and timing of these drugs in labor.

Current practice employs small doses of minimally depressant drugs administered intravenously early in labor. As discussed in Chapter 46, this leads to a minimum amount of placental transfer of these medications, and hence, a minimally depressed neonate.

The major group of drugs employed today are sedative-tranquilizers, narcotic analgesics, and dissociative anesthetics.

Sedative-tranquilizers. These drugs are administered to the parturient to diminish the adverse motivational-affective component of labor pain. Examples of such drugs are barbiturates, phenothiazines, and benzodiazepines.

Barbiturates. Secobarbital (Seconal) and pentobarbital (Nembutal) have been employed

Table 8-1. Narcotic Analgesics in OB Practice.

	Dosage	Onset	Duration
Meperidine	20–100 mg IM	40–50 min	3–4 hr +
	25–50 mg IV	5–10 min	3–4 hr
Alphaprodine	20–30 mg subcu	5–10 min	1–2 hr +
	10–20 mg IV	1–2 min	1–2 hr
Pentazocine	20–30 mg IM	10–20 min	3–4 hr +
	10–20 mg IV	2–3 min	3–4 hr
Fentanyl	50–100 μg IM	7–8 min	½–2 hr
	25–50 μg IV	3–5 min	½–2 hr

in obstetrics. Because of their prolonged effects, their principal use today is during the early latent phase of labor when delivery is not likely to occur before 12 to 24 hours.[27] Barbiturates have been described as having "anti-analgetic effects"; they may convert a minimally uncomfortable, controlled patient into a hyperventilating, confused, and unmanageable one.[28] For this reason, they are rarely used today.

Phenothiazines. Promethazine (Phenergan) and propiomazine (Largon) are the drugs in this class commonly employed in obstetrics. Hydroxyzine (Vistaril), although not a phenothiazine, has similar properties. These drugs are useful for relieving anxiety, and hence modify the response to painful stimulation. They are less likely than the barbiturates to cause "anti-analgesia," and they potentiate the actions of the narcotic analgesics.

In addition, they are useful in controlling nausea and vomiting, which may be severe enough in some labors to produce maternal dehydration. In the recommended intramuscular dosages (promethazine 50 mg IV, propiomazine 20 mg IV, hydroxyzine 50–100 mg IV), these drugs appear to have minimal depressant effects on both mother and fetus.[29–30]

Benzodiazepines. Diazepam (Valium) is the most widely prescribed drug in the world, and it is not surprising that it has been employed as an anxiolytic agent in obstetrics. Its use is controversial (see *Fetal effects*), but it is capable of reducing maternal anxiety, decreasing narcotic dosage, and antagonizing the convulsions associated with local anesthetic toxicity or eclampsia. When used in small doses (2.5–10 mg IV), diazepam appears to be without significant adverse fetal or neonatal effects.[31]

Narcotics. Narcotic analgesics are extremely effective antagonists of the motivational-affective and to a lesser extent, the sensory-discriminatory aspect of the pain of parturition. A wide variety of narcotics are currently available, but those most commonly in use in obstetrics include meperidine (Demerol), alphaprodine (Nisentil), pentazocine (Talwin), and fentanyl (Sublimaze). All narcotics share the same mechanism of action and similar side effects: nausea, vomiting, orthostatic hypotension, and respiratory depression. They differ chiefly in their potency, time of onset, and duration of action. (Table 8-1).

Narcotics are incapable of producing complete analgesia, however, except in doses that produce severe respiratory depression.[32] In addition, they are incompletely effective in blocking the sympathetic response to painful stimulation.[33] If this is deemed necessary (*e.g.*, in cardiac disease or toxemia), then more profound anesthetic techniques must be used, such as general anesthesia or regional anesthesia.

General Analgesia and Anesthesia

The further extension of the concept of systemic medication for the relief of labor pain is general analgesia and anesthesia. **General analgesia** consists of administration of subanesthetic concentrations of inhalational agents (nitrous oxide, methoxyflurane, trichoroethylene) which provide analgesia roughly equivalent to narcotic analgesics. The goal of general analgesia is that the patient remain awake and cooperative, and maintain protective laryngeal reflexes during the administration of the inhalational agent. **General anesthesia** further extends the scope of inhalational analgesia and provides profound analgesia, amnesia, hypnosis, and muscle relaxation.

Various types of general anesthesia and analgesia are available, using a wide variety of drugs. The techniques commonly applied to obstetrics include intermittent inhalational analgesia, dissociative general anesthesia (ketamine), and a general endotracheal anesthesia supplemented with neuromuscular blockers.

Intermittent Inhalational Analgesia. This technique was first applied by Simpson in 1847 and consists of the inhalation by the parturient of subanesthetic concentrations of inhalation agents. This technique may have an advantage over narcotics because of the rapid onset and reversibility of the analgesia produced.

The technique is simple in concept; the parturient self-administers an anesthetic agent from an inhaler device during the time of contractions. This apparent simplicity is a major hazard of the technique because the staffing of many obstetric units may lead to inadequate observation of the parturient. This is hazardous because the physiology of the pregnant state predisposes to overdosage with inhalation anesthesia.[34] The functional residual capacity of the lungs is reduced, and alveolar ventilation is increased, which, combined with the reduced anesthetic requirements noted in pregnancy,[35] leads to a rapid induction of the unconscious, *anesthetized* state, rather than the *analgesic* state desired. Thus, the major risk of inhalational analgesia is inadvertent, unobserved overdosage, with loss of consciousness and protective laryngeal reflexes. Maternal regurgitation, vomiting, and aspiration may then occur, leading to airway obstruction, asphyxia, and aspiration pneumonitis. It is estimated that approximately 5% to 15% of maternal deaths in the United States are attributable to anesthesia, with half of these being the sequelae of aspiration.[11,36] If the parturient is carefully observed, however, the risks of overdosage may be minimized, and inhalation analgesia safely administered.

Dissociative Analgesia. The intramuscular or intravenous administration of low-dose ketamine (Ketalar) produces a state known as dissociative analgesia. This state is characterized by an intense analgesia and amnesia, without loss of consciousness or protective airway reflexes.[37]

This is accompanied by a dreaming phenomenon which may be unpleasant. Used in doses less than 1 mg/kg, ketamine provides adequate analgesia for vaginal delivery and episiotomy repair, and has become widely used for this purpose.

General Anesthesia. General anesthesia is used in obstetric practice both for vaginal delivery and cesarian section. It should not be used without endotracheal intubation, because of the risks of aspiration of gastric contents. The technique consists of the administration of a combination of a muscle relaxant, a sedative, hypnotic drug, a narcotic or inhalational agent and nitrous oxide. Examples of commonly used drugs are listed in Table 8-2.

General anesthesia is frequently chosen for use in emergency obstetrics because of its rapidity and predictability. Used properly, general anesthesia is safe, with certain limitations which will be discussed under *Fetal effects.*

Major Regional Analgesia and Anesthesia

In many centers, regional analgesia and anesthesia for labor and delivery is the technique of choice. The parturient remains awake and cooperative, the risks of aspiration of vomitus are minimized, and excellent, predictable analgesia can be provided. The commonly employed methods of major regional anesthesia for parturition are subarachnoid (spinal) block and peridural (caudal or lumbar epidural) block.

Subarachnoid Block (Spinal Anesthesia). Spinal anesthesia is usually administered immediately before delivery. A small dose of a local anesthetic (*e.g.,* 4 mg tetracaine or 20 mg lidocaine) dissolved in a hyperbaric dextrose solution is injected into the subarachnoid space with the patient in the sitting position. This produces immediate analgesia of the lumbosacral nerve roots, and provides excellent anesthesia for episiotomy, forceps application, and delivery.

Peridural Block (Caudal, Epidural Anesthesia). Peridural block is usually performed early in labor, as soon as a satisfactory progress of labor is established (usually 6–8 cm cervical dilation in nulliparas, less in multiparas). A needle is placed by a variety of techniques and enters the potential space just outside the dura, the so-called peridural space. A plastic catheter is then introduced through the needle, the needle removed, and local anesthetic solutions injected through the catheter. By this means, analgesia may be attained and continued

Table 8-2. Drugs Commonly Used in General Anesthesia.

| Nitrous Oxide | A combination of | | |
	Muscle Relaxant	Sedative-Hypnotic	Analgesic Drug
N$_2$O 50%–70%	Succinylcholine 1.5 mg/kg IV; infusion of 0.1%	Thiopental 4 mg/kg IV	Narcotics (see Table 8-1)
	OR D-tubocurarine 0.1–0.6 mg/kg IV	OR Ketamine 1–2 mg/kg IV	OR Halothane .25–0.5%
	OR Pancuronium 0.05–0.1 mg/ kg IV		OR Methoxyflurane 0.1%
			OR Enflurane 0.5–0.75%

throughout the active phase of labor and delivery.

The drugs commonly employed for labor and delivery are described in Table 8-3.

Complication of Spinal and Peridural Block. *Hypotension* secondary to sympathetic blockade is the most common complication of major regional block for parturition.[38] Because uterine blood flow is reduced by hypotension, this complication must be avoided.[39] Prophylactic measures include adequate hydration, avoidance of the supine position, and displacement of the uterus off the abdominal great vessels. If hypotension occurs despite these measures, prompt treatment with further intravenous fluids, more uterine displacement, and vasopressor (ephedrine 10–20 mg IV) administration should be instituted. Transient hypoten-

Table 8-3. Drugs for Peridural Anesthesia.

| Drug | Concentration | Dosage | |
		Labor	*Delivery*
Bupivacaine (Marcaine)	0.125–0.5%	4–8 ml	10–12 ml
2-Chloro-procaine	1.5–3%	5–8 ml	10–15 ml

sion, if treated promptly, does not produce fetal depression or morbidity.[40]

Local Anesthetic Convulsions. High blood levels of local anesthetics may produce excitation of the central nervous system, seizures, and cardiovascular depression. High levels may occur from either overdosage or inadvertent intravascular injection of local anesthetic drugs. If these occur, the mother should have an airway secured and be given oxygen and small doses of barbiturates or diazepam. The circulation must be maintained and cardiopulmonary resuscitation initiated if required. Resuscitation and support of the mother will reestablish uterine blood flow and allow adequate fetal oxygenation and excretion of local anesthetic.[41] Unless the mother cannot be resuscitated, delivery of the fetus should not be attempted, because the neonate has an extremely limited ability to excrete local anesthetics and may have convulsions for many days.[41]

Hypoventilation. At any time during subarachnoid or peridural anesthesia, an excessive level of neural blockade may develop, leading to blockade of the motor nerves of the respiratory musculature. This paralysis may produce hypoventilation—the so-called "total spinal." Treatment of this complication consists of securing a protected airway (*e.g.*, endotracheal intubation) and ventilation with oxygen. This complication must be watched for at all times during major regional anesthesia because its onset may be insidious and go unnoticed until severe hypoxic damage occurs to both mother and fetus.

Minor Regional Anesthesia. Other regional anesthetic techniques have been employed for parturition. These techniques, including paracervical and pudendal block and local perineal infiltration, are commonly employed by obstetricians. Paracervical block is useful in the first stage of labor, and pudendal block and local infiltration are useful for delivery. Analgesia is not as profound as during major regional block, but complications such as hypotension and hypoventilation are avoided. Local anesthetic convulsions, however, may occur as a result of these techniques and their treatment should be as outlined above. In addition, paracervical block is associated with a high incidence of fetal bradycardia following the block.[42] The etiology of this phenomenon is unclear, but is probably due to a combination of decreased uterine blood flow secondary to the vasoconstrictor properties of local anesthetics, and from high fetal local anesthetic levels.[40] This bradycardia is associated with increased neonatal morbidity and mortality.[43] For this reason, this block is rarely performed, and should be employed only in low-risk pregnancies.

FETAL AND NEONATAL EFFECTS OF OBSTETRICAL ANESTHESIA

Maternal anesthetics may adversely affect the fetus and neonate by two mechanisms. First, drugs administered to the mother may diffuse from the maternal circulation to the fetal circulation causing **direct** drug effects. These are drug-specific effects, predictable from the pharmacology of the drug concerned, with treatment dependent on the particular drug. Second, an anesthetic drug or technique may **indirectly** affect the fetus, producing the signs and symptoms of fetal distress and asphyxia, and treatment is based upon restoring placental exchange, perfusion, and gas exchange. These two types of adverse interactions may coexist in the same patient and both effects may be observed in the neonates.

Direct Effects of Anesthetic Drugs

When a drug is present in sufficient concentration in the fetus it will exert direct pharmacologic effects. Chapter 46 discusses perinatal drug transfer, and Figure 8-1 summarizes this subject. It can be seen that serial dilutions and protein-tissue binding serve to protect the fetus from the effects of maternally-administered drugs. If, however, an excessive amount of any anesthetic drug is administered, or some of the serial dilutions are bypassed, (as in IV injection of local anesthetics, or injection directly into the uterine artery or fetus in paracervical blocks) then even a small amount of drug may exert profound effects. The effects observed vary with the specific drug concerned.

Sedative-Tranquilizers. Barbiturates. Barbiturates are highly lipid-soluble drugs which rapidly cross the placenta and produce a dose-related global depression in the neonate. Their primary use today occurs in low dosage for general anesthesia for cesarian section (thiopental 4 mg/kg). Maternal protein binding and maternal-fetal organ uptake usually prevent significant depression of the neonate. However, neonatal depression is found with higher dosages of barbiturates, (*e.g.*, thiopental 8 mg/kg), which must be treated by cardiorespiratory supportive techniques until the neonate can excrete the drug. This process may take up to 2 days.[43]

Phenothiazines. These drugs rapidly cross the placenta and have been noted to cause a decrease in fetal beat-to-beat variability. However, when used in the recommended dosages, these drugs do not seem to cause neonatal depression, at least as measured by Apgar scores.[29] An inadvertent overdosage of these medications should be treated similarly to barbiturate-induced depression.

Benzodiazephines. Diazepam (Valium), the most commonly employed member of this drug group, rapidly crosses the placenta, with approximately equal maternal and fetal blood levels within minutes of IV administration.[44] In addition, the neonate has a limited ability to excrete diazepam, and the drug and its active metabolite may persist in significant amounts in the neonate for a week.[45] The drug may produce hypotonia, lethargy, and hypothermia when used in large doses (30 mg).[45] However, when used in small doses 2.5–10

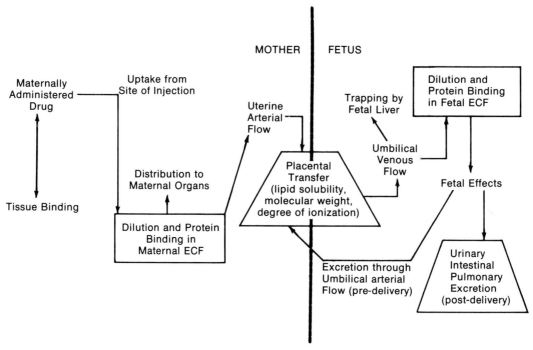

Fig. 8-1. *Perinatal drug transfer.* Maternally administered drugs are taken up by the maternal circulation from the site of administration at a rate dependent on perfusion of the administration site, tissue binding at the administration site, and the amount administered. In the maternal extracellular fluid (ECF), drugs are bound to protein and diluted by the volume of distribution of the drug. The amount present in the uterine arteries is available for placental diffusion. Depending on the physiochemical properties of the drug (*e.g.,* high lipid solubility, low molecular weight, and low ionization produce rapid placental transfer), the drug appears in the umbilical vein. After passage through the fetal liver and further dilution and protein binding in the fetal ECF, the drug can exert fetal effects. The effects of the drug are terminated by excretion—either placental (pre-delivery) or renal, intestinal, or pulmonary (post-delivery).

mg IV), minimal sedation and hypotonia have been observed.[31] It would appear, then, that low-dose diazepam is a safe anxiolytic drug, but that particular attention must be paid to providing a warm environment for these infants for at least 36 hours after delivery.

Narcotics. The lipid-soluble, poorly ionized narcotic analgesics rapidly enter the fetal circulation after maternal administration. Their chief fetal effect is a dose-related respiratory depression, as evidenced by a rightward shift in the carbon dioxide response curve. The amount of depression seen is a function of the amount of drug administered, the timing and route of administration.[41] IM administration appears to be associated with a high incidence of neonatal depression 2 to 4 hours after injection, which is the usual time when delivery may be expected. Therefore, IM injection of meperidine has, in many centers, been re-

placed by IV injection, which produces peak neonatal depression at 30 to 60 minutes post-injection, a time when delivery is less likely. If a neonate is suspected of narcotic-related depression, the administration of naloxone (Narcan), .01 mg/kg IV, will produce a reversal of the drug depression within 1 to 2 minutes and will last 1 to 2 hours. Because narcotic-induced respiration depression has been reported to last up to 5 hours,[47] the infant should be carefully observed, and later doses of naloxone administered if renarcotization occurs (Table 8-1).

General Anesthetics. Inhalational Agents. Placental transfer of inhalational agents is rapid, because these are nonionized, highly lipid-soluble substances of low molecular weight. The concentrations of these agents in the fetus is directly dependent on the concentration and duration of anesthetic in the mother. If excessive concentrations of anesthetic are given for inordinately long times, the incidence of fetal depression is increased.[48,49] If the anesthetic concentrations specified in Table 8-2 are exceeded or administered for induction to delivery times of greater than 20 minutes,[50] neonatal depression (evidenced by flaccidity, cardiorespiratory depression, and decreased tone) may be anticipated. Treatment should include effective cardiopulmonary resuscitation which will allow excretion of the inhalational anesthetic by the baby's lungs. Rapid improvement of Apgar scores should be expected, and, if not forthcoming in 5 to 10 minutes, a search for other causes of depression should be begun.

Neuromuscular Blockers. Nondepolarizing Neuromuscular Blockers. Under normal circumstances the poorly lipid-soluble, highly ionized, nondepolarizing neuromuscular blockers (d-tubocurarine, pancuronium) do not cross the placenta in significant amounts, and neonatal muscle weakness is not found.[51,52] This placental impermeability is only relative, however, and when large doses are given over long periods of time, as in the treatment of maternal tetanus or status epilepticus, neonatal neuromuscular blockade can occur.[53]

Depolarizing Neuromuscular Blockers. Succinylcholine, normally hydrolyzed in maternal blood by the enzyme pseudocholinesterase, does not usually interfere with fetal neuromuscular activity. However, if the hydrolytic enzyme is either present in low concentrations[54] or in a genetically determined atypical form,[55] prolonged maternal and neonatal respiratory depression secondary to muscular paralysis can occur.

Diagnosis and Treatment of Neonatal Neuromuscular Blockade. The diagnosis of neonatal depression secondary to neuromuscular blockade may be made on the basis of the maternal history (*e.g.,* prolonged administration of neuromuscular blockers or history of atypical psudocholinesterase), the response of the mother to neuromuscular blocking drugs, and the physical examination of the newborn. The paralyzed neonate will have normal cardiovascular function and good color, but no spontaneous ventilatory movements, muscle flaccidity, and no reflex responses. The anesthesiologist can place a nerve stimulator on the neonate and demonstrate the classical signs of neuromuscular blockade.[56]

Table 8-4. Local Anesthetics.

Ester	Amide
Procaine (Novocaine)	Mepivacaine (Carbocaine)
Chloroprocaine (Nesacaine)	Etidocaine (Duranest)
Tetacaine (Pontocaine)	Lidocaine (Xylocaine)
	Bupivacaine (Marcaine)

Treatment consists of respiratory support until the drug is excreted by the neonate, which may take 24 to 48 hours. Reversal of nondepolarizing relaxants with cholinesterase inhibitors may be attempted (*e.g.,* neostigmine .06 mg/kg), but adequate respiratory support should be the mainstay of treatment.

Local Anesthetics. The local anesthetic drugs in common use today are divided into two groups: ester and amide (Table 8-4). They differ in their mode of metabolism and in their fetal effects.

Ester Local Anesthetics are broken down in the maternal blood by pseudocholinesterase, the same enzyme responsible for the hydrolysis of succinylcholine. If normal levels of the enzyme are present, the half-life of these drugs in the maternal serum is extremely short (e.g., 21 sec for 2-chloroprocaine) and therefore, the amount available for placental transfer is limited.[57] If, however, the enzyme is deficient or atypical more local anesthetic is available for diffusion across the placenta, and fetal seizures and cardiorespiratory depression can occur.

Amide Local Anesthetics. The primary metabolic pathway for the excretion of these drugs is through the liver. This is a much slower process than the hydrolysis of esters, and significant maternal blood levels of these drugs may be produced during regional anesthesia. These drugs are arranged in Table 8-4 in the order of their placental permeability, with mepivacaine exhibiting the most placental transfer and bupivacaine the least.[58] In addition, bupivacaine and etidocaine are highly protein-bound in maternal tissues and serum, decreasing placental transfer.[40] If, however, a direct intravascular or intrafetal injection of any of the drugs occurs, significant depression can occur, exhibited by bradycardia and acidosis.

Treatment of Local Anesthetic Toxicity. The most important principle to follow if large amounts of any local anesthetic reach the fetus during regional anesthesia is *not* to attempt to deliver the baby immediately. If maternal cardiorespiratory support is provided, these reactions will be brief and the local anesthetic which has reached the fetus will diffuse back to the mother where the drugs can be redistributed, metabolized, and excreted. If delivery is effected, this route of excretion is lost. The neonate has an extremely limited ability to metabolize and excrete amide local anesthetics and prolonged seizures and cardio-respiratory depression can be expected.[40]

Indirect Effects of Anesthetic Drugs

In addition to the specific effects of the drugs listed above, all obstetric anesthetic techniques can also adversely affect the fetus and neonate by interfering with normal placental gas exchange. There are several mechanisms by which this can occur.

Decreased Arterial Oxygen Content. Any technique that produces maternal hypoxia will decrease maternal-fetal oxygen exchange and produce fetal distress. Examples of this phenomena include overdosage with narcotics or inhalational analgesia, total spinal anesthesia, or the maternal aspiration of vomitus.

Decreased Systemic Perfusion. Uteroplacental blood flow is dependent on an adequate maternal cardiac output and perfusion pressure. Anesthetic techniques which interfere with maternal cardiovascular integrity can produce fetal depression. This can be provoked by several mechanisms:

1. Decreased cardiac output secondary to decreased venous return can occur from vena cava compression by the gravid uterus (supine hypotension syndrome) or venodilation and bradycardia secondary to the sympathectomy accompanying spinal or peridural block.
2. Decreased cardiac output secondary to myocardial depression, usually produced by an overdose of potent inhalational anesthetic or local anesthetic drug
3. Decreased systemic blood pressure caused by the sympathectomy of high-spinal or peridural anesthesia

Uterine Arterial Vasoconstriction. Some local anesthetic drugs, notably lidocaine and mepivacaine, can cause constriction of uterine artery segments.[40] This is thought to be at least part of the etiology of fetal bradycardia following paracervical block and IV injections of local anesthetics.

The use of vasopressors to treat hypotension secondary to the sympathectomy of regional anesthesia can also cause uterine vasoconstriction. Drugs with primarily α-adrenergic activity should be avoided because the uterine arterial vasoconstriction they provoke worsens uterine blood flow. Drugs such as ephedrine and mephentermine, will have primarily β effects, restoring blood flow to normal values in this situation.[59]

Increased Uterine Tone. An increase in uterine muscular tone can decrease uteroplacental perfusion by impeding venous outflow from the intervillous space.[60] High levels of local anesthetics (*e.g.,* after intravascular injection) or α-adrenergic vasopressors may produce increased myometrial tone and fetal distress, particularly when combined with oxytocic stimulation.[61]

Diagnosis and Treatment of Indirect Fetal Depression. The decreases in uteroplacental perfusion caused by the above mechanisms all lead to the signs of fetal distress when fetal monitoring is employed.[62] For this reason, it is imperative when any obstetric anesthetic technique is employed, that continuous fetal heart-rate monitoring be likewise initiated. Detection of decreased beat-to-beat variability, late decelerations, or prolonged fetal bradycardia should prompt a search for the cause of the asphyxic insult. Treatment should then be directed at correcting the cause, by increasing cardiac output or systemic blood pressure with appropriate vasopressors, position changes, administrations of oxygen, decreasing oxytocic infusions, and so on.

CONCLUSION

The process of parturition is a painful process. The commonly employed methods of pain control in obstetrics have been presented. The fetal and neonatal effects of these techniques may be direct effects of the drugs employed, or produced indirectly via interference with placental gas exchange. Methods of recognizing and treating these adverse reactions have been proposed.

Although no method of obstetric pain control is totally devoid of fetal interaction, safe analgesia can be provided for the parturient if a skilled and alert perinatal team, consisting of obstetrician, anesthesiologist, and neonatologist, is available to treat the complications which may arise.

REFERENCES

1. **Crawford JS:** Principles and Practice of Obstetric Anaesthesia, p. 63. Oxford, Blackwell Scientific Publications, 1978
2. **Abouleish E:** Pain Control in Obstetrics, p. 15. Philadelphia, JB Lippincott, 1977
3. **Ueland K, Hansen J:** Maternal cardiovascular dynamics, II. Posture and uterine contractions. Am J Obstet Gynecol 103:1, 1969
4. **Shnider SM, Wright RG, Levinson G et al:** Uterine Blood flow and plasma norepinephrine changes during maternal stress in the pregnant ewe. Anesthesiology 50:524, 1979
5. **Myers RE:** Maternal psychologic stress and fetal asphyxia: A study in the monkey. Am J Obstet Gynecol 122:47, 1975
6. **Motoyama EK, Rivard G, Acheson F et al:** Adverse effect of maternal hyperventilation on the fetus. Am J Obstet Gynecol 122:47, 1975
7. **Ralston DH, Shnider SM, De Lorimer AA:** Uterine blood flow and fetal acid-base changes after bicarbonate administration in the pregnant ewe. Anesthesiology 40:348 1974
8. **Pearson JF, Davies P:** The effect of continuous epidural analgesia on maternal acid-base balance and arterial lactate concentration during the second stage of labour. J Obstet Gynaecol Br Commonw 80:225, 1973
9. **American Society of Anesthesiologists:** Guidelines for Anesthetic Practice, Chicago, American Society of Anesthesiologists, 1979
10. **American College of Obstetricians and Gynecologists:** National Survey of Maternity Care. Chicago, The American Society of Obstetricians and Gynecologists, 1970
11. **Bonica JJ:** Anesthetic Deaths. In Principles and Practice of Obstetric Anesthesia, p. 75. Philadelphia, FA Davis, 1972 p. 751
12. **Bonica JJ:** Anesthetic Deaths. In Principles and Practice of Obstetric Anesthesia, p. 752. Philadelphia, FA Davis, 1972
13. **Dick–Read G:** Childbirth Without Fear. New York, Harper and Row, 1959
14. **Jacobsen E:** How to Relax and Have your Baby. New York, McGraw–Hill, 1959
15. **Lamaze F:** Painless Childbirth: Psychoprophylactic Method. London, Burke, 1958
16. **Bradley RA:** Husband Coached Childbirth. New York, Harper and Row, 1974
17. **Beazley JM, Leaver EP, Morewood JHM et al:** Relief of pain in labour. Lancet 1:1003, 1967
18. **Doering SG, Entwisle DR:** Preparation during pregnancy and ability to cope with labor and delivery. Am J. Orthopsychiatry 45:825, 1975
19. **Saling E, Ligidas P:** The effect on the fetus of maternal hyperventilation during labour. J Obstet Gynaecol Br Commonw 76:877, 1969
20. **Zador G, Nillson BA:** Low dose intermittent epidural anesthesia with lidocaine for vaginal delivery. Acta Obstet Gynecol Scand [Suppl] 34:17, 1974
21. **Leboyer F:** Birth without Violence. London, Wildwood House, 1975
22. **Nelson NM, Enkin MW, Saigal S et al:** A randomized clinical trial of the Leboyer approach to childbirth. N Engl J Med 302:655, 1980
23. **Moya F, James LS:** Medical hypnosis for obstetrics. JAMA 174:2026, 1960
24. **Flowers CE, Littlejohn TW, Wells HB:** Pharmacologic and hypnoid analgesia. Obstet Gynecol 16:210, 1960
25. **Wahl CW:** Contraindications and limitations of hypnosis in obstetric analgesia. Am J Obstet Gynecol 84:1869, 1962
26. **Wallis L, Shnider SM, Palahniuk RJ et al:** An evaluation of acupuncture analgesia in obstetrics. Anesthesiology 41:596, 1974
27. **Levinson G, Shnider SM:** Systemic medication for labor and delivery. In Anesthesia for Obstetrics, p. 76. Baltimore, Williams and Wilkins, 1979
28. **Dundee JW:** Alterations in response to somatic pain associated with anesthesia, II. The effect of thiopentone and pentobarbitone. Br J Anaesth 32:407, 1960
29. **Powe CE, Kiem IM, Fromhagen C et al:** Propiomazine hydrochloride in obstetrical analgesia. JAMA 181:290, 1962
30. **Benson C, Benson RC:** Hydroxyzine-meperidine analgesia and neonatal response. Am J Obstet Gynecol 84:37. 1962
31. **Rolbin SH, Wright RG, Shnider SM et al:** Diazepam during cesarian section, p. 449. Abstracts of Scientific Papers, Annual Meeting, American Society of Anesthesiologists, New Orleans, 1977
32. **Levinson G, Shnider SM:** Systemic medication for labor and delivery. In Anesthesia for Obstetrics, p. 79. Baltimore, Williams and Wilkins, 1979
33. **Levinson G, Shnider SM:** Systemic medication for labor and delivery. In Anesthesia for Obstetrics. Baltimore, Williams and Wilkins, 1979
35. **Palahnuik RJ, Shnider SM, Eger EI II:** Pregnancy decreases the requirement for inhaled anesthetic agents. Anesthesiology 41:82, 1974
36. **Bond VK, Ragan WD:** Maternal mortality in Indiana as related to anesthesia, p. 13. Abstracts of Scientific Papers, Annual Meeting

Society for Obstetric Anesthesia and Perinatology, Seattle, 1977.

37. **Galloon S:** Ketamine for obstetric delivery. Anesthesiology 44:522, 1976

38. **Shnider SM:** Experience with regional anesthesia for labor and delivery. In The Anesthesiologist, Mother and Newborn, p. 38. Baltimore, Williams and Wilkins, 1974

39. **Wallis KL, Shnider SM, Hicks JS et al:** Epidural anesthesia in the normotensive pregnant ewe. Anesthesiology 44:481, 1976

40. **Ralston DH, Shnider SM:** The fetal and neonatal effects of regional anesthesia in obstetrics. Anesthesiology 48:34, 1978

41. **Morishima HO, Adamsons K:** Placental clearance of mepivacaine following administration to the guinea pig fetus. Anesthesiology 28:343, 1967

42. **Thiery M, Vroman S:** Paracervical block analgesia during labour. Am J Obstet Gynecol 113:988, 1972

43. **Villee CA:** Placental transfer of drugs. Ann NY Acad Sci 123:237, 1965

44. **Scher J, Hailey DM:** The effects of diazepam on the fetus. J Obstet Gynaecol Br Commonw 79:635, 1972

45. **Cree IE, Meyer J, Hailey DM:** Diazepam in labour. Br Med J 4:251, 1973

46. **Shnider SM, Moya F:** Effects of meperidine on the newborn infant. Am J Obstet Gynecol 89:1009, 1969

47. **Koch G, Wandel H:** Effects of pethidine on the postnatal adjustment of respiration and acid-base balance. Acta Obstet Gynecol Scand 47:27, 1968

48. **Moya F:** Volatile inhalation agents and muscle relaxants in obstetrics. Acta Anesthesiol Scand [Suppl] 25:368, 1966

49. **Fox FS, Smith JB, Namba Y et al:** Anesthesia for cesarian section. Am J Obstet Gynecol 133:15, 1979

50. **Marx GF, Joshi CW, Orkin LR:** Placental transmission of nitrous oxide. Anesthesiology 32:429, 1970

51. **Kivalo I, Saaroski S:** Placental transmission and foetal uptake of ^{14}C-dimethyltubocurarine. Br J Anesth 44:557, 1972

52. **Latto IP, Wainwright AC:** Anesthesia for cesarian section, Br J Anesth 44:1050, 1972

53. **Older PO, Harris JM:** Placental transfer of tubocurarine. Br J Anesth 40:459, 1968

54. **Shnider SM:** Serum cholinesterase activity during pregnancy, labor, and puerperium. Anesthesiology 26:355, 1965

55. **Barada A, Haroun S, Bassili M et al:** Response of the newborn to succinylcholine injection in homozygotic atypical mothers. Anesthesiology 43:115, 1975

56. **Ali HH, Savarese JJ:** Monitoring of neuromuscular function. Anesthesiology 45:216, 1976

57. **O'Brien JE, Abbey V, Hinsvaal O et al:** Metabolism and measurement of 2-chloroprocaine.

58. **Hyman MD, Shnider SM:** Maternal and neonatal blood concentrations of bupivacaine associated with obstetrical conduction anesthesia. Anesthesiology 34:81, 1971

59. **Martin CB, Gingerich B:** Uteroplacental physiology. J Obstet Gynecol Nurs [Suppl] 5:16, 1976

60. **Greiss FC, Still JG, Anderson SG:** Effects of local anesthetic agents on the uterine vasculature and myometrium. Am J Obstet Gynecol 124:889, 1976

61. **Vasicka A, Kretchmer H:** Effect of conduction and inhalation anesthesia on uterine contractions. Am J Obstet Gynecol 82:600, 1961

62. **Hon E:** Atlas of Fetal Heart Rate Patterns. New Haven, Harty Press, 1972

9

The Onset of Respiration

Nicholas M. Nelson

By the end of normal-term gestation the fetus and its lungs are well-prepared to assume responsibility for extrauterine gas exchange. The alveoli are developed by the 25th week, and, by the 35th week, the Type II great alveolar pneumocyte has begun to produce adequate quantities of the surface-active material upon which alveolar stability will later depend, once air breathing commences. *In utero* the alveoli are open and stable at nearly the normal neonatal lung volume, because they contain a fetal lung liquid, probably produced by ultrafiltration of pulmonary capillary blood, in addition to some secretion from alveolar cells.

The pulmonary and bronchial circulations are well-developed and thoroughly admixed by multiple mutual connections at the alveolar level. This combined circulation, then, is characterized by high pressure and low flow because of a high degree of pulmonary vascular resistance—both passive and active. The passive resistance most likely relates to compression of pulmonary capillaries by the fetal lung liquid, but there is also a high degree of active vasomotor tone resulting from the hypoxic level (P_{O_2} of 25 torr) of the pulmonary venous stream. This hypoxic increase in active pulmonary vasomotor tone is a dominant feature in the behavior of the pulmonary vasculature at all stages of development, but is more active in the fetus because of a relatively much larger vascular muscle mass than in the adult. These features are responsible for the key characteristic of the fetal circulation: namely, that pulmonary vascular resistance greatly exceeds systemic resistance (Table 9-1), so that nearly 50% of fetal cardiac output perfuses the placenta, whereas only 5% to 10% perfuses the lung (Tables 9-2 and 9-3). With the onset of inflation and ventilation of the lung at birth, these resistances will reverse, and it is the success of this reversal which principally determines the success of the cardiopulmonary adaptation to birth.

The neuromuscular controls of respiration are also laid down well before even premature birth. The fetus spends nearly 30% of its time engaged in a rapid, discoordinate form of "panting"—paradoxical motions of the chest and abdominal wall[1,2] associated with the rapid, irregular, and low-voltage electrocortical activity seen in rapid-eye-movement (REM), or "active," sleep.[3,4] In the human fetus near term, as much as 600 ml of amniotic fluid per day are inhaled through such activity.[5] Thus, the "first breaths of life" are now, perhaps, an inaccurate label, albeit a dramatic underscoring of the events which mark the perinatal shift from placental to pulmonary

Table 9-1. Hemodynamic Characteristics of the Perinatal Circulation.

	Resistances*			Conductances†		
	Fetal	*Neonatal*		*Fetal*	*Neonatal*	
	SHEEP	SHEEP	HUMAN	SHEEP	SHEEP	HUMAN
Pulmonary	530	85	140	1.9	11.8	7.1
Ductus	30	810	—	33.3	1.2	—
Systemic	170	220	300	5.9	4.5	3.3

* Units are torr $\times$ l^{-1} $\times$ kg $\times$ min
† Units are ml $\times$ kg^{-1} $\times$ min^{-1} $\times$ torr^{-1}
(From data of Arcilla et al,[70] Assali,[71] McMurphy et al,[72] and Wallgren et al[73-75])

Table 9-2. Distribution of Cardiac Output.

	Term Fetal Lamb			Human	
				Fetus	*Adult*
	R	*G*	F_{CO}	F_{CO}	F_{CO}
Vital Organs					
Brain	3.3	0.3	0.03	0.14	0.14
Heart	2.5	0.4	0.04	0.02	0.05
Lung	2.0	0.5	0.05	0.10	1.00
Placenta	0.25	4.0	0.40	0.33	0.00
Metabolic Organs					
Liver	0.56	1.8	0.18		
Gut	2.0	0.5	0.05	0.08	0.23
Spleen	5.0	0.2	0.02	0.02	
Kidney	5.0	0.2	0.02	0.05	0.22
Adrenal				0.04	
Carcass	0.27	3.7	0.37		
Bone					0.14
Muscle					0.18
Skin					0.04

R = resistance (torr/ml/kg/min)
G = conductance (ml/kg/min/torr)
F_{CO} = fractional cardiac output
(Values calculated from assumed mean blood pressure of 55 torr and data of Dawes,[76] Folkow and Neil,[77] Harned,[78] Rudolph and Heymann[79-81])

gas-exchange and from liquid to gaseous ventilation.

The First Breaths

The passive phase of these events during vaginal birth is shown in Figure 9-1, wherein the thoracic cage is compressed to pressures of 30-160 cm H_2O during passage through the birth canal, sometimes producing forcible ejection of as much as 30 ml of tracheal fluid through the airways.[6] The subsequent recoil of the chest wall after birth of the trunk may produce a small passive inspiration of air, perhaps accompanied by active glossopharyngeal forcing of some air into at least the proximal airways and introduction of some

Table 9-3. Organ Blood Flow

	ml/kg body weight/min			ml/100 g tissue/min		
	FETAL SHEEP	FETAL MAN	FETAL SHEEP	FETAL MAN	*Adult Man* REST	*Adult Man* MAX
Vital Organs						
Brain	16.5	51	132	25	50	130
Heart	22	7.3	291	165	70	400
Lung	27.5	36.3	126			
Placenta	220	120	130	11		
Metabolic Organs						
Liver	99		20		50	250
Gut	27.5	29	69	101	40	200
Spleen	11	7.3	240			
Kidney	11	18.2	173	155	400	550
Adrenal		14.5		340		
Carcass	204		26		2.5	260
Bone					3	15
Muscle					3	60
Skin					10	150
Total Cardiac Output *	550	363				

*Both ventricles
(From data of Dawes,[76] Folkow and Neil,[77] Harned,[78] Rudolph and Heymann[79-81])

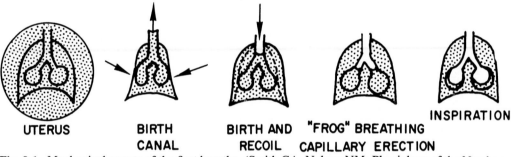

UTERUS   BIRTH CANAL   BIRTH AND RECOIL   "FROG" BREATHING CAPILLARY ERECTION   INSPIRATION

Fig. 9-1. Mechanical events of the first breaths. (Smith CA, Nelson NM: Physiology of the Newborn Infant, 4th ed. Springfield, (Ill), Charles C Thomas, 1976)[82]

blood into pulmonary capillaries ("capillary erection"). Thus, an air-liquid interface is established within the larger airways of the lung, and with it are established the surface retractive forces that would tend to collapse the smaller airways and alveoli, were it not for the presence of surface-active material in the alveolar lining layer. The first opening of these alveoli (and lung), however, will be easier if some fetal lung liquid is retained in at least the smaller airways of the lung before the "first" active breaths are taken (Fig. 9-2).

The reason for this is that inflation of the lung by air from the totally collapsed and gas-free state (**dashed line**) requires the exertion of considerable distending pressure across the lung—10 cm H_2O pressure is shown here for the first expansion, but levels up to 80 cm H_2O are not uncommon for the first full expansion—so that the spontaneous occurrence of alveolar rupture in term infants with healthy lungs becomes understandable. Note that "inflation" with liquid (**solid line**) requires rather less force, because of the lack of an air-liquid

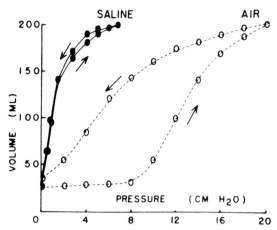

Fig. 9-2. Pressure-volume curves after air versus liquid expansion of the lung. (Radford EP: In Remington JW (ed): Tissue Elasticity, Vol 177. Washington, D.C., American Physiological Society, 1957)

interface. Note also that the deflation curve in air is not superimposable upon the inflation curve ("hysteresis") because mobilization and orientation of alveolar surfactant molecules during deflation decrease alveolar surface tension as the alveolar surface contracts. Hence, the transpulmonary (alveolus to intrapleural space) distending pressure required to maintain lung volume at 5 cc/g diminishes from 10 to nearly 0 cm H_2O.

Stimuli for Breathing

The precise reason(s) for the first extrauterine inspirations will probably remain somewhat obscure because the unfamiliar stimuli to which the newly born infant is subjected are multiple: cold, light, noise, gravity, and pain, all in addition to the hypercapnea, respiratory acidosis, and hypoxia (collectively called asphyxia) which result from normal labor and its accompanying intermittent cessation of maternal placental perfusion. Their possible interplay around the respiratory center is shown in Figure 9-3. The animal fetus at term has been demonstrated as responsive to all these stimuli, although there are certain inconsistencies. Thus, the fetal carotid body (the peripheral chemoreceptor) responds to hypoxia and to (particularly oscillatory) hypercapnea, and neuronal traffic from these influences is regularly recordable along the

carotid sinus nerve.[8] Moreover, although the acidity of the fetal cerebrospinal fluid, like that of the adult, appears to be regulated at pH levels lower than those of blood, the fetal central chemoreceptor responds poorly to the normal ventilatory drive of cerebrospinal fluid acidosis.[9] Throughout all of these observations has been noted the fact that the animal fetus will not breathe when warm and submerged, despite chemical stimuli for respiration, whereas when chilled and exposed, the fetus will breathe, despite the lack of chemical stimuli for respiration. The possibility thus arises of a well-tuned fetal respiratory center, quite responsive to the usual chemical stimuli, which is repressed *in utero* but derepressed by delivery.

The unaroused (? repressed) fetus is apneic and appears to have his respiratory rhythm generator switched off in expiration; that is, the inspiratory neurones are inhibited and the expiratory neurones are in tonic discharge.[10] In this state, the respiratory centers appear

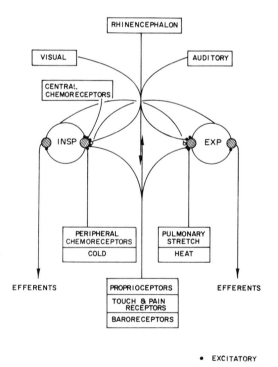

Fig. 9-3. Hypothetical functional organization of the respiratory center. (Adapted from Burns BD: Br Med Bull, 19:7, 1963)[7]

unresponsive to chemical or sensory stimuli. This refractory state can result from vagal (pulmonary stretch afferents)[11] or superior laryngeal (laryngeal taste afferents)[12,13] discharge in states of experimental manipulation, but in the normal fetus may more likely represent a hypoxic repression of facilitation from suprapontine centers. In any case, states of fetal arousal (such as REM sleep) appear to be linked, possibly through the reticular formation, to a rhythmic, alternating discharge of inspiratory and expiratory neurones. The accentuation of the normal fetal hypoxia by disruption of placental gas exchange during normal birth produces a gasping respiratory effort with resultant improved cerebral oxygenation, accompanied by decreasing tonic discharge of expiratory neurones. These effects, coupled with the general sensory arousal of birth, are evidently sufficient to restore the inherent rhythmicity of discharge in the respiratory centers.[14]

Figure 9-3 represents imaginary cross-connections that could explain these phenomena of possible interaction. This interactional concept portrays the inspiratory and expiratory centers as mutually inhibitory and, moreover, affected by neighboring neuronal "traffic" both from above and from below. Thus, the general "tone" of the respiratory neurons may well be enhanced or facilitated by nonrespiratory environmental stimuli such as pain, change in position or pressure, noise, and light.

Pulmonary Adaptation

In any case, the first active breaths of air, once taken and sustained, set in motion a nearly inexorable chain of events that

1. converts the fetal to the adult circulation.
2. empties the lung of liquid.
3. establishes the neonatal lung volume and the characteristics of pulmonary function in the newly born infant.

These events are outlined in Figure 9-4 and will be analyzed separately (although they occur concurrently) in the remainder of this chapter. The upper lefthand corner of Figure 9-4 is a reprise of the events diagrammed in Figure 9-1. Air entry into the respiratory system establishes the lung retractive forces of surface tension (Fig. 9-2) with consequent development of negative intrapleural and in-

terstitial pressure because the overlying chest wall resists collapse. These events, along with the increase in alveolar oxygen tension, are solidly established fact and are indicated as such by the solid boxes of Figure 9-4 (less well-established events are indicated by **broken line boxes**). The final and most dramatic events in the sequence are the great increases in blood and lymph flow through the lung that follow the onset of ventilation.

As some lung liquid is ejected from the airways and alveolar surfaces retractive forces become established, hydrostatic alveolar pressure upon the pulmonary capillaries decreases, and these compressible vessels with tone may open the "sluice gate" of the "alveolar waterfall" of blood flow through the lung.[15] Moreover, the increasing pulmonary venous oxygen tension of the air-breathing newborn serves to decrease active vasomotor tone in the precapillary pulmonary arterioles. Thus, for both reasons, intralumenal hydrostatic capillary pressure (Pc) rises as pericapillary interstitial (alveolar) pressure (Pif) decreases and Starling's equilibrium—

$$\text{Fluid transfer} = k \left[(Pc - \pi pl) - (Pif - \pi if) \right]$$

where k is the filtration constant (relating to pore size) and πpl is plasma osmotic pressure and πif is interstitial osmotic pressure. Positive values indicate transudation and negative values indicate fluid absorption.

—is perturbed, so that capillary fluid tends to transude into the interstitium, and alveolar fluid may well also be directly absorbed into the interstitial spaces at the alveolar corners.[16] These events are marked by a decrease in total plasma volume which reaches its nadir at 2 to 8 hours after birth, and by a dramatic increase in lung lymph drainage beginning promptly upon ventilation and subsiding by about 6 hours of age.[17] During this period after birth, lymphatic distension in the lung has been demonstrated both histologically[18] and radiologically.[19] It is of obvious clinical interest that infant rabbits delivered by cesarean section and immature lamb fetuses are both slow to clear their lung liquid; the one, presumably, denied the thoracic squeeze of vaginal birth and the other influenced by higher alveolar surface tensions because of lack of adequate alveolar surface-active material. Despite this, the "transient tachypnea" clinically ascribed to slow clearance of lung liquid has so far been

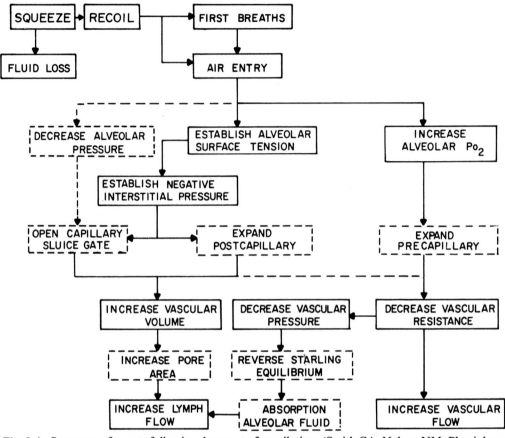

Fig. 9-4. Sequence of events following the onset of ventilation. (Smith CA, Nelson NM: Physiology of the Newborn Infant, 4th ed. Springfield, (Ill), Charles C Thomas, 1976)[82]

described only in the term human newborn and has not been related to cesarean section.[20]

Circulatory Adaptation

The magnitude of the passive and active increase in pulmonary blood flow following inflation and ventilation of the lung is shown in the experimental data of Figure 9-5. If the lung is inflated from the fetal state and ventilated with a gas mixture which does not change the fetal composition of the blood gases (approximately pH 7.35, P_{CO_2} 45, P_{O_2} 25), then an increase in pulmonary vascular conductance (decrease in resistance) can be achieved as shown by the increasing flow-pressure slopes of the two righthand curves in Figure 9-5. This increase in conductance is most likely caused by expansion of collapsible pulmonary capillaries (as mentioned above) as well as those vessels which are anatomically "tethered" to

the pulmonary parenchyma. Then, as the blood-gas composition is changed by increase in P_{O_2} and decrease in P_{CO_2} (similar to ventilation with air), further increases in vascular conductance are achieved as shown in the lefthand pair of curves in Figure 9-5.

The decrease in pulmonary vascular resistance thus set in motion, coupled with the increase in peripheral vascular resistance which follows increasing oxygenation, the loss of the umbilical circulation and the cold shock of birth, leads (as shown in Fig. 9-6) to closure of the foramen ovale within minutes of birth. The ductus arteriosus, however, remains open for some hours and, because systemic resistance is now higher than pulmonary resistance (the reverse of the fetal circumstance), blood flow through the ductus also reverses, now passing left to right. This is the "transitional" phase of the perinatal circulation, during which there may be reversion to the fetal pattern at any time pulmonary vascular resistance should again rise higher than peripheral vascular resistance. During this phase, there is also a considerable increase in the volume load presented to the left ventricle because of the vast increase in left ventricular input (*i.e.*, pulmonary venous return). The ductus arteriosus constricts under the influence of prostaglandins interacting with rising oxygen tension of the blood coursing through it.[21,22] This normally begins at about 4 to 12 hours postnatally and is completed by around 24 hours of age.

These events are diagrammed in Figure 9-7, along with blood flow data (in ml/kg/min) taken from experiments in fetal sheep. In this diagram, the ventricles are shown as (electric) generators in parallel with diodes (valves) to direct the flow of blood (as a diode directs the flow of electrons). The electrical symbol for

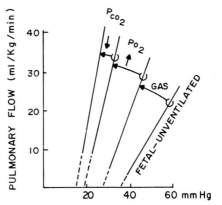

Fig. 9-5. Increase in pulmonary vascular conductance with the onset of ventilation. Separate curves are shown depicting the contributions of gaseous inflation, increased P_{O_2} and decreased P_{CO_2}. (Adapted from Strang LB: Arch Dis Child 40:575, 1965)

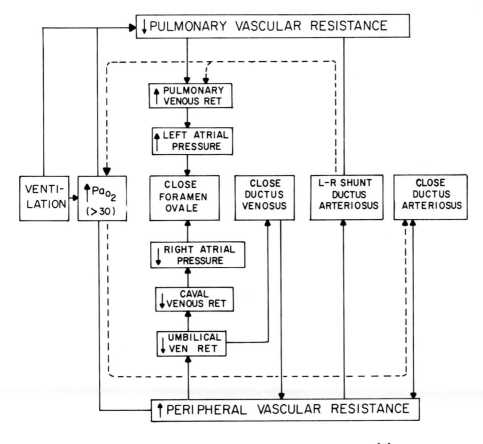

Fig. 9-6. Conversion of the perinatal circulation following the onset of ventilation. (Smith CA, Nelson NM: Physiology of the Newborn Infant, 4th ed. Springfield, (Ill), Charles C Thomas, 1976)[82]

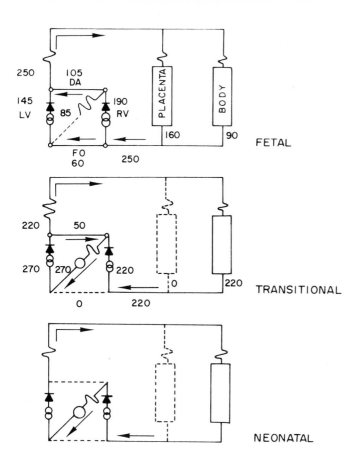

Fig. 9-7. Stages in the conversion of the perinatal circulation. (See text for symbols. Numbers refer to blood flow in ml/kg/minute). (Smith CA, Nelson NM: Physiology of the Newborn Infant, 4th ed. Springfield, (Ill), Charles C Thomas, 1976)[82]

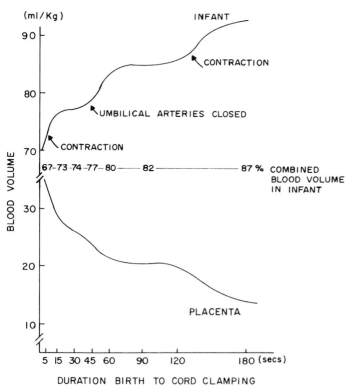

Fig. 9-8. The placental transfusion: sequence of events during the first 3 minutes of life. (Smith CA, Nelson NM: Physiology of the Newborn Infant, 4th ed. Springfield, (Ill), Charles C Thomas, 1976)[82]

resistance indicates relative resistances in the pulmonary and systemic circuits. The **large circle** in the center of the pulmonary circuit represents the expanding and established alveolus. The diagrammatic sequence makes obvious the conversion of the central circulation from that of two ventricles connected in parallel circuits, where volume loads may be unequal, to connection in series where the right ventricular output must equal left ventricular input (and, thus, output), except for some small amount of blood stored in the "capacitance vessels" (capillaries and veins) of the pulmonary circulation.

Much of the increase in peripheral vascular resistance is a result of the cessation of the umbilical circulation. The umbilical arteries constrict vigorously under the influence of increased oxygenation and, particularly, in response to longitudinal stretch on the umbilical cord. The balance of umbilical arterial inflow to and umbilical venous outflow from the placenta (aided by the positive force of uterine contractions and the negative force of neonatal thoracic inspiration[23-25]) determines the course of the transfusion of blood from the placenta to the infant, as shown in Figure 9-8. The umbilical arteries close very rapidly and in advance of closure of the umbilical vein, resulting in an average net transfer of about 15 to 20 ml/kg of blood to the infant within 3 minutes, if he is held below the introitus with the cord untouched. If one reflects that the primitive maternal posture for childbearing was kneeling (rather than the lithotomy position of modern obstetrics), one gains, perhaps, some insight into the intent of Nature regarding this "placental transfusion."

Apart from those shown in Figure 9-8 there are little human data to document these events, but those which are available are shown in Figures 9-9, and 9-10. Measurements of output from both ventricles, together with appropriate pressure data, permit calculation of the resistances shown in Figure 9-9 (fetal data are taken from the sheep). The dominant events depicted include (from the top)

1. the rise and subsequent fall in systemic resistance.
2. the vast decrease in pulmonary resistance.
3. the large, albeit transient, increase in left ventricular volume (and pressure) work.
4. the decrease in right ventricular pressure (and, transiently, volume) work.
5. closure of the ductus arteriosus (and equal-

ization of ventricular volume work) between 12 to 14 hours.
6. closure of the foramen ovale in the first minutes and hours after birth.

Human flow data (during the transitional phase of the perinatal circulation) are shown in Figure 9-10 and document that the left ventricle is pumping nearly two times the volume load of the right ventricle.

However, it is pressure work that chiefly determines the behavior of the electromotive forces of the beating heart. These are shown both in vector and scalar ECG form in Figure 9-11. Noticeable is that the QRS loop remains unchanged from its rightward-dominant orientation in the first days of life. This is a reflection of the dominance of right-over-left ventricular muscle mass as a result of the chronic "cor pulmonale" of the fetal state and will only slowly shift to the left-dominant picture of the adult over the first 3 to 6 months of life, as the ventricles become remodeled in response to decreasing right- and increasing left-ventricular pressure work. The only perinatal ECG indication of these shifting pressure/volume loads upon the ventricles is the change in orientation of the T-vector from *leftward,* inferior and anterior at birth to *rightward,* inferior and anterior at transition (about 6 hours) to *leftward,* inferior and *posterior* at restitution (12–24 hours).

Pulmonary Mechanics

To return to the first few extrauterine respirations, we note in Figure 9-12 that the first breath (**I**) begins with no (**air**) volume and no transpulmonary pressure gradient. As the chest wall (including the diaphragm) expands, the transpulmonary or distending pressure increases until it overcomes surface tension (compare with Fig. 9-2) in the smaller airways and alveoli, usually at transpulmonary pressures below 25 cm H_2O.[26] At this point actively inspired air begins to enter and does so with increasing ease as alveolar dimensions increase. The reason is contained in the La Place relation

$$P = 2T/R$$

which states that, if wall tension (*T*) of a spherical surface remains constant, the distending pressure (*P*) required to maintain equilibrium will decrease as the spherical radius (*R*) increases. An apt analogy is often drawn to this point by considering the increasing ease

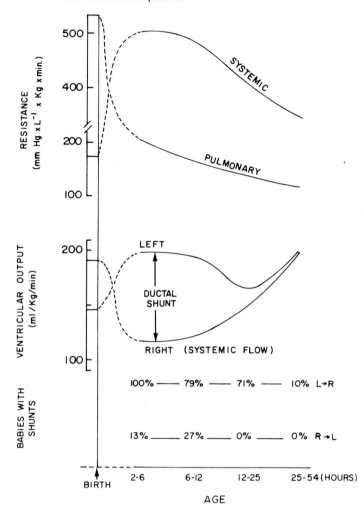

Fig. 9-9. Perinatal hemodynamics in the human showing changes in vascular resistance, ventricular output, and shunting. (Smith CA, Nelson NM: Physiology of the Newborn Infant, 4th ed. Springfield, (Ill), Charles C Thomas, 1976)[82]

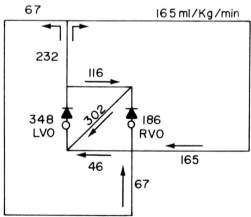

Fig. 9-10. The human perinatal (transitional) circulation. Flow data are in ml/kg/minute. (Smith CA, Nelson NM: Physiology of the Newborn Infant, 4th ed. Springfield, (Ill), Charles C Thomas, 1976;[82] flow data from Burnard ED et al: Clin Sci 31:121, 1966)[83]

with which a child's balloon is inflated, once first expanded.

At the maximum inspiratory level (of about 45 ml of air in this example) Breath I is actively exhaled (note negative transpulmonary pressure), but not to 0 volume. Evidently with great rapidity the alveolar lining layer, containing surface-active material, is able so to stabilize alveolar surfaces that surface tension *decreases* as alveolar dimensions decrease. Thus, both *T* and *R* decrease together in the La Place relation, so that the transpulmonary pressure required to maintain inflation is relatively stable and of small dimensions. These dimensions are indicated in Figure 9-13 which compares the pressure-volume characteristics of the infant lung, chest wall (and diaphragm) and total respiratory systems to those of the adult. Notable is the fact that, whereas the

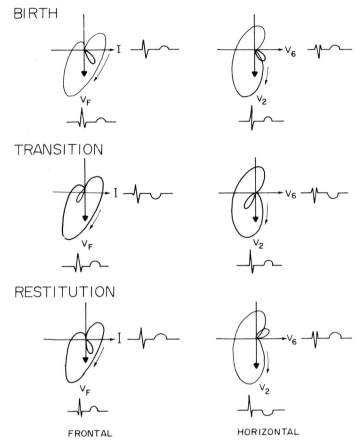

BIRTH

TRANSITION

RESTITUTION

FRONTAL   HORIZONTAL

Fig. 9-11. The perinatal ECG; vector and scalar. The scalar tracings are shown from leads I and aV_F in the frontal projection and from leads V_2 and V_6 in the horizontal projection. The vector pathway is indicated by the arrow. The orientational changes of the smaller T-loop are obvious, as is the relative stability of the larger QRS-loop. (Smith CA, Nelson NM: Physiology of the Newborn Infant, 4th ed. Springfield, (Ill), Charles C Thomas, 1976)[82]

relaxation pressure curves for the lung alone are remarkably similar across the age span, the infant's chest wall is almost infinitely distensible, or compliant. This results in large part, of course, from the nonossification of the infant thorax—a matter of thoughtful convenience during the high extrinsic pressures of vaginal birth. Indeed, even the adults of diving species, also subjected to high extrinsic thoracic pressures, have chest walls as compliant as the newborn human. However, it is the opposition of the retractive forces of the somewhat expanded lung against the expansive forces of the somewhat compressed chest wall that determines the rest (end-expiratory) volume of the total respiratory system, and the higher the compliance (nonstiffness) of the chest wall the lower will be the rest volume. Note in Figure 9-13, that the infant's rest volume is a good deal closer to the residual or "collapse" volume of the lung than is the case in the adult. Moreover, the transpulmonary pressure at rest is also less in the infant. This

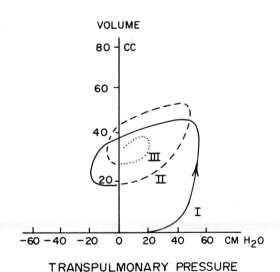

Fig. 9-12. Pressure-volume curves of the first 3 extrauterine breaths. (Smith CA, Nelson NM: Physiology of the Newborn Infants, 4th ed. Springfield, (Ill), Charles C Thomas, 1976)[82]

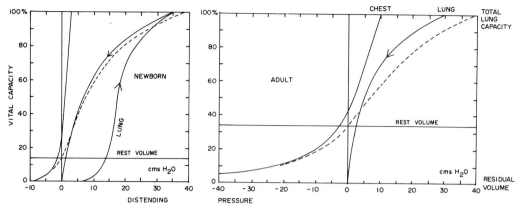

Fig. 9-13. Comparative mechanics of the infant and adult lung. (Smith CA, Nelson NM: Physiology of the Newborn Infant, 4th ed. Springfield, (Ill), Charles C Thomas, 1976)[82]

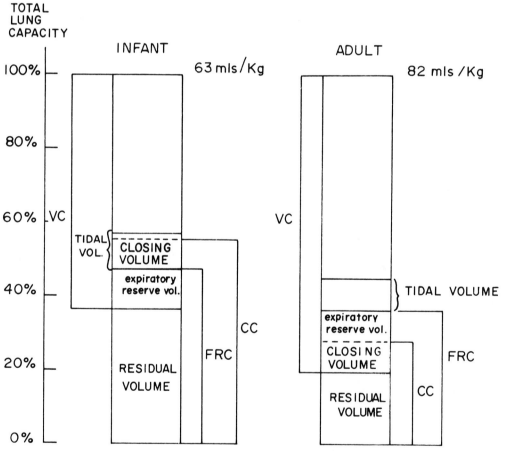

Fig. 9-14. Static lung volumes of the infant and adult. (Smith CA, Nelson NM: Physiology of the Newborn Infant, 4th ed. Springfield, (Ill), Charles C Thomas, 1976)[82]

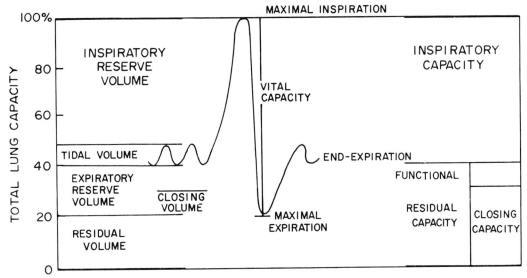

Fig. 9-15. Static lung volumes defined. A standard spirogram is shown for reference. (Smith CA, Nelson NM: Physiology of the Newborn Infant, 4th ed. Springfield, (Ill), Charles C Thomas, 1976)[82]

tenuous situation is further detailed in Figure 9-14, wherein it is seen that some smaller airways of the infant can close even within the range of the normal tidal volume and "trap" gas in the infant lung's periphery, so that it does not communicate with the trachea. By measuring total thoracic gas volume in comparison to functional residual capacity as much as 6 ml/kg of lung volume may be measured as trapped in the first 2 weeks of life.[27]

The facts that such gas-trapping is the more frequently observed in the first few postnatal days[28] and that intrapleural negative pressure increases to adult levels by 16 days after birth[29] suggest a developmental change in respiratory system equilibrium perhaps too rapid to be accounted for by ossification of the thoracic cage. It may be that this developmental change involves increasing tonus in the intercostal muscles (see below). This would serve to decrease the compliance of the chest wall, such that the rest volume of the lung may increase to a level at which smaller airways no longer collapse during quiet breathing.

Despite these qualifications, the standard static lung volumes as defined by Figure 9-15 have been measured frequently and reproducibly by many investigators of the newborn and are shown in Table 9-4. Infants delivered by elective cesarean section have decreased lung gas volume, presumably because they

have been denied the partial purging of fetal lung liquid provided by thoracic compression during passage through the birth canal.[30,31]

The decreased lung capacities (total, inspiratory, vital) may indicate an imperfect leverage exerted by a too compliant chest wall upon the underlying lung. The higher residual volume and lower expiratory reserve volume of the infant may relate to gas trapped behind smaller closed airways. In any case, the first few days of life, especially in the premature, are marked by disturbances in efficient gas exchange (requiring simultaneous and nearly equal ventilation and perfusion), which can be ameliorated by stabilization of the chest wall.[32]

It has recently become apparent that the stability of the chest wall, as well as many other integrative functions involving the respiratory system, depends upon the "sleep state" of the infant.[33-41] Active or REM sleep is the dominant state in the newborn and is one of relative arousal, characterized by intense low-voltage and fast electrocortical and reticular activity. It is associated with sucking, swallowing, and esophageal peristalsis, as well as glottic closure. Proprioceptive reflexes are generally depressed with resultant loss of postural tone. The precise mode of this depression is incompletely understood, but appears, peripherally at least, to involve an inhibition of monosynaptic muscle spindle ("gamma-

Table 9-4. Static Lung Volumes.

		Infant (ml/kg)	Adult (ml/kg)
Total lung capacity	(TLC)	63	82
Inspiratory capacity	(IC)	33	52
Thoracic gas volume	(TGV)	30–36	30
Functional residual capacity	(FRC)	30	30
Vital capacity	(VC)	30–40	66
Closing capacity	(CC)	35	23
Tidal volume	(V_T)	6	7
Expiratory reserve volume	(ERV)	7	14
Closing volume	(CV)	12	7
Residual volume	(RV)	23	16
ERV/FRC		0.23	0.47
RV/TLC		0.37	0.20
FRC/TLC		0.48	0.37
V_T/FRC		0.20	0.23

(From data of Chu et al,[84] Mansell et al,[85] Nelson,[86] Phelan, and Williams,[87] Polgar and Promadhat,[88] La Court and Polgar,[89] Milner et al,[90] Dahms et al[91])

loop") reflexes, which sense increased local muscular loads and, in response, increase alpha-motoneuron discharge.[33,34] Inhibition of the gamma-loop reflex apparently results in loss of intercostal muscle tone during REM sleep, so that stiffness ("elastance") of the thoracic cage decreases and diaphragmatic contraction deforms the ribs during inspiration, producing "paradoxical" respiration (Fig. 9-16). Such deformation is capable of triggering the intercostal phrenic (inhibitory) reflex which terminates early such an inspiration.[42–44] Thus, respiration in REM sleep is irregular and more rapid than in quiet sleep. Tidal volume is unchanged, but mean inspiratory air flow (tidal volume/inspiratory duration) is increased, as is minute volume. This is, however, a fatiguing form of respiration,[45] the more so for the premature infant whose respiratory muscle fibers resist fatigue poorly.[46] He is especially ill equipped, therefore, to compensate for extra respiratory loads during REM sleep. The Hering–Breuer reflex, especially strong in the premature, fosters recruitment of intercostal neurones under respiratory loads, but this reflex is inhibited during REM sleep. The diminished lung volume and arterial oxygenation observed in REM sleep[47] thus become more understandable.

During quiet breathing the infant's ventilatory efforts are opposed by several forces: the resistance of the lung and chest wall to stretch (elastic recoil), the resistance to movement (flow resistance) of air and tissue, and the inertial resistance offered by air and tissue at rest to any large change in their state of motion. An "equation of motion" states the relations among these variables:

$$P = V/C + R \cdot F$$

P = the muscular force (measured as transpulmonary pressure) applied to the respiratory system
V = the volume of gas in the system
C = the distensibility or compliance of the system
V/C = the force of elastic recoil
R = the flow resistance
F = air flow
R·F = the force required to overcome the resistance to flow. (During quiet breathing the inertial resistance is negligible.)

These forces, as currently measured, are set out in Table 9-5 wherein it is apparent that the muscular force to be generated by both infant and adult are really quite comparable (about 2 cm H_2O). Nonetheless, there are certain notable differences, including the lower proportional nasal resistance of the newborn. The

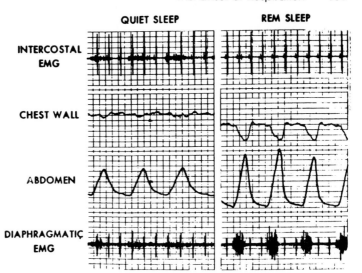

Fig. 9-16. Paradoxical respiration in REM sleep. As the abdomen expands (**upward deflection**) with diaphragmatic descent, the chest wall is drawn in (**downward deflection**). Large, brief EMG spikes are ECG artifact. Note tonic discharge of intercostal EMG throughout inspiration in quiet sleep, compared to brief, low-voltage phasic intercostal EMG, as well as intense phasic diaphragmatic EMG, in REM sleep. (Muller N et al: J Appl Physiol 46:688, 1979)[45]

Table 9-5. Forces Opposing Breathing.

	Infant		Adult	
Elastic recoil (V_L/C_L)	1.5 cm H_2O		1.5 cm H_2O	
Volume (V_L)	0.1 liters		2.1 liters	
Compliance (C_L)-total	0.0026*	0.029†	0.100*	0.03†
Chest wall	0.0236	0.262	0.200	0.06
Lung tissue	0.0050	0.055	0.200	0.06
Flow resistance ($R \cdot F$)	0.4 mean/1.9 max cm H_2O		0.4 mean/1.9 max cm H_2O	
Mean (pulmonary) resistance	35‡	—§	—‡	—§
Inspiratory (total) resistance	69	100%	5.5	100%
Chest wall	—	26%	—	16%
Pulmonary	25–50	—	4.5	—
Nose	10	21%	2.8	54%
Mouth-airway	16	34%	1.6	29%
Lung tissue	9	19%	0.1	1%
Expiratory (total) resistance	97	—	—	—
Chest wall	—	—	—	—
Pulmonary	35–70	—	—	—
Gas flow (mean)	.030–.050″		—	
Inspiration	.048		—	
Expiration	.037		—	

* l/cmH_2O
† l/cmH_2O/l lung volume
‡ cmH_2O/l/sec
§ % total resistance
″ l/sec

(From data of Chu, et al,[84] Nelson,[86] Polgar and Promadhat,[88] Lacourt and Polgar,[92] Sharp et al,[93] Milner et al[90])

Table 9-6. Pulmonary Ventilation.

	Symbol	Infant	Adult	Units
Respiratory frequency	(f)	34–35	13	BPM
Tidal volume	(V_T)	6–8	7	ml/kg
Alveolar volume	(V_A)	3.8–5.8	4.8	ml/kg
Dead space volume	(V_D)	2.0–2.2	2.2	ml/kg
Minute ventilation	$(\dot{V}_E)$	200–260	90	ml/kg/min
Alveolar ventilation	$(\dot{V}_A)$	100–150	60	ml/kg/min
Wasted (dead space) ventilation	(V_D)	77–99	30	ml/kg/min
Dead space/tidal volume	(V_D/V_T)	0.27–0.37	0.3	
Oxygen consumption	$(\dot{V}_{O_2})$	6–8	3.2	ml/kg/min
Ventilation equivalent	$(\dot{V}_A/\dot{V}_{O_2})$	16–23	19–25	
Alveolar ventilation	$(\dot{V}_A)$	2.3	2.4	l/m²/min

(From data of Chu et al,[84] Nelson,[86] Polgar and Promadhat,[88] and Lees et al[94])

much higher chest wall compliance of the newborn, again is most striking. Now, the product of the total compliance and resistance of the system is its "time constant," an expression of how rapidly the system, once perturbed by an active inspiration, will passively return to rest position under the force of elastic recoil operating against flow resistance. This time constant is about 0.29 seconds in the infant and 0.55 seconds in the adult, so that the resting respiratory rate of the infant (30–50 BPM) is necessarily about twice that of the adult (20 BPM). Further, any entity that reduces the total compliance (increases the "stiffness") of the system (such as fluid in the lung) must decrease the time constant and, hence, increase the resting respiratory rate.

Pulmonary Ventilation

It is this higher ventilatory rate that is chiefly responsible for the higher minute ventilation, alveolar ventilation, wasted ventilation and oxygen consumption (normalized for body weight) of the infant, as seen in Table 9-6. Yet, when compared on the basis of body surface area (generally held as a better basis for metabolic comparisons) the infant and adult are, again, strikingly similar.

The chemical and neuronal drivers of neonatal respiration are becoming better defined, but a number of mysteries remain. It is now clear that the respiratory centers of the newborn respond normally to CO_2 and that their response becomes more powerful with increasing postconceptional age.[48,49] Conceivably, this increasing respiratory response may represent,

in the human, the result of a postnatal increase in excitatory respiratory neuronal synapses, and consequent respiratory motor activity, as noted in other species.[50]

Responses to O_2 are more complex, probably because they involve suprapontine centers in the brain, as well as the peripheral chemoreceptors. Short-term (less than 90 sec) responses are like those in the adult, with hyperoxia producing immediate hypoventilation,[51,52] while hypoxia produces immediate hyperventilation,[53,54] thus demonstrating functional peripheral chemoreceptors. Prolonged (2–3 min) hypo- or hyperoxia, however, soon leads to reversal of both these responses (Fig. 9-17).[54] Postulated but unproven explanations for the biphasic hyperoxic response include cerebral vasospasm and impaired CO_2 carriage (by O_2-saturated hemoglobin), leading to local accumulation of carbonic acid and consequent direct stimulation of the respiratory centers. It also seems possible that hypoxia may impair presumed facilitation by higher centers of possibly inadequate synaptic contacts among the respiratory motor neurons (see Fig. 9-3). It may even prove to be the case that such an hypoxic lack of neuronal facilitation of quantitatively marginal respiratory synapses is responsible for fetal respiratory quiescence (fetal Pa_{O_2} is about 25 torr), apart from the fetal "respiration" seen to accompany the intense reticular activity of REM sleep. The interactional effects of CO_2 and O_2 breathing are, again, similar to the adult (*i.e.*, hypoxic enhancement of CO_2 responses, presumably caused by peripheral chemoreceptor dis-

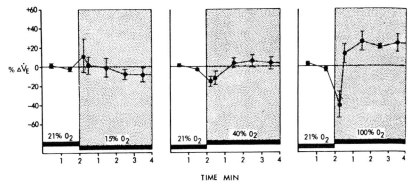

Fig. 9-17. Biphasic ventilatory responses to hypoxia and hyperoxia in the human newborn. The immediate ventilatory increase in hypoxic and decrease in hyperoxic environments (normal adult peripheral chemoreceptor responses) are not sustained. (Rigatto H et al: J Appl Physiol 39:896, 1975)[54]

charge), provided the experiments are short term.[53]

The association of chemical drives to and neuromuscular modulation of ventilation have come to be analyzed in the following equation:[55]

$$\dot{V}_E = \frac{V_T}{T_I} \times \frac{T_I}{T_{TOT}}$$

where $\dot{V}_E$ is total minute ventilation and V_T is the tidal volume of each breath. T_I is the duration of a given inspiration and T_{TOT} is the duration of a complete breath (inspiration + expiration).

V_T/T_I is the mean inspiratory gas flow per breath and a representative sum of chemical stimulation (principally CO_2 and H^+) and neuronal modulation (peripheral chemoreceptor signals, rapidly adapting vagal fiber signals from "irritant" receptors in the tracheobronchial epithelium, facilitative and inhibiting influences from suprapontine centers) of the inherent rhythmicity of respiratory neuronal discharge (Fig. 9-3),[56] as well as its neuromuscular expression in gas flow. The firing of these neurons requires a critical spatial and temporal summation of input impulses such that their resting potential may be raised above the firing threshold. T_I/T_{TOT} represents the "duty cycle," which determines the duration of firing of inspiratory neurons (i.e., T_I) or of expiratory neurons ($T_E = T_{TOT} - T_I$). These controls of frequency largely rest in the pulmonary submucosal stretch receptors (slow-adapting vagal fibers).[56]

All of these relations have recently come under intense scrutiny in the newborn, through detailed and critical analysis of the Hering–Breuer reflexes.[55,57–61] These are very well-developed in the premature in quiet sleep and allow him to recruit intercostal neurons when presented with a respiratory load (e.g., airway obstruction). They are not, however, active during REM sleep. With maturation, the strengths of these reflexes clearly decrease.[58,60,61] It seems possible, therefore, that maturational increases in respiratory neuronal synapses may render the respiratory centers less susceptible to the influences of vagal stretch and irritant receptors. As higher volitional centers develop to modulate an increasingly robust group of respiratory neurons, it appears that more primeval modulation through the vagus becomes less necessary to maintain constancy of ventilation under varying respiratory loads (e.g., speech, posture).

While none of this increasing attention to the role of the central nervous system, sleep state, and so on has yet produced a definitive explanation of the periodic respiration and apnea characteristic of the immature infant, it may at least have increased the quality of our speculations. Although earlier studies were conducted without knowledge of sleep state, there is strong evidence that hypoxia inhibits respiration in the newborn infant and that hyperoxia decreases the frequency of periodic respiration in the premature (despite its other dangers!).[62,63] In animals subjected to preterminal asphyxia, the evidence suggests that suprapontine centers become hypoxically de-

Table 9-7. Distribution of Pulmonary Ventilation ($\dot{V}_A$) and Perfusion ($\dot{Q}_C$) in the Infant.

Type of Alveolus	% Total Ventilation		% Total Perfusion		$\dot{V}_A/\dot{Q}_C$
Anatomically shunted	20		10		—
Atelectatic, perfused	0		15		0
Trapped gas, perfused	0		10		0
Silent (atelectatic, nonperfused)	0		0		0
Low $\dot{V}_A/\dot{Q}_C$ areas	2 ⎫		5 ⎫		0.4
Normal $\dot{V}_A/\dot{Q}_C$ areas	68 ⎬ 75		58 ⎬ 65		1.2
High $\dot{V}_A/\dot{Q}_C$ areas	5 ⎭		2 ⎭		2.5
Dead space (ventilated, nonperfused)	5		0		∞
Diffusion block	≪1		≪1		—

(Calculated from data of Nelson,[86] Polgar and Promadhat,[88] and Corbet, et al,[95,96] Kraus et al[97])

pressed, allowing activity of the respiratory neurons to be unmodulated from above and responsive, therefore, only to negative feedback from the peripheral chemoreceptors and vagal stretch receptors.[64,65] In such situations any defect in the "feedback loop" can lead to oscillatory behavior.[56,66] In REM sleep, there are multiple opportunities for disruption of feedback loops because of erratic respiratory timing. Premature infants, in addition, have in-phase oscillations of tidal volume and respiratory frequency during periodic breathing, suggesting an unstable total ventilation whereby CO_2 is either overblown or excessively retained.[66] Thus, the ancient observations that periodic respiration of the premature is relieved by O_2 breathing (restoring suprapontine facilitative neural influences) or CO_2 breathing (increasing pontine respiratory activity) become more understandable. Drugs such as caffeine and theophylline appear to facilitate respiration by increasing reticular activity, similar to that in REM sleep.

Ventilation-perfusion Imbalance

Exchange of respiratory gases between the tissues and the environment is, of course, the basic purpose of respiration, both cellular and pulmonary. It is thus obvious that adequate pulmonary respiration will be to no avail if the intervening circulation cannot carry and release oxygen to the tissues. Just as this principle applies to adequate distribution of arterialized blood to tissues, so also must the distribution of venous blood flow be well-matched to gaseous flow throughout the alveoli. Any inhomogeneity of the flow of gas and blood through the lungs must serve to reduce the efficiency of gas exchange. Such inhomogeneities are most frequently expressed as the ratio of ventilation/perfusion or V/Q within given groups of alveoli. Whereas the overall V/Q of the normal lung is nearly 1, there is a vast range of possible ratios from 0 (a "shunt") to infinity (a "dead space"). Presently available estimates for ventilation/perfusion ratios in the term newborn human at about 24 hours of age are shown in Table 9-7. It would appear from this that most ventilated areas are reasonably well perfused (i.e., little dead space or "wasted ventilation"), whereas significant amounts of perfusion are directed to atelectatic alveoli or are totally shunted around the lung. Probably little of this shunt flow passes through the foramen ovale and rather more passes right to left across the ductus arteriosus (even after reversal of dominant flow during the transitional phase of circulatory conversion). This occurs because of phasic pressure differences across the ductus during the cardiac cycle, the mean pressures on the pulmonary and systemic sides being essentially balanced for the first several hours (Fig. 9-9). A presently undocumentable amount of desaturated blood may also be shunted across the lung to the left atrium by way of bronchopulmonary anastomoses.

Alveolar-arterial Pressure Gradients

Such gas/blood flow relations are essentially responsible for the gas pressure differences established in the lung (Table 9-8). Further, the approximate relative contributions of the several components to the total arterial-alveo-

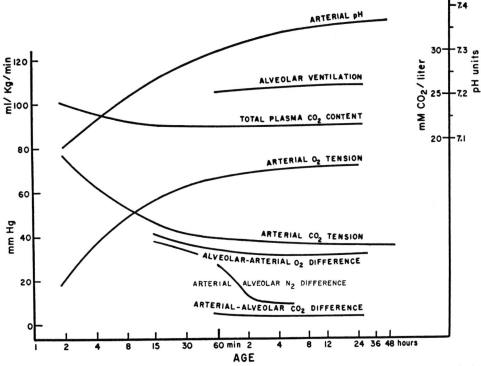

Fig. 9-20. Postnatal changes in blood gases. (Smith CA, Nelson NM: Physiology of the Newborn Infant, 4th ed. Springfield, (Ill), Charles C Thomas, 1976)[82]

related to alveolar instability, since the magnified blood gas differences of prematures diminish if the chest is stabilized at higher lung volume[32] and also during the first 2 weeks of life.

SUMMARY

To return in brief summation to the basic focus of this chapter, the *onset* of respiration, we may gain from Figure 9-18 an appreciation of just how rapidly the term newborn establishes respiration and recovers from the asphyxiating influence that is normal vaginal birth.

Finer indications of the components of this achievement are shown in Figure 9-19. The normal lung volume at rest (functional residual capacity) is essentially established by 8 to 10 minutes, albeit some of the dependent airways may be in intermittent collapse, as previously seen. The specific compliance (compliance normalized to lung volume) takes rather longer to achieve maximum. This most likely represents the rather slow clearance of fetal lung liquid from the parenchyma by way of the lymphatics. The airway conductance (reciprocal of resistance) increases somewhat slowly, possibly also representing clearance of fluid and "mucus" from airways and alveoli. If so, it should be possible to document a decrease in specific compliance and conductance in those infants felt to have "transient tachypnea of the newborn."

Figure 9-20 traces the development of respiratory gas pressure differences at the onset of respiration and indicates that, even as early as 60 minutes of age, there is insignificant wasted ventilation (*i.e.*, minimal aAD_{CO_2}). On the other hand, the large (35 torr) AaD_{O_2} in the first 2 hours appears mainly attributable to perfusion of poorly ventilated areas of the lung (*i.e.*, higher aAD_{N_2}). Subsequently, as lung volume becomes firmly established and compliance improves (? fluid clears) around 2 to 4 hours of age, low V/Q areas evidently become better ventilated (decreasing aAD_{N_2}). The high AaD_{O_2} remaining thus appears exclusively attributable to direct venoarterial shunting or to perfusion of persistently atelectatic areas of the lung.

REFERENCES

1. **Patrick J, Natale R, Richardson B:** Patterns of human fetal breathing activity at 34 to 35 weeks' gestational age. Am J Obstet Gynecol 132:507–513, 1978
2. **Boddy K, Mantell CD:** Observations of fetal breathing movements transmitted through maternal abdominal wall. Lancet 2:1219, 1972
3. **Merlet C, Hoerter J, Devilleneuve C, Tchobroutsky C:** Mise en évidence des mouvements respiratoires chez le foetus d'agneau in utero au cours du dernier mois de la gestation. C R Acad Sci [D] (Paris) 270:2462, 1970
4. **Dawes GS, Fox HE, Laduc BM, Liggins GC, Richards RT:** Respiratory movements and rapid-eye-movement sleep in the foetal lamb. J Physiol 220:119–114, 1972
5. **Duenhoelter JH, Pritchard JA:** Fetal respiration: quantitative measurements of amniotic fluid inspired near term by human and rhesus fetuses. Am J Obstet Gynecol 125:306–309, 1976
6. **Saunders RA, Milner AD:** Pulmonary pressure/volume relationships during the last phase of delivery and the first postnatal breaths in human subjects. J Pediatr 93:667–673, 1978
7. **Burns BD:** The central control of respiratory movements. Br Med Bull 19:7, 1963
8. **Purves MJ, Biscoe TJ:** Development of chemoreceptor activity. Br Med Bull 22:56, 1966
9. **Hodson WA, Fenner A, Brumley G, Chernick V, Avery ME:** Cerebrospinal fluid and blood acid-base relationships in fetal and neonatal lambs and pregnant ewes. Respir Physiol 4:322, 1968
10. **Bystrzycka E, Nail BS, Purves MJ:** Central and peripheral neural respiratory activity in the mature sheep foetus and newborn lamb. Respir Physiol 25:199–215, 1975
11. **Purves MJ:** Onset of respiration at birth. Arch Dis Child 49:333–343, 1974
12. **Lee JC, Stoll BJ, Downing SE:** Properties of the laryngeal chemoreflex in neonatal piglets. Am J Physiol 233:R30–R36, 1977
13. **Harned HS, Myracle, J, Ferreiro J:** Respiratory suppression and swallowing from introduction of fluids into the laryngeal region of the lamb. Pediatr Res 12:1003–1009, 1978
14. **Chernick V:** Fetal breathing movements and the onset of breathing at birth. Clin Perinatol 5:257–268, 1978
15. **Permutt S, Riley RL:** Hemodynamics of collapsible vessels with tone: the vascular waterfall. J Appl Physiol 18:924, 1963
16. **Bland RD, McMillan DD:** Lung fluid dynamics in awake newborn lambs. J Clin Invest 60:1107–1115, 1977
17. **Egan EA, Olver RE, Strang LB:** Changes in non-electrolyte permeability of alveoli and the absorption of lung liquid at the start of breathing in the lamb. J Physiol 244:161–179, 1975
18. **Aherne W, Dawkins MJR:** The removal of fluid from the pulmonary airways after birth in the rabbit, and the effect on this of prematurity and prenatal hypoxia. Biol Neonate 7:214, 1964
19. **Fletcher BD, Sachs BE, Kotas RV:** Radiologic demonstration of post natal liquid in the lungs of newborn lambs. Pediatrics 46:252, 1970
20. **Avery ME, Gatewood OB, Brumley G:** Transient tachypnea of newborn. Am J Dis Child 111:380, 1966
21. **Starling MD, Elliot RB:** The effects of prostaglandins, prostaglandin inhibitors and oxygen on the closure of the ductus arteriosus, pulmonary arteries and umbilical vessels *in vitro*. Prostaglandins 8:187, 1974
22. **Sharpe GI, Larsson KS:** Studies on closure of the ductus arteriosus, X. *In vitro* effects of prostaglandins. Prostaglandins 9:703, 1975
23. **Creasy RK, Drost M, Green MV, Morris JA:** Effect of ventilation on transfer of blood from placenta to neonate. Am J Physiol 222:186–188, 1972
24. **Marquis L, Ackerman BD:** Placental respiration in the immediate neonatal period. Am J Obstet Gynecol 117:358–363, 1973
25. **Philip AGS, Teng SS:** Role of respiration in effecting placental transfusion at Cesarean section. Biol Neonate 31:219–224, 1977
26. **Milner AD, Saunders RA:** Pressure and volume changes during the first breath of human neonates. Arch Dis Child 52:918–924, 1977
27. **Geubelle F, Francotte M, Beyer M, Louis I, Logvinoff MM:** Functional residual capacity and thoracic gas volume in normoxic and hyperoxic newborn infants. Acta Paediatr Belg 30:221–225, 1977
28. **Krauss AN, Auld PAM:** Pulmonary gas trapping in premature infants. Pediatr Res 5:10, 1971
29. **Agostoni E, Mead J:** Statics of the respiratory system. Handbook of Physiology, Vol. I. Washington, D.C. American Physiological Society, 1964
30. **Chiswick ML, Milner RDG:** Crying vital capacity. Measurement of neonatal lung function. Arch Dis Child 51:22–27, 1976
31. **Milner AD, Saunders RA, Hopkin IE:** Effects of delivery by Caesarian section on lung mechanics and lung volume in the human neonate. Arch Dis Child 53:545–548, 1978
32. **Thibeault DW, Poblete E, Auld PAM:** Alveolar-arterial O_2 and CO_2 differences and their relation to lung volume in the newborn. Pediatrics 41:574, 1968
33. **Bryan AC, Bryan MH:** Control of respiration in the newborn. Clin Perinatol 5:269–281, 1978
34. **Bryan MH, Knill RL, Bryan AC:** Chest wall instability and its influence on respiration in

the newborn infant. In Stern L, Fries–Hansen B, Kildeberg P (eds): Intensive Care in the Newborn. Masson-New York, 1976

35. **Finer NN, Abroms IF, Taeusch HW:** Ventilation and sleep states in newborn infants. J Pediatr 89:100–108, 1976

36. **Harding R, Johnson P, McClelland ME, McLeod CH, Whyte PL:** Laryngeal function during breathing and swallowing in foetal and newborn lambs. J Physiol 272:14P–15P, 1977

37. **Hathorn MKS:** The rate and depth of breathing in new-born infants in different sleep states. J Physiol 243:101–113, 1974

38. **Bolton DPG, Herman S:** Ventilation and sleep state in the new-born. J Physiol 240:67–77, 1974

39. **Frantz ID, Adler SM, Abroms IF, Thach BT:** Respiratory response to airway occlusion in infants: sleep state and maturation. J Appl Physiol 41:634–638, 1976

40. **Haddad GG, Epstein RA, Epstein MAF, Leistner HL, Marino PA and Mellins RB:** Maturation of ventilation and ventilatory pattern in normal sleeping infants. J Appl Physiol 46:998–1002, 1979

41. **Knill R, Andrews W, Bryan AC, Bryan MH:** Respiratory load compensation in infants. J Appl Physiol 40:357–361, 1976

42. **Knill R, Bryan AC:** An intercostal-phrenic inhibitory reflex in human newborn infants. J Appl Physiol 40:352–356, 1976

43. **Hagan R, Bryan AC, Bryan MH, Gulston G:** Neonatal chest wall afferents and regulation of respiration. J Appl Physiol 42:362–367, 1977

44. **Tusiewicz K, Moldofsky H, Bryan AC, Bryan MH:** Mechanics of the rib cage and diaphragm during sleep. J Appl Physiol 43:600–602, 1977

45. **Muller N, Gulston G, Cade D, Whitton J, Froese AB, Bryan MH, Bryan AC:** Diaphragmatic muscle fatigue in the newborn. J Appl Physiol 46:688–695, 1979

46. **Keens TG, Bryan AC, Levison H, Ianuzzo CD:** Developmental pattern of muscle fiber types in human ventilatory muscles. J Appl Physiol 44:909–913, 1978

47. **Henderson-Smart DJ, Read DJC:** Reduced lung volume during behavioral active sleep in the newborn. J Appl Physiol 46:1081–1085, 1979

48. **Frantz ID, Adler SM, Thach BT, Taeusch HW:** Maturational effects on respiratory responses to carbon dioxide in premature infants. J Appl Physiol 41:41–45, 1976

49. **Gosgrove JF, Neunburger N, Bryan MH, Bryan AC, Levison H:** A new method of evaluating the chemosensitivity of the respiratory center in children. Pediatrics 56:972–980, 1975

50. **Suthers GK, Henderson-Smart DJ, Read DJC:** Postnatal changes in the rate of high frequency bursts in inspiratory activity in cats and dogs. Brain Res 132:537–540, 1977

51. **Reinstorff D, Fenner A:** Ventilatory response to hyperoxia in premature and newborn infants during the first three days of life. Respir Physiol 15:159–165, 1972

52. **Krauss AN, Tori CA, Brown J, Soodalter J, Auld PAM:** Oxygen chemoreceptors in low birth weight infants. Pediatr Res 7:569–574, 1973

53. **Albersheim S, Boychuk R, Seshia MMK, Cates D, Rigatto H:** Effects of CO_2 on immediate ventilatory response to O_2 in preterm infants. J Appl Physiol 41:609–611, 1976

54. **Rigatto H, Verduzco RT, Cates DB:** Effects of O_2 on the ventilatory response to CO_2 in preterm infants. J Appl Physiol 39:896–899, 1975

55. **Wyszogrodski I, Thach BT, Milic-Emili J:** Maturation of respiratory control in unanesthetized newborn rabbits. J Appl Physiol 44:304–310, 1978

56. **Haddad GG, Mellins RB:** The role of airway receptors in the control of respiration in infants: A review. J Pediatr 91:281–286, 1977

57. **Olinsky A, Bryan MH, Bryan AC:** Influence of lung inflation on respiratory control in neonates. J Appl Physiol 36:426–429, 1974

58. **Olinsky A, Bryan MH, Bryan AC:** Response of newborn infants to added respiratory loads. J Appl Physiol 37:190–193, 1974

59. **Taeusch HW, Carson S, Frantz ID, Milic-Emili J:** Respiratory regulation after elastic loading and CO_2 rebreathing in normal term infants. J Pediatr 88:102–111, 1976

60. **Kirkpatrick SML, Olinsky A, Bryan MH, Bryan AC:** Effect of premature delivery on the maturation of the Hering-Breuer inspiratory inhibitory reflex in human infants. J Pediatr 88:1010–1014, 1976

61. **Adler SM, Thach BT, Frantz ID:** Maturational changes of effective elastance in the first 10 days of life. J Appl Physiol 40:539–542, 1976

62. **Rigatto H, Brady JP:** Periodic breathing and apnea in preterm infants: II. Hypoxia as a primary event. Pediatrics 50:219–228, 1972

63. **Fenner A, Schalk U, Hoenicke H, Wendenburg A, Roehling T:** Periodic breathing in premature and neonatal babies: incidence, breathing pattern, respiratory gas tensions, response to changes in the composition of ambient air. Pediatr Res 7:174–183, 1973

64. **Guntheroth WG, Kawabori I:** Hypoxic apnea and gasping. J Clin Invest 56:1371–1377, 1975

65. **Lawson EE, Thach BT:** Respiratory patterns during progressive asphyxia in newborn rabbits. J Appl Physiol 43:468–474, 1977

66. **Hathorn MKS:** Analysis of periodic changes in ventilation in new-born infants. J Physiol 285:85–99, 1978

67. **Parks CR, Woodrum DE, Alden ER, Standaert TV, Hodson WA:** Gas exchange in the immature

lung I. Anatomical shunt in the premature infant. J Appl Physiol 36:103–107, 1974

68. Koch G: Lung function and acid-base balance in the newborn infant. Acta Paediatr Scand [Suppl] 181:5, 1968

69. Dahms BB, Krauss AN, Auld PAM: Pulmonary function in dysmature infants. P Pediatr 84: 434–437, 1974

70. Arcilla RA, Oh W, Wallgren G, Hanson JS, Gessner IH, Lind J: Quantitative studies of the human neonatal circulation, II. Hemodynamic findings in early and late clamping of the umbilical cord. Acta Paediatr Scand 179:25, 1967

71. Assali NS: Some aspects of fetal life in utero and the changes at birth. Am J Obstet Gynecol 97:324, 1967

72. McMurphy DM, Heymann MA, Rudolph AM, Melmon K: Developmental changes in constriction of the ductus arteriosus: responses to oxygen and vasoactive agents in the isolated ductus arteriosus of the fetal lamb. Pediatr Res 6:231, 1972

73. Wallgren G, Hanson JS, Lind J: Quantitative studies of the human neonatal circulation, III. Observations of the newborn infant's central circulatory responses to moderate hypovolemia. Acta Paediatr Scan [Supp] 179:45, 1967

74. Wallgren G, Lind J: Quantitative studies of the human neonatal circulation, IV. Observations on the newborn infant's peripheral circulation and plasma expansion during moderate hypovolemia. Acta Paediatr Scan [Suppl] 179:57, 1967

75. Wallgren G, Hanson JS, Tabakin BS, Raiha NS, Vapaavuori E: Quantitative studies of the human neonatal circulation, V. Hemodynamic findings in premature infants with and without respiratory distress. Acta Paediatr Scand [Suppl] 179:71, 1967

76. Dawes GS: Fetal and Neonatal Physiology. Chicago, Year Book Publishers 1968

77. Folkow B, Neil E: Circulation. London, Oxford, 1971

78. Harned HS: Respiration and the respiratory system. In Stawe U (ed): Physiology of the Perinatal Period. New York, Appleton-Century-Crofts, 1970

79. Rudolph AM, Heymann MA: The circulation of the fetus in utero: methods for studying distribution of blood flow, cardiac output and organ blood flow. Circ Res 21:163, 1967

80. Rudolph AM, Heymann MA: Circulatory changes during growth in the fetal lamb. Circ Res 26:289, 1970

81. Rudolph AM, Heymann MA, Teramo KAW et al: Studies on the circulation of the previable human fetus. Pediatr Res 5:452, 1971

82. Nelson NM: Respiration after birth. In Smith CA, Nelson NM (eds): Physiology of the Newborn Infant. 4th ed. Springfield (Ill), Charles C Thomas, 1976

83. Burnard ED, Granang A, Gray RE: Cardiac output in the newborn infant. Clin Sci 31:121, 1966

84. Chu J, Clements JA, Cotton EK, et al: Neonatal pulmonary ischemia. Pediatrics 40:709, 1967

85. Mansell A, Bryan AC, Levison H: Airway closure in children. J Appl Physiol 33:711, 1972

86. Nelson NM: Neonatal pulmonary function. Pediatr Clin North Am 13:769, 1966

87. Phelan PD, Williams HE: Ventilatory studies in healthy infants. Pediatr Res 3:425, 1969

88. Polgar G, Promadhat V: Pulmonary Function Testing in Children: Techniques and Standards. Philadelphia, WB Saunders, 1971

89. LaCourt G, Polgar G: Development of pulmonary function in late gestation. The functional residual capacity of the lung in premature children. Acta Paediatr Scand 63:81–88, 1974

90. Milner AD, Saunders RA, Hopkin IE: Tidal pressure/volume and flow/volume respiratory loop patterns in human neonates. Clin Sci Mol Med 54:257–264, 1978

91. Tunell R, Copher D, Persson B: The pulmonary gas exchange and blood gas changes in connection with birth. In Stetson JB, Surger PR (eds): Neonatal Intensive Care, p. 99. Warren H Green, St. Louis, 1976

92. Lacourt G, Polgar G: Interaction between nasal and pulmonary resistance in newborn infants. J Appl Physiol 30:870, 1971

93. Sharp JT, Druz WS, Balagot RC, Bandelin VR, Danon J: Total respiratory compliance in infants and children. J Appl Physiol 29:775, 1970

94. Lees MH, Way RC, Ross BB: Ventilation and respiratory gas transfer of infants with increased pulmonary blood flow. Pediatrics 40: 259, 1967

95. Corbet AJS, Ross JA, Beaudry PH, Stern L: Ventilation-perfusion relationships as assessed by $aADN_2$ in hyaline membrane disease. J Appl Physiol 36:74, 1974

96. Corbet AJS, Ross JA, Beaudry PH, Stern L: Effect of positive-pressure breathing on $aADN_2$ in hyaline membrane disease. J Appl Physiol 38:33–38, 1975

97. Krauss AN, Klain DB, Auld PAM: Carbon monoxide diffusing capacity in newborn infants. Pediatr Res 10:771–776, 1976.

98. Avery ME, Fletcher BD: The Lung and Its Disorders in the Newborn Infant, 3rd ed. Philadelphia, WB Saunders, 1974

99. Nourse CH, Nelson NM: Uniformity of ventilation in the newborn infant; direct assessment of the arterial-alveolar N_2 difference. Pediatrics 43:226, 1969

III

Transition
and Stabilization

10

Thermoregulation in the Newborn

Jon W. Scopes

Although from time immemorial it has been considered a good thing to keep babies warm, it is only in the past two decades that a reasonable understanding of the physiology of thermoregulation in the newborn has made it possible to answer with any precision the question, "How warm is warm?"

Physiology of Temperature Control in the Infant

Adult mammals, including the human, have the attributes of a homeotherm. Over a fairly wide range of environmental temperature they maintain a remarkably constant deep body temperature, a vitally important aspect of sustaining a constant *milieu interieur*. Nonetheless, this homeothermy may be overwhelmed in extremes of cold or heat stress. It is only in the last 20 years that it has been demonstrated that the newborn baby has all the capabilities of a homeotherm, although the range of environmental temperature over which he can operate successfully is severely restricted when compared with the adult. He has disadvantages including a relatively large surface area, poor thermal insulation, and a small mass to act as a heat sink. Like the adult, his responses may be jeopardized by disease and adverse conditions such as hy-

poxia and drug intoxication. The understanding of his responses and the factors limiting them make up the physiology of thermoregulation in the newborn. As recently as 1957, there was little hard evidence that a baby in the first hours after birth was anything other than a temporary poikilotherm, although Day had in fact shown that the thriving baby, aged a week or two, had all the responses of a homeotherm.[2] In 1957 and 1958, Silverman and his coworkers deduced from their clinical trials that the newborn baby also had these responses,[1,3] and Bruck in 1961 produced unequivocal physiologic evidence that these responses applied in the first hours after birth even if prematurely born.[4]

Thus, the baby produces heat as a result of metabolic activity. In order to maintain a constant body temperature, he must dissipate this heat to the environment at a mean rate equal to that of its production. In cool conditions, he must conserve heat but, if, with maximal conservation, more heat is lost than produced, he must increase heat production (*i.e.*, display a metabolic response to cold). Conversely, in a very warm environment, he must dissipate more heat by vasodilation and sweating. To achieve all this, he must have a sensory system to appreciate temperature (an affector arc), a central control system, and the means of adjusting heat production and dissipation (an effector arc).

Affector Arc. As with the adult, cooling the skin produces a prompt and reproductible metabolic response in the baby showing the presence of skin receptors.[4] Also of interest is the demonstration that the trigeminus area of the face shows a marked sensitivity to heat and cold.[5] The existence of central cold receptors is difficult to demonstrate with precision in the human baby, although they can be inferred from the modification of response at different deep body temperatures. In the human baby, surface sensors are the more obviously dominant.[6] In the neonatal guinea pig, Brück and Wünnenberg have shown temperature receptors in the cervical part of the spinal cord.[7,8] The interaction of superficial and hypothalamic sensors have received special study by this group. A multiplicative evaluation of the signals in the hypothalamus seems likely. It is likely that as in the adult animal there are thermal sensors in the hypothalamic region and in the thorax.[9]

Central Regulating Mechanism. In the adult[10] and in newborn animals there is good evidence of a complex central regulating mechanism situated in the area of the hypothalamus. In the human infant such an area can be inferred, and confirmed by experiments of nature such as the studies of Cross and his coworkers on an anencephalic infant.[11] The central thermostat is not, however, set at a fixed and unvarying temperature; it certainly undergoes cyclic changes, falls about 0.5°C with the onset of sleep,[12] and is affected by pyrogens, drugs, and intrahypothalamic hormones such as noradrenaline.[13] Although set-point deviation can be considered as a form of cold adaptation, there is no good evidence to suggest that the set point (around which temperature is regulated) of a newborn is different from that in later life.[14] This control center can, of course, be rendered partially or totally ineffective by various drugs and by diseases such as intracranial hemorrhage, gross cerebral malformation, trauma, and severe birth asphyxia.

Effector Arc. Vasomotor Control. From birth there is a well-developed ability to control skin blood flow, even in very small infants.[4,15] It should be remembered that despite this ability, a baby's total thermal insulation is poor compared with that of the adult.[16]

Increased Heat Production. The ability to increase heat production (*i.e.*, achieve a metabolic response to cold) is a consistent phenomenon in the healthy baby, even if prematurely born.[17] Such heat may be produced by either shivering, together with other muscular activity, or by nonshivering thermogenesis. Large increases in heat production occur in babies in the absence of detectable shivering,[17] although, at very low environmental temperatures (15°C), shivering may be observed.[18] The evidence that brown fat is an important site of heat production in many newborn mammals is now well known.[19] In fact, catecholamine-mediated nonshivering thermogenesis in brown fat represents a physiologic effector organ quantitatively important to cold-adapted animals, to hibernating animals, and to the newborn. The evidence that it applies to the human infant is now incontrovertible.

1. The human infant has brown fat[20] and responds to infusions of noradrenaline with increased metabolism.[21]
2. In clinical situations in which this fat is depleted, his metabolic response is poor or absent.[22]
3. During a normal metabolic response to cold there is evidence of lipolysis.[23]
4. His metabolic response to cold is impaired by hypoxemia.[24]
5. During the metabolic response to cold, temperatures over the brown fat at the nape of the neck not only remain warm but on occasions exceed any other body temperature, which must mean heat production at that site.[25]

One can calculate, however, as Hey has done, that the amount of brown fat in babies is probably inadequate to explain the full observed increase in heat production, so that restlessness and other muscular activity must contribute.[26] The newborn guinea pig, as Brück and Wünnerberg have shown, is capable of both shivering and nonshivering thermogenesis.[7] If nonshivering thermogenesis is blocked by β-receptor blockade, heat is produced by shivering, and vice-versa, although shivering is less effective than nonshivering thermogenesis.

The dependence of the newborn on brown fat nonshivering thermogenesis has important practical consequences because this effector mechanism may be rendered useless by hy-

Table 10-1. Equilibrium Values for Heat Loss (k cal/m²hr) in a Week-Old 2 kg Baby Lying Naked on a Foam Mattress in Draught-free Surroundings of Uniform Temperature and Moderate Humidity

Heat loss	Environmental Temperature		
	30°C	33°C	36°C
Radiation	19 (43%)	12 (40%)	7 (24%)
Convection	15 (37%)	9 (33%)	5 (19%)
Evaporation	7 (16%)	7 (24%)	17 (56%)
Conduction	2 (4%)	1 (3%)	0 (1%)
Total (k cal/m²hr)	43	29	29

(Hey: In Recent Advances in Paediatrics. London, Churchill, 1971)[26]

poxia, certain drug blockade, and by lipid depletion. Nonshivering thermogenesis in animals is reduced with increasing age, although it can be preserved by exposure to cold (with *ad lib* feeding), such as one uses in producing a cold-adapted animal. In fasted newborn rabbits, brown fat deposits are maintained until death, when the rabbits are kept warm (35°C), but are depleted by the second day if kept in a cool environment (30°C or 25°C).[27] When the metabolic response fails, brown fat is virtually completely depleted of lipid.[27,28] No evidence is available to assess how long the response lasts in the human baby.

Sweating. Newborn term infants have six times more abundant sweat glands per unit area than do adults, but the peak response of each gland is only about a third of an adult gland.[29] One might therefore expect the baby's response to a warm stress to exceed that of an adult, but, in fact, the term baby only increases insensible water loss about fourfold when a warm environment has increased his rectal temperature to 37.8°C.[30] This only represents the dissipation of his basal metabolic rate; it follows that in a heat-gaining environment the risks of hyperthermia are great. Babies born about 8 weeks before term have virtually no ability to sweat, and even at 3 weeks before term sweating is severely limited and largely confined to the head and face.[30]

Physics of Heat Exchange in the Baby

The baby, like any physical body, exchanges heat by conduction, convection, evaporation, and radiation. Table 10-1 is Hey's schematic summary of the way heat loss is partitioned between these channels in the conditions that apply in a clinical warm air incubator.[26] Because conduction depends on the thermal conductivity of the substance in contact with the body, and because babies are usually laid on a mattress of low conductivity, thermal exchange through this channel is usually small. Convective exchange depends on air speed and air temperature and, with radiation, represents a major channel of heat loss, varying inversely with environmental air temperature. Evaporative loss depends on relative humidity and air speed, and represents a small but important fraction of heat dissipation in the ordinary circumstances of a clothed baby or one nursed in a regular air warmed incubator of moderate humidity. In very warm environments, or when nursed under a radiant overhead heater, or when a very immature baby with a thin skin is nursed in an environment of low relative humidity, it becomes a major fraction (latent heat of evaporation of water is large—540 cal/g, and, in this sense, a dry environment encouraging evaporation is "cool" and a saturated environment preventing evaporation is "warm"). In environments warmer than the body it represents the *only* means of heat dissipation. Draughts materially increase convective and evaporative losses.

Radiant heat loss depends on the presenting surface area (and thus to the geometry) and surface temperature of the body compared with the surface temperature of the receiving surface. From Table 10-1 it is seen that it represents a major proportion of heat dissipation in a naked baby in an incubator. It is important to remember that the radiant receiving surface is the *inside surface* of the Perspex canopy of the incubator which is

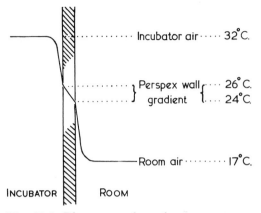

Fig. 10-1. Diagram to show the temperature gradient across the 9mm Perspex wall of a typical incubator. (Hey EN, Mount L: Lancet 2:202, 1966)[31]

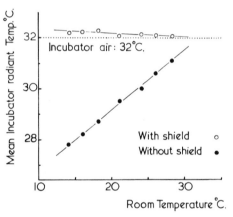

Fig. 10-2. The influence of room temperature on the mean inner wall temperature to which a baby will radiate *heat* within a series *111* incubator (Oxygenaire) whose air temperature was kept constant at 32°C. Hey EN, Mount L: Lancet 2:202, 1966)[31]

opaque to the thermal radiations of the baby's skin (wavelength 9,000–10,000 nm). The temperature of the canopy is so affected not only by incubator air temperature but also by room temperature that the inside canopy temperature may be very different from the temperature set on the incubator thermostat (Fig. 10-1). Thus, radiant exchange is profoundly affected by room temperature unless a second layer of Perspex is interposed between the baby and the canopy.[31] This second layer is warmed by the incubator air which is subject to the incubator's thermostat control. The effect is shown in Figure 10-2 from Hey and

Mount.[31] Heat can be captured in incubators from radiant sources which pass through Perspex, such as sunlight (the "greenhouse" effect). Radiant sources can, of course, be used to pour heat into a baby—the converse of his heat dissipation.

It follows from the above that, in strictly scientific terms, no single temperature is a full statement of the thermal environment of the baby. However, in draught-free surroundings of moderate relative humidity, in which the temperature of air, conductive surfaces, and radiant receiving surfaces are within a degree of each other, a single temperature such as air temperature is a reasonable statement of the "environmental temperature."

Optimal Thermal Environment

The clinical consequences of environments that are too hot or too cold are discussed below. In temperate zones, the more common failing in the past has been to provide too little warmth. With a better understanding of the physiology of the newborn it is possible to approach the question, "How warm is warm?" more scientifically than in the past.

The **neutral thermal environment** is that range of thermal environment in which a baby with a normal body temperature has a minimal metabolic rate and can maintain a constant body temperature by vasomotor and sudomotor control and by posture. Below this range, the lower end of which is termed the **critical temperature** (Fig. 10-3), a metabolic response

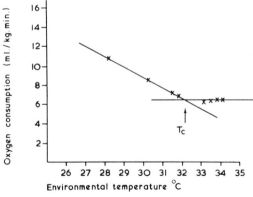

Fig. 10-3. Assessment of critical temperature when metabolic rate at several temperatures has been measured. The two lines are drawn by eye-to-intersect at T_c—the critical temperature. (Scopes JW, Ahmed I: Arch Dis Child 41:417 1966)[24]

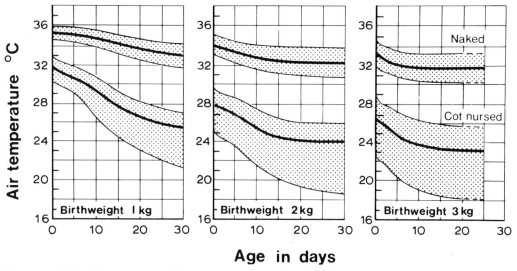

Fig. 10-4. This diagram summarizes the changes in optimal temperature that occur with age in babies weighing 1, 2, or 3 kg at birth. The **dark line** indicates the optimum and the **shaded area** the range within which a baby can be expected to maintain a normal body temperature without increasing either heat production or evaporative water loss by more than 25 percent. The upper range is for naked babies and the lower for those cot nursed. The "operative" temperature, in these cases, implies an air temperature, in a draught-free environment, of approximately 50% saturation and in which radiant receiving surfaces are the same as air temperature (*i.e.,* with a second layer of Perspex interposed between the baby and the single-walled incubator). For allowances to be made in other physical conditions, see text. (Courtesy of Dr. Edmund Hey; Adapted from Hey EN: In Hull D, Gairdner D (eds): Recent Advances in Paediatrics. London, Churchill, 1971)

to cold is necessary to replace lost heat. Above this range an increase of body temperature and thus of metabolic rate is inevitable. Thus, the neutral range represents the thermal range of minimal stress. It is very narrow with a naked baby (Fig. 10-4).

The lower end of the range can be assessed with precision in an individual baby if heat production (rates of oxygen consumption in Fig. 10-3) is measured at different environmental temperatures (Fig. 10-3). By measuring the critical temperatures for a large number of babies of different weights and ages, one can derive a table of *probable* critical temperatures for babies. By a knowledge of the baby's capacity to dissipate heat, one can derive an estimate of the upper border of the neutral range. Combining the information, Hey published Figure 10-4.[26]

There are some important *caveats* in the use of Figure 10-4. The temperatures are strictly appropriate only if the physical conditions defined in the legend apply. If relative humidity is higher (possible 75%) the temperatures predicted should be decreased by 0.5°C for naked babies and 1°C for clothed babies. If a single wall incubator is used, an allowance of 1°C should be made for every 7°C by which room temperature is below incubator air temperature. These data are derived from healthy babies and, on occasions when one may expect a low metabolic rate in a baby (in some very ill babies or in babies with cyanotic heart disease), temperatures should be slightly higher. Conversely, in restless babies, babies with frequent seizures and babies with large left-to-right shunts, slightly lower temperatures will be appropriate.

The figure emphasizes a number of important points. The neutral range is very narrow for naked babies and falls only a little with advancing age. All the temperatures are very warm by adult standards. *There is no single environmental temperature that is appropriate for all sizes and conditions of babies.* That which is appropriate for a lusty term infant is too cold for a tiny newborn preterm infant, and that which is appropriate for the latter is too hot for the term infant. When a baby is clothed and in a crib, the avenues of heat dissipation are all partially occluded; the temperatures required are lower, and the consequences of misjudging are less (see below).

It must be remembered that Figure 10-4 represents a guess (albeit a scientifically based guess) at an appropriate temperature for an untested baby. Because of the *caveats* mentioned above, it is still incumbent to monitor a baby's temperature to test whether the guess is working out in an individual case. This is, in fact, a form of **servocontrol** because the adult responsible adjusts the environmental temperature in response to a baby's temperature.

Servocontrol

The principle of servocontrol is an admission that it is so difficult to measure all the channels of heat exchange that one controls by using the baby's temperature as a measure of heat balance.[32] It is, therefore, a very sensible admission. The objections to servocontrol are that it deprives the temperature chart of its usual clinical value; that a baby with a fever (a high set point) could be subjected to cold stress; that a sensing thermistor failure could lead to hyperthermia; and that servocontrol adds to complexity and expense.

Proponents of servocontrol can muster a defense against each of these objections. Servocontrol is a very efficient and convenient means of controlling temperature in intensive-care situations and is the only reasonable method by which radiant heat sources can be employed. It is probably unnecessary when long, stable, situations exist, and must not be allowed to be a substitute for intelligent, thoughtful nursing. Servocontrol can be employed using either a body core temperature or a surface temperature as the sensing transducer on which the control is based. The disadvantage of a core sensor is that it does not detect a change until the baby's homeothermy is overwhelmed. (A very hot or a very cold skin producing a metabolic response may antedate a core temperature change.) A skin probe will sense an inappropriate temperature and allow adjustment of the thermal environment before the core temperature is changed. Theoretically, a number of skin sites should

be measured and a computerized weighted mean presented to the environmental control mechanism. In practice, the skin temperature of the exposed abdominal skin makes a good practical sensing site. Silverman and coworkers found minimal rates of oxygen consumption when abdominal skin temperatures were maintained at 36.0°C to 36.5°C.[33]

Using a skin temperature in this way assumes that the temperature measured is representative of the adjacent skin temperature. Belgaumkar and Scot have shown that this is an invalid assumption in the case of small premature infants nursed in a servocontrol environment of low relative humidity.[34] The very immature baby's skin allows evaporation to a marked degree (see also below under Overhead Heaters), even though sweating is not active. The skin sensor is applied by covering it with a piece of adhesive tape. Thus, the very site which is monitored is not subject to the large heat loss of evaporation and no longer represents the overall skin temperature. In consequence, the skin monitor "sees" a higher temperature than does the adjacent skin and the warming mechanism of the servocontrol incubator is not activated. In practical terms, the babies maintained in a servocontrol incubator with low humidity have a paradoxically low core temperature, and, as they further showed, an increased tendency to severe apnea.[35] It follows that a high relative humidity is essential to such babies nursed under servocontrol conditions.

Clinical Aspects

The clinical consequences of keeping a baby in too hot an environment are obvious. At the worst he may overheat and die, but at lesser extremes he may suffer heat stroke. Even if he survives, he may have cerebral damage or become dehydrated and even hypernatremic in prolonged conditions that are mildly too hot.

Very cold, freezing, temperatures have equally dramatic consequences. What is less obvious is that temperatures which feel hot to an adult may represent a dangerous cold stress to a baby, a stress that expresses itself in terms of morbidity and mortality. Even a moderately cool environment will inevitably require the baby to absorb more oxygen (threatening his life if he already has respiratory difficulty) and use more substrate as fuel (effectively creating artifical starvation). Thus, the effects of inadequate warmth have metabolic consequences, including metabolic acidosis, as well as purely physical effects.[18] Should he fail to produce an adequate metabolic response to cold, with its implied waste of oxygen and food substrate, his body temperature will fall, leading to the condition described by Elliott and Mann as the "neonatal cold injury syndrome." [36] Some of the dangerous consequences of neonatal hypothermia are now identified as being related to disseminated intravascular coagulation (DIC).[37]

In the 1950's, when hypothermia for organ surgery was in vogue, Silverman and his associates[1] and Jolly and his coworkers[38] conducted controlled trials on effects of warmth, demonstrating the descrease in mortality with extra warmth. In the former trial, survival in incubators maintained at 31.7°C was 93% (babies >1,500 g) 86% (1000–1500 g) and 50% <1,000 g) compared with survival in cooler incubators at 28.9° (which were 79%, 77%, and 14% respectively). Warmth alone tripled the chances of survival of the very small babies. Others have shown the favorable effect of using the higher incubator temperature (31.5°C) *plus* supplementary radiant heat to maintain body temperature at 36°C.[39,40] There can be no doubt that adequate warmth is a major factor in improving neonatal survival. Morevoer, evidence is accumulating that adequate warmth has a favorable effect on morbidity. In follow-up studies, Davis and Davies have produced evidence that slightly inadequate feeding and warmth impaired brain growth in babies.[41] In the same follow-up group, the interesting phenomenon of the disappearance of Little's disease (spastic diplegia—usually in grossly premature babies) has been noticed; the only obvious difference on review between those who suffered and similar babies who did not is that the former had lower body temperatures over the neonatal period, implying inadequate warmth by present-day standards.[42]

Possible advantages of minimal cold stress to healthy thriving babies have been investigated by Glass, Silverman, and Sinclair.[43] In a controlled comparison between a group of babies servocontrolled at 35°C (abdominal skin) and another servocontrolled at 36°C (abdominal skin), they showed a very minor growth retardation in the "cool" group which could be offset by increasing the feeds. The "cool" group, however, after 2 weeks had a better ability to withstand a minor cold stress. Stressing a baby continuously to "toughen" him must, however, await further animal work. It seems likely that intermittent short mild stress might achieve the same end at lesser risk because Ziesburger and his ascociates have shown that brown fat thermogenesis in the guinea pig can be preserved by intermittent exposures to cold.[44] It is interesting to speculate whether such "toughening" could be achieved by intermittent exposure of the face to cold.

Overhead Radiant Heaters

Overhead radiant heaters that pour heat back into a baby while he is losing it by other means have an important use in intensive care situations in which free access to airways, umbilical vessels and so on is essential. In such situations, it is impossible to continuously monitor heat loss and heat gain in the ordinary clinical situation. Therefore, monitoring the baby's temperature is the only practical way of assuring heat balance. The considerations discussed above under Servocontrol apply in particular detail and again a skin temperature *together with a core temperature* must be monitored. It has now been shown by Tafari and Gentz that this is a safe way of procuring heat balance, but it is not free from difficulty.[45] The heat flux into and out of the baby is so large that any mistake on the part of the adult attendant leads quickly to hypothermia or hyperthermia. Measurements by Robinson and Jones have shown the total heat input to be about twice the baby's own basal heat production.[46] The extra loss, which is compensated for by the large inpouring of heat, is, of course, largely evaporative loss from the moist, but not sweating, skin of the baby. Of secondary importance to the thermal considerations, but of vital importance in clinical terms, is that the water evaporated must be replaced in the baby. Various authors including Wu and Hodgeman have found that babies weighing less than 1 kg should be given an extra 90 ml/kg/day to replace insensible water loss: babies weighing 1 to 1.5 kg, an extra 60 to 75 ml/kg/day; and those over 1.5 kg, an extra 45 ml/kg/day.[47] These extra amounts of fluid constitute clinical problems of administration and of possibly aggravating persistent patent ductus arteriosus. It is certain that frequent determination of osmolality or serum sodium are important parts of monitoring babies under overhead heaters.

Risk Situations. The first risk situation to be borne in mind is the simple situation of a baby nursed naked in an incubator. The range of environmental temperature that he can tolerate is very narrow (Fig. 10-4), so his attendants must be wary. Furthermore, it has been shown that during the phases when supplement radiant heat is being given, the baby is more liable to apneic episodes.[48] Adults prefer to have their faces slightly cooler than their bodies and perhaps babies do also. In fact, the clothed baby in a crib is in a safer position than the naked baby in an incubator because his attendants need not control the environment quite so precisely. Clearly, control is still needed because extremes of cold or heat will damage him, but the latitude is greater. Exposing the face so that the infant can either sweat or vasoconstrict as the situation demands is an advantage.

The moments after birth, when a baby arrives naked, wet and partially asphyxiated is another period in which body temperature falls abruptly unless very special precautions are taken. If the delivery room temperature is about 25°C, even a lusty baby producing a maximal metabolic response to cold cannot match the rate of heat loss of about 200 kcal/kg/min. If he is small, ill, and asphyxiated, the rate of fall of body temperature is dramatic. Dabbing him dry to prevent evaporative loss and using a radiant heater to pour some heat back into him will help. The period of time that he is exposed to temperatures appropriate for adults must be minimized. As mentioned above, serious asphyxia may affect the baby's own homeothermy for many hours after birth. The suggestion that serious cooling at birth[49] led to aggravation of physiological jaundice was not confirmed by Reich and Martin.[50]

Other risk situations occur during major and minor surgery[51] (including exchange transfusion),[52] clinical examination, bathing, x-ray procedures, and transport. The risk of cooling when transporting a baby from one hospital to another is obvious; less obvious is the risk when transporting down a hospital corridor or elevator. There is no universal panacea applicable to all situations, and control of only a single temperature in the environment is inadequate. Means of occluding heat loss, such as conventional swaddling, the "silver swaddler,"[53] or transparent baby bag[54] should be considered. Certainly covering those parts of the baby that do not need to be seen, warming room air, and judicious use of radiant heat are all important. A useful source of warmth not often used in our sophisticated society is the baby's mother—a thermostatically controlled and affectionate heat sink.[55]

Taking the Infant's Temperature. The usual sites for taking a baby's temperature are the rectum, skin, and axilla. Rectal temperature is a reasonable measurement of core temperature; the esophageal or tympanic membrane temperatures are impractical for general use. The deeper a rectal probe is inserted—up to a depth of 10 cm—the higher is the temperature recorded. The major changes occur in the first 4 cm, the depth usually recommended. The disadvantages of rectal temperature measurement are the rare (but real) risk of perforation of the bowel and the risk of cross-infection contamination from repeated insertions.

Skin thermometers have the advantage of showing heat or cold stress early, with a minimal interference with the baby; in particular, they do not interfere with the baby's orifices. The main disadvantages are that skin probes are quite easily displaced, and skin temperatures may be misleading in rapidly changing situations.

The axillary temperature is an approximation to the core temperature, usually being lower than rectal, but occasionally, if brown fat is stimulated, reading higher. The advantages are again minimal handling and no interference with a baby's orifices, so that they are useful for routine monitoring when no obvious thermal problem exists.

The frequency with which a temperature is measured depends on the stability of the thermal situation and on the means used. When an electrical device such as a thermistor or a thermocouple is strapped in place it can be read as frequently as desired. When intermittent temperatures are taken, some compromise must be made to prevent unnecessarily frequent handling of the baby.[5] The mercury in glass thermometer is cheap and reliable if used properly, but it can break, and unless a special low reading thermometer is used, it may fail to record hypothermic situations.

Adequate Warmth

The demonstration that the provision of adequate warmth can cut mortality in small babies by a quarter is a powerful inducement to try to define what is meant by **adequate warmth.** There has been considerable advance in the last 20 years and there is more to be learned: for instance, understanding of the boundary layer of air at the skin, its thermal consequences, bacteriologic consequences, and its aerodynamics. Some fascinating work is already in progress.[56-58] The advantages of crib nursing are being rediscovered and a swing away from incubators may be expected.[51] Humidity, so important when airways are bypassed, has been shown to have comparatively little thermal consequence in air-heated incubators or in clothed babies.[59,60] Its far reaching consequences under conditions of servocontrol or of overhead heaters are discussed above.

The problem of how best to warm babies after severe accidental hypothermia still requires a detailed answer.[61] It seems that a baby acutely cooled may be warmed rapidly,[60] but this does not necessarily apply to a baby hypothermic after a prolonged cold stress.[62]

Also important are the effects on temperature control caused by the ever-increasing number of pharmacologic agents used in the present day. Diazepam, for instance, given to the mother, has recently been shown to impair her baby's metabolic responses.[63] It would not be surprising if other new sedative or anesthetizing agents given to the mother had similar effects on the baby.

It is interesting that sophisticated studies and techniques of warming have identified the advantages of traditional methods such as swaddling and crib nursing.

Thou, Nurse, in swadling Bands the Babe enfold,
And carefully defend its Limbs from Cold,
If Winter, by the chimney place thy Chair,
If Summer, then admit the cooling Air.
Old Quatrain

Moses was swaddled, and placed in a basket on the Nile. The swaddling and the basket are again acceptable modern practice; the advantages of the Nile as an enormous heat sink will no doubt be identified soon. I hope, however, that a baby's attendants would remain in closer contact over a critical period than were Moses' mother and sister.

REFERENCES

1. **Silverman WA, Fertig JW, Berger AP:** The influence of the thermal environment upon the survival of newly born premature infants. Pediatrics 22:876, 1958
2. **Day RL:** Respiratory metabolism in infancy and in childhood. Regulation of body temperature of premature infants. Amer J Dis Child 65:376, 1943
3. **Silverman WA, Blanc WA:** The effects of humidity on survival of newly born premature infants. Pediatrics 20:477, 1957
4. **Brück, K:** Temperature regulation in the newborn infant. Biol Neonate 3:65, 1961
5. **Mestyan I, Jarai GB, Fekete M:** Surface temperature versus deep body temperature and the metabolic response to cold of hypothermic premature infants. Biol Neonate 7:230, 1964
6. **Brück K, Schwennicke HP:** Interaction of superficial and hypothalamic thermosensitive structures in the control of non-shivering thermogenesis. Int. J Biometeorol 15:156,1971
7. **Wünnenberg W, Brück K:** Studies on the ascending pathways from the thermosensitive region of the spinal cord. Pfluegers Arch 321:233, 1970
8. **Wünnenberg W, Brück K:** Function of thermoreceptive structures in the cervical spinal cord of the guinea pig. Pfluegers Arch 299:1, 1968
9. **Mestyan J, Jarai GB, Fekete M:** The significance of facial skin temperature in the chemical heat regulation of premature infants. Biol Neonate 7:243, 1964
10. **Cooper KE:** Temperature regulation and its disorders. In Baron, Compston, Dawson (eds). Recent Advances in Medicine, 15th ed., p. 333. London, Churchill, 1968
11. **Cross KW, Gustavson J, Hill JR, Robinson DC:** Thermoregulation in an anencephalic infant as inferred from its metabolic rate under hypothermic and normal conditions. Clin Sci Mcl Med 31:449, 1966
12. **Day RL:** Regulation of body temperature during sleep. Am J Dis Child 61:734, 1941
13. **Zeisberger E, Brück K:** Central effects of noradrenaline on the control of body temperature in the guinea pig. Pfluegers Arch 322:152, 1971
14. **Brück K:** Which environmental temperature does the premature infant prefer? Pediatrics 41:1027, 1968
15. **Hey EN, Katz G:** The range of thermal insulation in the tissues of the newborn baby. J Physiol 207:667, 1970
16. **Hey EN, Katz G, O'Connell B:** The total thermal insulation of the newborn baby. J Physiol 207:683, 1970

17. **Scopes JW:** Metabolic rate and temperature control in the human baby. Br Med Bull 22: 88, 1966

18. **Adamsons K, Gandy GM, James LS:** The influence of thermal factors upon oxygen consumption of the newborn human infant. J Pediatr 66:495, 1965

19. **Hull D:** Brown adipose tissue. Br Med Bull 22:92, 1966

20. **Aherne W, Hull D:** The site of heat production in the newborn infant. Proc. R Soc Med 57: 1172, 1964

21. **Karlberg P, Moore RE, Oliver TK:** The thermogenic response of the newborn infant to noradrenaline. Acta Paediatr Scand 51:284, 1962

22. **Scopes JW:** Ph.D. thesis, London University, 1965

23. **Dawkins MJR, Scopes JW:** Non-shivering thermogenesis and brown adipose tissue in the human new-born infant. Nature 206:201, 1965

24. **Scopes JW, Ahmed I:** Range of critical temperatures in sick and premature newborn babies. Arch Dis Child 41:417, 1966

25. **Grausz JP:** The effects of environmental temperature changes on the metabolic rate of newborn babies. Acta Paediatr Scand 57:98, 1968

26. **Hey E:** The care of babies in incubators. In Hull D, Gairdner D (eds): Recent Advances in Paediatrics, p. 171. London, Churchill, 1971

27. **Cardasis C, Blanc WA, Sinclair JC:** The effects of ambient temperature on the fasted newborn rabbit. Biol Neonate 21:347, 1972

28. **Hardman MJ, Hey EN, Hull D:** The effect of prolonged cold exposure on heat production in new-born rabbits. J Physiol 205:39, 1969

29. **Foster KG, Hey EN, Katz G:** The response of the sweat glands of the newborn baby to thermal stimuli and to intradermal acetylcholine. J Physiol 203:13, 1969

30. **Hey EN, Katz G:** Evaporative water loss in the new-born baby. J Physiol 200:605, 1968

31. **Hey EN, Mount L:** Temperature control in incubators preliminary communications. Lancet 2:202, 1966

32. **Scopes JW:** A new look at thermoregulation in the newborn: servocontrol incubators. Proc RSM 70:207, 1977

33. **Silverman W, Sinclair JC, Agate FJ:** The oxygen cost of minor changes in heat balance of small newborn infants. Acta Paediatr Scand 55:294, 1966

34. **Belgaumbar TK, Scott KE:** Effects of low humidity on small premature infants in servoncontrol incubators. Biol Neonate 26:377, 1975

35. **Belgaumbar TK, Scott K:** Effects of low humidity on small premature infants in servo-control incubators. Biol Neonate 26:348, 1975

36. **Mann TP, Elliott RIK:** Neonatal cold injury due to accidental exposure to cold. Lancet 1: 229, 1957

37. **Chessells JM, Wigglesworth JS:** Secondary haemorrhagic disease of the newborn. Arch Dis Child 45:539, 1970

38. **Jolly H, Molyneux P, Newell DJ:** A controlled study of the effect of temperature on premature babies. J Pediatr 60:889, 1962

39. **Day RL, Caliguiri L, Kamenski C, Ehrlich F:** Body temperature and survival of premature infants. Pediatrics 34:171, 1965

40. **Buetow KC, Klein SW:** Effect of maintenance of "normal" skin temperature on survival of infants of low birth weight. Pediatrics 34:163, 1964

41. **Davies PA, Davis JP:** Very low birth-weight and subsequent head growth. Lancet 2:1216, 1970

42. **Davies PA :** Communication to European Society for Paediatric Research, Oct. 1943

43. **Glass L, Silverman WA, Sinclair JC:** Effect of the thermal environment on cold resistance and growth of small infants after the first week of life. Pediatrics 41:1033, 1968

44. **Zeisberger E, Brück K, Wünnenberg W, Wietasch C:** Das Ausmass der zitterfreien Thermogenese des Meerschweinchens in Abhángigkeit vom Lebensalter. Pfluegers Arch 296:276, 1967

45. **Tafari N, Gentz J:** Acta Paediatr Scandi 63: 595, 1979

46. **Robinson RO, Jones R:** Advantages and disadvantages of overhead radiant heaters. Proc RSM 70:209, 1977

47. **Wu PYK, Hodgman JE:** Pediatrics 54:704, 1979

48. **Perlstein PH, Edwards NK, Sutherland JM:** Apnoea in premature infants and incubator-air-temperature changes. New Eng J Med 282: 461, 1970

49. **Gernez L:** De la necessite de lutler centre l'hypothermie physiologique due noveaune. Bull Fed Soc Gynecol Obstet Lang Fr 4:11, 1952

50. **Reich J, Martin E:** Untersuchungen zur Beziehung zwischen Körpertemperatur und Serum-Bilirubinspiegel Frühgeborner. Z. Kinderheilk 95:217, 1966

51. **Silverman WA, Sinclair JC, Scopes JW:** Regulation of body temperature in pediatric surgery. J Pediatr Surg 1:321, 1966

52. **Hey EN, Kohlinsky S, O'Connell B:** Heat-losses from babies during exchange transfusion. Lancet 1:335, 1969

53. **Baum JD, Scopes JW:** The silver swaddler. Lancet 1:672, 1968

54. **Besch NJ, Perlstein PH, Edwards NK, Keenan WJ, Sutherland JM:** The transparent baby bag. New Engl J Med 284:121, 1971

55. **Davies PA, Robinson RJ, Scopes JW, Tizard JPM, Wigglesworth JS:** Medical Care of Newborn Babies. London, Spastics International Medical Publications, 1972

56. **Lewis HE, Foster AR, Mullan BJ, Cos RN, Clark RP:** Aerodynamics of the human microenvironment. Lancet 1:1273, 1969

57. **Clark RP, Cox RN, Lewis HE:** Particle transport within the human microenvironment. J Physiol 208:43, 1970

58. **Hey EN, O'Connell B:** Oxygen consumption and heat balance in the cot-nursed baby. Arch Dis Child 45:241, 1970

59. **Silverman WA, Blanc WA:** The effect of humidity on survival of newly-born premature infants. Pediatrics 20:477, 1957

60. **Hey EN, Maurice NP:** Effect of humidity on production and loss of heat in the newborn baby. Arch Dis Child 43:166, 1968

61. **Severe accidental hypothermia.** Lancet 237, Jan 1972

62. **Mann TP:** Hypothermia in the newborn. In Simpson K (ed): Modern Trends in Forensic Medicine. London, Butterworths, 1966

63. **Cree JE, Meyer J, Hailey DM:** Diazepam in labour: its metabolism and effect on clinical course and thermogenesis of the newborn. Br Med J 4:251, 1973

11

Delivery Room Management of the Newborn

Roderic H. Phibbs

Much of newborn intensive care is emergency medicine that requires rapid institution of appropriate diagnostic and therapeutic procedures. This is particularly true immediately after birth when the newborn infant may have cardiac arrest and apnea. The procedures undertaken to restore life constitute resuscitation (Latin, *resuscitare,* to arouse again) and include those actions necessary to help an infant make the transition from dependent fetal to independent neonatal life. Skillful resuscitation of the asphyxiated newborn infant can prevent brain damage and minimize subsequent neonatal disease.

The period of labor and delivery, as well as the first minutes following birth, carry a very high risk of asphyxia. This is so because of the arrangement of the fetal circulatory pathways, and because the newborn infant must successfully inflate his lungs and rearrange his circulation immediately after birth, if he is to adapt to extrauterine life.

THE FETAL CIRCULATION

In the fetus, it is the placenta, rather than the lung, that is the organ of oxygen uptake and CO_2 elimination. Blood flowing to the placenta by way of the umbilical arteries has a partial pressure of oxygen (P_{O_2}) in the range of 20 torr and of CO_2 (P_{CO_2}) in the range of 45 torr. By contrast, values for blood returning from the placenta through the umbilical vein are $P_{O_2} \simeq 35$ torr and $P_{CO_2} \simeq 40$ torr. This is the most highly oxygenated blood in the fetal circulation. The fetal circulatory pathways are shown in Figure 11-1. Note that this arrangement is essentially two circuits in parallel. The pulmonary circulation has a very high resistance because the pulmonary arterioles are tightly constricted. On the other hand, a major portion of the systemic circulation has a low resistance in the vascular bed of the placenta, which receives about 40% of the combined output of the two ventricles. Because of this arrangement, pulmonary arterial pressure exceeds aortic pressure, and the majority of the right ventricle's output passes through the widely patent ductus arteriosus into the descending aorta. Those tissues receiving their blood supply from the ascending aorta (*e.g.,* brain and myocardium) are perfused with more highly oxygenated blood than those supplied by the descending aorta below the ductus (*e.g.,* kidneys and intestine).

NEONATAL CIRCULATION

With the first breath, the lungs expand, the pulmonary vascular resistance decreases, and pressures in the pulmonary artery, right ventricle, and atrium begin to fall. Pulmonary blood flow increases as does pulmonary venous return to the left atrium. When the umbilical cord is clamped, the systemic vascular resistance increases. As a result, left atrial pressure exceeds the right atrial pressure and the foramen ovale closes, stopping blood flow through this orifice. Because systemic vascular pressure now exceeds pulmonary vascular pressure, flow through the ductus arteriosus changes from right-to-left to left-to-right. With these alterations in vascular resistances and flow, the course of the neonatal circulation becomes similar to that of the adult, with two circuits in series. This is shown in Figure 11-2. The establishment of this new pattern of circulation depends upon the responses of the pulmonary vascular bed to changes in P_{O_2} and pH.

Pulmonary vascular resistance is partly determined by the perivascular pH and oxygen tension because acidosis and hypoxia cause the release of vasoconstrictor substances into the tissue surrounding the pulmonary arterioles. In turn, the perivascular pH and P_{O_2} depend upon the alveolar oxygen and carbon dioxide tensions ($P_{A_{O_2}}$ and $P_{A_{CO_2}}$). In poorly ventilated areas, alveolar $P_{A_{CO_2}}$ rises, and $P_{A_{O_2}}$ falls, and the tissue pH and $P_{A_{O_2}}$ drop. This stimulates the release of vasoactive substances which constrict the precapillary arterioles. As pulmonary vascular resistance goes up, pulmonary blood flow may decrease as blood is shunted to areas of the lung with a lower vascular resistance or through the ductus arteriosus. After inflation and ventilation of a gasless lung with air, $P_{A_{O_2}}$ and pH rise, the pulmonary arterioles dilate, and pulmonary vascular resistance drops. Because pulmonary vascular resistance depends upon $P_{A_{O_2}}$, it drops more rapidly after inflation of the lungs with an oxygen-rich mixture. When newborn infants are acidemic, inflation of the lung causes a smaller decrease in pulmonary vascular resistance.

Perfusion with oxygenated blood causes constriction of the ductus arteriosus. It is likely that one or more vasoactive mediator substances are liberated into the periductal tissue when tissue oxygen tension rises. After the lung expands and the umbilical cord is clamped, pulmonary arterial pressure drops and systemic arterial pressure rises. This pro-

motes left-to-right shunting of oxygenated blood through the ductus arteriosus and leads to its closure. However, even when newborn infants are well oxygenated, complete closure does not always occur immediately. Persistent patency of the ductus arteriosus is particularly common in the prematurely born infants because of diminished constriction of the ductus in response to a rise in P_{O_2}.

If the newborn infant does not expand its lungs and establish effective ventilation and perfusion in the minutes following birth, the arterial blood P_{O_2} (Pa_{O_2}) will remain low, arterial blood P_{CO_2} (Pa_{CO_2}) will rise and pH will fall, causing constriction of pulmonary arterioles. This will cause either a persistence of the fetal circulatory pattern or a reversion to it, but without a functioning placenta in the circulation. This situation is illustrated in Figure 11-3. Once this process has started, it tends to be self-perpetuating with both progressive acidosis and hypoxia increasing the pulmonary vasoconstriction. The central process in this sequence of events is pulmonary vasoconstriction in response to hypoxia and acidosis. Because this response increases with gestation, the pathophysiology shown in Figure 11-3 is more likely to occur in the asphyxiated infant near or at term, than in the very prematurely born infant.

PATHOPHYSIOLOGY OF INTRAPARTUM ASPHYXIA AND RESUSCITATION

Asphyxia occurs when the organ of gas exchange fails. When this occurs, Pa_{CO_2} rises and pH falls. However, tissues continue to consume O_2 from blood until Pa_{O_2} reaches a very low level. Tissue hypoxia then occurs, and anaerobic metabolism produces large quantities of metabolic acids. These are buffered by the bicarbonate in the blood.

In practice, asphyxia is evaluated by measuring arterial blood to detect high P_{CO_2}, low pH, low P_{O_2}, low bicarbonate, and a large calculated base deficit. Arterial blood changes sometimes fail to reflect the full extent of the changes in tissues. This is particularly the case when blood flow to some tissues is markedly reduced. Such ischemia not only contributes to the asphyxial process, but also leaves CO_2 and metabolic acid pooled in the vasculature of the asphyctic tissues, rather than returning them to the central circulation where they can be detected.

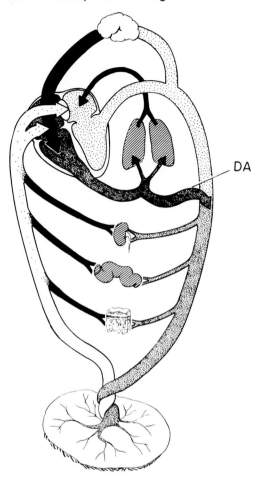

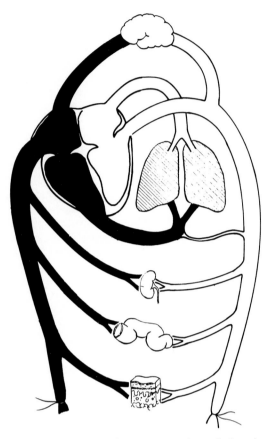

Fig. 11-1. A schematic representation of the fetal circulation. Oxygenated blood leaves the placenta by way of the umbilical vein (**vessel without stippling**). It flows into the portal sinus in the liver (not shown) and a variable portion of it perfuses the liver. The remainder passes from the portal sinus through the ductus venosus into the inferior vena cava where it joins blood from the viscera (represented by **kidney, gut, and skin**). About half of the inferior vena cava flow passes through the foramen ovale to the left atrium, where it mixes with a small amount of pulmonary venous blood. This relatively well-oxygenated blood (**light stippling**) supplies the heart and brain by way of the ascending aorta. The other half of the inferior vena cava stream mixes with superior vena cava blood and enters the right ventricle (blood in the right atrium and ventricle has little oxygen, which is denoted by *heavy stippling*). Because the pulmonary arterioles are constricted, most of the blood in the main pulmonary artery flows through the ductus arteriosus (**DA**), so that the descending aorta's blood has less oxygen (**heavy stippling**) than blood in the ascending aorta (**light stippling**).

Fig. 11-2. A schematic representation of the circulation in the normal newborn. After expansion of the lungs and ligation of the umbilical cord, pulmonary blood flow increases and left atrial and systemic arterial pressures rise while pulmonary arterial and right heart pressures fall. When left atrial pressure exceeds right atrial pressure, the foramen ovale closes so that all of the inferior and superior vena cava blood leaves the right atrium, enters the right ventricle, and is pumped through the pulmonary artery toward the lung. With the rise in systemic arterial pressure and fall in pulmonary artery pressure, flow through the ductus arteriosus becomes left-to-right, and the ductus constricts and closes. The course of the circulation is the same as in the adult.

The human infant is particularly vulnerable to asphyxia during labor, delivery, and immediately after birth. There are four basic mechanisms for asphyxia in these circumstances: (1) fetal asphyxia from interruption of umbilical blood flow, such as occurs with cord compression during labor; (2) fetal asphyxia from failure of exchange across the placenta because of placental separation, as in an abruption; (3) fetal asphyxia from inadequate perfusion of the maternal side of the placenta (*e.g.*, with severe maternal hypotension); and (4) neonatal asphyxia from failure to inflate the lungs and complete the changes detailed above in Figure 11-2 and leading to the changes shown in Figure 11-3. The fourth mechanism may occur because of airway obstruction, excessive fluid in the lungs, or weak respiratory effort. On the other hand, it may occur as a sequel of fetal asphyxia from one of the first three causes, because fetal asphyxia can result in an infant who is already acidotic at birth and apneic.

The blood gas changes will vary somewhat with the particular mechanism causing the asphyxia. With fetal asphyxia, the predominant changes are usually hypoxemia and secondary metabolic acidosis. Sufficient placental flow and exchange persist to provide adequate exchange for CO_2. The exception is complete occlusion of the umbilical cord. On the other hand, with neonatal asphyxia and inadequate lung inflation there is usually hypercarbia of a severity equivalent to the hypoxia.

Asphyxia in the fetus or newborn infant is a progressive process which is potentially reversible. The speed and extent to which it progresses are highly variable. Sudden severe asphyxia can be lethal in less than 10 minutes. Mild asphyxia may progressively worsen over a half an hour or more. There may also be repeated episodes of brief, mild asphyxia which reverse spontaneously over an hour or more, but which produce a cumulative effect of progressive asphyxia.

In the early stages, asphyxia may reverse spontaneously if the cause is removed. However, once asphyxia progresses to the very severe state, spontaneous reversal is unlikely because of the circulatory and neurologic changes that accompany it. Figure 11-4 is a schematic representation of the sequence of pathophysiologic changes that accompany asphyxia. There are some quantitative differences between the changes that occur in the fetus and those in the newborn infant. However, the scheme generally applies to both and it is useful to consider the changes in fetus and newborn infant together because many cases of neonatal asphyxia begin in the fetus and continue after birth.

Cardiac output is maintained early in as-

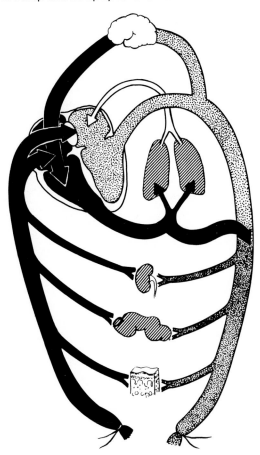

Fig. 11-3. A schematic representation of the circulation in an asphyxiated newborn with incomplete expansion of the lungs. Pulmonary vascular resistance is high, pulmonary blood flow is low (note small caliber of pulmonary vein) and flow through the ductus arteriosus large. With little pulmonary venous flow, left atrial pressure drops below right atrial pressure, the foramen ovale opens, and vena cava blood flows through the foramen into the left atrium. This partially venous blood goes to the brain by way of the ascending aorta. The descending aorta blood that goes to the viscera has less oxygen than the ascending aorta (**heavy stippling**) because of the right-to-left flow through the ductus arteriosus. The circulation is the same as in the fetus except that there is no oxygenated blood in the inferior vena cava from the umbilical vein.

phyxia, but its distribution changes radically. There is selective regional vasoconstriction with reduced blood flow to less vital organs and tissues such as gut, kidneys, muscle, and skin. Blood flow to vital organs, including brain, myocardium and adrenal glands, is

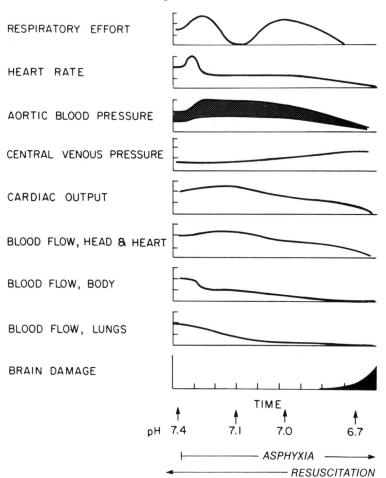

RESPIRATORY EFFORT

HEART RATE

AORTIC BLOOD PRESSURE

CENTRAL VENOUS PRESSURE

CARDIAC OUTPUT

BLOOD FLOW, HEAD & HEART

BLOOD FLOW, BODY

BLOOD FLOW, LUNGS

BRAIN DAMAGE

TIME

pH 7.4   7.1   7.0   6.7

ASPHYXIA →

← RESUSCITATION

Fig. 11-4. Schematic representation of the sequence of cardiopulmonary changes with asphyxia and resuscitation. Time is on the horizontal axis and asphyxia progresses from left to right while resuscitation proceeds from right to left. Units of time are not given. If there is complete interruption of respiratory gas exchange, the entire process of asphyxia from extreme left to right could occur in about 10 min. It could take much longer with an asphyxiating process that only partly interrupts gas exchange or does so completely, but only for repeated brief periods. With resuscitation, the process reverses beginning at the point to which the asphyxia has proceeded. (Adapted from Dawes G: Foetal and Neonatal Physiology. Chicago, Year Book Publishers, 1968)

maintained or increased. This high blood flow helps to maintain adequate oxygen delivery to the vital organs, even though the oxygen content of the arterial blood is reduced. In the fetus, blood flow is also maintained to the placenta unless the asphyxiating process is umbilical cord occlusion; this helps to maintain a supply of oxygen to the fetus. Pulmonary blood flow is low in the fetus and decreases for the reasons discussed above. This is of no immediate consequence in the fetus, but, in the newborn, it produces the changes shown in Figure 11-3.

Early in asphyxia, the newborn makes vigorous attempts to inflate its lungs. If successful, the lungs become adequately ventilated and perfused, but the mere presence of gasping does not ensure that this will happen. As asphyxia becomes more severe, the respiratory center is depressed and the chances of an infant spontaneously establishing effective ventilation and pulmonary perfusion diminish.

The myocardium depends upon its stored reserve of glycogen for energy as its supply of oxygen falls. Eventually, this reserve is consumed and the myocardium is simultaneously exposed to progressively lower P_{O_2} and pH levels. The combined effects lead to decreased myocardial function with a decreased blood flow to the vital organs. Brain injury begins late during this phase.

This sequence of cardiovascular events is manifested by changes of heart rate and aortic and central venous pressures (Fig. 11-4), which are all easily measured in the newborn immediately after birth. The early bradycardia and hypertension are due to the reflexes which shunt blood away from the nonvital organs.

Early in asphyxia, central venous (right atrial) pressure may rise slightly due to pulmonary hypertension and constriction of systemic capacitance vessels which also occur with asphyxia. When the myocardium finally fails, central venous pressure rises further, while aortic pressure falls and the heart rate falls even further.

Because the **physiology of resuscitation** is essentially a reversal of the pathophysiology of asphyxia, Figure 11-4 illustrates both processes. Asphyxia proceeds from left to right, and resuscitation from right to left, as indicated. It is crucial to determine where the infant is in this sequence of events when one starts resuscitation. If asphyxia has proceeded to myocardial failure, resuscitation must include restoration of cardiac output, as well as establishing effective ventilation and perfusion of the lungs. Generally, myocardial failure does not occur until both pH and Pa_{O_2} are extremely low, in the range of 6.90 and 20 torr, respectively. Cardiac output is reestablished by rapidly correcting the severe hypoxia and acidosis. Until this is done, output must be maintained by cardiac massage. As soon as pH is raised to the range of 7.10 and Pa_{O_2} to 50 torr, the myocardium responds rapidly, heart rate rises, aortic pressures rise, and pulse pressure widens while central venous pressure falls. These changes indicate that cardiac massage can be stopped. At this point, the infant will usually be hypertensive because the vasoconstriction in nonvital organs is still present. This is only relieved as adequate oxygenation is maintained and acidosis is relieved further. Then, pressures will fall toward normal. While the vasoconstriction is present, it is also manifested by intense pallor of the skin. As the vasoconstriction is relieved, the skin becomes pink and well perfused with rapid capillary refilling when blanched by pressure. As peripheral flow improves, lactic acid sequestered in these tissues enters the central circulation and a large base deficit, which may have been corrected earlier, now reappears.

If asphyxia is only moderately severe, resuscitation begins in the middle of the sequence depicted in Figure 11-4, and there is hypertension, indicating that the myocardium has not yet failed. Effective ventilation with a high oxygen concentration may be sufficient to correct acidosis by lowering the Pa_{CO_2} and to adequately oxygenate the blood and dilate the pulmonary vascular bed. However, if significant acidosis persists after alleviation of the hypercarbia, alkali should be given to partially correct the metabolic acidosis so as to relieve pulmonary vasoconstriction and establish good pulmonary perfusion. Generally, raising pH to the range of 7.25 is sufficient for this purpose.

When the changes of asphyxia are alleviated, **spontaneous respiratory efforts** return. The duration between the onset of resuscitation and reappearance of spontaneous respiratory efforts is directly proportional to the extent of brain injury that has occurred. In infants who had been severely asphyxiated with a pH in the range of from 6.95 to 7.00 but who were later proven to be free of brain damage, respiratory efforts usually reappeared within 10 to 20 minutes. Those who suffered severe brain damage remained apneic for hours after blood gases had been normalized.

Spontaneous respiratory efforts are not necessarily an indication to withdraw assisted ventilation. Often, the infant has some residual atelectasis and also lacks strong, regular respiratory efforts. Pa_{CO_2} may be normal and Pa_{O_2} may be rising to a dangerously high level while assisted ventilation is provided, but, as soon as it is withdrawn, effective ventilation falls and the whole process of asphyxia recurs. Such cases must be managed by gradual withdrawal of assisted ventilation and reduction of oxygen.

There may be major abnormalities of **blood volume** in the asphyxiated infant. Intrapartum asphyxia affects the distribution of blood volume between infant and placenta at the time of cord clamping. Asphyxia during labor usually causes a shift of fetal blood from the placenta to the infant. There are four exceptions in which infant blood volume will usually be reduced: (1) asphyxia from compression of the umbilical cord by the aftercoming head in a term breech delivery, in which the compression may selectively obstruct venous flow more than arterial, thereby trapping a large volume of blood in the placenta; (2) asphyxia from hemorrhage from the fetoplacental unit; (3) asphyxia from severe hypotension in the mother; and (4) asphyxia that only occurs at delivery.

Initially, it may be difficult to determine whether or not blood volume is adequate in the asphyxiated newborn. There are two main reasons for this. First, many of the circulatory responses to asphyxia are similar to those of blood volume loss. For example, either asphyxia or hypovolemia may cause an abnormal heart rate, metabolic acidosis, poor peripheral perfusion as manifested by pallor, slow capillary filling, and a large difference between core and skin temperature. A low aortic pressure could be due to either the end stage of asphyxia or to shock. Only changes in central venous pressure are in the opposite direction and even here the coexistence of the two processes could have offsetting effects. Secondly, the circulatory changes during asphyxia and resuscitation may determine the adequacy or inadequacy of the circulating blood volume. If an infant is moderately asphyxiated with systemic and pulmonary vasoconstriction (center of Fig. 11-4) and has a small blood volume, aortic and central venous pressures will be nearly normal. Giving a blood volume expander at this point would only overload the circulation. This would be even worse if the asphyxia were more severe with a component of myocardial failure. As asphyxia is relieved (moving to the left in Fig. 11-4), the vasoconstriction of resistance and capacitance vessels falls and the small blood volume which had been adequate may now become inadequate to support the circulation. In addition, with reperfusion of asphyxic and ischemic tissues, there is increased loss of intravascular water from these capillary beds leading to edema and reduced plasma volume.

During the recovery phase of asphyxia, several **metabolic abnormalities** appear. There may be hypoglycemia, probably because of depletion of carbohydrate reserves needed to maintain cardiac output during the asphyxia. This must be prevented as it may cause myocardial failure in a heart recently subjected to asphyxia. On the other hand, hyperglycemia due to administration of excessive glucose is very dangerous during asphyxia. It causes an increase in production of lactic acid which worsens the acidosis and also causes cerebral edema by an unknown mechanism.

Hypocalcemia develops from an unknown mechanism and it is also important because it, too, can lead to myocardial failure.

Hyperkalemia occurs during asphyxia. Hemoglobin is one of the buffers that reduces the fall in pH during acidosis. H^+ enters the red cell, and is bound by hemoglobin. In the process, K^+ is displaced from the binding site, leaves the red cell, and enters the plasma. Although the plasma K^+ is high during asphyxia, total body K^+ becomes depleted as some of the K^+ is excreted by the kidney. Upon relief of asphyxia, the buffering processes are reversed, K^+ leaves the plasma and enters the red cell, binding to hemoglobin, leading to hypokalemia. An exception to this process is asphyxia so severe that it produces severe renal ischemia and anuria.

HIGH-RISK PREGNANCIES

There are a number of situations during pregnancy, labor, or delivery in which serious neonatal disease can be anticipated. The fetus in these circumstances is regarded as being at high risk. If high-risk infants are identified *before* they are born, their progress during labor and delivery can be monitored and resuscitation can be started at birth. Some of the factors that should alert the physician to the advent of a high-risk infant are given in Table 11-1.

Optimal management of these cases requires good communication between obstetricians, anesthesiologists, and pediatricians. The physician responsible for care of newborn infants should always be aware of any potential problem patients in the labor and delivery areas.

If a severely asphyxiated infant is expected, a resuscitation team must be in the delivery area. Usually, there is time to assemble a team between identification of such an infant and its delivery. The team should have at least two persons: one member to intubate and ventilate the infant; and one to monitor heart rate, provide cardiac massage, and introduce catheters into the umbilical vessels, if they are required. Equipment and drugs must be assembled in advance, so that they are available to permit ventilation and support of the circulation. Body temperature must be maintained during resuscitation and a heat source is essential. Table 11-2 lists the necessary equipment, and a typical arrangement for neonatal resuscitation is shown in Figures 11-5 and 11-6. If a mother in labor with a high-risk pregnancy is laboring in a hospital lacking these facilities and personnel, she should be moved to a hospital with adequate resuscita-

Table 11-1. Some Factors Which Place the Newborn Infant at High Risk for Asphyxia

Maternal Conditions	Labor and Delivery Conditions	Fetal Conditions
Elderly primigravida (>35 years of age)	Forceps delivery other than low-elective or vacuum-extraction delivery	Premature delivery
Diabetes		Multiple births
Toxemia of pregnancy, hypertension, chronic renal disease	Breech or other abnormal presentation and delivery	Acidosis (fetal scalp capillary blood)
Low urinary estriol	Cesarian section	Abnormal heart rate or rhythm
Anemia (hemoglobin <10 g/dl)	Prolonged labor	Meconium-stained amniotic fluid
Blood type or group isoimmunization	(1st stage >24 hrs; 2nd stage >2 hrs)	Polyhydramnios
Abruptio placenta, placenta previa, or other antepartum hemorrhage	Prolapsed umbilical cord Cord compression (nuchal cord, cord knot, compression by aftercoming head in breech delivery)	Decreased rate of growth (uterine size or fetal size by ultrasound)
Narcotic, barbiturate, tranquilizer, psychedelic drug use, or ethyl alcohol intoxication		Immaturity of pulmonary surfactant system
History of previous neonatal death	Maternal hypotension	Fetal malformations (by ultrasound)
Prolonged rupture of membranes	Sedative or analgesic drugs given IV within 1 hr of delivery or IM within 2 hr of delivery	

tive facilities, if this can be done safely. Labor often can be stopped with drug therapy for a time long enough to carry out such transport.

INITIAL EVALUATION

The quantitative assessment of the newborn (Table 11-3) described by Dr. Virginia Apgar remains the simplest and best way to evaluate the condition of an infant at birth. If the score is 8 to 10 at 1 or 5 minutes of age, the infant usually does not require active resuscitation; if he has a score of 2 or less at 1 minute or less than 5 at 5 minutes of age, he requires resuscitation. One of the most ominous signs is a 5-minute Apgar score that is much lower than the 1-minute score.

RESUSCITATION OF THE ASPHYXIATED INFANT

The extent of the resuscitative measures needed initially can be determined only after the infant's condition is evaluated by someone with considerable clinical experience. In ad-

dition to infants with a low Apgar score, infants with any of the following signs or conditions will probably need resuscitation: moderate or severe erythroblastosis fetalis; birth weight < 1500 g; a negative test for pulmonary surfactant in the amniotic fluid; marked intrauterine growth retardation; intrapartum fetal distress; and a delivery preceded by vaginal bleeding. In almost all such cases, good communication between obstetricians and pediatricians will provide 30 minutes or more advance notice of the delivery of an asphyxiated infant. The actual steps in the resuscitation fall into three major phases.

Phase I

Maintain Body Temperature. When the cord is clamped, blot the infant dry with a sterile towel and place him under a radiant heater on a sterile table.

Clear the Airway. Gently suction the oropharynx and nose. If the infant's respiration is vigorous, nothing more may be necessary.

Insert ECG Electrodes and Monitor the Heart Rate.

Table 11-2. Equipment Required for Adequate Neonatal Resuscitation

Radiantly heated resuscitation platform with sterile drapes

Sterile bulb suction and vacuum suction with sterile catheters

Thermometer and thermal control for radiant heater

Laryngoscope

Oropharyngeal airways

Endotracheal tubes, sizes 8, 10, and 14, with stylets

Source of oxygen and air with an oxygen-air proportioner and heated nebulizer

Bennett face masks

Connectors from endotracheal tube or mask to soft 500-ml anesthesia bag and air-oxygen source

Aneroid manometer, for observing airway pressures during assisted ventilation

Oxygen analyzer

Sterile umbilical vessel catheterization tray, including small iris scissors, cord tie, and 3½ and 5F umbilical vessel catheters with 3-way stopcocks

Sterile syringes with flushing solutions and sterile 1 ml heparinized syringes for blood gas sampling

Spotlight

Pressure transducers and monitor for vascular pressures

ECG electrodes and heart rate monitor

Blood gas and pH electrodes

Clock with sweep second hand

Initiate Breathing. If the infant is apneic or the respiratory rate is slow and irregular, place a mask over the infant's face and ventilate with 60% oxygen, using intermittent positive pressure from the anesthesia bag, while continuously observing ventilation pressure on an aneroid manometer.

Ventilation should begin by slowly applying a pressure of 20 cm H_2O to the airway for term infants, and 30 cm H_2O to the airway for preterm infants. Maintain this inflating pressure for 1 to 2 seconds, then ventilate at a rate of 40 to 60 breaths per minute, using an inflation time of 0.25 to 0.50 seconds and just enough pressure to provide good expansion of the upper portion of the chest. Repeat the application of the initial inflating pressure pattern 3 to 4 times over the first 2 minutes. In mildly asphyxiated infants, this will produce a prompt increase in heart rate and the onset of regular, spontaneous respiration. If both do not occur, the trachea should be intubated and assisted ventilation continued. During intubation, bradycardia may reoccur from stimulation of the hypopharynx, but heart rate should increase again as soon as the intubation is completed and assisted ventilation is begun. With severe asphyxia, the experienced resuscitator may prefer to intubate the trachea immediately.

If the infant does not make strong respiratory efforts after the initial assisted ventilation, and the mother has received morphine or an equivalent narcotic within hours before delivery, a narcotic antagonist should be given (naloxone hydrochloride, 0.01 mg/kg).

Cardiac Massage. If there is no electrical activity on the ECG, no audible heart beat, or if the heart rate remains below 50 after onset of assisted ventilation, the heart must be massaged manually. Begin external cardiac massage by placing both hands around the infant's chest, with the fingertips towards the back, and the thumbs overlapping each other on the mid-sternum; then, quickly press down firmly with both thumbs at a rate of 80 to 100 strokes per minute. Coordinate the massage with the ventilation: 3 heart beats, pause for 1 breath; 3 heart beats, pause for 1 breath, and so on. Increase the inspired oxygen to 100% and

Table 11-3. The Apgar Score

Sign	0	1	2
Heart rate	Absent	<100/min	>100/min
Respiratory effort	Absent	Weak cry	Strong cry
Muscle tone	Limp	Some flexion	Good flexion
Reflex irritability (when feet stimulated)	No response	Some motion	Cry
Color	Blue:pale	Body pink; extremities blue	Pink

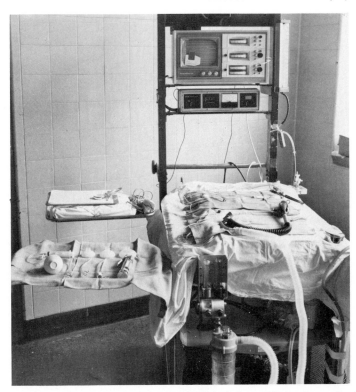

Fig. 11-5. A resuscitation cart for the delivery room. This unit is mobile and can also be used to transport infants within the hospital. Above the table is a radiant heat source which has an automatic servomechanism below the oscilloscope. In the foreground is an air/oxygen mixer which receives air and oxygen from small tanks on the bottom shelf of the cart. The gas mixture passes through a heated nebulizer and sterile white plastic corrugated tubing which is connected by a Norman elbow (modified T-piece) to either a mask or endotracheal tube. The other end of the Norman elbow is connected to a reservoir bag with an open tailpiece by means of a Sommers T-piece and black corrugated tubing. Side arms from the Norman elbow lead to an aneroid manometer **(right, foreground)** for measurement of ventilation pressures and to a 30 cm column of water **(attached to cart's right foreleg)** to prevent the creation of excessive pressures. The near tray has equipment for suctioning and intubating the airway (Fig. 11-6), and the far tray contains a sterile pack for umbilical vessel catheterization. On the platform **(left, front)** is tubing which goes to a pump on the lower deck of the cart which provides negative pressure for suctioning the airway. The surface of the platform is covered with sterile towels, and on these are 4 needle (26-gauge) ECG electrodes which are connected to a junction box below the mercury manometer. These can be placed beneath the infant's skin within 2 or 3 sec and allow an immediate visualization of the ECG on the oscilloscope. Pressure transducers that are calibrated with the mercury manometer by the nursing staff every 8 hr are mounted in plastic **(right, background)**. As soon as an umbilical artery or vein is catheterized, its pressure can be displayed on the oscilloscope. It is possible with this equipment and a skilled team to have, within 10 min of birth, a warmed infant intubated and ventilated, his progress monitored with an ECG, and both arterial and central venous pressures measured.

continue cardiac massage while proceeding with other resuscitative measures until the spontaneous heart rate is above 100 and the arterial pressure is normal. If there is no spontaneous heart rate, the infant needs intracardiac epinepherine (0.1 ml/kg of 1:10,000 solution). However, most cases of presumed cardiac arrest are actually profound bradycardia which respond to effective ventilation alone or to cardiac massage. The efficacy of massage and of return of adequate cardiac activity are best judged by monitoring aortic blood pressure. Massage can be discontinued for a few seconds to evaluate the spontaneous rate and blood pressure. Figure 11-7 shows such a case. Infants who do not respond rapidly to these

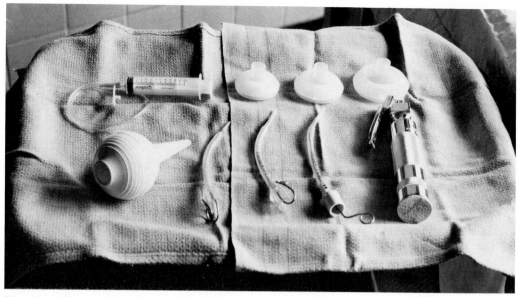

Fig. 11-6. Close-up view of a sterile tray for management of the airway. **Counterclockwise from top left:** a sterile disposable syringe and tube for suctioning the stomach; a bulb syringe for suctioning the mouth; Cole endotracheal tubes of 3 different sizes; an infant laryngoscope; and Bennet masks of three different sizes.

ıneasures will require prompt correction of acidosis (see below), atropine sulfate (0.01 mg/kg), and $CaCl_2$ (0.2 ml/kg of a 10% solution). Persistent bradycardia rarely requires treatment with isoproterenol, beginning with a dose of 0.5 μg/kg/minute.

Catheterize an umbilical artery and draw a sample of blood for determination of pH, Pa_{O_2}, and Pa_{CO_2} to evaluate efficacy of ventilation. Depending on the values obtained, adjust ventilatory rate, pressure, and inspired oxygen accordingly. Measure hematocrit, connect the catheter to a precalibrated pressure transducer, and measure blood pressure.

Marked Metabolic Acidosis. A pH less than 7.05 and a base deficit of 15 mEq/liter or more should be corrected by infusing 0.5 M* $NaHCO_3$ at a rate of 1 mEq/kg/minute or slower for a dose calculated by the formula

$$mEq = 0.3 \times \text{weight (kg)} \times \text{base deficit in mEq/liter.}$$

NO BICARBONATE SHOULD BE INFUSED UNLESS VENTILATION IS BEING ASSISTED EFFECTIVELY AND Pa_{CO_2} IS NEARLY NORMAL OR LOW. The ability of this buffer to raise pH depends upon the ability of the lungs to eliminate the CO_2 produced by the buffering process (H^+ + $NaHCO_3$ → Na^+ + H_2CO_3 → H_2O + CO_2). Figures 11-8 and 11-9 show data from two infants with severe mixed acidosis. In one, $NaHCO_3$ could be given early because CO_2 elimination was adequate. In the other, it had to be delayed until adequate CO_2 elimination was established.

Recent reports have called attention to an association between intracranial hemorrhage and sodium bicarbonate infusion in prematurely born infants. Whether the hemorrhages are caused by an increase in osmolarity, by the asphyxia for which the bicarbonate was given, or by an acute increase in Pa_{CO_2} from inadequate ventilation during $NaHCO_3$ therapy is not known. However, infusion of sodium bicarbonate at the rate of 1 mEq/kg/minute, for a total dose of up to 5 mEq/kg into the inferior vena cava, causes only a slight, transient increase in arterial sodium concentration. Until more information is available, $NaHCO_3$ should not be infused except when severe metabolic acidosis is judged to be life threat-

* $NaHCO_3$ is most commonly available as a 1.0 M solution. This should be diluted 1:1 with sterile distilled water, not 5% or 10% dextrose, to halve the osmolarity.

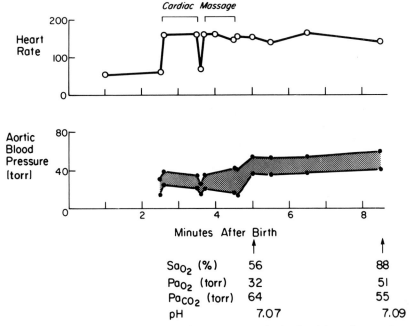

Fig. 11-7. Resuscitation, including cardiac massage, of a 2.1 kg, 34-week gestation infant delivered by cesarean section for signs of fetal asphyxia. (Sa_{O_2} = saturation of arterial blood hemoglobin with oxygen.) The infant was intubated and ventilated with 60% oxygen beginning 30 seconds after birth. ECG was recorded beginning at 1 min, and, at 2.5 min, an umbilical artery catheter connected to a pressure transducer and a recorder was passed into the descending aorta. Note persistent bradycardia despite assisted ventilation and low aortic pressure (Pao) with narrow phasic pressure. Cardiac massage raised heart rate and pressure. When briefly discontinued after 1 min, pressure and heart rate fell. After another minute of massage and assisted ventilation, good cardiac output had returned. This was manifested by a sustained higher heart rate and higher blood pressure with wider phasic pressure when massage was discontinued a second time at 5 min after birth. By 8.5 min, the infant was still acidotic, but there was adequate oxygenation and Pao was continuing to rise.

ening. The main objectives of alkali therapy are twofold: (1) to reverse the myocardial failure and low cardiac output that occurs with severe asphyxia; and (2) to relieve the intense pulmonary vasoconstriction that occurs in term infants with severe acidosis.

The other option for alkali therapy is tris-buffer.* This has the twofold advantage of reducing P_{CO_2} and buffering metabolic acid. However, experience with the use of this drug in newborns is quite limited. Its use should be considered in treating infants with severe

mixed metabolic and respiratory acidosis and also in those unfortunate situations of severe asphyxia with suspected severe acidosis in which blood gas measurements are not available. Tris-buffer may cause respiratory depression, but it would only be used in situations in which ventilation was already being assisted.

Phase II

Reevaluation of Assisted Ventilation. It is essential to watch for complications of assisted ventilation. The tracheal tube may advance into the right mainstem bronchus leading to nonventilation of both the entire left lung and the upper lobe of the right lung. Immediately

---

* The commercially prepared 0.3 M trimethamine (Tham) solution can be used without further dilution at the same infusion rate as $NaHCO_3$.

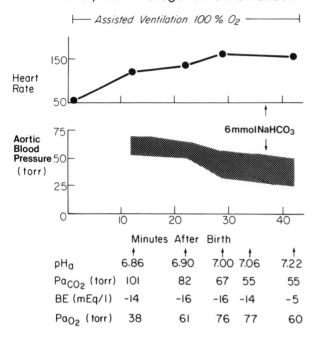

├── Assisted Ventilation 100 % O₂ ──────┤

Heart Rate
150
50

Aortic Blood Pressure (torr)
75
50
25
0

6 mmol NaHCO₃

10   20   30   40

Minutes After Birth

pHₐ	6.86	6.90	7.00	7.06	7.22
Pa$_{CO_2}$ (torr)	101	82	67	55	55
BE (mEq/l)	−14	−16	−16	−14	−5
Pa$_{O_2}$ (torr)	38	61	76	77	60

Fig. 11-8. Changes in heart rate, aortic blood pressure, and arterial blood gas tensions during the first 45 min after birth of a 1.2 kg premature infant with severe asphyxia complicated by bilateral pleural effusions. The child's trachea was intubated immediately after birth and he was manually ventilated with 100% oxygen throughout this time. Note the severe mixed acidosis in the first blood gas measurement at 11 min. Administration of NaHCO₃ at this point would have been inappropriate and ineffective because assisted ventilation had not yet achieved adequate elimination of CO₂. NaHCO₃ was only given after adequate CO₂ elimination was achieved. Note that there was no rise in Pa$_{CO_2}$ following this, indicating that all the CO₂ produced during the buffering process was eliminated and the only change was a reduction in base deficit from −14 to −5 mEq/ liter, which raised the pH from 7.06 to 7.22. Note the high Pao initially which was due to the vasoconstriction of asphyxia, indicating that myocardial failure had not yet developed. As asphyxia was relieved, Pao fell to normal.

after intubation, both sides of the chest should be auscultated to be sure breath sounds are equal and this should be repeated every few minutes until the tube is removed or secured in proper position. If breath sounds are absent or diminished on the left side, the tube should be withdrawn slowly while continuing ventilation until breath sounds are equal. Alternately, the tube may come out of the airway and pass into the esophagus, and this complication must be checked for by auscultating the chest for breath sounds.

The stomach should be aspirated during this phase of resuscitation. If a face mask was used for initial ventilation, the stomach will be distended with gas and will therefore restrict ventilation. On rare occasions, the stomach may be perforated during resuscitation. If it is, the resulting severe abdominal distention must be relieved to allow adequate ventilation.

Pulmonary function may change rapidly, leading to several complications. First, as ventilation and perfusion become better matched, Pa$_{O_2}$ will rise and may reach dangerously high levels. Hyperoxia is best managed by reducing inspired oxygen concentration rather than by withdrawing ventilatory assistance. Secondly, improved ventilation may lead to acute hypocarbia which will reduce cerebral blood flow. This is corrected by reducing the rate of assisted ventilation. Thirdly, as lung compliance increases, the ventilatory pressure which had been appropriate will now be excessive. If this mismatching is mild, the result will be hyperventilation and hypocarbia. However, if it is extreme, there will be tamponade of the pulmonary circulation producing right-to-left shunting at the atrial and ductal levels and low systemic blood flow. This is manifested by a low aortic pressure and extreme variations in aortic pressure, with pressure falling markedly during each positive pressure breath. The hypoxia from the shunt and the hypotension will improve almost instantaneously when ventilation pressure is reduced.

Tension pneumothorax may occur during ventilation of any infant but is most often a complication of meconium aspiration which is discussed below. A tension pneumothorax of small or moderate size may interfere with ventilation, causing asphyxia, and requires prompt treatment. It must be suspected whenever Pa$_{O_2}$ decreases, and a check of the ventilation system shows that the tracheal tube is properly located and that the oxygen delivery system has not failed. Sometimes the diagnosis is difficult to make by physical examination. Breath sounds may be unequal bilaterally, but often they are equal. The upper portion of the affected side of the chest tends to lag behind the unaffected side when they rise during inflation of the lungs. Transillumination with a cold fiberoptic light may show that the affected side glows brightly; however, the absence of this sign does not rule out pneumothorax, particularly in larger infants with thicker chest walls. The diagnosis can best be made by a cross-table lateral chest x-ray, but this is often impossible in the resuscitation area. If hypoxia and hypercarbia become severe, it may be necessary to perform a diagnostic thoracentesis with a small gauge needle and syringe (see below) before there is time to obtain an x-ray.

The situation changes when a tension pneumothorax is large. This will obstruct venous return to the heart and cardiac output may fall precipitously to an extremely low level. If blood pressure is being measured, this critical situation is very easy to diagnose because the onset of hypoxia and hypercarbia will be accompanied by severe hypotension, rather than by the expected hypertension of asphyxia. This situation requires almost as urgent treatment as a cardiac arrest. Figure 11-10 illustrates the diagnosis and successful treatment of such a case.

Satisfactory decompression of a tension pneumothorax usually requires a thoracostomy tube and continuous suction with an adequate-sized catheter and an underwater seal suction system. Aspiration with a needle and syringe usually gives only very brief relief. However, while assembling equipment for decompression, insert a No. 22 scalp-infusion needle connected to a three-way stopcock and large syringe. This is a convenient and safe way for temporary decompression.

Evaluate Circulatory Status. As discussed above, some asphyxiated infants may have an inadequate circulating blood volume. This will lead to underperfusion of tissues which should be corrected by an expansion of blood volume. On the other hand, many asphyxiated infants have a normal or greater than normal blood volume; expanding their blood volume is of no benefit and may actually be dangerous. Because some circulatory changes due to asphyxia may either mimic or mask shock, it is impossible to identify those infants who may need blood volume expansion until resuscitation has produced adequate oxygenation of arterial blood and a normal Pa_{CO_2}. It should be noted that hypocarbia may produce systemic

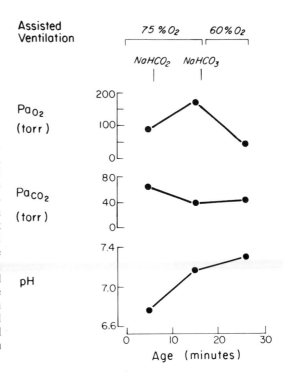

Fig. 11-9. Arterial blood gas tensions, pH, and therapy during the first 30 min after the birth of a 1.6 kg premature infant. There was a severe mixed acidosis initially. Unlike the case shown in Fig. 11-8, assisted ventilation achieved effective CO_2 elimination early in this infant; $NaHCO_3$ could be given earlier to begin correcting the metabolic component of the acidosis. The base excess on the first blood specimen was beyond the limits of calculation (more than -25 mEq/liter). The first infusion of $NaHCO_3$ was given between 6 and 10 min. When the second sample was drawn at 15 min, the calculated base excess was -22 mEq/liter. After the second infusion of $NaHCO_3$ the base excess was -6 mEq/liter, and no more alkali was given. Note that Pa_{CO_2} fell between the first and second measurements when $NaHCO_3$ was given.

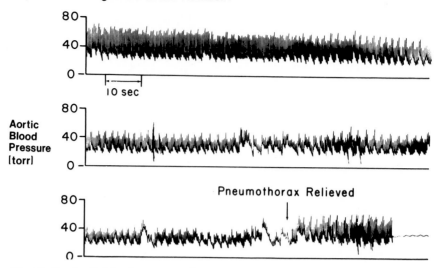

Fig. 11-10. Aortic blood pressure of a prematurely born infant (birth weight = 1.5 kg, gestational age = 32 weeks) during development of a tension pneumothorax. This is a continuous tracing at 2 hr of age. Because the patient's condition was rapidly worsening (as shown by hypotension, a narrow pulse pressure, and rapidly increasing cyanosis despite assisted ventilation with 100% oxygen) thoracentesis of the right pleural cavity was done (**arrow**) before radiologic confirmation of the pneumothorax was obtained. About 50 ml of air escaped when the pleural cavity was opened. The patient's color improved and his blood pressure promptly returned to normal.

hypotension, and severe overventilation may reduce systemic blood flow as discussed above. However, neither of these states requires blood volume expansion.

Signs that suggest an inadequate blood volume include the following: low aortic pressure (Fig. 11-11); low central venous pressure; falling hematocrit; persistent metabolic acidosis; low central venous P_{O_2} (<30 torr) after correction of arterial hypoxia; cold extremities; and delayed ($\geq$3 sec) filling of capillaries in the skin after they have been blanched under pressure (provided that core temperature is normal). Tachycardia is often absent in the early stages of severe shock and may be present from too many other causes to be a useful sign. If some findings suggest shock, but the diagnosis is uncertain, it is useful to connect a second catheter to a pressure transducer, then pass it through the umbilical vein and use direct pressure monitoring to locate the tip in the inferior vena cava or right atrium. Low central venous pressure and P_{O_2} are particularly reliable indicators of shock and therefore are valuable guides to follow during therapy.

Shock is best treated with repeated small infusions in group O Rh-negative whole blood, which has been cross-matched against the mother before delivery and is available in the resuscitative area at birth. If the blood is kept chilled in an insulated container, it can be returned to the blood bank if not used. Group O Rh-negative blood given to newborns without cross-matching against the mother's serum has occasionally produced fatal transfusion reactions due to incompatibility in minor blood groups and should not be used. Fresh frozen plasma is an acceptable alternate to whole blood, but the anemia it produces may require correction.

Plasma substitutes such as salt-poor albumin or plasma protein fraction (Plasmanate) are distinctly inferior. They produce only a transient expansion of plasma volume. Much of the colloid in them rapidly leaves the circula-

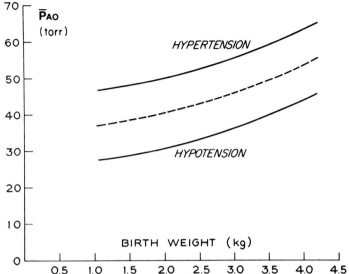

Fig. 11-11. Mean aortic blood pressure (PAO) obtained from an umbilical artery catheter is given in torr on the upright axis. Birth weight in kilograms is on the horizontal axis. The dashed line is the average blood pressure at each birth weight and the solid lines are the 95% confidence limits of this relationship. Blood pressure values below the lower confidence line are hypotensive. (Adapted from Kitterman JA, Phibbs R, and Tooley WH: Pediatrics 44:959, 1969, copyright American Academy of Pediatrics, 1969)

tion, taking water with it. This not only reduces plasma volume, but produces edema, including pulmonary edema.

The object of therapy is a prompt restoration of adequate tissue perfusion. This must be done rapidly enough to avoid the cumulatively harmful effects of prolonged underperfusion of tissues. The latter can lead to the secondary effects of shock, including increased capillary permeability and pulmonary disease, which make therapy more difficult. On the other hand, excessive speed in volume replacement is dangerous. Some vascular beds, such as that of the brain, vasodilate maximally in response to systemic hypotension. If systemic pressure is raised abruptly, there is no time for this vasculature to partially constrict, and the higher pressure is transmitted to the capillaries where it may cause capillary injury, edema, or hemorrhage.

In most cases, shock can be treated with repeated infusions of 5 ml/kg blood or plasma, given by a steady infusion over approximately 5 minutes. The response to each infusion must be carefully observed and therapy stopped as soon as tissue perfusion is judged adequate. Usually aortic pressure will rise following the first or first few infusions, but, as vasoconstriction is relieved with volume expansion, pressure falls again and further volume expansion may be given, provided other signs of

poor perfusion persist. Occasionally, when there has been massive hemorrhage, as with surgical incision of an anterior placenta at cesarean section, volume may have to be replaced more rapidly. In such a case, aortic pressure should be monitored continuously to avoid abrupt rises in pressure. Figure 11-12 shows the course of successful treatment during the first hour of life in an infant who lost approximately 50% of his blood volume during delivery and also suffered asphyxia. Figure 11-13 shows the course in an infant in whom hypovolemia did not become evident until assisted ventilation relieved asphyxia.

Phase III

Maintain Body Temperature. If a radiant lamp is used, have a nurse monitor the infant's axillary temperature. If a servocontrolled radiant heater is used, the temperature probe should be connected to the infant.

Prevent Hypoglycemia. When hypoxia and acidosis have been relieved, begin a steady infusion of 10% dextrose in water and begin screening for hypoglycemia with repeated testing of capillary blood with Dextrostix. For the reasons cited above, glucose infusion usually should not be started until hypoxia is relieved. Hypoglycemia can be corrected by temporarily increasing the infusion rate of the 10% dextrose to 5 ml/kg/hour, thereby providing 8 mg/kg/

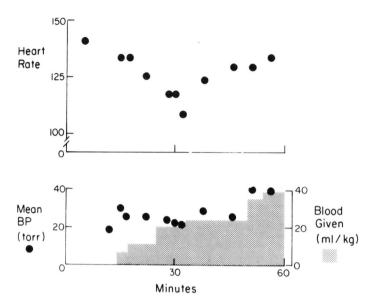

Fig. 11-12. Heart rate, Pao, and blood volume replacement during the first hour after birth in a 2.8 kg infant who suffered massive blood loss when the anteriorly placed placenta was incised deeply at cesarean section delivery. The shaded area shows the cumulative volume of whole blood given expressed as ml/kg body weight. The final volume, which produced a normal Pao and relieved signs of poor perfusion, was 40 ml/kg, approximately half of the total blood volume for a normal newborn infant. The blood was given as a series of small transfusions guided by the changes in blood pressure (**BP**). Note that the heart rate is not elevated at first, despite the extreme hypotension, and that, subsequently, heart rate does not consistently change in the opposite direction of blood pressure changes.

minute, which is more than sufficient in all but the most extreme cases of hypoglycemia following asphyxia. Rapid infusions of more concentrated solutions of dextrose are rarely needed to correct hypoglycemia and are dangerous because they are hyperosmolar and may produce serious vascular injury.

Adjust Respiratory Support and Inspired Oxygen Concentration. During recovery from asphyxia, the course of change in pulmonary function is highly variable and unpredictable. Some infants may go on to develop hyaline membrane disease, requiring increasing ventilatory support. In other infants, pulmonary function may improve slowly, requiring continued assisted ventilation at gradually decreasing pressure, rates, and inspired oxygen concentration for 12 to 24 hours. In still other infants, pulmonary function may improve so rapidly that the infant can safely be shifted to spontaneous breathing of room air by 20 to 30 minutes of age. Withdrawal of assisted ventilation and reduction of inspired oxygen must be exactly matched to the rate of improvement of pulmonary function. If reduction in therapy is too slow, dangerous hyperoxia may occur. If it is too fast, asphyxia may reoccur.

Figure 11-14 illustrates this repeated titering of therapy against improved pulmonary function in an asphyxiated infant in whom Pa_{O_2} was

measured continuously. When continuous monitoring is not available, blood gas measurements must be made every 15 to 20 minutes to guide adjustments of therapy during this unstable period. In preterm infants at risk for retrolental fibroplasia, it is generally better to maintain assisted ventilation, gradually reducing its rate so that the infant breathes spontaneously and every second or third breath is assisted as tolerated, while reducing inspired oxygen as rapidly as possible. Sometimes this requires decrements of as much as 10 to 20% at a time to prevent hyperoxia. After this, assisted ventilation can be reduced further, often by changing from mechanical ventilation to continuous positive airway pressure, and then extubation.

Maintain Electrolyte Balance. After initial resuscitation, add maintenance electrolytes to the parenteral fluid infusion. Because hypocalcemia and hypokalemia are common after successful resuscitation of neonatal asphyxia, electrolytes should include potassium chloride (2 mEq/kg/24 hr) and calcium gluconate (200 mg/kg/24 hr), in addition to sodium chloride (2 mEq/kg/24 hr). The potassium should be given only after the infant has urinated. In planning the sodium requirements, take into account any sodium given as $NaHCO_3$ during resuscitation.

MECONIUM ASPIRATION

Meconium aspiration presents a special problem in delivery room management. When a more mature infant is asphyxiated, it passes meconium. This response is rarely present before approximately 34 weeks of gestation. This material can be aspirated into the airway either from gasping efforts of the asphyxiated fetus or with the first breaths after birth.

If meconium is aspirated into the lower airways, it may cause pulmonary disease. This can vary from mild respiratory distress to respiratory failure and acute pulmonary hypertension with intracardiac shunting of blood. Amniotic fluid that is lightly stained with meconium rarely causes significant disease if aspirated, whereas thick meconium is more likely to do so. Severe disease is most likely when there has been heavy meconium staining of the amniotic fluid for more than 30 minutes before birth. Prompt suctioning of the airway at birth can often prevent or reduce the severity of disease. This is done by intubating the trachea immediately after delivery, then suctioning by mouth while withdrawing the tube. A face mask over the face of the person doing the suctioning catches the meconium. If meconium is obtained from below the vocal cords, the procedure should be repeated until all the meconium is cleared. The lungs should then be inflated by positive pressure.

The risk of pulmonary disease can be further reduced in vertex presentation infants if the upper airway is first suctioned after delivery of the head, but before delivery of the thorax. If the delivery can be halted briefly at this point, the obstetrician should use a sterile DeLee trap with a sterile suction tube to suction the hypopharynx. The delivery then proceeds and the airway is suctioned as described above.

These infants are often asphyxiated and one must proceed to the other steps in resuscitation after suctioning for meconium. Ten percent of all infants with meconium below the vocal cords develop pulmonary air leaks with pneumomediastinum, pneumothorax, or both.

COUNSELING OF PARENTS

Effective resuscitation requires a major disruption of contact between mother and infant at the time of birth. Several things can be done

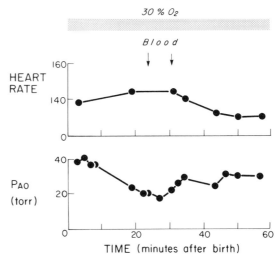

Fig. 11-13. Heart rate, Pao, and therapy during the first hour after the birth of a 1.5 kg second twin delivered by cesarean section. There had been a large abruption of the placenta. Initially, the infant was hypoxic and acidotic and aortic pressure was normal. As blood gas tensions normalized, aortic pressure fell and the infant continued to appear pale and poorly perfused. This is probably an example of the intense vasoconstriction of asphyxia keeping blood pressure at a normal level despite a subnormal blood volume. Relief of the asphyxia allowed sufficient vasodilation to unmask the hypovolemia.

to offset this. In most cases, there is sufficient advance warning to allow the person in charge of the resuscitation team to explain to the parents ahead of time what therapeutic measures may be needed. If the mother can be moved from the labor room and has a very high-risk infant who is certain to require intensive care, it is useful to give her and the father a tour of the intensive care nursery ahead of time. The attending physician must keep in mind that newborn infants may survive quite severe asphyxia (pH in the range of 7.00) without permanent brain injury, provided the insult is brief and resuscitation is prompt and effective. Parents need reassurance about this.

At delivery, it is usually safe to take at least a few seconds to show the mother her baby before taking the infant to the resuscitation area. The baby should be held face to face with the mother. Once resuscitation is initiated and the infant stabilized, mother, father and baby should be brought back together. This

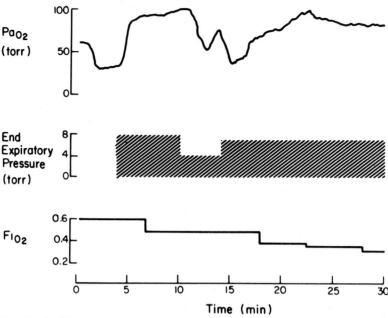

Fig. 11-14. Changes in assisted ventilation, inspired oxygen concentration ($F_{I_{O_2}}$) and Pa_{O_2} during the first 30 minutes after birth of an asphyxiated infant. Pa_{O_2} was recorded continuously after birth by a catheter with a micro-P_{O_2} electrode in its tip which was previously calibrated. It was then passed through the umbilical artery into the descending aorta 1 min. after delivery. The infant was breathing spontaneously, but Pa_{O_2} fell to 24 torr despite an $F_{I_{O_2}}$ of 0.6 (60% oxygen). The trachea was intubated and assisted ventilation with a PEEP was begun at 4 min. This produced a rapid rise in Pa_{O_2}. $F_{I_{O_2}}$ was lowered at 6.5 minutes to avoid hyperoxia. When assisted ventilation was continued, but end-expiratory pressure lowered at 10 min, Pa_{O_2} fell and rose again when end-expiratory pressure was raised again. Maintaining higher pressure allowed the succeeding reductions in $F_{I_{O_2}}$ while maintaining Pa_{O_2} at an adequate level.

can usually be done even in the most complicated cases. For example, a mother on a gurney following cesarean section can be positioned beside her infant receiving manually assisted ventilation on a resuscitation platform before the infant is moved to the intensive care unit.

SUGGESTED READINGS

Apgar V: A proposal for new method of evaluation of the newborn infant. Anesth Analg 32:260, 1953

Carson BS, Lasey BW, Bowes WA, Simmons MA: Combined obstetric and pediatric approach to prevent meconium aspiration syndrome. Am J Obstet Gynecol 126:712, 1976

Dahn LS, James LS: Newborn temperature and calculated heat loss in the delivery room. Pediatrics 49:504, 1972

Dawes G: Foetal and Neonatal Physiology. Chicago, Year Book Publishers, 1968

Gerhardt T, Bancalari E, Cohen H, Rocha LF: Use of naloxone to reverse narcotic respiratory depression in the newborn infant. J Pediatr 90:1009, 1977

Gregory GA, Gooding CA, Phibbs RH, Tooley WH: Meconium aspiration in infants: A prospective study. J Pediatr 85:807, 1974

Gluck L (ed): Intrauterine Asphyxia and the Developing Fetal Brain. Chicago, Year Book Publishers, 1977

James LS: Onset of breathing and resuscitation. J Pediatr 65:807, 1964

Kitterman JA, Phibbs RH, and Tooley WH: Catherization of umbilical vessels in newborn infants. Pediatr Clin North Am 17:895, 1970

Kitterman JA, Phibbs RH, Tooley WH: Aortic blood pressure in normal newborn infants during the first 12 hours of life. Pediatrics 44:959, 1969

Lawson EA, Birdwell RL, Huang PS, Taeusch HW

Jr: Augmentation of pulmonary surfactant secretion by lung expansion at birth. Pediat Res 13: 611, 1979

Linderkamp O, Versmold HT, Messow–Zahn K, Muller–Holve W, Riegel KP, Betke K: The effects of intrapartum and intrauterine asphyxia on placental transfusion in premature and full-term infants. Eur J Pediatr 127:91–99, 1978

Moya F, James L, Burnard L, Hanks EC: Cardiac massage in the newborn infant through the intact chest. Am J Obstet Gynecol 84:798, 1962

Ogata ES, Gregory GA, Kitterman JA, Phibbs RH, Tooley WH: Pneumothorax in the respiratory distress syndrome: incidence and effects on vital signs, blood gases and pH. Pediatrics 58:177, 1976

Thomson AJ, Searle M, Russell G: Quality of survival after severe birth asphyxia. Arch Dis Child 52: 620, 1977

Tunell R, Copher D, Persson B: The pulmonary gas exchange and blood gas changes in connection with birth. In Stetson JB, Swyer PR (eds): Neonatal Intensive Care. St. Louis, Warren H Green Inc, 1976

Volpe JJ, Pasternak JF: Parasagittal cerebral injury in neonatal hypoxic-ischemic encephalopathy: Clinical and neuroradiologic features. J Pediatr 91:472, 1977

IV
The Newborn Infant

12

Assessment of Weight and Gestational Age

Lula O. Lubchenco

GESTATIONAL AGE

The importance of birth weight in predicting problems in newborn infants is uncontested. One knows that the 1,000 g infant will have numerous problems and is best cared for in an intensive care nursery (ICN) and that the 2,000 g infant may develop the respiratory distress syndrome (RDS), jaundice or feeding problems. At the other end of the scale, one worries about the 4,000 g infant who may incur birth trauma or whose mother may have diabetes.

The role of gestational age is not quite so clear. Immaturity of various systems is to be expected in preterm infants and placental insufficiency occurs more often in postterm infants.

It is entirely logical that weight and gestational age are interrelated and that deviation in weight or gestational age, from a physiologic range, will result in increased neonatal morbidity.

This deceptively simple concept will be documented, step by step, in the following discussion.

Classification of Newborn Infants by Birth Weight and Gestational Age

The Academy of Pediatrics, through its Committee on the Fetus and Newborn, rec-ommended that all newborn infants be classi-fied by birth weight, gestational age and some standard for intrauterine growth.[1] This rec-ommendation followed years of experience with subdivisions of infants into two cate-gories: low birth weight (<2,500 g), and full birth weight (>2,500 g).

The low-birth-weight category was an im-portant one and served to identify 66% of the infants who died in the neonatal period. This relatively simple grouping made it possible to compare the incidence of low birth weight in various populations and thereby identify high-risk populations. It also was well known that the low-birth-weight designation included pre-term and term infants; but when it became apparent that approximately one-third of low-birth-weight infants were born at term, the need for a new classification was obvious. Intrauterine growth retardation (IUGR) im-plies a deviation in growth from some physi-ologic standard, and the recommendation by the American Academy of Pediatrics could not be carried out until such a measure became available. It also required a means of deter-mining gestational age in every infant.

One such classification can be seen in Figure 12-1; nine categories of infants emerge: three by pattern of intrauterine growth and three by gestational age. An explanation of these divi-sions follows.

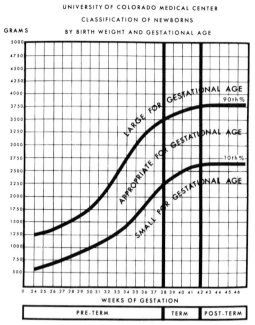

UNIVERSITY OF COLORADO MEDICAL CENTER
CLASSIFICATION OF NEWBORNS
BY BIRTH WEIGHT AND GESTATIONAL AGE

Fig. 12-1. University of Colorado Medical Center classification of newborns by birth weight and gestational age. (Battaglia FC, Lubchenco LO: J Pediatr 71:159, 1967)[2]

The Definition of Term Birth. The World Health Organization, with support from European pediatric groups, has set the dividing line between preterm and term birth at 37 weeks. One of the reasons for the division at 37 weeks, rather than 38 weeks, is the relatively large number of infants born between 37 and 38 weeks who would be designated as risk and require attention. Also, the mortality in this gestational age group is low. There is a clinical impression that infants born between 37 and 38 weeks of gestation, in some underdeveloped countries, behave as mature infants.

On the other hand, the decision to use 38 to 42 weeks to designate term birth was based on the scatter of birth around 40 weeks, which is a near normal distribution curve and includes 80% of the population when plus or minus 2 weeks is used; 38 to 42 weeks was considered to be a more physiologic distribution than 37 to 42 weeks, or 37 to 41 weeks. There is mounting evidence that the 37-week infant is not a low-risk infant. He has a higher neonatal morbidity,[3] and is not as healthy as mature infants in long-term follow-up studies.[4,5] Thus, infants born before 38 weeks are considered

preterm, those born between 38 and 42 weeks are **term,** and infants born at 42 weeks or later are considered to be **postterm.** The use of completed weeks of gestation is generally accepted (*i.e.,* an infant is 37 weeks of gestation even though he is 37 weeks and 6 days) as calculated from onset of the mother's last menstrual period (LMP). He becomes 38 weeks on the following day.

Intrauterine Growth Standards

Intrauterine growth standards are constructed from birth weights of infants born at different gestational ages and all of them have common problems. The population on which the standard is based presents the first problem.

What population should be used for the compilation of data? Should each community or institution have its own intrauterine growth curves or should one search for an optimal standard? Should there be different curves for each race? For males and females? For different parities? How should one correct for socioeconomic level, altitude, smoking, multiple births, disease in the mother, congenital anomalies in the fetus, and so forth?

One must question whether a pregnancy resulting in preterm delivery is ever normal and whether the condition resulting in preterm birth affects the growth of the fetus.

Intrauterine growth curves from Oregon[6] are based on a near optimal population for the United States. The infants were born to Caucasian mothers living at sea level who were cared for by private physicians. Only single births were included. The curves are based on 40,000 infants born from 1959 to 1966. Their disadvantage is that only intrauterine growth in weight has been presented; standards for growth in length and head circumference are not available.

The Colorado curves (Fig. 12-2) give percentiles of intrauterine growth for weight, length and head circumference. The Colorado data (altitude 5,280 feet) were based on infants born at the University of Colorado Medical Center from 1948 to 1961, plus low-birth-weight infants transferred to the Center from other hospitals. The population consisted of medically indigent persons with 30% being Mexican Americans, 15% Blacks, and the remainder Caucasians. The only infants excluded were those with gross congenital defects affecting birth weight and a small group

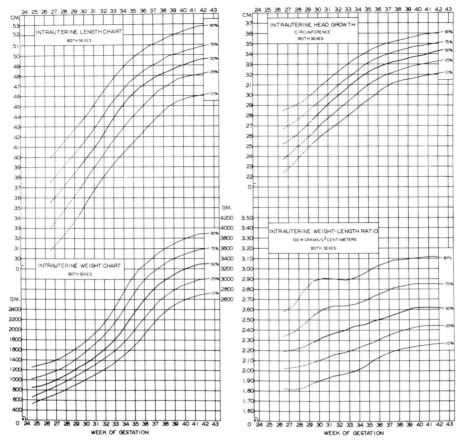

Fig. 12-2. The Colorado curves give percentiles of intrauterine growth for weight, length and head circumference. (Lubchenco LO, Hansman C, and Boyd E: Intrauterine growth in length and head circumference as estimated from live births at gestational ages from 26 to 42 weeks. Pediatrics 37:403, 1966, copyright American Academy of Pediatrics, 1966)

of large infants of short gestation which were considered to have the wrong gestational age.

This latter group of infants is of interest because every worker in this field has noted their occurrence when the gestational age is determined from the mother's menstrual history.[7] Studies that combine a clinical estimate of gestational age on the infant or a prenatal estimate of length of gestation based on serial maternal examinations, do not show this population.[8,9] It is likely that postconceptional bleeding accounts for this unusual group.

Comparison of the Portland, Baltimore, and Denver curves is seen in Figure 12-3. The Portland infants are larger than Denver infants although very little difference exists in the 90th and 50th percentiles at 34 to 36 weeks. The Denver curves flatten after this gestational age; the median weight of Colorado infants at 40 weeks is 3,230 g, compared to 3448 for Oregon infants. The difference is even greater at 43 weeks, being 3652 versus 3330. The tenth percentile, usually used to define small-for-gestational-age infants, is slightly but uniformly above the Denver tenth percentile from 32 to 44 weeks. At 40-weeks' gestation, the tenth percentile is 2800 g in Denver.

It is unclear whether one should prepare intrauterine growth curves for each specific population or use existing ones, and whether one should use the tenth and ninetieth percentiles or 2 standard deviations from the mean to designate high-risk infants. The important thing is to use some standard of intrauterine growth that makes it possible to select high-risk infants for close observation.

FETAL GROWTH

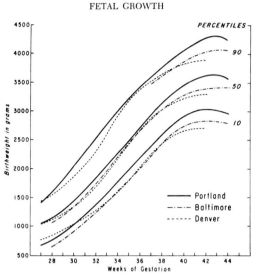

Fig. 12-3. Comparisons of fetal weight curves for different populations in the United States. (Babson SG et al: Pediatrics 45:937, 1970, copyright American Academy of Pediatrics, 1970)[6]

Pattern of Intrauterine Growth and Neonatal Morbidity

The large-for-gestational-age infant may be that of a diabetic mother (Fig. 12-4) with all the problems associated with maternal diabetes, or he may have congenital cyanotic heart disease. He may be erroneously classified as preterm and large for gestational age because the mother had postconceptional bleeding. Although physical characteristics and behavior are those of a term infant, he is known to have an increased mortality rate.

One worries about birth trauma or increased incidence of cesarean section in the large-for-gestational-age infant.

Morbidity in appropriately grown infants is determined more by the period of gestation than by birth weight. Preterm infants are subject to disturbances from immature organs, postterm infants from increased size or intrauterine asphyxia.

Intrauterine growth retardation (IUGR) may occur in the preterm, term, or postterm infant. The preterm infant with IUGR may be a discordant twin or an infant of a severely toxemic or hypertensive mother. Intrauterine viral infections cause retarded fetal growth, and congenital anomalies affect intrauterine growth in many infants. Malformations occur in a high percentage of small-for-gestational-

age infants. Some evidence of retarded growth may be present in "appropriately grown infants." The weight is disproportionate to length and head circumference, and the infants may appear wasted. IUGR in preterm infants is more difficult to recognize.

DETERMINATION OF GESTATIONAL AGE

There is much information to help determine the duration of pregnancy. The obstetrician uses the mother's history, his own observations, and a variety of laboratory aids to determine gestational age. The pediatrician has become proficient in estimating age from the physical characteristics and neurologic development of the infant. Together, the data make it possible to state within 1 to 2 weeks the age of the infant.

The Obstetrician's Estimate of Gestational Age. The last normal menstrual period still stands as the single most important basis from which gestational age is calculated. Many reasons have been given to cast doubt on its accuracy. The date is not always available because occasionally, no period occurs if the pregnancy follows closely after the birth of the previous infant, or sometimes the mother does not remember the exact date; or postconceptional bleeding may be confused with a normal menstrual cycle. Added to this list of problems is a new one relating to contraceptive drugs that complicate the estimation of gestational age because the ovulatory cycle is disrupted.

It is of particular significance that, when care is taken with the obstetrical history and when examinations occur early in pregnancy, the length of gestation can be determined in almost all pregnancies.

The obstetrician has available to him various tools to help determine the gestational age. For instance, McDonald's measurement (*i.e.,* the height of the uterine fundus above the symphysis pubis) is used to estimate gestational age in the normal fetus. It is not accurate, however, when there are 2 or more fetuses or when IUGR is present. Ultrasound scanning for size of the fetal head and/or thorax is used to confirm fetal size. Analysis of amniotic fluid for creatinine, bilirubin, and proportion of squamous to nucleated cells give further information on gestational age.

The Pediatrician's Estimate of Gestational Age. One can estimate the gestational age of the infant after birth from various physical characteristics that appear predictably with gestational age. Mitchell, Farr, and Dubowitz in England, and Usher in Canada have been instrumental in bringing these observations to the attention of neonatologists in the United States.[10-13] The neurologic devolopment of the preterm infant has been defined in relation to gestational age by the French group under the guidance of Minkowski.[14,15] Various combinations of the data of these investigators form the basis for the postnatal estimate of gestational age.

Data from these workers have been compiled into two charts—Figure 12-5 relates the findings to gestational age and lists the signs appropriate for the examination immediately after birth, and Figure 12-6 contains signs that are better delayed until after the infant has become stable. The signs in Figure 12-5 require very little manipulation of the infant and can be noted during the first hour after birth without undue stress to the baby. If there are gross discrepancies between calculated gestational age and the estimate based on these items, a complete neurologic examination is performed the next day.

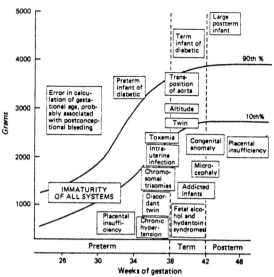

Fig. 12-4. Conditions associated with intrauterine growth related to birth weight and gestational age classification. (Battaglia FC: In Kempe CH, Silver HK, O'Brien D (eds): Current Diagnosis and Treatment, 5th ed. Los Altos, Calif., Lange, 1978)

Assessment of Individual Signs

The timing and method of making the observations in Figure 12-5 are described below.

1. **Vernix.** The amount and distribution of vernix must be observed as the infant emerges from the birth canal. The preterm infant is covered with a generous amount of vernix and as term approaches, it becomes sparse and remains only in the creases and hair. The post-term infant has none—he looks freshly bathed.

2. **Skin.** The thin, almost transparent appearance of the skin of the preterm infant becomes thick and more opaque with increasing age. Early in gestation, the skin is pink and venules are prominent over the abdomen. By 40 to 42 weeks, the skin is pale and few vessels are seen. As the vernix disappears, the skin becomes macerated and desquamation occurs. However, desquamation may not be apparent for an hour or more after birth.

3. **Nails.** Nails appear at about 20-weeks' gestation and cover the nail bed. Long nails, well beyond the fingertips, may be characteristic of postterm infants.

4. **Sole Creases.** The wrinkling of the soles of the feet first occurs on the anterior portion and extends toward the heel as gestation progresses. One or two creases are noted at about 32 weeks and they become more numerous, crisscrossed and cover the anterior two-thirds of the sole by 37 weeks. By 40 weeks, the entire sole is covered. The post-term infant has deeper creases and sometimes desquamation of the soles.

5. **Breast Tissue and Areola.** Although the nipple is present early in gestation, the areola is not evident until about 34 weeks. The areola first becomes raised and hair follicles are visible. At about 36 weeks, a 1 to 2 mm nodule of breast tissue is palpable. The nodule grows until it reaches 7 to 10 mm at 40 weeks. There is some increase postnatally at 2 to 3 days, and the nodule remains palpable for 2 to 3 months. Reproducible measurements are possible by palpation with the forefinger and comparing the size with a series of cardboard nodules. Size is not as consistently determined when the nodule is grasped between thumb and forefinger.

6. **Ear Form.** Incurving of the upper pinnae begins at about 33 to 34 weeks of gestation and, by 38 weeks, the upper two-thirds is complete. At 39 to 40 weeks, incurving has extended to the lobe. There may be differences

Examination First Hours

Physical Findings		Weeks Gestation (20–48) — progression of findings
Vernix		Appears (21) · Covers body, thick layer (24–28) · On back, scalp in creases (38) · Scant, in creases (40–41) · No vernix (43)
Breast tissue and areola		Areola and nipple barely visible, no palpable breast tissue (25) · Areola raised (34) · 1–2 mm nodule (36–37) · 3–5 mm (38–39) · 5–6 mm (40) · 7–10 mm (41) · ?12 mm (44)
Ear	Form	Flat, shapeless (21) · Beginning incurving superior (34) · Incurving upper 2/3 pinnae (36) · Well-defined incurving to lobe (39)
	Cartilage	Pinna soft, stays folded (24) · Cartilage scant, returns slowly from folding (33) · Thin cartilage, springs back from folding (37) · Pinna firm, remains erect from head (42)
Sole creases		Smooth soles without creases (25) · 1–2 anterior creases (33) · 2–3 anterior creases (35) · Creases anterior 2/3 sole (37) · Creases involving heel (41) · Deeper creases over entire sole (44)
Skin	Thickness & appearance	Thin, translucent skin, plethoric, venules over abdomen, edema (24–28) · Smooth, thicker, no edema (33) · Pink (37) · Few vessels (39) · Some desquamation, pale pink (40–41) · Thick, pale, desquamation over entire body (44)
	Nail plates	Appear (20) · Nails to finger tips (34) · Nails extend well beyond finger tips (44)
Hair		Appears on head (21) · Eye brows and lashes (24) · Fine, woolly, bunches out from head (29) · Silky, single strands, lays flat (38) · ?Receding hairline or loss of baby hair, short, fine underneath (44)
Lanugo		Appears (20) · Covers entire body (24) · Vanishes from face (34) · Present on shoulders (38) · No lanugo (44)
Genitalia	Testes / Scrotum	Testes palpable in inguinal canal (30) · Few rugae (28) · In upper scrotum (37) · Rugae, anterior portion (37) · In lower scrotum (42) · Rugae cover (41) · Pendulous (42)
	Labia & clitoris	Prominent clitoris, labia majora small, widely separated (30–32) · Labia majora larger, nearly cover clitoris (37) · Labia minora and clitoris covered (44)
Skull firmness		Bones are soft (24) · Soft to 1" from anterior fontanelle (29) · Spongy at edges of fontanelle, center firm (35) · Bones hard, sutures easily displaced (38) · Bones hard, cannot be displaced (42)
Posture	Resting	Hypotonic, lateral decubitus (22) · Hypotonic (27) · Beginning flexion, thigh (31) · Stronger hip flexion (32) · Frog-like (35) · Flexion, all limbs (36) · Hypertonic (39) · Very hypertonic (42)
Recoil	leg	No recoil (20) · Partial recoil (33) · Prompt recoil (40)
	Arm	No recoil (20) · Begin flexion, no recoil (34) · Prompt recoil, may be inhibited (37) · Prompt recoil after 30″ inhibition (42)

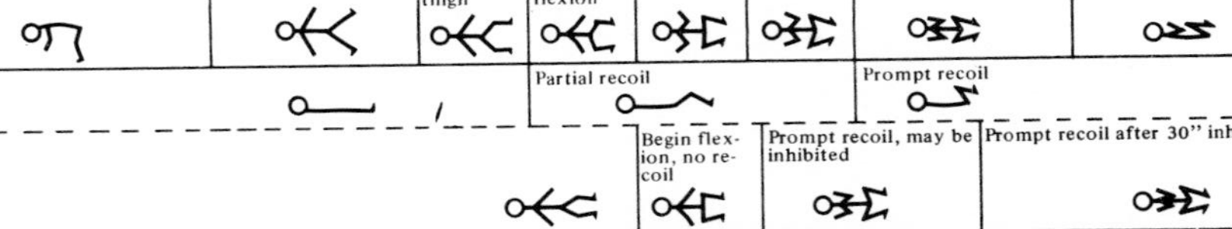

Week scale: 20 21 22 23 24 25 26 27 28 29 30 31 32 33 34 35 36 37 38 39 40 41 42 43 44 45 46 47 48

Fig. 12-5. Clinical estimation of gestational age. The examination in the first hours. (Kempe CH, Silver HK, O'Brien D (eds): Current Pediatric Diagnosis and Treatment, 3rd ed. Los Altos, Calif., Lange, 1974)

Confirmatory Neurologic Examination To Be Done After 24 Hours

Weeks Gestation

Physical Findings		20	21	22	23	24	25	26	27	28	29	30	31	32	33	34	35	36	37	38	39	40	41	42	43	44	45	46	47	48
Tone	Heel to ear	No resistance											Some resistance										Impossible							
	Scarf sign	No resistance													Elbow passes midline				Elbow at midline				Elbow does not reach midline							
	Neck flexors (head lag)	Absent																		Head in plane of body			Holds head							
	Neck extensors													Head begins to right itself from flexed position			Good righting cannot hold it			Holds head few seconds		Keeps head in line with trunk > 40			Turns head from side to side					
	Body extensors														Straightening of legs		Straightening of trunk				Straightening of head and trunk together									
	Vertical positions									When held under arms, body slips through hands						Arms hold baby, legs extended?			Legs flexed, good support with arms											
	Horizontal positions									Hypotonic, arms and legs straight									Arms and legs flexed			Head and back even, flexed extremities			Head above back					
Flexion angles	Popliteal	No resistance									150°			110°		100°				90°		80°			A pre-term who has reached 40 weeks still has a 40° angle					
	Ankle														45°			20°			30°		0								
	Wrist (square window)									90°				60°				45°												
Reflexes	Sucking								Weak, not synchronized with swallowing					Stronger, synchronized			Perfect			Perfect, hand to mouth					Perfect					
	Rooting								Long latency period slow, imperfect				Hand to mouth				Brisk, complete, durable									Complete					
	Grasp								Finger grasp is good, strength is poor					Stronger						Can lift baby off bed, involves arms							Hands open			
	Moro	Barely apparent							Weak, not elicited every time					Stronger			Complete with arm extension, open fingers, cry			Arm adduction added							?Begins to lose Moro			
	Crossed extension								Flexion and extension in a random, purposeless pattern					Extension, no adduction						Extension, adduction, fanning of toes				Complete					
	Automatic walk	Absent										Minimal		Begins tiptoeing, good support on sole			Still incomplete		Fast tiptoeing		Heel-toe progression, whole sole of foot					A pre-term who has reached 40 weeks walks on toes		?Begins to lose automatic walk		
	Pupillary reflex	Absent										Appears		Present																
	Glabellar tap	Absent												Appears			Present													
	Tonic neck reflex	Absent									Appears			Present																
	Neck-righting	Absent															Appears			Present after 37 weeks										

Fig. 12-6. Clinical estimation of gestational age. Confirmatory neurologic examination to be done after 24 hours. (Kempe CH, Silver HK, O'Brien D: Current Pediatric Diagnosis and Treatment, 3rd ed. Los Altos, Calif., Lange, 1974)

in the two ears and differences in individual infants. This sign is not as significant as others in estimating gestational age.

7. **Ear Cartilage.** Although the amount of cartilage deposited in the pinnae varies under different conditions, it is more reliable than ear form. Until 32 to 33 weeks, the pinnae stay folded, but by 36 weeks they spring back from folding. At term, they are firm and stand erect from the head.

8. **Hair.** The consistency of the hair can be determined after the bath. The strands are very fine early in gestation and tend to mat together, characteristic of wool. Little bunches will stick out from the head. By 40 weeks, the hair lies flat and is in single strands. This sign loses its significance in Blacks. In the postterm infant, a receding hairline is sometimes seen.

9. **Lanugo.** The body is covered with fine hair at about 20 weeks. It begins to disappear from the face, then trunk and extremities, and, by term, it is inconspicuous or present only over the shoulders.

10. **Genitalia.** Both male and female genitalia have characteristics which change with gestational age. The female genitalia depend, in part, upon fetal nutrition. The clitoris is prominent at 30 to 32 weeks and the labia majora are small and widely separated. The labia majora increase in size and fullness and, by term, completely cover the clitoris.

The testes descend into the external inguinal canal and can be palpated at the external inguinal ring at about 30 weeks. They gradually descend toward the scrotum and at 37 weeks are located high in the scrotal sac. By 40 weeks they are well descended. The postterm infant tends to have a pendulous scrotum covered with rugae. Rugae are first seen on the anterior scrotum at about 36 weeks and cover the entire sac by 40 weeks.

11. **Skull Firmness.** Sometimes this is included in the determination of gestational age. The bones of the preterm infant are soft, especially near the fontanelles and sutures. As gestation progresses, they become firm and the sutures are not easily displaced.

Neurologic Development

A great deal of the neurologic examination is related to the development of muscle tone. The development of tone has been shown to begin in the lower extremities and progress cephalad. This, in itself, is curious because all other neurologic functions begin to develop in the cephalad region and progress caudad. No clear explanation for these findings is available, but it is presumed that inhibitory and/or feedback controlling systems are in effect.[13] The relationship of muscle tone to gestational age has been summarized by Amiel–Tison.[15]

Resting Posture and Recoil of Extremities. Early in gestation, the infant lies on his side with arms and legs extended. Hypotonia is present until about 30 weeks of gestation when slight flexion of the feet and knees can be demonstrated. Flexion of the thighs and hips occurs at 34 weeks and results in the characteristic frog position of the legs, but the arms are extended. By 35 weeks, beginning arm flexion can be seen, and, at 36 to 38 weeks, the resting posture is that of total flexion. There is about a 2-week lag between the time that resting flexion of extremities is observed until the tone is sufficiently strong to result in recoil of the extremities after brief extension. At 36 to 37 weeks, the infant will lie in flexion, but if the arms are extended, they remain extended. By 40 weeks, there is prompt recoil of the arms, which is not inhibited by a 30-second period of extension.

These two responses are sufficient to give a reasonable estimate of neurologic development in the hour immediately following birth. The remainder of the neurologic examination (Fig. 12-6) is ideally carried out a day or two later in order to confirm the original findings.

Other criteria in the neurologic examination are described below.

State of the Infant. Because so much of the neurologic examination of the newborn depends upon muscle tone, it is important to perform the tests when the infant is neither too hungry nor too sleepy. Approximately 2 hours following a feeding has been found to be a satisfactory time.

Tests for Muscle Tone. Tests related to muscle tone are graphically portrayed in Figure 12-6. The first two tests, heel to ear and scarf signs, determine extremity tone by the resistance offered to passive movement; the next three test trunk tone; and the last two approach overall body tone in slightly different maneuvers.

Flexion Angles. The popliteal angle is indirectly related to muscle tone in the lower extremities—the greater the tone, the smaller the angle; whereas the last two angles, ankle and wrist, test for joint mobility. These angles become obliterated at term as the infant molds to the limited uterine space. When born preterm, the joints remain somewhat stiff and account for the preterm infant walking on his toes rather than flat on the soles at term.

Reflexes. Although the list of reflexes present in the newborn is significant, changes in the infant's appearance or the character of his response are not as clearly demarcated with age as the signs mentioned above. The signs that are helpful in determining gestational age are rooting and sucking movements, which occur early in prenatal life. The ability to take adequate nourishment with nipple feedings, however, occurs at about 34 weeks.

The crossed extension reflex, even though it is often difficult to elicit, is complete at term and, thereby, one can use this test to distinguish between preterm and term birth.

Eye Fixing and Following. These signs are important but they have not been standardized. The postterm infant is "wide-eyed" and fixes his gaze easily on a face.

Nursery Routines

Many conflicts exist between established nursery routines, the physician's responsibility to the infant, and the need of the mother. The first hour after birth is an optimal time for the mother and infant to be together. It is also the time when neonatal problems can be identifed and, ofttimes, prevented. The infant needs warmth and observation; both can be provided in the mothers's presence. It is important to know the gestational age and weight in order to screen for early morbidity, and this can be carried out with a minimum of disturbance to the infant by any trained nursery personnel.

Determining Gestational Age From the Individual Signs

One method of estimating gestational age is to assign a gestational age to each one. One may need to interpolate if the findings are between two landmarks. From these data, a mean age is obtained and expressed in even weeks or a range of 1 to 2 weeks. In practice, the clinical assessment is accurate only to within 2 weeks of the actual date and serves to support or refute the mother's dates.

The scoring system of Dubowitz, a weighted score, is one of the most accurate for determining gestational age.[12] It is widely used and accepted. It has the disadvantage of requiring evaluation of all 11 external and/or all 10 neurologic criteria in order to obtain a score. The scores do not provide the examiner with an appreciation of the age at which a finding occurs.

If a difference of 3 or more weeks exists between the clinical assessment and the mother's dates, one considers that there is a real discrepancy between the two estimates. Both estimates are used. Nursery care should be determined by the clinical estimate. If the infant, by clinical examination, is more immature than the dates indicate, he should be treated as a preterm infant and the problems associated with preterm birth anticipated. If the infant appears more mature than the dates, he should be treated accordingly. The mother's dates are used in classifying infants for outcome statistics because mortality data are customarily derived in this manner. Furthermore, one will miss an important high-risk population (*i.e.,* infants of short gestation with birth weights >2500 g) if the clinical assessment is used. Very little is known about these infants and why they have a high mortality rate, partly because they have not been recognized as a distinct group at increased risk.

One of the reasons for using a chart giving the gestational age at which a sign appears is that the examiner may detect irregularities in development. Uneven development may be a clue to some unusual or unfavorable fetal situation. For example, infants with IUGR show a wide scatter in gestational age of individual signs, but the mean values give a clinical estimate of gestational age that is close to the calculated gestational age based on the mother's dates. This means that some of the signs must appear less mature and others more mature than the actual age. The signs of advanced gestational age include skin desquamation, many sole creases, and loss of vernix, while immature signs include decreased size of the breat nodule, immature female genitalia, and less ear cartilage than expected. Appropriate-for-age male genitalia and neurologic development are noted.

When a pattern of development is recognized, one may then be curious about the reasons for the findings. Is there a differential perfusion of tissues *in utero* with fetal undernutrition? If so, is vernix production decreased or does it slough off the skin into the amniotic

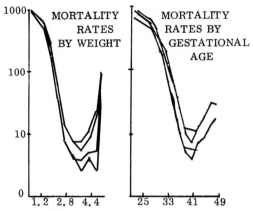

Fig. 12-7. Mortality rates by weight and gestational age. (Battaglia FC, Frazier TM, Hellegers AE: Birth weight gestational age, and pregnancy outcome, with special reference to high-birth-weight/low-gestational-age infant. Pediatrics 37:417, 1966, copyright American Academy of Pediatrics, 1966)

fluid? Without vernix, the skin would become wrinkled, macerated, and show deep sole creases and desquamation. One may ask why the breast nodule and ear cartilage are decreased. Are they related to a small placenta, lower estrogen levels, or another cause?

Neonatal Mortality by Birth Weight and Gestational Age

If one looks at mortality rates by birth weight or by gestational age, the rates are quite similar (Fig. 12-7). From these charts, it appears that one could choose either birth weight or gestational age to express risk. Mortality is high in infants born after a short gestation or in infants of very low birth weight. The rate decreases as the infant becomes more mature or heavier, and reaches its lowest level at 40 weeks or 3500 g. The rate increases again with prolonged gestation or excessive birth weight.

Because birth weight increases as gestational age advances, the mean values would be expected to be similar; but mean values do not show the effect of interaction of two conditions. Figure 12-8 gives mortality by large-birth-weight/gestational age blocks. In any weight range, mortality improves with advancing gestational age and for any gestational age the mortality improves with increasing weight until excessive size is reached.

Even though mortality data are usually collected and described by large groupings the

rates are, in fact, curvilinear, increasing in all directions from a low range (Fig. 12-9). This indicates that there is an optimal time and weight for delivery. In the Colorado data, the optimal weight is above the 50th percentile, and the optimal gestation is 38 to 42 weeks. There is an increased mortality if the infant's measurements fall outside this zone, either in weight or in gestational age.

NEONATAL MORBIDITY

Neonatal Morbidity by Birth Weight and Gestational Age

Neonatal morbidity of a significant nature follows the same pattern as mortality; it is lowest in the bull's eye and increases in every direction from it.[3] The lowest illness rate is 4%. Term, appropriate-for-gestational-age infants do not exceed 6%. Morbidity rate, rather than mortality rate, is a logical measure to estimate the need for nurses, ancillary personnel, and laboratory support for a nursery.

Incidence of Congenital Anomalies by Birth Weight—Gestational Age Groupings

Warkany's classical paper on IUGR showed the high incidence of congenital defects in

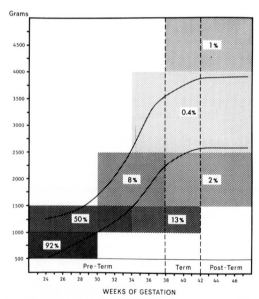

Fig. 12-8. Neonatal mortality by large-birth-weight-gestational-age blocks. (Battaglia, FC: Am J Obstet Gynecol 106:1103, 1970)

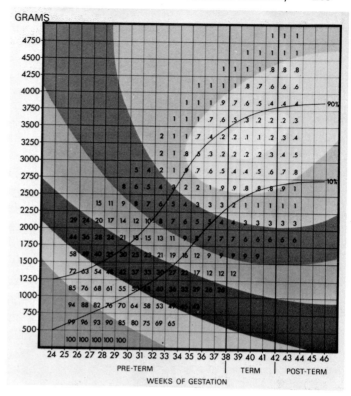

Fig. 12-9. Neonatal mortality by small-birth-weight/gestational-age blocks. (Lubchenco LO: J Pediatr 81:814, 1972)

small-for-gestational age infants.[16] Smith's review of syndromes associated with short stature further emphasizes the high incidence of IUGR in this population.[17] The increased anomaly rate in low-birth-weight infants of long gestation, compared to similar-weight, preterm infants, was also shown by Van Den Berg and Yerushalmy[18] and Yerushalmy.[19] These studies and those of Winick support the concept of decreased intrauterine growth of malformed fetuses.[20]

Not all anomalies are recognized at birth, so that minor or relatively insignificant abnormalities tend to be omitted. Reports give a 1 to 5% incidence of malformations in live-born infants, and an incidence as high as 35% in infants who die in the neonatal period. Chromosomal abnormalities are high, 25 to 50%, in first trimester spontaneous abortions.

A review of congenital anomalies of live-born infants for a 6-year period, at the University Hospital, Denver, showed some interesting relationships to birth weight and gestational age. The overall incidence was 3.3% (338/8996) with the highest incidence occurring at 28 to 29 weeks in infants of 1000 to 1500 g

birth weight. The next-highest incidence was in term, small-for-gestational age infants.

The incidence by year of birth was highest from 1963 to 1965, suggesting a relationship to environmental forces, such as the rubella outbreak prevalent during these years. It appeared that there were two populations of infants with congenital anomalies: a group of early preterm infants of very low birth weight and another of more mature small-for-gestational age infants.

Specific Congenital Malformations. Certain malformations tend to cluster by birth weight and gestational age. If the cluster is a tight one, the diagnosis can be anticipated from the infant's birth weight and gestational age. Some of the recognizable anomalies that may be suspected at birth, because of their relation to birth weight/gestational age patterns, are described below.

Congenital Heart Disease. An overall incidence of congenital heart disease by birth weight and gestational age was compiled by Yerushalmy (Fig. 12-10).[19] The incidence was the same in infants with birth weights <1500 g and in term, low-birth-weight infants (39.4/

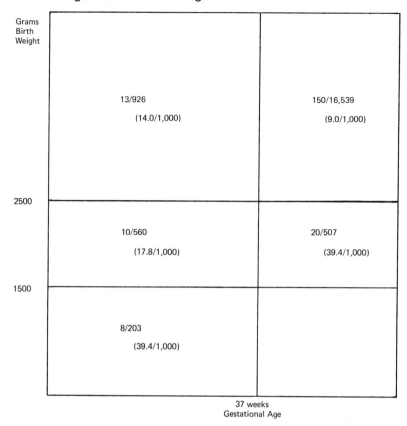

Grams
Birth
Weight

13/926

(14.0/1,000)

150/16,539

(9.0/1,000)

2500

10/560

(17.8/1,000)

20/507

(39.4/1,000)

1500

8/203

(39.4/1,000)

37 weeks
Gestational Age

Incidence of Preterm Versus Term = 18.3 Versus 9.9
Low Birth Weight Versus High Birth Weight = 29.9 Versus 9.3

Fig. 12-10. Incidence of congenital heart disease by birth weight and gestational age. (Yerushalmy J: Congenital Malformations, p. 299. In Fraser and McKusick [eds]: Excerpta Medica, Amsterdam and New York, 1969)

1000 live births). Mehrizi and Drash[20] and Naeye[22] noted that one type of congenital heart disease (*i.e.,* transposition of the aorta) was more common in large infants. The mean weight was 3450 g, compared to 3140 g for infants with all other congenital heart lesions.

Chromosomal Abnormalities. Important new information from banding techniques is available, and a relationship between small losses of genetic material or excess material to clinical syndromes is being made. The effect on fetal growth of trisomies has been studied. Trisomy of chromosomes of the E group (16–18) results in very small infants, having a mean weight of about 1800 g and a gestational age of 40 weeks. There is some evidence that they are postterm, even though most are reported as 40-weeks' gestation.

The weights and gestational ages of infants with Down's syndrome form a large, loose cluster with many large and mature infants, but the median gestational age is 37 weeks and the median birth weight is 2400 g.

Even though the physical and neurologic characteristics of infants with trisomy of the D group (13–15) are more severe than with infants with trisomy 16–18, the birth weights of the former are larger and the cluster by weight and gestational age is loose. The median birth weight is 2600 g at 40-weeks' gestation.[13]

Other syndromes. Seckel's bird-headed dwarf syndrome is noted for the very small birth weight and prolonged gestation it produces. Over half of the conditions resulting in short stature give evidence of onset of short stature prior to birth.[17]

Infants with osteogenesis imperfecta tend to be preterm as well as small-for-gestational age;

whereas, infants with anencephaly are characteristically well developed and well nourished and have greatly prolonged gestations.

Beckwith's syndrome is characterized by the large size of the infant, congenital anomalies, and hyperinsulinemia.

Data from The Collaborative Study showed an incidence of 0.9% single umbilical arteries.[23] The neonatal mortality rate was high (14.0%) and the incidence of major anomalies in those who died was 53.0%. Those who survived had essentially the same outcome as matched controls. Multiple gestations were not included in these data.

Morbidity Related to Gestational Age

There are specific problems that tend to occur in infants of various gestational ages. The severity of problems is indirectly related to gestational age, starting with lethal problems of immaturity in the shortest gestational ages to mild and even subtle problems near term. The type of morbidity appears to change from problems related to immaturity of organ systems in immature infants to intrapartum accidents and congenital anomalies in more mature infants. Intrapartum accidents occur in infants of all gestations, but they are more frequent at term because the other problems decrease. Postterm infants show evidence of IUGR even though they are in an acceptable weight range. There are more excessive-size infants as well.

Morbidity in Preterm Infants. The physiologic handicaps of preterm infants were described by Levine and Gordon in 1942, and are detailed in Chapter 14.[24] The age of viability has been pushed back, because ventilatory and metabolic support are available to the very immature infant. With this approach to care, both the immediate and long-term prognosis for these very immature infants has improved.

Problems of the Preterm Infant. (See also Chap. 14.) By 26 to 28 weeks of gestation, alveoli and capillaries have developed sufficiently that oxygen and carbon dioxide exchange make survival possible. Surfactant must be produced in sufficient quantities to maintain patent expanded alveoli; otherwise they will collapse. The immature infant dies with a clinical and pathologic picture of atelectasis; whereas, the more mature infant lives longer, develops typical HMD and may or may not survive.

The cardiovascular system, like the pulmonary system, is called upon to make immediate changes after birth. The lungs must act within minutes, while the cardiovascular system may take hours or even days to adjust to extrauterine life. When preterm birth occurs, there are additional hazards in this adjustment. Umbilical blood flow and blood pressure increase with gestational age and the term infant is prepared for the blood transferred from the placenta at birth. The preterm infant may not be able to handle the extra load.

There is a gradual transition from production of fetal hemoglobin in the young fetus to production of adult type hemoglobin near term. Fetal hemoglobin has a greater affinity for oxygen than does adult hemoglobin, but the effect of fetal hemoglobin on the preterm infant's ability to cope with extrauterine life is not clear.

Capillary fragility was considered to be a cause of bleeding in preterm infants, as were hypoprothrombinemia and defective hemopoiesis. The interest at present has turned to abnormal platelet function and disorders of coagulation. Platelets are important in producing a clot, in phagocytosis, or in clot retraction. These functions are diminished in preterm newborns and are thought to account for capillary fragility.

Hypercoagulability of blood is present in term infants and is especially prominent in preterm infants. A deficiency of an anticoagulant (antithrombin III) has been noted in newborns, and it is especially low in preterm infants with respiratory distress.

An optimal environmental temperature is essential for the survival of preterm infants. Energy requirements increase in a cool environment at the same time that nutrients are less available. Evaporative heat loss occurs in the newborn at birth. He also loses heat if there is little fat.

Evidence of vital central nervous system function can be seen early in prenatal life. The functions become less global and more and more complex as the fetus matures. Swallowing and sucking movements can be seen as early as 20 weeks and become strong enough to sustain nutrition at approximately 34 weeks.

Apnea in the infant of short gestation is thought to be a lack of responsiveness of the central nervous system to variations in blood gases.

The gastrointestinal tract develops early in

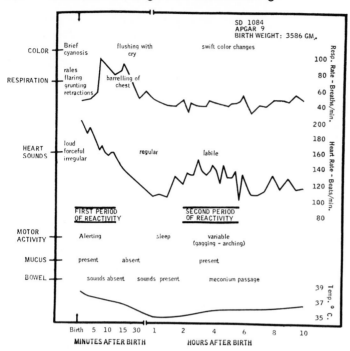

Fig. 12-11. A summary of the physical findings noted during the first 10 hours of extrauterine life in representative high-Apgar-score infant delivered under spinal anesthesia without prior premedication. (Desmond MM, Rudolph AJ, Phitaksphraiwan P: Pediatr Clin North Am 13:651, 1966)

fetal life. By 3 to 4 months of gestation, the stomach and the small and large intestines are well differentiated, and cells with specific functions can be found.

By 22 weeks of gestation, well-formed glomeruli and tubules are present. Glomeruli continue to increase in number until 36-weeks' gestation. Tubular development lags behind glomerular production and renal function is not comparable to the adult's until many months after term birth.

The term infant has relative undermineralized bones, and postnatal homeostasis is tenuous in the light of a transient hypoparathyroid state, decreased renal excretion of phosphorus, and the intake of cow's milk products. The preterm infant presents an exaggerated picture of the same metabolic problems.

The preterm infant is highly susceptible to acidosis. During fetal life, the acid-base status is largely controlled by the mother.

At birth, there may be immediate problems in regulating pH because of borderline respiratory sufficiency and limited renal function. Cow's milk formulas make acid-base regulation more difficult.

Although conjugation of bilirubin is functional, but at a reduced level in the fetus, it is temporarily insufficient to cope with the load presented to the liver after birth. In addition, hydrolysis of conjugated bilirubin in the gut results in unconjugation, reabsorption, and a still greater load to excrete.

Morbidity in the Term Infant

Physiologic Adaptation to Extrauterine Life. During intrauterine life, the fetus has grown, developed, and matured appropriately for extrauterine existence. There are many physiologic functions that are termed *immature* according to adult standards, yet they are not only adequate for the newborn but also necessary for his survival. For example, the term infant appears to have a decreased reactivity to various stresses at birth. He tolerates a low glucose level without signs or symptoms characteristic of the adult with hypoglycemia. If he responded as the adult, he would utilize all available energy sources and would not survive.

The immediate adjustment of the term healthy infant is described by Desmond (Fig. 12-11). To the average observer the infant is doing well, and is alert and pink; yet the respiratory and cardiac rates are high, oral mucus and regurgitation are present, he is apprehensively alert, and there is a fall in body temperature. Within a few hours, the majority of the vital signs are stable.

Morbidity in Term Infants Caused by Congenital Anomalies. Although the incidence of congenital anomalies is low in term infants, the actual number of children with malformations is greater than at any other gestational age.

Intrapartum Accidents. The neonatal morbidity and mortality in term, appropriate-for-gestational-age infants is low, especially in the "bull's eye." However, 4% of infants in the lowest morbidity zone have significant illness in the neonatal period.

Congenital anomalies and intrapartum accidents are the major causes of morbidity. Postnatal infections, isoimmunization and infants of diabetic mothers contribute to term morbidity.

Morbidity in Postterm Infants. Clifford's article in 1954 on the postmaturity syndrome caused obstetricians and pediatricians to reconsider the possibility that prolonged gestation could be clinically important.[25] The patients he described were postterm, but their weights ranged from 2400 to 4100 g. Mortality was especially high in primigravidas and in babies of mothers who were more than 35 years of age, whether multiparas or primiparas. Hypertension was a bad omen. Intrapartum deaths were increased in primiparas. Postterm, small-for-gestational age infants have the same problems as term, small-for-gestational age infants, except that certain congenital anomalies occur more frequently (trisomy 16–18 and Seckel's syndrome). In one series (Lucas et al.),[26] the morbidity of infants with birth weights >4,000 g doubled as did cesarean sections for cephalopelvic disproportion.[26]

Although aging of the placenta or placental insufficiency has been postulated, morphologic examination of placentas and correlation with morbidity has not been found to be significant.

Prolonged pregnancy in anencephalic infants is well known and probably related to the lack of fetal pituitary–adrenal complex which initiates labor.

Morbidity by Pattern of Intrauterine Growth

Morbidity in the Large-for-Gestational-Age Infant. The best-known relationship to excessively sized infants is maternal diabetes. Infants of diabetic mothers have been shown to have hyperinsulinemia as have large infants with other conditions. Infants with Beckwith's syndrome are large-for-gestational-age and have hyperinsulinemia in addition to the other malformations. Infants with Rh isoimmunization may have hyperinsulinemia as well. Whether or not insulin is responsible for the excessive growth or whether an increase in insulin affects other growth parameters is not clear.

Infants of diabetic mothers often have hypoglycemia following birth, and they also have a higher incidence of congenital malformations and problems associated with hypercoagulability of blood. If the infant of the diabetic mother is preterm, he also has problems associated with immaturity. Because elective preterm delivery has been customary in the past, many of the morbidities ascribed to maternal diabetes are not related to her metabolic state but to preterm delivery.

The question arises as to whether all large-for-gestational-age infants should be considered at risk. It is known that large parents will have large newborn infants and that these large-for-gestational-age infants will have no special problems. The incidence of such a population in the large-for-gestational-age group is not clear.

When large-for-gestational-age infants born to mothers without evidence of diabetes or without a family history of diabetes are followed for hypoglycemia, about 20% respond with a clinically significant fall in glucose levels. Whether these mothers later develop diabetes is not known. Large-for-gestational-age infants, whether or not they are born to diabetic mothers, may have difficulty in being delivered because of their size. It is interesting to note the trend toward a low morbidity in large-for-gestational-age infants.

Mothers with a menstrual history of very short gestations, but who have term-sized infants, are discussed in the section on intrauterine growth.

Racial characteristics must also be considered. Some tribes of American Indians, such as the Crow and Cheyenne Indians in Montana, have large babies. The tenth percentile of birth weights of these tribes fell in the twenty-fifth percentile of the Colorado intrauterine growth curves, and their fiftieth percentile was greater than the Colorado seventy-fifth percentile. This increased fetal weight is all the more

Table 12-1. Infections Affecting the Fetus or Newborn.

Maternal Infection	Effects on Fetus or Newborn
Specific viral infections	
Herpes simplex	Generalized herpes, encephalitis, death
Mumps	Fetal death, endocardial fibroelastosis (?), and malformations (?)
Rubeola	Increased abortions and still-births
Western equine encephalitis	Encephalitis
Chickenpox—''shingles''	Chickenpox or ''shingles,'' increased abortions, and stillbirths
Smallpox	Smallpox, increased abortions, and stillbirths
Vaccinia	Generalized vaccinia, increased abortions
Influenza	Malformations (?)
Poliomyelitis	Spinal or bulbar poliomyelitis
Hepatitis	Hepatitis
Coxsackie B viruses	Myocarditis
Nonspecific viral infections	
Upper respiratory infections	None
Severe viral infections	Prematurity
Bacterial infections	
Spirochetal infections: syphilis	Congenital syphilis
Acute bacterial infections	Prematurity
Tuberculosis	Congenital tuberculosis
Listeriosis	Abortions, stillbirths, septicemia, meningoence-phalitis, habitual abortion (?)
Protozoan infections	
Malaria	Low birth weight and increased mortality (?)

(Sever JL: In Waisman HA, Kerr GR (eds): Fetal Growth and Development. New York, McGraw-Hill, 1970)[27]
See also Chapter 33 for congenital infections of the TORCHES group.

surprising because of the low socioeconomic status of these Indian tribes.

Morbidity in the Small-for-Gestational-Age Infant (see also Chap. 15)

Many more conditions are related to IUGR than to excessive growth *in utero*. The etiologies are varied and the mechanisms responsible for decreased growth are numerous.

Unlike the large-for-gestational-age infant, very few small-for-gestational-age infants are normal, small infants of small parents. The possibility that the small-for-gestational-age infant may be normal should not be dismissed, but a high priority should be placed on anticipating the problems likely to occur in abnormal small-for-gestational-age infants.

Congenital Malformations. In the discussion on congenital malformations, it is clear that the anomaly rate is high among small-for-ges-tational-age infants. An abnormality in the fetus itself will prevent normal development of tissues and organs and result in reduced size of the fetus or infant at birth.

Congenital Infections. Chronic intrauterine infections usually inhibit growth of the fetus and several etiologies are recognized. In Table 12-1, Sever lists maternal infections that have an effect on the fetus or newborn.[27]

The organisms most often associated with congenital malformations are rubella virus, cytomegalovirus, and toxoplasmosis. Actually, if one considers the widespread effect of sepsis in causing meningoencephalitis, chorioretinitis, hepatitis, and invasion of bone marrow, the findings at birth are more related to sepsis than to congenital malformation. One could argue that microcephaly is an expected consequence of meningoencephalitis rather than being a true congenital defect.

Small-for-gestational-age infants with congenital infections have characteristic findings of sepsis and hematologic problems if the disease is severe. More subtle infections are suspected when jaundice and irritability are present and when the head circumference is disproportionately small. In the case of rubella, length is appropriate, but weight and head circumference are low.[28]

Fetal Undernutrition. The majority of small-for-gestational-age infants do not have congenital malformations or intrauterine infections. However, they are presumably undernourished because of inadequate nutrients reaching them.

Many conditions which have been shown to decrease mean birth weight are frequently cited as causes for small-for-gestational-age infants. The following conditions do affect fetal weight but the proportion of infants who are small-for-gestational-age may be relatively small.

Maternal Nutrition. Under severe conditions of near starvation for the mother, fetal growth is reduced on an average of about 200 g at term. The effects of specific nutritional deficiencies must be important, but they are not recognized as clinical entities.

Altitude. Infants born at high altitudes are smaller than those born at sea level. Term infants average 3400 g at sea level, 3200 g at 5000 feet, and 2900 g at 10,000 feet altitude.

Low Socioeconomic Status. There is an increased incidence of low birth weight among the poor, but how much is due to preterm birth and how much to intrauterine growth retardation is not clear.

Toxemia. A reduction in size, comparable to the above conditions, is noted in pure toxemia.

Smoking. A reduction in fetal size accompanies heavy smoking in the mother (>20 cigarettes per day), but does not result in premature birth.

Maternal alcohol consumption may result in infants with IUGR. These infants have low birth weights and lengths, and small head circumferences. The facies are characteristic with small palpebral fissures, long upper lips, and other minor anomalies. The outlook is poor for normal growth and development. Information to date indicates the effect on the fetus is related to alcohol and not to dietary or other deficiencies.[29]

There is some evidence to suggest that a cumulative effect on birth weight occurs if several of these conditions are present. Then the incidence of small-for-gestational-age infants may be increased significantly.

The following maternal diseases or conditions result in significant morbidity in the infant.

Hypertensive Cardiovascular Disease. Whenever hypertensive disease occurs and is of long duration, the fetus is likely to be small-for-gestational-age. The diseases in this category include Class V diabetic mothers and severe or prolonged toxemia.

Small or Diseased Placenta. These situations are not usually known prior to delivery. Why a placenta is small is not clear. Some workers believe that the size of the placenta depends on fetal factors and that a small fetus produces a small placenta. Others believe that the size depends on the uterine environment and especially vascular perfusion. When disease processes (infection, infarction, tumors) involve the placenta, failure of growth of the fetus is expected.

Twins. Twins at term have a median weight on the tenth percentile so that half of the twins delivered at term will be small for gestational age. If the twins have unequal sized placentas, the smaller twin may be much smaller and present with severe IUGR.

Other. The majority of small-for-gestational-age infants are not suspected prior to birth and the etiology for their growth retardation is not clear. A prospective study by obstetricians at the University Hospital, Denver, aimed at diagnosing the small-for-gestational-age infant prenatally, resulted in identifying only one-half of the infants.

The following conditions are clinically significant in small-for-gestational-age infants (see also Chap. 15).

1. Small-for-gestational-age infants do not tolerate labor and delivery well, so that fetal distress, aspiration of meconium, and even intrapartum deaths are likely.
2. Small-for-gestational-age infants have, in addition to fetal distress, an inability to conserve heat. There is no wonder that hypoglycemia is frequent in these infants who have an increased need for energy sources and yet have small glycogen and fat reserves (Fig. 12-12). Small-for-gestational-age infants are not able to build up

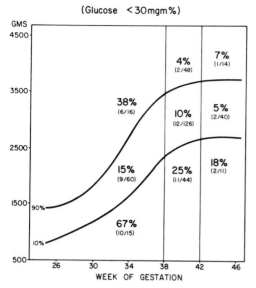

Fig. 12-12. Incidence of hypoglycemia prior to first feeding. (Lubchenco LO, Bard H, Goldman A et al: Dev Med Child Neurol 16:421, 1974)[31]

large stores of glycogen or fat *in utero.* When labor occurs, fetal distress is frequent and meconium passage and aspiration may complicate the already precarious situation. Fetal distress has already mobilized the small available stores of glycogen so that very little is available after birth. Hypoglycemia developing in this setting is a critical situation for the infant and, if a source of exogenous glucose is not supplied promptly, central nervous system damage is likely to occur.

3. Small-for-gestational-age infants are often polycythemic, probably because of chronic intrauterine hypoxia. The hyperviscosity syndrome is a serious condition for the infant and symptoms of central nervous system abnormality may appear.[30]

LONG-TERM FOLLOW-UP (See also Chap. 19)

Most of the older reports of long-term follow-up of "premature" infants are given by birth weight, without reference to gestational age. With the appreciation of the problems of the small-for-gestational-age infants, reports are appearing which show a poor prognosis for this group, as well as for preterm infants. Very

few reports cover all birth weight-gestational age categories.

One such study gives IQ by birth weight and gestational age.[4] These infants were born during 1952 and were 8 years old when followed. Unusual care was taken with the testing and a large sample was studied: 500 low-birth-weight infants and 492 term infants by weight. When the IQ was related to birth weight and gestational age, interesting results were noted (Fig. 12-13).

The IQ improves with birth weight. However, at birth weights >2500 g and gestational ages <38 weeks, children had significantly lower IQs than those born after 38 weeks. The reason is not apparent for the less than optimal neurologic outcome of the large, slightly preterm infants. Other data confirm the finding of an increased incidence of central nervous system handicaps in preterm infants, even though their birth weights were >2500 g.[31]

Of singular importance is the changing prognosis for infants born in the late 1960s and 1970s. Rawlings and coworkers show an improved neonatal mortality and improved long-term outcome in infants cared for in more recent years in an ICN.[32] Findings from other intensive care nurseries confirm this trend.[33,34] The provision of supportive measures could be correlated with outcome. In the former paper, administration of intravenous glucose and/or bicarbonate in the first hours after birth was related to a better outcome; and in the

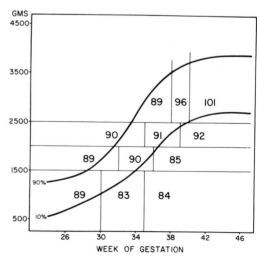

Fig. 12-13. IQ by birth weight and gestational age. (Weiner G: J Pediatr 76:694, 1970)[4]

latter study, the immediate correction of hypotension apparently resulted in improved central nervous system function. Infants with severe respiratory distress, who were given ventilatory support, were found to have good long-term prognosis.[35]

Efforts at supporting the high-risk infant (*i.e.,* providing warmth, fluid, calories, and maintaining metabolic homeostatis), support of the pulmonary and cardiovascular systems, and early recognition and treatment of disease are resulting in an increased survival of infants; and the infants who survive are, in great part, developmentally normal.

REFERENCES

1. **Silverman WA:** Nomenclature for duration of gestation, birth weight and intrauterine growth. Pediatrics 39:935, 1967
2. **Battaglia FC, Lubchenco LO:** A practical classification of newborn infants by weight and gestational age. J Pediatr 71:159, 1967
3. **Lubchenco LO, Brazie JV, Searls DT:** Perinatal events and neonatal morbidity: A predictive model. In preparation.
4. **Weiner G:** The relationship of birth weight and length of gestation to intellectual development at ages 8 to 10 years. J Pediatr 76:694, 1970
5. **Lubchenco LO, Little GA:** The outcome of large pre-term infants: An unexpected high-risk population, Abstract. Pediatr Res 6:412, 1972
6. **Babson SG, Behrman RE, Lessel R:** Liveborn birth weights for gestational age of white middle class infants. Pediatrics 45:937, 1970
7. **Gruenwald P:** Growth of the human fetus. I. Normal growth and its violation. Am J Obstet Gynecol 94:1112, 1966; II. Abnormal growth in twins and infants of mothers with diabetes, hypertension, or isoimmunization. Am J Obstet Gynecol 94:1120, 1966
8. **Usher R, McLean F:** Intrauterine growth of liveborn Caucasian infants at sea level: Standards obtained from measurements in 7 dimensions of infants born between 25 and 44 weeks of gestation. J Pediatr 74:901, 1969
9. **Wong KS, Scott KE:** Fetal growth at sea level. Biol Neonate 20:175, 1972
10. **Mitchell RG, Farr V:** The Meaning of Maturity and the Assessment of Maturity at Birth in Gestational Age, Size and Maturity. Dawkins, McGregor (eds). Lavenham, Suffolk, England, Lavenham Press, Ltd., 1965
11. **Farr V, Mitchell RG, Neligan GA, Parkin JM:** The definition of some external characteristics in the assessment of gestational age in the newborn infant. Dev Med Child Neurol 8:507, 1966
12. **Dubowitz LMS, Dubowitz V, Goldberg C:** Clinical assessment of gestational age in the newborn infant. J Pediatr 77:1, 1970
13. **Usher R, McLeon F, Scott KE:** Judgment of fetal age. II. Clinical significance of gestational age and an objective method for its assessment. Pediatr Clin North Am 13:835, 1966
14. **Minkowski A:** Development du Systeme Nerveux Central de la Periode Foetal au Terme. Paris, Service du Filme de Recherche Scientifique, 1964
15. **Amiel-Tison C:** Neurologic examination of the maturity of newborn infants. Arch Dis Child 43:89, 1968
16. **Warkany J, Monroe BB, Sutherland BS:** Intrauterine growth retardation. Am J Dis Child 102:249, 1961
17. **Smith DW:** Recognizable Patterns of Human Malformation. Philadelphia, W. B. Saunders, 1970
18. **Van Den Berg BJ, Yerushalmy J:** The relationship of the rate of intrauterine growth of infants of low birth weight to mortality, morbidity and congenital anomalies. J Pediatr 69:531, 1966
19. **Yerushalmy J:** The California child health and development studies. Study design and some illustrative findings on congenital heart disease, congenital malformations. Fraser and McKusick (eds): Proc 3rd Internat'l Conf, p. 299. The Hague, Netherlands, Excerpta Medica, Amsterdam, New York, 1969
20. **Winick M:** Cellular growth of human placenta, III. Intrauterine growth failure. J Pediatr 71:390, 1967
21. **Mehrizi A, Drash A:** Birth weight of infants with cyanotic and acyanotic congenital malformations of the heart. J Pediatr 59:715, 1961
22. **Naeye RL:** The Influence of Glucose Metabolism on Prenatal Development. Presented at the 36th annual meeting of the Society for Pediatric Research. Program and Abstracts, p. 79, 1966
23. **Froehlich LA, Fujikura T:** What prognosis with single umbilical artery? Pediatrics 52:6, 1973
24. **Gordon HH, Levine SZ:** Physical handicaps of the premature infant. I. Their pathogenesis; II. Clinical applications. Am J Dis Child 64:274, 297, 1942
25. **Clifford SH:** Postmaturity—with placental dysfunction: Clinical syndrome and pathologic findings. J Pediatr 44:1, 1954
26. **Lucas WE, Anctil AO, Callagan DA:** The problem of post-term pregnancy. Am J. Obstet Gynecol 91:241, 1965
27. **Sever JL:** Infectious agents and fetal disease. In Waisman HA, Kerr G (eds): Fetal Growth

and Development, p. 223. New York, Mc-Graw-Hill, 1970

28. **Desmond MM, Montgomery JR, Melnick JL et al:** Congenital rubella encephalitis. Effects on growth and early development. Am J Dis Child 118:30, 1969

29. **Erb L, Andressen BD:** The fetal alcohol syndrome (FAS). Clin Pediatr 17:644, 1978

30. **Wirth FH, Goldberg KE, Lubchenco LO:** Neonatal hyperviscosity: I. Incidence. Pediatrics 63:833, 1979

31. **Lubchenco LO, Bard H, Goldman AL et al:** Newborn intensive care and long-term prognosis. Dev Med Child Neurol 16:421, 1974

32. **Rawlings G, Stewart A, Reynolds EOR, Strang LB:** Changing prognosis for infants of very low birth weight. Lancet 1:516, 1971

33. **Usher R:** Changing mortality rates with perinatal intensive care and regionalization. Semin Perinatol 1:309, 1977

34. **Thompson T, Reynolds J:** The results of intensive care therapy for neonates, J Perinatol Med 5:59, 1977

35. **Stahlman M:** Long time results of respirator therapy. Biol Neonate 16:133, 1970

13

Needs of the Term Infant

Ernest N. Kraybill

More than 80% of all infants are born after a full-term gestation, are of normal birth weight and have no obvious congenital defect or illness. The purpose of this chapter is to review the principles that should govern their care in the hospital.

Delivery Room Care

Cord Clamping. The clamping of the umbilical cord profoundly influences cardiovascular and pulmonary adjustments that must take place in the first minutes of life. Infants whose cords are clamped late (usually defined as after cessation of pulsation) have an initially higher blood volume, reflected at 3 days of age by a larger red cell mass, smaller plasma volume, and higher hematocrit, compared with infants whose cords are clamped immediately. These late-cord-clamped infants have a faster respiratory rate, higher pulmonary artery pressure, higher Pa_{CO_2}, lower Pa_{O_2}, lower pulmonary compliance, and smaller functional residual capacity. As a result of the larger red cell mass, there is a larger iron reserve, a larger turnover of bilirubin, and a somewhat greater tendency toward hyperbilirubinemia. It has been suggested, but not proven, that excessive placental transfusion to the low-birth-weight infant may be an important factor in causing transient tachypnea.[1]

Despite this wealth of information, the optimal time for cord clamping remains unsettled. Certain apparent advantages of late clamping are counterbalanced by distinct disadvantages. Perhaps in the full-term, nonasphyxiated infant, the issue is not of great consequence. It is unlikely that survival is affected and there is no information concerning the importance of the differing physiologic consequences of early and late clamping.

With present information, it seems reasonable to avoid both the extremes of immediate and of very late clamping. The first 30 to 60 seconds after delivery are well spent in suctioning the airway and drying the infant. The normal newborn invariably cries during this interval. The cord should then be clamped and the 1-minute Apgar score assigned. In the event of asphyxia and failure to cry, the cord should also be clamped at no later than 1 minute in order to begin resuscitation. Except in rare instances of placental bleeding with obvious hypovolemia of the infant, there appears to be no justification for stripping of the umbilical cord.

Thermoregulation. The transition from the warm aqueous environment of the uterus to the air-conditioned delivery room represents a potentially damaging thermal stress to the newborn. If unprotected, he will sustain large heat losses, mainly by evaporation and radiation, but by conduction and convection as well. He responds to this stress by vasoconstriction, an attempt to reduce heat loss, and by metabolism of brown fat (nonshivering thermogenesis). These adaptive mechanisms are metabolically expensive, resulting in depletion of energy stores and an increase in oxygen consumption to nearly three times the basal level. Despite these responses, the unprotected infant cannot fully counter the massive heat loss and his core temperature falls to unphysiologic levels. Consequences of this negative thermal balance may include hypoglycemia, metabolic acidosis, and, indirectly, decreased pulmonary perfusion.

The provision of a microenvironment using a radiant heat source has been widely accepted as an effective method of minimizing the infant's heat loss in the delivery room. Equally important, and less expensive, is the prompt and thorough drying of the infant to reduce evaporative heat loss. If he is then wrapped in a warm blanket, heat loss is reduced to an amount approaching that achieved with a radiant heat source.[2] Because of the potential heat loss during circumcision, this procedure, if done in the delivery room, must be performed under a radiant heat source.

Gonococcal Prophylaxis. The recent increase in gonococcal infections among young adults appears to be accompanied by an increased incidence of gonococcal ophthalmia neonatorum.[3] Prenatal care should include the routine culturing of cervical secretions for gonococci and treatment of those women who are infected. Even when this is consistently done, the routine use of a prophylactic agent in the eyes of newborns remains a necessary precaution.

A solution of 1% silver nitrate has had widespread acceptance and efficacy. Despite reported failures and proposals of various substitutes, no clearly superior alternative has emerged. The eyes should not be irrigated immediately afterward. The chemical conjunctivitis frequently associated with silver nitrate may interfere with the quiet alert state during the first hour of life and thus unfavorably affect maternal response to the infant. For this reason, instillation of silver nitrate is delayed for an hour in some centers. This seems a reasonable compromise but the safety of such a delay has not been carefully tested. Chemical conjunctivities can be resolved by frequent bathing

of the eyes with sterile saline and need not be confused with gonococcal ophthalmia.

Vitamin K Administration. The newborn, especially if he is premature, breast-fed, or fasted more than 12 hours, has a deficiency of vitamin K-dependent coagulation factors, a prolonged prothrombin time, and an increased risk of significant bleeding. The prothrombin time can be corrected toward normal, and hemorrhagic disease can be prevented by the routine administration of vitamin K_1. A single parenteral dose of 0.5 to 1.0 mg or an oral dose of 1.0 to 2.0 mg has been recommended by the Committee of Nutrition of the American Academy of Pediatrics. This dose has not been reported to be associated with side effects, although larger doses used previously caused hemolysis in glucose-6-phosphate-dehydrogenase(G-6-PD)-deficient infants.

Identification Procedures. It is of utmost importance to establish with certainty the identification of each newborn infant. The time-honored routine of footprinting has been challenged as useless. Fingerprint experts insist, however, that if properly taken, absolute identity *can* be established from a newborn's footprint. Yet it is apparent that in many hospitals the footprint as usually taken would be of no value in establishing identity. Therefore, emphasis must be placed on other measures. A wrist or ankle bracelet, containing data including the mother's name and hospital number, if prepared in advance, can be attached in seconds. Even in an emergency, the infant should not leave the delivery room without it.

Prevention of Infection

In recent decades, changing patterns of bacterial infections have been observed in hospital nurseries. Before the antibiotic era, gram-positive organisms, particularly β-hemolytic streptococci, were predominant. Gradually, and subsequent to widespread use of antibiotics, gram-negative organisms came to the fore. The late 1950s and early 1960s were marked by epidemics of staphylococcal disease throughout hospitals as well as in newborn nurseries. The decline in serious neonatal staphylococcal disease seen in the late 1960s was popularly attributed to the routine use of hexachlorophene for infant bathing in hospitals. This conclusion seemed to be confirmed in 1972 by reports of epidemics occurring in hospitals which had discontinued routine use of hexachlorophene for infant bathing. However, this was called into question by the observation that hospitals that had never routinely used hexachlorophene were also experiencing an increase in neonatal staphylococcal disease in 1972.

In recent years, group B streptococci have become the leading cause of sepsis and a major cause of morbidity and mortality in the newborn period.[4] Up to one-third of mothers harbor the organism in their vaginal tracts during the third trimester and a similar fraction of newborns may be colonized. About 1% of colonized infants develop serious infection. There is evidence of nosocomial spread of the organism in newborn nurseries. Suggestions for prophylactic antibiotic treatment of both mother and infant have been made but no effective program has been demonstrated. Triple dye (a solution containing gentian violet, brilliant cresyl green, and proflavin hemisulfate), if applied to the umbilical cord at birth, appears to decrease colonization rates due to staphylococci but not due to group B streptococci or *Escherichia coli*. Silver sulfadiazine has a broader spectrum of activity.

There is sufficient evidence of hexachlorophene toxicity to warrant the recommendation that preparations containing this compound not be used for routine bathing of infants. Reliance must be placed on more basic epidemiologic principles for prevention of spread of pathogenic organisms in nurseries. The chief route of bacterial contamination of the newborn is by direct contact, rather than airborne. Careful scrubbing of the hands and arms to elbows before handling of each infant is the most important element in reducing transmission by human contact. There appear to be no grounds at present for prohibiting the use of hexachlorophene as a hand-washing preparation for nursery personnel, although iodophor-containing preparations are also widely used and effective. Most nurseries have nonhuman points of common contact such as scales and examining tables; precautions must be taken to avoid transmission of organisms by these sources.

In obstetric units large enough to justify several nursery modules, the "cohort system" of caring for newborns is remarkably effective in preventing spread of pathogenic organisms. Even two modules, if used in this manner, can allow frequent interruptions in the overlapping tenures of "old" and "new" babies and allow for thorough cleaning of the room. If only one nursery module exists, it may be necessary to control an epidemic by a temporary period of "rooming in," to break the cycle of potential transfer of organisms from old to new babies.

Following the discovery of hexachlorophene toxicity there has been increased use of topical preparations such as triple dye, for local application to the umbilical stump. This has some logic because the umbilical cord appears to become colonized first.

Feeding Routines

The first few hours after birth are a time of stabilization of the infant's temperature, respiration, and cardiovascular dynamics. For the healthy, alert infant there is no contraindication to suckling soon after birth and there are important psychological advantages. Artificial feeding, however, is usually both unnecessary and undesirable at this time. The interval until the first feeding generally need not exceed 8 hours, but there is considerable variation among babies. Nurses accustomed to newborns are aware of these variations and are quick to recognize clues about readiness to feed.

Glucose water, long considered a safe liquid for the first feeding, has been shown to be as damaging (to rabbit's lung) as is milk.[5] The first artificial feeding for bottle-fed infants should therefore be sterile water. If this is swallowed and retained without difficulty, milk should be given at the next feeding.

The nutritional, immunologic and psychological superiority of human milk over cow's milk formulas is well established. Breast feeding should be given unanimous support by physicians and nurses who care for mothers and their infants. Mothers ambivalent about nursing are often influenced by subtle attitudes on the part of medical and nursing staffs. Routines must be flexible enough to permit mother and infant to establish their own rhythms. It is important, particularly after discharge, to avoid too frequent a feeding schedule that is exhausting to the mother.

Screening Procedures

Determination of Cord Blood Type, Group, and Coombs' Reaction. The frequency of idiopathic jaundice in the newborn period justifies this study as a routine to rule out isoimmune hemolytic disease. Parents also should be given this information for future reference.

Test for Syphilis. Unless a routine exists for performing a serologic test for syphilis on each mother at the time of delivery, cord blood should be used for this purpose. Failure to detect and treat this disease may result in permanent handicap or death.

Test for Phenylketonuria (PKU). Mass screening programs for PKU have been successful in detecting affected infants in the newborn period, while dietary control can be effective in preventing mental retardation. Criticisms of the high-cost-to-yield ratio do not seem warranted. The cost to society of PKU screening is lower than the cost of caring for the phenylketonuric persons who would become mentally retarded if undetected and untreated. More important, the value to the family of discovering this treatable disease is unquestioned.

Emphasis has been placed on assuring a significant milk intake before PKU testing. Some screening programs have included repeat testing at 4 to 6 weeks of age to avoid missing affected infants who are discharged early. There appears to be poor correlation between milk intake and early diagnosis of PKU by screening tests. Some infants (siblings of known PKU patients) have been tested before any milk was given and have had abnormal (though not diagnostic) results; other infants were "missed" by screening tests after significant milk intake.[6]

Test for Hypothyroidism. Several studies have demonstrated the feasibility and cost-effectiveness of mass newborn screening programs for hypothyroidism.[7] The high incidence of this disorder (1 in 4000) and the efficacy of early replacement therapy in preventing mental retardation make this an ideal screening test. Like PKU testing, thyroid screening programs detect benign variants (thyroid-binding globulin deficiency) which do not require treatment. Careful followup of abnormal test results is mandatory and most efficiently done by a single center for a large geographic area.

Screening Procedures Not Recommended as Routine. Urinalysis and Urine Culture. The difficulty in obtaining uncontaminated specimens, the significant likelihood of false-positives, and the low eventual yield all support the view that urine examinations and cultures

are not useful routines for apparently well newborns.[8]

Hemoglobin Concentration and Hematocrit. Unless there is abnormal bleeding during labor, perinatal asphyxia, respiratory distress, or pallor, routine hemoglobin concentrations and hematocrit determinations are of little value in the full-term, normal-size singleton. Twins should routinely have these studies done to detect twin-to-twin transfusion syndrome.

The Infant—family Relationship

It may well be that the most important contribution physicians and nurses can make to the welfare of newborn infants is the fostering of a healthy relationship between the infant and his family. Hospital routines sometimes seem at odds with this purpose. There is evidence that early and increased contact between mother and infant is associated with differences in the quality of mothering.[9] Little investigation has been reported regarding the father's role in the immediate neonatal period. While much more information is needed, there appears to be no justification for nursery routines that arbitrarily limit contact between mother and infant, or prohibit direct contact by the father.

It is both feasible and desirable for mothers to have contact with their infants as soon as the infant's condition permits and the mother is awake. A modified "rooming-in" plan permits the infant to remain in the mother's room as long as she is awake and desires to have him there. Responsibility for observation and care of the baby is shared between the mother and the nursing staff. During the times when the mother wishes to sleep or is otherwise occupied, the infant should be returned to a central nursery. Such a system requires flexibility on the part of nursery personnel and limits visiting in the mother's room. After practicing the same technique for prevention of cross-contamination required of hospital personnel having similar contact with the baby, the father should be encouraged to spend time together with the mother and baby.

The hospital setting provides unequaled opportunity for important early counseling. The specific instructions needed by the well-educated, middle- or upper-class mother are relatively few and are readily available in printed form from many sources. The less-advantaged mother, particularly if she is young and unmarried, asks few questions, is not likely to have read about baby care, and usually needs specific instructions about formula, bathing, and so forth. With all mothers it is important to avoid the implication that there is a specific, correct pattern of infant rearing that is clearly superior to others. It should be recognized that there is legitimate variation in infant rearing and feeding practices, just as adults express infinite variety in their life-styles and eating patterns.

The role of the counselor should be to support development of the mother's self-confidence and reliance on her own instincts and common sense. This "grandmotherly" role need not necessarily be filled by a physician. A temperamentally suited nurse or physician's assistant, particularly if she is herself a mother, usually spends more time at this task and is more effective.

Duration of the Hospital Stay

The period of hospital confinement for mothers and their newborn infants has become progressively shorter in recent years. Many newborns now leave the hospital with their mothers at 48 hours of age and it is not rare for infants to be discharged 24 hours after birth. So short a period of hospital observation, while having certain undeniable advantages, poses potential problems. There is minimal time for leisurely counseling of the mother. Many cases of significant jaundice will not have become apparent and feeding problems are often not identified and dealt with. Other provisions must be made for these families to insure that the health of the infant is not compromised by early discharge. An essential element is an informed family member (usually the mother, but not necessarily so) who is aware of danger signals and knows how to obtain help. The other essential is easy accessibility of a physician familiar with the family or better yet, home visits by a nurse or physician's assistant.

The traditional 4- to 6-week interval between discharge and first check-up should be shortened to 2 weeks, not only for early-discharge infants, but routinely. At this time, many problems not apparent in the newborn nursery (*e.g.,* congenital heart disease, prolonged jaundice, and feeding problems) can be recognized.

REFERENCES

1. **Richardson DW:** Transient tachypnea of the newborn associated with hypervolemia. Can Med Assoc J 103:70, 1970
2. **Dahm LS, James LS:** Newborn temperature and calculated heat loss in the delivery room. Pediatrics 49:504, 1972
3. **Snowe RJ, Wilfert CM:** Epidemic reappearance of gonococcal ophthalmia neonatorum. Pediatrics 51:110, 1973
4. **Franciosi RA, Knostman JD, Zimmerman RA:** Group B streptococcal neonatal and infant infections. J Pediatr 82:707, 1973
5. **Olson M:** The benign effects on rabbits' lungs of the aspiration of water compared with 5% glucose or milk. Pediatrics 46:538, 1970
6. **Dontanville VK, Cunningham GC:** Effect of feeding on screening for PKU in infants. Pediatrics 51:531, 1973
7. **Fisher DA, Dussault JH, Foley TP, Klein AH, LaFranchi S et al:** Screening for congenital hypothyroidism: Results of screening one million North American infants. J Pediatr 94:700, 1979
8. **Edelmann CM Jr, Ogwo JE, Fine BP, Martinez AB:** The prevalence of bacteriuria in full-term and premature newborn infants. J Pediatr 82:125, 1973
9. **Klaus MH, Jerauld R, Kreger NC, McAlpine W et al:** Maternal attachment: Importance of the first post-partum days. New Eng J Med 286:460, 1972

14

The Special Problems of
the Premature Infant*

Robert H. Usher

INTRODUCTION

Infants who are delivered prior to term, irrespective of their birth weight, are subject to various disorders which complicate their neonatal course. Neonatal mortality rises progressively with increasing degrees of prematurity.[1] Sequelae may affect the growing ex-premature infant for many months or years after birth.[2,3]

Optimal management of premature infants, although complex and difficult, is often effective. Most, if not all, of the disorders associated with prematurity are potentially treatable and the sequelae preventable. Failure to apply appropriate therapy, or (as happens not infrequently) inappropriate use of therapeutic agents, may be fatal or permanently damaging.

Different degrees of prematurity present different problems as follows:

1. **Borderline Premature (37–38 weeks).** Such infants are usually of normal birth weight but many manifest their borderline prematurity by excessive jaundice or slowness to feed. They occasionally develop life-threatening respiratory distress syndrome.

2. **Moderately Premature (31–36 weeks).** The many physiologic handicaps of the infant born 1 to 2 months prematurely can be dealt with effectively using modern therapeutic techniques. Rare prematurity-related deaths are the result of specific disease entities, either respiratory distress syndrome or severe infection.

3. **Extremely Premature (24–30 weeks).** These infants are at the borderline of viability. Although until recent years few survived, and then often with impaired physical or neurologic function, it is now possible using sophisticated methods of management to achieve good results with almost all infants of 28 to 30 weeks. The outlook for infants of 24 to 27 weeks is still gloomy, but it seems to be improving with new advances in understanding of pathogenetic mechanisms in this age group. At these early gestational ages, infants develop a multitude of complex and interrelated problems, requiring expert nursing and medical care for optimal results.

* This chapter overlaps with many other portions of the book dealing with particular conditions. It represents the particular views and policies of Dr. Usher, and is supplied to bring together in one place the multiple problems faced by prematures and to illustrate how they are handled in his fine neonatal service. (G.B.A., ed)

BORDERLINE PREMATURE INFANTS

Infants of 37- to 38-weeks' gestation usually weigh 2500 to 3250 g at birth and comprise 16% of all live births. They are usually considered to be normal full-term deliveries and are cared for in the regular newborn nursery.

Functional Disorders

The attention of nurses is usually drawn to these borderline premature infants because of their occasional inability to stabilize body temperature without the aid of external heat after admission to the nursery, or they may not suck well enough to obtain adequate milk intake during the neonatal period and show prolonged weight loss or require gavage feeding. Sometimes they suck well initially but then become tired and require gavage feeding 2 or 3 days after birth.

Jaundice is the feature which most often distinguishes the borderline premature infant from his similar size full-term counterpart. Many infants who develop worrisome bilirubin levels in the regular nurseries are 2 to 3 weeks premature by gestational age. Characteristically, their hyperbilirubinemia does not develop until the third day and persists until the fourth or fifth day of age before declining. Treatment with phototherapy or exchange transfusion is the same as for full-term infants using similar criteria for intervention.

Respiratory Distress Syndrome (RDS)

RDS (hyaline membrane disease) does not develop in infants delivered after 38½ weeks (270 days) of gestation. Infants who are 37 to 38 weeks, however, develop it frequently (8% incidence) if delivered by cesarean section. Its incidence in vaginal deliveries at this gestational age is rare (less than 1%).[1] It is interesting to note that the male-to-female ratio among infants with RDS is high (about 5:1) in infants of 37- to 38-weeks' gestational age, but it gradually declines to become equal in the infants of 28 weeks or less.[4] Infants with respiratory distress syndrome, if not carefully observed for early clinical signs of chest retraction, grunting, and alar flaring during their first day of life, may deteriorate gradually to a depressed, cyanotic, and acidotic state before the seriousness of their condition is recognized. For this reason, infants who are of 38-weeks' gestation or less should be observed carefully during their first 12 hours of life, even though their birth weight is usually normal.

Clinical Diagnosis of Borderline Prematurity

Distinguishing the borderline premature infant from his full-term nursery mates is therefore of value in clinical management. Temperature instability, feeding problems, or hyperbilirubinemia suggest sepsis or other pathology in the full-term infant, but they usually represent functional immaturity in the borderline premature.

Fortunately, the borderline premature infant can readily be distinguished from this full-term counterpart by the comparative paucity of creases on the sole of the foot (Fig. 14-1), the smaller breasts, fuzzy hair on the head, lanugo, and less developed genitalia.[5]

MODERATELY PREMATURE INFANTS

Infants of 31- to 36-weeks' gestational age comprise 6% to 7% of all newborn infants. Although premature, many (about one-half) have birth weights exceeding 2500 gm,[5] particularly those born at 35 to 36 weeks. Birth weight of the smallest infants in this 31- to 36-week gestation category is usually 1500 g.

The different problems in management presented by premature infants of 31- to 36-weeks' gestation are discussed individually. With appropriate management, these difficulties can be successfully handled, with the exception of severe RDS,[6] which usually causes the only deaths from functional causes among infants of this age.[6]

Premature Rupture of Membranes

Because premature deliveries are sometimes preceded by several days of rupture of the membranes, the potential for intrauterine infection, especially pneumonia, is present more often than at term.[7,8]

The indications for induction of labor for premature rupture of the membranes depend on the relative risk of infection versus the risk of premature delivery itself. Significant as is the risk of infection with premature rupture of membranes, it is seldom as great as that of RDS with preterm birth prior to 35 weeks of gestation.[1] Only if there are signs of intrauter-

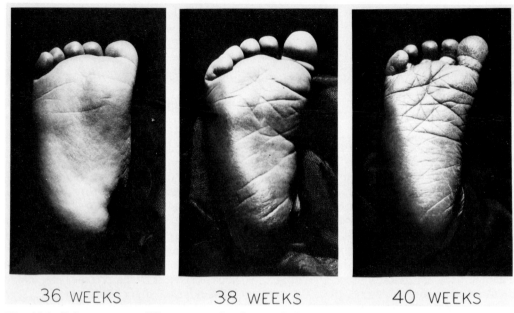

36 WEEKS   38 WEEKS   40 WEEKS

Fig. 14-1. Sole creases at different gestational ages. Only an anterior transverse crease is present before 36 weeks, some creases about the instep develop by 38 weeks, and the whole sole is covered with creases at 40 weeks, in Caucasian infants. (Usher R, McClean F, Scott KE: Judgment of fetal age. Pediatr Clin North Am 13:835, 1966)

ine infection, signalled by maternal fever or leukocytosis, foul smelling amniotic fluid, fetal tachycardia, or contractions resistant to tocolytics, is the balance of risk in favor of premature delivery before 35 weeks. Antibiotics are not of use unless there is evidence of infection, and in such cases labor should also be stimulated.[9,10]

At birth, cultures are taken of throat or ear canal, blood is cultured, and acute phase reactants are determined. The placenta, membranes, and gastric aspirate are examined for inflammatory cells.[11]

If the infant is ill or distressed, or if acute phase reactants are abnormal, then broadspectrum antibiotic therapy should be commenced. With the increased prevalence of group B streptococci, penicillin or ampicillin must be employed along with either gentamicin or chloramphenicol. The latter is of use against anaerobes such as Bacteroides, which are especially a problem in infections of intrauterine origin, when the fastidious anaerobe is often impossible to culture despite severe leukocytosis and chorioamnionitis.

Iatrogenic Prematurity

All too often, infants are delivered prematurely in error. Elective inductions at what was considered by the obstetrician to be full term are discovered in retrospect to have been done early because ovulation was delayed by contraceptive pills in the previous menstrual cycle, or because the woman had unusually long or irregular cycles. Such errors can be avoided by more careful history taking, and by corroborating the gestational age by amniotic fluid analysis of creatine concentration,[12] fat cells,[13] lecithin/sphingomyelin ratio,[14] or by the bubble stability shake test for surfactant.[15] Ultrasound measurement of head size does not determine gestational age when done in the last trimester, but routine ultrasound measurements of biparietal diameter at 15 to 18 weeks accurately reflect gestational age.

The danger of errors in gestational assessment prior to elective induction, especially prior to elective repeat cesarean section, is that the infant in this situation may develop RDS. When premature delivery is indicated for a condition of high fetal risk (*e.g.*, fetal malnutrition, isoimmunization, or maternal diabetes), vaginal induction is preferable to cesarean section whenever this is practicable, in order to reduce the incidence and severity of RDS.

Placental Transfusion

Placental transfusion is a controversial aspect of delivery which, although of little significance to the full-term infant, may have greater importance to the premature. As circulating red cell volume is expanded up to 50% with a 2- to 5-minute delay in cord clamping,[16] there is a like increase in hemoglobin mass and, with it, circulating iron (the majority of the body's iron). This reduces the severity of anemia of prematurity, while neonatal hyperbilirubinemia is markedly increased.[16]

The cardiorespiratory effects of placental transfusion in the premature are not agreed upon. There is still considerable dispute concerning the possible role of placental transfusion, or its denial, on the development of respiratory distress syndrome.[17,18]

The premature infant who receives a full placental transfusion (2–5 minutes) runs a risk of cardiorespiratory distress of another form, referred to as **symptomatic neonatal plethora.** Premature infants who are affected seldom show high hematocrits, but have very expanded blood volumes which they seem incapable of contracting. These infants, during the first hours of life, are a beet-red, plethoric color, very depressed to the point of apneic spells, or tachypneic with shallow breathing. Chest films show pulmonary congestion and edema rather than a reticulogranular pattern of RDS, slightly enlarged cardiac size, and excess pleural fluid in the fissures and costophrenic angles. Hypotension and metabolic acidosis reflect decreased cardiac output with the volume overload, and in the most severe cases hypoxemia develops. Blood volume determinations are required to establish the diagnosis of hypervolemia (usually 100–125 ml/kg). The clinical and radiologic symptoms are dramatically relieved with a phlebotomy of 20% of the blood volume.[19] Milder cases of this volume overload syndrome constitute many of the infants diagnosed as transient tachypnea of the newborn.[20]

As a result of the foregoing considerations, it seems advisable to allow sufficient delay in cord clamping (30–60 seconds) to reduce the risk of RDS and anemia, without creating an excessive risk of hyperbilirubinemia or symptomatic plethora.

Neonatal Asphyxia

Asphyxia at birth is a major hazard of premature delivery. Severe birth asphyxia (Apgar score 0–3, requiring more than 3-minutes' artificial ventilation) occurs in 1 in 200 infants weighing more than 2500 g, in 1 in 20 infants of 1001 to 2500 g, and in 1 in 2 infants weighing 1000 g or less.[21] The immature respiratory center is the underlying cause, with antepartum hemorrhage, intrauterine infection, breech delivery, and protracted desultory labor often contributory factors. Inasmuch as possible, analgesic agents and general anesthesia are to be avoided in premature births in which conduction (*e.g.,* epidural) analgesia and anesthesia achieve their greatest value.

Principles of Treatment. The major therapeutic principles in treatment of the asphyxiated premature are

1. anticipation of impending asphyxia, with attendance at all premature deliveries of personnel skilled in resuscitation.
2. provision of adequate heat to the infant during resuscitation either by overhead radiant heaters or by a warm (34–36°C) incubator in the delivery room.
3. avoidance of trauma and usage of the simplest measures first in resuscitation (most cases respond to bag and mask; only the most severe require endotracheal intubation). Although there is controversy as to whether birth asphyxia predisposes to RDS, its association with RDS certainly increases mortality.

Temperature Control
(See also Chap. 10)

Cold exposure greatly increases metabolic rate and oxygen consumption,[22] and, in the hypoxemic infant, aggravates lactic acidosis.[23] It is therefore not surprising that maintenance of adequate environmental temperature is one of the most effective means of reducing premature infant mortality.[24–26]

With modern equipment, adequate environmental temperature is obtained by servocontrolled heating of the environment sufficient to maintain a "normal" skin temperature measured by a skin thermistor. Unfortunately, the skin probe under a piece of tape does not bear a constant relationship to the core (rectal) temperature. In infants in low humidity, in fact, skin probe temperature may be above the rectal temperature because the remainder of the skin not covered by tape is experiencing rapid evaporative heat loss not occurring from the tape-covered skin under the thermistor.[27]

It is therefore so important to maintain servocontrolled temperature conditions that rectal temperature is held constant at 37°C, with the skin probe setting adjusted to whatever temperature is required to maintain the desired rectal temperature. This usually means a skin temperature somewhere between 36.5 and 37.5°C. Infants more mature than 33 weeks (over 2000 g) usually do not need an incubator to maintain adequate core temperature, although an overhead radiant heater is often necessary during the first day(s) of life.

Feeding

Premature infants of 31 to 36 weeks usually cannot suck effectively and require gavage or indwelling nasogastric tube feedings. Other than those who are sick (usually with RDS), these infants have adequate gastric capacity, intestinal motility and absorption to accept the minimal requirements of fluids (100 ml/kg/day) by the second or third day, and adequate calories (120 cal/kg/day) by the fourth to sixth day. They therefore seldom require intravenous supplementation of fluids or calories. Occasional premature infants (and more particularly low-birth-weight, full-term infants) accept gastric feedings very readily, but diarrhea results from malabsorption if feedings are advanced too rapidly. (More than 100 cal/kg/day before 72 hours of age usually exceeds the intestinal absorptive capacity.)

Because one factor limiting milk intake is a small gastric volume which usually expands considerably during the first 2 weeks of life, it is useful to feed premature infants more frequently than the full-term infant (*i.e.*, every 3 hours instead of 4) and with milk of higher concentration (24 instead of 20 cal/oz). As gastric capacity increases prior to discharge from hospital, the feedings are offered 4-hourly, and their concentration reduced to 20 cal/oz. In order to remain within the limited renal capacities of the premature, the concentrated milk is usually of lower electrolyte and protein content than cow's milk. The animal fat of cow's milk is replaced by vegetable oils to improve intestinal fat absorption, which is limited in the premature.

Mothers with premature infants often desire to breast feed their infants when they come home. Such women can maintain their milk production by expressing breast milk while the infant is in the hospital and nursing the infant once or twice a day for several days before discharge from hospital. If the breast milk is to be fed to the infant during the hospital stay, great efforts must be made to prevent bacterial contamination, and ideally it should be pasteurized. Once the infant begins to develop a strong suck reflex, the mother should be encouraged to nurse her baby at the breast as frequently as she can visit. On discharge, the mother should be advised to gradually increase breast feeds as her milk supply allows, with decreasing bottle feeds.

Vitamin supplementation with 50 mg of vitamin C and 400 units of vitamin D is necessary as the infant begins to grow. In addition to the antiscorbutic property of vitamin C, it is of value in the premature for its action in increasing the activity of tyrosine oxidase.[28] This enzyme is deficient in premature infants resulting in transient hypertyrosinemia, probably benign, which can be avoided by receiving large doses of vitamin C.

Growth

Growth during the postnatal period should ideally parallel the growth rate which is expected *in utero,* in which nutritional support is normally optimal. Infants *in utero* average a 30 g weight gain per day after 30 weeks of gestation, and add 1.2 cm to their length and 0.9 cm to their head circumference every week.[29]

After birth, it is usually not possible to provide sufficient calories for weight gain until the infant is 5 to 10 days of age, during which time there is a 5% to 10% weight loss. Once the infant is taking 120 cal/kg/day of milk, he usually gains at the intrauterine rate. Those who require larger caloric intakes for adequate weight gain may be acidotic, septic, or simply malabsorbing more than the 20% of ingested calories which the average premature infant appears to lose. Conversely, unusually large weight gains for caloric intake, or failure to lose weight during the first days of life when caloric intake is inadequate, usually means that excessive fluid retention is occurring, although this is more particularly a problem for the infants of less than 31-weeks' gestational age.

Respiratory Problems

Aside from the rare instances of premature infants with lethal infections, those of 31 to 36 weeks, who are normally formed and in good condition after birth, should always do well and survive unless they develop RDS. During the first few hours of life, it is therefore possible to distinguish those at risk from those for whom the prognosis can be considered excellent.

RDS develops in approximately 12% of 31- to 36-week infants delivered vaginally, the incidence rising from 5% at 35 to 36 weeks to 35% at 31 to 32 weeks. Infants delivered by cesarean section 2 to 6 weeks preterm have an eight- to ten-fold greater frequency of respiratory distress syndrome than those delivered vaginally.[1] However the recent trend to deliver all breech presentations by cesarean section has led to a surge of cesarean deliveries for very preterm babies, who often present by the breech. The associated increase in RDS has been very slight (Table 14-1).

Glucocorticoid (*e.g.,* betamethasone) administration to the mother for 24 to 48 hours prior to preterm delivery was shown by Liggins to greatly reduce the incidence of RDS, and our experience supports this (Table 14-2). The difficulty now is to delay preterm labor for 24 to 48 hours in order to provide adequate time for glucocorticoid action. Pregnant women should be informed of the need to come to hospital or see their doctor as soon as labor contractions begin or membranes rupture or bleeding starts more than 4–6 weeks before term. Success of glucocorticoid prophylaxis depends upon early initiation of tocolytic therapy before cervical dilatation is too far advanced.

Although periodic breathing is commonly noted in this gestational age group of infants, particularly in the latter half of the first and into the second or third weeks of life, it is rare to see apneic spells.[31] Respiratory and car-

Table 14-1. Incidence of RDS by Mode of Delivery, Royal Victoria Hospital, 1978.

Gestational Age	Cesarean*		Vaginal*	
	No.	%	No.	%
28–31 weeks	5/20	25	3/17	18
32–33 weeks	3/17	18	5/35	14

* 71% of cesarean and 61% of vaginal deliveries were preceded by 24–48 hours of betamethasone therapy.

diac monitoring are therefore not usually indicated in the absence of RDS. Chronic pulmonary disease (Mikity–Wilson) is rarely seen after 30-weeks' gestation, nor is patent ductus arteriosus with congestive pulmonary failure. Oxygen therapy and measurements of blood oxygen tension are therefore seldom required, except in the treatment of RDS.

Hyperbilirubinemia

Bilirubin concentrations rise higher in premature infants than in full-term because of impaired ability to conjugate bilirubin in the liver. This functional defect is manifested in equal degree among premature infants of all gestational ages until 37-weeks' gestation, beyond which much lower bilirubin concentrations develop.[16] In nurseries with bright general lighting conditions, premature infants who are not bruised or plethoric and who are fed early seldom develop worrisome levels of hyperbilirubinemia. Their relative hypoproteinemia (4–5 g/dl) and acidemia make them candidates for low bilirubin kernicterus, however;[32-34] and phototherapy should be employed when bilirubin concentrations exceed 10 mg/dl, with exchange transfusion indicated for bilirubin concentrations somewhere between 15 and 20 mg/dl, depending upon the particular infant's condition.[35,36]

Table 14-2. Livebirths, 28–33 weeks, with Betamethasone Therapy, Royal Victoria Hospital, 1978.

Therapy	<24 hours	24–47 hours	48+ hours
No.	30	21	35
Incidence RDS	12 (40%)	3 (15%)	1 (3%)

Metabolic Disorders

Late Metabolic Acidosis. The commonest metabolic problem in the management of premature infants is late metabolic acidosis.[37] This usually develops after the first 3 days of life when feedings are being tolerated in larger amounts, and, probably in large part, derives from an acid-loading property of the diet itself.

It is uncertain at the present time to what degree the acidosis is contributed to by sulfur-containing amino acids requiring renal acid excretion, by malabsorption of disaccharides resulting in lactic acid formation in the intestine, by malabsorption of fats with resultant fatty acids in the intestine, and by impaired renal ability to excrete hydrogen ions.[38] Although the latter explanation is attractive, in view of the relative inability of the premature infant to develop a normal urine-to-plasma hydrogen ion gradient, as well as an additional inability to excrete adequate amounts of ammonia,[39] there seems to be little correlation between renal acid excretion and degree of late metabolic acidosis in the premature infant. It is interesting to note that replacing prepared formula diets by human breast milk abruptly corrects the tendency to acidosis, implicating dietary factors.

Late metabolic acidosis can be defined as an excessive acidosis (base excess minus 7 to minus 15 mmol/liter) developing after the third day of life, unrelated to asphyxic accumulation of lactic acid or other known acid-producing disorders such as gastroenteritis. If untreated, this condition usually responds spontaneously within 3 to 10 days in premature infants of more than 30-weeks' gestation. Late metabolic acidosis is also found at times in full-term infants, particularly in those who are underweight for gestational age. The incidence of the condition seems to be inversely related to gestational age as well as to postnatal age and directly related to caloric intake ingested, although not to concentration of feeding employed.

Clinical suspicion of late metabolic acidosis should be raised when the following symptoms present:

1. Inadequate weight gain or weight loss on an adequate or large caloric intake
2. Watery stools
3. Lethargy leading in the more premature infants to apneic spells
4. A gray pallor not due to anemia or hypoxemia

Presence of these symptoms in association with metabolic acidosis is adequate indication to treat with alkali. Treatment consists of addition of sodium bicarbonate in a quantity sufficient to neutralize the base deficit, considering the acid-base space of the body to be 60% of body weight. An infant weighing 2000 g with a 10 mmol/liter base deficit would therefore be given 12 mmol of sodium bicarbonate mixed with the milk feedings spaced over a 24-hour period.

Concomitant with this treatment there is usually a rapid weight gain, which may amount to 100 to 200 g over a 2-day period. This weight gain occurs without edema formation and the weight remains and the infant usually continues to gain after the bicarbonate is discontinued, indicating that it is not caused by excess fluid retention. There is usually a remarkable improvement in tone, activity, and color with correction of acidosis. Loose stools, if previously present, return immediately to normal, suggesting that metabolic acidosis produces malabsorption. If acidosis persists or recurs following initial correction, maintenance bicarbonate therapy is occasionally employed, although this is seldom necessary for infants beyond 30-weeks' gestation.

Compensation for metabolic acidosis by hyperventilation with lowering of carbon dioxide tensions to 20 to 30 torr is usually noted in full-term infants in whom blood pH is thereby maintained at an almost normal level in spite of the metabolic acidosis. Premature infants, however, have diminished respiratory response to late metabolic acidosis. Their blood carbon dioxide tensions are usually normal (35 to 45 torr) even though blood pH may drop to 7.25 to 7.15 during the process.

Hypocalcemia, Hypoglycemia. (See also Chaps. 26 and 27.) Premature infants are frequently hypocalcemic[40] or hypoglycemic,[41] although seldom are symptoms related to their abnormal biochemical status. Hypocalcemia (total serum calcium below 7.0 mg/dl) often develops during the first 3 days of life and responds spontaneously over the next few days even if untreated. If the infant becomes excessively jittery, 500 mg/kg of calcium gluconate may be given daily for several days.

Blood glucose concentrations below 25 mg/

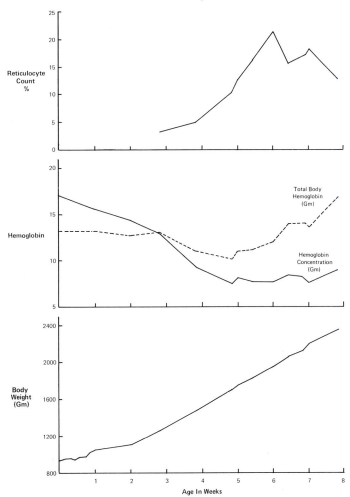

Fig. 14-2. Changes in reticulocyte count, hemoglobin concentration, and total body hemoglobin with increase in weight during the first 8 weeks of life in an infant of 925 g birth weight, 32-weeks' gestational age, who received no blood transfusions.

dl or plasma glucose concentrations below 35 mg/dl are sometimes found in premature infants, but they are difficult to relate to symptoms and usually return to normal after a few feedings. It is reasonable to treat for blood glucose levels below 20mg/dl with intravenous 10% glucose/water infusions, even though hypoglycemia in premature infants who are of normal weight for gestational age is usually asymptomatic and perhaps innocuous.

Other Metabolic Disorders Seldom does azotemia develop to a severe or persistent degree in premature infants of more than 30 weeks. Sodium imbalances and fluid retention, common in less mature infants, are rarely a problem. Hyperphosphatemia, relative hypoproteinemia, tyrosinemia, and elevated alkaline phosphatase levels are all characteristic of the

growing premature in the first weeks of life but are of little clinical importance.

Anemia (Fig. 14-2)

The fetus *in utero* at preterm gestation has slightly lower hemoglobin concentration than his full-term counterpart (14 instead of 17 g/dl hemoglobin in cord blood). If cord clamping is delayed 1 to 1½ minutes after birth, there is a 25% increase in circulating red cell volume,[16] which becomes apparent by concentrations which rise from cord values to 15 to 18 g/dl in the first days of life. These hemoglobin values are for venous blood, capillary values being 2 to 4 g/dl higher. The total body iron content of the premature infant is much less than that of the full-term infant, not because of diminished "stores," but because the premature baby is smaller and therefore has less blood volume and less circulating hemoglobin iron. Iron content per kilogram body weight is only slightly less in the premature than in the term infant.[42] Hematopoiesis is active at birth with reticulocyte counts commonly above 5% and normoblasts evident for the first day or two of life.

After the first week of life, away from the hypoxic intrauterine environment, the premature baby enters a stage of inactive red cell production and reticulocytes typically fall to 2% or less. Hemoglobin concentration therefore falls because of inactive erythropoiesis, exacerbated to some degree by a slightly shorter red cell life span than at term.

As the infant starts to grow, hemoglobin concentration falls more rapidly because of the expanding blood volume. A 2000 g baby growing 30 g/day will in 1 week add 10% to his body weight and thereby to his blood volume, producing a progressive dilutional anemia. There is no evidence of accelerated hematopoiesis until the hemoglobin concentration falls below 10 g/dl.

The hemoglobin concentration therefore declines steadily during the first weeks of life, the rate of decline being proportional to the rate of growth, and there is during this period no reticulocytosis. As the hemoglobin concentration falls below 10 g/dl, reticulocytes appear, rising usually to between 5% and 15% over a 2-week period. The initial reticulocytosis must be especially pronounced, because the red cell population at this time has a very short life span, few new red cells having been produced during the first weeks of life and the average age of red cells being, for a premature, advanced.

After 2 weeks of active reticulocytosis, hemoglobin concentration stabilizes. It must be remembered that total body hemoglobin is increasing rapidly, even though hemoglobin concentration is stable, because active growth is occurring in weight and blood volume. Following a period of stable hemoglobin concentration, it then rises over several weeks to between 10 and 12 g/dl, where it remains throughout the first year of life. As this rise is accomplished, reticulocytosis decreases. Seldom does the rise in hemoglobin occur above 10 g/dl while the infant remains in the hospital because relative rates of growth are usually too rapid for hematopoiesis to do much more than keep abreast of the growth rate until the infant weighs more than 2500 g.

Iron is released during red blood cell destruction over the first weeks of life. It is not lost from the body but stored in the reticuloendothelial system to be reutilized when reticulocytosis commences. When reticulocytosis restores the total body hemoglobin mass to the quantity that existed at birth, this stored iron supply is depleted. At this point the infant must rely upon external sources of iron to maintain red cell production and to allow reticulocytosis to continue.

In a premature infant who has 16 g/dl hemoglobin during the first week of life, and ultimately develops active reticulocytosis to maintain a 10 g/dl hemoglobin concentration, the iron stored from initial red cell breakdown will be sufficient until the infant has grown to 16/10 or 1.6 times his original birth weight. It can therefore be calculated that infants of 2500 g birth weight will usually need supplemental iron when they weigh 4000 g; those of 2000 g birth weight when they attain 3200 g; and those of 1500 g birth weight when they reach 2400 g.

Iron need will develop earlier in infants with lower cord blood hemoglobin concentrations, in those denied placental transfusion, and in those who have lost hemoglobin by sampling or exchange transfusion. Gestational age and postnatal age of the infant are not independently related to iron need, except by their relationship to birth weight and to relative rate of postnatal growth.

It is possible to calculate the amount of supplemental iron needed from external sources to supply the new hemoglobin required for an expanding blood volume during active growth once the reticuloendothelial iron is utilized. With a growth rate of 30 g/day, of which 8% is blood volume, 2.4 ml of new blood will be formed daily, which optimally contains 12 g/dl hemoglobin or 0.3 g of new hemoglobin per day. The iron content of this amount of new hemoglobin is 1.0 mg/day which must be derived from external sources. With a 20% absorption of dietary iron, this means that an intake of 5 mg of elemental iron per day is required.

Because it is difficult to be certain at which point each premature infant has depleted his particular iron stores, it is customary to provide iron-fortified milk to all premature infants from birth, the usual fortification providing 2 mg of elemental iron per 100 cal, or about 2.4 mg/kg body weight per day. This should be adequate for infants of birth weight over 1500 g because they would rarely require supplemental iron until they weigh at least 2000 g at which point they would be ingesting almost 5 mg daily. The usual iron-fortified prepared formula therefore have sufficient iron for most infants of 31-weeks' gestation or more.

The role of vitamin E deficiency in the development of anemia of prematurity, and the possible hemolytic effect of supplemental iron, has led some to use vitamin E supplementation and delay of iron fortification for the first weeks.[43]

Blood transfusions may be required to treat anemia in a premature infant who becomes symptomatic. Symptoms of anemia usually take the form of lethargy and apneic spells rather than of congestive heart failure. Such symptoms are rare in infants beyond 30-weeks' gestation whose hemoglobin concentrations are above 8 g/dl, unless there is accompanying chronic pulmonary disease or patent ductus arteriosus with left-to-right shunting. These conditions impair the infant's ability to increase cardiac output to compensate for the anemia, resulting in lethargy or apneic spells even at hemoglobin concentrations of 8 to 12 g/dl, which can be relieved by blood transfusion.

When blood transfusions are indicated, they can be given in the form of packed red blood cells in volumes of 7 ml/kg body weight/day in order to avoid cardiac overload, until a hemoglobin concentration of 10 to 12 g/dl is achieved. Each such transfusion usually elevates hemoglobin concentration by 1.0 to 1.5 g/dl. Sometimes there is no rise in hemoglobin following the transfusions, even though the infant becomes much pinker and more active, indicating an expansion of blood volume which is often reduced in anemia of prematurity. Because blood transfusion depresses the infant's own hematopoietic response, it should be employed only when anemia is progressive or persistent in the absence of a reticulocyte response, and when the infant is symptomatic. This usually means that transfusions are given for hemoglobin concentrations below 7 to 8 g/dl, or in symptomatic infants for concentrations of less than 10 to 12 g/dl.

Infection (See also Chap. 32.)

Pneumonia of intrauterine origin and septicemia, meningitis, or urinary tract infection acquired postnatally, are conditions that afflict premature infants much more often than those delivered at term. Clinical signs of infection are notoriously difficult to evaluate during the newborn period, particularly in the premature. Laboratory tests are therefore more important in the diagnosis of infection in these infants than in other age groups.[9]

Blood cultures are of great value when positive; however, they are somewhat traumatic to obtain, are often negative even when other evidences of systemic infection are clearly present, and when positive may represent contamination. Lumbar punctures have the advantage of immediately demonstrating meningitis when it is present by the combination of pleiocytosis (usually hundreds of polymorphonuclear leukocytes), bacteria on smear and culture, and very low cerebrospinal fluid sugar concentrations (usually less than 20% of blood levels). When the cerebrospinal fluid is normal except for the presence of bacteria, it is advisable to repeat the tap in 12 to 24 hours to confirm the diagnosis of meningitis, which in the newborn invariably produces a severe and protracted cellular response, persisting for days after antibiotics have been started. Urinary infections may be diagnosed by suprapubic bladder tap yielding a high colony count and pyuria.

We have found it useful to investigate all premature infants with signs suggestive of infection with noninvasive tests of acute-phase reaction—white blood count and differential, C-reactive protein, and erythrocyte sedimentation rate—as well as a urinalysis of a specimen collected in a bag.

Abnormal white blood counts exceed 30,000/mm³ in the first day of life, 20,000 the second day, and 17,000 thereafter.[44] Band counts exceeding 1500/mm³ are abnormal, and provide the most sensitive index of infection in our experience, though much higher band counts (up to 4000) may be normal during the first day of life. C-reactive protein does not usually exceed 1 mm of sedimentation (1+ positive) except with infection. The sedimentation rate (capillary or venous) corrected to a 50% hematocrit is abnormal if over 3 mm/hour in the first 4 days of life, or 8 mm/hour thereafter.

Table 14-3. Survival by Weight.

Birthweight (g)	No. livebirths	Percent survival
501–750	35	8.6
751–1000	40	35.0
1001–1250	38	73.7
1251–1500	52	92.3
1501–2000	141	95.0
2001–2500	474	99.6
over 2500	11018	99.93

Survival rates to discharge home alive
Royal Victoria Hospital births by weight group, 1971–1975 (excludes lethal
malformations)

Urinalyses show fewer than 5 leukocytes per high-power field on a centrifuged specimen in the absence of urinary tract infection or external contamination. Seldom does an infant who is infected fail to show at least one of these tests as positive. Acute phase reactants are also useful in following the course of an infection under treatment. They cannot replace cultures and lumbar punctures, but they provide a useful screening battery to indicate which mildly symptomatic infants should be cultured and investigated more thoroughly. Infants with pronounced symptoms suggestive of infection require complete investigation from the outset.

Antibiotic treatment is standardized with a particular broad-spectrum antibiotic regimen for a particular nursery. The treatment is altered later depending upon culture results.

The technique used in our intensive care nursery to prevent spread of infection is based primarily on adequate washing of hands and forearms between the handling of each infant. Masks are not employed, although we continue to use gowns in the nursery. Because the toxicity of absorbed hexachlorophene was discovered in premature infants, local applications of antiseptics to the umbilical cord area (such as triple dye) have taken its place. One such application after birth effectively maintains a low staphylococcal colonization rate in the nursery.[45–48]

Isolation of infected premature infants is effectively accomplished by the incubator isolation technique, the infant being kept in the intensive care nursery using the incubator as an isolation chamber. This permits the infant to benefit from the skilled nursing and medical care available there, and it allows him to remain under continuous careful observation while being treated for an infection.

Increasing confidence has developed in the effectiveness of adequate handwashing in preventing spread of infection among premature and sick newborn infants. Now, neonatal intensive care centers encourage the active involvement of consultants, medical students, and particularly parents in the nursery, without any indication that these additional personnel increase the risk of bacterial spread or of infection, providing that proper technique is followed in the nursery.

Discharge

Premature infants are usually discharged when they are feeding well enough by bottle to gain weight normally on a 4-hourly schedule. In most instances, this coincides with a gestational age of 36 to 37 weeks, and a body weight of about 2500 g. Infants who are underweight for gestational age may be ready for discharge at lower birth weights. Conversely those who are large for gestational age or who have had a prolonged course of chronic chest disease may require hospitalization until they are 3000 g or more. It is important to delay discharge of infants who are weak because cyanotic spells and severe infections are hazards to the ex-premature during his first weeks at home.

Parents of a premature infant should at discharge be counseled that their infant was born prior to full maturation and that they should expect him to behave like a full-term newborn only when he reaches the date when he was originally expected. All future development, physical and mental, should be evaluated from that date, rather than from the date

Table 14-4. Survival by Gestational Age.

Gestational age (weeks)	No. Livebirths	Percent survival
21–22 (147–160 days)	2	0
23–24 (161–174 days)	14	0
25–26 (175–188 days)	33	24.2
27–28 (189–202 days)	40	52.5
29 (203–209 days)	33	81.9
30 (210–216 days)	20	85.0
31 (217–223 days)	35	88.6
32 (224–230 days)	37	100.0

Survival rates to discharge home alive
Royal Victoria Hospital Births by gestational age, 1971–1975 (excludes lethal malformations)

of birth, because the infant does not develop or mature faster outside the uterus than inside. Unless the infant has sustained some brain-threatening insult, as with severe birth asphyxia, parents should be given every reason to hope for and expect a child with normal physical and mental capacities, even though it is not possible for the physician to guarantee this for any particular infant.

The parents should be assured that although special care was needed in the hospital for their infant because of his prematurity, after discharge excessive concern is unwarranted and potentially harmful. Their child does not require overprotection. The only special precautions are to maintain iron therapy for several months until a full diet adequate in iron is being given, to have hemoglobin checks if the value is low or still falling at discharge, and to attempt to prevent respiratory infections during the first months of life and to have them treated early if they should develop.

EXTREMELY PREMATURE INFANTS

Infants of 24- to 30-weeks' gestation (usually 500 to 1500 g) comprise only 0.8% of the live-born population, but account for almost all neonatal deaths and neurologic sequelae not attributable to malformations. Survival rate by weight group is indicated in Table 14-3, where the unexpectedly high incidence of very low-birth-weight infants is caused by antenatal referral of mothers in premature labor. From 1971 to 1975, occasional infants weighing less than 750 g, one-third of those weighing 751 to 1000 g, three-quarters of those weighing 1001 to 1250 g, and 92% of those weighing 1251 to 1500 g survived.

During the period of from 1971 to 1975 at our hospital, the least mature infant who survived delivered at 24-weeks' gestation. Survival rates excluding lethal malformations reached 25% by 26 weeks, 50% by 27 to 28 weeks, 80% by 29 weeks, and above 90% by 32 weeks (Table 14-4).

Four causes of death were common among these extremely premature infants, all potentially treatable: (1) some infants died after being severely asphyxiated at birth, never developing sustained respirations in an effective manner; (2) others had been infected *in utero* after a period of prolonged rupture of the membranes and usually died in the first day of life; (3) many died of respiratory distress syndrome; and (4) others, who survived the first days of life, became debilitated, developed apneic spells, and after a period of gradual deterioration died between 3 and 20 days of life. Occasional deaths among these extremely premature infants were caused by patent ductus arteriosus with congestive pulmonary failure, necrotizing enterocolitis, or postnatal meningitis or septicemia. Those infants requiring endotracheal intubation and positive pressure respirator therapy were also at risk of dying from intraventricular hemorrhage or bronchopulmonary dysplasia.

The major therapeutic challenge in managing these very immature infants is not so much the specific treatment of disease entities as it is the control of the many pathophysiologic derangements resulting from marked immaturity itself. Although many of these disorders are discussed elsewhere, this section will deal with special considerations related to the 24- to 30-week infant.

For practical purposes this group of infants

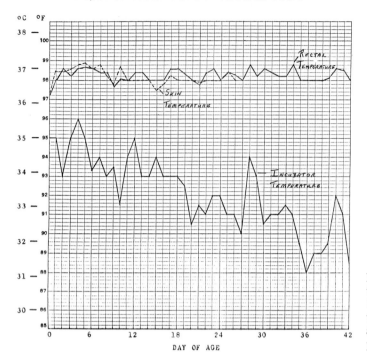

Fig. 14-3. Rectal, skin, and incubator temperatures for a premature infant of 1110 g birth weight, 27-weeks' gestation, during the first 6 weeks of life. No added humidity or radiant heat was provided.

can be subdivided into those of 28 to 30 weeks (1000 to 1500 g) for whom treatment, though very complex at times, is usually successful, and those of 24 to 27 weeks (650 to 1000 g) where problems in management are often insuperable. For instance in our service in 1978, survival to discharge occurred in 18 of 19 livebirths (95%) of 28- to 30-weeks' gestation and in only 5 of the 22 infants (23%) of lesser gestational age.

Neonatal Asphyxia

This may be severe, requiring endotracheal intubation. Such infants should be resuscitated in a very warm environment (we use an incubator with an ambient temperature of 36 to 38°C), and even then they often lose body heat by the time they have been brought to the nursery. It is a constant challenge to the resuscitator to enable the extremely premature infant to arrive in the neonatal unit with a rectal temperature above 36°, a feat we succeeded in doing only 26 times in the 41 infants less than 31 weeks gestation (63%) treated in 1978.

Although acidosis may be profound following asphyxia, we prefer to see it corrected (usually over a 12-hour period) with the help of slow infusions of glucose and bicarbonate (no more than 0.5 mmol/kg of bicarbonate/hour) while providing adequate ventilation, oxygenation, and heat rather than employing rapid infusions of alkali, which run the risk of hyperosmolarity and brain hemorrhage.

Temperature Control

Ambient temperatures required to maintain a normal rectal temperature of 37.0°C are often as high as 37 to 38°C during the first hours of life, and incubator temperatures of 35 to 37°C may be necessary for days thereafter. Additional incubator humidity to prevent evaporative losses, radiant heat from an overhead lamp, and placement of a transparent plastic shell over the infant to reduce radiant heat loss[49] may be necessary as thermal supports during the first day(s) of life to maintain a normal rectal temperature. By recording incubator temperature along with skin and rectal temperatures, it is possible to note widening of the gap between incubator and rectal temperature indicative of clinical improvement in the infant, or narrowing of this "homeothermic gap" often presaging deterioration (Fig. 14-3). Although overheating has been considered a factor in the development of apneic spells,[50,51] our experience indicates that extreme prematures require sufficient ambient heat to provide a rectal temperature of 37.0°C if they are to remain in good condition.

Initial Handling

Extremely premature infants tolerate handling poorly. All interventions must be assessed as to the relative value of the procedure versus the disturbance entailed. Especially during the first hours of life, the less handling the better for the infant. Other than weighing the infant on entry to the nursery, starting a scalp vein infusion, and placing cardiac monitor leads and temperature skin probe, further handling (such as bathing, x-rays, blood cultures unless antibiotics are to be started), is postponed for several hours to allow regular respirations to become sustained and the temperature to stabilize. Blood gases and hemoglobin from a heel prick are usually obtained at 30 minutes of age.

Although this "hands-off" technique has been a practice of our unit for years, many services are much more therapeutically active in the immediate neonatal minutes and get excellent results with umbilical artery catheters, respiratory assistance, and many diagnostic studies performed right after birth.

Respiratory Distress and Oxygen Therapy

Although RDS is very frequent in this group of infants, the most immature infants (less than 28 weeks) may have a lower incidence than those of 28 to 30 weeks. Treatment for RDS is similar to that used in more mature infants (see Chaps. 20 and 22).

Oxygen therapy is regulated at first by skin color, which is relatively easy to assess in extremely premature infants in the first hours of life because the skin circulation is very flushed. Cyanosis can usually be prevented with 25% to 30% oxygen in the first hours of life, and the temptation to use higher concentrations (because of the extremely small size and immature appearance of the infant) must be resisted, unless the infant requires higher ambient oxygen concentrations to remain thoroughly pink. Blood gases, either from arterialized capillary (after 5 minutes of heating the heel in 42 to 43°C water), or umbilical arterial indwelling catheter, are obtained to ensure that ambient oxygen is enough to maintain an adequate oxygen tension Pa_{O_2} of 45 torr, which provides a hemoglobin oxygen saturation of 85% to 90% if pH is above 7.25) but not excessive (Pa_{O_2} above 80). The respective optimal arterialized capillary values are a minimum of 35 and a maximum of 50 torr oxygen tension. These infants are highly susceptible to the development of retrolental fibroplasia.

We would insist that whenever capillary blood gases are used (and possibly with transcutaneous oxygen monitors and arterial sampling also), that the endpoint for adequate oxygenation should be expressed as hemoglobin-oxygen saturation rather than oxygen tension. On the steep part of the dissociation curve, a shift in pH from 7.10 to 7.50 can increase oxygen saturation of the hemoglobin leaving the lungs by more than 20%, at the same arterial oxygen tension. We find no tendency to lactic acidosis when capillary oxygen saturations are maintained at 80% to 90%, or arterial at 90% to 95%, and are concerned that higher levels require greatly enhanced inspired oxygen concentrations, thus increasing pulmonary oxygen toxicity and enhancing the risk of developing retrolental fibroplasia. Arterial saturations are calculated from a measured P_{O_2} and acid-base balance.

Many extremely premature infants require little or no oxygen during their first days of life, although oxygen need often increases gradually after 3 days of age. Because some oxygen need may persist in these small infants for weeks or even months, we have found capillary sampling or transcutaneous oxygen monitoring a more practical means of controlling oxygen therapy than arterial gases.

Nutrition and Hydration (See also Chap. 42)

The intestinal tract of an infant of less than 31-weeks' gestation is usually incapable of accepting and absorbing an adequate milk intake until the infant has attained 32 weeks gestational age. This places a large reliance upon intravenous feeding to provide not only fluid and electrolyte support but also most or all of the nutritional needs for the first 10 to 60 days of life. It is now possible to meet these needs through peripheral (scalp) vein infusion of solutions that need not be irritatingly hyperosmolar because intravenous lipid solutions have become available.[51]

The program of intravenous nutritional supplements presented in Table 14-5 has been developed to provide nutrients as quickly as

Table 14-5. Parenteral Nutrition for Infants <1500 g, Royal Victoria Hospital, Montreal.

Day of age	10% Dextrose (40 cal/dl)	Dilute Amino Acid 2 g AA, 8 g glucose 1.4 mmol/dl Na 1.2 mmol/dl K (40 cal/dl)	Standard Amino Acid 3 g AA, 10 g glucose 5 mmol/dl Na 3 mmol/dl K (52 cal/dl)	10% Lipid (110 cal/dl)	Total Volume
		Component Solutions			
1	80–120*	0	0	0	80–120
2	0–10	100	0	10–20†	120
3	0–10	110	0	15–25	135
4	0–10	0	95	20–30	135
5 on	0–10	0	105	25–35	140

* Larger volumes for smaller infants (using added distilled water to limit glucose to 8g/kg/d).
† Smaller lipid volumes for smaller and sicker infants, the difference in volume being made up by 10% dextrose. Lipid solution is pumped from a separate infusion joining the clear solution in a Y tube just before the scalp vein needle.

most extremely premature infants are able to metabolize them. Using this approach, which entails the use of a fat emulsion, amino acids and glucose as intravenous supplements to milk feeds, the maximal intravenous nutritional contribution is advanced from 80 to 120 ml and 32 cal/kg, day one, to 140 ml and 93 cal/kg/day on and after day five. Over this 5-day period, the intake/kg/day of glucose is increased from 8 to 10.5 g, amino acid from nil to 3.1 g, fat from nil to 3.5 g, sodium from nil to 5 mmol, and potassium from nil to 3 mmol. Not all infants are able to tolerate even this graduated approach. Particularly the less mature or sicker infants require reduction in protein intake for azotemia, in glucose intake for hyperglycemia, in fat intake for visible lipemia, and in fluid intake for excessive weight gain and edema formation. On occasion, infants will demonstrate dehydration by excessive weight loss in the early days, requiring increased fluid intake.

Hypernatremia during the first 3 days of life may require a reduction in sodium intake, and hyponatremia after 3 days of age an additional supplement of sodium chloride. Nutrition is continued and sodium bicarbonate added, as is described later, when metabolic acidosis develops, which is an almost constant finding in extremely premature infants.

Infants who are unable to tolerate any milk intake are at maximal intravenous nutrition receiving 10.5 g of carbohydrate, 3.0 g protein hydrolysate, and 3.5 g fat/kg body weight/day. The 93 cal/kg body weight provided intrave-

nously usually produces adequate growth in all dimensions at the expected intrauterine rate from the fifth day onward. An example of a 27-week infant's postnatal growth is shown in Figure 14-4.

We have not mentioned the difficulty of beginning to meet the enormous calcium and phorphorus needs of the rapidly growing premature, as these substances can be provided in only limited concentrations in IV fluids without precipitating. They precipitate especially easily in the presence of sodium bicarbonate if this is also needed. Their relative deficiency results in bone demineralization during growth on IV nutrition. In addition, vitamins and trace metals are added.

In order to ascertain that intravenous nutrients are being biochemically tolerated, infants on this program are assessed by the tolerance checks outlined in Table 14-6. Specific intolerances are managed by reduction of the appropriate nutrient, the provision of bicarbonate for acidosis, and the alteration of electrolyte intake.

The infant of less than 31-weeks' gestation is limited in his ability to receive milk feedings by a small gastric capcity. It may be many days after birth before the infant's feeding volume can be increased from 2 to 5 ml at a time, and gastric emptying can be very slow. For these reasons we have used continuous, hourly, or 2-hour feeding intervals of concentrated (27 cal/oz) milk for these smallest infants because the stomach is volume limited rather than calorie limited. Other units may have

Usher, R., and McLean F.

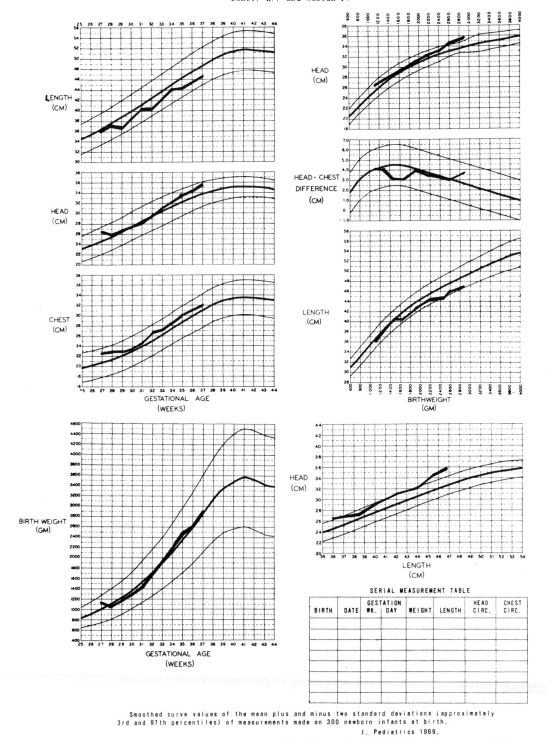

Smoothed curve values of the mean plus and minus two standard deviations (approximately 3rd and 97th percentiles) of measurements made on 300 newborn infants at birth.

J. Pediatrics 1969.

Fig. 14-4. Postnatal growth of an 1110-g-birth-weight, 27-week-gestational-age premature infant during the first 9 weeks of life plotted on an intrauterine growth grid for Caucasian infants at sea level. The infant was given intravenous supplements to milk feedings until 12 days of age. (Usher R, McClean F: Intrauterine growth of live-born Caucasian infants at sea level. J Pediatr 74:901, 1969)

Table 14-6. IV Nutrition Tolerance Check.

Test	Interval	Acceptable limits
Blood acid-base	Daily	pH>7.30
Glycosuria	q8h	0
Plasma glucose	prn glycosuria	<125 mg/dl
Plasma lipemia	Daily (more often with deterioration)	0
Serum sodium	Daily × 4 days, then twice weekly	135–145 mmol/liter
Serum potassium	Daily × 4 days, then twice weekly	3.5–5.5 mmol/liter
Blood urea nitrogen	Daily × 4 days, then twice weekly	<25 mg/dl
Body weight	q12h × 1 week, then daily	Initial weight loss 5%–10%; weight gain 20–35g/day on full nutrition
Pitting edema of feet	Daily	None

success in increasing feedings more rapidly after birth using unboiled human milk, but this remains an open question at the present time.

In addition to the gastric limitations (which some have attempted to overcome by naso-jejunal tube feedings),[52] extremely premature infants almost routinely develop a paralytic ileus manifested by obstipation and abdominal distention with diminished bowel sounds. Small saline or mineral oil enemas are sometimes useful when there have been no stools for a 12- to 24-hour period. It is extremely risky to feed these immature infants beyond a point of mild distension because regurgitation is a major risk with overfeeding, as is necrotizing enteorcolitis. Overfeeding diarrhea does not occur in infants of less than 31 weeks fed by the gastric route, presumably because gastric limitations prevent overloading of intestinal absorptive capacity. Nasojejunal feeds, however, can readily produce diarrhea if progression is too rapid.

For these reasons, it often takes many days before milk feedings can be increased to 100 to 125 cal/kg/day, which we have found necessary for adequate growth. This is greater than the intravenous nutritional requirements because some of the milk calories are lost by malabsorption. As milk feeds are increased, intravenous intake is reduced by an equivalent volume so that the infants are never offered more than 140 ml/kg/day. Using these nutritional substances, we have found 140 ml/kg/day to be an upper limit of fluid tolerance for immature kidneys. When excessive weight gain and edema occur, the fluid intake may have to be reduced, some infants being unable to accept more than 115 ml/kg/day without abnormal fluid retention.

Dietary Requirements for Growth

It has been customary to feed extremely premature infants the same diet on a per kilogram body-weight basis as that fed to the full-term infant, or for that matter, to the 3 month old. A moment's reflection indicates that this may not be the most appropriate diet for the very small infant.

Dietary needs can be divived into two components:

1. Growth requirements for deposition into new tissue
2. Maintenance requirements to replace daily body losses, and energy needs.

The growth needs must satisfy an average 30 g weight gain each day, which is approximately the same for all ages from 28-weeks' gestation to 2-months' postnatal life. These needs bear no relation to the infant's body weight and should be calculated in absolute terms. Maintenance needs may be expressed on a body-weight basis. (Growth needs, in fact, increase *in utero* from about 20 g/day at 27 weeks to 30 g/day at 33 weeks [Table 14-7]; but catch-up postnatal growth to make up for first-week losses often means that extremely premature infants are gaining 30 g/day in the nursery from 7 days of age onward.)

Using calcium as an example, an infant taking 120 cal/kg/day is ingesting 120 mg calcium/kg/day, of which some two-thirds or 80 mg/kg/day may be absorbed. Growth of 30 g/day requires 0.7% calcium uptake in new tissue or 210 mg of calcium deposition/day in absolute terms, most of which goes to bone mineralization.[42]

The 2-month old infant weighing 5000 g can absorb 400 mg calcium/day of which 210 mg is needed for growth and the remaining 190 mg can be malabsorbed or used for maintenance (urinary excretion). A 3000-g, full-term infant, if also growing 30 g/day, can absorb up to 240 mg, and will need 210 of that for growth. The 1,000 g extreme premature will, on the other hand, absorb only 80 mg and still require 210 mg for growth if maintaining 30 g/day. This growth deficit of calcium may be responsible for the deminineralization of bone and tendency to pathologic rib fractures seen in some extreme prematures as they grow.

The same type of calculation suggests that standard prepared formulas are deficient in protein, iron, phosphorous, sodium, and chloride.[42] This may be one reason why the actively growing extreme premature so readily develops hyponatremia. It should be evident that fluid retention problems of the extreme premature should usually not be treated by provision of a low-sodium or low-solute formula; the normal formulas provide insufficient sodium and other electrolytes for adequate growth and maintenance when taken in the small quantities ingested by the 1000 g growing premature.

As the 1000 g premature grows and reaches 2500 g, all of the elements required for normal growth can be found in his regular formula diet with the exception of iron. By this time, however, he has developed deficits, most readily apparent for calcium, which require further weeks of feeding to replenish. These deficits are most marked when very low-birth-weight infants are fed human milk.

From these considerations it seems clear that dietary preparations specially designed for the extreme premature are required if nutrition of these smallest of infants is to become optimal. Such diets must contain increased concentrations of each of the growth factors (protein, calcium, phosphorus, and sodium particularly) for each 100 cal of formula to meet the disproportionate growth:maintenance ratio of their needs.

Control of Acidosis

The infant of 24- to 30-weeks' gestation, unlike the premature infant beyond 30 weeks,

Table 14-7. Expected Intrauterine Daily Weight Gain.

Fetal Weight (g)	Average Gestational Age (Weeks)	Daily Weight Gain (g)
500	$22^0/_7$	
		11
750	$22^5/_7$	
		17
1000	$27^3/_7$	
		22
1500	$30^5/_7$	
		26
2000	$33^3/_7$	
		31
2500	$35^5/_7$	
		38
3000	$37^4/_7$	

may develop a profound respiratory acidosis. Characteristically, this is not present during the first 3 days of life, unless the infant is suffering from RDS or intrauterine pneumonia. (It is often amazing to see how a lung of a 26-week old infant, which at autopsy is almost glandular, with cuboidal alveolar epithelium, could have allowed normal ventilation with P_{CO_2} of 40 torr and adequate oxygenation with only low concentrations of ambient oxygen during much of the infant's life.)

Alveolar ventilation must markedly diminish in many extremely premature infants in the latter half of the first week and through the second week of life, however. During this time, the carbon dioxide tension usually rises to 50 torr or higher, and the baby shows decreased lung volume and a diffuse grey opacification on x-ray film. In some infants, this hypercapnea is associated with congestive pulmonary failure from patent ductus arteriosus, but there is no evidence of ductus patency in many. Usually the elevated carbon dioxide tensions subside by 10 to 20 days of age to values between 45 and 50 torr, and then gradually fall to normal neonatal levels of 35 to 40 torr over the next month or two.

The kidney of the extremely premature infant does not respond to this respiratory acidosis by increased acid excretion, probably because there is a marked incapacity to excrete ammonia as well as hydrogen ion at this gestational age. Compensatory metabolic alkalosis therefore does not develop; and the base excess, instead of becoming positive, as in a hypercapneic adult, is negative, aggravating the severity of the acidosis.

Metabolic acidosis often develops in the extremely premature infant. As in the more mature infant, it is rare to see significant metabolic acidosis until 2 or 3 days of age, when nutritional intake is increasing, and it seems to make little difference whether the nutrients are in the form of milk or of intravenous fat and amino acids.

The 24- to 30-week premature infant may be unable to excrete an acid urine for several weeks (sometimes 2 months) after birth, the urine pH varying from 6.0 to 7.5, even though blood pH is acidemic. Late metabolic acidosis in the extreme premature is therefore not a transient problem that needs correction, but a persisting situation which requires maintenance support with sodium bicarbonate. This need for alkali support may continue when intravenous nutrition is replaced by milk feedings. Unless such support is provided, a persistent state of metabolic or combined respiratory and metabolic acidosis is maintained. It has been our experience that infants who are allowed to develop acidosis and to remain acidotic have difficulty in gaining weight on a good caloric intake, become lethargic, and develop more frequent and severe apneic spells.

Our practice has, therefore, been, when necessary, to supplement the intravenous fluids (or when any milk is being tolerated, the gastric feeds) wih adequate amounts of sodium bicarbonate to maintain arterialized capillary blood pH between 7.30 and 7.35. In conditions of elevated carbon dioxide tension, this means producing a positive base excess of 3 to 10 mmol/liter and an actual serum bicarbonate of 30 to 40 mmol/liter. When the P_{CO_2} is normal, the resultant base excess is usually minus 3 to 6 mmol/liter. The quantity of sodium bicarbonate required to maintain a normal blood pH varies from 2 to 8 mmol/kg body weight/day, and the duration of bicarbonate need may be from 1 to 10 weeks.

There seems to be little correlation between bicarbonate administration and the tendency to abnormal fluid retention, which is a separate although coexisting problem in most extreme prematures. Stopping the the use of bicarbonate does not result in diuresis. Serum sodium concentrations are characteristically not elevated but rather are low, in spite of the bicarbonate supplement. Where then does the bicarbonate go? Some of it is excreted in the urine. Urine with a usual pH of 7.0 contains 10 mmol/liter of sodium bicarbonate. The remainder may neutralize the acids released from new bone formation which the immature kidney is incapable of excreting.

Other Metabolic Disorders

Blood Sugar. The extreme premature behaves like a diabetic.[54] Carbohydrate tolerance appears to be no more than 8 g/kg/day in the first day, rising to 10 to 12 g/kg/day by the end of the first week. These values are low compared with those of 1-month-old, full-term infants, who are usually able to tolerate 20 to 30 g/kg of carbohydrate/day. Not only is carbohydrate tolerance of the 24- to 30-week premature limited, it becomes still more diminished with ill health and particularly with infection. The development of hyperglycemia is therfore an omnious sign if carbohydrate intake is not excessive. For this reason, it is useful to monitor spot urines for glucose 2 or 3 times daily in order to know when to measure the blood sugar, remembering that sugar spill into the urine may occur at lower serum levels in extremely premature infants (usually about 125 to 150 mg/dl).

Development of hyperglycemia has not in our experience resulted in an osmotic diuresis, but concentrations of blood sugar above 150 mg/dl (and they may rise to 300 mg/dl or even higher if not monitored) cause hyperosmolarity and cerebral depression with apneic spells. It is therefore necessary to control carbohydrate intake to prevent glucose concentrations rising above 125 mg/dl.

Hypoglycemia is rarely a problem of the extreme premature who is fed intravenously from birth in the manner described here, blood sugar levels usually averaging 100 mg/dl.

The limited glucose tolerance of the small premature means that nutritional needs of 90 to 100 cal/kg per day cannot be met from protein and carbohydrate alone, and that fat is required to provide adequate calories in such infants. Although one might attempt to treat these infants as diabetics, using higher carbohydrate intakes with supplemental insulin injections, they prove very labile indeed and insulin need changes rapidly, producing hypoglycemic crises. Thus, this approach to nutrition is difficult.

Azotemia. All infants develop some degree

of azotemia during the first 3 days of life because of catabolism from inadequate nutrition and relative renal insufficiency. Azotemia is more severe in premature infants, and especially in extreme prematures, as well as in infants who are stressed by RDS or infection and undergo increased catabolic rates. Although the azotemia may not be harmful, elevated levels of serum amino acids and ammonia may accompany urea in these infants. We have therefore usually withheld protein from the intravenous nutrition when blood urea nitrogen exceeds 25 mg/dl. This is seldom a problem after the first week of life, even in the least mature infant, provided protein intake is not excessive.

Hypocalcemia. Serum calcium concentrations normally run lower in the extreme premature than in other newborn infants, because of their lower serum protein concentrations. Healthy infants of 24 to 30 weeks average serum calcium values of 6.0 to 7.5 mg/dl, and we have not treated them with supplemental calcium gluconate unless concentrations fall below 6.0 mg/dl. Such levels may develop in the first 3 days of life and usually correct spontaneously by 7 days. They are not usually associated with symptoms of hypocalcemia such as tremors, irritability, convulsions, or apneic spells. Treatment may therefore be more to assuage the physician's need to do something "therapeutic" than to correct a real problem in the infant. (See also Chap. 27.)

Hyper- and Hyponatremia. Infants of 24 to 30 weeks, particularly those below 28 weeks, tend after birth to have a rising serum sodium concentration up to or above 150 mmol/liter by 3 days of age. The initial rise may occur with little sodium intake either in the form of bicarbonate or chloride. This sometimes severe hypernatremia is the result of rapid insensible water loss right after birth when there is little urine output, as if the skin at this time is very permeable. There is a close correlation between the amount of first-day weight loss and the degree of hypernatremia. Severe neonatal hypernatremia is a preventable condition if adequate fluids are given to avoid excessive weight loss the first 24 to 48 hours, a period when the infant should be weighed every 12 hours. These fluids should not contain electrolytes because they are replacing mainly insensible water loss, which is pure water.

There is a rapid decline in serum sodium toward 130 mmol/liter over the next few days as the infant starts to grow. This later hyponatremia is a more persistent and difficult problem to treat. We have found that sodium bicarbonate used to correct metabolic acidosis does not produce a rise in serum sodium when it is low, and that sodium chloride must be provided to keep the serum sodium within the normal range. The usual neonatal maintenance need of 2 to 3 mmol of sodium chloride/kg/day is rarely sufficient for the extreme premature, especially the infant of 24 to 27 weeks in severe respiratory insufficiency or on a respirator. As much as 4 to 8 mmol/kg/day of sodium chloride may be needed to keep abreast of the sodium need in such infants.

When extremely premature infants are allowed to develop hyponatremia below 125 to 130 mmol/liter, it is almost impossible to increase the serum sodium concentrations without a period of severe fluid restriction.

Disturbances of serum sodium concentration in either direction are associated with deterioration in the infant's status, and with apneic spells, which are relieved as the serum sodium concentration is corrected.

Hypoproteinemia. The low serum protein concentration at birth of extremely premature infants (3.0–4.5 g/dl) is a sign of their prematurity and is not pathologic. It must be taken into consideration in assessing kernicterus risk at bilirubin levels which would not be dangerous for infants with higher serum protein concentrations available for bilirubin binding. It explains the usual physiologic hypocalcemia of these infants, although not the extremely low calcium levels (down to 4 mg/dl) seen at times.

Hypoproteinemia, which persists for many weeks after birth in some extremely premature infants, suggests chronic fluid overload or inadequate protein in the diet.

Abnormal Fluid Retention. This represents one of the most important disturbances found in the 24- to 30-week infant. It is not always possible to distinguish clearly between the inability to excrete solutes and the inability to excrete water itself as the cause of fluid retention in these infants, but the latter seems the more important factor.

The sequence of events that all too often occurs is as follows. Some time after 5 days of age, occasionally as late as 1 or 2 months of age, the baby is noted to gain weight excessively on a normal caloric intake. Pitting edema of the feet is first noted and the whole body starts to appear slightly swollen. Chest retractions become apparent, air entry is diminished on auscultation, and, occasionally, there may be rales. Oxygen need rises, as does the carbon dioxide tension in marked cases. The chest film shows a streaky increase in lung markings and pulmonary congestion.

Only in recent years with the advent of effective diuretic agents has it become clear that this syndrome is a result of abnormal fluid retention rather than a primary pulmonary disorder. When such an infant is treated with furosemide or ethacrynic acid, there is a remarkable diuresis, a weight loss of up to 150 g and clearing of the pedal edema and generalized puffiness. Most striking, the respiratory pathology clears up simultaneously, retractions subside, oxygen need disappears, P_{CO_2} returns to normal, and the chest film clears.

Fluid retention seems to pose a greater problem for the more premature infants (particularly those less than 29 weeks). Other less premature infants who have a patent ductus arteriosus with borderline heart failure, or bronchopulmonary dysplasia following respirator therapy, also have a fluid retention problem.

In order to keep extremely premature infants within reasonable limits of fluid intake, we have restricted intakes almost invariably to 140 ml/kg/day of either the intravenous fluid regime described, or 27 cal/oz/milk, until the infants reach about 32 weeks of gestational age. When occasional infants start to gain excessively or become edematous on this intake, diuretics are utilized and the fluid intake restricted. Some infants, particularly those with patent ductus arteriosus or bronchopulmonary dysplasia, cannot be given more than 110 to 125 ml/kg/day without accumulating excess fluid with concomitant severe cardiorespiratory distress. In such situations, the intake may have to be kept to these levels for several weeks, temporarily sacrificing some growth to keep within the limited renal capacities of the particular infant, until gradually the tolerance of the infant for fluids increases.

Fluid retention in these very premature infants must not be treated by restricting sodium, of which they are already in short supply. We have found that many infants who require repeated diuretic therapy soon become resistant to furosemide, but that ethacrynic acid remains very effective. These drugs are potentially ototoxic and should not be given along with aminoglycoside antibiotics.

Apneic Spells. Extremely premature infants have a disturbing tendency to develop periodic respiratory arrests whenever their clinical condition deteriorates.[50,55] Death from any cause in these infants is usually preceded by a downhill course marked by apneic spells of increasing frequency and severity. Most infants of 24- to 30-weeks' gestation who survive also develop apneic spells at a time when they are weakest, usually between 4 days and 2 weeks of age. These occur at a time when alveolar ventilation is reduced and carbon dioxide tensions elevated.

Apneic spells do not strike unexpectedly. The infant who has one spell tends to have several during the same day. They often occur at a time when the infant has become generally lethargic with poor tone. They seem to be an ominous extension of the periodic respirations seen in healthy premature infants of more advanced gestational age. Usually apnea is preceded by a few minutes of limp inactivity (which may follow handling or a crying episode). Respirations become slower and shallower, the heart rate slows from 140 to 100 beats/minute, and then respirations stop. If the infant is still in fair general condition prior to the spell, tone, color, and heart rate remain fairly good for about 1 minute and the infant is fairly easy to revive with gentle stimulation. In an infant who has been in poorer condition, the onset of apnea is quickly followed by a pale, dusky appearance, the heart rate falls quickly, and positive-pressure ventilation with oxygen by bag and mask is required for 1 or more minutes before spontaneous respirations are reestablished. During this resuscitation period, continuous positive airway pressure applied manually by means of the bag and mask is of value in improving oxygenation. It also helps to maintain and enhance the early feeble respiratory efforts when the infant starts to breathe again. The head should be lifted from the bed and slightly hyperextended with the neck on a slight stretch to avoid airway occlusion and give optimal chest dynamics to the hypotonic baby who is making weak efforts to breathe.

The earlier in the spell intervention is begun, the less resuscitative efforts are needed. For this reason, cardiac and/or respiration monitors are employed in the management of all infants of 30-weeks' gestation or less, from birth until apneic spells have ceased to occur, usually by 4 weeks of age. A nurse moves to the baby to stimulate him as soon as respirations or heart rate slow. Bag and mask ventilation is employed by the nursing staff if stimulation alone is ineffective.

Two additional modes of therapy for apnea have been discovered in the past few years that are often very effective in stopping or reducing the apneic spells. One is the use of respiratory stimulants. We have had much experience with intravenous caffeine citrate (20 mg/kg initially and then 5 mg/kg/day starting 48 hours later), as developed by Aranda.

Equally effective is the distension of the lungs, either by continuous positive pressure (CPAP) on the upper airway (through nasal catheter or endotracheal tube) or by continuous negative thoracic pressure by placing the baby in a negative-pressure ventilator. In either case, an airway distending pressure of 5 cm water is usually efficacious and safe from the standpoint of pneumothorax.

Our preference is to start with continuous airway distending pressure, if apneic spells start to require bag and mask resuscitation, and to add caffeine therapy if apneic spells recur on airway distending pressure. If apneic spells break through both forms of therapy, positive-pressure mechanical ventilation through an endotracheal tube must be initiated as the last resource.

Several factors contribute to the development of apneic spells in the extremely premature infant. Prevention or early treatment of these conditions can diminish the severity of apneic spells. These predisposing factors include: anemia, acidosis, lipemia, hyperglycemia, hypoglycemia or undernutrition, hypothermia, hypoxemia, infection, patent ductus arteriosus, sodium disturbances, or abdominal distension.

Infants who start to develop apneic spells therefore are given blood transfusions if they are needed to raise the hemoglobin concentration to 12 g/dl. Supplementary sodium bicarbonate is provided to maintain the blood pH between 7.30 and 7.35. Adequate ambient oxygen is provided. Incubator temperature is kept at whatever level is needed to maintain rectal temperature at 37° C. Acute phase reactants, urinalysis, and sometimes a blood culture are obtained; if these suggest that an infection is present, broad-spectrum antibiotics are begun. If there is a murmur of patent ductus arteriosus, full pulses, and evidence of congestive pulmonary failure, diuretics, fluid restriction, and sometimes digoxin are employed to control the heart failure. Abdominal distension, which may be exacerbated by bag and mask ventilation, is treated with continuous gastric suction.

It is a rare infant who can tolerate sufficient milk feedings while manifesting apneic spells, and intravenous supplements are provided to allow for as optimal nutrition as the infant has the metabolic capacity to handle. Care is taken to avoid hyperglycemia or hyperlipemia during intravenous supplementation because either can produce or exacerbate apneic spells. If either should develop, intravenous sugar or fat intake is temporarily discontinued until serum levels readjust and is recommenced at lower levels of intake. The infant whose condition deteriorates can quickly become intolerant to intakes of intravenous lipid or glucose which were previously well tolerated, and a vicious cycle of **apnea → lipid/glucose intolerance → more apnea** is produced. Hyper- or hyponatremia can cause apneic spells, and sodium chloride intake is varied accordingly when either develops.

As should be clear from the foregoing, apneic spells are regarded as a nonspecific manifestation of ill health in the extremely premature baby. Every effort is made to maintain the susceptible infant in optimal condition to prevent the development of apneic spells. When they do develop, a rapid search is made for correctable conditions which may be contributing to the spells, and any disorders found are immediately treated.

Patent Ductus Arteriosus. Infants recovering from RDS often develop the characteristic heart murmur of a patent ductus arteriosus. The variable, long, systolic murmur at the upper left sternal border, ending as a crescendo at the second heart sound or passing through it, loudest in expiration, hypoventilation, or during apnea, indicates patent ductus arteriosus. In premature infants of more than 30-weeks' gestation who have had RDS, this murmur may be heard for several days without concomitant indications of failure or distress.

Less mature infants of 24 to 30 weeks, with or without RDS, frequently develop a murmur of patent ductus arteriosus which is often associated with congestive pulmonary failure.[57,58] This murmur usually has its onset about the third to fifth day of age, perhaps associated with the postnatal decline in pulmonary vascular resistance allowing increased left-to-right flow across the patent ductus. After several days, the aortic run-off increases, causing bounding pulses to the extent that the dorsalis pedis and palmar pulses become quite perceptible.

As left-to-right ductal shunting increases, the left ventricle, which must pump the shunted blood, becomes progressively strained until pulmonary congestion and edema develop. This state of congestive pulmonary failure becomes manifest by chest retractions, diminished breath sounds on auscultation, and moist rales in the most severe cases. Mild cyanosis is easily relieved by 25% to 30% ambient oxygen concentrations because the shunt is left-to-right and not right-to-left. The heart rate may increase slightly to 160/minute, and a gallop rhythm is occasionally heard. Cardiac activity on palpation and auscultation becomes very hyperdynamic.

The ECG is normal for an extreme premature; that is to say, it shows a left-axis deviation with left-ventricular dominance rather than the right-sided dominance of the full-term infant. Chest films may be impressive, with pronounced pulmonary congestion and edema, although seldom with pleural effusions. The pulmonary edema affects upper lobes more than lower. It may be difficult at times to distinguish the severe pulmonary congestion and edema from pneumonia, though the other aspects of the clinical picture, the murmur, and negative acute phase reactants usually permit enough confidence to avoid unnecessary use of antibiotics. Carbon dioxide tension may be elevated, presumably from poor lung compliance. There is a frequent correlation between the degree of hypercapnea and the severity of failure and pulmonary edema.

The most ominous clinical sign in a premature infant with a patent ductus arteriosus is the development of apneic spells, especially if progressive in severity. These indicate an aortic run-off sufficient to deprive the brain of its normal share of the cardiac output.

Surgical treatment of extremely premature infants with patent ductus arteriosus is possible, even in the smallest infants.[58] The decision to ligate the ductus arteriosus is usually made

on clinical grounds alone without cardiac catheterization. The diagnosis of patent ductus arteriosus as distinguished from other forms of congenital heart disease is based on the degree of prematurity, the typical time of presentation, the characteristics of the murmur and full pulses, the x-ray findings, and hypercapnea, all in the absence of ECG abnormalities. With echocardiography, it is possible to assess the degree of left-ventricular failure by the demonstration of left-atrial enlargement. Postoperatively, within 2 days the infant is often markedly improved, demonstrating clear lungs on x-ray film and a normal P_{CO_2}.

However, anesthesia and surgery in an infant who is often 27 weeks and 1000 g in congestive pulmonary failure has a high mortality rate. Medical management is therefore preferable whenever possible, and increased experience with this condition has led to better understanding of therapeutic measures capable of tiding the infant over and controlling heart failure until the patent ductus arteriosus closes spontaneously, usually 2 to 6 weeks after birth.

The most important principles of medical management are fluid restriction, diuresis of excess fluid, maintenance of normal blood pH with supplemental sodium bicarbonate, oxygen as needed, and, of greatest value, the maintenance of adequate hemoglobin concentration (over 12 g/dl). Digitalization is reserved for those infants who cannot be controlled by these measures because it is not too effective and may be difficult to maintain without toxicity.

Today, it is possible, using a prostaglandin inhibitor, indomethacin, to close the patent ductus arteriosus in many infants without recourse to surgery. Although this agent is most effective when used in the first week of life, its potential toxicity has led us to administer it only when there is evidence of failure, apneic spells, or respirator dependency in the presence of a patent ductus.

There is a possibility that a hyperdynamic precordium and the other clinical, radiologic, and blood gas evidences of a patent ductus arteriosus may present in the absence of a murmur: the "silent duct." Echocardiography may help delineate such cases.

Evidence is accumulating that administration of excessive fluid, and particularly colloid, to extremely premature infants may be an important factor in causing duct patency. Volume loading certainly can play a major role in producing heart failure in the presence of a patent ductus arteriosus.

Chronic Pulmonary Disease (Mikity–Wilson). (See also Chap. 21.) Until recent years, it was thought that premature infants had problems with respiratory distress only during the first few days of life, and thereafter respirations, although sometimes irregular, were not labored. It is now clear that extremely premature infants (usually 30 weeks or less) sometimes develop a chronic form of respiratory distress, which in its most severe degree appears pseudocystic on x-ray film and is called Mikity–Wilson disease.[59,60]

This condition occurs in infants who may or may not have had RDS during the first days of life. Their pulmonary function is relatively normal to 1 to 2 weeks of age, and they develop an insidious type of respiratory distress. This takes the form of gradually increasing chest retractions, decrease in air entry on auscultation, slowly increasing oxygen need to about 30% to 40% and a characteristic streaky pattern of infiltrations on x-ray film. The lungs develop increasing densities which start to show small, cystic lucencies, and later a pattern of soap-bubble pseudocysts appears in those most severely affected. At peak severity, lung fields become overinflated and the right atrium of the heart enlarges because of cor pulmonale.

Blood gas changes are relatively minor compared to the radiologic signs, carbon dioxide tension rarely rising above 55 torr and arterialized capillary P_{O_2} remaining about 45 torr in less than 40% oxygen. This chronic pulmonary disease picture tends to improve after 4 to 8 weeks of age.

In recent years, with extremely premature infants limited in their fluid intake to 140 ml/kg/day and diuretics employed as soon as there is any evidence of fluid retention, chronic pulmonary disease of the premature with and without cyst formation has all but disappeared in our nursery. The only cases of chronic chest disease seen during this period have been infants suffering from bronchopulmonary dysplasia after long periods of positive-pressure mechanical ventilation.[61] We therefore consider chronic pulmonary disease of the extreme premature to be a preventable disorder caused by abnormal fluid retention which, if it develops, is usually responsive to fluid restriction and diuretics.

Anemia. Anemia of the extreme premature is of relatively earlier onset and greater severity. Initial hemoglobin concentrations in extremely premature infants are sometimes only 12 to 14 g/dl and there is proportionately larger blood loss from sampling. Relative body growth is more rapid, so that a 900 g infant triples his birth weight during his 10 weeks in the hospital. Dependence on external iron sources may therefore begin as early as 2 weeks of age. Absorption of supplemental iron in milk (2 mg/100 cal) is excellent and evidence of iron deficiency is very rare even though the infant's growth need for iron may almost equal his ingested iron intake until he attains 2 kg in weight.

The tendency to more rapid and more severe degrees of anemia, coupled with the increased concern about anemia because of the often associated apneic spells, patent ductus arteriosus, or bronchopulmonary dysplasia, lead to transfusion of most extremely premature infants. This is done in aliquots of 7 ml/kg as packed red blood cells. Usually blood is taken in a heparinized syringe (5–10 units of heparin per millilter of blood) from a "walking donor" on the nursing or medical staff, or from a parent, who is cross-matched to the baby. The blood is allowed to sediment in the syringe, the plasma removed, and the cells infused by pump. The same walking donor is used for serial transfusions to avoid the need for repeated cross-matching. Indications for transfusion are hemoglobin concentrations of less than 7 to 8 g/dl in a healthy infant, or less than 12 g/dl in the presence of apneic spells, patent ductus arteriosus, or bronchopulmonary dysplasia.

Though it is tempting in an ill infant to try to attain higher hemoglobin concentrations than 12 gm/dl with blood transfusion, volume overload is an ever-present hazard and this temptation should be resisted. We often consider it useful to administer a diuretic at the onset of a transfusion.

Infection. Pneumonia or septicemia at birth, from prolonged rupture of the membranes, occurs most frequently in infants of less than 31-weeks' gestation. Intrauterine as well as postnatally acquired infections represent major causes of death in these infants, and are exceedingly difficult to diagnose. Fortunately, the extremely premature infant does respond to infection with a marked acute phase reac-

Table 14-8. Frequency of Therapy.

Treatment	Frequency (%)
Resuscitation bag and mask at birth	34
Resuscitation endotracheal tube at birth	7
Mechanical respirator (Pos.)	25
Continuous negative pressure or CPAP	16
Oxygen: Total	54
>60%	25
>7 days	25
Umbilical artery catheter	12
Antibiotics	59
Caffeine for apnea	12
Diuretics	25
Tolazoline	5
Pharmacologic Agents for PDA	5
Phototherapy	65
Exchange transfusion	3
Transferred to Children's Hospital for surgery/cardiology	5
For survivors only	
Duration IV nutrition (<30 weeks)	36 days
Duration IV nutrition (30–33 weeks)	11 days
Hospital stay (<30 weeks)	85 days
Hospital stay (30–33 weeks)	36 days

Treatment in 110 preterm infants of less than 34-weeks' gestation born in Royal Victoria Hospital, 1978

tion, so that white blood cell and differential counts, and erythrocyte sedimentation rates are useful as diagnostic tools. If ethacrynic acid or furosemide diuretic therapy is used, the aminoglycoside antibiotics (gentamicin and kanamycin) entail a risk of synergistic toxicity to hearing.

Necrotizing Enterocolitis. (See also Ch. 42.) The extreme premature is susceptible to necrotizing enterocolitis, a catastrophic form of intestinal disorder of uncertain etiology.[62] It usually strikes after intestinal feeds have been started, occurring either during the build-up phase or within the first week of attaining full feeds. The timing suggests that it is caused by overdistension of a poorly functioning intestine during a period when it is being called upon to function earlier than it is capable of doing.

The infant suddenly develops severe, acute abdominal distension, vomits, passes blood by way of the rectum, and becomes toxic and borders on shock. X-ray films of the abdomen demonstrate distended bowel loops, streaks of intramural air in the bowel wall, and sometimes peritoneal air from perforation. Death may follow shortly after from shock or sepsis, or recovery may occur gradually with bowel function returning after several weeks. Sometimes a palpable abdominal mass develops some days later, or foci of bowel obstruction develop. Surgical treatment consists of removal of necrotic or perforated segments of bowel, but it is very dangerous in "shocky," septic, 1000 g infants. This condition also occurs at times in infants beyond 30-weeks' gestation.

Prevention of necrotizing enterocolitis consists, in part at least, of limiting intestinal feeds to the volumes that can be tolerated without producing abdominal distension, even though this may mean that many days pass with intravenous nutritional supplements required. At the first sign of acute abdominal distention, gastric suction should be employed and feedings should be discontinued until normal bowel function is restored, with loss of distension and development of bowel sounds and bowel movements.

Respirators and Mechanical Aids

As is evident from the foregoing sections, this author has attempted to avoid endotracheal intubation and mechanical aids whenever possible because of their complications. The survival rates under 1500 g reported in Tables 14-3 and 14-4 were obtained with fewer than 10% of surviving infants having been treated on a positive-pressure respirator. The infrequent sequelae found in our experience and that of others when infants do not require respirators for survival and the higher sequelae rate following respirator therapy have supported us in this conservative view.

It is becoming increasingly apparent, however, that some centers employing respirators and CPAP for the majority of their under 1500 g infants are now obtaining spectacular results. Andrew Shennan of Womens' College Hospital, Toronto, has obtained a 96% survival to discharge of infants weighing 1001 to 1500 g, 93% at 751 to 1000 g, and 46% at 501 to 750 g, among 112 infants without lethal malformations born in his hospital in 1979, most of whom received positive-pressure ventilation by endotracheal tube.

Bronchopulmonary dysplasia, intraventric-

Table 14-9. Frequency of Conditions.

Disorders	Incidence	Mortality
Prolonged rupture membranes (24 hours)	25%	11%
Asphyxia: Apgar, 1 min = 0–3	25	54
Apgar, 1 min = 4–6	29	13
Hypothermia on admission (< 36.0° C)	24	38
Respiratory distress syndrome	20	29
Infection: meningitis	0	—
septicemia	5	80
other systemic	16	11
Convulsions	5	80
Apneic spells	29	34
Extraalveolar air	4	60
Bronchopulmonary dysplasia	6	33
Other chronic chest disease	2	0
Obstructive jaundice (IV nutrition)	10	27
Surgical necrotizing enterocolitis	5	80
Nonsurgical necrotizing enterocolitis	6	14
PDA in failure	10	27
PDA without failure	9	10
Retrolental fibroplasia	2	0
Hyperbilirubinemia (12 mg/dl)	12	8
Hypoglycemia (< 40 mg/dl plasma)	12	15
Hyperglycemia (> 150 mg/dl plasma)	14	40
Hypocalcemia (< 7 mg/dl)	24	23
Hyponatremia (< 130 mmol/liter)	5	50
Hypernatremia (> 150 mmol/liter)	10	64
Late metabolic acidosis (BE, 8 mmol/liter > 3 days)	43	13
Thrombocytopenia (< 100,000/mm³)	11	42
Anemia (Hgb < 10 g/dl)	28	6
Polycythemia after birth (Hgb 21 g/dl)	36	8
TOTAL*	100%	25%

* Some infants had more than one condition.
Disorders in 110 preterm infants of less than 34-weeks' gestation born in Royal Victoria Hospital, 1978

ular hemorrhage, hydrocephalus, and protracted courses with emotionally draining and extremely costly late deaths have made us approach the respirator with dread, particularly for the infant under 900 g. Others are now beginning to prove that these outcomes can be avoided, Shennan having lost only two nonmalformed infants out of those who survived the first week. Future experience will have to determine whether earlier intervention with airway distending pressure and intermittent mandatory ventilation, which Shennan often initiates at birth, may avoid the extended respirator courses and poor outcomes we often experience when respirator therapy is initiated later, after considerable deterioration has occurred.

Frequency of Disorders and Treatments

In an attempt to provide an order-of-magnitude understanding of the incidence and associated mortality of the different disorders, and the frequency of the treatments that have been discussed, the recent experience of our unit is tabulated for 110 infants of 33-weeks' gestation or less (Tables 14-8, 14-9). These included 58 infants of 31 weeks or less (19 died) and 52 of 32 to 33 weeks (5 died).

Emotional Aspects

Being the parent of a 24- to 30-week premature infant is one of the most emotionally draining experiences of a lifetime. The infant looks like nothing on earth to the new parents. There are tubes and wires all over, and the treatment area is often a frightening hubbub of emergencies. It is difficult to relate to the son or daughter in the incubator and almost impossible to imagine taking "it" home 2 months later as a healthy infant. The physician can give no assurance of survival, and the parents are afraid to ask about sequelae. Then follow days or weeks of sudden ups and downs, with every telephone call or personal contact with nurses or doctors beginning with a moment of fright that the news may be bad.

Gradually, the realization dawns that all really might be all right, that the fears are over, and that they can realistically hope for the best in the years ahead. Ideally, a sound, warm relationship should be established between parents and baby prior to his leaving the hospital.

How can the nurse and doctor help to support the parents through this series of crises and encourage healthy bonding to their child? All parents, as part of their prenatal classes, should be shown the neonatal intensive care area and told that many infants spend some time there after birth for observation or treatment. When premature labor starts, at least the father should be shown around the intensive care unit and introduced to the equipment and procedures and to other infants similar to his own. The neonatologist should discuss the situation with both parents and answer their questions. He should deal with any misconceptions they may have before they deliver, and indicate why tocolytic agents, prolonged hospitalization, and glycocorticoids are of value. The baby can be shown to the parents in the delivery room and encouraging features pointed out. The father can be brought into the nursery by the doctor an hour later and the infant felt to be warm, human, responsive to the touch, and not a breakable glass doll.

From then on parents are to consider the nursery theirs to be in as often as desired. Positive steps forward are clearly indicated at each visit. Open discussion of all of the parents' questions is forthcoming from *every* member of the nursing and medical staff involved with the infant's care. **Good news** consists of first feedings, first weight gain, less oxygen need, graduation from the respirator, and increased physical activity. **Discouraging news** may be of need to discontinue feedings and of decreased vigor to account for apneic spells. **No news** includes laboratory results, medical minutiae, vital signs, and all the other information of vital interest to physicians but of no value to parents, except when required to account for changes in the baby's condition or in his treatment program, and then always in terms understandable to laymen.

As long as there is reasonable hope for survival, the attitude must be to foster hope in the parents. Parents do not need to obtain a comprehensive report of all the hurdles the baby is having to get over. Their interest is in learning that the baby is coming through all right. Apneic spells become "pauses in breathing when the infant falls asleep and needs to be awakened" and that "they are expected in all infants of his degree of prematurity during the first few weeks." RDS is "slowness to open the lungs because the baby is premature and this usually takes 3 or 4 days of deep breathing for the baby to overcome." Words such as **critical period,** or being **in danger** are superfluous and are usually said to provide the doctor an "out" if the infant should die.

If an infant dies, there is sufficient time during the period of deterioration to warn the parents that things are not going well and to allow them to prepare for the loss. Having established a hopeful relationship to the infant in life does not make the death harder to take in the long run. Grief will be more acute but more real and can be worked out completely over the next days and weeks.

It should always be remembered that most infants over 1000 g birth weight do survive. As to their future, the parents should be given the feeling that they have every reason to plan for a healthy normal child. Nothing is to be gained by cataloging the potential long-term hazards of prematurity that they are likely never to have to face. Modern medical care for the premature has changed the outlook of the 1000 g infant for the better. The parents should be counseled in the brighter context, even though the physician cannot guarantee it.

Parents in the nursery also help the staff's attitude. The look of joy or concern on a mother's or father's face at seeing the baby puts a completely different texture to working with prematures. As nurses or doctors in the nursery, frustrations mount from the inability to "relate" meaningfully to the uncommunicative patient. Relating to the parents of that patient provides an alternative satisfaction. Good relations with parents are easier when the physical setting of the nursery is planned with a view to their needs. Rocking chairs in the nursery, bright pictures on the walls, and a parents' visiting area within the nursery proper are physical aids to happy parent contact. Follow-up pictures of ex-1000 g infants riding their tricycles at 3 years of age are priceless. A parent information sheet on each medical record allows different staff members to keep a log of parent counseling. Keeping a log of telephone calls and visits indicates when parents have gotten out of touch and might benefit from some encouragement.[63]

As the physical needs of the premature infant become more readily resolved with recent medical advances, the greater challenge today in caring for an extremely premature infant is often the emotional needs of both parents and staff.

Social workers are of great help to parents and become involved with all of our long stay or very ill infants' parents. They can provide a calm, expert counsel and a listening ear, not distracted by the urgent demands of acute care which compete for the attentions of nurse and doctor.

Having one attending neonatologist in charge of the case who will take time to review the changing situation periodically with the parents and whom the parents realize is aware of and responsible for the care being given, is a most important reassuring element.

PREMATURE INFANT SEQUELAE AND MORTALITY RATES

Effectiveness of premature infant care must be gauged by neonatal mortality rates and by reduction of sequelae in later life. The latter is more difficult and takes longer to measure, but recent reports are most encouraging, with about 90% of under 1500 g survivors mentally and neurologically intact on follow-up.[64]

Follow-up of 95% of the under 1500 g survivors of our hospital by Dr. Diana Willis is showing that of 152 infants seen at 1 to 5 years of age, 2% are unlikely to be able to lead independent lives, 7% have specific deficits which are amendable to aids and training, and 91% are totally normal with normal developmental quotients. Retrolental fibroplasia was severe in 2% and left milder injury in 2% more, these severe cases accounting for two of the three infants with severe developmental delays. Hydrocephaly (one mild case), cerebral palsy (one mild case) and deafness (one partial case), are much less frequent than expected. Epilepsy and child battering have not been seen, hospital readmissions and chronic chest disease are very rare, there has been one death after discharge from hospital, and the incidence of marriage break-up among parents is almost nil. Physical growth after 2 years is above the third percentile in weight in 90% and in head circumference in 95%.

From these data and those of others it is now possible to have an optimistic long-term outlook for premature infants. Greatest concern must be for those of less than 1000 g birth weight, those requiring respirator care, and those who were growth retarded at birth or who grew poorly in their first 2 months.

Mortality rates should be available yearly in each center and are much simpler to assess. Those existing at one maternity hospital-based neonatal intensive care service are presented by gestational age in Table 14-4 and by birth weight in Table 14-3 for the years 1971 to 1975.

The changes in neonatal mortality by weight group over the past few years have been striking (Fig. 14-5). For the Province of Quebec, where approximately 100,000 infants are born yearly, the neonatal mortality among low-birth-weight infants of 1000 to 2500 g fell from 9.8% to 5.9% between 1968 and 1974. There was a decrease of 32% to 53% within each 500-g weight group in this range.[65]

Comparing province-wide with perinatal intensive care center results (the "optimal" hospitals of Fig. 14-5) shows the gap that continues to exist between the prevailing results and those that potentially could be obtained if all premature infants were delivered where intensive care was available. This gap is greatest for the infants to 1001 to 1500 g, who had a 36% mortality throughout the province and an 18% mortality in the intensive care centers.

In Figure 14-6, the Quebec mortality rates among 1001 to 1500 g infants for 1974 are analysed by hospital of birth grouped according to type of neonatal care available. Among

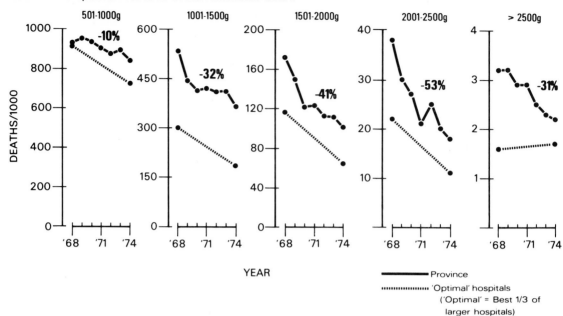

Fig. 14-5. Changes in neonatal mortality by weight group in the Province of Quebec between 1968 and 1974 (approximately 100,000 births/year), with the percent decrease in each weight group indicated (data from the Quebec Perinatal Committee). For comparison, the mortality rates from the best third of the larger hospitals (those providing intensive care) are shown.

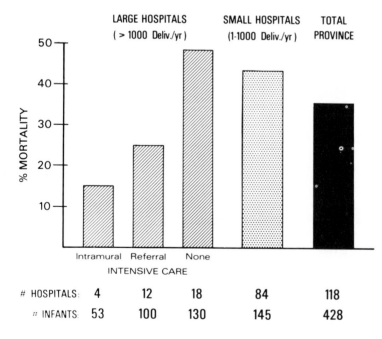

Fig. 14-6. Neonatal mortality for very low-birth-weight infants by hospital of birth according to size of obstetrical service and utilization of neonatal intensive care. **Intramural** = obstetrical services with their own neonatal intensive care units; **Referral** = obstetrical services routinely referring high-risk newborn infants to other neonatal intensive care units; and **None** = no intramural neonatal intensive care unit and little or no referral of sick newborns. (Data for the whole Province of Quebec, 1974, collected by the Quebec Perinatal Committee)

large obstetric services, hospitals providing intramural neonatal intensive care after birth lost 15%, those routinely referring sick infants to pediatric centers lost 25%, and those using neither form of intensive care lost 48% of their infants. Infants born in small obstetric services had 45% mortality rate.

From this experience, it became evident that groups of hospitals should organize their care so that one perinatal intensive care service could serve the population in need from several hospitals. At McGill University, such regionalized planning took place from 1973 to 1974 and now the high-risk pregnancies (mainly premature labor) from 14,000 births usually deliver in the two of six obstetrical services providing perinatal intensive care.[65] The results show a decrease by more than half in neonatal mortality among the 1001 to 1500 g weight group (Table 14-10).

The borderline viable (501–1000 g) infant mortality rates have also been improving dramatically with time, though not as striking as the figures quoted earlier from Andrew Shennan. Because the risk of post-1-week death is high in this group of infants, we have analysed survival rates until discharge home alive (Table 14-11).

OVERVIEW

The special needs of the premature infant, especially infants born before 31 weeks, now clearly require a very complex system of care provided by full-time subspecialists in well-equipped and well-staffed units wherever possible. The complexity of care and the rarity of need (1% of births), lend themselves to a regionalized approach with specialized centers providing care for referrals from neighboring hospitals. Results are much better when the mother is used as the transport incubator and

Table 14-10. Neonatal Mortality (0–7 days) Among Livebirths 1001–1500 g (McGill University obstetric services).

1971–73	1974–76*	1978*
32.6%	14.1%	13.0%

* After regionalization. In 1972, 26% of infants 1001–1500 g were born in intensive care centers; in 1976, 73%; and in 1978, 85%.

Table 14-11. Survival to Discharge Home Alive of 501–1000 g Livebirths

	Province of Quebec	McGill University Intramural Intensive Care Centers		
	1970–72	*1966–70 (One Center)*	*1971–75 (One Center)*	*1978 (System)*
No. livebirths	1011	73	75	49
% Survived	6	11	23	37

intensive care begins before delivery, rather than when the baby is transferred for intensive care only after his birth.

The day is almost here when normally formed infants beyond 28 weeks, or 1000 g, should seldom need to die or become damaged as a result of their early birth. For the 24- to 27-week, or 600- to 999-g infants, cautious optimism can begin to be expressed, though extreme difficulties remain inherent in their care.

REFERENCES

1. **Usher RH, Allen AC, McLean FH:** Risk of respiratory distress syndrome related to gestational age, route of delivery, and maternal diabetes. Am J Obstet Gynecol 111:826, 1971
2. **Drillien CM:** The incidence of mental and physical handicaps in school-age children of very low birth weight. Pediatrics 27:452, 1961
3. **Lubchenco LO, Horner FA, Reed LH, Hix IE, Jr, et al:** Sequelae of premature birth. Evaluation of premature infants of low birth weights at ten years of age. Am J Dis Child 106:101, 1963
4. **Shanklin, DR:** The sex of premature infants with hyaline membrane disease. South Med J, 56:1018, 1963
5. **Usher R, McLean F, Scott KE:** Judgment of fetal age. II. Clinical significance of gestational age and an objective method for its assessment. Pediatr Clin North Am 13:835, 1966
6. **Usher RH:** Clinical implications of perinatal mortality statistics. Clin Obstet Gynecol 14: 885, 1971
7. **Blanc WA:** Amniotic infection syndrome. Pathogenesis, morphology, and significance in circumnatal mortality. Clin Obstet Gynecol 2: 705, 1959

8. **Lebherz TB, Boyce CR, Huston JW:** Premature rupture of the membrane. A statistical study from 7 U.S. Navy hospitals. Am J Obstet Gynecol 81:658, 1961

9. **Davies, PA:** Bacterial infection in the fetus and newborn. Arch Dis Child 46:1, 1971

10. **Lebherz TB, Hellman LP, Madding R, et al:** Double-blind study of premature rupture of the membranes. Am J Obstet Gynecol 87:218, 1963

11. **Benirschke K, Clifford SH:** Intrauterine bacterial infection of the newborn infant. Frozen sections of the cord as an aid to early detection. J Pediatr, 54:11, 1959

12. **Pitkin RM, Zwirek SJ:** Amniotic fluid creatinine. Am J Obstet Gynecol 98:1135, 1967

13. **Brosens IA, Gordon H., Baert A:** Prediction of fetal maturity with combined cytological and radiological methods. J Obstet Gynecol Br Commw 76:20, 1969

14. **Gluck L, Kulovich MV:** Lecithin/sphingomyelin ratios in amniotic fluid in normal and abnormal pregnancy. Am J Obstet Gynecol, 115:539, 1973

15. **Clements JA:** Respiratory distress syndrome: rapid test for surfactant in amniotic fluid. New Engl J Med 286:1077, 1972

16. **Saigal S, O'Neill A, Surainder Y et al:** Placental transfusion and hyperbilirubinemia in the premature. Pediatrics, 49:406, 1972

17. **Yao AC, Lind J:** Placental transfusion. Am J Dis Child 127:128, 1974

18. **Usher R, Saigal S, O'Neill A et al:** Estimation of red blood cell volume in premature infants with and without respiratory distress syndrome. Biol Neonate 26:241, 1975

19. **Saigal S, Usher, R:** Symptomatic neonatal plethora. Biol Neonate 32:62, 1977

20. **Avery ME, Gatewood OB, Brumley G:** Transient tachypnea of newborn: Possible delayed resorption of fluid at birth. Am J Dis Child 111:380, 1966

21. **O'Brien JR, Usher RH, Maughan GB:** Causes of birth asphyxia and trauma. Can Med Assoc J 94:1077, 1966

22. **Bruck K:** Temperature regulation in the newborn infant. Biol Neonate 3:65, 1961

23. **Gandy GM, Adamsons K Jr, Cunningham N, et al:** Thermal environment and acid-base homeostasis in human infants during the first few hours of life. J Clin Invest 43:751, 1964

24. **Silverman WA, Fertig JW, Berger AP:** The influence of the thermal environment upon the survival of newly born premature infants. Pediatrics 22:876, 1958

25. **Jolly H, Mollyneux P, Newell DJ:** A controlled study of the effects of temperature on premature babies. J Pediatr 60:889, 1962

26. **Day RL, Caliquiri L, Kamenski C, et al:** Body temperature and survival of premature infants. Pediatrics 34:171, 1964

27. **Belgaumkar TK, Scott KE:** Personal communications

28. **Light IJ, Berry HK, Sutherland JM:** Aminoacidemia of prematurity. Am J Dis Child 112:229, 1966

29. **Usher R, McLean F:** Intrauterine growth of live-born Caucasian infants at sea level: Standards obtained from measurements in 7 dimensions of infants born between 25 and 44 weeks of gestation. J Pediatr 74:901, 1969

30. **Liggins GC, Howie RN:** A controlled trial of antepartum glucocorticoid treatment for prevention of the respiratory distress syndrome in premature infants. Pediatrics 50:515, 1972

31. **Chernick V, Heldrich F, Avery ME:** Periodic breathing of premature infants. J Pediatr 64:330, 1964

32. **Stern L, Denton RL:** Kernicterus in small premature infants. Pediatrics 35:483, 1965

33. **Gartner LM, Snyder RN, Chabon S, et al:** Kernicterus: High incidence in premature infants with low serum bilirubin concentrations. Pediatrics 45:906, 1970

34. **Ackerman BD, Dyer GY, Leydorf MM:** Hyperbilirubinemia and kernicterus in small premature infants. Pediatrics 45:918, 1970

35. **Behrman RE, Brown AK, Currie MR, et al:** Preliminary report of the committee on phototherapy in the newborn infant. J Pediatr 84:135, 1974

36. **Lucey J, Ferriero M, Hewitt J:** Prevention of hyperbilirubinemia of prematurity by phototherapy. Pediatrics 41:1047, 1968

37. **Kildeberg P:** Disturbances of hydrogen ion balance occurring in premature infants, II. Late metabolic acidosis. Acta Paediatr 53:517, 1964

38. **Svenningsen NW:** Renal acid-base titration studies in infants with and without metabolic acidosis in the postneonatal period. Pediatr Res 8:659, 1974

39. **Allen AC, Usher R:** Renal acid excretion in infants with the respiratory distress syndrome. Pediatr Res 5:345, 1971

40. **Tsang RC, Light J, Sutherland JM, et al:** Possible pathogenic factors in neonatal hypocalcemia of prematurity. J Pediatr 82:423, 1973

41. **Baens GS, Lundeen E, Cornblath M:** Studies of carbohydrate metabolism in the newborn infant, III. Levels of glucose in blood in premature infants. Pediatrics 31:580, 1963

42. **Widdowson EM, Spray CM:** Chemical development in utero. Arch Dis Child 26:205, 1951

43. **Melhorn DK, Gross S:** Vitamin E-dependent anemia in the premature infant: Effects of large doses of medicinal iron. J Pediatr 79:569, 1971

44. **Akenzua GI, et al:** Neutrophil and band counts in the diagnosis of neonatal infections. Pediatrics 54:38, 1974

45. **Kimbrough RD, Gaines TB:** Hexachlorophene effects on the rat brain. Arch Environ Health 23:114, 1971

46. **Curley A, Kimbrough RD, Hawk RE, et al:** Dermal absorption of hexachlorophene in infants. Lancet 2:296, 1971

47. **Kopelman AE:** Cutaneous absorption of hexachlorophene in low-birth-weight infants. J Pediatr 82:972, 1973

48. **Powell H, Swarner O, Gluck L, et al:** Hexachlorophene myelinopathy in premature infants. J Pediatr 82:976, 1973

49. **Fanaroff AA, Wald M, Gruber HS, et al:** Insensible water loss in low birth weight infants. Pediatrics 50:236, 1972

50. **Daily WJR, Klaus M, Meyer HB:** Apnea in premature infants: Monitoring incidence, heart rate changes, and an effect of environmental temperature. Pediatrics 43:510, 1969

51. **Perlstein PH, Edwards NK, Sutherland JM:** Apnea in premature infants and incubator air temperature changes. New Engl J Med 282:461, 1970

52. **Cashore W, Sedaghatian M, Usher R:** Nutritional supplements with intravenously administered lipid, protein hydrolysate and glucose in small premature infants. Pediatrics 56:8, 1975

53. **Loo SWH, Gross I, Warshaw JB:** Improved method of nasojejunal feeding in low-birth-weight infants. J Pediatr 85:104, 1974

54. **Dweck HS, Cassady G:** Glucose intolerance in infants of very low birthweight, I. Incidence of hyperglycemia in infants of birthweights 1,100 grams or less. Pediatrics 53:189, 1974

55. **Rigatto H, Brady JP:** Periodic breathing and apnea in preterm infants, I. Evidence for hypoventilation possibly due to central respiratory depression. Pediatrics, 50:202, 1972

56. **Aranda J, Gorman W, Bergsteinson H, Gunn T:** Efficacy of caffeine in the treatment of apnea in the low-birth-weight infants. J Pediatr 90:467, 1977

57. **Auld PAM:** Delayed closure of the ductus arteriosus. J Pediatr 69:61, 1966

58. **Kitterman JA, Edmunds LH Jr, Gregory GA, et al:** Patent ductus arteriosus in premature infants: Incidence, relation to pulmonary disease and management. New Engl J Med 287:473, 1972

59. **Wilson MG, Mikity VG:** A new form of respiratory disease in premature infants. Am J Dis Child 99:489, 1960

60. **Burnard ED:** The pulmonary syndrome of Wilson and Mikity, and respiratory function in very small premature infants. Pediatr Clin North Am 13:999, 1966

61. **Northway WH Jr, Rosan RC, Porter DY:** Pulmonary disease following respirator therapy. New Engl J Med 276:357, 1967

62. **Mizrahi A, Barlow O, Berdon W, et al:** Necrotizing enterocolitis in premature infants. J Pediatr 66:697, 1965

63. **Fanaroff AA, Kennell JH, Klaus MH:** Follow-up of low birth weight infants: The predictive value of maternal visiting patterns. Pediatrics 49:287, 1972

64. **Rawlings G, Stewart A, Reynolds EO, et al:** Changing prognosis for infants of very low birth weight. Lancet 1:516,1971

65. **Usher R:** Changing mortality rates with perinatal intensive care and regionalization. Sem Perinatol 1:309, 1977

15

The Small-for-Date Infant

George Cassady

HISTORY AND INTRODUCTION

> *"Nature is but
> a name for an effect."* [342]

Scattered references to the growth-retarded fetus have appeared in the literature for more than 30 years.[1,2] Söderling was one of the first to take issue with judging the degree of maturity by birth weight.[3] He noted that some low-birth-weight (LBW) infants were much more advanced in motor ability, reflexes, alertness, and appetite than other infants of like birth weight. He suggested the need for different neonatal management for these "pseudopremature" infants. But it was Gruenwald who, in the early 1960s, called attention to this common neonatal problem.[4,5]

Until 1961, the World Health Organization (WHO) defined as prematures all infants weighing 2500 g or less at birth. With the recognition that birth weight alone does not take cognizance of gestational age and maturity, WHO amended its earlier definition and, in 1961, suggested that infants weighing 2500 g or less at birth be termed "infants of low birth weight."[6] Birth weight could then be related to independent assessments of gesta-

tional age and the intrauterine-growth-retarded fetus, or small-for-date infant, could be defined.

Following these early reports, many terms have been used to designate the fetus whose growth is impaired: pseudopremature, small for dates, dysmature, fetal malnutrition syndrome, chronic fetal distress, intrauterine growth retarded, and small for gestational age (SGA). In the following discussion, the generally accepted abbreviation SGA will be used.

SIGNIFICANCE OF THE PROBLEM

Studies in the United States and Great Britain show that about one-third of all infants whose birth weight is less than 2500 g (LBW) are not truly premature but are small for gestational age.[5,7] Recent evidence however, suggests that in developing countries more than eight in ten LBW infants are born at term.[8] Such observations have led some authors to speculate that much of the variance in LBW rates is due to population differences in the incidence of SGA.[9]

The magnitude of this problem is second only to prematurity as a cause of perinatal mortality. While the preterm infant has an increased neonatal mortality, the SGA baby has a vastly increased fetal death rate.[10,117] The overall neonatal mortality for SGA infants

The author acknowledges the contributions of Marilyn L. Renfield, M.D., who authored a chapter dealing with this subject matter in the first edition of *Neonatology* and is largely responsible for the general outline of this chapter and many of the thoughts presented here.

(3.2%) is less than for appropriately grown prematures but more than for appropriately grown term infants.[10] However, death from intrapartum asphyxia alone is ten times higher than for appropriately grown infants,[11] with 14% of all stillbirths and 6% of all neonatal deaths occuring in infants whose birth weights are below the third percentile for gestational age.[12]

If the child is born alive, the infant's quality of life may be compromised. Congenital anomalies occur more frequently in SGA infants.[10,12] The SGA term infant has a 5% to 7% incidence of congenital anomalies,[2,10] and compromised physical as well as neurodevelopmental growth appears to be common in many of these babies.[13,14]

DEFINITION

There is *no* uniform definition of SGA. Once normal intrauterine growth is defined for a given population, one may then compare deviations from normal and define growth as abnormal by using arbitrary statistical limits. However, enormous variations in defining the arbitrary **limits of normal** (*i.e.*, <3rd percentile, <10th percentile, <2 standard deviations), **measurements to be compared** (*i.e.*, birth weight, length, birth weight × 100/length,[3] head circumference, length/head circumference), and **characteristics of the population studied** (race, sex, altitude, genetic growth potential) characterize most reports on this topic. These variations, which affect "growth" values, together with clinical inaccuracies in values for gestational age, account for much of the scatter within and discrepancies among studies which purport to establish "normal" and "abnormal" growth patterns.

For example, Lubchenco and coworkers define any infant whose birth weight is at the tenth percentile or less for gestational age as SGA.[15] These Denver intrauterine growth curves were constructed using only Caucasian infants born at high altitude; use of the curves seldom takes into account the sex of the infant. On the other hand, Gruenwald prefers to define as SGA any infant whose birth weight is more than two standard deviations below the mean for any given week of gestation, corresponding approximately to the third percentile on the intrauterine growth curves.[4,16] While the data of Freeman and associates allow definition of

such factors as race and sex, problems of population selection limit the uncritical, routine clinical use of their data.[17] These are but three examples from a large number of studies concerning the correlation of birth weight with duration of gestation. Nearly all were performed before evaluation of physical and neurologic characteristics of the neonate to assess gestational maturity was in routine use.[18,19] They are noted here to underscore the uncertainty of that basic premise, or definition, on which much of our presumed knowledge of the SGA infant is based.

Low birth weight for gestational age is the most commonly employed index for diagnosis. Because a neonate of any gestational age may have an unusually low birth weight, preterm, term, and post-term infants may be SGA. Of concern are an unknown number of newborns whose birth weights may fall along "normal" percentiles for gestational age but who, nonetheless, have not achieved their full growth potential. For example, some infants have the genetic potential to be unusually large. They may manifest wasting and fetal asphyxia even though their weights do not fall below the norm for gestational age. These infants, often called dysmature, may be recognized by their clinical appearance.[20,21] At death, they may show alterations in organ weights typical for the SGA infant.[22] Because our usual definition is based on a low weight for gestational age, their condition may escape clinical notice. As a consequence, such infants have not been carefully evaluated. Attention has recently been directed toward evaluation of physical measurements other than weight in distinguishing impaired from normal fetal growth.[23-35] While these will be discussed in detail in the following section, it is important to recognize that we broaden considerably our operational definition of fetal growth retardation by accepting dysproportionate body growth in babies who are not "light-for-dates" as evidence of altered or impaired fetal growth.

DIAGNOSIS

Fetal

A variety of methods have been proposed in the search for early and precise diagnosis of impaired fetal growth. These techniques have been evaluated, nearly without exception, on a retrospective basis; prospective,

Table 15-1. Fetal Diagnosis of SGA by Ultrasound.

Measurement	Predictive Accuracy (%)	Reference
Head circ./abdomen circ.	71	65
Crown-rump length × trunk area	68	66
Trunk circumference	94	67
Abdomen circumference	63–87	70
Intrauterine volume	75	71
Head area/chest area	72	73

randomized clinical trials have not been performed. It is not surprising, therefore, that usefulness of these methods is uncertain and varies widely from one report to another. Clinical assessment of **risk factors in the maternal or pregnancy history** may be useful in as few as one-third or as many as two-thirds of these cases.[36,37] History of maternal renovascular disease, multiple pregnancy, or previous SGA births accounts for most of these successful (retrospective) predictions. Use of such **simple clinical methods** as manual estimation of fetal weight, maternal assessment of fetal activity, or serial measurement of fundal height are lauded by some and condemned by others.[38–41] Several **biochemical indices of (feto) placental function** have been proposed as useful; none are proven by prospective, controlled trial. Among these are diminished levels of crystine aminopeptidase, oxytocinase, human placental lactogen, β_1-glycoprotein and estriol, as well as elevated levels of α-fetoprotein, heat-stable alkaline phosphatase, N-acetyl-β-glucosaminidase and α-aminonitrogen in maternal serum.[42–51,185,200] Measurement of amniotic fluid hydroxyproline as an index of fetal collagen turnover and growth activity makes physiologic sense but is clinically unproven.[52,53]

Studies by Metcoff and others have clearly shown **biochemical changes in leucocytes** obtained from maternal venous and umbilical cord blood obtained at delivery of SGA babies.[54,55] Among the changes observed have been diminished contents of pyruvic kinase, adenylic kinase, ATP and total adenine nucleotides, and an increased protein/DNA ratio. These findings, interpreted as demonstrating a diminished "energy capacity" and increased size for these cells, have also been observed in maternal venous leucocytes prior to birth of SGA babies.[56] Other changes include a decreased content of RNA polymerase and impaired activation of fructose-1-6-phosphate, as well as altered kinetic characteristics of pyruvic kinase in maternal leucocytes and increased amino acid (leucine and proline) incorporation into protein in placental polysomes.[56–60] In addition, the same group has demonstrated a modest but statistically significant relation of maternal serum carotene (r = +0.31), plasma zinc (r = +0.21) and a number of serum amino acid concentrations (r = +0.41 to +0.59) to birth weight.[59] The clinical usefulness of these observations in the accurate prediction or precise postnatal diagnosis of impaired fetal growth is untested and awaits further study.

Ultrasonic cephalometry has been helpful in determining rate of growth of the biparietal diameter (BPD) of the head. When growth rate is less than optimal, 53% to 82% of such infants have been found to have birth weights below the tenth percentile for gestational age.[61–63] Use of serial changes in BPD appears to have a low false-negative rate but an unacceptably high false-positive rate; specificity is good but sensitivity is poor.[64] Recently, sophisticated sonar evaluation providing measurements of crown-rump length; chest, trunk, abdominal, and head circumferences and areas; intrauterine volume; and a variety of ratios, products and other combinations of these measurements has improved the sensitivity of ultrasound as a predictor of impaired fetal growth.[64–73] It now appears possible to accurately predict patterns of impaired fetal growth with a better than 70% accuracy using these techniques, as summarized in Table 15-1.

Neonatal

Reduced birth weight for gestational age ("light-for dates") is the simplest and oldest method of diagnosis. Observations, however,

Table 15-2. Neonatal Diagnosis of SGA by Physical Examination.

Measurement	Result	Reference
Birth weight	light	35
Crown-heel, femoral, foot length	short	23, 24, 28, 30
Head, chest, abdominal, thigh circ.	small	23, 24, 30
Breast tissue	reduced	35
Epiphyseal development	delayed	28, 34
Skin-fold thickness	reduced	23, 26, 29, 33
Anterior fontanelle	large	28
Head circ./weight	reduced	35
Crown-heel length/head circ.	< 1.36	24
Birth weight × 100/crown-heel length³	< 2.0 to 2.3	24, 29, 30, 32

suggesting that some infants of appropriate weight may demonstrate **evidences of wasting** or disproportionate growth, as well as speculations that the presence, absence, or nature of **altered body proportions** in these infants may provide a clue to the timing and cause of impaired fetal growth has recently led to more careful assessments of physical findings at birth (Table 15-2). Soft tissue wasting, diminished skin-fold thickness, decreased breast tissue and reduced thigh circumference have been cited as evidence for recent wasting and have been suggested, by some, as useful measurements for neonatal diagnosis.[23,26,29,35] Widened skull sutures and large fontanelles, diminished foot, femoral, and crown-heel length and delayed development of epiphyses have been cited as failures in bone growth.[12,23,24,28,30,32,34] Combinations of measurements such as weight/head circumference, crown-heel length/head circumference, and birth weight/crown-heel length have been used with increasing frequency to assess disproportionate patterns of growth.[24,29,30,32,35] More careful attention to these as well as other measures of quality of fetal growth seems certain to expand our knowledge of this condition. Unquestioning acceptance of the currently popular use of these observations as describing "types" as well as "causes" of SGA,[25,27,30,31] however, does not appear to be justified.[28] Clinical simplifications appear to have preceded a sound knowledge of cause-and-effect relationships in this regard.

CAUSES

Normal intrauterine growth for body weight, length, and organ weights progresses in a systematic fashion between 28 and 38 weeks of gestation. From about 38 weeks onward, growth of the fetus and placenta departs from this previous pattern.[75] Stated simply, two major factors influence fetal growth: the inherent growth potential of the fetus and the growth support it receives by way of the placenta from the mother.[76] Certain factors which have been suggested to cause or accompany impaired fetal growth are summarized in Table 15-3.

Altered Growth Potential

Most current writing ignores the extraordinary variations in birth weight observed between populations. The classic study of Meredith[77] reviews these data in detail and brings to our attention that mean birth weights may vary from 2400 g (in New Guinea)[78] to 3880 g (in the West Indies).[79] Of particular interest are certain data which demonstrate striking ethnic differences in birth weight, regardless of current socioeconomic status or geographic location.[76,80-82] Whether such observations are the consequence of genetic variation, prior intrauterine experience on the part of the mother, or whatever, is unclear.[83] What is clear, however, is that racial, ethnic, and population differences in expected birth weight at a given gestational age are considerable.

Retardation of growth *in utero* may be caused by factors inherent in the fetus itself. Subnormal embryonic growth may then be viewed as a form of maldevelopment. Examples of causes include certain genetically determined dwarfs, fetal infections, chromosomal syndromes, several congenital anomalies and some inborn errors of metabolism.[12,76,84-98,201] In certain of these forms of

Table 15-3. Factors Suggested to Cause (or be Associated with) Impaired Fetal Growth (References in Text).

Altered Growth Potential	Impaired Support for Growth
I. Genetic/Racial/Ethnic/Population	I. Placental
II. Fetal	A. Anatomic
A. Genetic dwarfs/leprechauns	1. infarcts
B. Osteogenesis imperfecta	2. partial separation (occult abruptio/abdominal implantation)
C. Congenital infection	3. hemangioma
1. rubella	4. aberrant cord insertions
2. cytomegalovirus	5. single umbilical artery
3. toxoplasmosis	B. Microscopic
D. Chromosomal syndromes	1. umbilical vascular thrombosis
E. Congenital anomalies	2. avascular terminal villi
1. cardiac	3. diffuse fibrinosis
2. anencephaly	
3. Cornelia de Lange syndrome	II. Maternal
4. gastrointestinal atresia and obstruction	A. Reduced uteroplacental blood flow
5. Potter syndrome	1. pregnancy-induced hypertension
6. pancreatic agenesis	2. chronic renovascular disease
7. parabiotic twins	3. smoking
F. Inborn errors of metabolism	B. Primiparity/grandmultiparity
1. transient neonatal diabetes	C. Multiple gestation
2. galactosemia	D. Small stature/low weight/socioeconomic
3. phenylketonuria	E. Drugs
G. Female sex	1. narcotics, alcohol, x-ray, teratogens
	F. Hypoxemia
	1. hemoglobinopathies (esp. SS)
	2. altitude
	G. Behavioral

SGA, reduced cell number has been demonstrated.[92,93,99,100] It is fascinating to speculate what clues these cruel experiments of nature may provide us. For example, retarded fetal growth in the infant with intestinal or central nervous system anomalies which preclude normal swallowing may suggest that amniotic fluid is a more important source of nutrients than currently suspected.[75,337–339] Of equal interest is the presence of profoundly impaired growth in infants with end-organ insensitivity to insulin,[96] as well as in infants with pancreatic agenesis,[94] observations which provide a tantalizing glimpse of the importance of insulin/cell relationships in the growth process. Despite these as well as other provocative associations, precise sequences for these events are poorly understood. While most of these "inherent" forms of SGA have an early onset, and therefore might be expected to result in "proportionate" undergrowth, exceptions are striking and common.[84,85,89,94]

Impaired Support for Growth

Before the third trimester of pregnancy, supply far exceeds needs of the fetal organism and growth is determined by inherent fetal potential. By the third trimester, the adequacy of the supply line becomes the limiting factor in fetal growth. Multiple pregnancy is an example of this. In this situation, each fetus may have a normal growth potential, but the placenta is inadequate to meet the full supply demands of multiple fetuses. Unrestricted growth of twins occurs until a cumulative weight of about 3000 g, and growth retardation begins at about 1500 g body weight for each twin. Few cases of growth retardation occur in the early weeks of the third trimester, but after 32 to 34 weeks of gestation abnormalities in fetal growth are more common, becoming prominent as pregnancy continues past term.[21,101,102] The functional reserve of the placenta, so abundant early in pregnancy, becomes insufficient. The development of chronic fetal distress, with its attendant growth retardation, then depends on the duration of intrauterine life beyond the capacity of a placenta to nurture. Such a situation, often termed "placental insufficiency," is recognized most often in post-term gestations but may occur at any time during gestation.

A wide variety of anatomic abnormalities have been described in the SGA placenta.[103,104,111] It appears probable that many of these—gross or microscopic infarctions, hemangiomas, aberrant cord insertions, single umbilical artery, or umbilical vascular thrombosis—may impair fetal growth. Premature placental separation (occult abruptio), avascular terminal villi, and diffuse fibrinosis, all factors which may reduce placental surface area for exchange, may also be reasonably suspected of having a more than casual relation to an SGA outcome.[105] Interpretation of these findings is difficult. Placental tissue, as examined and analyzed at birth, is fetal tissue. As such, it shares the same reduced potentials for growth as the fetus. An unpleasant intrauterine environment is likely to affect placental as well as fetal development. It is therefore not surprising that SGA babies have small placentas; in most instances, however, the fetal/placental weight ratio is normal.

The most commonly recognized associations with SGA are those which affect the fetus by way of the mother. Perhaps most commonly discussed and best proven is the association of SGA with maternal vascular compromise. Although it is not proven that **reduction in uteroplacental blood flow** is a cause of impaired fetal growth in the human, maternal conditions that reduce placental blood flow (preeclampsia, toxemia, and chronic hypertensive vascular disease) are often associated with SGA.[112] Diminished clearance of radioactive sodium and obliterative-degenerative lesions in the spiral arteries of the myometrium and decidua have been described in toxemia and chronic hypertension, suggesting reduced uteroplacental blood flow.[113] A provocative case report by Theobald describes *in utero* death of an SGA fetus in a mother with iliac artery hypoplasia and hypertension.[114] Following denervation of the iliac vessels, subsequent pregnancies were accompanied by normal fetal growth and outcome. Diabetes mellitus with severe microangiopathy also causes reduced placental flow and growth-retarded babies.[92,115]

Living at high **altitudes,** with lowered oxygen environment, reduces birth weight.[116] **Teratogens,** such as antimetabolites or alkylating agents, and irradiation may also lower birth weight during pregnancy.[84] Other maternal factors associated with subnormal birth weight include maternal **small stature, smoking, low socioeconomic class, low maternal age, primiparity, grand multiparity, and low prepregnancy weight.**[92,124] Effects of maternal short stature, low socioeconomic class, multiparity, and smoking reduce birth weight at term by about 200 g or less.[101,102] Smoking reduces length as well as weight of the baby.[243]

Maternal **narcotic** usage in pregnancy is clearly associated with poor fetal growth.[118] Maternal **alcohol** intake, even in socially acceptable quantities, appears to be accompanied by serious compromise in both quantity and quality of fetal growth.[119,120] **Hemoglobinopathies,** especially with sickle cell hemoglobin, also commonly result in SGA babies.[121] In addition, offspring of mothers with **phenylketonuria** consistently show growth retardation and are often microcephalic at birth.[122] Observations of diminished platelet life span in pregnancies with SGA babies suggest the relation of a **thrombocytolytic state** in the mother with poor fetal growth.[123] A reported relation between birth weight and **maternal hematocrit** is convincing ($r = +0.64$),[125] at least until one reads of evidence to the direct contrary.[126] Preliminary data suggest an impact of asymptomatic **pyelonephritis,** as detected by antibody-coated bacteria in maternal urine, on fetal growth.[127] Recent evidence of poor mothering and other improper behavioral characteristics in many women who deliver SGA infants deserves careful attention and further study.[128] The suggestion that inappropriate **maternal behavior** during pregnancy may be a major factor in impaired fetal growth may alter our view from that of the mother as a passive funnel through which the ravages of disease and a hostile environment affect the fetus, to one of the mother as the cause, by her inappropriate actions or inactions, of compromised fetal growth.

Whether or not improper **maternal nutrition** during human pregnancy has any appreciable effect on the birth of the fetus is entirely uncertain, despite the volume of views supporting this theory which have been published recently.[129–138] War famines have been clearly shown to result in a modest decline in birth weight.[139–142] The most profound effect of such disasters (during which, incidently, poor nutrition is but one of a multitude of hurtful events) would appear to be infertility and an increase in spontaneous abortions. It is important to note that an effect on birth weight is seen only when starvation occurs during the last trimester of pregnancy. The observations made during these studies confirm, rather than deny, the concept of the fetus as a true parasite, living off maternal nutrient stores, despite her lack of proper intake.

The role of chronic maternal malnutrition, which precedes conception and continues throughout gestation, on the production of SGA is even less well understood. Data from human studies are limited and difficult to interpret. The clinical meaning, for example, of statistically significant relations between diet quality (an artificial, retrospective index) and birth weight ($r = +0.30$),[137] between calories supplemented and birth weight ($r = +0.13$),[134] or between maternal protein levels and birth weight,[143] are open to serious question.[144] Altered essential/nonessential amino acid ratios in the SGA infant and between the infant and mother at birth have been suggested by some[51,129,147–149] but denied by the carefully done studies of others.[145,146] Sinclair and Saigal have noted that "it is a central problem of perinatal medicine to know the relative contributions of heredity and environment to the variance in fetal growth rate, and, among the environmental factors, to know the effect of maternal undernutrition."[138] The problem of clearly defining the weighted roles of nature and nurture in the SGA infant remains unresolved.

COMPOSITIONAL CHANGES IN SGA

Animal Models

Many of our clinical and pathophysiologic views of SGA have their origin in animal experimental work.[150–184,186–199,202–208,211–213] While it is unclear how much can be "transposed" from these animal data, it is important that we understand the methods and models employed as well as the variations and occasional contradictions in results. Details from

selected examples are summarized in Table 15-4. As will be seen, some findings in these animal models are similar to those observed in human SGA infants while some are different. For most of these animal data, however, parallel observations in the human SGA baby are not available—the work has not yet been done.

Animal models have included hamsters, rabbits, sheep, guinea pigs, mice, pigs, and monkeys, but the rat has been studied most frequently. Methods employed to hamper fetal growth have included maternal administration of immunosuppressants, alloxan or narcotics, diet restriction both during later pregnancy as well as from the time of conception, fetal pancreatic and partial intestinal ablation, placental embolization with microspheres, partial surgical ablation of the placenta, ligation of placental vessels leading to the secondary placental disc, unilateral umbilical artery ligation, unilateral or bilateral uterine vascular clamping or ligation, unilateral maternal nephrectomy with contralateral renal artery constriction or contralateral nephrectomy, induction of post-term delivery, fetal streptozotocin, or even decapitation or removal of fetal brain by aspiration. In one instance, natural runts have been studied. Timing of these insults has varied from study to study and relation of the compromise to specific developmental and growth sequences in both the animal model and the (extrapolated) human are, for the most part, uncertain.[202,203]

The Human SGA Infant

When comparing SGA infants of greater gestational age to premature infants of the same birth weight, one finds that brain and heart remain large in proportion to the reduction in body weight, while the liver, spleen, adrenals, placenta, and thymus are smaller.[21,92,101] A variety of compositional differences have been reported in the human SGA infant. Some of these are summarized in Table 15-5.

The **placenta** has been studied most often.[56,60,106–110,209,210,214,215,217,231] Enhanced protein synthesis, aromatizing capacity, and glycogen utilization have been observed but diminished oxygen consumption has also been reported. Increased RNA polymerase activity and reduced RNA content have been found. Decreases in DNA and nitrogen content are compatible with a reduced cell number in the

Table 15-4. Animal Models of Impaired Fetal Growth

Animal	Procedure/References	Fetal Effects
Hamster	Maternal narcotics[150]	↓ weight
Rabbit	Maternal/fetal narcotics[186]	↓ weight
		↑ pulmonary maturation
	Fetal alloxan[191]	↓ weight
	Decapitation[212]	**no change** in weight
Sheep	Single umbilical artery ligation[151−153]	↓ weight
		placental infarction
		↓ glucose uptake
		↓ umbilical blood flow:
		? ↑ birth asphyxia but normal placental gas exchange
	Placental embolization with 15 μ microspheres[154−156]	↓ weight
		↓ placental gas exchange; hypoxemia
		↑ fibrinogen, hematocrit
		↓ cardiac output and blood flow to lung; ↑ flow to brain and heart
	Dietary restriction[194,208]	↓ weight (esp. liver and spleen)
	Fetal pancreatic and partial intestinal ablation[190]	↓ weight
	Partial surgical ablation of placenta[207]	↓ weight
Guinea Pig	Dietary restriction[196,206]	↓ weight
		↓ brain weight, cholesterol, cerebroside, and sulfatide
		↓ cerebellar weight, DNA, and protein
		↓ cerebral DNA, weight/DNA, and protein/DNA
		↓ muscle DNA, protein/DNA
Monkey	Fetal streptozotocin[192]	↓ weight
	Ligation of placental vessels leading to 2° placental disc[183,184,193]	↓ weight
		↓ organ weight (esp. liver and spleen)
		↑ brain/body and brain/liver weight
		↓ cerebral DNA
		↓ cerebellar DNA, RNA, and protein; ↑ H_2O
		↓ liver DNA, RNA, protein, fat, and glycogen
		↓ muscle DNA, RNA, protein, protein/DNA, and protein/RNA; ↓ water
Pig	Natural runts[182,189,197,206]	↓ weight
		↓ organ weight (esp. liver and small intestine)
		↑ brain/body weight
		no change in brain DNA, RNA, protein, or ganglioside
		↓ liver CHO, protein
		↓ muscle protein/DNA
		↓ renal protein/DNA
		↓ bone growth and development

(Continued on next page)

Table 15-4. Animal Models of Impaired Fetal Growth – (Continued)

Animal	Procedure/References	Fetal Effects
Mouse	Irradiation of hypophysis[211]	**no change** in weight
Rat	Immunosuppressants[157]	↓ weight
		↓ placental weight
	Post-term birth[177,178]	↓ weight
		↑ brain/body and brain/liver weight; ↑ % dry mass
		↓ liver % dry mass
		↓ renal % dry mass
	Unilateral renal artery constriction and contralateral nephrectomy[179]	**no change** in weight
	Unilateral nephrectomy and contralateral heminephrectomy[180]	**no change** in weight so long as nutrition adequate
	Narcotics[188]	**no change** in weight
	Brain removal by aspiration[181]	↓ weight
		no change in placental weight
	Decapitation[213]	**no change** in weight
	Dietary restriction[175,176,198,199,204,205,209,210]	↓ weight
		↑ N loss after birth
		no change in maternal glucagon or neonatal/maternal glucose
		↓ insulin
		↓ placental weight, DNA; ↑ RNA/DNA; **no change** in protein DNA
	Bilateral uterine vascular ligation[174]	↓ weight
		↓ neonatal/maternal glucose
		↑ insulin
		↓ maternal glucagon
	Uterine vascular clamping[158,159]	↓ weight
		↑ malformation, depending on timing
	Unilateral uterine vascular ligation[152,160–173,208–210]	↓ weight
		↓ or **no change** in placental weight
		↓ organ weights (esp. liver)
		↑ brain/body and brain/liver weight
		↑,↓ or **no change** in brain, RNA, DNA and protein
		↑ or **no change** in brain protein/DNA
		↓ or **no change** in brain RNA/DNA
		↓ DNA synthesis from thymidine (esp. in cerebellum)
		↓ synaptosomal sphingomyelin, cephalin, protein, DNA and RNA
		↑ synaptosomal γ-aminobutyric acid, glutamine, and glutamic acid
		maldistribution of succinate dehydrogenase between synaptosomes and mitochondria
		↓ liver glycogen, glucose, total lipids, phospholipids, protein, DNA, and fructose-1-6-disphosphate
		↓ hepatic gluconeogenesis; ↑ glycogen synthesis

(Continued on next page)

Table 15-4. Animal Models of Impaired Fetal Growth—(Continued)

Animal	Procedure/References	Fetal Effects
Rat (*continued*)	Unilateral uterine vascular ligation (*continued*)	↑ or **no change** in total body water ↓ or **no change** in carcass dry fat-free solids ↓ or **no change** in total body fat ↓ glucose, total protein and free fatty acids ↑,↓ or **no change** in hematocrit ↓ DNA synthesis from thymidine (esp. in cerebellum) ↓ or **no change** in placental weight or DNA; **no change** or ↑ in placental RNA and RNA/DNA **no change** or ↓ placental protein/DNA, depending on timing ↓ histamine decarboxylase

organ. It is important to recognize that these disturbances are not consistent findings in placentas from all SGA babies. For example, many of these changes are apparently absent in placentas from SGA infants with malformations.

Several studies of **muscle** composition have been performed.[86,93,99,100,195,216,218,219,222,223] Wide variations in patient selection, study age, and methods of analysis have contributed to discrepancies in the results. At present, it is uncertain under what circumstances of impaired fetal growth a reduced cell number, size, or both occur in the human fetus. Studies of **visceral organs** are scant and results must be judged as preliminary at this time.[74,92,100,216,221]

Biochemical alterations found in **brains** from SGA human infants include a decreased cerebroside-sulfatide content and galactolipid sulfotransferase enzyme activity. These components are necessary in myelin lipid formation. Because myelin is formed primarily postnatally in the human, it is possible that these deficits may be reversible after birth. Lipids found mainly in neuronal tissue (phospholipid and ganglioside) are not reduced in term SGA infants.[220] Significant reductions in mucopolysaccharides (hyaluronic acid, chondroitin sulfate, and heparin sulfate) have also been reported.[224]

In vivo studies of body water and its distribution in SGA babies demonstrate a sizable

Table 15-5. Compositional Changes in Human SGA Infants (references in text)

Organ	Findings
Placenta	↓ or **no change** in weight ↓ or **no change** in DNA ↓,↑ or **no change** in RNA; ↑ RNA polymerase ↑ or **no change** in RNA/DNA **no change** in protein/DNA ↓ or **no change** in protein or N ↓ glycogen; ↑ glycogen utilization ↓ oxygen utilization ↑ aromatizing capacity ↑ protein synthesis (from leucine and proline) ↓ heat-stable alkaline phosphatase ↑ inhibition of urokinase-induced fibrinolysis
Muscle	↓ or **no change** in total water; ↑ ICW and ↓ or ↑ ECW ↑,↓ or **no change** in DNA; ↓ RNA; ↓ protein/DNA; ↓ RNA/DNA

(*Continued on next page*)

Table 15-5. Compositional Changes in Human SGA Infants (references in text)—(Continued)

Organ	Findings
Muscle (*continued*)	↓ protein
	↓ Zn, K, Mg; ↑ Na
	↓ fat
Adipose tissue	↓ protein and collagen
Brain	↓ weight (esp. cerebellar)
	↓ DNA (cell number) in cerebellum
	↓ myelin lipids (cerebroside and sulfatide)
	↓ galactolipid sulfotransferase
	↓ glycosaminoglycans in protein/DNA
Liver	↓ weight
	no change in DNA or protein/DNA
	↓ glycogen
Heart	**no change** in DNA or protein/DNA
	↓ sarcoplasmic mass
	↓ glycogen
Adrenal	↓ fetal zone
Water compartments	↑ TBW (esp. ECW)

increase in body water per kilogram of body weight.[225–230] Expanded plasma volume and cell water spaces are particularly prominent in infants studied soon after birth and in those with the most severe degrees of growth retardation. Prompt, downward adjustments return these spaces to normal within 4 to 6 hours of birth, while more sluggish adjustments are observed in extracellular and total water compartments. All of these studies, to date, have been cross-sectional. Sequential studies, accompanied by concurrent estimations of acid-base balance, will be required to determine whether the early excess in cell water is a consequence of impaired cellular metabolism and increased cellular acidity in the SGA fetus.

FUNCTIONAL CHANGES IN SGA

Biochemical and metabolic consequences of impaired fetal growth have been studied extensively. While a number of these changes would appear to be real, having been noted by several authors, their exact pathophysiologic sequences and consequences are still open to some speculation. Selected observations are summarized in Table 15-6.

Elevated blood levels of **serum nitrogen products** (ammonia, urea, and uric acid) may reflect diminished caloric reserves and a protein catabolic state in the SGA baby.[232–234] Low **urine hydroxyproline/creatinine ratios** at birth and a rapid rise in this ratio as well as in **glycosaminoglycan excretion** during the first postnatal week have been interpreted by some to reflect poor fetal but rapid postnatal growth in these babies.[235–238] While observations of reduced amniotic fluid hydroxyproline in these same infants[52,53] tend to confirm these thoughts, there is some disagreement.[239] There are many reports of disorders in **serum protein levels;** low total protein, prealbumin, and IgG (especially IgG$_1$) levels have been found.[240–242,244–248] Again, not all authors agree.[241,242] Reduced humoral as well as cellular **immunocompetence** has also been reported in SGA babies.[249–253] Whether these altered protein levels are caused by impaired placental transfer or by compromised production is unclear. A relation between elevated IgM levels and intrauterine infection seems more certain.[262]

A number of **hematologic disturbances** have been documented. Elevated hematocrits and increased red cell volumes[12,226,254,255] may be consequent to acute placental-fetal transfusion during episodes of fetal hypoxia[256] or to an elevation of erythropoietin from chronic fetal hypoxemia.[257] As expected, increased viscosity is a further consequence of this polycythemia,[258] and there is some evidence that high hematocrits in the SGA baby lead to coagulation disturbances.[259–260] Unexpectedly, the reticulocyte counts in these babies are normal but the "reticulocyte index" (corrected for hematocrit) is elevated.[255,261]

Altered **oxygen consumption** has been noted by several authors.[263–270] An increased metabolic rate in these infants may be a consequence of imbalances between organs with a high oxygen utilization (such as brain, the growth of which is least reduced in the SGA baby) and other organs with a lower consumption (thymus, spleen, and liver, whose weights are reduced the most). More recent

early detection and prompt intervention. Proof of the clinical utility of early enteral feeding in stabilizing blood glucose levels or the ability of hydrocortisone to correct the defective gluconeogenesis in these babies awaits prospective clinical trial.[305] Also unclear are the clinical implications of animal data showing reduced CSF glucose in spite of elevated plasma glucose levels[306] and the diagnostic usefulness of elevated plasma pressors, triglycerides, plasma and urine xanthines, or CSF lactate levels in defining the severity of asphyxia in some of these infants.[306–311]

Prior to discharge from the nursery, an especially thorough **search for anomalies** should be made. This should include appropriate **screening for intrauterine infections,** most of which are clinically silent.[262]

OUTCOME (See also Chap. 19)

The ultimate developmental prognosis certainly depends on the cause of impaired fetal growth. A fetus with a normal growth potential whose growth is impaired by an insult of limited severity and duration may have a more happy outcome than one whose compromise may predate conception or may have begun in early fetal life. Recent data suggest, however, that while these views seem logical, they may not necessarily be correct.[28] Furthermore, follow-up studies require meticulous design for results to be more than anecdotal. There must be controls, matched at least in terms of socioeconomic status and perinatal morbidity. Adequate numbers are required and factors of selection, details of perinatal care received, illnesses suffered, and treatments provided require precise and complete description. Ideally, methods should be reproducible, employing hard data concerning motor and neurologic development, auditory and visual capabilities, EEG changes, growth measurements and so forth, rather than using impressionistic soft data such as IQ/DQ tests, personality or behavioral deviations, speech development, perceptual or reading disorders, and so on. The studies should be prospective; attrition rate should be so low that it cannot possibly affect the results; methods used should be standard, proven, and reproducible; and the examiners should be "blinded" as to whether each baby is a study or control subject. As there are not follow-up studies of SGA infants which meet even these minimum requirements, our views of outcome for these infants must be considered tentative and preliminary at this time.

There appears to be general agreement that many SGA babies will ultimately be **more slim and less tall** than their gestational or weight peers.[13,28,76,312–319,335] Not all authors agree on this point, however.[320–322,325] Of particular interest is one recent report which suggests a return to normal body proportions (ponderal index) in certain SGA babies.[320] These discrepancies make it difficult to interpret the clinical meaning of reports suggesting a beneficial effect on growth patterns of human growth hormone therapy in SGA babies.[323,324] Degree of fetal growth impairment appears to predict postnatal growth achievement poorly,[13,28] but velocity of growth in the early months after birth may be an important indicator of ultimate size.[13,313,316] Particularly fascinating are recent studies suggesting a critical role for insulin in "catch-up" growth.[325,326] A significant, positive correlation between linear growth velocity and insulin release after glucose load,[325] and the impact of insulin on growth patterns in transient neonatal diabetes[94,326] suggest an important role for this hormone in the postnatal growth of an SGA baby. Delayed eruption of teeth and enamel hypoplasia have been found in SGA infants and appear related to impaired fetal skeletal growth.[319] The pattern of **head circumference** growth may parallel that of weight and height.[327] However, Babson found an accelerated rate of head growth over the first 4 years of life, with weight and length following the same growth percentile present at birth.[328]

Most studies demonstrate **normal IQ/DQ** results when infants with overt anomalies and clinically detectable congenital infections are excluded.[14,315,321,328,333,336] Major **neurologic problems have been infrequent** in the term SGA,[14,315] and recent data are conflicting as to whether significant defects are present in the preterm, undergrown baby.[314,321] **Motor behavior** after birth is significantly reduced.[332] Other behavioral changes are difficult to interpret,[315,329,330] especially in view of the important observation that improper "mothering" behavior is common after birth of SGA infants.[331] This **altered maternal acceptance** of the SGA baby is perhaps most evident in the significant increase in adoptions in SGA babies.[331] It is particularly important to note the wide variety in outcomes for these babies. Available data clearly demonstrate that the infant is not doomed to damage by virtue of being SGA alone. In fact, degree of impairment of fetal growth has shown no correlation with subsequent development in all studies where this factor has been examined. Most important in this regard are recent studies suggesting that severe perinatal asphyxia may play a major role in the outcome of these infants.[314,334,336]

REFERENCES

1. **McBurney RD:** The undernourished full-term infant: A case report. West J Surg 55:363, 1947

2. **Colman HI, Rienzo J:** The small term baby. Obstet Gynecol 19:87, 1962

3. **Söderling B:** Pseudoprematurity. Acta Paediatr 42:520, 1953

4. **Gruenwald P:** Chronic fetal distress and placental insufficiency. Biol Neonate 5:215, 1963

5. **Gruenwald P:** Infants of low birth weight among 5,000 deliveries. Pediatrics 34:157, 1964

6. Public Health Aspects of Low Birth Weight. World Health Organization Technical Report, Series 217, 1961

7. **Walker J:** Small-for-dates—clinical aspects. Proc R Soc Med 60:877, 1967

8. **Mata L, Urrutia JJ, Mohs E:** Implicaciones de bajo peso al nacer para la salud publica. Arch Latinoam Nutr (Suppl. 1) 27:198, 1977

9. **Belizán JM, Lechtig A, Villar J:** Letter: Distribution of low-birth-weight babies in developing countries. Am J Obstet Gynecol 132:704, 1978

10. **Lugo G, Cassady G:** Intrauterine growth retardation: Clinicopathologic findings in 233 consecutive infants. Am J Obstet Gynecol 109:615, 1971

11. **Gruenwald P, Dawkins M, Hepner R:** Panel discussion: Chronic deprivation of the fetus. Sinai Hospital Journal 11:51, 1963

12. **Usher RH:** Clinical and therapeutic aspects of fetal malnutrition. Pediatr Clin North Am 17:169, 1970

13. **Fitzhardinge PM, Steven EM:** The small-for-date infant, I. Later growth patterns. Pediatrics 49:671, 1972

14. **Fitzhardinge PM, Steven EM:** The small-for-date infant, II. Neurological and intellectual sequelae. Pediatrics 50:50, 1972

15. **Lubchenco LO, Hansman C, Dressler M, Boyd E:** Intrauterine growth as estimated from liveborn birth-weight data at 24 to 42 weeks gestation. Pediatrics 32:793, 1963

16. **Gruenwald P:** Growth of the human fetus, I. Normal growth and its variation. Am J Obstet Gynecol 94:1112, 1966

17. **Freeman MG, Graves WL, Thompson RI:** Indigent Negro and Caucasian birth-weight, gestational age tables. Pediatrics 46:9, 1970

18. **Usher RH, McLean F, Scott KE:** Judgement of fetal age, II. Clinical significance of gestational age and an objective method for its assessment. Pediatr Clin North Am 13:835, 1966

19. **Dubowitz LMS, Dubowitz V, Goldberg C:** Clinical assessment of gestational age in the newborn. J Pediatr 77:1,1970

20. **Sjöstedt S, Engleson G, Rooth G:** Dysmaturity. Arch Dis Child 33:123, 1958

21. **Gruenwald P:** The fetus in prolonged pregnancy. Am J Obstet Gynecol 89:503, 1964

22. **Gruenwald P:** Deprivation of the human fetus: Forms, causes, and significance. In Adamsons E (ed): Diagnosis and Treatment of Fetal Disorders, pp 1–14. New York, Springer-Verlag, 1968

23. **McLean F, Usher R:** Measurements of liveborn fetal malnutrition infants compared with similar gestational and with similar birth-weight normal controls. Biol Neonate, 16: 215, 1970

24. **Miller H, Hassanein K:** Diagnosis of impaired fetal growth in newborn infants. Pediatrics 48:511, 1971

25. **Urrusti J, Yoshida P, Velasco L, Frenk S et al:** Human fetal growth retardation, I. Clinical features of sample with intrauterine retardation. Pediatrics 50:547, 1972

26. **Brans YW, Sumners JE, Dweck HS, Cassady G:** A non-invasive approach to body composition in the neonate: Dynamic skinfold measurements. Pediatr Res 8:215, 1974

27. **Rossa P, Winick M:** Intrauterine growth retardation: A new systematic approach based on the clinical and biochemical characteristics of this condition. J Perinat Med 2:147, 1974

28. **Philip AGS:** Fetal growth retardation: Femurs, fontanelles, and follow-up. Pediatrics 62:446, 1978

29. **Roord JJ, Ramaekers LHJ:** Quantifications of intrauterine malnutrition. Biol Neonate 33:273, 1978

30. **Woods DL, Malan AF, deV.Heese H:** Patterns of retarded fetal growth. Early Hum Dev 3: 257, 1979

31. **Daikoku NH, Johnson JWC, Graf C, Kearney K, Tyson JE, King TM:** Intrauterine growth retardation, I. Patterns. Obstet Gynecol 54: 211, 1979

32. **Lubchenco LO:** Assessment of gestational age and development at birth. Pediatr Clin North Am 17:125, 1970

33. **Gampel B:** The relation of skinfold thickness in the neonate to sex, length of gestation, size at birth, and maternal skinfold. Hum Biol 37:29, 1965

34. **Scott KE, Usher RH:** Epiphyseal development in fetal malnutrition syndrome. New Engl J Med 270:822, 1964

35. **Brans YW, Cassady G:** Intrauterine growth and maturation in relation to fetal deprivation. In Gruenwald P (ed): The Placenta, pp 307–334. Lancaster, Medical and Technical Publishing Co, 1975

36. **Tejani N, Mann LI, Weiss RR:** Antenatal diagnosis and management of the small-for-gestational-age fetus. Obstet Gynecol 47:31, 1976

37. **Galbraith RS, Karchmar EJ, Piercy WN, Low JA:** The clinical prediction of intrauterine growth retardation. Am J Obstet Gynecol 133:281, 1979

38. **Mathews DD:** Maternal assessment of fetal activity in small-for-dates infants. Obstet Gynecol 45:488, 1975

39. **Belizán JM, Villar J, Nardin JC, Malamud J, Vicuña LS:** Diagnosis of intrauterine growth retardation by simple clinical method: Measurement of uterine height. Am J Obstet Gynecol 131:643, 1978

40. **Beazley JM, Underhill RA:** Fallacy of the fundal height. Br Med J 4:404, 1970

41. **Ong HC, Sen DK:** Clinical estimation of fetal weight. Am J Obstet Gynecol 112:877, 1972

42. **Chapman L, Burrows-Peakin R, Rege VP, Silk E:** Serum cystine aminopeptidase and the small-for-dates baby in hypertensive pregnancy. Br J Obstet Gynaecol 83:238, 1976

43. **Pathak S, Himaya A, Mosher R:** The small-for-dates syndrome: Some biochemical considerations in prenatal diagnosis. Am J Obstet Gynecol 120:32, 1974

44. **Hensleigh PA, Cheatum SG, Spellacy WN:** Oxytocinase and human placental lactogen for prediction of intrauterine growth retardation. Am J Obstet Gynecol 129:675, 1977

45. **Spellacy WN:** Human placental lactogen and intrauterine growth retardation. Obstet Gynecol 47:446, 1976

46. **Daikoku NH, Tyson JE, Graf G, Scott R, Smith B, Johnson, JWC, King TM:** The relative significance of human placental lactogen in the diagnosis of retarded fetal growth. Am J Obstet Gynecol 135:516, 1979

47. **Arias F:** The diagnosis and management of intrauterine growth retardation. Obstet Gynecol 49:293, 1977

48. **Burnard WP, Logan RW:** The value of urinary oestriol estimation in predicting dysmaturity. J Obstet Gynaec Brit Cwlth 79:1091, 1972

49. **Campbell S, Kurjak A:** Comparison between urinary oestrogen assay and serial ultrasonic cephalometry in assessment of fetal growth retardation. Br Med J 4:336, 1972

50. **Petrucco DM, Cellier K, Fishtall A:** Diagnosis of intrauterine fetal growth retardation by serial serum oxytocinase, urinary oestrogen, and serum heat stable alkaline phosphatase (HASP) estimations in uncomplicated and hypertensive pregnancies. J Obstet Gynaec Brit Cwlth 80:499, 1973

51. **Clemetson CAB, Churchman J:** The placental transfer of amino-acids in normal and toxaemic pregnancy. J Obstet Gynaec Brit Cwlth 61:364, 1954

52. **Wharton BA, Foulds JW, Fraser ID, Pennock CA:** Amniotic fluid total hydroxyproline and intrauterine growth. J Obstet Gynaec Brit Cwlth 78:791, 1971

53. **Shah SI, Alderman M, Queenan JT, Brasel JA, Winick M:** Nondialyzable peptide-bound hydroxyproline in human amniotic fluid: An indicator of fetal growth. Am J Obstet Gynecol 114:250, 1972

54. **Metcoff J, Yoshida T, Morales M, Rosada A, Urrusti J, Sosa A, Yoshida P, Frenk P, Velasco L, Ward A, Y-Al-Ubaidi:** Biomolecular studies of fetal malnutrition in maternal leukocytes. Pediatrics 47:180, 1971

55. **Yoshida T, Metcoff J, Morales M, Rosado A et al:** Human fetal growth retardation, II. Energy metabolism in leukocytes. Pediatrics 50:559, 1972

56. **Metcoff J, Wikman-Coffelt J, Yoshida T, Bernal A, Rosado A, Yoshida P, Urrusti J, Frenk S, Madrazo R, Velasco L, Morales M:** Energy metabolism and protein synthesis in human leukocytes during pregnancy and in placenta related to fetal growth. Pediatrics 51:866, 1973

57. **Metcoff J:** Maternal leukocyte metabolism in fetal malnutrition. Adv Exp Med Biol 49:73, 1974

58. **Mameesh MS, Metcoff J, Costiloe P, Crosby W:** Kinetic properties of pyruvate kinase in human maternal leukocytes in fetal malnutrition. Pediatr Res 10:561, 1976

59. **Crosby WM, Metcoff J, Costiloe JP, Mameesh M, Sanstead HH, Jacob RA, McClain PE, Jacobson G, Reid W, Burns G:** Fetal malnutrition: An appraisal of correlated factors. Am J Obstet Gynecol 128:22, 1977

60. **Rosado A, Bernal A, Sosa A, Morales M et al:** Human fetal growth retardation, III. Protein, DNA, RNA, adenine nucleotides, and activities of the enzymes pyruvic and adenylate kinase in placenta. Pediatrics 50:568, 1972

61. **Campbell S, Dewhurst CJ:** Diagnosis of the small-for-dates fetus by serial ultrasonic cephalometry. Lancet 2:1002, 1971

62. **Dewhurst CJ, Beazley JM, Campbell S:** As-

sessment of fetal maturity and dysmaturity. Am J Obstet Gynecol 113:141, 1972

63. **Whetham JCG, Muggah H, Davidson S:** Assessment of intrauterine growth retardation by diagnositc ultrasound. Am J Obstet Gynecol 125:577, 1976

64. **Queenan JT, Kubarych SF, Cook LN, Anderson GD, Griffin LP:** Diagnostic ultrasound for detection of intrauterine growth retardation. Am J Obstet Gynecol 124:865, 1976

65. **Campbell S, Thomas A:** Ultrasound measurement of the fetal head-to-abdomen circumference ratio in the assessment of growth retardation. Br J Obstet Gynaecol 84:165, 1977

66. **Wittmann BK, Robinson HP, Aitchison T, Fleming JEE:** The value of diagnostic ultrasound as a screening test for intrauterine growth retardation: Comparison of nine parameters. Am J Obstet Gynecol 134:30, 1979

67. **Higginbottom J, Slater J, Porter G, Whitfield CR:** Estimation of fetal weight from ultrasonic measurements of truck circumference. Br J Obstet Gynaecol 82:698, 1975

68. **Waldimiroff JW, Bloemsma CA, Wallenburg HCS:** Ultrasonic assessment of fetal head and body sizes in relation to normal and retarded fetal growth. Am J Obstet Gynecol 131:857, 1978

69. **Sabbagha RE:** Intrauterine growth retardation: Antenatal diagnosis by ultrasound. Obstet Gynecol 52:252, 1978

70. **Campbell S, Wilkin D:** Ultrasonic measurement of fetal abdomen circumference in the estimation of fetal weight. Br J Obstet Gynaecol 82:689, 1975

71. **Gohari P, Berkowitz RL, Hobbins JC:** Prediction of intrauterine growth retardation by determination of total intrauterine volume. Am J Obstet Gynecol 127:255, 1977

72. **Wladimiroff JW, Campbell S:** Fetal urine production rates in normal and complicated pregnancy. Lancet 1:151, 1974

73. **Wladimiroff JW, Bloemsma CA, Wallenburg HCS:** Ultrasonic assessment of fetal growth. Acta Obstet Gynecol Scand 56:37, 1977

74. **Naeye RL:** Cardiovascular abnormalities in infants malnourished before birth. Biol Neonate 8:104, 1965

75. **Brans YW, Cassady G:** Fetal nutrition and body composition. In Ghadmi H (ed): Total Parenteral Alimentation: Premises and Promises. Philadelphia, J. Wiley and Sons, 1974

76. **Ounsted M, Ounsted C:** On Fetal Growth Rate: Its Variations and Their Consequences. Clinics in Developmental Medicine #46, Spastics International Medicine Publications, Philadelphia, JB Lippincott, 1973

77. **Meredith HV:** Body weight at birth of viable human infants: A worldwide comparative treatise. Hum Biol 42:217, 1970

78. **Wark L, Malcolm LA:** Growth and development of the Lumi child in the Sepik district of New Guinea. Med J Aust 2:129, 1969

79. **Ashcroft MT, Buchanan IC, Lovell HG, Welsh B:** Growth of infants and preschool children in St. Christopher-Nevis-Anguilla, West Indies. Am J Clin Nutr 19:37, 1966

80. **Salber EJ, Bradshaw ES:** Birth weights of South African babies. Brit J Soc Med 5:113, 1951

81. **Salber EJ, Bradshaw ES:** Birth weights of South African babies: II. Effect of birth rank on birth weight. Brit J Soc Med 5:247, 1951

82. **Barron SL, Vessey MP:** Birthweights of infants born to immigrant women. Brit J Prev Soc Med 20:127, 1966

83. **Johnstone F, Inglis L:** Familial trends in low birth weight. Brit Med J 3:659, 1974

84. **Warkany J, Monroe BB, Sutherland BS:** Intrauterine growth retardation. Am J Dis Child 102:249, 1961

85. **Cassady G:** Anencephaly: A six year study of 367 cases. Am J Obstet Gynecol 103:1154, 1969

86. **Naeye RL, Blanc WA:** Pathogenesis of congenital rubella. JAMA 194:1277, 1965

87. **Naeye RL:** Cytomegalic inclusion disease. The fetal disorder. Amer J Clin Pathol 47:738, 1967

88. **Siegal M, Fuerst HT:** Low birthweight and maternal virus diseases. JAMA 197:680, 1966

89. **Cozzi F, Wilkinson AW:** Intrauterine growth rate in relation to anorectal and oesophageal anomalies. Arch Dis Child 44:59, 1969

90. **VandenBerg BJ, Yerushalmy J:** The relationship of the rate of intrauterine growth of infants of low birth weight to mortality, morbidity and congenital anomalies. J Pediatr 69:531, 1966

91. **Levy RJ, Rosenthal A, Fyler DC, Nadas AS:** Birth weight of infants with congenital heart disease. Am J Dis Child 132:249, 1978

92. **Naeye RL, Kelly JA:** Judgment of fetal age, III: The pathologist's evaluation. Pediatr Clin North Am 13:849, 1966

93. **Naeye RL:** Unsuspected organ abnormalities associated with congenital heart disease. Am J Pathol 47:905, 1965

94. **Hill DE:** Effect of insulin on fetal growth. Semin Perinatol 2:319, 1978

95. **Donohue WL, Uchida I:** Leprechaunism—A euphamism for a rare familial disorder. J Pediatr 45:505, 1954

96. **D'Ercole AJ, Underwood LE, Groelke J, Plet A:** Fetal growth retardation (FGR) and hyperinsulinism: Evidence for an aberrant intracellular response to insulin (Abstr). Pediatr Res 11:513, 1977

97. **Schiff D, Colle E, Stern L:** Metabolic and growth patterns in transient neonatal diabetes. N Engl J Med 287:119, 1972

98. **Young DG, Wilkinson AW:** Mortality in neonatal duodenal obstruction. Lancet 2:18, 1966

99. **Cheek DB:** Muscle cell growth in abnormal children. In Cheek DB (ed): Human Growth: Body Composition, Cell Growth, Energy and Intelligence, Chapt. 25, p. 352. Lea & Febiger, Philadelphia, 1968

100. **Hill DE, Arellano C, Izukawa T, Holt AB, Cheek DB:** Studies in infants and children with congenital rubella: Oxygen consumption, body water, cell mass, muscle and adipose tissue composition. Hopkins Med J 127:309, 1970

101. **Gruenwald P:** Growth and maturation of the foetus and its relationship to perinatal mortality. In Butler NR, Alberman ED (eds): Perinatal Problems, pp. 141–162. Edinburgh, E and S Livingstone, 1969

102. **Gruenwald P, Funakawa H, Mitani S, Nishimora T, Takeuchi S:** Influence of environmental factors on foetal growth in man. Lancet 1:1026, 1967

103. **Shanklin DR:** The influence of placental lesions on the newborn infant. Pediatr Clin North Am 17:25 1970

104. **Gruenwald P:** Fetal deprivation and placental pathology: Concepts and relationships. In Rosenberg HS, Bolande RP (eds): Perspectives in Pediatric Pathology Vol 2, pp 101–149. Chicago, Year Book Medical Publishers

105. **Cefalo RC, Simkovich JW, Abel F, Hellegers AE, Chez, RA:** Effect of potential placental surface area reduction on fetal growth. Am J Obstet Gynecol 129:434, 1977

106. **Tremblay PC, Sybulski S, Maughan GB:** Role of the placenta in fetal malnutrition. Am J Obstet Gynecol 91:597, 1965

107. **Sybulski S, Tremblay PC:** Placental glycogen content and utilization in vitro in intrauterine fetal malnutrition. Am J Obstet Gynecol 103:257, 1969

108. **Sybulski S:** In vitro estrogen biosynthesis from testosterone by homogenates of placentas from normal pregnancies and pregnancies complicated by intrauterine fetal malnutrition and diabetes. Am J Obstet Gynecol 105:1055, 1969

109. **Iyengar L:** Chemical composition of placenta in pregnancies with small-for-date infants. Am J Obstet Gynecol 116:66, 1973

110. **Winick M, Noble A:** Cellular growth in human placenta, I, Normal placental growth. Pediatrics 39:248, 1967

111. **Altshuler G, Russell P, Ermocilla R:** The placental pathology of small-for-gestational age infants. Am J Obstet Gynecol 121:351, 1975

112. **Gruenwald P:** Growth of the human fetus, II, Abnormal growth in twins and infants of mothers with diabetes, hypertension, or isoimmunization. Am J Obstet Gynecol 94:1120, 1966

113. **Dixon HG, Browne JCM, Davey DA:** Choriodecidual and myometrial blood-flow. Lancet 2:369, 1963

114. **Theobald GW:** Sympathetic nerves and eclampsia. Br Med J 1:422, 1953

115. **Naeye RL:** Infants of diabetic mothers: A qualitative, morphologic study. Pediatrics 35:980, 1965

116. **Lichty JA, Ting RY, Bruns PD, Dyar E:** Studies of babies born at high altitude, I Relation to birth weight. Am J Dis Child 93:666, 1957

117. **Butler NR, Alberman ED:** Perinatal problems: Second report of the 1958 British Perinatal Mortality Survey, pp. 47–71. Edinburgh, E and S Livingstone, 1969

118. **Wilson GS, Desmond MM, Verniaud WM:** Early development of infants of heroin-addicted mothers. Am J Dis Child 126:457, 1973

119. **Naeye RL, Blanc W, Leblanc W, Khatamee MA:** Fetal complications of maternal heroin addiction: Abnormal growth, infections and episodes of stress. J Pediatr 83:1055, 1973

120. **Hanson JW, Jones KL, Smith DW:** Fetal alcohol syndrome: Experience with 41 patients. JAMA 235:1458, 1976

121. **Anderson M, Went LN, MacIver JE, Dixon HG:** Sickle–cell disease in pregnancy. Lancet 2:516, 1960

122. **Frankenburg WK, Duncan BR, Coffelt W, Koch R, et al:** Maternal phenylketonuria: Implications for growth and development. J Pediatr 73:560, 1968

123. **Wallenburg HCS, VanKessel PH:** Platelet life span in pregnancies resulting in small-for-gestational age infants. Am J Obstet Gynecol 134:739, 1979

124. **Edwards LE, Alton IR, Barrada MI, Hakanson EY:** Pregnancy in the underweight woman: Course, outcome and growth patterns of the infant. Am J Obstet Gynecol 135:297, 1979

125. **Harrison KA, Ibeziako PA:** Maternal anemia and fetal birthweight. J Obstet Gynaecol Brit Cwlth 80:798, 1973

126. **Koller O, Sagen N, Ulstein M, Vaula D:** Fetal growth retardation associated with inadequate haemodilution in otherwise uncomplicated pregnancy. Acta Obstet Gynecol Scand 58:9, 1979

127. **Harris RE, Thomas UL, Shelokov A:** Asymptomatic bacteriuria in pregnancy: Antibody-

coated bacteria, renal function and intra-uterine growth retardation. Am J Obstet Gynecol 126:20, 1976

128. **Miller HC, Hassanein K, Henaleigh P:** Effects of behavioral and medical variables on fetal growth retardation. Am J Obstet Gynecol 127:643, 1977

129. **Lindblad BS, Zetterström R:** Causes of impaired fetal growth. Proc 2nd Europ Congr Perinatal Med, London, 1970, p 181. Basel, Karger, 1971

130. **Naeye RL:** Malnutrition: Probable cause of fetal growth retardation. Arch Pathol 79:284, 1965

131. **Bergner L, Susser MW:** Low birth weight and prenatal nutrition: An interpretive review. Pediatrics 46:946, 1970

132. **Lechtig A, Yarbrough C, Delgado H, Habicht, J–P, Martorell R, Klein RE:** Influence of maternal nutrition on birth weight. Am J Clin Nutr 28:1223, 1975

133. **Lechtig A, Delgado H, Lasky R, Yarbrough C, Klein RE, Habicht J–P, Béhar M:** Maternal nutrition and fetal growth in developing countries. Am J Dis Child 129:553, 1975

134. **Lechtig A, Habicht J–P, Delgado H, Klein RE, Yarbrough C, Martorell R:** Effect of food supplementation during pregnancy on birth weight. Pediatrics 56:508, 1975

135. **Page EW:** Human fetal nutrition and growth. Am J Obstet Gynecol 104:378, 1969

136. **Osofsky HJ:** Antenatal malnutrition: Its relationship to subsequent infant and child development. Am J Obstet Gynecol 105:1150, 1969

137. **Phillips C, Johnson N:** The impact of quality of diet and other factors on birth weight of infants. Am J Clin Nutr 30:215, 1977

138. **Sinclair JC, Saigal S:** Nutritional influences in industrial societies. Am J Dis Child 129:54, 1975

139. **Smith CA:** Effects of maternal malnutrition on fetal development. Am J Dis Child 73:243, 1947

140. **Smith CA:** The effect of maternal undernutrition upon the newborn infant in Holland (1944–45). J Pediatr 30:229, 1947

141. **Smith CA:** Effects of the hunger winter (1944–45) in Holland upon pregnancy and the new–born infant. Maandschrift voor Kindergeneeskunde 15:1, 1947

142. **Antonov AN:** Children born during the siege of Leningrad in 1942. J Pediatr 30:250, 1947

143. **Stein H:** Maternal protein depletion and small-for-gestational-age babies. Arch Dis Child 50:146, 1975

144. **Ancri G, Morse EH, Clarke RP:** Comparison of the nutritional status of pregnany adolescents with adult pregnant women, III, Maternal protein and calorie intake and weight gain in relation to size of infant at birth. Am J Clin Nutr 30:568, 1977

145. **Hibbard ED, Kenna AP:** Valine/glycine ratio in newborn infants. Biol Neonate 27:56, 1975

146. **Young, M, Prenton MA:** Maternal and fetal plasma amino acid concentrations during gestation and in retarded fetal growth. J Obstet Gynaecol Brit Cwlth 76:333, 1969

147. **Lindblad BS, Baldesten A:** The normal venous plasma free amino acid levels of non-pregnant women and of mother and child during delivery. Acta Paediatr Scand 56:37, 1967

148. **Lindblad BS, Zetterström R:** The venous plasma free amino acid levels of mother and child during delivery, II, After short gestation and gestation complicated by hypertension with special reference to the "small-for-dates" syndrome. Acta Paediatr Scand 57:195, 1968

149. **Lindblad BS, Rahimtoola RJ, Said M, Haque Q, Khan N:** The venous plasma free amino acid levels of mother and child during delivery, III, In a lower socio-economic group of a refugee area in Karachi, West Pakistan, with special reference to the "small-for-dates" syndrome. Acta Paediatr Scand 58:497, 1969

150. **Geber WF, Schramm LC:** Postpartum weight alteration in hamster offspring from females injected during pregnancy with either heroin, methadone, a composite drug mixture or mescaline. Am J Obstet Gynecol 120:1105, 1974

151. **Emmanouilides GC, Townsend DE, Bauer RA:** Effects of single umbilical artery ligation in the lamb fetus. Pediatrics 42:919, 1968

152. **Kwong MS, Moore TC, Lemmi CAE, Oh W, Thibeault DW:** Histidine decarboxylase activity in fetal intrauterine growth-retarded rats. Pediatr Res 10:737, 1976

153. **Hobel CJ, Emmanouilides GC, Townsend DE, Yoshiro K:** Ligation of one unbilical artery in the fetal lamb. Obstet Gynecol 36:582, 1970

154. **Creasy RK, Barrett CT, deSwiet M, Kahanpää KV, Rudolph AM:** Experimental intrauterine growth retardation in the sheep. Am J Obstet Gynecol 112:566, 1972

155. **Creasy RK, deSwiet M, Kahanpää KV, Young WP, Rudolph AM:** Pathophysiological changes in the fetal lamb with growth retardation. In Foetal and Neonatal Physiology: Proc of the Sir Joseph Barcroft Centenary Symposium. Cambridge, Cambridge Univ. Press, 1973

156. **Pickart LR, Creasy RK, Thaler MM:** Hyperfibrinogenemia and polycythemia with intrauterine growth retardation in fetal lambs. Am J Obstet Gynecol 124:268, 1976

157. **Scott JR:** Fetal growth retardation associated

with maternal administration of immunosuppressive drugs. Am J Obstet Gynecol 128: 668, 1977

158. Franklin JB, Brent RL: The effect of uterine vascular clamping on the development of rat embryos three to fourteen days old. J Morphol 115:273, 1964

159. Brent RL, Franklin JB: Uterine vascular clamping: New procedure for the study of congenital malformations. Science 132:89, 1960

160. Wigglesworth JS: Experimental growth retardation in the foetal rat. J Path Bact 88:1, 1964

161. Dahlquist G, Persson B: Effect of intrauterine growth retardation on the postnatal development of D-β-hydroxybutyrate dehydrogenase activity in rat brain. Biol Neonate 28: 353, 1976

162. Bernal A, Morales M, Feria–Velasco A, Chew S, Rosado A: Effect of intrauterine growth retardation on the biochemical maturation of brain synaptosomes in the rat. J Nutr 104: 1157, 1974

163. Lugo G, O'Neil L, Cassady G: Carcass water, fat and chloride in the fetal growth retarded rat. Am J Obstet Gynecol 110: 358, 1971

164. Hohenauer L, Oh W: Body composition in experimental intrauterine growth retardation in the rat. J Nutr 99:23, 1969

165. Brans YW, Ortega P: Water content and distribution in intrauterine growth-retarded newborn rats. Biol Neonate 31:166, 1977

166. Nitzan M, Groffman H: Hepatic gluconeogenesis and lipogenesis in experimental intrauterine growth retardation in the rat. Am J Obstet Gynecol 109:623, 1971

167. Nitzan M, Groffman H: Metabolic changes in experimental intrauterine growth retardation in rats: Blood glucose and liver glycogen in dysmature and premature newborn rats. Isr J Med Sci 6:697, 1970

168. Oh WH, D'Amodio MD, Yap LL, Hohenhauer L: Carbohydrate metabolism in experimental intrauterine growth retardation in rats. Am J Obstet Gynecol 108:415, 1970

169. Oh W, Guy JA: Cellular growth in experimental intrauterine growth retardation in rats. J Nutr 101:1631, 1971

170. Chanez C, Tordet–Caridroit C, Roux JM: Studies on experimental hypotrophy in the rat. II. Development of some liver enzymes of gluconeogenesis. Biol Neonate 18:58, 1971

171. Nitzan M, Groffman H: Glucose metabolism in experimental intrauterine growth retardation. In vitro studies with liver and brain slices. Biol Neonate 17:420, 1971

172. Roux JM, Jahchan, T, Fulchignoni MC: Desoxyribonucleic acid and pyrimidine synthesis in the rat during intrauterine growth retardation: Responsiveness of several organs. Biol Neonate 27:129, 1975

173. Roux JM, Tordet–Caridroit C, Chanez C: Studies on experimental hypotrophy in the rat, I, Chemical composition of the total body and some organs in the rat foetus. Biol Neonate, 15:342, 1970

174. Levitsky LL, Speck SM, Shulman R: Metabolic response to fasting in experimental intrauterine growth retardation: A comparison of two models. Biol Neonate 30:11, 1976

175. Chow BF, Lee CJ: Effect of dietary restriction of pregnant rats on body weight gain of the offspring. J Nutr 82:10, 1964

176. Adlard BPF, Dobbing J, Smart JL: An alternative animal model for the full-term small-for-dates human baby. Biol Neonate 23:95, 1973

177. Bührdel P, Willgerodt H, Keller E, Theile H: The postnatal development of rats after preterm and post-term birth, I, Body weight. Biol Neonate 33:184, 1978

178. Bührdel P, Keller E, Willgerodt H, Theile H: The postnatal development of rats born preterm and post term, II, Liver, brain, heart and kidneys. Biol Neonate 33:240, 1978

179. Sybulski S, Toth A, Maughan GB: The influence of experimental renal hypertension on pregnancy in the rat. Am J Obstet Gynecol 110:314, 1971

180. Nitzan M, Ofloff S, Chrzanowska BL, Schulman JD: Intrauterine growth retardation in renal insufficiency: An experimental model in the rat. Am J Obstet Gynecol 133:40, 1979

181. Swaab DF, Honnebier WJ: The influence of removal of the fetal rat brain upon intrauterine growth of the fetus and the placenta and on gestation length. J Obstet Gynaecol Brit Cwlth 80:589, 1973

182. Widdowson EM: Intrauterine growth retardation in the pig, I, Organ growth and cellular development at birth and after growth to maturity. Biol Neonate 19:329, 1971

183. Myers RE, Hill, DE, Holt AB, Scott RE, Mellits ED, Cheek DB: Fetal growth retardation produced by experimental placental insufficiency in the Rhesus monkey, I, Body weight, organ size. Biol Neonate 18:379, 1971

184. Hill DE, Myers RE, Holt AB, Scott RE, Cheek DB: Fetal growth retardation produced by experimental placental insufficiency in the Rhesus monkey, II, Chemical composition of the brain, liver, muscle and carcass. Biol Neonate 19:68, 1971.

185. Gordon YB, Grudzinskas JG, Jeffery D, Chard T, Letchworth AT: Concentration of pregnancy-specific β_1-glycoprotein in maternal blood in normal pregnancy and in intra-

uterine growth retardation. Lancet 1:331, 1977

186. **Taeusch HW, Carson SH, Wang NS, Avery ME:** Heroin induction of lung maturition and growth retardation in fetal rabbits. J Pediatr 82:869, 1973

187. **Friedler G, Cochin J:** Growth retardation in offspring of female rats treated with morphine prior to conception. Science 175:654, 1972

188. **Zagon IS, McLaughlin PJ:** Effect of chronic maternal methadone exposure on perinatal development. Biol Neonate 31:271, 1977.

189. **Dickerson JWT, Merat A, Widdowson EM:** Intrauterine growth retardation in the pig, III, The chemical structure of the brain. Biol Neonate 19:354, 1971

190. **Liggins GC. Quoted in Hill DE:** Effect of insulin on fetal growth. Semin Perinatol 2:319, 1978

191. **Harding PGR, Young A, Possmayer F:** The effect of hypoinsulinemia on the fetus (abstr). Clin Res 23:611A, 1975

192. **Cheek DB, Hill DE:** Changes in somatic growth after ablation of maternal or fetal pancreatic beta cells. In Cheek DB (ed): Fetal and Postnatal Cellular Growth, Chapter 19. New York, Wiley, 1975

193. **Hill DE:** Experimental growth retardation in rhesus monkeys. In Size at Birth, Ciba Foundation Symposium #27, Excerpta Medica, Amsterdam, 1974.

194. **Wallace LR:** Effect of diet on fetal development (Abstr). J Physiol (Lond) 104:34P, 1945–46.

195. **Brans Y, Ortega P, Bailey P:** Water contents of human muscles in relation to fetal growth (abstr). Clin Res 24:72A, 1976

196. **Chase HP, Dabiere CS, Welch NN O'Brien D:** Intrauterine undernutrition and brain development. Pediatrics 47:491, 1971

197. **Adams PH:** Intrauterine growth retardation in the pig, II, The development of the skeleton. Biol Neonate 19:341, 1971

198. **Zamenhoff S, van Marthens E, Margolis FL:** DNA (cell number) and protein in neonatal brain: Alteration by maternal dietary protein restriction. Science 160:322, 1968

199. **Venkatachalam PS, Ramanathan KS:** Severe protein deficiency during gestation in rats on birth weight and growth of offspring. Indian J Med Res 54:402, 1966

200. **Brock DHJ, Barron L, Jelen P, Watt M, and Scrimgeour JB:** Maternal serum-alpha-fetoprotein measurements as an early indicator of low birth-weight. Lancet 2:267, 1977

201. **Ounstead C:** Effect of Y chromosome on fetal growth rate. Lancet 2:857, 1970

202. **Dobbing J:** The later growth of the brain and its vulnerability. Pediatrics 53:2, 1974

203. **Dobbing J:** The developing brain: A plea for more critical interspecies extrapolation. Nutr Rep Int 7:401, 1973

204. **Lee CJ, Chow BF:** Protein metabolism in the offspring of underfed mother rats. J Nutr 87:439, 1971

205. **Winick M:** Cellular growth of the placenta as an indicator of abnormal fetal growth. In Adamsons K (ed.): Diagnosis and Treatment of Fetal Disorders, p. 83. New York, Springer, 1968

206. **Widdowson EM:** Harmony of growth. Lancet 1:901, 1970

207. **Alexander G:** Studies on the placenta of the sheep (Ovis aries L.): Effect of surgical reduction in the number of caruncles. J Reprod Fertil 7:307, 1964

208. **Wigglesworth JS:** Foetal growth retardation. Br Med Bull 22:13, 1966

209. **Winick M:** Cellular changes during placental and fetal growth. Am J Obstet Gynecol 109:166, 1971

210. **Brasel JA, Winick M:** Maternal nutrition and prenatal growth. Experimental studies of effects of maternal undernutrition on fetal and placental growth. Arch Dis Child 47:479, 1972

211. **Raynaud A, Frilley M:** Destruction des glandes génitales, de l'embryon de souris, par une irradiation au moyen des rayons x, a l'age de treize jours. Ann Endocrinol (Paris) 8:400, 1947

212. **Jost A. Quoted in Deanesly R:** Foetal endocrinology. Br Med Bull 17:91, 1961

213. **Wells LJ:** Progress of studies designed to determine whether the fetal hypophysis produces hormones that influence development. Anat Rec 97:409, 1947

214. **Winick M:** Cellular growth of human placenta, III, Intrauterine growth failure. J Pediatr 71:390, 1967

215. **Dayton DH, Filer LJ, Canosa, C:** Cellular changes in the placentas of undernourished mothers in Guatemala. Fed Proc 28:488, 1969

216. **Widdowson EM, Crabb DE, Milner RDG:** Cellular development of some human organs before birth. Arch Dis Child 47:652, 1972

217. **Winick M:** Cellular growth in intrauterine malnutrition. Pediatr Clin North Amer 17:69, 1970

218. **Cheek DB, Graystone J, Mehrizi A:** The importance of muscle cell number in children with congenital heart disease. Hopkins Med J 118:140, 1966

219. **Cheek DB, Brasel JA, Elliott D, Scott R:** Muscle cell size and number in normal children and in dwarfs (pituitary, cretins, and primordial) before and after treatment (Preliminary observations). Hopkins Med J 119:46, 1966

220. **Chase HP, Welch NN, Dabiere CS, Vasan NS,**

Butterfield LJ: Alterations in human brain biochemistry following intrauterine growth retardation. Pediatrics 50:403, 1972

221. Shelley HJ, Neligan GA: Neonatal hypoglycaemia. Br Med Bull 22:34, 1966

222. Naeye RL: Organ and cellular development in congenital heart disease and in alimentary malnutrition. J Pediatr 67:447, 1965

223. Plotkins SA, Boué A, Boué JG: The in vitro growth of rubella virus in human embryo cells. Am J Epidemiol 81:71, 1965

224. Vasan NS, Chase HP: Brain glycosaminoglycans (mucopolysaccharides) following intrauterine growth retardation. Biol Neonate 28:196, 1976

225. Cassady G: Body composition in intrauterine growth retardation. Pediatr Clin North Amer 17:79, 1970

226. Cassady G: Plasma volume studies in low birth weight infants. Pediatrics 38:1020, 1966

227. Cassady G: Bromide space studies in infants of low birth weight. Pediatr Res 4:414, 1970

228. Cassady G, Milstead RR: Antipyrine space studies and cell water estimates in infants of low birth weight. Pediatr Res 5:673, 1971

229. Friis-Hansen B: Care and hazards of the small-for-dates infant. In Proc 2nd Europ Congr Perinatal Med, London, 1970, pp 223–234. Basel, Karger, 1971

230. Bhakoo ON, Scopes JW: Weight minus extracellular fluid as metabolic reference standard in newborn baby. Arch Dis Child 46:483, 1971

231. Elder MG, Myatt L: Coagulation and fibrinolysis in pregnancies complicated by fetal growth retardation. Br J Obstet Gynaecol 83:355, 1976

232. Marks JF, Kay J, Baum J, Curry L: Uric acid levels in full-term and low-birth-weight infants. J Pediatr 73:609, 1968

233. Rubaltelli FF, Formentin PA, Tatò L: Ammonia nitrogen, urea and uric acid blood levels in normal and hypodystrophic newborns. Biol Neonate 15:129, 1970

234. Rubaltelli FF, Peratoner L: Ammonia nitrogen in "small-for-dates" newborn babies. Lancet 1:208, 1969

235. Younoszai, MK, Kacic A, Dilling L, Haworth JC: Urinary hydroxyproline/creatinine ratio in normal term, pre-term and growth-retarded infants. Arch Dis Child 44:517, 1969

236. Younoszai MK, Haworth JC: Excretion of hydroxyproline in urine by premature and normal full-term infants and those with intrauterine growth retardation during the first three days of life. Pediatr Res 2:17, 1968

237. Klujber L, Mestyán G, Sulyok E, Soltész G: Urinary hydroxyproline excretion in normally grown and growth retarded newborn infants. Biol Neonate 20:196, 1972

238. Klujber L, Sulyok E: Urinary glycosaminoglycan excretion in normally grown and growth retarded neonates, I, Total glycosaminoglycan excretion. Acta Paediatr Acad Sci Hung 13:81, 1972

239. Brans Y, Bailey P, Blake M, Cassady G: Urinary hyroxyproline/creatinine ratio and perinatal growth. (abstr). Pediatr Res 9:275, 1975

240. Bazso M, Asztalos M, Kassai L: Serum proteins in foetal growth retardation. In Horsky J, Stembra ZK (eds): Intrauterine Dangers to the Fetus, p. 585. Excerpta Medica Foundation, Amsterdam, 1967

241. Jacobsen BB, Peitersen B, Andersen HJ, Hummer L: Serum concentrations of thyroxine-binding globulin, prealbumin and albumin in healthy full-term, small-for-gestational age and preterm newborn infants. Acta Paediatr Scand 68:49,1979

242. Eggermont E, Socha J, Bhavani S, Carchon H: Letter to the Editor, Plasma prealbumin in the newborn. Acta Paediatr Scand 68:613, 1979

243. Miller HC, Hassanein K: Maternal smoking and fetal growth of full term infants. Pediatr Res 8:960, 1964

244. Yeung CY, Hobbs JR: Serum-γG-globulin levels in normal, premature, post-mature and "small-for-dates" newborn babies. Lancet 1:1167, 1968

245. Papadatos C, Papaevangelou G, Alexion D, Mendris J: Immunoglobulin levels and gestational age. Biol Neonate 14:365, 1969

246. Papadatos, C, Papaevangelou G, Alexion D, Mendris J: Serum immunoglobulin G levels in small-for-date newborn babies. Arch Dis Child 45:570, 1970

247. Catty D, Seger R, Drew R, Ströder J, Metze H: IgG-subclass concentrations in cord sera from premature, full-term and small-for-dates babies. Eur J Pediatr 125:89, 1977

248. Hyvarinen M, Zeltzer P, Oh W, Stiehm ER: Influence of gestational age on serum levels of alpha-l-fetoprotein, IgG globulin, and albumin in newborn infants. J Pediatr 82:43, 1973

249. Prokopowicz J, Ziobro J, Iwaszko–Krawczuk W: Bactericidal capacity of plasma and granulocytes in small-for-dates newborns. Acta Paediatr Acad Sci Hung 16:267, 1975

250. Iwaszko–Krawczuk W, Prokopowicz J: Phagocytosis in small-for -dates newborns. Acta Paediatr Acad Sci Hung 14:47, 1973.

251. Iwaszko–Krawczuk W: Serum lysozyme activity in small-for-dates newborn .Acta Paediatr Acad Sci Hung 14:135, 1973

252. Chandra RK: Immunocompetence in low-birth-weight infants after intrauterine malnutrition. Lancet 2:1393, 1974

253. **Chandra RK:** Fetal malnutrition and postnatal immunocompetence. Amer J Dis Child 129:450, 1975

254. **Haworth JC, Dilling L, Younoszai MK:** Relation of blood-glucose to hematocrit, birth weight and other body measurements in normal and growth-retarded newborn infants. Lancet 2:901, 1967

255. **Humbert JR, Abelson H, Hathaway WE, Battaglia FC:** Polycythemia in small for gestational age infants. J Pediatr 75:812, 1969

256. **Oh W, Omori K, Emmanouilides GC, Phelps DL:** Placenta to lamb fetus transfusion in utero during acute hypoxia. Am J Obstet Gynecol 122:316, 1975

257. **Finne PH:** Erythropoietin levels in cord blood as an indicator of intrauterine hypoxia. Acta Paediatr Scand 55:475, 1966

258. **Bergquist G:** Viscosity of the blood in the newborn infant. Acta Paediatr Scand 63:858,1974

259. **Rivers RPA:** Coagulation changes associated with a high haematocrit in the newborn infant. Acta Pediatr Scand 64:449, 1975

260. **Perlman M, Dvilansky A:** Blood coagulation status of small-for-dates and postmature infants. Arch Dis Child 50:424,1975

261. **Lochridge S, Pass R, Cassady G:** Reticulocyte counts in intrauterine growth retardation. Pediatrics 47:919, 1971

262. **Alford CA, Schaefer J, Blankenship WJ, Straumfjord JV, Cassady G:** A correlative immunologic, microbiologic and clinical approach to the diagnosis of acute and chronic infections in newborn infants. N Eng J Med 277:437, 1967

263. **Sinclair JC, Silverman WA:** Intrauterine growth in active tissue mass of the human fetus, with particular reference to the undergrown baby. Pediatrics 38:48, 1966

264. **Sinclair JC, Scopes JW, Silverman WA:** Metabolic reference standards for the neonate. Pediatrics, 39:724, 1967

265. **Sinclair JC:** Heat production and thermoregulation in the small-for-date infant. Pediatr Clin North Am 17:147, 1970

266. **Scopes JW, Ahmed I:** Minimal rates of oxygen consumption in sick and premature newborn infants. Arch Dis Child 41:407, 1966

267. **Bhakoo ON, Scopes JW:** Minimal rates of oxygen consumption in small-for-dates babies during the first week of life. Arch Dis Child 49:583, 1974

268. **Lees MH, Younger EW, Babson SG:** Thermal requirements of undergrown human neonates. Biol Neonate 10:288, 1966

269. **Rubecz I, Mestyán J:** The partition of maintenance energy expenditure and the pattern of substrate utilization in intrauterine malnourished newborn infants before and during recovery. Acta Paediatr Acad Sci Hung 16:335, 1975

270. **Gentz J, Kellum M, Persson B:** The effect of feeding on oxygen consumption, RQ and plasma levels of glucose, FFA, and D-β-hydroxybutyrate in newborn infants of diabetic mothers and small for gestational age infants. Acta Paediatr Scand 65:445, 1976

271. **Scott K, Usher R, MacLean F:** Postnatal study of fetal malnutrition syndrome. J Pediatr 63:734, 1963

272. **Phillips L, Lumley J, Paterson P, Wood C:** Fetal hypoglycemia. Am J Obstet Gynecol 102:371, 1968

273. **Melichar V, Novak M, Zoula J, Hahn P, Koldovsky O:** Energy sources in the newborn. Biol Neonate 9:298, 1965

274. **deLeeuw R, deVries IJ:** Hypoglycemia in small-for-dates newborn infants. Pediatrics 58:18, 1976

275. **Salle B, Ruitton–Uglienco, A:** Glucose disappearance rate, insulin response and growth hormone response in the small for gestational age and premature infant of very low birth weight. Biol Neonate 29:1, 1976

276. **Horváth I, Tóth P, Méhes K:** The predictive value of glucose utilization rate in neonatal hypoglycaemia of small-for-gestational-age infants. Acta Paediatr Acad Sci Hung 16:143, 1975

277. **Gentz JCH, Warrner R, Persson BEH, Cornblath M:** Intravenous glucose tolerance, plasma insulin, free fatty acids and β-hydroxybutyrate in underweight newborn infants. Acta Paediatr 58:481, 1969

278. **Pildes RS, Patel DA, Nitzan M:** Glucose disappearance rate in symptomatic neonatal hypoglycemia. Pediatrics 52:75, 1973

279. **LeDune MA:** Response to glucagon in small-for-dates hypoglycaemic and non-hypoglycaemic newborn infants. Arch Dis Child 47:754, 1972

280. **Schiff D, Lowy C:** Carbohydrate metabolism in the newborn. Lancet 1:475, 1968

281. **Pagliara AS, Karl IE, Haymond M, Kipnis DM:** Hypoglycemia in infancy and childhood, Part I. J Pediatr 82:365, 1973

282. **Haymond MW, Karl IE, Pagliara AS:** Increased gluconeogenic substrates in the small-for-gestational-age infant. N Eng J Med 291:322, 1974

283. **Williams PR, Fiser RH, Sperling MA, Oh W:** Effects of oral alanine feeding on blood glucose, plasma glucagon and insulin concentrations in small-for-gestational-age infants. N Eng J Med 292:612, 1975

284. **Stern L, Sourkes TL, Raiha N:** The role of the adrenal medulla in the hypoglycemia of foetal malnutrition. Biol Neonate 11:129, 1967

285. **Melichar V, Novák M, Hahn P, Koldovsky O:**

Free fatty acid and glucose in the blood of various groups of newborns. Preliminary report. Acta Paediatr 53:343, 1964

286. **Melichar V, Drahota Z, Hahn P:** Ketone bodies in the blood of full term newborns, premature and dysmature infants and infants of diabetic mothers. Biol Neonate 11:23, 1967

287. **Săbata V, Znamenáček K, Přibylová H, Melichar V:** The effect of glucose in the prenatal treatment of small-for-date fetuses. Biol Neonate 22:78, 1973

288. **Rautenbach M, Beyreiss K:** Absorption rates of fructose and influence of fructose on the glucose blood level in preterm and term newborns appropriate for gestational age as compared to preterm and term newborns small for gestational age. Biol Neonate 30: 123, 1976

289. **Tsang RC, Gigger M, Oh W, Brown DR:** Studies in calcium metabolism in infants with intrauterine growth retardation. J Pediatr 86: 936, 1975

290. **Dewhurst CJ, Dunham AM, Harvey DR, Parkinson CE:** Prediction of respiratory-distress syndrome by estimation of surfactant in the amniotic fluid. Lancet 1:1475, 1973

291. **Dyson D, Blake M, Cassady G:** Amniotic fluid lecithin/sphingomyelin ratio in complicated pregnancies. Am J Obstet Gynecol 122:772, 1975

292. **Lindback T:** Amniotic fluid lecithin concentrations in pregnancies complicated by hypertensive disorders and intrauterine growth retardation. Acta Obstet Gynecol Scand 55: 355, 1976

293. **Pichler E:** 11-Hydroxycorticosteroids in maternal, umbilical cord and neonatal plasma. In Proc 2nd Europ Congr Perinatal Med London, 1970, p 252. Basel, Karger, 1971

294. **Robertson AF, Sprecher HW, Wilcox JP:** Total lipid fatty acid patterns of umbilical cord blood in intrauterine growth failure. Biol Neonate 14:28, 1969

295. **Chance GW, Bower BD:** Hypoglycaemia and temporary hyperglycaemia in infants of low birth weight for maturity. Arch Dis Child 41: 279, 1966

296. **Gentz JCH, Cornblath M:** Transient diabetes of the newborn. Adv Pediatr 16:345, 1969

297. **Madsen A:** Spontaneous hypoglycaemia with convulsions and deficient adrenalin reaction. A case occurring in one of uniovular twins. Acta Paediatr Scand 54:483, 1965

298. **Dahms BB, Krauss AN, Auld PAM:** Pulmonary function in dysmature infants. J Pediatr 84:434, 1974

299. **Gluck L, Kulovich MV:** Lecithin/sphingomyelin ratios in amniotic fluid in normal and abnormal pregnancy. Am J Obstet Gynecol 115:539, 1973

300. **Haymond M, Karl I, Pagliara A:** Defective gluconeogenesis (GNG) in small for gestational age infants. (SGAI) (abstract). J Pediatr 83:153, 1973

301. **Freeman RK, Goebelsman U, Nochimson D, Cetrulo C:** An evaluation of the significance of a positive oxytocin challenge test. Obstet Gynecol 47:8, 1976

302. **Gregory GA, Gooding CA, Phibbs R, Tooley WH:** Meconium aspiration in infants—a prospective study. J Pediatr 85:848, 1974

303. **Ting P, Brady JP:** Tracheal suction in meconium aspiration. Am J Obstet Gynecol 122:767, 1975

304. **Carson BS, Losey RW, Bowes WA, Simmons MA:** Combined obstetric and pediatric approach to prevent meconium aspiration syndrome. Am J Obstet Gynecol 126:712, 1976

305. **Sann L, Ruitton A, Mathieu M, Lasne Y:** Effect of intravenous hydrocortisone administration on glucose homeostasis in small for gestational age infants. Acta Paediatr Scand 68:113, 1979

306. **Holowach-Thurston J, Hauhart RE, Jones EM, Ikossi MG, Pierce RW:** Decrease in brain glucose in anoxia in spite of elevated plasma glucose levels. Pediatr Res 7:691, 1973

307. **Holden KR, Young RB, Piland JH, Hurt WG:** Plasma pressors in the normal and stressed newborn infant. Pediatrics 49:495, 1972

308. **Tsang R, Glueck CJ, Evans G, Steiner PM:** Cord blood hypertriglyceridemia. Am J Dis Child 127:78, 1974

309. **Andersen GE, Friis-Hansen B:** Neonatal hypertriglyceridemia: A new index of antepartum-intrapartum fetal stress. Acta Paediatr Scand 65:369, 1976

310. **Saugstad OD:** Hypoxanthine as a measurement of hypoxia. Pediatr Res 9:158, 1975

311. **Mathew OP, Bland H, Boxerman SB, James E:** CSF lactate levels in high risk neonates with and without asphyxia. Pediatrics (in press)

312. **Beck GJ, VandenBerg BJ:** The relationship of the rate of intrauterine growth of low-birth-weight infants to later growth. J Pediatr 86:504 1975

313. **Cruise MO:** A longitudinal study of the growth of low birth weight infants, I, Velocity and distance growth, birth to 3 years. Pediatrics 51:620, 1973

314. **Commey JOO, Fitzhardinge PM:** Handicap in the preterm small-for-gestational age infant. J Pediatr 94:779, 1979

315. **Low JA, Galbraith RS, Muir D, Killen H, Worthington D, Karchmar J, Campbell D:** Intrauterine growth retardation: A prelimi-

nary report of long term morbidity. Am J Obstet Gynecol 130:534, 1978

316. **Martell M, Falkner F, Bertolini LB, Diaz JL, Nieto F, Tenzer SM, Belitzky R:** Early postnatal growth evaluation in full-term, preterm, and small-for-dates infants. Early Hum Dev 1:313, 1978

317. **Beargie RA, James VL, Greene JW:** Growth and development of small-for-dates newborns. Pediatr Clin North Am 17:159, 1970

318. **Fancourt R, Campbell S, Harvey D, Norman AP:** Follow-up study of small-for-dates babies. Br Med J 1:1421, 1976

319. **Wedgwood M, Holt KS:** A longitudinal study of the dental and physical development of 2–3-year-old children who were underweight at birth. Biol Neonate, 12:214, 1968

320. **Davies DP, Beverley D:** Changes in body proportions over the first year of life: Comparisons between "light-for-dates" and "appropriate-for-dates" term infants. Early Hum Dev 3:263, 1979

321. **Vohr BR, Oh W, Rosenfield AG, Cowett RM, Berstein J:** The preterm small-for-gestational age infant: A two-year follow-up study. Am J Obstet Gynecol 133:425, 1979

322. **Chamberlain R, Davey A:** Physical growth in twins, postmature and small-for-dates children. Arch Dis Child 50:437, 1975

323. **Foley TP Jr, Thompson RG, Shaw M, Baghdassarian A, Nissley SP, Blizzard RM:** Growth responses to human growth hormone in patients with intrauterine growth retardation. J Pediatr 84:635, 1974

324. **Lanes R, Plotnick LP, Lee PA:** Sustained effect of human growth hormone therapy on children with intrauterine growth retardation. Pediatrics 63:731, 1979

325. **Colle E, Schiff D, Andrew G, Bauer CB, Fitzhardinge P:** Insulin responses during catch-up growth of infants who were small for gestational age. Pediatrics 57:363, 1976

326. **Schiff D, Colle E, Stern L:** Metabolic and growth patterns in transient neonatal diabetes. N Eng J Med 287:119, 1972

327. **Davies P, Davis J:** Very low birth weight and subsequent head growth. Lancet 2:1216, 1970

328. **Babson SG, Kangas J:** Preschool intelligence of undersized term infants. Am J Dis Child 117:553, 1969

329. **Als H, Tronick E, Adamson L, Brazelton TB:** The behavior of the full-term but underweight newborn infant. Dev Med Child Neurol 18:590, 1976

330. **Michaelis R, Schulte FJ, Nolte R:** Motor behavior of small-for-gestational age newborn infants. J Pediatr 76:208, 1970

331. **Miller HC, Hassanein K:** Fetal malnutrition in white newborn infants: Maternal factors. Pediatrics 52:504, 1973

332. **Schulte FJ, Schrempf G, Hinze G:** Maternal toxemia, fetal malnutrition and motor behavior of the newborn. Pediatrics 48:871, 1971

333. **Parmelee AH, Schulte FJ:** Developmental testing of pre-term and small-for-date infants. Pediatrics 45:21, 1970

334. **Dweck HS, Huggins W, Dorman LP, Saxon SA, Benton JW Jr, Cassady G:** Developmental sequelae in infants having suffered severe perinatal asphyxia. Am J Obstet Gynecol 119:811, 1974

335. **Ounstead M:** Post-natal growth of children who were S.F.D and L.F.D. Dev Med Child Neurol 13:121, 1971

336. **Babson SG, Henderson NB:** Fetal undergrowth: Relation of head growth to later intellectual performance. Pediatrics 53:890, 1974

337. **Renaud R, Kirschtetter L, Koehl C, Boog G, Brettes JP, Schumacher JC, Vincendon G, Willard D, Gandar R:** Amino-acid intra-amniotic injections. In Persianinov LS, Chervakova TV, Presl J (eds): Recent Progress in Obstetrics and Gynaecology, Proc VII World Cong Obstet Gynaecol, pp 234–256, Moscow, 1973. Amsterdam, Excerpta Medica, 1974

338. **Saling E, Dudenhausen JW, Kynast G:** Basic investigations about intra-amniotic compensatory nutrition of the malnourished fetus. In Persianinov LS, Chervakova TV, Presl J (eds): Recent Progress in Obstetrics and Gynaecology, Proc VII World Cong Obstet Gynaecol, pp 227–233, Moscow, 1973. Amsterdam, Excerpta Medica, 1974

339. **Heller L:** Intrauterine amino acid feeding of the fetus. In Bode HH, Warshaw JB (eds): Parenteral Nutrition in Infancy and Childhood, pp 206–213. New York, Pleneum Press, 1974

340. **Stanley CA, Anday EK, Baker L, Delivoria-Papadopolous M:** Metabolic fuel and hormone responses to fasting in newborn infants. Pediatrics, 64:613, 1979

341. **Huddleston JF, Sutliff G, Carney FE Jr, Flowers CE:** Oxytocin challenge test for antepartum fetal assessment: Report of a clinical experience. Am J Obstet Gynecol 135:609, 1979

342. **Cowper W:** The Task. Book IV, The Winter Walk at Noon, line 223.

16

The Infant of the Diabetic Mother

Anne B. Fletcher

Reports of pregnancy in the diabetic woman date back to the early 1800s, but mortality was extremely high for both the mother and the infant. Only in the last 40 years could a diabetic woman expect to bear live children. It has been estimated that infants of diabetic mothers (IDMs) occur in 4 in 1000 pregnancies; while 6 in 1000 infants will be born to mothers with gestational diabetes.[1] Thus, 1 in 100 live-born infants will be subjected in some manner to "the intrauterine indiscretions of which we know nothing," so well-stated by Farquhar.[2] This problem, therefore, is of considerable significance to the practicing neonatologist.

When one speaks of the IDM, one thinks of the classic fat, plethoric infant with gigantism. Yet we must also consider the infant born to the gestational diabetic mother (IGDM), the small-for-dates infant with placental insufficiency born to the mother with diabetes of long duration, and the infant who is normal yet whose mother has diabetes.

THE DIABETIC MOTHER AND HER PREGNANCY

Pregnancy has been known to impose some carbohydrate intolerance on the normal mother. Renal glucosuria, impaired glucose utilization in response to a glucose load despite increased insulin-like activity, accelerated insulin degradation, and elevated fasting-free fatty acid serum levels have all been reported in nondiabetic pregnancies.[3] Human chorionic somatomammotropin (HCS), also known as HPL, rises throughout pregnancy and probably plays a major role in these findings because it facilitates the transfer of glucose, free fatty acids, and amino acids to the fetus for use as substrate.[4] Estrogen, progesterone, and cortisol may also be responsible to a lesser degree for these abnormalities which are particularly magnified in the diabetic pregnancy.

During pregnancy, variation in the severity of the diabetic state is seen probably in relation to the increasing HCS levels. Silenkow has reported higher than normal HCS levels in diabetic pregnancies.[4] Beginning with the 10th week and lasting from 2 to 3 months, an improvement in carbohydrate tolerance is frequently manifested. Insulin requirements may drop by as much as 34%, and hypoglycemic attacks or shock sometimes occur. On occasion, pregnancy in the diabetic has been diagnosed in this way. At approximately the 24th to 28th week, carbohydrate tolerance decreases and insulin requirements may increase by as much as 75%, at times resulting in

Table 16-1. Major Maternal Complications During Pregnancy

	Toxemia	Eclampsia	Pyelonephritis	Polyhydramnios	Urinary Tract Infection
Kitzmiller[6] *(1978)*	19%*	—	1%	31%	—
Pedersen[7] *(1965)*	23%	0.2%	6%	25%	16%
Kyle (1963)[8]	25%	—	—	19%	—
Normal Population	5.9%	.05%	—	0.7%	—

* Edema, preeclampsia, hypertension

diabetic coma. This change coincides with the rising and then peaking of HCS levels in the mother. It is from this time on that the effect of diabetes is felt most by the fetus, and the typical changes of the IDM occur.[5] Though there may be some improvement of the diabetic state prior to delivery, an abrupt fall in insulin requirements may be ominous for the well-being of the infant. During lactation, insulin requirements remain lower than in the pre-pregnant state. Six to nine months following the pregnancy, the diabetic woman has returned to her usual insulin dosage.

Problems that may complicate other pregnancies are greater threats to the diabetic mother. These include toxemia, eclampsia, polyhydramnios and urinary tract infections with or without pyelonephritis (Table 16-1).

Outcome of the Diabetic Pregnancy

Fetal wastage and perinatal mortality are higher in the diabetic owing to the increased incidence of complications during pregnancy, stillbirths, cesarean sections and prematurely born infants. Some investigators have found an increased incidence of abortions, although this is not universal. Some of these deaths are related to the gestational age of the infant (i.e., hyaline membrane disease and other respiratory problems); others are secondary to severity and classification of the diabetic state in the mother and to Pedersen's bad prognostic signs of pregnancy (Tables 16-2, 16-3). Table 16-4 shows trends in the course of pregnancy by class. With improved perinatal care for the infant and our presently improved management of the pregnancy, overall mortality has

Table 16-2. White's Classification of Diabetes.
Classification of Pregnant Diabetic Women

Class	Diabetes		Insulin or Oral Agent Needed	Calcified Arteries	Retinopathy		Nephropathy
	Onset Age	*Duration*			*Benign*	*Malignant*	
A (GTT+)	Any	Any	0	0	0	0	0
B	>20	<10	+	0	0	0	0
C	10–19 or	10–19	+	0	0	0	0
D	<10 ‖≅	>20	+	+			
				(legs and/or	+	0	0
E	Any	Any	+	pelvis)	±	0	0
F	Any	Any	+	±	±	0	+
R	Any	Any	+	±	±	+	0
FR	Any	Any	+	±	±	+	+
G—Multiple failures in pregnancy							

(Tables 16-2 and 16-4 from Marble, A. (ed.): Joslin's Diabetes Mellitus. Lea & Febiger, 1971)[10]

Table 16-3. Prognostic Bad Signs in Pregnancy (PBSP)[9]

1. Clinical pyelonephritis
2. Precoma or severe acidosis
3. Toxemia
4. "Neglectors"

been drastically reduced. The neonatal mortality for all classes of diabetes has decreased from 40% to between 5 and 10% (Table 16-5). It is unclear whether the IGDM is at greater than normal risk. Warrner and Cornblath, in a small series, found no increase in abortions or stillbirths;[1] while Dekaban, in an older but larger group, found increased abortions, stillbirths, and abnormal survivors, but no increased neonatal mortality.[12]

Any comparison of figures for overall mortality and fetal wastage must be done with great care because series differ according to size of population, gestational ages of the infants, classification of the diabetic state, and inclusion of infants weighing less than 1000 g.

THE INFANT OF THE DIABETIC MOTHER
Body Composition

For many years, it was a common misconception that the characteristic appearance of the IDM was caused by increased body water. In fact, a decreased total body water, particularly in the extracellular space, has been found.[13] With better maternal diabetic control, though still larger than their normal counterparts, total body weight of IDMs has decreased. Their appearance is still typical, with an abundance of hair, fat and the presence of plethora (Fig. 16-1).

While all agree that the IDM is fat rather than edematous, other organs also share in the excess to varying degrees, particularly the heart and the fetal adrenal cortex, with the liver and kidneys enlarged to a lesser extent.[14] In contrast, the brain and thymus are small in relationship to weight and gestational age controls.[14–16] The ovaries may show cystic follicles; the testes, hyperplasia of the interstitial cells of Leydig.[14,15] The pancreas demonstrates definite beta-cell hyperplasia, a decrease in the number of alpha cells, along with an undefined eosinophilia and occasional fibrosis.[17] Naeye

Table 16-4. Trends of Course of Pregnancy by Class.

Class	Spontaneous Abortion Rate	Hydramnios Degree	Excessive Weight Gain	Preeclampsia	Large Placenta	Heavy Birth Weight
A	N	+	+	+ + + +	+ + + +	+ + + +
B	N	+ + + +	+ + + +	+ + + +	+ + + +	+ + + +
C	N	+ + +	+ + +	+ + +	+ + +	+ + +
D	+	+ +	+ +	+ +	+ +	+ +
E	+ + + +	+ +	+ +	+ +	+	+
F	+ + + +	+	0	?	0	0
R	+ + + +	+	0	Superimposed?	0	0

Class	Fetal Loss Intrauterine	Fetal Loss Intrapartum	Fetal Loss Neonatal	Congenital Anomalies	Diabetes Intensification
A	+	+ + + +	+	+	+
B	+ +	+ + + +	+	+	+ + + +
C	+	+ +	+ +	+	+ +
D	+ + +	+		+	+
E	+ + + +	+	+ + + +	+	+
F	+ + + +	+	+ + + +	+	±
R	+ + + +	+	+ + + +	+	±

Table 16-5. Perinatal Mortality Based on PBSP and White's Classification (1959–1972)

White's Class	PBSP Present % Mortality		PBSP Absent % Mortality	
A	14.3		3.0	
B	19.1	17.1	3.8	3.4
C	29.4		9.0	
D	25.2	26.7	10.5	9.8
F	37.5		30.8	
Total	25.9		7.5	

(Adapted from Pedersen J, Mølsted–Pedersen L, Anderson B: Assessors of fetal perinatal mortality in diabetic pregnancy. Diabetes 23:302, 1974)[11]

in 1965, comparing IDMs with controls in a quantitative morphologic study, demonstrated that the body weight of the infant could be correlated with the mass of pancreatic islet tissue.[18] Other organs are compared in Table 16-6.

Infants who are born to Classes D through F diabetic women tend to be of more normal weight, but up to 10% may be small for gestational age. When small, their organ weights are reduced as in infants with placental insufficiency. Infants of gestational diabetic women have not had direct analysis.

METABOLIC ABNORMALITIES IN THE IDM

Insulin

Over the years, measurement of insulin levels in infants of insulin-dependent mothers has been difficult and misleading due to the passage of insulin antibodies across the placenta. With newer methods for measuring C-peptide immunoreactivity, it has been shown that IDM cord, venous, and arterial serum insulin levels vary from normal to high.[19] While no good correlation has been shown between maternal insulin or glucose levels and infant insulin levels, a direct relationship does exist between large birth weight, higher cord insulin levels,[20] and higher maternal glycohemoglobin (HbAlc) levels (an indicator of long-term maternal control).[21]

Because of these problems, much of the work to show that IDMs do indeed have excess insulin in their environment *in utero* has been done in infants whose mothers were not taking insulin during pregnancy.[22] Demonstration of increased insulin secretion has also been shown in an indirect fashion by excessive glucose utilization in these infants. When measuring insulin levels after a 0.5 g/kg glucose load, IDMs show an immediate high peak while normal infants show a slow rise with a peak at approximately 1 hour.[23]

Free Fatty Acids (FFAs). In the fasted normal newborn, cord FFA levels have been found to be lower than maternal values. The FFA level gradually rises in the first few hours of life, equaling adult values by 12 hours and peaking higher, between 24 to 48 hours, probably in response to generally lowered blood sugars.

Compared to normal infants, several studies have shown that IDMs and IGDMs as a group have similar or slightly lower mean FFA levels at birth, and do not have as large a rise in subsequent hours. This failure of the usual

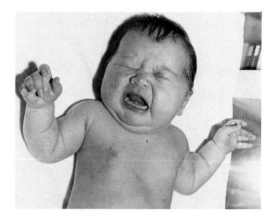

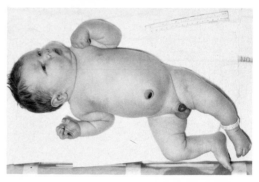

Fig. 16-1. The infant of a diabetic mother showing typical features.

Table 16-6. Body Composition of IDMs

	IDMs 36 weeks (%)	Gestational Age Controls (%)	Underweight IDMs 36 weeks (%)
Body weight	141	100	60
Length	112	100	87
Brain weight	97	100	none weighed
Heart	174	100	51
Lung	127	100	86
Liver	179	100	83
Spleen	127	100	68
Thymus	137	100	70
Pancreas,	110	100	48
islets	10.8 (300)	3.5 (100)	5.4 (153)
Kidney	105	100	83
Adrenal	158	100	54
	(inc. fetal zone)		
No	21	14	4

(Naeye RL: Pediatrics 35:980, 1965, copyright American Academy of Pediatrics, 1965)[18]

inverse FFA to glucose relationship is relatively worse in infants of insulin-dependent mothers.[24] Pildes and coworkers also found lower fasting FFAs in the IGDM.[22] The composition of FFAs in IDMs is normal.[24]

Human Growth Hormone (HGH) and Adrenocorticosteroids. HGH has not been extensively studied in either normal infants or infants of diabetic mothers. It has been reported that both premature and full-term newborns, have a rise in HGH levels, in response to hyperglycemia, that is different from the inverse relationship seen in older infants, children, and adults.[25,26] This temporary pattern disappears after the first few days of life. Cord and infant fasting HGH levels are much higher than maternal values. IDMs show a similar picture, but levels appear to be somewhat lower. More data are needed in this area.

Controversy concerning adrenal function in the IDM has not been entirely settled. Aarskog[27] and Migeon[28] have shown that cord and postnatal cortisol levels are similar to normal newborns, both premature and full term. Others have reported urinary excretion of corticosteroid metabolites in nondistressed IDMs to be increased over that of control infants.[29,30] A further increase is seen in IDM's with respiratory distress compared to nonIDM distressed prematures. This increased response to stress in the IDMs may be related to the larger size of the fetal adrenal cortex. Aarskog

has also looked at cortisol production per 24 hours, and, although IDMs fall into a slightly higher range, the difference from normal infants was not significant.[31] More recently, Chattoraj showed that IDMs may suffer from a state of hyperadrenocorticism during fetal life by demonstrating that, with all modes of delivery, the concentrations of cortisone are much higher in the umbilical arteries than in normal controls.[32] What this means in terms of symptomatology or presentation is unknown.

Glucagon

Glucagon is a hormone important in maintaining glucose homeostasis by way of glycogenolysis and gluconeogenesis. At birth, normal infants and IDMs have similar plasma glucagon levels. However in response to early hypoglycemia,[33] followed by alanine stimulation,[34] IDMs do not have significantly elevated glucagon levels when compared to normal and small for gestational age infants with hypoglycemia. This, along with pathologic evidence of decreased alpha cells, suggests a blunted response of glucagon, further disabling glucose metabolism in these infants.

Epinephrine

Catecholamine excretion in IDMs varies from normal to very low levels.[35-37] In normal subjects, epinephrine releases FFAs, induces

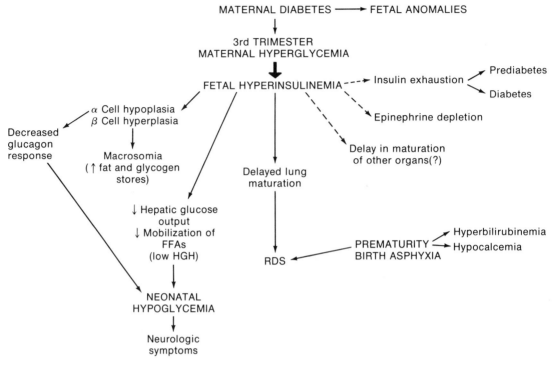

Fig. 16-2. Proposed pathophysiology of the IDM.

hyperglycemia, inhibits peripheral utilization of glucose, and may lower serum insulin. Although epinephrine excretion is not consistently low, its depletion may contribute to the metabolic derangements seen in these infants.

Plasma Proteins and Amino Acids

Plasma proteins in the IDM are generally lower than those of normal infants of an equivalent gestational age, indicating a functional immaturity of the IDM.[38] Only transferrin has been found to be elevated, the significance of which is unknown.

The plasma amino acid pattern of IDMs has been studied in only small numbers of patients. Some researchers have found the pattern no different from that of normal infants; others have found it to be both abnormally high and low, with respect to certain amino acids.[39-41] Asphyxiated infants were found to have elevated levels of alanine and glycine.[41] Another group of infants had a pattern consistent with that seen in infants with Kwashiorkor.[40] Although it is unlikely that IDMs have protein malnutrition or that the amino acid pattern plays an important part in glucose homeosta-

sis, the hyperinsulinemic state may cause a rapid and imbalanced transfer of amino acids into the tissues. Further study is warranted in this area.

Pathophysiology of the IDM

Though hyperadrenocorticism and elevated levels of HGH have been implicated in the past to explain the pathophysiology of the IDM, it appears that neither plays a significant role in the somatic appearance or the metabolic abnormalities of these infants. Though no one theory explains all the problems that these infants encounter in their early postnatal period, maternal hyperglycemia and fetal hyperinsulinemia best elucidate their typical appearance and metabolic alterations. A nonresponsiveness to glucagon and epinephrine depletion are likely, secondary to the hyperinsulinism (Figure 16-2). Further problems in these infants will be discussed individually later in the chapter.

Neonatal Problems of the IDM

Hypoglycemia. Early hypoglycemia is the most common problem seen in the IDM, with rapid decreases in glucose, particularly in those infants whose mothers are insulin dependent during pregnancy. Blood sugar also falls in IGDMs, but not to the same degree. Glucose utilization is far more rapid in the IDM immediately after birth than in either the normal infant or the IGDM.[23] McCann and coworkers showed the percent glucose disappearance per minute to be 0.77% in normal infants, 1.31% in IGDMs, and 2.57% in infants of insulin-dependent mothers.[42]

Less clear is the actual incidence of hypoglycemia in these infants; a 2 to 75% occurrence has been reported. These discrepancies may well be caused by variable maternal care and control of diabetes, early versus late feeding of the infants, differences in maternal blood sugars at the time of delivery, length of labor, the class of maternal diabetes, and variations in blood sugar measurement techniques.

The importance of asymptomatic hypoglycemia has also not been settled. A number of infants with extremely low blood sugars show no symptoms at all and some authorities feel that their outcomes will be normal. Farquhar states that "babies of both diabetic and normal women can, in my experience, be both asymptomatic and undamaged at blood glucose levels below 20 mg or even 10 mg per 100 ml."[43] However, because adequate follow-up studies of infants with asymptomatic hypoglycemia are not available, many practicing neonatologists are reluctant to allow the blood sugar to remain low. This is particularly true in view of the frequency of neurologic sequelae after symptomatic hypoglycemia.

While controversy exists concerning the percentage of IDMs having hypoglycemia, many of these infants do indeed become symptomatic with blood sugars less than 20 mg/dl. Their symptoms include jitteryness, tremors, convulsions, sweating, cyanosis, weak or high-pitched cry, refusal to feed, and limpness. When these are present, the blood sugar must be treated, though central nervous system abnormalities, infection, heart disease, and other metabolic problems must also be ruled out.

Hypocalcemia. IDMs are well known for their neuromuscular irritability. Although it is not always explained by either hypoglycemia or hypocalcemia, the latter has been noted to occur in up to 60% of these infants.[44] Certainly, IDMs have many reasons to become hypocalcemic: they are usually premature to some degree; there is often a history of difficult

pregnancy, labor, and delivery; or a history of repeated abortions. It is postulated that increased maternal calcium levels result in functional hypoparathyroidism and transient hypocalcemia in the infant. An increased incidence of hypomagnesemia has also been reported in one small series, though others have failed to record this finding. Hypomagnesemia, if present, may be due to hypocalcemia, decreased maternal magnesium levels, or neonatal hyperphosphatemia.[45]

Hyperbilirubinemia. Elevated bilirubin levels at 48 to 72 hours occur more often in IDMs than in other infants of similar weight or gestational age. An increased rate of hemolysis or immune incompatibility has not been seen. Hematocrits on the third day of life in IDMs are higher than controls, whether the cords were clamped early or late.[46] The decreased extracellular volume present in IDMs may contribute to this problem. Complicated vaginal deliveries predispose to elevated bilirubin values. IDMs, with their large size and greater tendency toward enclosed hemorrhage, are certainly in this category more frequently than other premature infants. All these factors have probably contributed to the fact that IDMs, particularly those between 33 to 36 weeks of gestation, have required significantly more exchange transfusions than other infants. However, the use of bilirubin lights has changed this incidence considerably.

Respiratory Function and HMD

Many studies have been done to see whether respiratory physiology *per se* is abnormal in the IDM. With the exception of a slightly higher respiratory rate and a minimally greater degree of acidosis in the first few hours of life, respiratory function is very similar to that of other premature or full-term infants.

Respiratory distress due to HMD still is a major cause of death in these infants during the perinatal period. The overall percentage of IDMs having the disease however has decreased because of better perinatal care, fetal monitoring, and allowing the infant to remain *in utero* as long as possible.

A 31% incidence of HMD in 711 infants was reported by Gellis and Hsia from the Joslin Clinic in 1959.[47] An overall incidence of from 3 to 8% is now reported from the same clinic.[6] Two conflicting studies exist: one that has found the incidence when compared to infants of the same gestational age to be greater in

IDMs only after 38 weeks; the other reported a 5.6 times greater incidence in IDMs only from 32 to 38 weeks, when controlled for other perinatal difficulties.[48,49]

Gluck and Kulovich have shown that for a particular gestational age, Classes A through C diabetes during pregnancy seems to delay lung maturation as measured by L/S ratios.[50] It has since been noted by many that a classically "mature" L/S ratio of greater than 2:1 does not necessarily mean that the lungs are genuinely mature in the IDM. This has lead to further animal investigation of the effects of hyperinsulinemia and hyperglycemia on lung maturation *in utero*.

When insulin is added to rat liver enzymes, it antagonizes the effects of glucocorticoids.[51] Similarly, insulin added to type II alveolar cells in culture causes a slight increase in baseline incorporation of choline into lecithin but eliminated the marked choline incorporation that occurs when steroids were given.[51] When added to rat lung in organ culture, insulin slowed morphologic maturation and delayed appearance of lamellar bodies.[53] Finally, in rhesus monkey fetuses whose mothers were made diabetic by streptozotocin, there was a difference in the ability of the hyperglycemic fetus to synthesize, store, and release lecithin.[54] Therefore, it appears that the IDM comes from a highly abnormal and complex *in utero* environment.

Most recently, it was shown that while IDMs have the normal phospholipids that make up surfactant, guidelines used for prediction of fetal maturity may not be accurate in these and other complicated pregnancies.[55] Thus care must be taken in determining lung maturity of the IDM, and greater than 2:1 ratios may be required to predict mature function. Certainly, more work is warranted in this area.

Renal Vein Thrombosis

Avery and her coworkers first described renal vein thrombosis in the IDM, and, since then, there have been a number of similar reports.[56] This entity, as well as other thromboses, has also occurred in IGDMs and in infants who were large for gestational age but when the diabetic status of the the mother was unknown.[57] These findings have been reported in stillbirths as well as in the perinatal period and, as yet, the etiology is not known. Polycythemia, decreased extracellular fluid, and transient dehydration in the first days of life have been suggested as causes. Palpable flank masses with hematuria and proteinuria should suggest the diagnosis. Thrombosis in the brain, if suspected, may require identification by CT scan.

Infection

Infections are always a hazard in the neonatal period. Although infants are not immunologically incompetent, they have been shown to have decreased components of complement, chemotactic factor, opsonin activity, and cellular immunity.[58] IDMs often born prematurely, would be expected to share in this decreased immunity, though this has not been demonstrated directly. In addition, diabetic mothers have a higher incidence of urinary tract infections and expose their infants to a greater risk of infection by passage of bacteria across the placenta. The diagnosis of sepsis is often difficult to make because of the varied presenting picture. The IDM who is jittery, jaundiced, and who has some respiratory distress must always be suspect. Work-up should proceed accordingly; treatment may be withheld if the infant's general condition is good and if he can be observed closely.

Congenital Anomalies

Despite some controversy, the bulk of evidence suggests an increased incidence of congenital anomalies among IDMs compared with the normal population. Only a small series have shown no difference. Two large and fairly comprehensive compilations, though varying slightly in their conclusions, have been reported.

Pedersen,[59] in 1964, compared 853 IDMs with 1212 nonIDMs and has since increased these numbers in a more recent publication to 1452 IDMs and 8789 normal infants.[60] Table 16-7 shows not only the comparison for total numbers of anomalies, including major and multiple defects, but also points out that, despite improved maternal care, the incidence appears to have increased. Chung, using 48,437 pregnancies of the Collaborative Perinatal Project and 339 patients from the Joslin Clinic, has shown that there is essentially no increased risk for mothers with gestational diabetes. However the risk for white mothers with overt diabetes, whether treated with insulin or not, is double that of the normal population, with

Table 16-7. Congenital Anomalies

	No.		Total Anomalies (%)		Major (%)		Multiple (%)	
	1964	*1977*	*1964*	*1977*	*1964*	*1977*	*1964*	*1977*
Total IDM	853	1452	6.4	8	5.2	6.1	1.6	2.1
Class								
A–C	573	948	4.4	4.9				
D–F	280	504	10.7	13.7				
NonIDM	1212	8789	2.1	2.8	1.2	1.6	0.2	0.4

(Pedersen LM: Lancet, 1:1124, 1964;[59] Pedersen J: The Pregnant Diabetic and her Newborn, pp. 192–193. Baltimore, Williams and Wilkins, 1977[60])

incidences of 17.94% and 10.94% respectively for major and minor malformations. In Black mothers, the incidence for major malformations was greater than in the normal mothers (13.64%), but no increase was seen for minor anomalies.[61] In necropsy material, congenital anomalies have been found to account for from 19.5 to 26% of deaths in IDMs versus 6.6% in controls.[62,59]

Because total numbers are actually small, it has been difficult to draw conclusions as to which anomalies are most common. Cardiac defects, particularly transposition of the great vessels, ventricular septal defect and patent ductus, spinal anomalies varying from simple hemivertebrae to the syndrome of caudal regression, and anencephaly are reported to occur with greater frequency in the IDM. Chung has found anomalies to be generally distributed throughout all organ systems.[61]

The factors causing these malformations are unclear. However, a few generalizations can certainly be made. First, the teratogenic effects of diabetes must have to derange early embryonic development because multiple anomalies are frequently seen. Secondly, it appears that insulin therapy does not have an effect despite animal studies which show teratogenicity. Thirdly, the risk of malformation of the fetus appears to increase with the length of maternal disease. Genetic factors have not been proven because infants of diabetic fathers do not have an increased incidence of anomalies. First trimester hypoglycemia and oral hypoglycemic agents, though mentioned as causes, probably do not play much of a role. All these observations suggest that it is truly maternal diabetes, *per se,* through its adverse effects on metabolism, that is responsible for increased malformations in the IDM.

Treatment of the IDM

Care of the Mother. By far, the most important treatment of the IDM is the very careful monitoring and supervision of the diabetic mother. Her health, particularly during the last trimester of pregnancy, will have great bearing on the outcome of the infant. Recent publications have suggested the following model.[6,63,64] The Class A mother, providing she remains in that class, needs only to be followed in the diabetic clinic weekly. Classes B through F mothers should be hospitalized briefly for regulation when first seen and then followed for control on a weekly basis until the 34th week of gestation. They should then be hospitalized for bedrest, careful control, a creatinine clearance, urine cultures, daily 24-hour urine estriol determinations, weekly OCTs or nonstress tests, weekly amniocentesis for L/S ratio and creatinine concentration, and weekly ultrasonic fetal biparietal diameter determinations. If all is well, the fetus can be allowed to proceed to 38- to 39-weeks' gestation. When a large fetus is suspected, the delivery may be done by cesarean section. If a nonmacrosomic infant is expected, delivery is managed by induction with oxytocin and careful monitoring. The liberal use of cesarean section has been suggested to avoid birth injury. Following such a regimen will in general allow the best possible infant to result from a diabetic pregnancy.

While much attention has been placed on the treatment of the overtly diabetic mother, there is less dealing with the gestational diabetic mother. There is now some evidence to suggest that treatment with low-dose insulin rather than diet alone after 32 weeks of pregnancy may have some effect on the outcome of these infants. A decreased perinatal mortality in infants of women over 25 years of age was shown in one study[65] and in another a significant decrease in infant weight was reported in mothers who had had a previously large infant.[66] Both authors suggest caution and further study before this treatment is universally used.

Care of the Infant: General. Treatment of the IDM differs only in a few minor ways from the specialized care that many premature infants need in the first few days of life. Much of this is detailed in other chapters.

Once the infant is delivered, he should be observed closely for at least 24 hours, monitoring for changes in acid-base status, respiratory distress, temperature, glucose, calcium, and bilirubin levels. Watching for infection is of equal importance.

Early feedings of glucose, then formula, in the first 4 to 6 hours have been suggested by most for the asymptomatic infant, and are usually tolerated well. Hubbell has observed early- and late-fed IDMs and found that early-fed infants had a slightly higher mortality rate, though the difference was not significant.[64] The early-fed infants had lower bilirubin values at 48 and 72 hours. Overall, the large majority of both the IGDM and IDM will be asymptomatic and feedings seem advisable as soon as the infant is stabilized.

Hypoglycemia

The monitoring of glucose should begin shortly after birth because levels less than 20 mg/100 ml will often appear in the first few hours of life. Dextrostix can be used easily and quickly by the nursing staff. Single doses of glucagon, 300 μgm/kg, for the transiently asymptomatic hypoglycemia have been used, but this effect will last only for 2 to 3 hours in most infants. Glucagon should not be given repeatedly, nor is it the usual mode of therapy.

Symptomatic hypoglycemia requires immediate attention. While intravenous glucose is extremely important for the infant, the use of 25% and 50% dextrose as a rapid infusion is *contraindicated* in the IDM because it may lead to severe rebound hypoglycemia following a brief initial increase. A constant infusion of 10 to 15% glucose at the volume of fluids necessary for the infant, or a glucose infusion at the rate of 4 mg/kg/min (0.24 g/kg/hr), may be adequate to maintain normoglycemia. The more concentrated the solution, the more care

must be given to infuse through a central vein or artery because these solutions are hypertonic. If the glucose is abruptly stopped for any reason, blood sugar must be monitored because hypoglycemia may rapidly occur. Once the glucose is stabilized for 24 hours, the solution is then decreased in concentration while the glucose level is watched. When the infant's condition permits, oral feedings may be started. Positioning of an umbilical artery catheter just above the level of the celiac axis may have an inordinate influence on the amount of glucose delivered to the pancreas and thus may increase the insulin secretion. Should difficulty in raising blood sugars occur, repositioning the catheter tip at the aortic bifurcation should be considered. If, despite the above, there is persistent hypoglycemia, hydrocortisone 5 mg/kg/24 hours, given in fractional doses every 8 hours, may be used. In an occasional infant, the dosage of hydrocortisone needs to be doubled.

Other more controversial therapies exist but cannot be recommended. McCann and co-workers[27] have postulated a state of epinephrine depletion in some IDMs and suggest the use of epinephrine HCl (Sus-Phrine)† 0.01 ml/kg, diluted 1:10 to be given every 6 hours to infants who show accelerated glucose utilization in response to an intravenous glucose load. In treated infants, they found more normal blood sugars, respiratory rates, and a decreased incidence of HMD.[67] The use of epinephrine HCl (Sus-Phrine) in IDMs in another study failed to show normalization of glucose levels.[68]

Infusion of fructose during labor, at a rate of 0.25 to 0.5 g/kg as a 10% solution has been found to give less of a fall in blood glucose in the infant following delivery.[69] Fructose causes minimal stimulation of insulin secretion. It probably equilibrates in the extracellular fluids of the fetus during delivery, and thereafter diffuses gradually back into the infant's circulation, with hepatic uptake and conversion to glucose. Direct infusion of fructose into the infant results in more rapid utilization, and, in some infants, the initial hypoglycemia is postulated to result from transient suppression of hepatic glucose output. However, symptoms have not appeared until glucose levels dropped below 10 mg/dl. It may be that fructose relieves systemic symptoms while glucose is sent to the brain for consumption.[69] At present, fructose is not as readily available in most centers as is dextrose; it is more costly; the initial hypoglycemia may be harmful; and there is some evidence in animals that infusion of fructose depletes liver ATP, causes marked elevations of uric acid, and, concomitantly, incorporation of leucine into liver protein is almost completely inhibited.[70] Therefore, fructose cannot be recommended as treatment for the infant.

Hyperbilirubinemia

The treatment of hyperbilirubinemia in the IDM is fundamentally similar to its management in any premature infant who may require an exchange transfusion at relatively lower bilirubin levels to prevent kernicterus. However, consideration should be given to the type of preservative in the blood. Acid-citrate-dextrose (ACD) blood has largely been replaced by citrate-phosphate-dextrose (CPD) blood. Both contain large amounts of dextrose, which has been shown to cause significant rebound drops in the blood sugar of normal infants.[71] For the IDM with increased glucose utilization, the blood sugar may fall to hypoglycemic levels after the exchange transfusion unless closely monitored. Heparinized blood, though low in dextrose, may decrease binding of bilirubin to albumin, thus giving an increased risk of kernicterus.[72] Though there is no set rule for the type of blood to be used, and institutional practices vary, the close observation of blood sugars is important during and after exchange transfusion. In the past few years, the use of blue light to break down bilirubin in the skin to water-soluble products has greatly decreased the necessity for exchange transfusions.

Oddities of the IDM

A number of unexplainable but relatively minor abnormalities may occur in the IDM. In the face of normal blood sugars and calcium levels, these infants are often jittery for the first 4 to 7 days of life. This condition has been attributed to cerebral hypofunction, perhaps secondary to enzymatic immaturity, lack or excess of certain amino acids, or long chain fatty acids in the brain.[73] EEGs done on these infants show only physiologic immaturity.[74]

Occurring less frequently is the neonatal small left colon syndrome described in 1975 by David and Campbell.[75] These infants may present with abdominal distension and vomiting, without delay in the passage of meconium stools; some are completely asymptomatic. A barium enema shows a uniform narrowing of the left colon and no other abnormalities. Treatment should be symptomatic only, as this entity disappears in a short period of time. The etiology is completely unknown.

Transient hypertrophic subaortic stenosis has been reported in a few cases proved by angiography and echocardiography.[76] Treatment with digoxin and diuretics was ineffective, but propranolol appeared to improve the condition. In all reported cases, resolution occurred by 6 months of age.

Finally, some of these infants show cardiomegaly on routine x-ray films without evidence of organic heart disease. A number of etiologies including hypoxia during labor and delivery, organomegaly due to hyperinsulinemia, and hypoglycemia can be postulated but are hard to prove because the cardiomegaly also disappears. Thus, in a number of ways, the IDM still remains an enigma.

Follow-up of the IDM

Because immediate complications for pregnant diabetics and their infants have decreased, what then does this mean for the future? Will these children be mentally normal? Will they have an increased risk of diabetes at an earlier age, and thus a shortened life span? Will they have an increased incidence of obesity? Most important will the diabetic gene be perpetuated and perhaps increase as a result of increased childbearing?

Some data on the outcome of IDMs are summarized in Table 16-8. It appears that, as a group, they are mentally normal. The incidence of congenital anomalies following the neonatal period is increased, and there is a discrepancy in their future growth. White[78] and Breidahl[81] have indicated that there is excessive growth in both height and weight in later years, while others have found a tendency toward being shorter and heavier.[80,82]

The outcome with respect to factors in pregnancy was examined by Churchill and associates who found a significant correlation with decreased IQ in IDMs whose mothers had experienced acetonuria during pregnancy.[84] There was no correlation with insulin reactions. Decreased IQs have also been de-

Table 16-8. Follow-up in Infants of Diabetic Mothers

Series	Number of Patients	Age at Follow-up (years)	% Normal	% Retarded	% Late Anomalies	Growth Weight	Growth Height	Comments
Pedersen[77] 1948	91	0.5—15.0	94	2.2	2.2	—	—	Nearly ⅓ birth asphyxia
White[78] 1960	129	Up to 30	—	—	9.0	50% were 30 pounds overweight	60% were 3–11 inches above average	Bone age increased in 48%
Fredrikson[79] 1957	123	Two series: mean 6 and 19	100	—	0.81	—	—	—
Hagbard[80] 1959	514	27% > 11	—	1.4	5.4	Heavier*	Shorter*	—
Breidahl[81] 1966	200	Up to 28	—	—	20	21% > 90th percentile	7% > 90th percentile	—
Farquhar[82] 1969	260	Up to 18	97.7	2.3	8.8	Essentially normal	Essentially normal	Slight tendency to be overweight
Yssing[83] 1975	749	Up to 26	78 (completely normal)	5.7	5.5	—	—	36% with cerebral dysfunction (18% major)

*If born after onset of maternal diabetes

298

Table 16-9. Incidence of Diabetes in IDM

Series	No.	Overall Incidence (%)	Borderline or Abnormal G. T. T. (%)	Age at F.U. (years)
Control population (US) 0–25 yr		0.16		
Control population (Sweden) 5–10 yr		0.11		
White,[78] 1960	129	7*		30
Breidahl,[81] 1966	200	0.5		1–28
Hagbard,[80] 1959	87	0.19		5
Fredrikson,[79] 1957	123	0.81	8.1	5
White,[85] 1953	105	10.5	26	1–20
Pedersen,[77] 1948	91	1.1		6 mo–15
Yssing,[83] 1975	749	1.0		1½–26
Bibergeil,[86] 1975	352	0.7	34.3	≤ 15

*2% in infants of diabetic fathers; 8% in infants of diabetic mothers

scribed with more severe diabetes and with the bad prognostic signs of pregnancy.

There is wide disparity among various published series in the later development of diabetes in children of diabetic mothers (Table 16-9). However, all show an increased incidence (up to 225-fold). Studies with the longest follow-up report the most clear-cut increase when compared to the general population under 25 years of age. The incidence of borderline or abnormal glucose tolerance tests has been reported to be as high as 34%.

It is not known whether there will be significant shortening of the life span of IDMs or whether their childbearing will cause an increased incidence of the diabetic gene in the population. Long-term follow-up is not extensive in the literature. More information will still be needed concerning subsequent generations. However, it would seem that, with the present information, diabetic women should be encouraged to have at least a limited family as early as possible, with proper genetic counselling.

REFERENCES

1. **Warner RA, Cornblath M:** Infants of gestational diabetic mothers. Am J Dis Child 117: 678, 1969
2. **Farquhar JW:** The child of the diabetic woman. Arch Dis Child 34:76, 1959
3. **Pedersen J:** The pregnant diabetic and her newborn, p 22. Baltimore, Williams & Wilkins, 1977
4. **Silenkow HA, Varma K, Younger D, White P, Emerson K:** Patterns of serum immuno reactive human placental lactogen (IR-HPL) and chorionic gonadotropin (IR-HCG) in diabetic pregnancy. Diabetes 20:696, 1971
5. **Fee BA, Weil WB Jr:** Body composition of infants of diabetic mothers by direct analysis. Ann NY Acad Sci 110:869, 1963
6. **Kitzmiller JL, Cloherty JP, Younger MD et al:** Diabetic pregnancy and perinatal morbidity. Am J Obstet Gynecol 131:560, 1978
7. **Pedersen J, Pedersen LM:** Prognosis of the outcome of pregnancies in diabetics. A new classification. Acta Endocrinol (Copenh) 50: 70, 1965
8. **Kyle GC:** Diabetes and pregnancy. Ann Intern Med 59:(No. 11, Pt. 2, Suppl. 3), 1963
9. **Pedersen J, Molsted-Pedersen L:** Prognosis of the outcome of pregnancies in diabetics. A new classification. Acta Endocrinol (Copenh) 50:70, 1965
10. **White P:** Pregnancy and diabetes. In Marble A et al (eds.) Joslin's Diabetes Mellitus, 11th ed p 588, Philadelphia, Lea & Febiger, 1971
11. **Pedersen J, Mølsted-Pedersen L, Anderson B:** Assessors of fetal perinatal mortality in diabetic pregnancy. Diabetes 23:302, 1974
12. **Dekaban A, Baird R:** The outcome of pregnancy in diabetic women. 1. Fetal wastage, mortality, and morbidity in the offspring of diabetic and normal control mothers. J Pediatr 55:563, 1959

13. **Osler M, Pedersen J:** The body composition of newborn infants of diabetic mothers. Pediatrics 26:985, 1960

14. **Driscoll SG:** The pathology of pregnancy complicated by diabetes mellitus. Med Clin North Am 49:1053, 1965

15. **Cardell BS:** The infants of diabetic mothers. A morphological study. J Obstet Gynecol Br Emp 60:834, 1953 (b)

16. **Gruenwald P:** Growth of the human fetus II. Abnormal growth on twins and infants of mothers with diabetes, hypertension, or isoimmunization. Am J Obstet Gynecol 94:, 1120, 1966

17. **Mølsted-Pedersen L, Tygstrup I:** Cell infiltrations in the pancreas of newborn infants of diabetic mothers. Acta Pathol Microbiol Scand 73:537, 1968

18. **Naeye RL:** Infants of diabetic mothers: A quantitative morphologic study. Pediatrics 35:980, 1965

19. **Block MB, Pildes RS, Mossabhoy MD et al:** C-Peptide Immunoreactivity (CPR): A new method for studying infants of insulin-treated mothers. Pediatrics 53:923, 1974

20. **Shima K, Price S, Foa PP:** Serum insulin concentration and birth weight in human infants. Proc Soc Exp Biol Med 121:55, 1966

21. **Widness JA, Schwartz HD, Thompson D et al:** Glycohemoglobin (HbAlc): A predictor of birth weight in infants of diabetic mothers. J Pediatr 92:8, 1978

22. **Pildes RS, Hart RJ, Warner R, Cornblath M:** Plasma insulin response during oral glucose tolerance tests in newborns of normal and gestational diabetic mothers. Pediatrics 44:76, 1969

23. **Baird JD, Farquhar JW:** The insulin secreting capacity of the pancreas in the newborn infants of normal and diabetic women. Lancet 1:71, 1962

24. **Chen CH, Adam PAJ, Laskowski DE et al:** The plasma FFA composition and blood glucose of normal and diabetic pregnant women and of their newborns. Pediatrics 36:843, 1965

25. **Cornblath M, Parker ML, Reisner SH et al:** Secretion and metabolism of growth hormone in premature and full term infants. J Clin Endocrinol 25:209, 1965

26. **Wolf H, Stubbes P, Sabata V:** The influence of maternal glucose infusions on fetal growth hormone levels. Pediatrics 45:36, 1970

27. **Aarskog D:** Cortisol in the newborn infant. Acta Paediatr Scand (Suppl.) 158:1, 1965

28. **Migeon CJ, Nicolopoulos D, Cornblath M:** Concentration of 17-hydroxycorticosteroids in the blood of diabetic mothers and in blood from the umbilical cords of their offspring at the time of delivery. Pediatrics 25:605, 1960

29. **Smith EK, Reardon HS, Field SH:** Urinary constituents of infants of diabetic and non diabetic mothers. J Pediatr 64:652, 1964

30. **Cathro DM, Forsyth CC:** Excretion of corticosteroids in infants of diabetic and pre-diabetic mothers. Arch Dis Child 40:583, 1965

31. **Aarskog D:** Cortisol production rate in newborn infants of diabetic mothers. J Pediatr 62:807, 1963

32. **Chattoraj SC, Carroll CJ, Turner AK et al:** Carbohydrate intolerance: Its influence on maternal and fetal levels of cortisol and cortisone. Obstet Gynecol 44:646, 1974

33. **Bloom SR, Johnston DI:** Failure of glucagon release in infants of diabetic mothers. Br Med J 25:453, 1972

34. **Williams PR, Sperling MA, Racasa Z:** Blunting of spontaneous and alanine-stimulated glucagon secretion in newborn infants of diabetic mothers. Am J Obstet Gynecol 133:51, 1979

35. **Light IJ, Sutherland JM, Loggie JM et al:** Infants of diabetic mothers. N Engl J Med 277:394, 1967

36. **Stern L, Ramos A, Leduc J:** Urinary catecholamine excretion in infants of diabetic mothers. Pediatrics 42:598, 1968

37. **McCann ML, Miyazaki Y, Guthrie RA et al:** A new therapeutic rationale for the infant of the diabetic mother. Mo Med 65:275, 1968

38. **Davidsen O:** Serum proteins in newborn infants of diabetic mothers. Am J Obstet Gynecol 111:934, 1971

39. **Cockburn F, Blagden A, Michie EA et al:** The influence of pre-eclampsia and diabetes mellitus on plasma free amino acids in maternal, umbilical vein and infant blood. J Obstet Gynecol Br Commw 78:215, 1971

40. **Vejtorp M, Pedersen J, Klebe JG et al:** Low concentration of plasma amino acids in newborn babies of diabetic mothers. Acta Paediatr Scand 66:53, 1977

41. **Soltesz G, Schultz K, Mestyan J et al:** Blood glucose and plasma amino acid concentrations in infants of diabetic mothers. Pediatrics 61:77, 1978

42. **McCann ML, Katigbak EB, Kotchen J et al:** The prevention of hypoglycemia in infants of diabetic mothers. Presented at meeting of Society for Pediatric Research, May 5, 1965

43. **Farquhar JW:** Metabolic changes in the infant of the diabetic mother. Pediatr Clin North Am, 12:743,1965

44. **Tsang RC, Kleinman LI Sutherland JM et al:** Hypoglycemia in infants of diabetic mothers. J Pediatr 80:384, 1972

45. **Tsang RC, Strub R, Brown DR et al:** Hypomagnesemia in infants of diabetic mothers: perinatal studies. J Pediatr 89:115, 1976

46. **Taylor PM, Wolfson JH, Bright NH, et al:**

Hyperbilirubinemia in infants of diabetic mothers. Biol Neonate 5:289, 1963

47. **Gellis SS, Hsia DY-Y:** The infant of the diabetic mother. Am J Dis Child 97:1, 1959

48. **Jones MD, Burd LI, Bowes WA et al:** Failure of association of premature rupture of membranes with respiratory distress syndrome. N Engl J Med 292:1253, 1975

49. **Robert MF, Neff RK, Hubbell JP et al:** Association between maternal diabetes and the respiratory distress syndrome in the newborn. N Engl J Med 294:357, 1976

50. **Gluck L, Kulovich MV:** Lecithin/sphingomyelin ratios in amniotic fluid in normal and abnormal pregnancy. Am J Obstet Gynecol 115:539, 1973

51. **Weber G, Singhal RL, Stamm NB et al:** Hormonal induction and suppression of liver enzyme biosynthesis. Fed Proc 24:745, 1965

52. **Smith BT, Giroud CJP, Robert M et al:** Insulin antagonism of cortisol action on lecithin synthesis by cultured fetal lung cells. J Ped 87:953, 1975

53. **Gross I, Smith GJW:** Insulin delays the morphologic maturation of fetal rat lung in vitro (abstr). Pediatr Res 11:515, 1977

54. **Epstein MF, Farrell PM, Chez RA:** Fetal lung lecithin metabolism in the glucose-intolerant rhesus monkey pregnancy. Pediatrics 57:722, 1976

55. **Torday JS, Demottaz V, Frantz ID:** Prediction of fetal pulmonary maturation in complicated pregnancies (abstr). Pediatr Res 13:542, 1979

56. **Avery ME, Oppenheimer EH, Gordon HH:** Renal vein thrombosis in newborn infants of diabetic mothers. N Engl J Med 256:1134, 1957

57. **Ward TF:** Multiple thromboses in an infant of a diabetic mother. J Pediatr 90:982, 1977

58. **Dossett JH:** Microbial defenses of the child and man. Pediatr Clin North Am 19:355, 1972

59. **Pedersen LM, Tygstrup I, Pedersen J:** Congenital malformations in newborn infants of diabetic women. Lancet 1:1124, 1964

60. **Pedersen J:** The pregnant diabetic and her newborn pp 192–193. Baltimore, Williams & Wilkins, 1977

61. **Chung CS:** Effect of maternal diabetes on congenital malformations. Birth Defects 11:23, 1975

62. **Hubbell JP, Muirhead DM Jr, Drorbaugh JE:** The newborn infant of the diabetic mother. Med Clin North Am 49:1035, 1965

63. **Freeman RK, Kreitzer MS:** Current Problems in Pediatrics, Current Concepts in Antepartum and Intrapartum Fetal Evaluation, Vol. II, No. 9. Chicago, Year Book, July, 1972

64. **Gabbe SG, Mestman JH, Freeman RK et al:** Management and outcome of pregnancy in diabetes mellitus, classes B to R. Am J Obstet Gynecol 129:723, 1977

65. **O'Sullivan JB, Mahan CM, Charles D et al:** Medical treatment of the gestational diabetic. Obstet Gynecol 43:817, 1974

66. **Harding PGR, Tevaarwerk G:** The metabolic adaptation to pregnancy and the prevention of fetal macrosomia in the gestational diabetic. In The Diabetic Pregnancy and Its Outcome, p. 53. Mead Johnson Symposium on Perinatal and Developmental Medicine, No. 13, 1978

67. **McCann ML, Likly BF:** The role of epinephrine prophylactic therapy in the infant of a diabetic mother. Atlantic City, NJ, Society for Pediatric Research, 1967

68. **Haworth JC, Dillings LA, Vidyasagar D:** Hypoglycemia in infants of diabetic mothers: Effect of epinephrine therapy. Pediatrics 82:94, 1973

69. **McCann ML, Chen CH, Katigbak EB et al:** On hypoglucosemia in the infants of diabetic mothers. N Engl J Med 275:8, 1966

70. **Maenpaa PJ, Raivio KO, Kekomaki MP:** Liver adenine nucleotides: Fructose-induced depletion and its effect on protein synthesis. Science 161:1253, 1968

71. **Schiff D, Aranda JV, Colle E, et al:** Metabolic effects of exchange transfusions. II. Delayed hypoglycemia following exchange transfusion with citrated blood. J Pediatr 79:589, 1971

72. **Schiff D, Aranda JV, Chan G, Colle E, Stern L:** Metabolic effects of exchange transfusion. I. Effect of citrated and of heparinized blood on glucose, nonesterified fatty acids, HBABA binding and insulin. J Pediatr 78:693, 1971

73. **Pedersen J:** The Pregnant Diabetic and Her Newborn, p. 191. Baltimore, Williams & Wilkins, 1977

74. **Pildes RS:** Infants of diabetic mothers. N Engl J Med 289:902, 1973

75. **David WS, Campbell JB:** Neonatal small left colon syndrome. Am J Dis Child 129:1024, 1975

76. **Gutgesell HP, Mullins CE, Gillette PC et al:** Transient hypertrophic subaortic stenosis in infants of diabetic mothers. J Pediatr 89:120, 1976

77. **Pederson J:** Follow-up examinations of children of diabetic mothers (abstr). Acta Paediatr Scand (Suppl) 77:203, 1948

78. **White P:** Childhood diabetes. Diabetes 9:345, 1960

79. **Fredrikson AH, Hagbard L, Olow L et al:** Efterundersokning af barn till diabetiska Modrar. Nord Med 57:669, 1957

80. **Hagbard L, Olow I, Reinand T:** A follow-up study of 514 children of diabetic mothers. Acta Paediatr Scand 48:184, 1959

81. **Breidahl HD:** The growth and development of

children born to mothers with diabetes. Med J Aust 1:268, 1966

82. **Farquhar JW:** Prognosis for babies born to diabetic mothers in Edinburgh. Arch Dis Child 44:36, 1969

83. **Yssing M:** Long-term prognosis of children born to mothers diabetic when pregnant from early diabetes in early life. In Camerini–Davalos RA, Cole HS, (eds): Early Diabetes in Early Life, p 575. New York, Academic Press, 1975

84. **Churchill JA, Berendes HW, Nemore U:** Neu-
ropsychological deficits in children of diabetic mothers. Am J Obstet Gynecol 105:257, 1969

85. **White P, Koshy P, Duckers J:** The management of pregnancy complicating diabetes and of children of diabetic mothers. Med Clin North Am 37:1481, 1953

86. **Bibergeil H, Godel E, Amendt P:** Diabetes and pregnancy: Early and late prognosis of children of diabetic mothers. In Camerini-Davalos RA, Cole HS (eds): Early Diabetes in Early Life, p 427. New York, Academic Press, 1975

17

Psychological Needs of the Mother in Early Mother-Infant Interactions

Arnold J. Sameroff

The natural process of a mother rearing her infant has been so taken for granted as a current social value that attention is exclusively focused on the "how" of this caretaking. Professional concern has been related to the best techniques for assuring the physical well-being of the infant. However, recent trends have shifted from an exclusive concern with physical care of the child to an increasing interest in the psychological care of the infant. The ability of medical technology to minimize the physical disabilities associated with the birth process has permitted the physician to begin attending to the psychological variables which contribute to normal developmental outcomes.

Concern with the emotional environment of the child has been given added impetus by the discovery of two syndromes which seem to be related to poor caretaking practices: failure-to-thrive and the battered child. These situations, in which the parent does not appear to be interested in the "how" of adequate child-rearing have raised questions about the "why" of caretaking. As long as one assumed that child-rearing was a natural process, one could wonder about its occurrence, but one was not forced to explain it. However, when the clinician is confronted with a number of situations in which child-rearing is approached in an unnatural way, he is forced to look at parenting in a larger context. Only by seeing normal child-rearing in the perspective of other possible parenting behavior, can one understand "why" parents tend to take care of their infants. Within this larger view one can then attempt to manipulate and remedy the situations in which deviancies in child-rearing occur.

This chapter treats both the "why" and "how" of child-rearing. The data on animal studies in mother-infant caretaking behavior will be first reviewed in an evolutionary context. Then the literature on the nature of human caretaking behavior will be reviewed to see what can be learned from the animal model. Finally, the distinctly human characteristics for child-rearing will be discussed with an emphasis on how these qualities may be maximized through both parent education and medical practice.

MOTHER-INFANT ATTACHMENT

The term "attachment" has been given currency by Bowlby as a general term to include those behaviors that serve to maintain proximity to another individual.[1] Although Bowlby's use of the term refers mainly to the infant's attachment to the mother. This chapter will focus more on the mother's attachment to the child, which permits her to engage in the necessary caretaking behavior.

Bowlby has described an evolutionary shift from lower species, in which the infant takes all the initiative in keeping contact with the mother, to higher species, in which the mother takes all the initiative. This shift is particularly evident in the decreasing capacity of the newborn infant to take care of itself, as seen in the most advanced members of the primate order: gorilla and man. The behavior of birds that are able to follow their mothers within hours after hatching is an example of the former case in which the infant maintains attachment. Closer to man are mammals, and, especially, primates. Among the lowest primates, such as the lemur and marmoset, the infant must cling to his mother from birth, the mother providing no support whatever. More advanced primate infants, such as the baboon and rhesus monkey, must do most of the clinging, although the mother gives some assistance in the first hours or days of life. Among the most advanced primates, the gorilla and man, the infant is incapable of hanging on to his mother during the first month and she must carry him instead.

Whereas lower species learn only minor aspects of caretaking practice, the socialization and caretaking practices of mammals, especially primates, are strongly affected by the developmental experiences of the mother herself.

Important correlates to the "caretaking" behavior of the mother are the "care-eliciting" behavior of the infant. In general, the infant must provide cues to the mother so that his needs will be met at the appropriate time and in the appropriate way. In lower species, such as rats and mice, these care-eliciting behaviors such as clinging, sucking, and crying are important in helping the mother identify her offspring. It will be seen that the absence of care-eliciting behaviors will reduce caretaking behavior in the mothers, while the presence of care-eliciting behaviors will produce maternal behavior even in nonmothers (*e.g.,* adult virgin females and even males).

Care-eliciting Behavior (Animal Studies)

Attempts to explain the caretaking behavior of the mother toward her young have been based on both physiologic and psychological variables. Physiologic explanations have focused on the hormonal changes that occur following parturition or in connection with lactation, which were assumed to make the mother more sensitive to her offspring. Rosenblatt, in an extensive analysis of maternal behavior in rats, has shown that, although biochemical effects do exist, they are secondary in significance to the eliciting effects of the behavior of the infant rats.[2] Groups of ovariectomized and hypophysectomized females, in addition to intact and castrated males were exposed to young pups. The typical maternal behaviors of retrieving, crouching to nurse, and nest building appeared in all the groups. The duration of exposure to the infant mice required to elicit the maternal behavior was similar for all of these groups including the males.

The behavior of the young rats appeared to be a necessary condition to elicit maternal behavior in their mothers. Rosenblatt found that the mother was most prepared to be maternal during the first few days after parturition. After that period, it was more difficult to elicit maternal behavior. The maintenance of maternal behavior was also most vulnerable during the first few days after birth. If the pups were removed after the initiation of maternal behavior in the first day or two this behavior quickly waned. After 3 days, there was only a slight reduction of maternal responsiveness following a 4-day separation from the infant rats. It appeared to be important for the mother rats to spend time with their offspring in the period immediately following delivery if later maternal behavior was to be maintained in reunions after separation from the young.

It has been difficult to separate the effects of biochemical changes in the mother from those eliciting properties of the offspring in fostering the caretaking relationship. In another attempt to study the effects of the infant's characteristics alone, Noirot placed infant mice 1 to 20 days of age with virgin adult female mice.[3] The virgin mice responded with the typical maternal behavior of retrieving, licking, nest building, and crouching in a lactation position. This behavior occurred at high levels in response to infants of 1 to 10 days of age. Beyond that age, there was a decline in this behavior. Some characteristic of the appearance of external behavior of these new-born mice served to elicit maternal behavior even in these virgin female mice.

Animal research provides an evolutionary context into which human behavior can be placed. Rosenblatt has hypothesized that a synchrony exists in the activities of mother and infant that follows a transactional model of development.[4] The behavior of both the mother and the infant mutually affect each other. The infant's initial helpless movements give rise to caretaking in the mother. The caretaking by the mother increases the infant's abilities to suckle and eliminate. As the infant increases in mobility and independent action, he again alters his mother's behavior by reducing the amount of caretaking she engages in. The mother's reduction in maternal behaviors moves her offspring in the direction of independence and maturity.

To draw analogies to the human situation requires the identification of the specific characteristics of the offspring, both physical and behavioral, which elicit maternal behavior. Although the specificity of these characteristics may be quite different for man and animals, the general organizational principles may be quite similar.

Separation (Animal Studies)

Rodent research has demonstrated that separation from the mother shortly after birth strongly reduces the caretaking activities of the mother even after the infants are returned. Another example of the effects of the interruption of the mother-infant synchrony can be found in a study of goats reported by Moore.[5] The typical behavior of goats following birth is for the mother to lick off the amniotic fluid from her newborn kid, after which she pushes the kid toward her udder where suckling is initiated. The mother then establishes a territory including herself and her kid but excluding all other members of her herd. If the kid is removed before having a chance to begin sucking, the mother does not establish this relationship to her own particular infant. If the kid is returned as quickly as an hour later, the mother has already become indifferent to him and will allow herself to be suckled by any kid in the herd. The completion of the initial suckling experience appears to be important for the maintenance of a specific mother-child relationship.

In addition to the immediate reduction of the mother's caretaking produced by separation from her young shortly after birth, there are long-range effects on the offspring's capacity for child rearing. Moore reported that the separated kids were much less effective as mothers after reaching adulthood than kids who had not been separated from their mothers. Much more dramatic evidence of the deleterious effect of having been raised without a mother is seen in the research of the Harlows.[6] When infant monkeys were separated from their mothers and reared alone, they were severely handicapped in the performance of many adult functions including sexual intercourse and motherhood. As mothers they were indifferent or even brutal to their offspring.

In contrast to the negative effects of separation on the mother's attachment to her infant are the positive effects of a strong mother-infant attachment. In order to establish a strong mother-infant attachment, the care-eliciting behaviors of the infant are extremely important. But once initiated, the absence of these care-eliciting behaviors does not appear to reduce the mother's attachment. Studies of non-human primates have shown that even after the infant has died, the mother will continue to hold it, in some cases even after the body has begun to decompose.

Human Mother-Infant Attachment

The manner in which a human mother and her infant relate in normal development can be placed in the evolutionary context described above. A mother may be seen to acquire appropriate caretaking practices from her own experience of being cared for as an infant, from her observations of other mothers' child-rearing, from education in appropriate child-rearing techniques, and from practice experiences with younger siblings or children of others.

The goals of professional perinatal care should be (1) to maximize the strengths of the mother's abilities for and sensitivity to the caretaking of her child, (2) to produce a child who is maximally capable of signaling his needs and responding to this mother, and (3) to provide the setting in which the initial bonding between mother and infant can take place. In the next section the variables interfering with these goals will be examined and suggestions made for practices by which the reaching of these goals can be maximized.

THE MOTHER

The ability of the mother to produce the required attachment and caretaking behaviors is related to a complex of socioeconomic, educational, and personality factors. In general, mothers from middle or upper socioeconomic classes, with better than high-school education, a secure personal identity, and a stable family emotional life are at a relative advantage. On the other hand, especially when the infant has suffered some reproductive complication which alters its appearance or causes it to require greater attention, mothers who are from lower socioeconomic strata, who have poor education or emotional problems, will tend more often to produce children who will have later developmental deviancies.[4,7] To this list must be added the experience the mother had while being raised herself. In studies of children who have suffered abuse or neglect as manifested in the battered-child or failure-to-thrive syndromes, it has been found that their parents have often had similar experiences as children. The parents' experiences of abuse as children tend to set the norms for their own child-rearing behavior.[8]

Socioeconomic Status

Social and economic influences do not directly affect development but must be mediated through the behavior of the mother. Circumstances of poverty create pressures that do not permit the mother to devote herself fully to either her childbearing or child-rearing. Birch and Gussow have presented impressive evidence documenting the full range of poor medical consequences resulting from impoverished living conditions.[9]

Accompanying these economic conditions are additional stresses associated with poor social conditions. The social class scale does not represent a continuous spectrum of social organization. Poor families can have strong cultural and social values that act to maintain and support the family. However, in families at the lowest socioeconomic stratum, a significant increase occurs in the level of family disorganization. In this subculture, absence of one or both parents is the rule rather than the exception.[10] A hand-to-mouth economic existence seriously affects the mother's capacities to deal with anything other than the "here-and-now" circumstances of life. The inability to financially or socially plan for the future is reflected by accompanying cognitive inadequacies that are not remedied by the mother's educational background.

Cognitive Level

Cognitive and intellectual development is seen, by such figures as Piaget, as a shift from dealing with the concrete to dealing with the abstract.[11] Whereas an adult can think in the hypothetical terms required to systematically plan for the future, a child cannot. The child overdepends on the appearance of things for his thinking and finds it extremely difficult to take or appreciate the view of others.[12] However, the shift from the concrete thinking of the child to the abstract conceptualizations of the adult does not occur automatically. He is faced with the problem of responding to the demands of an environment in which concrete solutions do not solve problems. This conflict or disequilibrium forces the child to alter his thinking toward a system in which the concrete can be placed in a larger abstract context with a wide range of possible solutions.

In lower social strata, these steps may not occur. The disorganization found in social settings accompanied by a paucity of available social roles do not provide the stimuli for the child that enable him to reach higher levels of cognitive functioning. Even the school system, which would normally lead the child to the necessary levels of competence, is inadequate in these settings. Many such children do not complete their education and even many of those who do are at significantly lower levels of functioning than children from comparable schools in other social settings.

How do cognitive deficiencies affect the mother's ability to rear her child? In the face of a normal pregnancy outcome there is little that the neonatologist can contribute to the system. The mother will have as good an attachment to her child and rear him as adequately as her resources allow. However, given a child with some evident abnormality, the consequences of the mother's cognitive deficiencies become manifest. Prematurity, anoxia, plus a variety of other reproductive complications may be seen as defects which invariably produce later intellectual or tempermental deficits, rather than as disorders of infancy which need not have direct influence upon the developmental outcome of the child.[4] Indeed, this concrete view is not restricted to those who have poor formal education, but can be found as an expression of concrete thinking at all educational levels.

Experience As a Child

Child-rearing styles have been categorized into a variety of systems. Authoritarian and permissive practices are usually seen as two endpoints of a scale, with other styles such as neglectful, laissez-faire, democratic, accommodative, and authoritative in between. These categorizations give the impression that each of these styles is practiced by a large number of parents. However, Chamberlin in a survey of middle-class families found that the vast majority practiced some variation of authoritarian child rearing.[13] Consistent permissive or accommodative styles existed in less than 10% of the homes surveyed.

Because of the dominant use of authoritarian child-rearing techniques in our culture, one can gain an overview of how most children are reared by an analysis of the authoritarian style. The parents tend to control and evaluate the child's behavior by defined standards of conduct. Obedience is valued along with respect for authority and work. The parents are punitive and discussion is discouraged when there is a conflict between the wishes of the parents and those of the child.[14]

Despite the pejorative connotations of the above descriptions of authoritarian child rearing, it must be understood that such parents are proceeding in behaviors which they believe to be in the best interest of the child. They are intent on producing offspring who will accept and follow the parents' social, moral, and intellectual values. The way in which the demands of the authoritarian parent are enforced range from persuasion to severe physical punishment. Yet even the most severe physical abuse is frequently an expression of the parents' child-rearing beliefs. Children who have been reared under such regimens may come to see these techniques as acceptable for bringing up their own children.

As a consequence of this role definition, there are set expectations as to what a baby does and set techniques as to how the baby should be reared. These set expectations are met by the average full-term infant. However, when a child requires some degree of specialized treatment, the system breaks down. Because of the inflexibility of the authoritarian child-rearing system, the special needs of the child may go unmet.

Thomas, Chess, and Birch have been most explicit in their emphasis on the individualized needs of infants.[15] Reviewing the history of child-rearing techniques, they have found that no matter what the societal norms, there are always deviant outcomes among some children. They attribute these to the fact that no one mode of child-rearing works for the entire spectrum of temperamental characteristics found among young infants. This holds true especially for the cluster of characteristics that typify the "difficult" child. The parents must be aware that there are a variety of techniques that must be adapted to the temperament and requirements of their infant. This need for adaptability runs counter to the typical rigidity found in standard child-rearing behavior.

At the concrete level of thinking, the parent places variations in temperamental or physical characteristics into one of two categories—normal or abnormal—which have serious implications for later development. At the abstract level of thinking, the same infant variations are seen as part of a wide range of reproductive outcomes that may or may not have negative consequences for later development.

Emotions

To the list of factors playing a role in the mother's attachment to her infant and caretaking must be added her mental health and emotional status. In order to focus on the needs of her child, the mother must be able to separate the child's demands from her own personal concerns and needs. When the mother has problems with her own self-identity, she will tend to focus on her own needs, anxieties, and emotions rather than on those of the infant. Even if all other factors are positive, none can operate if the mother is too involved with her own concerns to be able to focus on the child.

Emotional factors, however, begin taking their toll on developmental outcomes even before the mother has an opportunity to care for her child. Several reviews have shown that emotional factors play a role in producing obstetric complications that affect the duration and the quality of the pregnancy.[16,17] Mac-Donald found, despite shortcomings of research in this area, that consistent differences appeared between the emotional characteristics of women who had complications and those who had none.[18] The groups of women with abnormal consequences had significantly higher levels of anxiety. Sameroff and Zax found that, in general, the more chronic the mother's mental disorder, the greater the incidence of delivery complications.[19]

A vicious cycle can thus result from the mother's poor emotional state during pregnancy. The anxiety of the mother worsens her physiologic experience of pregnancy, which in turn worsens her attitudes toward the pregnancy, and eventually affects its outcome. There is some additional evidence that the effects of these emotional disturbances during the pregnancy and delivery even affect the product of the pregnancy. Stress on the mother can increase the incidence of both major and minor physical anomalies in the offspring,[20] as well as behavioral anomalies such as fussiness and crying.[21]

Summary of Antecedent Maternal Variables

Four factors play significant roles in the mother's ability to take care of the infant. These include her socioeconomic background, her educational training, her own experiences as a child, and her emotional stability. Although these factors have been dealt with separately, they often are closely linked with each other and also with the character of the infant. Low socioeconomic status is frequently associated with poor mental health, lower educational outcomes, and poor childhood experiences. As a consequence, those mothers who suffer from one of these factors often suffer from all of them.

THE CHILD

In the preceding section, the mother's attachment to her child was related to factors in her own social history and upbringing. Once the infant is born, a new array of variables begins to influence her behavior. These vari-ables have been treated earlier under "care-eliciting behavior" of the infant. In the present section, normal care eliciting behavior of the human infant will be described, followed by a discussion of the individual differences in these behaviors. The section will be concluded with an analysis of iatrogenic factors contributing to the disruption of these care-eliciting behaviors in the infant.

Human Care-eliciting Behaviors

Humans who have been normally reared are prepared to engage in maternal caretaking behavior when placed in a situation with a young infant. As was noted in the review of the animal literature, this ability to demonstrate caretaking behavior is not limited to mothers, but also applies to other adults of the species including males and virgin females.[22]

How the characteristics of the young infant act to attach his mother to him has been the subject of a growing research interest. Influenced by the work of ethologists, John Bowlby speculated on the instinctual basis of the infant's behavior.[1] Recently he has interpreted attachment behavior in terms of a control system emphasizing the reciprocal nature of the mother-infant bond. Despite the increased plasticity and variability of human behavior when generally contrasted with that of other species, attachment behavior in the young is seen as the most environmentally stable behavioral system across all species.[23]

What then are the properties of the infant that produce this attachment effect on other members of his species? The immediately evident characteristics of the infant are related to his physical appearance. He is tiny and "cute." Some ethologically oriented investigators have argued that the facial configuration of the infant, with its large head in relation to body and large forehead in relation to face, elicits maternal responses in adults.[24]

Moving from appearance to performance, two aspects of the newborn infant's behavior can be distinguished. The first aspect can be interpreted as a signal to his environment that he needs attention. The infant's ability to differentiate between animate and inanimate objects, and then between mother and other animate objects, is a process that will be acquired over a period of some months.[11] Although initially these signals are restricted to crying, with age other behaviors such as visual tracking, smiling, and reaching become additional components. After about 3 months, the intentional aspects of the signaling increase and are specifically directed to bring the mother into closer proximity. In the newborn period, these behaviors can only be considered as built-in expressions of the child's feelings of comfort or discomfort.

The second aspect of the infant's behavior is his responsivity to the ministrations of his environment. An initial repertoire of sucking, clinging, and looking expands to include smiling and babbling after a few months, and still later the addition of locomotor activities such as crawling and walking. These establish a reciprocal relationship with the mother whereby either partner can initiate a sequence to be completed by the other. The baby's cry is the most frequent starting point; it causes the mother to respond with a variety of caretaking behaviors such as diaper changing, feeding, or rocking the child.[25] The infant in turn, responds by quieting and going to sleep, or by becoming alert and looking around, or by sucking and grasping the mother.

The important ingredient for the mother in these behavior chains is the infant's response to her ministrations. Most contemporary formulations of motivation subscribe to an "effectance" concept (*i.e.,* what motivates and reinforces behavior is the effectiveness of that behavior in predictably causing something to happen).[26] Initially, most efforts of the mother are devoted to quieting the crying baby. As the infant's increasing wakefulness permits him to look around and smile, the mother, especially when primiparous, tends to begin behavior chains by poking or rocking the child or by presenting visual or auditory stimuli in an attempt to evoke a response. In these instances, the mother's positive feelings toward the child appear to be a function of how readily the child will respond to the mother's behavior.

In summary, the normal mother, imbued with the cultural traditions of her society, finds herself in the situation of taking care of a newborn infant. Whether the experience is a pleasure or a displeasure depends on how effective she is at controlling her infant's behavior. The more effective the mother is, the happier she will be, and the more willing she will be to continue to interact with the child. On the other hand, if she is not effective in controlling her child's behavior, she will tend to become insecure in her feelings of competence as a mother and unhappy in the caretaking situation.

Individual Differences in Infancy

Although a number of researchers over the past half century have been involved in studies assessing variability in early behavior, it is the work of Thomas, Chess, and their associates, at New York University which has most explicitly dealt with the relation of these individual differences to the quality of mother-infant interaction.[27] The NYU group attended to a number of behavioral categories which composed the reactive style of the infant. The word "temperament" was used to describe the individuality of each infant's style and at the same time to separate these styles from issues related to the origins of individuality. Each child's temperament was described in terms of nine categories of behavior which included

1. Activity level.
2. Rhythmicity (regularity of biologic functioning).
3. Approach-withdrawal (positive or negative initial response to new stimulation).
4. Adaptability (the ease with which behavior was changed when the situation changed).
5. Positive or negative quality of mood.
6. Intensity of mood.
7. Sensory threshold (intensity of stimulation required to elicit a response).
8. Distractability or soothability.
9. Persistence (attention span).

When the temperament of infants in the first few months of life was assessed using these categories, two major clusters emerged: "the easy child" and "the difficult child." The larger group of **easy** children were typified by regularity, rapid adaptability, approach behavior, and positive moods of moderate intensity. About 10% of the infants studied were considered **difficult** and were typified by irregularity, slow adaptability, and frequent negative moods of high intensity.

The major emphasis of this research on temperament was to demonstrate that childrearing practices are not the sole determinants of developmental outcome. The identical "normal" practices would produce different outcomes for children who had initially different temperamental makeups. Where demand feeding schedules and a general permissiveness might be fine for an "easy" child, they would lead to increased disorganization in the already disorganized "difficult" child. Chess argues that the responsibility of parents and their advisors is to become aware of the infant's temperament and modify their child-care rules to be appropriate for that infant.[28]

Although behavior deviancies can occur in children of any temperament, when given inappropriate child-rearing the group of "difficult" infants seem to be most vulnerable in this respect. For parents who are exceptionally tolerant of the child's lengthy adjustment period, who are patient with negative moods, and who are not embarrassed by tantrums in public, the initial difficult temperament dissipates as the child moves out of infancy. But for parents who become angry or insecure in reaction to the child's behavior, or who resent and avoid the child, the difficult temperament can be perpetuated into a continuing behavioral disturbance throughout development. Faced with an average infant, these latter parents might have been quite adequate, but faced by the exceptional demands for accommodation required by the difficult child, they are unequal to the task.

The temperamental variations found in newborn infants can affect their interaction with their parents. One of the major requirements for the satisfaction of the mother during this period is a responsive baby. To the extent that the infant's temperament interferes with his ability to be responsive, it will adversely affect his mother's feelings toward him, if the mother cannot quiet her crying baby, her competence as a caretaker may be brought into question. Initially the failure to elicit eye-to-eye contact and later to elicit smiling fosters further feelings of inadequacy. An infant with a high threshold to stimulation creates other problems for the mother, because her mode of behavior may not be strong enough to elicit a response from the infant. Some children provide no opportunity for mothers to interact with them because they are always insulated from their environment. Either they are sound asleep or, when awake, are so agitated with crying that nothing the mother does can break through to them.[29]

The mother's feelings of maternal competence and security derive in large measure from her capacity to make her infant respond to her. To the extent that the infant's temperament denies her that experience, the attachment process is made that much more difficult. She is left with only the cultural training and social expectations of motherhood to maintain her caretaking behavior.

Sources of Newborn Behavioral Differences

Hereditary factors are given as a standard explanation for individual differences. However, from the genetic point of view, little is known about the inheritance of personality.

Other mechanisms of a nongenetic nature have been suggested by which the behavior of the parents is transmitted to their offspring. A mother with a poor emotional state during pregnancy can affect the behavior of the infant both *in utero* and after birth.[21] Women with poor attitudes toward pregnancy or who suffered undue emotional stress tend to have infants who are "difficult" or have deviant or abnormal behavior.[30] The mechanism by which the mother's distress is translated into the infant's behavior is still a subject for speculation. Biochemical changes in the mother caused by her upset have been the most common of these hypothesized etiologic agents.[17]

Another source of variation in newborn behavior can be found in the delivery process itself. Duration of labor, amount and type of medication, and instrumental deliveries have all been implicated as factors influencing the newborn's behavior. Narcotics have been found to decrease the infant's sucking abilities.[31] Sensitivity to the environment, as reflected by the infant's ability to habituate to stimulation was reduced by high medication levels.[32] In some reports, long labor seemed to account for more of the disruption of the infant's behavior than did medication.[33]

Although the influence of delivery variables on infant behavior has been discussed apart from the effect of the mother's emotional state on her pregnancy, the two factors frequently act together. The mother with poor attitudes and anxiety during pregnancy often has a greater number of complications during delivery. The anxious mother creates the impression that she needs more medication. Once the medication is administered, she is less competent to help in the delivery, and the duration of her labor as well as her chances for an instrumental intervention are increased. The product of such a delivery is often a newborn who initially is less responsive to his mother and thereby less able to provide her with early rewards for her caretaking behavior.

Summary of the Infant's Role

The infant's contribution to the mother's pleasure in her caretaking role is to be responsive to her ministrations. By signaling her when he needs care and by being receptive to that care, the infant provides the mother with a basis for confidence in her ability to nurture her child and in her ability to fulfill the social and cultural expectations related to motherhood. Responsivity to its mother is reduced in an infant whose temperament makes him or her insensitive to care either because of high threshold to stimulation or of constant inconsolability. The "difficult" child is a category used to describe such an infant. The chance of having a difficult child may be increased by a mother's poor emotional state during pregnancy. The infant's responsivity can also be reduced by complications of the delivery process.

THE MATERNITY SETTING

It has been argued that perinatal hospital care over the last century has moved in the direction of an environment's minimizing the attachment between mother and infant.[34] The professionalization of obstetric practice and concerns about infectious disease have moved the mother further from participation in or even knowledge of the childbirth experience. In the early days of the century, the mother learned about childbirth through participating in the delivery of others and was awake for her own deliveries. Later the ideal was to make the mother as oblivious as possible to the birth process through medication during delivery. Previously, the mother received and cared for the baby immediately after delivery with no period of separation. In recent times, the mother of the normal infant is immediately separated from her child for as long as a day, while the mother of the infant who is born prematurely or with other special problems may be separated from her child up to 3 months.

Of course, there have been justifications for these changes in perinatal practices; infant mortality and morbidity have been reduced. The great successes in fighting medical illnesses now are permitting the neonatologist to turn to issues relating to the mental health of his charges: the mother and her newborn infant.

Prematurity and Deviant Caretaking

Increasingly, neonatologists have become concerned with the effects of separating mother and child in the newborn period. These concerns have been made especially salient by studies that have found that a large number of premature infants are abused and neglected later in infancy.[35] Many of the battered children who were of normal birth weights had contracted a variety of other illnesses that could have affected their relationship to their parents. Studies have been made of infants with failure-to-thrive syndrome, identified as a "growth and developmental failure accompanied by psychosocial disruption followed by improvement on placement in a nurturing environment." Although somatic symptomatology clouded the diagnosis in many of these cases, the clinical manifestations generally cleared up early in the hospitalization. In one study of failure-to-thrive more than half of the mothers had suffered some complication of pregnancy or delivery, while 41% of the infants had weighed less than 2,500 g at birth.[36] Analyses of the family situations of these patients disclosed a variety of psychosocial stresses ranging from poor and disruptive caretaking to the death of close relatives. The developmental consequences of neglect and abuse are not restricted to physical disorders. Many intellectual and emotional deviancies may be found in these children. The long-term consequences of childhood abuse were studied by Elmer and Gregg by following up 20 battered children 1 to 16 years after discharge from the hospital.[37] At the time of the follow-up only 2 of the 20 children were found to be normal in physical, mental, and emotional development.

The developmental prognosis for abused children is poor indeed, unless massive interventions are made into the social environment of the child. If premature infants and infants who suffer other illnesses can be identified as a group at high risk for later neglect or abuse, early prophylactic programs might serve to reduce not only the incidence of these problems but also the need for massive intervention treatments after the fact. Such early programs, require an understanding of the variables affecting early mother-infant interaction.

Separation of the Mother from Her Premature Infant

The issue of mother-infant attachment comes to the center of attention when the care of premature infants is studied. When the mother of the premature who is placed in the special-care nursery is finally permitted to take the infant home, she often reports her experience as one of receiving a stranger. Her feelings about the infant appear to be quite different from those of the mother of the full-term infant. Attempts have been made to assess the consequences of separation on the behavior of mothers who are kept from their infants placed in special care nurseries.

At Stanford University, Leiderman and his coworkers have been engaged in a series of studies in which three groups of mothers were observed: two groups with premature infants and one group with full-term infants.[38] The two groups of premature infants were separated from their mothers after birth and placed in an intensive care nursery (ICN) from 3 to 12 weeks until they weighted 2100 g. At that point the infants were transferred to a discharge nursery until they weighed 2500 g, which took from 7 to 10 days, after which they were discharged. The mothers of one of the premature groups followed normal hospital procedures and were "separated" from their infants in the ICN. Only visual contact occurred between these mothers and their infants. The second group of mothers of premature infants were allowed to be in "contact" with their infants in the ICN. They handled their infants in the incubators and participated as much as possible in the normal caretaking of the infants. When the infants were transferred to the discharge nursery, both the "separated" and "contact" groups of mothers were permitted to be with their infants as much as they desired. The premature infants in the separated group were handled by the nursing staff to assure that the infants of the two groups would not receive differing experiences. The mothers in the full-term group saw their infants at the normal feeding times during their 3-day hospital stay.

The mother-infant interactions of the three groups were observed at three points: the first time just before leaving the hospital, the second a week after discharge, and the third a month after discharge. During these observations it was seen that the "full-term" mothers smiled at their infants more often and held them close to their bodies more than both groups of mothers of the prematures. There were no major differences in the behavior of the mothers of the prematures to their infants between the separated and contact groups.

The differences between the behavior of mothers of premature and full-term infants can be attributed to the separation from their infants experienced by these mothers. The incubator prevented even the mothers in the contact group from cuddling their infants close to their bodies. They could only manipulate the infant with their hands. Furthermore, an explanation which cannot be completely ruled out is that, as with animals, the mother's hormonal state when contacting her infant makes a difference in her behavior. The full-term mothers had full contact with their infants right after birth; the mothers of the premature infants did not have full contact until a few weeks after delivery, when any biochemical changes associated with birth would have been dissipated.

Although no differences in behavior toward their infants was noted between the separated and contact groups, a number of differences were found in their subsequent attitudes of self-confidence and in their marital situations. In the group of mothers allowed to be in contact with their premature infants, only 1 out of 22 subsequently became divorced. In contrast, in the separated group, there were five divorces and two of the infants were given up for adoption. These findings may reflect the stressful situation created by having an ill child in the hospital.

In follow-up of this white, middle-class sample through 8 years of age, no differences were found between the contact and separated children. Leiderman concluded that contact within the first 2 days does not produce major changes in maternal behavior and attitudes that have lasting effects. He argued that socioeconomic status, parity of the mother, and gender of the child play a much greater role in predicting later mother and infant behavior.

Other factors associated with separation have been identified which act to undermine the mother's self-evaluation as a caretaker.[39] By placing the child in the ICN, the hospital staff communicates to the mother that her infant needs more care than the mother can provide. Further feelings of inadequacy may result from her knowledge that she was unable to carry her infant to term. In addition, the difference in physical appearance between the premature and the full-term infant continually confronts the mother.

When the mothers in the separated and contact groups in the study described earlier were interviewed, reduced levels of caretaking self-confidence were found among the primiparous women in the separated group. The previous successful childbirth experience of multiparous mothers seemed to insulate them from the debilitating effects of being separated from the premature offspring of their current pregnancy. In the group of mothers who were allowed to visit in the ICN, the initial deficits in self-confidence were reduced by the time the infant was ready to go home. Only one of the mothers in the separated group showed such a positive change. It would appear from this data that allowing mothers, especially primipara, to be in contact with their premature infants reduces their feelings of inadequacy.

The data from the Stanford studies indicated that mothers of full-term infants handled them differently than mothers of premature infants. The full-term group showed more smiling toward their infants and more ventral body contacts. A possible explanation for the reduced physical contact can be found in the studies of Klaus, Kennell, and their associates at Case–Western Reserve University.[40] In observations of the first physical interactions of a mother with her full-term baby, the mother would be seen to begin tentatively touching the extremities of the infant with her fingertips. She would then move from the extremities to the trunk and eventually touch the baby with her full hand. The mother appeared to be testing the baby's fragility and as she became more assured that the infant would not be harmed she increased the amount of contact, eventually cuddling and hugging the infant. Mothers of premature infants proceed more slowly in this process. The mother is reinforced in her feelings that the infant is fragile by his appearance and also by the special care setting. It could be expected then that these findings would be carried over into the home, where the mother would continue to handle her prematurely born infant relatively gingerly.

Recent studies have examined the interactions of mothers and their premature infants during the first year.[41,42] A consistent finding is that while the total amount of interaction is similar in families with conceptional-age matched preterm and full-term infants, the quality of the interaction is different. Mothers of preterm groups tend to be much more active in initiating and maintaining the interaction. Because the preterm infant tends to be hypoactive, the mother must pick up the slack to keep a relationship active. In addition, the interaction with preterm infants tended to be more stereotyped and less varied than interactions with full-term infants. Surprisingly these differences in early mother-infant interactions did not relate to the social or cognitive ability of the child at age 3. Bakeman and Brown suggest that the baby may be buffered against long-term effects of early interactional problems.[41]

Maternal Stress Following Premature Delivery

The stress associated with premature birth can cause maladaptive responses in individuals who are considered to be well within the normal range of personality adjustment. Kaplan and Mason, after studying 60 families following the birth of a premature child, noted many contrasts to a normal birth.[43] Normal deliveries occur in an atmosphere in which a mother desires to complete the pregnancy and produce the normal infant that she is expecting. Following delivery, she is encouraged to feel happy and proud. The happiness is then shared with the infant and acts to heighten her relationship with the child.

In contrast, the woman about to deliver a premature infant receives a completely different set of experiences. She lies in the hospital attempting to delay the delivery until term is completed. Instead of the routine hospital procedure, there is an atmosphere of emergency conditions with a general apprehensiveness about the infant's fate. Following delivery, the mother has a heightened concern about the normality of her infant who is immediately removed from her and placed in a special-care nursery. The hospital staff acts to maintain these concerns by not being able to respond to her with exact prognostications. It is generally difficult to get a good view of the child in the incubator, and the tiny creature that the mother does see only supports her feeling of having had a deviant pregnancy outcome. When the mother of the premature goes home she is typically empty-handed and feels disappointed and deprived. When the infant eventually joins her, he is greeted with continued apprehension about his appearance, smallness, and the mother's adequacy to care for such a fragile creature. The mother of the premature thus faces the future with the feeling of having failed in her pregnancy, a concern for her ability to care for her infant, and an expectation that in the future there will be abnormality showing up in the infant as a consequence of his premature birth.

Kaplan and Mason proposed four tasks that the mother of the premature must resolve if she is to make a satisfactory adjustment to her child.[43] The *first* task is the preparation for the possible loss of the child at delivery by an anticipatory grief and emotional withdrawal from the child. The *second* task is to acknowledge her failure to deliver a normal full-term baby. The grief and depression accompanying these two tasks are positive signs that the mother is struggling with these issues. They are healthy responses until the baby's chances of survival are seen as secure. The *third* task for the mother is to resume the interrupted task of relating to her baby. This task involves her preparation for the baby's homecoming and the now renewed possibility of a positive outcome for her pregnancy. The *fourth* task concerns her future attitudes and involves understanding the special caretaking needs of the premature infant while at the same time being aware that prematurity is a *temporary* state which in time will yield to normality. Kaplan and Mason see the completion of these four tasks as requirements for normal adaptation to the stress of the premature delivery.

Separation of the Mother from Her Full-term Infant

Little surprise should be evoked by the data showing that the long-term separation of the mother from her premature infant would affect their later relationship. However, even short separations from their infants may have similar effects on mothers of full-term infants. The effect of increased mother-infant contact was studied in a group of lower class, primarily black primiparous mothers of full-term infants who had high school education or less.[44] One group of mothers who were allowed to play with their nude infants for an hour right after birth and then for 5 hours during each day of the hospital stay, was compared with another group of mothers given the standard hospital regimen of separation from the infant immediately following birth, a short visit 6 to 12 hours later, and then visits of 30 minutes every 4 hours for the infant's feedings.

The mothers in both groups returned to the hospital a month later and again a year later for an interview and observation. After 1 month, the mothers in the extra-contact group appeared to be more positively involved with their infants than did the control group. Extra-contact mothers stayed closer to their infants and tended to soothe them more when the infants became distressed. The results of a questionnaire indicated that these women engaged in the same behaviors more often at home, never ignoring their infant when crying, and tending to be concerned about the child's welfare whenever away from him. During the observation of the mother-infant interaction at the hospital, mothers in the extra-contact group showed substantially more fondling and eye-to-eye contact with their infants.

Follow-up studies done at 1, 2, and 5 years examined the long-term effects of increased neonatal contact. During a pediatric examination at 1 year of age, the extra-contact mothers were more involved with their infants, more soothing in responses to infant crying, and more likely to kiss them. At 2 years, a subsample of five extra-contact mothers were found to speak in a manner suggestive of closer social bonding than five control mothers. At 5 years, the children in the extra-contact group were more advanced in language development and had higher IQs.

Because the Klaus and Kennell findings are from a sample of lower social status, predominantly unmarried, black women, it is important to know if these results could be obtained from other samples. In a study of middle-class Swedish mothers, de Chateau gave a group of mothers the opportunity for tactile contact with their babies for the first 30 minutes after birth.[45] After 3 months, these mothers breastfed for longer periods and were more affectionate in their interactions than a control group that did not have the early contact experience.

The data from these two studies suggest that as little as 30 minutes of extra contact can affect later behavior of the parents, and, possibly, the intellectual outcomes for the children. It is not clear from the results of these studies which variables played the major role in producing the effects of the intervention, or whether the same effects would be found in other samples of women. Whether the crucial element was the prolonged contact with the infant immediately after birth, or the longer periods of contact during each of the early days, or the mother's possible feeling of being in a special group with special responsibilities for her infant, is less important than the striking finding that the caretaking behavior of these mothers could be altered by hospital practice for long periods afterward.

What is clear is that these mothers are given the impression that what they do makes a difference—that parents can have an impact on outcomes for their children. It is this attitude, conveyed by professionals to the mothers, that may influence them far beyond the neonatal period, especially young mothers from economically deprived groups in which these attitudes are not generally prevalent.

Rooming-in

The paucity of research on the effects of various nursery practices is striking. In the quarter century that has elapsed since the publication of the original description of the Yale Rooming-In project, there have been few reports in the literature on such nursery practices.[46] Before the turn of the century, nurseries were almost nonexistent, and "rooming-in" was the only mode of newborn care. From the early 1900s through the 1930s, the concern of the medical profession for preventing infections combined with the antispoiling psychology of John B. Watson to create the sterile, antisocial nurseries of the 1930s and 1940s. The psychoanalytic movement which placed great emphasis on the importance of the early experience of the mother and her child began to assert its effect in the 1940s with the loosening up of nursery care.

In reaction to the quarter century of increasing separation of mother and infant in the newborn nursery, a pioneering "rooming-in" unit was established at the Grace–New Haven Hospital. The research group at Yale felt that a contributing factor to psychological disturbance in the mother and child was rooted in the frustration of mothers who wanted to be with their infants right after delivery, combined with the imposition of a rigid schedule during the newborn period which set the tone for later caretaking behavior. The widespread lack of regard for individual variations among babies as well as among mothers was communicated as the accepted caretaking practice. The Grace–New Haven unit had four mothers and their infants living together. In general, the mothers found the presence of other mothers an advantage. Infants tended to cry less in the rooming-in units than in the nursery because their needs were rapidly attended to. The mothers noted that knowing whose baby was crying was to be preferred over wondering whose baby was crying, as in the standard nursery situation.

The importance was emphasized of only accepting women in rooming-in who were willing to participate.[47] In addition, there must be a supporting and sympathetic nursery staff. It was recommended that for the first two nights the infant be returned to the regular nursery to allow the mother a gradual adjustment to providing the complete care of the infant. The requirements for participation included a well child, no emotional disturbance in the mother, and the desire to breast-feed. Of the women with these qualifications who were invited to participate, 54% were willing. Among the 46% of the mothers at Grace–New Haven who were opposed or undecided, the major objection was that they would not receive enough rest. However, the mothers who participated in the rooming-in program and had had previous infants in the regular nursery reported that they were as well or better rested in the rooming-in unit.

An example of what can happen when rooming-in is made mandatory without the support of an adequate nursing staff was reported when a threat of epidemic diarrhea closed the nursery. There was a spate of complaints to the hospital administration by mothers who had to take care of their infants with insufficient preparation or help.

The reactions of mothers who did agree to

go through the rooming-in experience was reported as overwhelmingly favorable. One of the major advantages was the opportunity it gave the father to share in the caretaking of the infant. After discharge, both parents were prepared for relatively confident care of the infant. A questionnaire sent to the mothers a year after delivery asked if they would like rooming-in again; 95% reacted positively.

The extent to which popular demand was moving in the direction of more mother-infant contact in a more permissive nursery setting can be seen by the fact that, based on the Yale study, the American Academy of Pediatrics recommended rooming-in nursery units as a standard requirement. The standards and recommendations for hospital care of newborn infants of the American Academy of Pediatrics outline the special features of rooming-in as (1) providing the mother and her infant with a natural interactive experience as soon after delivery as the mother is capable for caring for her infant; (2) fostering infant feeding on a permissive plan; (3) facilitating the instruction of both mother and father in infant care; and (4) reducing the incidence of cross-infection among infants.[48] These recommendations were made on the basis of studies with no control groups and no major follow-up to demonstrate the importance of these early experiences.

Skin-to-skin Contact and Breast-feeding

Breast-feeding is another example of a nursery practice which waxes and wanes with the general social climate irrespective of any evidential base. The literature on breast-feeding is filled with controversial medical claims such as aiding the mother's uterine functioning or passing antibody protection to the infant. Holt, in reviewing the reasonable advantages attributed to breast-feeding, listed four:[49]

1. It is safer.
2. It is nutritionally superior.
3. It is more convenient.
4. It is of psychological value to the mother and infant.

He concludes that the last factor, the psychological value of breast feeding, appears to be the most important one but also the most difficult to evaluate.

There is little doubt that the mother's experiences can be made more emotionally satisfying through successful breast-feeding. While artificial feeding may not directly emotionally deprive the infant, the satisfaction the mother derives from the breast-feeding experience may act to increase the pleasure she derives from the infant and, as a consequence, increase her attachment to the infant. Holt claims that more than any other factor, the general psychological state of the mother can facilitate or impede her success in nursing her infant.

Laupus' review of breast-feeding is more specific about the mother's emotional advantages from breast-feeding.[50] These include the greater personal involvement of the mother in nurturing her infant, her increased feeling of being essential to the child's well-being, and her increased physical involvement with the infant through tactile contact and stimulation. Both Holt and Laupus emphasize the importance of the mother's attitude to the success of breast-feeding. Both caution that a mother who does not desire to breast-feed should not be made to feel compelled to do so, or to feel inadequate as a mother if she does not or cannot. There is no reason that positive psychological outcomes cannot be obtained from the ample opportunities for security and affection in the bottle-feeding situation.[47,51]

Mothers who have been content with their breast-feeding experiences often report that the feelings which they get from breast-feeding are sexually pleasurable and somewhat arousing.[52] It would appear that if a goal is to make the mother comfortable with her infant, then it must be left to the mother to decide on her most comfortable mode of feeding.

Animal research has placed strong emphasis on the infant's need for tactile stimulation in normal development.[53] Breast-feeding can provide both mother and child with tactile stimulation over large portions of their bodies. The mutual skin-to-skin contact provides a responsive environment for both mother and infant. While the infant's capacities for responsive eye-to-eye contact with the mother are not fully functional until a month of age, and although responsive smiling will require yet another 2 months, the possibility of skin-to-skin contact exists from birth. For the normal mother who does not breast-feed, there is still the range of possible interactions that run from hugging the swaddled infant against her bathrobe to hugging the naked baby against her

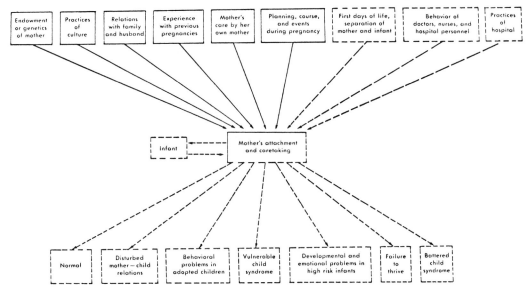

Fig. 17-1. Disorders of mothering: a hypothesis of their etiology. **Solid lines** indicate determinates which are ingrained: **dashed lines** indicate factors which may be altered or changed. (Klaus M, Kennell J: Pediatr Clin N Amer 1970)[54]

naked breast. Klaus and his associates have placed emphasis on the mother being able to play with her naked baby immediately after birth.[44] Their study showed the potential positive changes in mother-infant attachment that may be fostered by such an experience.

The advantages of breast-feeding therefore, are rooted neither in pseudomedical benefits nor in mystical properties of motherhood, but rather in the additional opportunity to provide the mother with an experience in which she can competently take care of her responsive infant.

FOSTERING MOTHERHOOD

Klaus and Kennell[54] have outlined the factors playing a role in disorders of mothering.[54] Figure 17-1 can serve as a basis for the current discussion of these variables. Although many of these factors (enclosed in **solid lines**) are fixed before the mother enters the hospital, neonatologists should be aware of these variables, and, to the extent that influence can be exerted beyond the newborn nursery setting, should educate the patients in specific, and society in general, of their consequences.

Prenatal Variables

Prenatal factors that need fostering at the societal level are the general mental, physical, and economic health of the populace, so that the mother need not experience stresses in these areas during her pregnancy and delivery. The expectant mother should be educated as to the possible effect of stresses that are specific to her own pregnancy. Both education in planned parenthood and childbirth can play a valuable role in these areas. The mother and father may then attempt to choose a time to have a child when social factors would interfere the least. Childbirth education which focuses on helping parents control themselves both physically and mentally appears to serve the mother by lessening her fears of an unknown situation and her needs for obstetric medication and intervention.

Obstetric Variables

Successful infant-mother attachment has been described as the ability of the infant to elicit and to be responsive to the caretaking behaviors of his mother. It then follows that the most successful products of the delivery are an infant awake, alert, and responsive to a mother in the same condition. The awareness of obstetricians of the importance these factors have in the successful attachment of the mother to her child should tend to make them less prone to overmedicate the mother and, through her, the infant. Indeed, obstetricians should attempt to maximize the mother's ability to deal successfully, both physically and emotionally, with a delivery in which their roles are minimized. The preceding review has tried to demonstrate a basis for this obstetric attitude, not in the putative emotional "high" of the natural childbirth experience, but rather in the strengthening of the mother's satisfaction with her child.

Neonatal Variables

There is an apparent consensus of opinion based on both research and sentiment in determining what kind of treatment is appropriate for the mother and child during the newborn period. The more positive experiences the mother has in competent caretaking of her child, the better she will feel and the more she will be willing to take care of the child. Mothers who are allowed to see and touch their babies immediately after birth are more attached to their infants than mothers who see their babies later. Mothers who have their babies with them longer during the day are more attached to their infants than mothers who see their infants only at feeding time.

During these togetherness experiences, the mother, especially the primipara, has to feel capable of coping with the needs of her infant. The hospital staff has the task of making sure that the mother is prepared, and of being supportive and sympathetic to her efforts. If too many demands are placed on an unprepared mother, the togetherness experience can have negative consequences.

Most nursery practices related to the mother-infant relationship are based on sentiment and common sense rather than on research data. Although it may be apparent that more contact makes for a different mother-infant relationship later, neither the magnitude nor the duration of these effects is yet known, nor is it known how much of what kind of contact would produce the optimal effects.

Positive and Negative Reciprocal Cycles

One of the major stumbling blocks to studying the separate effects of prenatal, delivery, or neonatal variables is that they are frequently confounded. The mother who begins her pregnancy under stressful emotional conditions starts a cycle which may lead to a poor attachment after delivery. Her prenatal stress tends to be associated with more delivery complications and a higher incidence of difficult temperament in the offspring. The difficult temperament places more demands on the mother's adaptive ability and caretaking skill that may result in reduced affection and attachment to the child. At what point in this negative cycle interventions should occur, and what kind of interventions are the most effective, are still major research questions.

In contrast to the stress-laden situations described above is the positive reciprocal cycle of the mother prepared for her pregnancy, who suffers a minimum of stress, trains for her delivery, and requires a minimum of intervention, immediately begins caretaking for a child with a normal temperament, feels effective in her caretaking, and is able to enter a responsive, affectionate relationship with her infant.

Dealing with Deviancy

The definition of deviancy in the newborn period must center on the mother and child as a dyadic unit. In terms of abnormal developmental outcomes, a focus on the characteristics of the infant alone has been the least adequate predictive variable.[4] The crucial factor has been the environmental context in which the child's characteristics are nurtured or hindered. From the perspective of the child's development, deviancy during the newborn period is truly in the eye of the beholder, because the consequences for a child who is temperamentally or physically different need not be later aberrant behavior.

The task for the neonatal specialist is to convert the mother's attitude from one of seeing the child as different from the normal to that of seeing him as part of a continuous spectrum of developmental maturity or temperament. The professional has two tasks to achieve with the new mother: the *first* relates to her attitudes toward the child and the *second* relates to her competence at taking care of her infant. In her attitudes, the mother should feel that the differences between her child and what she would consider a normal child may be only temporary. With age, children outgrow their prematurity and colic, and recover from their illnesses. The mother's susceptibility to perceiving her infant as different often goes beyond the child's appearance. Mothers of seemingly normal infants often think of their children as different either through their own ignorance or through some casual remark of the hospital staff. The impulse to treat these fears lightly or even to ignore them may not be helpful to a mother whose future attitudes toward the child may be strongly colored by her initial impressions.

The second task is to assure the mother that she can be a competent caretaker of her infant. The mother's fears and self-doubts about her ability to care for her infant may stem from her lack of experience. These fears occur in nearly every primiparous mother, but having a child in a special care unit would give pause even to an experienced mother. The best way to assure a mother of her caretaking competence is not through verbal instruction but rather through the actual experience of caring for her infant. The maximal experience of this kind for the mother of the full-term infant is a "rooming-in" arrangement, while for the mother of the premature infant, similar experiences can be had by being allowed into the special-care nursery to tend to her child.

For some mothers, even allowing them into the premature nursery is not sufficient contact for promoting the necessary attachment to their infants. An additional period of intensive contact before leaving the hospital may be desirable, with the mother given primary responsibility for the infant's care. Nurses would be permitted to intervene only at the mother's request. An exploratory study using this procedure found that the mother's confidence in her caretaking ability increased by the end of the second day.[55] Whether these effects would carry over into the mother's behavior at home is a subject for further study. Many of the major problems in the mother's response to a premature infant are resolved in this type of setting. The mother has the feeling that the hospital staff has confidence in her ability as she successfully cares for the infant, while at the same time she has resource people readily available.

Postneonatal Variables

Until the child does appear and act in accord with the mother's view of normality, there is still the potential of later caretaking problems. For this reason, the family requires follow-up care to assure that the mother will not be overwhelmed by a child who may give little satisfaction in return for meeting his many caretaking demands. These problems may occur in those families with the fewest economic, educational, or emotional resources to deal with such burdens. How best to provide this aftercare is a problem to which the medical profession must address itself.

The Father

The role of the father has not been emphasized in this review of factors related to the neonatal period. This neglect does not mean that the father has a minor role, but rather that until recently, very little research has been done on the possibilities of his role.[56] Increasing importance has recently been given the father's role in support of the mother and in the actual caretaking of the child. Childbirth education groups have emphasized the father's sharing in the psychological experience of bearing a child. Because he does not experience the somatic problems associated with the pregnancy or delivery, he can maintain a view of the child unbiased by ancillary issues. He may thus be able to support the mother through any problems she may have, while maintaining a broader perspective.

After the delivery, the father can play an important role in relieving the mother's responsibilities by participating in the caretaking of the infant, especially in the early period while the mother is still recuperating. In those situations where the infant has extra care demands, the father's role gains in importance by allowing the mother to share her insecurities, and by giving her respite in a stressful situation which may extend for several months into the postnatal life of the child.

The training of the father as a caretaker during the neonatal period may be as important as the training of the mother. Similar positive consequences can be expected from his increased self-confidence in being able to deal with his infant's needs. A father emotionally involved in the welfare of both the mother and the child, and who is competent to aid and care for them can be very helpful in the aftercare situation.

Although the father's ability to *give* support to the mother and infant has been emphasized above, a more beneficial aspect exists in the father's ability to *take* pleasure in the new infant. The same psychological analysis of the pleasure that the mother gains from being effective in eliciting responses from her infant applies to the father. The pleasures of participating in skin-to-skin, eye-to-eye, or smiling contact with the baby are equally applicable. The magnitude of these rewards is a function of the magnitude of the father's and the mother's positive emotional investment in the infant. The fostering of this emotional investment is the task of the professionals concerned with the newborn period.

REFERENCES

1. **Bowlby J:** Attachment and loss. Attachment, vol 1. New York, Basic Books, 1969
2. **Rosenblatt JS:** The basis of synchrony in the behavioral interaction between the mother and her offspring in the laboratory rat. In Foss BM (ed): Determinants of Infant Behavior, vol 3. London, Methuen, 1965
3. **Noirot E:** Changes in responsiveness to young in the adult mouse: The effect of external stimuli. J Comp Physiol Psychol 57:97, 1964
4. **Sameroff AJ, Chandler M:** Reproductive risk and the continuum of caretaking casualty. In Horowitz FD, Hetherington M, Scarr–Salapatek S, Siegel G (eds): Review of Child Development Research, vol 4. Chicago, University of Chicago, 1975
5. **Moore AV:** Effects of modified maternal care in the sheep and goat. In Newton G, Levine S (eds): Early Experience and Behavior, pp 481–529. Springfield, Ill, Charles C Thomas, 1968
6. **Harlow HF, Harlow MK:** Effects of various mother-infant relationships on rhesus monkey behaviors. In Foss BM (ed): Determinants of Infant Behavior, vol 4. London, Methuen, 1969
7. **Werner EE, Bierman JM, French FE:** The Children of Kauai. Honolulu, University of Hawaii, 1971
8. **Galdston R:** Dysfunction of parenting: The battered child, the neglected child, the emotional child. In Howells, JG (ed): Modern Perspectives in International Child Psychiatry. New York. Brunner/Mazel, 1971
9. **Birch H, Gussow GD** Disadvantaged Children. New York, Grune & Stratton, 1970
10. **Lorion RP:** Socioeconomic status and traditional treatment approaches reconsidered. Psychol Bull 4:263, 1973
11. **Piaget J:** Psychology of Intelligence, New York, Harcourt, Brace & World, 1950
12. **Chandler MJ:** Egocentrism and antisocial behavior: The assessment and training of social perspective-taking skills. Dev. Psychol 9:373, 1973
13. **Chamberlin RA:** Authoritarian and accommodative child rearing styles: Their relationships with the behavior patterns of two-year-old children and other variables. J Pediatr 84:287, 1974
14. **Baumrind D:** Current patterns of parental authority. Dev Psychol Mon 4:(No. 1), 1971
15. **Thomas A, Chess S, Birch H:** Temperament and Behavior Disorders in Children. New York, New York University, 1968
16. **Joffe JM:** Prenatal Determinants of Behavior. Oxford, Pergamon, 1969
17. **Ferreira A:** Prenatal Environment. Springfield, Ill, Charles C Thomas, 1969
18. **McDonald RL:** The role of emotional factors in obstetric complications: A review. Psychosom Med, 30:222, 1968
19. **Sameroff AJ, Zax M:** Perinatal characteristics of the offspring of schizophrenic women. J Nerv Ment Dis, in press
20. **Stott DH:** The child's hazards in utero. In Howells JG (ed): Modern Perspectives in International Child Psychiatry. New York, Bruner/Mazel, 1971
21. **Sontag LW:** Fetal behavior as a predictor of behavior in childhood. Paper presented at the meetings of the American Psychiatric Association, Toronto, 1962
22. **Parke RD:** Perspectives on father–infant interaction. In Osofsky JD (ed): Handbook of Infant Development. New York, Wiley, 1978
23. **Ainsworth MDS:** Object relations, dependency, and attachment: A theoretical review of the infant–mother relationship. Child Dev 40:969, 1969
24. **Lorenz K:** The cross-cultural approach to child development problems. In Tanner JM, Inhelder B (eds): Discussion on Child Development, Vol 1, pp 222–223. New York, International University Press, 1953
25. **Stechler G, Carpenter GC:** A viewpoint on early affective development. In Hellmuth J (ed): The Exceptional Child, Vol 1, The normal infant. New York, Brunner/Mazel, 1968
26. **White RW:** Motivation reconsidered: The concept of competence. Psychol Rev 66:297, 1959
27. **Thomas A, Chess S, Birch HG, Hertzig M, Korn S:** Behavioral Individuality in Early Childhood. London, University of London, 1963
28. **Chess S:** Genesis of behavior disorder. In Howells JG (ed): Modern Persepctives in International Child Psychiatry. New York, Brunner/Mazel, 1971
29. **Bell RO:** Stimulus control of parent or caretaker behavior of offspring. Dev Psychol 4:63, 1971
30. **Turner EK:** The syndrome in the infant resulting from maternal emotional tension during pregnancy. Med J Aust 1:221, 1956
31. **Brazelton TB:** Effect of prenatal drugs on the behavior of the neonate. Am J Psychiatry 126:1261, 1970

32. **Bowes WA, Brackbill Y, Conway E, Stein-schneider A:** The effects of obstetrical medication of fetus and infant. Monographs of the Society for Research in Child Development, Vol 35 (serial No. 137), 1970

33. **Kraemer CH, Korner A, Thoman E:** Methodological considerations in evaluating the influence of drugs used during labor and delivery on the behavior of the newborn. Dev Psychol 6:128, 1972

34. **Klaus MH, Kennell JH:** Maternal–Infant Bonding. St. Louis, Mosby, 1976

35. **Klein M, Stern L:** Low birthweight and the battered child syndrome. Am J Dis Child 122:15, 1971

36. **Shaheen E, Alexander D, Truskowsky M, Barbero GJ:** Failure to thrive—A retrospective profile. Clin Pediatr 7:255, 1968

37. **Elmer E, Gregg CD:** Developmental characteristics of the abused child. Pediatrics 40:596, 1967

38. **Leiderman PH:** Human mother to infant social bonding: Is there a critical phase? In Immelmann K, Barlow GW, Main M, Petrinovich LF (eds): Behavorial Development: An Interdisciplinary Approach. Cambridge, Cambridge University Press, 1980

39. **Seashore MJ, Leifer AD, Barnett CR, Leiderman PH:** The effects of denial of early mother-infant interaction on maternal self-confidence. J Pers Soc Psychol 26:369, 1973

40. **Kennell JH, Klaus MH:** Care of the mother of the high-risk infant. Clin Obstet Gynecol 14:926, 1971

41. **Brown JV, Bakeman R:** Relationships of human mothers with their infants during the first year of life: Effects of prematurity. In Bell RV, Smotherman WP (eds): Maternal Influence and Early Behavior. Holliswood, Spectrum, 1979

42. **Field TM:** Interactions of high risk infants: Quantitative and qualitative differences. In Sawin DB, Hawkins RC, Walker LO, Penticuff JH (eds): Exceptional Infant, Vol 4: Psychosocial risks in Infant–Environment Transactions. New York, Brunner/Mazel, 1980

43. **Kaplan DM, Mason EA:** Maternal reactions to premature birth viewed as an acute emotional disorder. Am J Orthopsychiatry 30:539, 1960

44. **Kennell JH, Jerauld R, Wolfe H, Chester D, et al:** Maternal behavior one year after early and extended post-partum contact. Dev Med Child Neurol 16:172, 1974

45. **de Chateau P:** Neonatal care routines: Influences on maternal and infant behavior and on breastfeeding. Umea University Medical Dissertations, New Series #20. Umea, Sweden, 1976. Cited in Klaus MH, Kennell JH: Maternal–Infant Bonding. St. Louis, Mosby, 1976

46. **Jackson EB, Olmstead RWW, Foord A, Thomas H, Hyder K:** A hospital rooming-in unit for four new-born infants and their mothers. Pediatrics 1:28, 1948

47. **Jackson EB:** Pediatric and psychiatric aspects of the Yale rooming-in project. Conn State Med J 14:616, 1950

48. **American Academy of Pediatrics:** Standards and recommendation for hospital care of new-born infants. Evanston, (Ill), American Academy of Pediatrics, 1964

49. **Holt LE Jr:** Feeding techniques and diets. In Barnett HL (ed): Pediatrics, 15th ed. New York, Appleton–Century–Crofts, 1968

50. **Laupus WE:** Feeding of infants. In Nelson WE, Vaughan VC III, McKay RJ (eds): Textbook of Pediatrics, 9th ed. Philadelphia, WB Saudners, 1969

51. **Newton N, Newton M:** Psychologic aspects of lactation. N Eng J Med 277:1179, 1967

52. **Salber EJ, Feinleib M:** Breast feeding in Boston. Pediatrics 37:299, 1966

53. **Prescott JW:** Early somatosensory deprivation as an ontogenetic process in the abnormal development of the brain and behavior. In Goldsmith JE, Moor-Jankowski J (eds): Medical Primatology. Basle S Karger, 1971

54. **Klaus MH, Kennell JH:** Mothers separated from their newborn infants. Pediatr Clin North Am 17:1015, 1970

55. **Kennell JH, Klaus MH, Wolfe H:** Nesting behavior in the human mother after prolonged mother–infant separation. In Stetson A, Swyer P (eds): Proceedings of the Congress of Neonatal Intensive Care. St. Louis, WH Green, (in press.)

56. **Lamb ME (ed):** The Role of the Father in Child Development. New York, Wiley, 1976

18

Behavioral Competence of the Newborn Infant

T. Berry Brazelton

It is important that we begin to value the neonate's contribution to his new environment. Because the parents' inclination is to nurture the newborn and to value his reactions to their handling, to voice, to vision, it is belittling to these reactions if we as physicians do not value them in the neonate. If we do attend to them by changing neonatal nurseries and lying-in arrangements to value and capture the neonate's best periods of alert responsiveness, we place a stamp of approval both on the parents' attention to the neonate and on the newborn as an important, interactive person from the start. We are providing new, confused parents with a way of communicating with their infants. We are showing them that the neonate can lead them when they are confused.

The demands of a complex, undirected society, coupled with the lack of support (often even negative input) of new parents by our present nuclear family system, leave most parents insecure and at the mercy of tremendous internal and external pressures. They have been told that their infant's outcome is to be shaped by them and their parenting: at

This chapter was written with the support of The Robert Wood Johnson Foundation, Carnegie Corporation, and the National Institute of Mental Health.

the same time, there are few stable cultural values on which they can rely for guidance in setting their course as new parents.

An infant is not as helpless as he seems, and there are rewards as well as messages from an infant that can guide a new mother and new father as they become faced with their new roles. The infant comes well equipped to signal his needs and his gratitude to his environment. In fact, he can even make choices about what he wants from his parents, and shut out what he doesn't want in effective ways. He can be seen as a powerful force, stabilizing and influencing those around him.

Compared to any other species, the human neonate is relatively helpless in the motor sphere and relatively complex, even precocious, in the sensory sphere. This causes a motor dependence and a freedom for acquisition of the many patterns of sensory and affective information that are necessary for the child and adult human to master and survive in a complex world.

From a medical standpoint, it becomes more and more important to evaluate infants at risk as early as possible with an eye to more sophisticated preventive and therapeutic approaches. Premature and minimally brain-damaged infants seem to be less able to compensate in disorganized, depriving environments than are well-equipped neonates, and the problems of the former with organization in development are compounded early.[1] Parents of children admitted to the wards of the Children's Hospital in Boston for clinical syndromes, such as failure to thrive, child abuse, repeated accidents and poisonings, and infantile autism, are often successful parents of other children. By history, they associate their failure with the one child to an inability to "understand" him from the neonatal period onward, and they claim a difference from the other children in his earliest reactions to them. If we are to improve the outcome for such children, assessment of the risk in early infancy could mobilize preventive efforts and programs for intervention.

We need more sophisticated methods of assessing neonates and for predicting their part in the possible failure of the environment-infant interaction. We also need to be able to assess "at-risk" environments, because the impracticality of spreading resources too thin requires the selection of target populations for our efforts at early intervention. Minimally brain-damaged babies do make remarkable compensatory recoveries in a fostering environment.[2]

The behavioral responses of the neonate can be used as a means to understand the organization of the central and autonomic nervous systems at birth. Also, as we examine and understand the individual differences in neonatal behaviors, we have been able to see that behavioral responsiveness reflects the genetic endowment and the intrauterine influences on the genotype. As the neonate is influenced by labor, delivery, and recovery in the new environment, we can begin to predict both what his new environment will do to him through experience and learning, and we can also get an idea of how he will cause his environment to interact with him.

EFFECTS OF IN UTERO ENVIRONMENT

Early attempts looked at single perinatal factors that placed an infant at risk. Studies from the Collaborative Child Development Study, which focused on a single prenatal or perinatal event to discover its effect on development, revealed that a clear one-to-one association rarely could be established.[3,4]

Researchers have begun to develop at-risk scores that are based on multiple factors. Table 18-1 is an example of such a risk score.[5] This at-risk score not only delineates historical factors, but it also weighs these factors to refine the more general notion of at riskness into a measure of "degree of at riskness."

Lubchenco, at the University Hospital in Denver, Colorado, has acquired extensive experience with the implementation of an at-risk scoring system in newborn care (Fig. 18-1).[6] Her system is less detailed and the content is easily taught to nurses and house staffs. The nurses, being the stable personnel in the nursery, have the major responsibility for collecting and recording the data included in their at-risk scoring system. This information then is used to triage babies into different groups requiring different levels of intensity of care. Using this system, Lubchenco has been able to document an important decrease in mortality and long-term morbidity of a group of "borderline babies"—babies who formerly have been offered little additional observation and care, but who, by virtue of being considered at higher risk on the basis of a detailed obstetric and perinatal history, are now placed under closer supervision, which allows for earlier detection and intervention.[6]

This system allows for an economy of time, money, and effort by channeling care to those who need it and by freeing the caretakers from extensive care of the low-risk babies.

A standardized at-risk score makes data collecting more efficient, encourages immediate collection, and promotes a form of record keeping that facilitates data analysis when assessing effectiveness of neonatal care.

Undernutrition: Small-for-Dates Baby

Prenatal nutrition has been shown to have significant differential effects on the growing fetus. Winick has pointed out that organ growth occurs as two general phases.[7] The initial phase is cellular division with a resultant increase in the number of cells. The subsequent but overlapping phase is an increase in cell size. Significant malnutrition during cell division will irreversibly result in a smaller organ because new cells will not be made regardless of subsequent nutrition. In contrast, malnutrition during the period of increase in cellular size is sometimes reversible. The brain is not spared these nutritional insults, but their timing affects it differently. These data suggest

Table 18-1. Prenatal Risk Factors

	Score
I. Cardiovascular and renal	
1. Moderate to severe toxemia	10
2. Chronic hypertension	10
3. Moderate to severe renal disease	10
4. Severe heart disease, Class II–IV	10
5. History of eclampsia	5
6. History of pyelitis	5
7. Class I heart disease	5
8. Mild toxemia	5
9. Acute pyelonephritis	5
10. History of cystitis	1
11. Acute cystitis	1
12. History of toxemia	1
II. Metabolic	
1. Diabetes ≥ Class A-II	10
2. Previous endocrine ablation	10
3. Thyroid disease	5
4. Prediabetes (A-I)	5
5. Family history of diabetes	1
III. Previous histories	
1. Previous fetal exchange transfusion for Rh	10
2. Previous stillbirth	10
3. Post-term > 42 weeks	10
4. Previous premature infant	10
5. Previous neonatal death	10
6. Previous cesarean section	5
7. Habitual abortion	5
8. Infant > 10 pounds	5
9. Multiparity > 5	5
10. Epilepsy	5
11. Fetal anomalies	1
IV. Anatomic abnormalities	
1. Uterine malformation	10
2. Incompetent cervix	10
3. Abnormal fetal position	10
4. Polyhydramnios	10
5. Small pelvis	5
V. Miscellaneous	
1. Abnormal cervical cytology	10
2. Multiple pregnancy	10
3. Sickle cell disease	10
4. Age ≥ 35 or ≤ 15	5
5. Viral disease	5
6. Rh sensitization only	5
7. Positive serology	5
8. Severe anemia (< 9 g Hgb)	5
9. Excessive use of drugs	5
10. History of TB or PPD ≥ 10 mm	5
11. Weight < 100 or > 200 pounds	5
12. Pulmonary disease	5
13. Flu syndrome (severe)	5
14. Vaginal spotting	5
15. Mild anemia (9–10.9 g Hgb)	1
16. Smoking ≥ 1 pack per day	1
17. Alcohol (moderate)	1
18. Emotional problem	1

(Hobel CJ, Hyvarinen MA, Okada D, Oh W: Prenatal and intrapartum high-risk screening, Am J Obstet Gynecol 117:1, 1973)

UNIVERSITY OF COLORADO MEDICAL CENTER   Date
Newborn and Premature Infant Center   Ward
    Name
MORBIDITY MODEL   Hosp. No.
Encircle the scores which apply and add to get morbidity score.

Variable		Score
1. Birth weight	1500 grams or less	61.7
	1501 to 2000	55.0
	2001 to 2500	15.8
	2501 to 3500	4.3
	3501 or more	5.0
2. Gestational age	27 weeks or less	21.6
	28 - 31	18.4
	32 - 33	15.0
	34 - 35	9.0
	36 - 37	3.8
	38 weeks or more	1.1
	unknown	2.7
3. Mother's age	Less than 15 years	7.4
	15 - 19	1.9
	20 - 34	0
	35 years or more	3.9
4. Condition at birth	good (Apgar 8-10)	0
	fair (Apgar 5-7)	3.1
	poor (Apgar 0-4)	11.0
5. Toxemia		4.5
6. Diabetes		34.7
7. Fetal distress		4.2
8. Saddle, Spinal, Caudal anesthesia		2.4
9. Labor complications*		4.1
10. PROM (24 hours or more before delivery)		6.3
11. Abnormal delivery		5.3
12. Positive pressure resuscitation		6.4
13. Stimulants in delivery room		11.8
14. Habitual aborter (3 or more)		10.4
15. If male baby		4.1

Fig. 18-1. Morbidity model. (Klaus MH, Fanaroff AA: Care of the High Risk Neonate. Philadelphia, WB Saunders, 1973; courtesy of L Lubchenco)

Total score equals percentage risk of morbidity

* Induction, pitocin stimulation, uterine inertia, prolapsed cord, contracted pelvis, transverse arrest, antepartum hemorrhage, other.

strongly that the timing of malnutrition is important to neonatal function.

An initial assessment of such a depleted newborn, who demonstrates a decrease in weight with respect to height, slightly decreased head circumference, loss of subcutaneous tissue and relatively poor behavioral responses, is not adequate for an understanding of the infant's specific *in utero* nutritional experience and future capacities. But a repeated evaluation of his behavior might assess his potential for recovery and tell us a great deal more.

In a study of ten 2.42 kg small-for-gestational-age babies on days 1, 5, 10,[8] we found that newborns who differed from their full-weight peers only in terms of Ponderal Index (see below),[9] and who were considered normal pediatrically, were found to behave substantially differently from their full-weight peers. Although their organization of state was comparable and their physiologic stability nearly comparable with that of the full-weight babies, they differed markedly in motor behavior and in interactive behaviors. The typical underweight newborn tended to have poor tone, very low activity levels, poor hand-to-mouth coordination, poor defensive reaction, and jerky or cogwheel-like movements of the limbs with restricted arcs. He was floppy on the pull-to-sit maneuver and did not show good crawling, walking, sucking or rooting, nor motor tone when his limbs were moved passively. Although he came to an alert state, his responsiveness was poor. He did not lock into social stimuli easily and did not interact in a focused and modulated manner with the animate or inanimate environment. He did not mold to the examiner and did not need to be consoled because he did not cry easily. He was extremely difficult to console when he began to cry. He gave the overall impression of stress when handled and his facial expression when brought to an alert state signaled strain, discomfort, and exhaustion; he wanted to be left alone. If this signal was not followed, he would often start to gag and turn blue around the mouth; he would frown intensely yet could not muster enough energy either to go to sleep or to begin to cry and thereby terminate unwelcome stimulation. We felt that he was easily overwhelmed by the environment, and, if put down after even a brief interaction session, he looked exhausted, but in fact often was too exhausted to go to sleep.

What implications this behavior has for the caretaking adult can only be hypothesized. During the newborn period, the parents of the underweight babies emphasized how undemanding their baby was. They stressed that he rarely cried, that he did not seem to want to be played with or fed, and that he was happiest if left alone. The poor motor performance and the general lack of vigor puzzled mothers, who felt uneasy with their babies.

Because the underweight babies did not behave like full-weight babies on day 10, they were reassessed informally at a later date.

Their age at follow-up ranged from 6 to 9 months. The infants were assessed with the Denver Developmental Screening Test[10] and the mothers were interviewed as to their babies' sleeping and eating patterns, and their general temperamental and behavioral characteristics.

They were difficult babies all along. They were easily overstimulated, continuously on the go, unpredictable in their sleeping habits, difficult feeders, and generally overreactive and overactive. Three had developed severe food allergies, two had real sleep disorders. All ten performed adequately on the mental and motor tests, but they had had a stormy 9 months.

Zambian Infants. The importance of multiple assessments and the pattern of recovery is dramatically evidenced in another study of Zambian infants.[11] Twenty Zambian infants were examined in days 1, 5, and 10 with an earlier version of the Brazelton Scale.[12] Their mothers were multiparous, had used no birth control measures, and had experienced a series of pregnancies in rapid succession (reportedly at 10–11 month intervals). The infants were seen as having suffered from their mothers' protein malnutrition in pregnancy because histories from the mothers substantiated inadequate intakes of eggs, meat, or fish, with low-calorie intakes.

On day 1, the infants showed all the signs of dysmaturity indicating recent intrauterine depletion suggestive of placental dysfunction. Their skin was dry and peeling. Subcutaneous tissue was sparse throughout their bodies, the neonates' faces were wizened, and their eyes were glazed. The cord stumps were yellow as if this had resulted from intrauterine stress in the last trimester of the pregnancy. These depleted babies lacked muscle tone, had poor head control in pull-to-sit maneuvers, did not cuddle when held, and were irritable. They had low scores in all elicited responses, especially in such complex responses as alerting and following an object with their eyes (Table 18-2). This pattern of response, as well as their depleted appearances, certainly would have put them in a high-risk category in a U.S. group, and parents would have responded to them with an anxious, overprotective approach.

By day 10, breast feeding had rehydrated the depleted infants, and they seemed to have

Table 18-2. Mean Scores of Brazelton Examination
for Zambian Infants*

Significant Measures	Day 1 Zambians	Day 5 Zambians	Day 10 Zambians
Motor activity	3.00	5.89	4.60
Tempo at height	3.20	5.90	4.40
Rapidity of build up	3.22	5.62	3.50
Irritability	2.50	4.40	3.80
Consolability	6.60	5.00	6.12
Social interest	4.20	6.20	6.70
Alertness	3.40	6.30	7.40
Follow with eyes	2.40	4.60	4.67
Reactivity to stimulation	3.35	5.30	6.14
Defensive movements	3.20	5.11	4.90
Cuddliness	3.30	5.22	6.30

*Scores were obtained from 11 items of the Brazelton Neonatal Behavioral Assessment Scale. Each of the items was scored on a 9-point scale.
(Tronick ET, Brazelton TB: Clinical Uses of the Brazelton Neonatal Scale. In Friedlander BZ, Sterritt GM, Kirk GE (eds): Exceptional Infant, Vol 3. New York, Brunner/Mazel, Inc 1975)

recovered in all observable respects from the intrauterine physiologic stress. The infants showed no sign of dehydration or depletion at 10 days, and their performance exhibited remarkable recovery. They were consolable and alert, and they participated actively when cuddled. Their irritability had decreased and their muscle tone had improved. Most striking was their interest in social stimuli and their capacity to control interfering motor behaviors. They now were appropriately active and vigorous.

This dramatic recovery pattern emphasized the importance of making multiple assessments for at-riskness during the neonatal period. Several examinations allow for the dissipation of transient stresses and allow the infant to manifest his capability for recovery. At no time did the Zambian mothers treat their infants as though they were at risk. They took their infants out of the hospital on day 1, carrying them upright against their sides, wrapped in a dashiki, and did not even provide support for the shoulders and head. The mothers placed the limp infants in the dashiki by swinging them over their shoulders while holding the infant by one arm. To arouse the infant, a mother would joggle and bounce her baby. Mothers left these infants out on the bed to be played with by other siblings and visitors. In short, they handled their infants as if they were strong and vigorous on day 1 when it

looked inappropriate to us to do so, but, by day 10, this was perfectly suited to their now vigorous and responsive infants.

Parents in poor families in urban America, stressed with significant socioeconomic factors, have a relatively high proportion of dysmature and depleted infants. Their neonatal behavior is affected as well. When the infants are quieter, difficult to arouse, and difficult to bring to responsive states for interaction, it is easy to imagine that they will elicit fewer responses and maybe even less nourishment from their stressed mothers. We can see that the cycle of chronic minor undernutrition can start in *in utero* undernutrition and then be mediated and continued by the effects of resultant neonatal behavior on the family. Unlike the Zambian mothers, isolated ghetto mothers may not have the same historic or cultural knowledge of recovery, or they may be too stressed to feed and energize a relatively lethargic, poorly interacting baby to optimal recovery.

Postnatal Undernutrition. Another factor adversely influencing behavioral recovery in the neonate can be a lack of nutritional resources to maintain adequate nutrition after birth. Chavez, in a study of infants during their first 2 years, has empirically illustrated the cycle of improved nutrition → increased activity → greater demands → greater interaction.[13] The supplemented child slept less and played more. Not only was the greater interaction seen in more time spent in caretaking activities, but mothers also spoke almost twice as much to these infants compared to the nonsupplemented group. They spoke in sentences with adjectives and adverbs and used explanations rather than commands. Also, fathers became more involved earlier. When the infant became a toddler, the greater activity of the nutritionally supplemented group was manifested by increased exploratory behavior and toddlers were more mischievous, demanding, and disobedient. The family needed to respond with greater supervision and more limit setting. In general, the nonsupplemented malnourished child was found "predominantly negative, passive, withdrawn and timid; and at certain ages, especially when signs of evident deficiency are shown, an attitude of apathy was manifest, mixed with certain attitudes of anxiety when separated from the mother."[13]

Drug Effects in Gestation

The importance of drug effects on a neonate's behavior and his subsequent adaptation now is being recognized. These effects are most prominent in babies whose mothers are addicted to narcotics or alcohol during pregnancy. Besides a high incidence of congenital anomalies, narcotic addiction results in severe withdrawal symptoms in the neonatal period.[14] Well-recognized signs of withdrawal include clonus, convulsions, decreased sleeping time, diarrhea, high-pitched cry, sweating, sneezing, nasal congestion, and so on. When behaviors were looked at, addicted babies demonstrated extreme irritability, inability to be comforted except by constant oral activity or swaddling, and they demonstrated an overreaction to all stimuli from the environment with violent agitated motor activity. Lability of state behaviors and an inability to quiet or control themselves make them extremely difficult infants for which to care.[15]

Alcohol abuse in pregnancy causes similar effects on the fetus. Congenital anomalies are now recognized as being associated with excessive alcohol use during pregnancy.[16] Cases of withdrawal symptoms in these infants have been described.[17] They are also jittery, slow to react but overreactive when roused, and then difficult to quiet and unpredictable. Many of these infants are small-for-gestational age because of associated nutritional deficiencies.

We can wonder what effects other drugs may have on systems involving learning, attention, motor control, emotional lability, or the like. Newborn behavioral effects of *in utero* exposure to LSD have not as yet been assessed. Another drug with unknown but probable effects on the developing nervous system presently is being used with frequency by pediatricians. Theophylline has unequivocally been demonstrated to reduce the frequency of primary apnea of premature infants.[18] Pharmacologically, theophylline inhibits the phosphodiesterase activity that normally metabolizes cyclic AMP to an inactive form. Theophylline, therefore, results in increased levels of cyclic AMP, and this is how it mediates its therapeutic effect on the respiratory system. We must now ask ourselves what effects cyclic AMP may have on developing systems, such as the nervous system of the premature infant. Assessing neonatal behavior and subsequent development of infants exposed to theophylline *in utero* may provide insights that will supplement laboratory data.

Perinatal Use of Medication

Maternal anesthesia and analgesia, with their rapid transport across the placenta, are known to have a pharmacologic effect on the fetus and, subsequently, on the newborn. Studying maternal drug effects in an animal model, Moya and Thorndike concluded that these drugs had a greater effect on the fetus because of increased permeability of the blood-brain barrier, inefficient metabolism in the liver, and the asphyxia and physical trauma of normal deliveries.[19] Specific neurobehavioral responses of these intrapartum drugs have been investigated. We have observed and described a 1 to 2 day prolongation of CNS depression or disorganization following birth in babies of more heavily medicated mothers.[20] In addition, mothers of these babies reported greater difficulty in breast feeding for 40 hours, longer than a comparison group in which minimal sedation had been used. Neonatal weight gain was delayed by 24 hours in the heavily premedicated group. By affecting neonatal behaviors, these intrapartum drugs could easily influence the early mother-infant relationship. Mothers who have any postpartum depression might easily see the baby's disorganization around feeding as amounting to a rejection of their efforts to reach them.

Using sucking as a modality to study, Kron described the effects on nutritive sucking of 200 mg of IV secobarbital given from 10 minutes to 3 hours before delivery.[21] Compared to infants whose mothers received no sedatives, these infants had a significantly decreased sucking rate, with an associated decrease in consumption over the first 4 days.

Using visual attention as an outcome measure, Stechler and Latz concluded that the more drugs administered around delivery the less attentive the infant is likely to be.[22] They measured attention as the total time spent starting at or scanning a visual stimulus, as opposed to nonattention behaviors such as looking away, closing eyes, or fussing.

Brackbill and Conway have also investigated the effects of medication, both analgesic and anesthetic, on a number of behaviors.[23] Significant differences as a function of medication were seen in items measuring muscle tension on days 2 and 5, on the ability to visually fix and follow on day 5, and a greater inability to habituate to an auditory signal as late as 4 weeks.

Our view is that previous studies have not paid sufficient attention to the additive or synergistic effects of medication with other stress factors, such as labor, delivery, and entrance into a new environment, which affect the infant's behavioral recovery.

To meet these objections, a sample was studied comprised of a homogeneous group of 54 infants who were full-term and healthy and whose mothers had problem-free pregnancies, labors, and deliveries. This selection carefully excluded all infants who had experienced prenatal and perinatal stress factors which would have produced poorer behavioral organization. These results then do not negate the behavioral effects seen in studies using more typical, heterogeneous populations. Repeated behavioral assessments were made on each infant after the first 10 days of life. Within the first 12 hours after birth, each infant was examined with the Neurobehavioral Examination developed by Scanlon and coworkers.[24] This examination was designed to evaluate the initial behavioral effects of drugs by assessing the infant's motor organization and responsiveness to external events. The motor behaviors assessed are pull-to-sit, arm recoil, truncal tone, body tone, moro, placing, rooting, and sucking. Items assessing responsiveness are initial response and the decrement of the response to repeated pin-pricks, initial response to sound, decrement in response to repeated sounds, decrement in response to repeated light flashes, and overall alertness. Following this assessment, the infants were examined with the Neonatal Behavioral Assessment Scale[12] on days 1, 2, 3, 4, 5, 7, and 10.

The results of this study demonstrated that low dosages of certain medications administered to women during labor and delivery have minimal effects on the behavior of their newborn infants. Local anesthesia and analgesic premedication produced few significant behavioral changes. Epidural anesthesia produced an initial diminution in the infants' motor organization but this effect was quite transient.

These data provided a picture of the behavioral recovery of a group of neonates in whom the effects of medication were minimized through the control of a multiplicity of stress variables. Their recovery is characterized by a definite improvement over the first 10 days of life in major areas of their behavioral functioning. During this initial recovery period, the infants became more alert and capable of orienting to external, particularly animate, stimuli. Their motor maturity, muscle tone, and integrated motor performances also improved. On behavioral items reflecting their psychological adjustment, there was a clear improvement with a decrease in their numbers of startles and amounts of tremulousness. Items reflecting state control appeared to remain relatively stable over the first 10 days, which probably reflects their well-organized condition at birth.

NEONATAL BEHAVIORAL ASSESSMENTS
Apgar Score[25]

The Apgar score is the traditional and most universal criterion for assessing the newborn's well-being in the delivery room. Its primary effect has been to focus attention on the neonate. The five categories—color, respiratory effort, cardiac effort, body tone, and responsiveness to aversive stimuli—measure the functions necessary to sustain life. The score reflects the neonate's capacity to respond to the stresses of labor and delivery. The score is influenced to a certain extent by any perinatal event, such as moderate hypoxia, drugs, or anesthesia given the mother; prolonged labor; cesarean section; and so on. However, as the score is done 1, 5, and 15 minutes after delivery, it basically measures the immediate capacity of the neonate for an "alarm" reaction. The kind and depth of depression that may follow later, representing the depleted resources of the baby, is not predicted by the Apgar score. Subtle effects of insults, such as hypoxia or drugs are easily overlooked by the Apgar score because it is necessary to have a substantial insult to impair the gross functioning of neuromuscular, cardiac, or respiratory systems.

The limited ability of the Apgar score to predict long-term outcome has been a disappointment to pediatricians and pediatric neurologists. However, as an initial screening device, it is important. Drage and coworkers reported a fourfold increase in neurologic abnormalities at 1 year in infants with low 5-minute Apgar scores compared to those with high scores.[26] However, only 4.3% of those with low 5-minute Apgar scores had gross neurologic abnormalities. More subtle effects identifiable at outcome were suggested by Lewis and associates, who studied visual attentiveness at 3, 9, and 13 months of age in babies with normal Apgar scores at 1 minute.[27] In this group, the researchers differentiated between those with scores of 7 to 9 and those with scores of 10 in their capacities to respond to complex visual tasks. Their results suggest that the Apgar score in some way reveals a spectrum of behavior that may predict future functioning, if we use more sensitive outcome tests along with it.

Scanlon Assessment[24]

Scanlon has further emphasized the importance of measuring immediate postnatal adaptation by developing a neurobehavioral scale that assesses the infant during the first 8 hours after birth. His scale includes a number of reflexes, the use of response decrement in 2 sensory modalities, and an observation of the infant's state and state lability. The scale was developed to detect the influence of subtle and transient perinatal influences. Using his scale, Scanlon found that infants of mothers who were given continuous lumbar epidural blocks with either lidocaine or mepivacaine had significantly lower scores on muscle strength and tone. A significantly greater number of infants failed to decrease a response to repetitive pinprick. Such an assessment provides the clinician with additional data to evaluate his methods of managing mothers during labor.

Graham—Rosenblith Scale of Neonatal Behavior[28]

A newborn **behavioral** examination was first devised by Graham in the mid1950s. It was she who first introduced the concept of the arousal state as important in evaluating muscle tone and reflex responses. Items in her scale included motor activity and strength, responses to auditory, visual and tactile stimulation and two behavioral items: irritability and tension (muscle tone). Using her scale to study anoxic infants, she found that newborn behavioral depression correlated well with infants who had a history of anoxia. The children with anoxia and depressed neonatal behavior were still judged neurologically, behaviorally, and intellectually abnormal at 3 years of age, but, by 7 years, there was no difference in neurologic and psychological outcome measures between the anoxic and control groups. This study illustrates an important point: that there is an amazing amount of plasticity and ability to recover in the neonatal brain, even after acute anoxia.

Rosenblith subsequently has revised Graham's scale to improve reliability, the degree of quantification, and external consistency.[29] Using this revision in a prospective study, she found significant correlations between the score on her neonatal scale and the 8-month motor score on a Bayley examination. There are also a number of correlations with 3-year hearing examinations and 4-year psychologic evaluations.

Ponderal Index

A unique and helpful measurement to define the adequacy of fetal nutrition is the ponderal index, a ratio of birth weight to body length.[30]

$$\frac{\text{weight (g)}}{[\text{length (cm)}]^3} \times 100$$

Miller and Hassanein describe the use of the ponderal index to identify fetal malnutrition, defined as either the relative decrease in soft tissue accumulation or as the increase in its utilization.[9,31] Unlike birth weight, the ponderal index was shown, in term babies, not to be confounded by race, sex, fetal age, or parity when defining malnutrition. By taking length into consideration, babies who are long, with a relatively small amount of soft tissue mass, can be seen as having experienced a late gestation nutritional insult. The ponderal index was not shown to change after 37-weeks' gestation, thus making an evaluation of chronologic age unnecessary. Between 29 and 37 weeks, it increases slightly with age, and malnutrition is defined as a ponderal index of 2.00 or less, as opposed to 2.20 at 37 weeks. In a study utilizing the ponderal index, factors associated with fetal malnutrition were poor maternal weight gain, absence of prenatal care, pre-eclampsia, and major chronic illness.[31]

Neonatal Behavioral Assessment Scale (Brazelton Scale)[12]

In order to record and evaluate some of the integrative processes in neonatal behavior, we have developed a behavioral evaluation scale that tests and documents the infant's changing state of consciousness and his response to various kinds of stimulation.

Because the neonate's reactions to all stimuli are dependent on his ongoing state, any interpretation of reactions must be made with this in mind. His use of state to maintain control of his reactions to environmental and internal stimuli is an important mechanism and reflects his potential for organization. State no longer need be treated as an error variable, but instead sets a dynamic pattern to allow for the full behavioral repertoire of the infant. Specifically, our examination tracks changes in state over the course of the examination, and its lability and direction. The variability of state indicates the infant's capacities for self-organization. His ability to quiet himself as well as his need for stimulation also measures this adequacy.

The behavioral examination tests for neurologic adequacy with 20 reflex measures, and for 26 behavioral responses to environmental stimuli, including the kind of interpersonal stimuli that mothers use in their handling of the infant. Best performance is accepted to overcome variability. In the examination, there is a graded series of procedures—talking, hand on belly, restraint, holding, and rocking—designed to soothe and alert the infant. His responsiveness to animate stimuli (*e.g.*, voice, face) and to inanimate stimuli (*e.g.*, rattle, bell, red ball, white light, temperature change) is assessed. Estimates of vigor and attentional excitement are measured, and an assessment is made of motor activity, tone, and autonomic responsiveness as he changes state. With this examination, given on successive days, we have been able to outline (1) the initial period of alertness immediately after delivery; (2) the period of depression and disorganization that follows; and (3) the curve of recovery to optimal function after several days. The period of depression and disorganization lasts 24 to 48 hours in infants with uncomplicated deliveries and no medication effects, but it persists for 3 to 4 days in infants compromised by medications given during the delivery. The curve of recovery may be the best single early predictor of individual potential function, and it seems to correlate well with the neonate's ability on retest at 30 days.[32]

A condensed list of the behavioral items is indicated in Table 18-3. In addition to the 26 items of behavior, assessed on a nine-point scale, there are 20 reflex responses that are also evaluated.

We feel that the behavioral items elicit important evidences of cortical control and responsiveness, even in the neonatal period. The neonate's capacity to manage and overcome the physiologic demands of this adjustment period in order to attend to, to differentiate, and to habituate to the complex stimuli of an examiner's maneuvers may be an important predictor of the baby's future central nervous system (CNS) organization. Certainly, the curve of recovery of these responses over the first neonatal week must be of more significance than the midbrain responses detectable in routine neurologic examinations.

Included in this examination are behavioral tests of such important CNS mechanisms as (1) habituation, or the neonate's capacity to shut out disturbing or overwhelming stimuli; (2) choices in attention to various objects or human stimuli (a neonate shows clear preferences for female versus male voices, and for human versus nonhuman visual stimuli); and (3) control of his state in order to attend to information from his environment (the effort to complete a hand-to-mouth cycle in order to attend to objects and people around him). These are all evidenced in the neonate and even in the premature infant and seem to be more predictive of CNS intactness than are reflex responses.[33]

Assessment of Behavioral States

There are predictable, directed responses from a neonate when he is in a social interaction with a nurturing adult or as he responds to an attractive auditory or visual stimulus. When positive rather than intrusive stimuli are utilized, the neonate has amazing capacities

Table 18-3. Neonatal Behavioral Assessment

Behavioral Items

---

1. Response decrement to repeated visual stimuli
2. Response decrement to rattle
3. Response decrement to bell
4. Response decrement to pinprick
5. Orienting response to inanimate visual stimuli
6. Orienting response to inanimate auditory stimuli
7. Orienting response to animate visual—examiner's face
8. Orienting response to animate auditory—examiner's voice
9. Orienting response to animate visual and auditory stimuli
10. Quality and duration of alert periods
11. General muscle tone in resting and in response to being handled (passive and active)
12. Motor Maturity
13. Traction responses as he is pulled to sit
14. Cuddliness—responses to being cuddled by the examiner
15. Defensive movements—reactions to a cloth over his face
16. Consolability with intervention by examiner
17. Peak of excitement and his capacity to control himself
18. Rapidity of buildup to crying state
19. Irritability during the exam
20. General assessment of kind and degree of activity
21. Tremulousness
22. Amount of startling
23. Lability of skin color (measuring autonomic lability)
24. Lability of states during entire exam
25. Self-quieting activity—attempts to console self and control state
26. Hand to mouth activity

(Brazelton, TB: Neonatal behavioral assessment. National Spastics Monograph # 50. London, William Heinemann & Sons, 1973)

for alerting and attention, for suppressing interfering reflex responses in order to attend, and, with very predictable behaviors, he responds to and interacts with his environment from birth.[12] But this predictability requires a knowledge of his ongoing state of consciousness.* When state is accounted for, most of his reactions are predictable, both to negative and to positive stimuli, from internal as well as external sources. State becomes a matrix

* State of consciousness or "state" of the infant becomes a most important matrix for interpretation of neonatal behavior. His reactions to all stimuli, internal and external, are dependent on his ongoing state of consciousness. Using **state** as a matrix, behavioral responses become quite predictable. State depends on physiologic variables such as hunger, nutrition, degree of hydration, and the timing within the wake-sleep cycle of the infant. Our criteria for state throughout this chapter are based on the descriptions by Prechtl and Beintema.[35]

for understanding his reactions. It qualifies stimulation as appropriate or inappropriate to the infant's organization. Thus, for almost any maturational level, the behavior produced by appropriate stimuli in appropriate states will demonstrate the complexity of an intact and adaptable CNS.

The matrix of state as a concept for organization in the neonate has become important since its use as a background for neurologic responses in Prechtl's assessment.[34] Within the context of an optimal state of alertness, Prechtl was able to demonstrate that the newborn could show better reflexive behavior and that the neurologic examination became a better predictive measure.[35]

If the sleeping or awake state of the baby is accounted for, an experienced examiner can make a fairly accurate prediction of how a baby will respond to any given stimulus. For example, within a deep sleep state, a baby will respond very slightly to a moderately loud, brief rattle, and although his breathing will change and he may blink, he probably will stir very little. In lighter sleep, he will startle, he may even begin to rouse, his face may become alert, and his respirations will change markedly. In a state in-between sleep and awake, he probably will startle briefly, but the startle will be followed by a slower movement of his arms and legs, and a writhing of his trunk, and he will open his eyes to look dully for the next stimulus. In a semialert state, he will become more alert, will begin to move about a bit, and may even search for the rattle, respirations becoming slower and more regular. In a wide-awake state, a newborn infant often will become quiet, look surprised but remain wide awake and alert, and then shift his eyes and then his head to turn toward the rattle, as if he were searching for it. Unless it is a very loud or insistent rattle, he may not stop crying in a crying state to respond to the sound. Thus, the state of arousal becomes not only a matrix for predictable responses but may be seen as the infant's way of defending himself from the world around him in the case of sleep states and of controlling arousal in order to attend to his environment in waking states. The parameters of state are relatively easy to determine by simple observation.

Thoman has devised an eight-state matrix, which she uses for observing neonatal behavior.[36] The categories of behavioral states and the criteria for their definition are as follows:

Quiet Sleep A. The infant's eyes are firmly closed and still. There is little or no motor activity, with the exception of occasional startles or rhythmic mouthing. Respiration is abdominal and relatively slow (average around 36/minute), deep, and regular.

Quiet Sleep B. All of the characteristics of Quiet Sleep A apply except for respiration, which deviates somewhat from the slow regularity seen in A. In this state, the respiration may be relatively fast, above 46, and show some irregularities; or the respiration may be slower but with irregularities. Respiration is primarily abdominal in this state.

Active Sleep without Rapid Eye Movements (REMs). The infant's eyes are closed, but slow, rolling movements may be apparent. Body activity can range from minor twitches to writhing and stretching. Respiration is irreg-

ular, costal in nature, and generally faster than that seen in Quiet Sleep (average of 46/min). Facial movements may include frowns, grimaces, smiles, twitches, mouth movements, and sucking (although face movements are not often seen in this category of Active Sleep).

Active Sleep with REMs. The infant's eyes are closed and REMs occur during a 10-second interval; other respiration and movement characteristics are the same as those described for Active Sleep without REMs, except that the facial activity is highly likely to accompany REMs or to be interspersed between groups of REMs.

Drowsy State. The infant's eyes either may open and close or they may be partially or fully open, but very still and dazed in appearance. There may be some generalized motor activity, and respiration is fairly regular, but faster and more shallow than that observed in regular sleep.

Alert Inactivity. The infant's body and face are relatively quiet and inactive, and the eyes are bright and shining in appearance.

Fussing. The characteristics of this state are the same as those for Alert Inactivity, but mild, agitated vocalizations are continuous or one cry burst may occur.

Crying. The characteristics of this state are the same as Alert Inactivity, but generalized motor activity is more intense, and cry bursts are continuous.

During 8 hours of daytime observations in the home, Thoman and coworkers found that these states have a rather predictable pattern, both in the amount of time neonates spend in each state, and in the probabilities of moving from one of these states to another (Figs. 18-2, 18-3).[36] Thus, they became a way of assessing CNS integrity by simple observational techniques; for when they were not following predicted patterns, they were found to be associated with CNS disorders.

Sleep Cycles. The length of sleep cycles (REM-active and quiet sleep) changes normally with maturation of the CNS. At term, cycles occur in a periodicity of 45 to 50 minutes, but immature babies have even shorter less well-defined cycles. Newborn infants have as much active REM in the first half of the deep period as in the second half. Initial brief, individual sleep and wake patterns coalesce as the environment presses the neonate to develop diurnal patterns of daytime

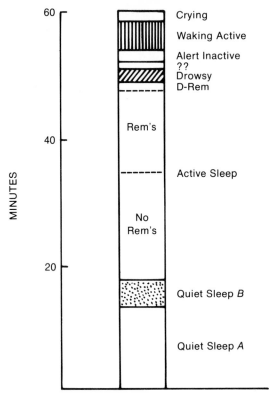

Fig. 18-2. Amount of time the neonate spends in each of eight states during an 8-hr observation. (Thoman EB: In Ellis NR (ed): Aberrant Development in Infancy. New York, John Wiley & Sons Inc., 1975)

anoxia, maternal drugs, or other disorganizing factors, one might expect a delay in a clear differentiation of sleep states, and these infants may be at risk for prolonged CNS disorganization. Steinschneider suggested that this kind of sleep disorganization may be a predictor for the apneic attacks found in sudden infant death syndrome.[39]

Anders has proposed a diagnostic sleep polygram in which the proportions of quiet and active-REM sleeps, as well as their rhythmicity, are measured against standards that now are fairly well determined by EEG. He has found that there is a lack of expected slower cyclical shifts from active to quiet, with unusually frequent and irregular shifts in CNS-damaged babies. Sleep states are not well organized in premature infants and quiet sleep is difficult to determine by EEG or by observing behavior. There is less observable quiet, regular sleep. Quiet sleep should increase over time in relation to REM sleep, and Thoman has found that a 1-hour observation when the baby is quiet can provide reliable information about this proportion.[36] Perhaps this may prove to be an important method for assessing the integrity of the CNS.

Differentiating characteristics that may help to predict future temperament and environmental adjustments include (1) the difficulty in rousing certain infants from sleep states to an alert or crying state with disturbing stimuli; (2) the rapidity with which others go from sleep to crying and down again; (3) the lability that certain newborns demonstrate as they move rapidly from one state to another; (4) those who console easily from crying; and (5) the self-quieting efforts on the part of other infants in order to maintain alert or quiet states.

Crying serves many purposes in the neonate, not the least of which is to shut out painful or disturbing stimuli. Hunger and pain are also responded to with crying, which brings the caretaker to him. And there is a kind of fussy crying that occurs periodically throughout the day, usually in a cyclic fashion, that seems to act as a discharger of energy and an organizer of the states that ensue.[40] After a period of such fussy crying, the neonate may be more alert and he may sleep more deeply.

As a behavior for organizing the day and for reducing disturbance within the CNS, crying seems to be of real importance in the neonatal

wakefulness and night sleep.[37] Appropriate feeding patterns, diet, absence of excessive anxiety on the part of the parents, sufficient nurturing stimulation, and a fussing period prior to a long sleep have all been implicated as reinforcing the CNS maturation necessary for the development of diurnal cycling of sleep and wakefulness.

Anders suggests that REM sleep is regulated by brainstem mechanisms that constitute an autoregulating and stimulating system of the CNS.[38] This state contributes to the growth and maintenance of neural tissue by cyclic excitatory activation of developing neuronal structures, which increases their differentiation. Without well-differentiated REM cycles, the neurophysiologic structures may be delayed in their development of differential responses. Thus, in immature organisms or neonates whose brainstems have been stressed by

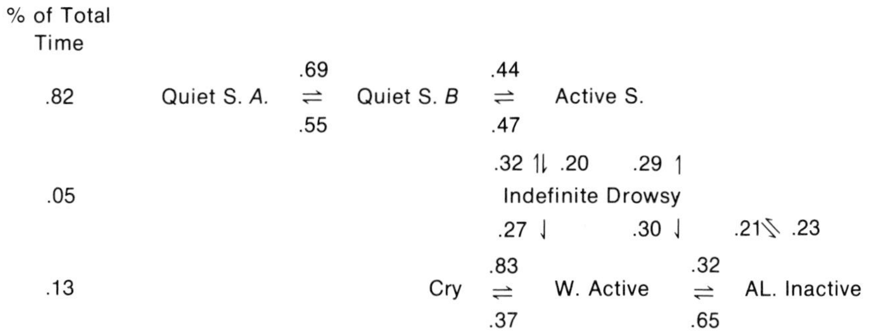

% of Total
Time

		.69		.44	
.82	Quiet S. *A.*	$\rightleftharpoons$	Quiet S. *B*	$\rightleftharpoons$	Active S.
		.55		.47	

.32 ⇅ .20   .29 ↑

.05   Indefinite Drowsy

.27 ↓   .30 ↓   .21↘ .23

		.83		.32	
.13	Cry	$\rightleftharpoons$	W. Active	$\rightleftharpoons$	AL. Inactive
		.37		.65	

Fig. 18-3. Probabilities of the neonate moving from one state to another. (Thoman EB: In Ellis NR (ed): Aberrent Development in Infancy. New York, John Wiley & Sons Inc., 1975)

period. Most parents can distinguish cries of pain, hunger, and fussiness by 2 to 3 weeks and learn quickly to respond appropriately.[41] So the cry is of ethologic significance to elicit appropriate caretaking for the infant.

Studies of the cry patterns of infants with various clinical syndromes or diseases suggest that there are cry features that distinguish damaged or sick infants from controls.[42] The cry can be used to aid in the differential diagnosis of certain diseases.[43] Down's syndrome is associated with a low-pitched, hoarse, gutteral cry, a higher threshold for the production of the cry and a longer latency from stimulation to cry onset. On the other hand, infants with maladie du cri de chat and those with 13–15 trisomy have a fundamental frequency which is high-pitched, averaging 850 Hz in contrast to the 400 to 600 range in healthy infants.

Lester found that malnourished infants had a longer cry duration, longer cry latency, higher fundamental frequency, lower amplitude of the fundamental frequency, and fewer harmonics than well-nourished infants.[44] These cry features were correlated with the magnitude of heart rate deceleration in a study of the habituation of the cardiac-orienting response.

Usefulness of State Assessments

We have used neonatal state observations to increase our capacity to help parents in several ways. With an overresponsive, rapidly upset, intensely motor-reactive neonate, we let the parents know that we have observed this and tell them that we expect the baby to cry for unpredictable reasons and not console as easily as they might hope. Often we suggest such soothing measures as swaddling, pacifiers, cradles, and rocking chairs. But our main effort is to establish the fact that this difficulty in state control is a part of the baby and not the result of their inadequate reading of the baby. Most new parents believe that they should be able to handle any crying, and therefore believe that it is their fault if they cannot soothe their new baby. Their guilt and anxiety build up, and as they transmit it to the infant, a normal amount of crying increases to long periods of "colic" or inconsolable crying.[45] If parents can be forewarned, they can be kept from participating in such a build-up. They can be given a new and more appropriate role with such an infant: that of helping him to learn state controls and to bring himself down from such an upset state.

In the same way, a difficult-to-rouse, unresponsive neonate will produce another kind of stress in his environment. We studied a group of full-term infants weighing greater than 2700 g whose ponderal indices[31] showed that they had suffered from mild placental insufficiency and were small-for-gestational age. These infants were difficult to rouse from sleep states. When they finally came to an awake state, they still were realtively inactive and difficult to alert. They reacted dully to visual and auditory cues to which an average baby would have responded in an excited, intense way. After they were awakened, they maintained a dull awake state for long periods, which seemed to prevent them from getting back down into normal sleep. These rather poorly organized states inevitably affected their environments. Mothers reported that they found their babies "unpredictable" and "difficult to understand." They complained that they were never sure that they were reaching them, and their inclination was to leave the babies alone. Because such babies may set the tone for a failure in interaction, it is no surprise that many of the failure-to-thrive infants as well as many abused infants have these characteristics. One of our jobs as pediatricians could be to note these difficulties in state behavior in our neonatal examination and to alert the parents to this as a part of their baby. Their role with such an infant could be introducing more stimulation rather than less, thus gradually teaching the infant to respond with more appropriate alerting behavior. As the physiologic status of the infant improves with rehydration and nutrients, his responsiveness and his capacity to interact with his environment will increase also.[11] Parents will see this improvement as an indication of their success in their role, and the parent-infant relationship will be reinforced.

In the neonatal period, state behavior can be assessed and used to predict normalcy or developmental delay, and may even predict other difficulties such as apnea and problems in organization that could lead to failure in the parent-child interaction.

SENSORY CAPACITIES
Visual

The newborn is equipped at birth with the capacity for processing complex visual information and for demonstrating ocular movements to track an object in space. Even more important to his survival is the fact that he can defend himself from visual stimuli that might otherwise force him to make excessive demands on his immature physiologic system. When a bright light is flashed into a neonate's eyes, not only do his pupils constrict but he also blinks, his eyelids and whole face contract, and he withdraws his head by arching his whole body, often setting off a complete startle as he withdraws. His heart rate and respirations increase and there is an evoked response registered on his visual occipital EEG. Repeated stimulation of this nature induces diminishing responses because of his capacity to shut down his responses. For

example, in a series of 20 bright light stimuli presented at 1-minute intervals we found that the infant rapidly habituated and damped out the behavioral responses.[46] By the tenth stimulus, he had decreased not only his observable motor responses but also his cardiac and respiratory responses. The latency to evoked responses, as measured by EEG tracings, was increasing, and, by the 15th stimulus, the EEG reflected the induction of a quiet, unresponsive behavioral state accompanied by trace alternans and spindles. The infant's capacity to shut out repetitious, disturbing visual stimuli protects him from having to respond to visual stimulation and at the same time frees his energy to meet physiologic demands.

This capacity of the neonate has been considered a kind of neurologic habituation,[47-49] and is present in neonates with intact CNSs.[50] The capacity to habituate to visual stimuli is decreased, although it is present, in immature infants.[51] It is affected by medication such as barbiturates, given to mothers as premedication at the time of delivery. This has led Brazier to postulate that the primary focus for this mechanism is in the reticular formation and midbrain.[52] The infant finally becomes deeply asleep; with tightened, flexed extremities; with little movement except jerky startles; no eye blinks; deep, regular respirations; and rapid, regular heart rate. This state of habituation seems to signal a defensive state against the assaults of the environment.

In a practical way, it is important to realize that any newborn baby in a brightly lit, noisy nursery is likely to be in such a habituated state. In such a state, he is unlikely to be as responsive to loud noises or a flashlight if they are used as a test stimulus. And if one wanted to test his vision or hearing, it would be necessary to move him to a darker, quieter room. Then complex visual responses can be captured more easily and reliably. The only justification that we can find for those who claim that newborns cannot see, or do not respond with real behavioral preference to various visual stimuli, is that they have tested them in an overlit, inappropriate setting. For, just as he is equipped with the capacity to shut out certain stimuli, the newborn demonstrates the capacity to alert to, turn his eyes and head to follow, and fix on a stimulus that appeals to him. Fantz first pointed out neonatal preference for certain kinds of complex visual stimuli.[53] For instance, he found that sharply contrasting colors, larger squares, and medium-brightly lit objects were appealing to the neonate, and brought him to a prolonged alert state of fixation. Fantz and others found that the neonate preferred an ovoid object, and one in which there were eyes and a mouth.[22] Furthermore, the kind of attention and the length of fixation were markedly reduced if mothers had been medicated prior to delivery.

More recently, Goren showed that, immediately after delivery, a human neonate would not only fix on a drawing that resembled a human face, but would also follow it, with eyes and head turning, for 180° arcs. A scrambled face did not demand the same kind of attention, nor did the infant completely follow the distorted face with his eyes and head; the head turned to follow only half of the arc. We found that the capacity of neonates to fix on and follow a red ball was a good predictive sign of neurologic integrity.[55] However, its absence is not a serious predictor because it is so dependent on whether the infant is in an alert state. Many conditions interfere with the neonate's capacity to come to an alert state: the CNS depression that follows delivery; hypoxia, or any of the stress of delivery; premedication given the mother; transient effects of metabolic derangement or even illness in the neonate; and normal conditions of hunger, fatigue, and an overlit nursery. But newborns are capable of visual fixing and following during alert periods, and this may be a sensitive predictor of neurologic and visual integrity.[33]

Visual acuity of the newborn still is difficult to determine. Gorman, Cogan, and Gellis used the neonate's opticokinetic responses to a moving drum lined with stripes and found that 93 of 100 infants responded preferentially to stripes subtending a visual angle of only 33.5 minutes of arc.[56] We found that prematures were less reliable but could also fix on and follow the same lined drum.[55] Dayton and coworkers found at least 20/150 vision in newborns by this same technique.[57] It does not seem, however, that newborns are able to accommodate well but rather that they have a fixed focal length of about 19 cm.[58] In order to capture visual interest, an examiner must present a bright object at this distance.

Extremes of brightness and noise in the environment have been found to interfere with the neonate's capacity to respond. In a noisy, overlighted nursery, the neonate tends to shut down his capacity to attend, but in a semidarkened room, a normal neonate in an alert state can be made to respond to the human face as well as to a red or shiny object.

The involvement of the neonate's state behavior as well as the coordination of visual motor and head turning seem to point to the entrainment of rather complex nervous system pathways. It is difficult not to believe that his cortex is maintaining this alert state of consciousness and controlling interfering motor behavior. The visual and motor cortices certainly are involved in the following motions of the head and eyes. In a recent long-term study, Sigman, Parmelee, and coworkers found that visual behavior may be one of the best predictors of intactness of the CNS in the neonate.[59] They found that summary scores on the neonate's neurologic examination were significantly related to the length of first fixation on a black-and-white checkerboard as a visual stimulus. This capacity to stare at a complex object was, of course, related to an alert state, and, when infants could not be brought to such a state, the prediction was more ominous.

An optimal response to visual stimulation in a neonate can be described as (1) an initial alerting, (2) attention that increases but which is followed by (3) a gradual decrease in interest, and (4) a final turning away from a monotonous presentation.

Tronick and Clanton have experimentally demonstrated this remarkable coordination of head and eye movements.[60] Using electro-oculogram recordings of eye movements and transducer-recorded head movements, they examined the pattern of head and eye movements in 3-week-old infants. They found that when infants were in an upright position both head and eyes became aimed at the target. When the infant moved his line of sight from one target to another, the eyes typically moved first, with a rapid saccadic shift, followed by a slower head movement. They found four basic patterns. First, a rapidly shifting pattern in which a fairly rapid head movement was integrated with a brief saccadic movement of the eyes to one side. Second, a search pattern involving a slow movement of the head with a series of fixations and saccades of the eyes. Third, a focal pattern in which the head remained stable while a series of fixations scanned a portion of the visual field. Last, a compensatory pattern in which the line of sight could be maintained by the eyes even when the head moved in an opposite direction. These complex patterns appeared to be quite organized in the normal newborn and they suggested that the infant has a cortically controlled visual system at birth that coordinates head and eyes for the extraction of information from the environment.

Several observers have demonstrated that neonates prefer moving and somewhat complex visual patterns to stationary ones.[22,61] If the moving object can be moved slowly parallel to the natural, lateral movements of the eyes, it is more likely to capture the baby's interest. Furthermore, the duration and degree of his attention may be correlated with both a middle range of complexity and the similarity of the target to the ovoid shape and the structures involved in the human face.

Auditory

The neonate's auditory responses are also specific and well organized. Too commonly, assessments are not sensitive to the complexity of the newborn's behavior. For example, the loud clackers used on the Collaborative Project of NINDB for Early Detection of CNS Defects were ineffective in loud, noisy nurseries. A large percentage of neonates tested with such a routine were unresponsive; they appeared to have shut out or habituated to the ambient auditory stimuli. Another approach under these conditions would have been to use a soft rattle.

With an interesting auditory stimulus, such as a rattle, we see an infant move from a sleeping state to an alert state. His breathing becomes irregular, his face brightens, his eyes open, and, when he is completely alert, his eyes and head will turn toward the sound. In the case of a well-organized neonate, head turning will be followed by a searching look on his face, a scanning of his eyes to find a source for the auditory stimulus. In order to find out whether the neonate can respond this way, a full test of hearing should include several stimuli, animate as well as inanimate, with careful attention to the neonate's ongoing state of consciousness so that it will break into his state. For example, one should use a rattle in light sleep, a voice in awake states, and a handclap in deep sleep. Respirations and eyeblinks can be monitored for change as he responds, as can more obvious behavioral startles to auditory stimuli.[12]

Eisenberg has determined the differential responses to different ranges of sound that are available to the infant.[62] In the range of human speech (500–900 Hz) the neonate will inhibit motor behavior. He often will demonstrate cardiac deceleration as an evidence of his attention, and will orient with head turning toward the source of sound. Outside this human range, there is a less complex behavioral response. With a high-pitched or too-loud sound, the infant will startle initially, turn his head away from the sound, his heart rate and breathing will accelerate, and his skin will redden. He will attempt to shut out the repetitious sound by habituation, and, if that is unsuccessful, he will start to cry in order to control the disturbing effects of such auditory input. The strikingly narrow range of stimuli for positive, attending responses can be demonstrated by linking devices for recording sucking to the auditory input.[63] Within this narrow human range, sucking will cease as an initial response to the stimulus, and be followed by a burst-pause pattern of sucking, as if the infant were pausing off and on to receive more of the interesting auditory input.

Lower and higher frequencies have different functional properties. Signals above 4000 Hz are more effective in producing a response, even in crying or sleep states, but they are likely to produce distress. Lower intensities (35–40 db) are effective inhibitors of distress, especially as continuous white noise.[64] White noise at these levels will most often induce a sleep state after a time period, even in a crying neonate.[41] Kearsley has demonstrated the importance of the rise time of the sound on the neonate's behavioral responses.[65] Sounds with prolonged onset times and low frequencies produced eye opening and cardiac deceleration followed by an attentive look whereas sounds with rapid onset and high frequency produced eye closing, cardiac acceleration, increased head movements, and aversion.

As one defines the neonate's behavioral response to an appropriate sound, one sees a series of regular steps. As the sound is localized,[63] cardiac rate first increases and may be accompanied by a mild startle.[66] If the auditory stimulus is attractive to the infant, his face will brighten, his heart rate will decelerate, his breathing will slow, and he will alert and search with his eyes until the source of the sound is localized to the *en face* midline of the baby. This behavior, which occurs as a response to an attractive auditory stimulus (*e.g.,* rattle or the human voice), becomes a measure of the neonate's capacity to organize his central and autonomic nervous systems.

Habituation to repeated auditory stimuli becomes a further test of CNS function. When there is a damaged cortex, behavioral inhibition is not likely to occur. Bronstein and Petrova found that 2-hour-old to 8-day-old infants ceased sucking on a pacifier initially, but after repeated sounds of 60 to 70 db, they resumed sucking.[67] Bridger found that the heart rate acceleration as an initial response to an auditory stimulus ceased after several trials, and the baby essentially habituated behaviorally and autonomically to this repetitive stimulus.[48] But, a change in frequency or a tonal change brought about an immediate increase in motor activity, as well as a change in heart rate (representing dishabituation). In other words, cardiac response can be used to study the infant's mental organization for repetitive, novel, and contingent responses. A paradigm of habituation registers his response to the repetition of auditory, visual, and tactile stimuli. Not only does the change in heart rate decrease as the same stimulus is presented repeatedly to a newborn, but he also begins to lose interest and actively shuts out the repeated stimulus by going to sleep or by crying. He seems to have appreciated and learned about the similarity. If the stimulus is varied slightly, he begins to become interested again, he rouses or quiets, begins to brighten and his heart rate changes return to the new stimulus. One can document his capacity to detect differences in duration, intensity, and rise time by monitoring his heart rate at such a time.

Cairns and Butterfield have documented the differences in the neonate's responses to human versus nonhuman sounds by using a sucking paradigm to detect subtle information-processing differences (discussed in the section under sucking).[68] They believe that monitoring for a burst-pause pattern in sucking as one changes auditory stimuli can differentiate between CNS impairments of receptive process-ing from the kind of peripheral impairment that is found in nerve deafness of rubella, congenital malformations, hyperbilirubinemia, and other disorders.

Olfactory

Engen and coworkers have demonstrated observably differentiated responses to odors in the neonate, and one can conclude that the newborn is set up with a highly equipped sense of smell, ready to pick up the odors that will help him adapt to his new world.[69] For example, he acts as if he were offended by acetic acid, asafetida, and alcohol in the neonatal period, but is attracted to sweet odors such as milk and sugary solutions. More recently, MacFarlane has shown that 5-day-old neonates can reliably distinguish their own mother's breast pads from those of other lactating mothers, although this discrimination was not present at 2 days.[70] They turn their heads toward their own mother's breast pads with 80% reliability, after controls for laterality are imposed. In other words, the neonate's sense of smell perceived the differential odor of his mother as a learned response by the fifth day.

Taste

The newborn has fine differential responses to taste. Nelson has observed different sucking responses to sugar and decreased sucking to other tastes.[71] More recently, Johnson and Salisbury have reported that a newborn's taste preferences are expressed in an even more complex fashion.[72] An infant is fed different fluids through a monitored nipple and his sucking pattern is recorded. Saline causes such resistance that the baby is likely to aspirate. With a cow's milk formula, he will suck in a rather continuous fashion, pausing at irregular intervals. If breast milk then is fed to him by this same system, he will register his recognition of the change in taste after a short latency, then suck in bursts with frequent pauses at regular intervals. The pauses seem to be directly related to the taste of breast milk, and his burst pause pattern seems to indicate that he changes to a kind of program for other stimuli (such as social communication) to be added to the feeding situation in the pauses.

Newly developed procedures for recording various parameters of sucking behavior have enabled the documentation of fine discriminations which infants make.[73] A sucking apparatus connected to a polygraph has been used for recording the infant's sucking behavior under conditions in which the presentation of drops of fluid is made contingent upon that behavior. When sucking on a blank nipple, the infant sucks in short bursts separated by long pauses, and sucking within those bursts is quite rapid. When a sweet fluid (*e.g.*, 15% sucrose) is delivered contingent upon sucking, the infant engages in more sucks per minutes, invests more sucks per burst, takes shorter rest periods, and sucks more slowly within each sucking burst. Moreover, all of these parameters are affected by sweetness along a continuum from 0 through 15% sucrose, as well as by the amount of fluid received per suck.[74] Thus, with either increasing concentrations or amounts of sucrose, infants tend to suck more slowly within bursts.

Crook has recently capitalized upon the sensitivity of sucking parameters, such as length of sucking burst, to study the neonate's response to mildly aversive as well as to pleasant taste stimuli.[75] By administering three drops of either a sweet or salty fluid, one drop at a time, and by recording the length of the immediately subsequent sucking burst, Crook was able to demonstrate that increased concentrations of sweet fluid produce larger sucking bursts, whereas increased concentrations of salt produce shorter bursts. The technique has considerable potential for the careful study of the psychophysics of taste in infancy.

Tactile Stimuli

The sensitivity of the infant to handling and to touch is apparent. A mother's first response to an upset baby is to contain him, to shut down his disturbing motor activity by touching or holding him. By contrast, fathers are more likely to tap in a playful, rhythmic fashion or to use tactile methods to excite the infant in an interaction. Touch becomes a message system between the caregiver and the infant, both for calming him down and for building him up in order to attend to cues. We found that a patting motion of three times per minute was soothing whereas five to six times per minute becomes an alerting stimulus.[76] As with auditory stimuli, the law of initial values seems to be of primary importance. When a baby is quiet, a rapid, intrusive tactile stimulus serves to bring him up to an alert state. When he is upset, a slow, modulated tactile stimulus seems to serve to reduce his activity.

Swaddling is used in many cultures to replace the important constraints offered first by the uterus and then by mothers and caretakers. As a restraining influence on the overreactions of hyperactive neonates, the supportive control that is offered by a steady hand on a baby's abdomen or by holding his arms so that he cannot startle reproduces the swaddling effects of holding or wrapping a neonate. This added control of disturbing motor responses allows the neonate to attend and interact with his environment.

When an infant cannot use soothing tactile stimuli to help him to adapt his state behavior one must consider a diagnosis of CNS irritability. A baby with CNS irritation from a bleed or from infection demonstrates constantly increasing irritability with stimuli, especially tactile. Such a response should signal the examiner to investigate him further for evidence of CNS difficulties.

Sucking

An awake, hungry newborn exhibits active searching movements in response to tactile stimulation in the region around the mouth, and even as far out on the face as the cheek and sides of the jaw and head.[77] This is called the **rooting reflex,** and it is present in the premature even before sucking itself is effective.[78] Peiper described three sets of oral pads in the cheeks and mouth, which help maintain and establish negative pressure.[77] Sucking is facilitated by the thorax in inspiration[79] and by fixing the jaw to maintain it between respirations. A second mechanism, **expressing,** is made by the tongue as it moves up against the hard palate and from the front to the back of the mouth. Swallowing and respirations must be coordinated, and the depth and rate of respiration are handled differently in nutritive and nonnutritive sucking. Peiper argues for a hierarchical control of swallowing, sucking, and breathing in which swallowing controls sucking, and sucking controls breathing. The absence of coordination between these three systems in the neonate is indicative of discoordination within the CNS, and it may be seen in damaged infants and in the very immature infant.

Gryboski describes a technique of monitoring three components of sucking with three transducers: one, a lapping mechanism, at the front of the tongue; another, a milking feeling at the base of the tongue; and a third, a suction component in the upper esophagus.[80] The timing of the three components becomes a measure of the maturity of the CNS of a premature infant. There is a latency before they become coordinated in an effective milking mechanism; the more prolonged the latency the more immature the baby. One can feel these three by a finger in the mouth. A nurse who is familiar with premature infants can tell clinically whether they are coordinated. When there is CNS irritation, one can feel the disruption of the central processes that control these mechanisms by insertion of a finger into the neonate's mouth, and when the infant is sucking, an examiner can determine for himself the presence and coordination of the three components. This, then becomes an easily available and valuable measure of the infant's stage of relative maturity and of his CNS coordination.

The infant sucks in a more or less regular pattern of bursts and pauses.[41] Bursts seem to occur in packages of 5 to 24 sucks per burst.[81] The pause between bursts has been considered a rest and recovery period as well as a period during which cognitive information is being processed by the neonate.[75] Kaye found that the pauses were important ethologically because they are taken by mothers as signals to stimulate the infant to return to sucking.[82] Mothers tend to look down at, talk to, and stimulate a baby when he pauses in a sucking burst. As a result, the mother's jiggling actually prolongs the pause as the infant responds to the stimulating information given to him by his mother.

Sucking, because of the stability produced through central control early in gestation, is used by infant researchers to measure all sorts of behaviors: sensory discrimination, conditioning, and learning,[83] orienting and attention.[63,81] The importance of sucking as a way of regulating himself can be seen in a newborn as he begins to build up from a quiet state to crying. His attempts to achieve hand-to-mouth contact in order to keep his activity under control are fascinating to watch. When he is finally able to insert a finger into his mouth, suck on it and quiet himself, he seems rewarded. The sense of satisfaction and of gratification at having achieved this self-regulation are so striking that one can see that he has achieved a goal. His face softens and alerts as he begins to concentrate on maintaining this kind of self-regulation. This is the most obvious evidence that the baby has goal-oriented behaviors that he can achieve for himself. A pacifier can achieve this same quieting in an upset baby, but a pacifier may not serve the self-regulating feedback system as richly as the baby's own maneuver.

Pairing sucking with other modalities, auditory, visual, or tactile, has been too neglected in most neonatal nurseries. The variations and complexity of this system as it reflects CNS functions are well studied by psychologists and psychophysiologists.[84]

For example, Cairns and Butterfield found that when a neonate was sucking on a nonnutritive pacifier, he presented a rich set of responses to human and nonhuman auditory signals.[68] After hearing a human voice, he would increase his sucking rate as a signal to bring it on again, and he could be conditioned in 20 minutes to suck harder or to pause in order to produce a second vocal signal. However, with white noise or pure-tone (nonhuman) signals, he sucks less hard after the signal, and learns to suck only to reduce the noise, *not* to repeat it or increase it.

In the same way, when a human vocal sound was introduced to a neonate who was monitored by a nonnutritive pacifier, he began to produce a burst-pause pattern with prolonged pauses as if he were waiting for the human signals to repeat themselves. Cairns and Butterfield suggest that pairing nonnutritive sucking with auditory stimulation can differentiate forms of CNS difficulty by the ability of the neonate to discriminate between paired signals that differ only in this way (human versus nonhuman).[68] Cairn's group has been able to discriminate between the central and peripheral forms of impairment in auditory receptiveness that are residual of rubella, hyperbilirubinemia, prematurity, and hypoxia.

The suggestion of pairing two separate modalities of CNS function, such as sucking and sensory receptors, to test for fine discrimination tasks, for habituation and dishabituation to repetitive signals, and for conditioning and learning tasks, suggests new and excitingly innovative methods for evaluating the neonate's CNS function.

ORGANIZATION OF MOTOR BEHAVIOR

One of the most neglected and illuminating sources of information about a neonate's status is gathered from simple observation of how he moves his extremities, what kind of movements he makes, and, in particular, whether his movements are simple random startles or whether they seem to be purposeful. For instance, one of the most exciting behaviors one can observe in the neonatal period can be seen in a well-organized neonate. As he begins to rouse from sleeping and when he begins to startle and become upset, he may attempt to bring his hand up to his mouth. In this effort, he may turn his head to one side, immediately controlling one side of his body by the central monitoring effects of the tonic neck reflex (TNR). The face and arm first extend and then slow down in extension; an observer can see the infant work to bring his hand up to his mouth with flexion at the elbow. As it reaches his mouth, the infant's body begins to relax, his face softens and he makes real efforts to insert his clenched fist. When these efforts are successful, he will maintain a quiet state of semialertness, sucking loudly on the fist. Even when he cannot actually insert the hand or a finger, he remains in a rewarded peaceful state, ready to listen to a sound or look at a presenting stimulus. In other words, he has demonstrated to the observer that he can achieve a complex motor act by first, shutting out interfering reflex startles; second, completing a cycle of lateralizing his motor energy, bringing his hand up to his mouth, and; third, using this activity to maintain a quiet and alert state, receptive to information from the environment. This complex behavior embedded in the goal-oriented achievement of wanting to listen or to look becomes powerful evidence in the neonate of optimal CNS organization.

When such behavioral organization is not observed in a particular interval, does it mean that the neonate cannot perform as well as this? Not necessarily. One must constantly be aware of the conditions that influence his performance. These include

1. his ongoing state of arousal; for if he is too deeply asleep or too upset during such an observation period, the likelihood of organized behavior is reduced.
2. environmental conditions such as temperature (too low or too high) or sound or light levels that reduce him to a relative shutout state
3. ongoing chemical or humoral imbalances, such as mild dehydration, hypocalcemia, or hypoglycemia, which render him hypersensitive and jittery or too sleepy.
4. his state of well-being (illness or stress); his relative motor disorganization may be a primary symptom of an impending illness.
5. his degree of recovery from the stresses of labor and delivery.
6. perinatal stresses of hypoxia, maternal medication, and so on.

In other words, disorganization of motor activity may become an important symptom of stress in a neonate, and should therefore be assessed carefully. Repeated examinations as he recovers over the neonatal period become most important in this regard.

There are maneuvers which should be used for assessment of muscle tone and the balance of flexor and extensor muscles. The range that is possible for a given baby may be more important than any one sample of motor performance. Resting, spontaneous posture gives one an idea of preferred position. A normal full-term baby spontaneously prefers a position of flexion for both arms and legs. His extremities may flatten out into extension from time to time, but in general he will be found in flexed postures. A baby who lies in full extension may be seen as hypotonic. Hypertonicity is signaled by tightly flexed extremities with few spontaneous movements except brief, jerky startles. Thus, one can observe in the first few minutes the most likely category to which the baby will be assigned. A few simple passive maneuvers of extending then flexing arms, legs, neck, and trunk confirm the degree of hypertonicity or hypotonicity. Hypertonicity is accompanied by jerky snapback of extremities or overshooting into tight flexion after the limbs are released. Hypotonicity is signaled by floppy, hyperextensive limbs, with little resistance or spontaneous movement after they are released. One then must attempt to account for the time observed in terms of the infant's degree of maturity as well as for the variables listed above, which can be expected to influence his motor responsivity. Organized reflex motor responses—such as motor stepping, placing, and prone responses; crawling movements and attempts to lift his head; traction of his neck and shoulder; and girdle musculature in a pull-to-sit maneuver—confirm and bring out even more information about his motor strength and the balance between flexor and extensor groups. Jerky, clonic movements and the snapback described above point to an imbalance of flexor and extensor muscle groups. Smooth movements of a neonate are an indicator of good balance between these groups and point to a well-organized CNS.

Restricted arcs of movement of the extremities are a sign of relative hypertonicity or of immaturity. A full-term infant should demonstrate smooth, free cycles of arm and leg movements, which denote an ideal balance of flexors and extensors. Recovery from stress of delivery, maternal medication, dehydration, or illness can be determined by the infant's motor progress over time toward a free, smooth, balanced motor performance.

Defensive reactions to a cloth over the face or to a painful stimulus to any part of the body bring out structured motor patterns, and the baby's effectiveness in approaching and removing an obtrusive stimulus becomes a way of testing for intact motor pathways and their organization. For example, covering his face with a cloth elicits a series of motor maneuvers. First he roots, then twists his head from side to side, stretches his neck backward in active arching, and finally brings each arm up to swipe at the offending cloth. Many newborns effectively push the cloth off the face. These responses (hand-to-mouth, defensive movements or other sequential motor acts) may be of equal value as elicited reflexes as one assesses the upper extermities for neurologic adequacy.

An integrated motor act that is useful in an assessment is the combined hand-grasp and traction response in the shoulder girdle as one pulls the baby to sit. His repeated attempts to control his head in an upright position bring out his vigor, his motor integration and the strength of motor groups in his upper extremities.

LEARNING IN THE NEONATAL PERIOD

Because the neonate is equipped with such remarkable capacities for responsiveness, we can now begin to devise better assessments of CNS integrity at birth. Static neurologic assessments have not been particularly fruitful in predicting future function. Perhaps a model of assessment based on his capacity to use stimulation from the environment would offer us a better chance for prediction of his outcome.

Classic Conditioning

One of the most obvious signs of newborn learning can be seen by using classic conditioning techniques, in which the infant is presented with a neutral stimulus (conditioning stimulus) in association with a stimulus effective in eliciting an observable response (unconditioned stimulus). Over a series of presentations in which the stimuli are paired, the neutral stimulus comes to elicit the response under investigation and demonstrates the infant's capacity to retain these associations. For instance, Denisova and Figurin first demonstrated that newborns could be conditioned by being placed in the feeding position to which they had become accustomed.[86] After only a few days, they exhibited anticipatory sucking movements.

The Babkin response[85] has been successfully conditioned by Kaye.[87] This reflex involves several components, including gaping, sucking, turning the head to midline, raising the head, and , in some instances, eyelid closure and forearm flexion. The congenital stimulus for this behavior is pressure on the baby's palms. Kaye utilized tactile-kinesthetic stimulation, involving movement of the arms from the infant's sides up to his head, just before the application of the pressure. This procedure resulted in classic conditioning of the Babkin response, a finding subsequently replicated.[88] The latter researchers successfully demonstrated the acquisition of this response to an auditory conditioning stimulus as well as to kinesthetic stimulation.

Lipsitt and Kaye used the presentation of a low-frequency, loud tone (93 db) in association with the insertion of a nipple in the mouths of infants 3 and 4 days old.[89] To a control group, the tone and nipple were presented noncontiguously. On every fifth trial, the tone was presented alone as a test for conditioning, and, after training was completed, all babies received a series of extinction trials with the test tone alone. Evidence was found for classic appetitional conditioning, although the effects of training did not manifest themselves until the extinction condition.

Other investigators have also been able to obtain such conditioning.[90]

Papousek[91] and Siqueland and coworkers[92] have studied the effect of contingent reinforcement of head turning to a touch at the side of the mouth. Such stimulation produces the rooting reflex and head turning in 30% of preconditioning trials. After 5% dextrose solution was offered upon the neonate's successful head turning, the head turning was significantly increased by the reinforcement. By associating a tone with the positive condition, one could enhance their head turning to 83%. If on alternate trials the head turns were not reinforced with dextrose solution, there was a gradual behavioral shift down to 30% head turning. These studies demonstrated that reflexive behavior could be altered by contingent reinforcement.

Operant Conditioning

Sameroff showed that the subsystems of the general sucking pattern of infants can be altered by specific environmental conditions.[93] He was able to demonstrate that when the delivery of fluid is made directly contingent upon the negative pressure component of the sucking response, the infant uses more negative pressure than when this contingency is not in effect. Such a demonstration is possible because there are two major components of sucking behavior in the newborn: one consisting of negative pressure in the buccal cavity; and the other simply the positive pressure created by the gum action with which the infant engages the nipple. The Sameroff study showed that these two components may be reinforced differentially to enhance one or the other of them.

Habituation

Fantz's work suggests that visual habituation of infants presents an opportunity for assessing the CNS status of the newborn.[94] He demonstrated that the infant's gaze duration may be used over repetitive trials to assess the infant's diminishing interest in specific visual stimuli. Forty newborns were presented with two checkerboard targets: one with four squares, the other with 144 squares. Both males and females showed response decrements over trials, but males demonstrated this phenomenon to the less dense visual (4-square) stimulus, and females to the denser (144-square) stimulus.

In typical studies of auditory habituation, the stimuli are presented in a time-locked fashion, once every 30 seconds, with some indicator response serving as the measure of response strength over repetitive presentation trials. It has been shown that acceleration of heart rate declines with repetitive presentations; it declines more quickly the shorter the inter-stimulus interval. Also, dishabituation can be seen in the newborn by an increase in the intensity of the test stimulus over the familiarization stimulus, or by a change in the tonal pattern of the recovery stimulus.[95] It has also been shown that response diminution following repeated stimulation may still be present even after a 1-day interval in newborns.

In one study of neonatal sensitivity to olfactory stimuli, and of habituation of response to such stimuli, infants were presented with ten trials of an odorant, half of the infants receiving asafetida first and the other half receiving anise oil first. Initial response levels to these odorants based upon a combined respiration and stabilimeter index were about 90%, and response levels dropped to approximately 25% by the tenth trial. At the conclusion of the trials, the alternate odorant was capable of producing response recovery, although not to the level at which the infant first responded.[69] In subsequent studies, further refinements in method ruled out sensory fatigue as the basis of the response decrement obtained. This was done by showing that there may occur a response recovery to odorants which were present in a solution to which habituation had been previously obtained.

Inasmuch as habituation relates to memory function, which is mediated by the brain, it should be possible to refine techniques for improved assessment of impairment of the CNS by including indices of habituation.[12] In fact, Lewis has shown that impaired infantile habituation is related to low Apgar scores and other indices of brain damage.[96] Other workers have shown that hydrocephalic and anencephalic infants may show no habituation at all.[97]

A study of averaged auditory evoked responses made of infants with Down's syndrome showed that, relative to normal infants matched in age (from 8 days to 13 months), the infants with Down's syndrome showed no significant response decrement.[98] As a byproduct of the study, it was also demonstrated that none of the babies under one month of age, normal or otherwise, showed evoked response habituation.

Effects of Stimulation upon Recovery

If these learning paradigms are capable of indicating sensory and neurologic integrity, perhaps a clinical test of the baby's future function could be based on a curve of behavioral improvement. Using the Neonatal Behavioral Assessment Scale,[12] we have seen that in a low-risk group of babies, there was a significant improvement over the first 10 days in major areas of behavior function.[99] The infants became more alert and capable of orienting to animate and inanimate stimuli. They turned significantly more to the voice and rattle, and followed the human face and a red ball with significantly more head turning and alerting. Their motor maturity, muscle tone, and integrated motor performances also improved. On behavioral items reflecting their physiological adjustments, such as startles and termulousness, they improved significantly, as well. This pattern of behavioral recovery on the items on the Neonatal Behavioral Assessment Scale[12] seemed to serve as an important evaluative system of intactness.

There is increasing evidence that sensory input that is *appropriate* to the state of physiologic recovery of that neonate may further his weight gain, his sensory integrity, and even his outcome. Unless we pay more attention to appropriate stimulation for the infant, we may well be retarding or even interfering with his optimal sensory development. For example, Pettigrew found that for kittens specific visual input was necessary to develop the specificity of initially undifferentiated cells.[100] Blakemore and Cooper found that visual cortex neurons responded predominantly to stimuli that were equivalent to the environment in which the kittens were reared.[101] However, in both cases these effects were found only after a given level of CNS maturity had been achieved. Before that time, exposure had no effect because it did not appropriately fit the organism's level of development.

Most of the studies on early stimulation have not been individualized to the subjects. We have evidence that leads us to feel that each premature or recovering neonate *must* be examined for the possibility of sensory overloading. A premature infant will respond to a soft rattle by turning his head away from the rattle (and other means of shutting it out), whereas a normal neonate will turn toward the rattle and search for it.[102] We feel that the finely defined thresholds for appropriate sensory stimuli, as opposed to those that must be coped with or shut out, must be taken as seriously as whether or not we offer stimulation. In the recovery phase, a high-risk baby may be too easily overwhelmed, and routine stimulation may force him into an expensive coping model: whereas grading the stimuli to his particular sensory needs may further his recovery as well as his ultimate CNS outcome.

How can we tell when he is being overloaded? We can tell by watching his color changes, his kind of respirations, his state of alertness, by looking for evidences of fatigue. Using Kearsley's ideas[65] about the relative degree of attention to a stimulus as measured against physiologic demands, we have a clearly defined area of "appropriate" versus "inappropriate" properties of all stimuli that can be applied to each neonate individually, permitting estimation of the amount and the quality of stimulation that can be offered to every at-risk neonate without undue expense.

The studies by Sander and coworkers show that the infant shapes his motility and his state behavior to the environment, *particularly* if it is sensitive to him and to his individual needs.[103] Two models of regulation occurred with the neonates and caretakers they studied. The first related to basic regulation of endogenous biorhythmicity and was entrained by specific extrinsic cues in relation to the neonate's endogenous rhythm. Entrainment was most effective when the exogenous cue approximated the point in time at which a shift in the endogenous cycle was occurring. With the repeated establishment of contingent relationships between state changes in the infant and specific configurations in caretaking events, entrainment was favored. The second model depended on the caretaker and infant achieving a regulatory balance based on mutual readiness of states, and with this the stage was set to facilitate initial cognitive development. As the partners appreciated a mutual regulation of states of attention, they began to learn about and from each other, and a kind of reciprocity or affective interaction ensued.

These demonstrations of behavioral and sensory responsiveness not only serve to assess the neonate, but also enable us to enhance the parent-infant interaction by sharing this assessment with the parent. The nonverbal communication between parent and infant in the initial stages of attachment is built upon the infant's behavior. As pediatricians interested in enhancing the parent-infant bond, we would do well to observe, assess, and participate in the marvelous responsive capacities of the newborn infant.

REFERENCES

1. **Greenberg NH:** A comparison of infant-mother interactional behavior in infants with atypical behavior and normal infants. In Hellmuth J (ed): Exceptional Infant, vol 2, p. 390. New York, Brunner Mazel, 1971
2. **Sigman M, Parmelee AH:** Longitudinal evaluation of the preterm infant. In Field TM (ed.): Infants Born at Risk. New York, Spectrum Publications Inc., 1979
3. **Buck C, Gregg R, Stavraky K et al:** The effect of simple prenatal and natal complications upon the development of children of mature birth weight. Pediatrics 43:943, 1969
4. **Niswander KR, Friedman EA, Hoover OB et al:** Fetal morbidity following potentially anoxigenic obstetrical conditions: I. Abruptio placenta. II. Placenta previa. III. Prolapse of the umbilical cord. Am J Obstet Gynecol 95:838, 1966
5. **Hobel CJ, Hyvarinen MA, Okada D, Oh W:** Prenatal and intrapartum high risk screening. Am J Obstet Gynecol 117:1, 1973
6. **Lubchenco LO, Bard H, Gordman AL, Loyer WE, McIntyre C, Smith D:** Newborn intensive care and long term prognosis. Dev Med Child Neurol 16:421, 1974
7. **Winick M et al:** Effects of prenatal nutrition upon pregnancy risk. Clin Obstet and Gynecol 16:1, 1973
8. **Als H, Tronick E, Adamson L, Brazelton TB:** The behavior of the full term but underweight newborn infant. Dev Med Child Neurol 18:590, 1976
9. **Miller HC, Hassanein K:** Fetal malnutrition—white newborn infants: Maternal factors. Pediatrics 52:4, 1973
10. **Frankenberg WK, Dodds JB, Fandal AW:** Denver Developmental Screening Test. Denver, University of Colorado Medical Center, 1970
11. **Brazelton TB, Tronick E, Koslowski B:** Neonatal behavior among urban Zambians and Americans. Journal of the Academy of Child Psychology 15:97, 1976
12. **Brazelton TB:** Neonatal behavioral assessment. National Spastics Society Monographs Clinics in Developmental Medicine #50.

London, William Heinemann & Sons, 1973; Distributed in the U.S. by JB Lippincott Company, Philadelphia
13. **Chavez A, Martinez C, Yashine T:** Nutrition, mother-child relations and behavioral development in the young child from a rural community (unpublished data).
14. **Rothstein P, Gould JB:** Born with a habit. Pediatr Clin of North America 21:307, 1974
15. **Kaplan SL, Kron RE, Litt MD, Finnegan LP, Pheonix MD:** Behavioral assessment of passively addicted infants. Presented at Society for Research in Child Development, Denver, Col, 1975
16. **Jones KL, Smith DW:** Recognition of the fetal alcohol syndrome in early infancy. Lancet 2:999, 1973
17. **Streissguth AP, Herman CS, Smith OW:** Intelligence, behavior and dysmorphogenesis in the fetal alcohol syndrome. J Pediatr 92:363–367, 1978
18. **Shannon DC et al:** Prevention of apnea and bradycardia in low birthweight infants. Pediatrics 55:5, 1975
19. **Moya F, Thorndike V:** Passage of drugs across the placenta. Am J Obstet Gynecol 84:1778, 1962
20. **Brazelton TV:** Psychophysiologic reaction in the neonate II. J Pediatr 58:513, 1961
21. **Kron R:** Newborn sucking behavior affected by obstetric sedation. Pediatrics 37:1012, 1966
22. **Stechler G, Latz E:** Some observations on attention and arousal in the human infant. Journal of the Academy of Child Psychology 5:517, 1966
23. **Brackbill Y, Conway E:** Delivery medication and infant outcome: An empirical study. Monogr Soc Res Child Dev 35:4, 1970
24. **Scanlon JW, Brown WJ Jr, Weiss JG, Alper NH:** Neurobehavioral responses of newborns after maternal anesthesia. Anesthesiology 40:121, 1974
25. **Apgar VA:** A proposal for a new method of evaluation of the newborn infant. Anesthesia and Analgesia 32:260–267, 1953
26. **Drage JS, Kennedy C, Berendes H et al:** The Apgar score as an index of infant morbidity: A report from the Collaborative Study of Cerebral Palsy. Developmental Medicine and Child Neurology 8:141–48, 1966
27. **Lewis M, Bartels B, Campbell H et al:** Individual differences in attention. Am J Dis Child 113:461–465, 1967
28. **Graham FK, Matarazzo RG, Caldwell BM:** Behavioral differences between normal and traumatized newborns. Psychol Monogr 70:427–448, 1956
29. **Rosenblith JF:** The modified Graham behav-

ior test for neonates. Biol Neonate 3:174, 1961

30. **Anders TB, Roffwarg H:** The effects of selective interruption and total sleep deprivation in the human newborn. Dev Psychobiol 6:79, 1973

31. **Miller HC, Hassanein K:** Diagnosis of impaired fetal growth in newborn infants. Pediatrics 48:511, 1971

32. **Horowitz FD, Self PA, Paden LN et al.:** Newborn and four week retest on a normative population using the Brazelton newborn assessment procedure. Presented at the annual meeting of the Society for Research in Child Development, Minneapolis, 1971. Unpublished

33. **Tronick E, Brazelton TB:** Clinical uses of the Brazelton Neonatal Behavioral Assessment. In Friedlander BZ, Sterritt GM, Kirk GE (eds): Exceptional Infant, Vol 3, Assessment and Intervention. New York, Brunner Mazel, 1975

34. **Prechtl H, Beintema O:** The Neurological Examination of the Full Term Newborn Infant. London, William Heinemann, 1964

35. **Prechtl H, Dykstra J:** Neurological diagnosis of cerebral injury in the newborn. In Berge TS (ed): Proceedings of Symposium on Prenatal Care. Groningen, Nordhoff, 1959

36. **Thoman EB:** Early development of sleeping behavior in infants. In Ellis NR (ed): Aberrant Development in Infancy, pp. 123–138. New York, John Wiley & Sons Inc, 1975

37. **Michaelis R, Parmelee AH, Stern E, Haber A:** Activity states in premature and term infants. Dev Psychobiol 6:209, 1973

38. **Anders TF, Weinstein P:** Sleep and its disorders in infants and children: A review. Pediatrics 50:312, 1972

39. **Steinschneider A:** Nasopharyngitis and prolonged deep apnea. Pediatrics 56:967, 1975

40. **Brazelton TB, Koslowski B, Main M:** Origins of reciprocity. In Lewis M, Rosenblum L (eds): Mother-Infant Interaction, pp. 49–76. New York, John Wiley & Sons Inc., 1974

41. **Wolff P:** The causes, controls, and organization of behavior in the neonate. Psychology Monograph, V, No. 7, 1966

42. **Lester BM:** The organization of crying in the neonate. Journal of Pediatric Psychology 3: 122, 1978

43. **Wasz-Hockert O, Lind J, Vuorenkoski V, Partanen T, Valanne E:** The Infant Cry. England, Lavenham Press, 1968

44. **Lester BM:** Spectrum analysis of the cry sounds of well-nourished and malnourished infants. Child Dev 47:237, 1976

45. **Brazelton TB:** Crying in infancy. Pediatrics 29:579, 1962

46. **Brazelton TB:** Observations of the neonate. J Am Acad Child Psychiatry 1:38, 1962

47. **Bartoshuk AK, Tennant JM:** Human neonatal correlates of sleep wakefulness and neural maturation. J Psychiat Res 2:73, 1964

48. **Bridger WH:** Sensory habituation and discrimination in the human neonate. Am J Psychiatry 117:991, 1961

49. **Jeffrey WE, Cohen LB:** Habituation in the human infant. Child Dev 46:163, 1975

50. **Ellingston RV:** Cortical electrical responses to visual stimulation in the human infant. Electroencephalography Clinics in Neurophysiology 12:663, 1960

51. **Hrbek A, Mares, P:** Cortical evoked responses to visual stimulation in full term and premature infants. Electroencephalograph Clinics in Neurophysiology 16:575, 1964

52. **Brazier MAB (ed):** The Central Nervous System and Behavior trans. 2nd Conference. New York, Josiah Macy Foundation, 1959

53. **Fantz RL:** Visual perception from birth as shown by pattern selectivity. Annual New York Academy of Science 118:793, 1965

54. **Goren CC, Sarty M, Wie PYK:** Visual following and pattern discrimination by newborn infants. Pediatrics 56:544 1975

55. **Brazelton TB, Scholl ML, Robey JS:** Visual responses in the newborn. Pediatrics 37:284, 1966

56. **Gorman JJ, Cogan DG, Gellis SS:** An apparatus for grading the visual acuity of infants on the basis of opticokinetic nystagmus. Pediatrics 19:1088, 1957

57. **Dayton GO Jr, Jones MH, Aiu P, Rawson RA, Steele B, Rose M:** Developmental study of coordinated eye movements in the human infant. Arch Ophthalmol 71:865, 1964

58. **Haynes H, White, BL, Held R:** Visual accommodation in human infants. Science 148:528, 1965

59. **Sigman M, Kopp CB, Parmelee AH, Jeffrey WE:** Visual attention and neurological organization in neonates. Child Dev 44:461, 1973

60. **Tronick E, Clanton C:** Looking patterns. Vision Res 11:1479, 1971.

61. **Hershenson M:** Visual discrimination in the human newborn. J Comp Physiol and Psychol 58:270, 1964

62. **Eisenberg RB:** Auditory behavior in the human neonate: Methodologic problems. J Aud Res 5:159, 1965

63. **Lipsitt LP:** Learning in the human infant. In Stevenson HW, Rheingold HL, Hess E (eds): Early Behavior: Comparative and Behavioral Approaches, pp. 225–247. New York: John Wiley & Sons Inc, 1967

64. **Lipton EL, Steinschneider A, Richmond J:**

Auditory sensitivity in the infant: Effect of intensity on cardiac and motor responsivity. Child Dev 37:233, 1966

65. **Kearsley RB:** The newborn's response to auditory stimulation: A demonstration of orienting and defensive behavior. Child Dev 44:582, 1973

66. **Drillien CM:** Aetiology and outcome in low birthweight infants. Dev Med Child Neurol 14:563, 1972

67. **Bronstein AI, Petrova EP:** The auditory analyzer in young infants. In Brackbill Y, Thompson GC (eds): Behavior in Infancy and Early Childhood, pp 163–172. New York, Free Press, 1967

68. **Cairns GF, Butterfield EC:** Assessing infant's auditory functioning. In Friedlander BZ, Sterritt GM, Kirk GE (eds): Exceptional Infant, Vol 2, p 84. New York, Brunner Mazel, 1975

69. **Engen T, Lipsett LP, Kaye H:** Olfactory responses and adaptation in the human neonate. Journal of Comprehensive Physiology and Psychology 56:73, 1963

70. **MacFarlane A:** Olfaction in the development of social preferences in the human neonate. In Parent-Infant Interaction, p. 103. Oxford, Elsevier Press, 1975

71. **Pratt KC, Nelson AK, Sun KH:** The behavior of the newborn infant. Ohio State University Student Contributions in Psychology, Vol 10, 1930

72. **Johnson P, Salisbury DM:** Breathing and sucking during feeding in the newborn. In Parent-Infant Interaction, p. 119. Oxford, Elsevier Press, 1975

73. **Lipsitt LP:** The synchrony of respiration, heart rate, and sucking behavior in the newborn. In Perinatal and Developmental Medicine: Biological and Clinical Aspects of Brain Development, 6:67, 1964

74. **Crook CK, Lipsitt LP:** Neonatal nutritive sucking: Effects of taste stimulation upon sucking rhythm and heart rate. Child Development 47:518, 1976

75. **Bruner JS:** Eye, hand and mind. In Elkind D, Flavell JH (eds): Studies in Cognitive Development, p 223. New York, Oxford University Press, 1969

76. **Brazelton TB, Tronick E, Adamson L, Als H, Wise S:** Early mother-infant reciprocity. In Parent-Infant Interaction, p. 33. Oxford, Elsevier Press, 1975

77. **Peiper A:** Cerebral function in infancy and childhood. In Naglei B, Naglei H (eds): Consultants Bureau, 1963

78. **Blankfield A:** The optimum position for childbirth. Med J Aus 2:666, 1965

79. **Jensen K:** Differential reactions to taste and temperature stimuli in newborn infants. Genetic Psychology Monograph 12:361, 1932

80. **Gryboski JD:** The swallowing mechanism of the neonate: Esophageal and gastric motility. Pediatrics 35:445, 1965

81. **Kaye K:** Infant sucking and its modification. In Lipsitt LP, Spiker CC (eds): Advances in Child Development and Behavior, Vol 3. New York, Academic Press, 1967

82. **Kaye K, Brazelton TB:** The ethological significance of the burst pause pattern in infant sucking. Presented at the Society for Research in Child Development, Minneapolis, April, 1971

83. **Haith MM, Kessen W, Collins D:** Response of the human infant to level of complexity of intermittent visual movement. Journal of Experimental Child Psychology 7:52, 1969

84. **Lipsitt L:** The study of sensory and learning processes of the newborn. Clin Perinatol 4: 163, 1977

85. **Babkin PS:** The establishment of reflex activity in early postnatal life. In U.S. Department of Health, Education, and Welfare, Public Health Service (trans): The Central Nervous System and Behavior, pp 24–32. Washington, D.C., U.S. Government Printing Office, 1960

86. **Denisova MP, Figurin NKL:** Voprosu o pervykh sochetatelnykh pishchevykh refleksakh u grudnykh detei. Vop Genet Refleks Pedol 1:81, 1929

87. **Kaye H:** The conditioned Babkin reflex in human newborns. Psychonomic Science 2: 287, 1965

88. **Connolly K, Stratton P:** An exploration of some parameters affecting classical conditioning in the neonate. Child Dev 40:431, 1969

89. **Lipsitt LP, Kaye H:** Conditioned sucking in the human newborn. Psychonomic Science 1:29, 1964

90. **Abrahamson D, Brackbill Y, Carpenter Y et al:** Interaction of stimulus and response in infant conditioning. Psychosom Med 32:319, 1970

91. **Papousek H:** Conditioned motor digestive reflexes in infants. II. A new experimental method for the investigation. Csek Pediatr 15:981, 1960

92. **Siqueland ER, Lipsitt LP:** Conditioned head turning in human newborns. Journal of Experimental Child Psychology 3:356, 1966

93. **Sameroff AJ:** Learning and adaptation in infancy: A comparison of models. In Reese HW (ed) Advances in Child Developmental Behavior 7:170–214, 1972

94. **Fantz RL, Miranda SB:** Newborn infant attention to form of contour. Child Dev 46:224, 1975

95. **Bartoshuk AK:** Response decrement with repeated elicitation of human neonatal cardiac acceleration to sound. Journal of Comprehensive Physiology and Psychology 55:9, 1962

96. **Lewis M:** The meaning of a response, or why researchers in infant behavior should be oriental metaphysicians. Merrill-Palmer Quarterly 13, 1967

97. **Brackbill Y:** The role of the cortex in orienting: Orienting reflex in an anencephalic human infant. Developmental Psychology 5: 195, 1971

98. **Barnet AB, Olrich ES, Shanks BS:** EEG evoked responses to repetitive stimulation in normal and Down's syndrome infants. Developmental Medical and Child Neurology 5:612, 1974

99. **Tronick E, Wise S, Als H, Adamson S, Scanlon J, Brazelton TB:** Regional obstetric anesthesia and newborn behavior: Effect over the first 10 days of life. Pediatrics 58:94–100, 1977

100. **Pettigrew JD:** The effect of visual experience on the development of stimlulus specificity by kidden cortical neurones. J Physiol 237: 49–74, 1974

101. **Blakemore C, Cooper GF:** Development of the brain depends on the visual environment. Nature 228:477–478, 1970

102. **Als H, Tronick E, Brazelton TB:** Manual for the behavioral assessment of the premature and at-risk newborn (an extension of the Brazelton Neonatal Behavioral Assessment Scale). Presented at the Annual Meeting of the American Academy for Child Psychiatry, Toronto, 1976. Unpublished

103. **Sander LW, Chappell PF, Gould SB et al:** An investigation of change in the infant-caretaker system over the first week of life. Presented at the Annual Meeting of the Society for Research in Child Development, Denver, 1975. Unpublished

19

Follow-up Studies of the High-Risk Newborn

Pamela M. Fitzhardinge and
Karen E. Pape

Over the past 15 to 20 years a great deal of time, energy, and money has been directed towards acute care of the sick newborn resulting in a steady decline in neonatal mortality. Most striking has been the improved survival rate of babies treated with mechanical ventilation for primary lung pathology and for apnea of prematurity. At the Hospital for Sick Children in Toronto, the mortality rate for infants under 1500g birth weight has dropped from 85% in 1968 to 32% in 1977 (Table 19-1). Lowering the mortality for these high-risk infants has resulted in an increased number of normal survivors but has also, in some instances, resulted in an absolute increase of children with handicapping sequelae. It now becomes imperative that centers which provide neonatal intensive care also provide a mechanism to ensure continuing care and evaluation of their high-risk survivors.

ORGANIZATION OF A FOLLOW-UP PROGRAM

Objectives

The scope and emphasis of a follow-up program depends upon the needs of the hospital center and upon the over-all aims set for the program. In general, follow-up programs are designed to meet one or more of the following objectives:

1. Quality Control of the Intensive Care Nursery ICN. Perinatal or neonatal mortality figures provide only a partial evaluation of the activities of the ICN and need to be supplemented by a constant monitoring of the quality of the survivors. Mortality and morbidity figures do not always parallel each other. An excellent survival rate does not necessarily mean that a high proportion of the survivors will be normal. In fact, the reverse situation sometimes occurs: low mortality may be achieved by very aggressive and prolonged ventilatory support of neonates who have sustained severe hypoxia, intracranial hemorrhage or both, who later develop severe handicapping neurologic and intellectual deficits. Such was the case when ventilation was first used extensively for the very low-birth-weight infant (VLBW $\leq$ 1500g). Mortality rates dropped from levels of approximately 75% to 80% in the 1960s to levels of 45% to 50% in the 1970s. However, the neurologic defects in the survivors of the 1970s tended to be more severe and more frequently associated with retardation than those in the survivors of the 1960s. On the other hand, preliminary reports on the outcome of VLBW born and treated in high-risk

Table 19-1. Premature Mortality.*

	Mortality
Prior to 1960	85%
1960–1970	70%
1970–1973	52%
1974	35%
1975–1976	40%
1977	32%

* Changing mortality rate for neonates with birthweight ≤ 1500 g admitted to ICN at the Hospital for Sick Children, Toronto

perinatal centers suggest that the improved survival in such centers is also accompanied by a higher proportion of non-handicapped survivors.

2. *Provision of Ongoing Primary or Secondary Care to the Infants After Discharge.* High-risk infants, especially those with VLBW and those with chronic lung disease, require close medical supervision during their first year of life and often need specialized investigation or treatment. In addition, many families will present with social and/or parenting problems requiring counseling and utilization of community resources. The service aspects of the follow-up program can become overwhelming in terms of time, personnel, and funding. It is important that such services do not duplicate services of equal merit already provided in another area of the medical community. In many instances, primary care can best be provided by the family physician, pediatrician, or community clinic with interval consultations with the specialized personnel of the follow-up team. Such an approach has a number of positive side effects. The follow-up personnel can devote their efforts to the problem areas in which they have special expertise and will then have the time to extend such services to a larger number of high-risk infants. Recognition of the important role of the primary physicians tends to reduce the threat of the "ivory tower" and encourages the community medical services to support the specialized function of the follow-up program. Ongoing communication between the follow-up center and outside physicians helps to emphasize the importance of growth and development in general and to disseminate up-to-date information on the particular problems encountered during the early years of life in the high-risk infant. The net results are better care to more patients and fewer patients lost to long term follow-up.

3. *Specific Research Studies.* For years, investigators in neonatology have concerned themselves only with the immediate neonatal period, largely ignoring the fetus in the uterus or the infant after discharge. This approach has the same disadvantages of attending only the second act of a three-act drama: one is unfamiliar with the cast and setting and one is ignorant of the outcome and overall purpose of the drama. An important function of research in follow-up is not only to determine the success and failure rates associated with neonatal complications and therapy, but also to complete the studies on normal and abnormal development. For example, the neonatal studies on lung development and the control of respiration have been extended in one direction to study respiratory physiology in the fetus and in the other direction to study the maturation of respiratory control in the young infant. Research in follow-up of the high-risk newborn need not be limited to a description of the neurologic and intellectual status of the survivors. It should be extended to include such fields as the variable patterns of growth in the LBW infant; the impact of early nutrition on subsequent growth and development; the effect of premature birth and respiratory complications on subsequent lung growth and function; and the effects of intervention programs on subsequent development. Obviously, any one of these studies requires a multidisciplinary approach, but a well-organized follow-up program can provide a controlled study population and can guarantee the collection of longitudinal data, as well as adding expertise in the neurodevelopmental and epidemiologic aspects of the studies.

4. *Training Program.* There is a very real need for good training programs in developmental pediatrics, especially as applied to prospective studies on growth and development in high-risk infants. Many centers with a level II or III ICN are attempting to establish a creditable follow-up program but are faced with the problem of finding adequately trained personnel.

Personnel

The size and complexity of the follow-up team depends upon the scope of the program and the size of the patient population. One or more members must provide expertise in neonatal physiology and pathology, developmental neurology, psychometric assessment, and biostatistics and epidemiology. The director may be trained in one or all of these areas but he must be intimately involved in all aspects of the program. It is his responsibility to determine the overall objectives and to see that these objectives are met.

Relegation of specific duties varies and depends upon the budget and the personnel available. A key member of the team is the individual who relates most closely with the patients, that is, the person involved with the initial referral to the program. He or she will be responsible for maintaining subsequent contact, organizing return visits, helping to interpret results, and, in general, encouraging and supporting the patient and family. This role is frequently filled by a nurse-coordinator but has been done well in some centers by a social service worker or by a trained secretary. Regardless of past training, this individual must be a warm, concerned person who relates well to patients and medical staff and is dedicated to the success of the follow-up program. Organizational ability and an ease in adaptation to changed schedules, missed appointments, and distraught parents are a major help to the smooth functioning of the program.

An important question facing the director is the training required by the person interviewing and examining the patients. A basic rule to follow is that this person have more skill at the particular task at hand than someone who might be providing the same service in an outside physician's office or in a community clinic. A trained nurse-practitioner and a physiotherapist together can give a good assessment of the infant in terms of growth, general health, and neuromuscular development by using basic screening tools such as the Denver Developmental Screening Test.[1] However, at least once during each year, the child should also be assessed by a physician who is competent in developmental neurology.

Another important feature of the total evaluation is the psychometric assessment. Many centers do serial tests at frequent intervals during infancy and then yearly thereafter. However, the value of the tests, at any age, varies directly with the experience and skill of the person conducting the test. How a child approaches a task often yields much more valuable information than his actual success or failure rate. For the tests to be of use, they must be performed by a fully trained psychometrician. The services of a first-class psychometrician do not come cheaply and repeated testing can result in a serious drain of the operating budget. We have found the most practical solution has been to limit the frequency of the tests to those ages that yield the most useful and valid results: once at 18 months and again at 5 and 7 years of age. When performing the first test in prematurely born infants, the age should be calculated from the expected date of delivery. This correction is not necessary at school age.

At regular intervals, the results of the separate examinations must be pooled by some mechanism such as a joint conference. Interpretation of all the findings in terms of the child's present performance and potential is the responsibility of the director. He must be prepared to make the decisions regarding future management of the patient and to provide a concise, meaningful interpretation for both the patient's family and the primary physician.

Selection of Patients for Follow-up

At our present stage of expertise, the risk for major neurodevelopmental defects is greater than 10% for only one-third of the patients discharged from a referral ICN[2] An even smaller proportion of the infants discharged from an inborn ICN face such a risk. The proportion increases in perinatal units that function exclusively as high-risk maternal transfer centers, as well as in units in which the majority of patients are in a low socioeconomic level. A follow-up program that has limited budget and personnel would do well to restrict its patient population to those infants with a risk factor greater than 10%, realizing that a few defects will occur in the children not in the program but that the majority of sequelae will occur in the selected patients. Table 19-2 outlines the risk factors for various categories of neonates. At highest risk are infants with (1) birth weight under 1500 g or gestational age less than 33 weeks; (2) gestation less than 37 weeks and birth weight more than 2 standard deviations below the mean for gestational age; (3) meningitis; (4) seizures or persistent abnormal neurologic behavior; (5) evidence by computed tomography or ultra-

Table 19-2. Risk Factors for Major Neurologic and/or Cognitive Sequelae.[2]

Birthweight	Category	Risk Factor (%)
>2500	All admissions	<5
	RDS	5
	Post-asphyxia seizure	30–50
	Meningitis	30–50
1501–2500 g	All admissions	10
	SGA	<10
	RDS	<10
	BPD	20–30
	Postasphyxia seizure	30–50
	Meningitis	30–50
≤1500 g	All admissions	10–30
	AGA, nonventilated	10–15
	AGA, ventilated	30–40
	SGA	30–50
	Seizures, decerebrate posture	75–80

RDS—respiratory distress syndrome
BPD—bronchopulmonary dysplasia
AGA—appropriate weight for gestational age
SGA—small for gestational age

sound of hemorrhage into the ventricles, cerebrum or cerebellum; and (6) bronchopulmonary dysplasia (BPD). With the exception of cases of BPD, most of these infants can be diagnosed as high risk by the second week of life and plans can then be made for enrollment in the follow-up program. The early identification of the patients ensures that a prospective compilation of their clinical, laboratory, and therapeutic data can be made before discharge. In addition, the follow-up team can take advantage of the weeks before discharge to become acquainted with the families, explaining the purpose of the program, and laying the groundwork for continued support after discharge of the neonate from the nursery.

Schedule for Clinic Visits

The timing of clinic visits should coincide with the periods of parental concern and with the stages at which developmental defects first become obvious. The sequence of visits should not be rigid but should be tailored to the expected problems for the individual neonate. For example, hydrocephalus usually becomes clinically apparent during the first 3 months post-term (PT). Dilatation of the ventricles can

be identified even earlier by ultrasound or computed tomography. The infants at risk for hydrocephalus are those who sustain intraventricular hemorrhages or meningitis. Such babies should be seen at frequent (at least monthly) intervals after discharge until they are over 3 months PT. On the other hand, the cardiorespiratory problems associated with BPD are at peak levels for 6 to 9 months after discharge, and these patients need frequent (occasionally, monthly) monitoring during that period.

The LBW babies without the neonatal complications mentioned above need much less supervision. Most can be managed with only three to four visits the first year, two the second year, and then once yearly thereafter. It should be noted, however, that irrespective of the severity of the neonatal course of their infant, parental concern is at its peak during the first few weeks following discharge of the child from the nursery. We have made it a policy to schedule the first return visit to the clinic at the term date (expected date of delivery). This is usually about 2 to 3 weeks after discharge, at which time the parents have many questions regarding the care of the infant and can discuss the preceding neonatal course in a more relaxed manner. Visits are then scheduled from the term date, thus simplifying the correction for gestational age in subsequent visits. Table 19-3 gives a suggested outline for scheduling visits and special investigations.

Reliability of Early Assessment

The care of the sick neonate is in a constant state of flux; many new methods of treatment are introduced each year. Evaluation of benefits or hazards of therapeutic changes should take place as soon as possible after the institution of the change.

How reliable are the developmental assessments made in the first 2 years of life? We have just completed a prospective 6-year study of 133 children with birth weights less than 1501 g.[2] Neurologic assessments were made at 1 and 2 years of life, and were reassessed at 6 years. Psychometric testing was performed at 6-month intervals for a 2-year period after the term date (Bayley Developmental Scale[3]) and then repeated at 6 years (Wechsler Intelligence Scales for Children[4]). The children with major neurologic defects (hydrocephalus and/or cerebral palsy) were diagnosed by 1

Table 19-3. Schedule of Visits*

Assessment	Interval
General	Every 3 months until 1 year
Interim history	(prematures: first visit at
Measurements (weight, length, head circumference)	term), 18 months, 24 months,
Physical examination including CNS	yearly until 7 years
Clinical developmental assessment	
Psychometry	18–24 months, 6–7 years
Assessment of school performance	7 years
CNS	
Skull transillumination	Each visit to 6 months
Brain ultrasound or computed tomography	1, 2, 3 months for postmeningitic and post-IVH patients
EEG	1 year, 5 years for postseizure patients
Hearing	
Screening	6 months
Audiogram	4 years
Speech assessment	
Clinically	Each visit
Therapy	2 years if necessary
Ophthalmology	
Eye movements	
Indirect fundoscopy	6–9 months for VLBW infants
Cycloplegic refraction	
Full examination with refraction	4 years
Chest film	Every 6 months until normal for BPD, Postventilator
ECG	6–12 months; repeat every 6 months until normal (BPD patients only)

* Timing of visits for all premature patients should be referenced to post-term age until 2 years. Other investigation is done when clinically indicated.

year PT. No new cases were discovered after that age. The degree of handicap imposed by the defect remained constant from 2 to 6 years, except for two patients with mild cases of spastic diplegia who did not present with any handicap by school age. Although a positive correlation existed between the Bayley scores at all ages and the Wechsler scores at 6 years, the correlation was not highly significant until 18 to 24 months PT. At that age it was possible to predict whether the child would score above or below 85 on the Wechsler test in 80% of the cases. Thus, by 2 years of age, we can, with good reliability, identify the children with major defects, whether the defects be neurologic or cognitive, or a combination of both. On the other hand, minor neurologic defects, minor degrees of retardation, or learning disabilities could not be predicted at this early age.

OUTCOME FOR SPECIFIC CATEGORIES OF NEONATES

The VLBW Infant: Birthweight Less than 1501 g

The prognosis for the VLBW infant will be discussed under seven major headings: general health, growth, vision, hearing, speech development, neurologic integrity, and intellectual status.

General Health. The death rate for the VLBW infant during the first year after discharge from the nursery is considerably higher than for the full-term infant. Reported mortality varies from 3% to 5%, with about half of the deaths associated with major neurologic defects or with acute respiratory illness.[5] The remainder of the deaths are sudden or unexplained—typical crib deaths. Sudden Infant Death Syndrome (SIDS) occur four to five times as frequently in the VLBW infants as in full-term children.[6] The commonest age of death varies from 1 to 3 months from term. There is no relationship between the severity of the neonatal course and later crib death, although persistently recurring apnea must be viewed with suspicion.

Apart from the above, the major health concerns for the VLBW relate to surgery for developmental defects and pathology of the lower respiratory tract. The former consist mainly of inguinal hernia repair, ocular muscle resection and, much less frequently, ligature of a persistent patent ductus. Intermittent signs of lower respiratory tract disease are common among the VLBW infants during the first year of life and are usually precipitated by an upper respiratory infection. The signs consist of tachypnea, chest retractions, wheezing, and prolongation of the expiratory phase. The chest film may be normal or show varying degrees of air trapping. Infants with bronchopulmonary dysplasia are most frequently affected. They are rarely entirely symptom-free the first year and are prone to recurrent exacerbations requiring supplementary oxygen therapy. The incidence of respiratory disease in the remainder of the VLBW infants varies from center to center. Table 19–4 summarizes the results of follow-up studies we have conducted on four groups of infants who received neonatal intensive care in three different centers.[7] Mechanical ventilation and immaturity of the lung are associated with a greater risk for recurrent chest infections during the first year, but respiratory distress syndrome (RDS) itself does not seem to be a specific predisposing factor. Studies of lung volume, airway resistance and compliance have been done by Stocks and coworkers at 2 and 7 months of age in 19 premature infants, 11 of whom had required ventilation as neonates.[8] Values for all infants were normal at 2 months, but by 7 months, the ventilator survivors showed significantly greater airway resistance. Comparison of the initial and follow-up test results revealed that, as in term controls, all infants showed a decrease in airway resistance with age, but the rate of decrease was far slower in the ventilated infants. Using flow-volume curves, Coates has also reported increased airway resistance in school-aged, prematurely born children, compared with full-term children of the same age.[9] Both studies suggest that injury to the airway at a critical stage in development can, in some manner, impede its growth, resulting in a failure to increase airway conductance at a normal rate as lung volume increases with age. Presumably, the more immature the airway at the time of the insult, the greater the effect on airway growth. Delay in airway growth would explain the prevalence of small-airway disease (bronchiolitis, bronchitis) in young exprematures, especially in those who had sustained the extra stress of mechanical ventilation. With continued growth of alveoli and airways over the first few years of life, these children become asymptomatic and apparently normal.

Growth. The healthy premature infant whose birth weight is appropriate for gestational age (AGA) can be expected to grow at the same velocity as a full-term infant of the same postconceptional age. Standard growth charts can be used if the premature infant's age is calculated from his expected date of delivery or term date. Even infants with very low birth weight, appropriate for gestational age, born prior to 32 weeks, follow this pattern.[10] Unless

Table 19-4. Lower Respiratory Tract Infection (LRTI)*

No. patients	Birth Weight	Year	% Ventilated	% LRTI	Association of LRTI with RDS
32	≤ 1250	1960–1966[19]	3	50	none
44	≤ 1500	1970–1972[10]	27	5	none
62	≤ 1500	1970–1973[37]	100	18	none
42	≤ 1000	1974[14]	74	19	none

* Data for very low birthweight infants. All cases of BPD have been excluded.[10,14,19,37]

very ill, such an infant usually regains birth weight by 2 to 3 weeks. During this period, linear growth is usually zero but head growth continues. For the next few weeks, if intake is sufficient, growth in all parameters continues at the normal intrauterine rate. From about the 34th to 36th postconceptional week, accelerated growth occurs until normal size for age is reached, usually at 40- to 42-weeks' postconceptional age. Figure 19-1 shows linear growth for 67 premature infants during the first year of life of each. All were appropriate weight for gestational age and were born before the 33rd week of gestation. At their term dates, the mean length fell on the 50th percentile of the Stuart grid. The velocity of linear growth for the ensuing year was equivalent to that of normal full-term infants. The growth pattern for weight was similar although the average weight tended to be slightly below the 50th percentile. This discrepancy between weight and linear growth may become more marked in ensuing years so that the preschool, very low-birth-weight infant usually is slender although of normal height.

Head growth also follows normal velocity curves after the term date. Figure 19-2 shows serial head circumference measurements for the same 67 infants plotted on the Nellhaus grid. Except for the first 2 to 3 months, the mean head circumference is at the 50th percentile. The early discrepancy is probably due to the greater occipitofrontal diameter of the premature head, producing a spuriously greater head circumference for volume. This scaphocephaly gradually returns to a more normal shape by 3 to 4 months PT.

Growth failure occurs in two types of low-birth-weight infants: those who are SGA at birth, and those who, although appropriately sized at birth, fail to grow during the first 4 to 6 weeks of postnatal life because of inadequate nutrition. Early growth patterns in these two types of infants differ but the end result seems to be similar.

The baby who is small for gestational age usually begins growing soon after birth.[11] Head growth occurs at a greater velocity than either linear or weight growth, especially if the baby is also preterm. Sutures appear to split and it is often difficult to distinguish this baby from one with developing hydrocephalus. Accelerated linear and weight growth then occur, so that by the term date, although the head is still

disproportionately big, head and linear growth are occurring at the same velocity. Rarely, however, are the measurements for head and length above the 10th percentile by the term date. Weight is usually below the 3rd percentile.

The extremely premature infant, with birth weight appropriate for gestational age, who is very ill and unable to tolerate adequate nutrition orally or parenterally, loses weight for 2 to 3 weeks, and then either fails to gain or gains very slowly. Linear growth is usually static during this period. Head growth may also apparently cease. Alimentation with amino acid and glucose solutions seems to provide sufficient nutrients for normal head growth but not for linear or weight growth. Supplementation of the alimentation with Intralipid, when tolerated, does seem to provide sufficient nutrients for weight and linear growth, although our data on this are still at a very preliminary stage. When these sick infants recover and can tolerate adequate nutrition, they show accelerated growth in a manner similar to that described for the immature infant born SGA, although the acceleration is occurring at a later age. These infants, like the SGA infants, are still undersized at the term date.

Growth from term for both types then appears to proceed in a manner similar to that described for infants born at term with a weight well below the third percentile (*i.e.*, the term SGA infant).[12] Accelerated velocity of growth continues for the first year, although it is most rapid 6 to 9 months PT. The rate of growth after 1 year is similar to that of normal full term children. If acceleration of growth has been sufficient, the child's size will be within normal limits. If the acceleration has been insufficient, he will stay small.

Factors regulating the degree of catch-up growth are not completely understood. A prospective study of 17 full-term infants with birth weights more than 2 standard deviations below the mean showed that the degree of growth deficit at birth was critical in terms of final height.[13] A significant negative correlation occurred between birth length and growth velocity in the first year of life. A positive correlation was shown between incremental linear growth during the first 6 months and insulin release following an intravenous bolus of glucose at 6 months. The authors concluded that growth

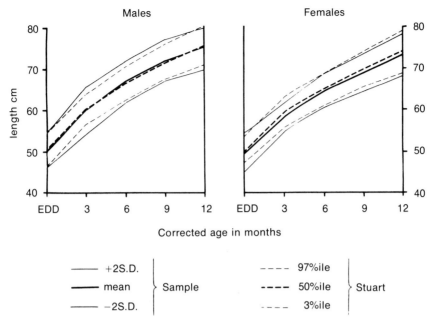

Fig. 19-1. Linear growth is shown for 67 infants (AGA) born prior to 33-weeks' gestation. The mean length ± 2 SD is shown for the boys and girls for 12 months post-term (after expected date of delivery [EDD]) and superimposed upon the Stuart percentiles.

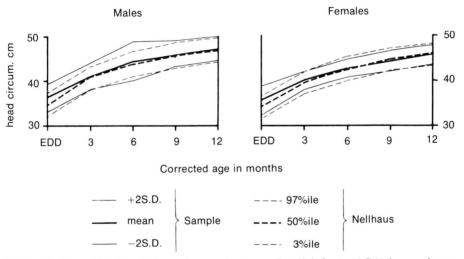

Fig. 19-2. Growth in head circumference is shown for 67 infants (AGA) born prior to 33-weeks' gestation. The mean head circumference ± 2 SD is shown for the boys and girls for 12 months post-term and superimposed upon the Nellhaus standards.

velocity during catch-up growth was related to the degree of preceding growth retardation, but that insulin might play a permissive role. Early nutrition for the SGA infant or the ill premature baby with AGA birth weight thus becomes of paramount importance during this critical period to allow for sufficient "catch-up" growth in the central nervous and skeletal systems.

Vision. The detection and treatment of visual

disturbance is a major concern in the management of a VLBW child. Refractive errors and ocular muscle imbalance account for the majority of the abnormalities, which may be present in as many as 44% of the smallest of premature survivors.[14] Retrolental fibroplasia still accounts for a significant proportion of the defects, especially in infants weighing less than 1000 g at birth. Retinal neovascularization with tortuosity of the retinal arteries is present in a high proportion of infants with birthweight less than 1000 g. Usually one eye is more affected than the other. The process remains active for a variable period of weeks, followed by a regression in activity or development of cicatricial changes. Apparent healing occurs in most cases except when marked retinal hemorrhage is accompanied by retinal scarring. This scarring and distortion of the retina persists and may result in retinal detachment and blindness. Less severe retinal scarring results in severe myopia. Because these defects are usually much worse in one eye, the visual abnormality often presents as a squint with loss of fixation of the affected eye. Corrective lenses should be prescribed early to prevent amblyopia in the most severely affected eye.

Although most babies with mild to moderate degrees of retinopathy of prematurity will have an apparently normal retina when examined at 1 year, a significant number will present with varying degrees of myopia.[15] As myopia tends to worsen in the preschool period, repeated refraction should be done and corrective lenses prescribed when indicated.

Strabismus is the next most common eye

disorder seen in the VLBW. Some cases are due to pure muscle imbalance; most are associated with an imbalance in visual acuity. Table 19-5 outlines the types and frequencies of eye defects reported in two prospective follow-up studies performed in our unit.

It is extremely important that all visual defects be detected as early as possible and appropriate treatment instituted. Persistent nystagmus, failure to fixate and persistent squint are absolute indications for a full ophthalmologic examination anytime after the term date. Infants depend upon visual stimulation for normal development. The blind infant requires extra auditory, tactile, and postural stimulation to develop to his full potential. Blind infants and children are often mistakenly diagnosed as mentally retarded because of a failure to employ specific teaching methods and adapted tests for assessment.

Hearing. Prior to 1960, severe hearing loss was reported in 10% of VLBW survivors.[16,17] The reported incidence in VLBW born in the 1960s dropped as low as 1% to 2%.[18,19] However, studies on current survivors are now reporting clinically significant sensorineural hearing loss in the range of 8 to 9%.[20]* The initial decrease was probably related to better control of neonatal hyperbilirubinemia and to discontinued use of streptomycin. The recent increase in incidence seems to be related to increased survival of hypoxic VLBW infants rather than to ototoxic medication or ambient noise level.[20-22] At highest risk for subsequent deafness are the infants who sustained severe asphyxia or recurrent apnea in the neonatal period. In a recent review of 62 ventilated VLBW survivors whom we have followed to school age, clinical hearing loss was diagnosed in 30% of those with major neurologic defects compared with an incidence of 12% in those without neurologic defects.*

Hearing loss is usually most marked in the high frequency range. Deafness is very rarely absolute; most affected infants can hear low- and midfrequency tones. Consequently they will startle at noise, locate towards a sound of mixed frequency, and thus do not appear to be deaf to the casual observer. Screening tests should employ only pure tones with special attention to the high frequencies. The examiner should suspect deafness in all cases of delayed

Table 19-5. Eye Defects in VLBW Infants.*

	≤1000 g	≤1500 g
Number	43	105
Age	1 year	4 years
Normal	61%	85%
RLF		
blind	5%	1%
scarring	12%	1%
Myopia	22%	9%
Amblyopia	—	5%
Cataract	—	3%

* ≤1000 g examined at 1 year[14] and ≤1500 g examined at 4 years (Fitzhardinge PM, FitzSimons R: Unpublished data). Some children presented with more than one visual defect.

* Fitzhardinge PM, FitzSimons R: unpublished data

speech development. This is especially true for the infant who demonstrates normal vocalization at three months PT but then fails to develop the normal babbling pattern by 6 to 9 months PT. Speech development requires constant reinforcement, which is normally provided by a positive vocal response from the caretaker and by hearing the self-produced sounds. Failure of reinforcement results in loss of speech or arrested development of speech. Early use of a hearing aid is the only hope for reasonably normal speech development in the child who sustains a severe hearing loss as a neonate.

Children with partial hearing also present with delayed speech patterns with characteristic loss of sibilant sounds. Unless routine audiometric screening is performed, these children are usually not diagnosed until 18 to 24 months of age. Because of difficulty in verbal comprehension, they are often thought to be retarded or, occasionally, autistic.

Speech Development. An assessment of speech development must consider the onset and enrichment of nonverbal sounds as well as the use and comprehension of the spoken word. The VLBW develops nonvocal communication early; he fixes and brightens before term, smiles socially at or slightly after the term date. Vocal communication begins with a single syllable repetitive sound (ga, ga) at the second to third month PT. A two-syllable sound (ah-goo) should be present by 6 months PT and should be presented in a give-and-take conversational manner. Inflection, changes in tone, and more variety in consonant and vowel sounds are established by the ninth month PT. Single words (Mama, Dada) used in an appropriate manner should appear at 12 to 13 months PT. However, expressive speech development frequently lags behind in the VLBW child. Only a few recognizable words may be used by 18 to 24 months PT. Normal speech can be predicted to develop at a later date if early preverbal speech patterns were normal, if verbal comprehension is normal, or if the child communicates well with his own jargon. Mental retardation, hearing deficit, or parental neglect should be excluded. Speech delay due to mental retardation is accompanied by delayed or abnormal development in other areas, particularly play behavior and nonverbal comprehension.

The incidence of delayed speech uncompli-cated by global retardation, deafness, or poor parenting has been poorly reported but appears to be high. We followed to school age 32 infants born between 1960 and 1966 with birth weights less than 1250 g.[19] Only 15 of the 32 had begun to speak by 2 years of age. Six of the seventeen with delayed speech ultimately developed good speech. Eleven others had speech deficits persisting into school age and scored less than 80 on standard intelligence tests. A similar study of VLBW born between 1970 and 1972 showed a decrease in the incidence of expressive delay from 13% at 2 years to less than 3% at school age.* In a more recent 2-year prospective study of 209 children with birth weights under 1500 g born in 1974, 74 (35%) showed a significant delay in speech development at 24 months of age.† These studies emphasize the prevalence of speech delay in the young VLBW child. The results suggest, however, that, for a good proportion of children, the speech defect is temporary and is not apparent by school age.

Neurologic Integrity. The neurologic sequelae to VLBW are divided into major and minor abnormalities. The major defects are frequently handicapping and consist of cerebral palsy, hydrocephaly, and seizure disorders. The minor defects include a variety of abnormalities which may impair function to some extent but do not impose any significant handicap. Most commonly included in this group are alterations in muscle tone, impaired balance, and poor fine or gross motor coordination.

Major Defects. The predominant form of cerebral palsy in the expremature child is spastic diplegia, characterized by a nonprogressive spasticity of the legs. The arms and trunk may also be involved, but always to a lesser degree. Cognitive development may be normal or impaired but the severity of the impairment is not necessarily related to the severity of the motor disability. Occasionally, the expremature infant presents with true quadriplegia or hemiplegia in which the muscles of the arms, hands, and trunk are predominantly affected. Cognitive impairment in these cases is usually proportional to the severity of the motor defect.

One of the earliest signs of cerebral palsy is

* Fitzhardinge PM, FitzSimons R: unpublished data
† Fitzhardinge PM: unpublished data

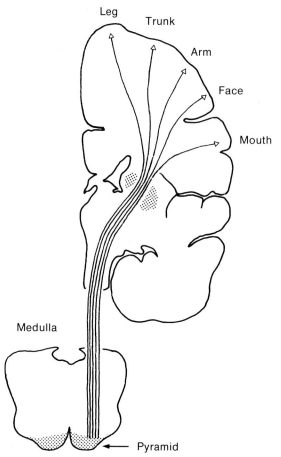

Fig. 19-3. Diagrammatic representation of the motor tracts from the cortex to the medulla showing proximity of the leg fibers to the periventricular area.

increased extensor tone of the muscles of the neck and shoulder girdle. This tone change first becomes apparent at term and lasts 2 to 3 months.[23] However, it is not a specific indicator for cerebral palsy.[24] In our experience, approximately one-half of infants so affected progress to some form of neurologic or intellectual defect but the remainder improve and are later free of major abnormality.[25] The first specific sign of spastic diplegia is extensor hypertonicity and hyperreflexia of the legs with subsequent delay or abnormality in sitting and crawling. The most severely affected cases are apparent by 6 months PT; milder cases may not be diagnosed with certainty until 12 months PT. Quadriplegia and hemiplegia can usually be detected prior to 6 months PT. The most reliable early signs of quadriplegia are impaired positioning and de-

layed function of the hands and arms together with persistent extensor hypertonicity of the shoulder girdle muscles.

Infarction of the periventricular white matter with or without hemorrhage has long been considered the underlying cause of spastic diplegia in the premature infant.[26] The extent of these lesions is variable. They occur in the boundary zone between the centrifugal and centripedal arterial branches to the periventricular area.[27] The descending tracts of the motor cortex course through this area, thus explaining the characteristic leg involvement. More extensive lesions will result in progressive involvement of the trunk and arm (Fig. 19-3). With asymmetric lesions, the clinical signs may mimic a classic hemiplegia, but careful examination will reveal a more severe impairment of the leg compared with the arm. Widespread destruction of the white matter results in loss of association and commissural fibers that produce cognitive defects as well as motor impairment of the upper limb and trunk.

Hydrocephalus is difficult to diagnose in the very young infant without special procedures. Apart from head size, the clinical signs are nonspecific. Disproportionate increase in head circumference is a late sign of increased intraventricular pressure.[28,29] Early diagnosis depends upon a high index of suspicion and monitoring of ventricular dilatation in suspect cases either by serial ultrasounds[30] or by computed tomography. The latter method has the obvious disadvantage of repeated irradiation.

The ventricular dilatation results from intraventricular hemorrhage and is caused by obstruction of CSF flow or to impaired CSF absorption. The dilatation may occur acutely after the hemorrhage or follow a latent period of 1 to 3 months. Many infants with hydrocephalus also have evidence of cerebral palsy and cognitive impairment.

The incidence of major defects in the VLBW varies considerably from study to study. At highest risk are the infants sustaining hypoxic-ischemic insults whether *in utero,* during delivery, or postnatally. The proportion of these high-risk infants in a particular study population will determine the incidence of sequelae in that population. The best results have been reported from perinatal centers that have the facilities for fetal monitoring and a team of experienced perinatologists to manage the intrapartum period and immediate resuscitation and stabilization of the infant. Such centers report only 4% to 6% of their VLBW survivors to have major neurologic defects.[31,32] In an outborn unit, where babies are referred from many different hospitals with varying degrees of perinatal expertise and where transport facilities may be suboptimal, the incidence of defects ranges from 13% to 15%.[2,33]

Most workers in rehabilitative medicine recommend intervention at the first persistent sign of neurologic defect. This intervention consists of minimizing extensor positioning, teaching the young infant means of achieving developmental milestones within the limits of his capabilities, and maintaining joint flexibility. Such treatment will, in most cases, prevent the secondary complications of muscle contracture and joint instability. Another major benefit of treatment is to enable the child to explore his environment and develop his cognitive ability to its fullest potential.

In a 6-year prospective study of 133 VLBW, all cases of major neurologic abnormality were diagnosed by 1 year. The degree of handicap remained constant from ages 2 to 6 except for improvement in the mild cases of diplegia.[2]* Table 19-6 lists the proportion of major defects seen in these children at school age.

Minor Neurologic Defects. The incidence of minor defects has not been well reported. In the prospective study of 133 children mentioned above, 13% had one or more minor problems at 2 years of age. The most common types of problems at that time were hypertonicity (9%), hyperreflexia (11%), and/or fine motor delay (13%). By 6 years, the incidence of minor defects was 11%, but there was no consistency in the type of defect over the years.

Intellectual Status. In most studies, the intellectual or cognitive status is evaluated solely by psychometric tests. While such tests give an objective measure of intelligence they must be interpreted with caution. Marked variations in scores for verbal and nonverbal items and problems with visuomotor coordination and spatial orientation may be more predictive of cognitive deficiency than is the global IQ. The full assessment of cognitive ability should include an evaluation of performance at school and at home, but objective measurement in these areas is difficult.

Psychometric tests administered at different

* Fitzhardinge PM, FitzSimons R: Unpublished data

Table 19-6. Neurologic Defects.*

Hydrocephalus	7
Quadriplegia	2
Hemiplegia	5
Diplegia	4
Convulsions	1
Total	19 (14%)

* Present at 6 years in 133 infants with birth weights ≤1500 g, born in 1970, 1971. One hydrocephalic and two quadriplegic children died between 1 and 3 years of age.

ages measure different aspects of intelligence. Infant tests tend to stress motor activities; preschool tests:—a combination of verbal and motor activities; school age tests—concept formation, problem solving, and visuomotor coordination. The practice of combining scores obtained by different tests at different ages to give a group result should be condemned.

For the same reasons stated in the previous section, the mean and range of IQ scores in any one group of VLBW children depends upon the population sample being studied. Factors to be considered are the proportion in the sample of the highest risk infants: intrauterine growth retardation, extreme prematurity, neonatal asphyxia, and post-natal hypoxia. Other factors influencing outcome are the standards of obstetric care, whether neonatal transport was necessary and the quality of such transport, the standards and philosophy of the neonatal unit, and the predominant socioeconomic level and parenting abilities of the families. Because of population differences and the above factors, outcome results vary considerably from study to study. In general, however, the mean school-age global IQ tends to be about 10 points below the mean for the general population, with the distribution skewed towards the lower scores. Figure 19-4 represents the distribution of the global scores for the 133 VLBW children followed to school age from our unit. Although two-thirds of the children scored over 85 on the Wechsler, only one-half had a satisfactory report from school at the end of 1 year. These infants were referred at birth from a total of 56 hospitals with varying expertise. Transport was managed by doctors or nurses largely unskilled in neonatology. These results are compared in Table 19-7 with two other centers. One study was on children with birthweights ≤1250 g who were born and treated in the same unit during the early 1960s.[19] The other study was

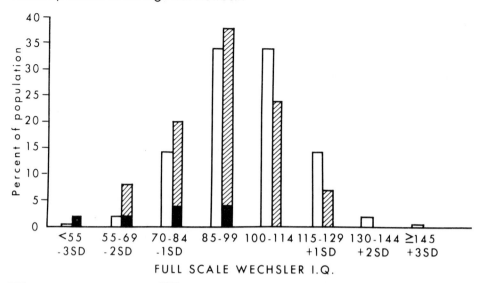

□ Population at large ▨ ≤1500g Normal CNS ■ ≤1500g Abnormal CNS

Fig. 19-4. Global IQ scores obtained at 6 years in 133 children with birthweights ≤ 1500 g; mean IQ is 91. Children with major neurologic defects all scored below 90.

on slightly heavier children (≤1500 g), about half of whom were referred after birth from other hospitals to the NICU.[34] No information is available for these other two studies concerning school performance.

SPECIFIC NEONATAL COMPLICATIONS IN FULL-TERM AND PREMATURE INFANTS

The preceding discussion reports the outcome of a rather heterogeneous group of infants selected only by birth weight. The risk factor for major deficit varies within the group depending upon the maturity of the infant and the amount of insult to the brain. The prognoses for some specific neonatal complications are discussed below.

Intrauterine Growth Retardation (IUGR)

Even when infants with chromosomal defects and intrauterine infection are excluded, the infant with significant IUGR (birth weight >2 SD below the mean) has a poor prognosis especially when born prior to 37 weeks' gestation. In a recent study, 49% of 71 preterm SGA babies born in 1974 and 1975 presented with major neurologic and/or cognitive handicap at 2 years of age.[11] An early onset of generalized CNS depression was highly predictive of late handicapping sequelae, reflecting the twin problems of perinatal asphyxia, and postnatal stabilization. All SGA babies appear to be particularly vulnerable to superimposed hypoxic-ischemic injury and this vulnerability is magnified when the problem is combined with immaturity. Full-term SGA children have a low incidence of major neurologic and cognitive defects but frequently have major school problems related to specific learning disabilities.[35,36] Because effective diagnosis of these learning problems is still only possible after 5 years of age, short-term follow-

Table 19-7. IQ at School Age*

Type of ICN	Year of Birth	Birth Weight	N	Global IQ
Inborn[19]	1960–1966	≤1250 g	32	90
Mixed[34]	1961–1968	≤1500 g	105	97
Outborn[2]	1970–1972	≤1500 g	133	91

* Full-scale or global IQ at school age of VLBW studies in three different centers.

Table 19-8. Mechanical Ventilation.*

Year of Birth	1970–1972[37]	1974–1975†
Admissions to ICN	640	340
No. ventilated	339 (53%)	201 (59%)
Ventilator survivors	72 (21%)	99 (49%)
Normal at 2 years	40 (56%)	71 (72%)
Handicap at 2 years	32 (44%)	28 (28%)

*Outcome for VLBW infants treated in the same ICN with mechanical ventilation in two distinct time periods showing a marked reduction in mortality and morbidity in the group born in 1974–1975.
†Fitzhardinge PM: Unpublished data.

up of SGA infants will tend to underestimate the extent of the disability.

Mechanical Ventilation

Mechanical ventilation was introduced to the care of the neonate in the mid1960s and is now used widely on even the smallest of infants. Since 1970, improved techniques have been associated with improved survival and decreased morbidity (Table 19-8). The primary pathology precipitating the need for ventilatory assistance may be pulmonary disease, defective central respiratory control, or a combination of both. The reported follow-up studies are composed of a heterogeneous mixture of primary pathology. This makes interpretation of their outcome results difficult (Table 19-9). In general, infants weighing more than 1500 g tend to require ventilation either for pulmonary disease (RDS, meconium aspiration, pneumonia) or following severe asphyxia, with the latter group showing a much higher proportion of developmental sequelae. In the VLBW, combined pathology is much more frequent. Neurologic handicap in both term and preterm infants is related to the degree of brain insult rather than to the process of ventilation *per se*.

Asphyxia

There are numerous problems in the definition of asphyxia. Improvements in our understanding of the pathophysiology of ante- and intrapartum asphyxia has led to a better identification of high-risk mothers before labor and delivery. The delivery process has been described as a period of repetitive stress which some infants are better able to tolerate than others. Following from this, the development of non-stressed antepartum fetal monitoring

has led to a more rational use of cesarean section. Intrapartum monitoring of the fetal heart rate has identified at an early stage those infants suffering early asphyxial insults. Recently, Adamson and Myers have confirmed, in a monkey model, that late deceleration of the fetal heart rate is an early indication of fetal compromise and does not necessarily reflect permanent neurologic damage.[38] With appropriate intervention, permanent neurologic sequelae should be avoidable in a large percentage of cases. Significant degrees of intrapartum asphyxia are associated with fetal acidosis.[39,40] Used in conjunction with fetal heart rate monitoring, low fetal pH aids the obstetrician in selecting the optimum time for intervention. These methods have all been developed with the aim of preventing severe birth asphyxia. They reflect abnormalities of fetal homeostasis but not necessarily damage. As such, these methods, aimed at prevention, cannot be used to define a population of asphyxiated infants.

The classical definition of asphyxia at birth has been a low Apgar score. Early studies demonstrated a good correlation of a low 5-minute score with later developmental handicap.[41] The major problem with such scoring systems is that they represent only a few isolated points in time. The actual score is easily modified by variations in scoring skill, maternal sedation, cerebral concussion, and immaturity. Even zero Apgar scores at birth have been shown to be compatible with reasonable survival with efficient, prompt resuscitation.[42,43] A recent report from the Collaborative Perinatal Project has emphasized this point. The 1-year outcome of 50,000 infants has been related to low Apgar scores at 1, 5, 10, and 20 minutes. The incidence of cerebral

Table 19-9. Ventilator Outcome, Six Studies.

	Johnson[50]	Brown[51]	Dinwiddie[52]	Marriage[53]	Fitzhardinge[37]	Kalman[54]
Year of birth	1962–1969	1968–1971	1964–1968	1966–1973	1970–1973	1974–1975
Type ICN	Inborn	Both	Inborn	Both	Outborn	Outborn
Ventilator mortality	72%	67%	63%	79%	75%	51%
No. followed	55	27	37	73	72	99
Birth weight (g)	2319*	1996*	2010*	1921*	≤1500	≤1500
RDS	85%	70%	58%	49%	45%	67%
Age assessed (years)	3–9	1–5	5–8	6	2	2
Neurologic defect	22%	15%	20%	?	29%	11%
IQ or equivalent	110*	?	88*	?	87†	84†
Handicap ‡ (%)	11	30	14	16	44	28

* Mean
† Mean MDI, PDI of Bayley Scale
‡ Handicap refers to major neurologic defect and/or IQ <80.

palsy increased with late low scores to a peak of 38% in infants with Apgar scores of 0 to 3 at twenty minutes. The neurologic lesion in these infants was severe and often associated with profound mental retardation and seizures.[44] It is important to recognize, however, that this study has not included the diagnosis of mental subnormality in the absence of cerebral palsy.

The preceding data support the value of the Apgar score as a screening method for identifying infants at risk for hypoxic-ischemic complications, but it must be recognized that the high number of false positives invalidates its use as an accurate predictor of late neurologic sequelae.

Asphyxia resulting in a prolonged period of abnormal behavior in the neonatal period is associated with a more defined prognosis in the term infant. The prognosis for later development is good for the infant whose neurologic examination has returned to normal by the end of the first week.[45,46] Persistent severe neurologic abnormalities and/or a persistent EEG pattern of status epilepticus in the full-term infant is associated with abnormal outcome in 60% to 90% of cases.[45,47−49] Approximately 75% of VLBW infants presenting with decerebrate posturing or seizures have major handicaps by 2 years.[33,37]

Vulnerable brain areas. The areas of the brain most vulnerable to hypoxic-ischemic insult are different in preterm and full-term infants. In preterm, the major site of pathology is in the periventricular region producing hemorrhage and/or infarction. In the full-term brain, bleeding is much less common and is rarely restricted to the periventricular area. Cerebral edema, parasagittal cortical infarction, and necrosis of the thalamic and brain stem nuclei are the major foci of injury. The types of neurologic sequelae are determined by the site of injury. Thus, the asphyxiated preterm infant is subject to hydrocephalus or spastic diplegia, the asphyxiated full-term to microcephaly, quadriplegia, hemiplegia, seizure disorder, or athetosis, all of which are usually associated with mental retardation.

REFERENCES

1. **Frankenburg WK, Dodds JB:** The Denver developmental screening test. J Pediatr 71: 181, 1967

2. **Fitzhardinge PM:** Current outcome of NICU population. In Brann AW, Volpe JJ (ed): Neonatal Neurological Assessment and Outcome: Report of the Seventy-seventh Ross Conference on Pediatric Research. Columbus, Ross Laboratories, 1980

3. **Bayley N:** Bayley Scales of Infant Development, p 15. New York, Psychological Corporation, 1969

4. **Wechsler D:** The Wechsler Intelligence Scale for Children. New York, Psychological Corporation, 1949

5. **Fitzhardinge PM:** Follow-up studies on the low birthweight infant. Clin Perinatol 3:503, 1976

6. **Weitzman ED, Graziani L:** Research planning workshops on the sudden infant death syndrome: neurophysiological factors. Bethesda, U.S. Department of Health, Education and Welfare, No. (NIH) 75-580, 1972.

7. **Fitzhardinge PM:** Follow-up studies of infants treated with mechanical ventilation. Clin Perinatol 5:451, 1978

8. **Stocks J, Godfrey S:** The role of artificial ventilation, oxygen and CPAP in the pathogenesis of lung damage in neonates: assessment by serial measurements of lung function. Pediatrics 57:352, 1976

9. **Coates AL, Bergsteinsson H, Desmond K et al:** Long term pulmonary sequelae of premature birth with and without idiopathic respiratory distress syndrome. J Pediatr 90:611, 1977

10. **Fitzhardinge PM:** Early growth and development in low birthweight infants following treatment in an intensive care nursery. Pediatrics 56:162, 1975

11. **Commey JOO, Fitzhardinge PM:** Handicap in the preterm small-for-gestational-age infant. J Pediatr 94:779, 1979

12. **Fitzhardinge PM, Stevens EM:** The small-for-date infant: 1. later growth patterns. Pediatrics 49:671, 1972

13. **Colle E, Schiff D, Andrew G et al:** Insulin responses during catch-up growth of infants who were small for gestational age. Pediatrics 57:363, 1976

14. **Pape KE, Buncic RJ, Ashby S et al:** The status at two years of low birthweight infants born in 1974 with birthweights of less than 1001 g. J Pediatr 92:253, 1978

15. **Baum JD:** Retinal artery tortuosity in ex-premature infants. Arch Dis Child 46:247, 1971

16. **Drillien CM:** The incidence of mental and physical handicaps in school age children of very low birth weight. Pediatrics 39:238, 1967

17. **Lubchenco LO, Delivoria-Papadopoulos M, Butterfield LJ et al:** Long term follow-up studies of prematurely born infants: 1. Relation-

ships of handicaps to nursery routines. J Pediatr 80:501, 1972

18. **Davies PA, Tizard JPM:** Very low birthweight and subsequent neurologic defect. Dev Med Child Neurol 17:3, 1975
19. **Fitzhardinge PM, Ramsay M:** The improving outlook for the small prematurely born infant. Dev Med Child Neurol 15:447, 1973
20. **Abramovich SJ, Gregory S, Slemick M, Stewart A:** Hearing loss in very low birthweight infants treated with neonatal intensive care. Arch Dis Child 54:421, 1979
21. **Stennert E, Schulte FJ, Vollrath M:** Incubator noise and hearing loss. Early Hum Dev 1:113, 1977
22. **Finitzo-Hieber T, McCracken GH, Roeser RJ et al:** Ototoxicity in neonates treated with gentamycin and kanamycin: results of a four year controlled follow-up study. Pediatrics 63:443, 1979
23. **Amiel-Tison C, Korobkin R, Esqué-vaucouloux MT:** Neck extensor hypertonia: a clinical sign of insult to the central nervous system. Early Hum Dev 1:181, 1977
24. **Drillien CM:** Abnormal neurologic signs in the first year of life in low birthweight infants: possible prognostic significance. Dev Med Child Neurol 14:575, 1972
25. **Pape KE, Fitzhardinge PM:** Reliability of the neurological assessment at 6 months post-term in the infant ≤1500 g birthweight (abstract). Pediatr Res 10:451, 1976
26. **Armstrong D, Norman MG:** Periventricular leukomalacia in neonates: complications and sequelae. Arch Dis Child 49:367, 1974
27. **Van den Bergh R, Vender Eecken H:** Anatomy and embryology of cerebral circulation. Prog Brain Res 30:1, 1968
28. **Korobkin R:** The relationship between head circumference and the development of communicating hydrocephalus in infants following intraventricular hemorrhage. Pediatrics 56:74, 1975
29. **Volpe JJ, Pasternak JF, Allan WC:** Ventricular dilatation preceding rapid head growth following neonatal intracranial hemorrhage. Am J Dis Child 131:1212, 1977
30. **Pape KE, Blackwell R et al:** Ultrasound detection of brain damage in preterm infants. Lancet 1:1261, 1979
31. **Brown ER, Taeusch W:** In Letter to editor. Lancet 2:362, 1979
32. **Stewart AL, Reynolds EOR:** Improved prognosis for infants of very low birthweight. Pediatrics 54:724, 1974
33. **Fitzhardinge PM, Kalman E, Ashby S et al:** Present status of the infant of very low birthweight treated in a referral neonatal intensive care unit in 1974. Major Mental Handicap:

methods and cost of prevention. Ciba Foundation Symposium 59:139, 1978

34. **Francis-Williams J, Davies PA:** Very low birthweight and later intelligence. Dev Med Child Neurol 16:709, 1974
35. **Fitzhardinge PM Stevens EM:** The small-for-date infant: II. neurological and intellectual sequelae. Pediatrics 50:50, 1972
36. **Rubin RA, Rosenblatt C, Balow B:** Psychological and educational sequelae of prematurity. Pediatrics 52:352, 1973
37. **Fitzhardinge PM, Pape KE, Arstikaitis M et al:** Mechanical ventilation of infants of less than 1501 grams birthweight: health, growth and neurologic sequelae. J Pediatr 88:531, 1976
38. **Adamson K, Myers RE:** Late decelerations and brain tolerance of the fetal monkey to intrapartum asphyxia. Am J Obstet Gynecol 128:893, 1977
39. **Beard RW, Mours ED, Clayton SG:** pH of fetal capillary blood as an indicator of the condition of the fetus. Br J Obstet Gynaecol 74:812, 1967
40. **Hon EH, Khazin AF:** Biochemical studies of the fetus: I. the fetal pH-measuring system, II. fetal pH and Apgar scores. Obstet Gynecol 33:219, 1969
41. **Drage JS, Kennedy C, Berendes H et al:** The apgar score as an index of infant morbidity. Dev Med Child Neurol 8:141, 1966
42. **Scott H:** Outcome of very severe birth asphyxia. Arch Dis Child 51:712, 1976
43. **Thomson AJ, Searle M, Russel J:** Quality of survival after severe birth asphyxia. Arch Dis Child 52:620, 1977
44. **Nelson KB, Ellenberg JH:** Neonatal signs as predictors of cerebral palsy. Pediatrics 64:225, 1979
45. **Amiel-Tison C:** Neurologic disorders in neonates associated with abnormalities of pregnancy and birth. Curr Probl Pediatr 3:3, 1973
46. **Volpe JJ:** Perinatal hypoxic-ischemic brain injury. Pediatr Clin North Am 23, No. 3:383, 1976
47. **Ziegler AL, Calame C, Marchand, C et al:** Cerebral distress in full term newborns and its prognostic value: a follow-up study of 90 infants. Helv Pediatr Acta 31:299, 1976
48. **Calame A, Reymond–Goni I, Maherzi M et al:** Psychological and neurodevelopmental outcome of high risk newborn infants. Helv Pediatra Acta 31:287, 1976
49. **Dennis J:** Neonatal convulsions: aetiology, late neonatal status and long-term outcome. Dev Med Child Neurol 20:143, 1978
50. **Johnson JD, Malachowski NC, Grobotein R:** Prognosis of children surviving with the aid of mechanical ventilation in the newborn period. J Pediatr 84:272, 1974

51. **Brown JK, Cockburn F, Forfar JO et al:** Problems in the management of assisted ventilation in the newborn and follow-up of treated cases. Br J Anaesth (Suppl) 45:808, 1973

52. **Dinwiddie R, Mellor DH, Donaldson SHC:** Quality of survival after artificial ventilation of the newborn. Arch Dis Child 49:703, 1974

53. **Marriage KJ, Davies PA:** Neurological sequelae in children surviving mechanical ventilation in the neonatal period. Arch Dis Child 52: 176, 1977

54. **Kalman EA, Pape KE, Ashby SA et al:** Mask ventilation in premature infants: association with severe retardation (abstract). Pediatr Res 12:527, 1978

V

Particular Problems and Considerations

20

Acute Respiratory Disorders in the Newborn

Mildred T. Stahlman

In caring for the newborn with respiratory distress, it is well to remember that not all such distress is caused by pulmonary disease. Labored and abnormal breathing may result from CNS disorders and from severe metabolic acidosis. A variety of congenital malformations cause respiratory distress, some of them surgical emergencies such as diaphragmatic hernia, tracheo-esophageal fistula, and congenital lobar emphysema (see Chap. 34). In some instances, congenital heart disease may be difficult to distinguish from primary lung disease (see Chap. 23). Perhaps the most important principle is to make every effort at the outset to establish a specific diagnosis, and not to blindly treat the symptoms without understanding the pathophysiology.

Many of the respiratory disorders which present themselves in the newborn are unique to that period of development. Understanding their incidence, pathogenesis, and natural history depends upon an understanding of lung maturation and differentiation. Our knowledge of the anatomic sequences of the developing lung is reasonably well established at present, but our understanding of the biochemical events involved in differentiation of the various tissues which make up the lung is just beginning

to unfold. (See Chap. 22 for details of pulmonary therapy.)

DEVELOPMENT OF THE LUNG[1]

Anatomic. Around the 24th day of human embryonic life, an outpouching of the endodermal-lined gut appears, and proceeds by dichotomous branching to invade the mesenchymal tissue surrounding it. These divisions are accompanied at 10-weeks' gestation by the appearance of cartilage. The antenatal formation of new bronchi is complete by about 16 weeks. The branching bronchial tree is originally accompanied in its evagination from the gut by paired segmental arteries arising from the dorsal aorta caudal to the aortic arches, ending in a capillary plexus in the developing lung.

The pulmonary vein develops as an endothelial diverticulum from the posterior surface of the left atrium at about 30 days; it extends dorsally and joins other endothelial channels within the lung buds. The pulmonary arteries descend from the inferior surface of the sixth pharyngeal arch arteries ventrolateral to the trachea and ramify within the lung buds. The pattern of branching of the pulmonary arteries follows that of the airways, ending in a rich capillary bed with anastomotic connections to the bronchial blood supply. Only the bronchial arteries persist as remnants of the first segmental dorsal aortic arch with connections to the pulmonary capillaries.

The epithelial mass invading the mesenchyme early in embryonic life has a solid, glandular appearance and canalization first appears at around 18- to 20-weeks' gestation. The cells surrounding primitive air sacs are columnar or cuboidal in shape and are rich in intracellular glycogen. As further budding progresses, the cytoplasm of some of these cells appears to undergo a transformation from being largely glycogen-filled to an appearance more typical of great alveolar Type II epithelial cells, with lamellar inclusions characteristic of storage sites for surface-active material and with microvilli on the free edge. At about this same time, budding capillaries invade the walls of terminal airways, which are lined with cuboidal cells. At free surfaces, flattened cells with scant cytoplasm, no glycogen, and no lamellar inclusions are seen. These cells have the characteristic appearance of Type I lining epithelial cells, which in the mature lung serve as a barrier for diffusion of gas between alveolar air and capillary blood. It seems likely that both Type II and Type I epithelial cells are differentiated from the glycogen-filled primitive lining cells.

At around 24 to 26 weeks of gestation, most of the epithelial lung tissue is made up of glycogen-rich cuboidal cells with only a few typical Type I cells presenting themselves over a few capillary loops. The airblood surface area for gas diffusion is therefore very limited, and, should the fetus be delivered at this gestational age, survival would be extremely difficult. In addition, there is some question whether those Type II cells developing lamellar inclusions have the ability to discharge their surface-active lipids onto the alveolar surface at a rate commensurate with lung stability on continuous air breathing. It is at this critical stage of intrauterine growth and development that there seem to be factors affecting the fetus as a whole which may be capable of speeding up lung differentiation. Until we fully understand the mechanisms involved in normal lung differentiation, we can only speculate why some infants undergo rapid lung maturation, while others differentiate more slowly.

Normally, between 26- and 32-weeks' gestation, small, terminal air sacs give way to air spaces with the branching pattern of alveolar ducts. The lining layer of cells shows a transition from glycogen-filled cuboidal cells to a mixture of cuboidal cells, an increasing number of which contain lamellar bodies, and typical Type I alveolar cells. The proportion of interstitial tissue decreases, and capillary loops are found in increasing abundance. The cells containing lamellar inclusions appear clustered at the branch-points of the alveolar ducts, and the number of inclusions per cell increases.

From 32 to 36 weeks, further budding occurs from these alveolar ducts, and true alveoli, with walls made up, for the most part, of many anastomosing capillaries covered with typical Type I alveolar lining cells, become more and more numerous. The remaining cuboidal cells are two types: those still richly filled with glycogen, lining respiratory bronchioles and alveolar ducts down to the atria, now called Clara cells; and typical Type II great alveolar cells with lamellar inclusions. These present themselves in clusters of two and three at junctional sites, each cell oriented with its free surface toward an airspace.

Concomitant with the development of the pulmonary circulation is the development of a rich pulmonary lymphatic tree, which can readily be seen in the newborn surrounding bronchi down to the alveolar ducts and immediately adjacent to pulmonary arteries and veins.

Biochemical Events

As these anatomic events progress during normal intrauterine growth, biochemical changes are also occurring. Farrell and coworkers have recently summarized current thought concerning the biochemistry of fetal lung development.[2] It has long been recognized that a combination of surface active phospholipids line the mature lung terminal airspaces and are extremely important in maintaining alveolar stability, especially at low transmural pressures. The two principal components of surfactant are now thought to be phosphotidylcholine (PC), and phosphotidylglycerol (PG); the acyl component of both is esterified palmitic acid.

In the human fetus two pathways develop for the production of surface-active phospholipids: (1) Cytidine diphosphate choline (CDP choline) + D-α, β-diglyceride $\rightarrow$ lecithin (choline incorporation pathway); and (2) phosphatidylethanolamine (PE) + 2CH$_3$ $\rightarrow$ PDME (phosphatidyldimethylethanolamine) + 2CH$_3$ $\rightarrow$ lecithin (methylation pathway). *De novo* synthesis of disaturated phosphatidylcholine is achieved primarily through the CDP-choline pathway. The second pathway is of minor importance in both fetal and adult lung.[3] The CDP-choline pathway results in the formation of predominantly unsaturated phosphatidylcholine. Two transformation reactions are possible to convert it to dipalmitoyl phosphatidylcholine: deacylation-reacylation[4] and deacylation-transacylation.[5] The production of saturated PC increases with increasing gestational age, and with the appearance of mature alveolar Type II cells containing lipid-filled lamellar bodies. The biochemical changes in surfactant production and composition are reflected by quantitative increases in the amount of surface-active phospholipids that appear in human amniotic fluid at successive stages of gestation. The fetal lung contributes to the amniotic fluid, and material discharged from cells lining potential air sacs eventually finds its way into the amniotic contents by means of the fluid produced within the developing lung. The changing pattern of amniotic fluid phospholipids can therefore be used to assess the maturation of the biochemical pathways of surfactant production. As reported by Gluck and coworkers, phosphotidylcholine concentration increases as gestation progresses, while sphingomyelin remains fairly stable in concentration with a small peak at 28 to 30 weeks.[6] The ratio of lecithin to sphingomyelin (L/S ratio) in amniotic fluid has been widely used as an index of fetal lung maturity, a ratio greater than 2 being considered compatible with relatively mature lung function. More recently, Gluck and associates have suggested that the relative values of phosphotidylinositol and phosphotidylglycerol may be helpful in refining this evaluation. Phostidylinositol is found in very low concentrations until 26- to 30-weeks' gestation, after which time its concentration rise parallels that of lecithin, peaking at about 36 weeks and declining to about half that value at term. However, phosphotidylglycerol does not appear in amniotic fluid until 35- to 36-weeks' gestation, and its concentration increases as that of phosphotidylinositol falls.[7] Prediction of the degree of lung maturity may be improved with increasing use of combinations of data, such as these.

Role of Steroids

The length of gestation in animals may be normally and artificially influenced by the secretions of the pituitary-adrenal axis. Liggins has shown that ablation of the pituitary or adrenal glands in fetal sheep extends the length of gestation, and that ACTH or glucocorticoid infusion into the fetus over several days results in premature delivery.[8] The startling finding was that steroid-treated lambs had more mature lungs, both biophysically and histologically, than their untreated twins. These observations are paralleled in man. Anencephalic infants without pituitary glands have immature lungs, and infants with adrenal cortical hyperplasia, on the other hand, may be prematurely born with lungs which appear to be mature for their gestational age. It is not recognized that many types of pregnancies which result in chronic fetal stress, such as maternal toxemia, may be associated with premature delivery of infants who are both small for gestational age and who have lungs resembling those of infants with more advanced gestational ages. They are also remarkably nonsusceptible to the development of hyaline membrane disease (HMD). In addition they have evidence of small thymuses and big adrenal glands, both facts suggestive of fetuses which have had high glucocorticoid levels *in utero*.

These observations have been extended to a controlled trial of glucocorticoids, given to women in premature labor by Liggins[9] and coworkers with evidence that lung differentiation and maturation can be artificially induced in humans.[9] These studies have been extended by others, with equally encouraging results.[10–14] However, the effectiveness of this regimen in preventing respiratory distress has largely been shown to be limited to (1) fetuses treated between 27- and 34-weeks' gestation; (2) at least 48 hours before delivery; and (3) delivery no more than 7 days after treatment.

It is thought, both from these studies in humans and from studies in animals, that effective pharmacologic induction of lung maturation is a reasonable approach toward the prevention of problems related to immaturity of the newborn lung, such as hyaline membrane disease, if the fetus can be shown to be at risk (such as by an immature L/S ratio), if it is within a susceptible period for induction, and if labor can be prevented for 48 hours. The question of repeated treatment after seven days without delivery is still under discussion.

Other fetal organs are almost surely affected by steroid treatment and the overall effects may not be wholly salutory for the fetus. There is also increasing evidence that other mechanisms may be involved in lung maturation, both *in utero* during stress, and with repeated specific maternal states such as heroin use. This is a rapidly expanding field of investigation and we hope to know more about the advantages and disadvantages of accelerated lung maturation in the future.

CIRCULATORY ADAPTION AND ITS EFFECTS ON NEONATAL RESPIRATORY DISTRESS[15]

The principal characteristic of the circulatory pattern of the fetus is that the two ventricles work in parellel rather than in series as in the normal adult. The newborn circulation therefore has a transition between these two patterns and its progression may be arrested under adverse circumstances.

During fetal life, the pulmonary vascular resistance is high with respect to the total systemic vascular resistance, maintained primarily by the low P_{O_2} of the blood perfusing the fetal lung. This level of P_{O_2} (around 20 torr in the pulmonary artery) causes marked pulmonary arterial vasoconstriction despite a reasonably high oxygen saturation achieved by fetal hemoglobin, a "normal" pH (7.40), and a relatively low P_{CO_2} (35 torr). The lower total systemic resistance is caused in large part to the available run-off into the placenta, which is a low-resistance system functioning as the fetal lung to allow for oxygen and CO_2 diffusion. Blood returning to the fetus from the placenta is thus well saturated with oxygen (85–90%) despite a low P_{O_2} (about 30 torr) resulting from the shift to the left of the oxygen dissociation curve of fetal blood. The importance of this left shift cannot be overemphasized because it places the fetus in jeopardy of drastic decrease in saturation with small drops in P_{O_2}, due to the steep slope of the hemoglobin dissociation curve. Also the high affinity for O_2 of fetal hemoglobin forces tissue P_{O_2}s to very low levels before O_2 release is

accomplished. Thus the fetus is particularly vulnerable to hypoxia.

Fetal stress, such as that associated with asphyxial states, is thought to induce additional redistribution of blood flow in the "dive" pattern, with preservation (indeed, increases) of flow to brain, myocardium, adrenals, and placenta, at the expense of liver, lung, gut, kidneys, muscles, and skin. These reflex effects are exaggerated in the presence of an open foramen ovale and widely patent ductus arteriosus, both shunting right to left.

After placental separation and the assumption of gas exchange by the lung, the fetal circulatory pattern undergoes profound adjustments. Normally, pulmonary blood flow is increased manyfold as a consequence of mechanical lung expansion and of progressively better oxygenation of the blood perfusing it. Both mechanisms reduce pulmonary vascular resistance. Simultaneously, there is a rise in systemic vascular resistance as the result of removel of the large placental run-off. The net effect of these changes is to lower the pulmonary arterial pressure at the same time that the systemic pressure is increased, bringing about a reversal of the pressure gradient across the ductus arteriosus. Bidirectional shunting through the ductus arteriosus may occur for a short time in normal infants, and during this time a small right-to-left shunt may persist through the foramen ovale. As these changes progress in the normal infant, the shunt through the ductus arteriosus becomes directionally left to right, further increasing the pulmonary venous return to the left atrium. This reverses the small pressure gradient at the atrial level and acts to close the valve of the foramen ovale. With increasing oxygenation associated with better pulmonary perfusion, the ductus arteriosus begins to constrict. Shunting through the ductus is progressively diminished and functionally ceases in normal-term infants about 24 hours after birth.

Patent Ductus Arteriosus (PDA). There is increasing evidence that the oxygen-responsive vasoconstrictive mechanisms of the mature infant may not be completely operative in the immature infant and that persistence of ductus is the rule rather than the exception in very immature infants who have not been subjected to chronic stress and accelerated maturation *in utero*. A symptomatic PDA is especially common if the infant is under 1500 g birth weight and has clinical HMD.

An interesting group of compounds, referred to as prostaglandins, have been shown to affect various vascular beds with either vasoconstriction or vasodilitation. Certain of these, such as prostacyclin (PGI_2) have been shown to decrease pulmonary vascular resistance in the fetus. This compound is in high concentration in ductal strips. Others, such as PGE_2, have been shown to maintain ductal patency when infused into the pulmonary artery. These observations have led to the hypothesis that intraductal production of prostaglandins, presumably PGI_2, plays a role in normal ductal closure. Therefore, blockers (*e.g.*, indomethacin) of prostaglandins production from its precursor, arachidonic acid, are being tried to induce pharmacologic closure of the ductus arteriosus in small preterm infants in whom its continued patency threatens congestive heart failure, recurrent pulmonary edema, and oxygen and ventilator dependency. Not all ductus respond to indomethacin treatment, especially those in very low-birth-weight infants, but carefully controlled and closely monitored use may be indicated with symptomatic PDA as an alternative to surgical closure.

In the infant with a transitional circulation, the ductus arteriosus is anatomically open and potentially capable of shunting blood in either direction. Also the foramen ovale valve is unsealed and "can readily be held open to allow right-to-left shunting of blood" from the inferior vena cava into the left atrium when a pressure gradient exists in that direction (via sinistra). Whether the open ductus arteriosus will allow shunting to occur right-to-left or bidirectionally depends largely on the differential pressure gradient between the aorta and the pulmonary artery, and on the relative resistances in the pulmonary and systemic circulations. Shunting between the atria, on the other hand, appears to depend largely upon venous return and the different elasticity characteristics of the atria.

Persistent Transitional Circulation

Situations in the neonatal period which either increase pulmonary vascular resistance, such as hypoxia, or lower systemic vascular resistance, such as hypotension, or both, promote the fetal direction of shunting through both the foramen ovale and the ductus arteriosus. Pulmonary pathology or central depression of ventilatory drive, which themselves lead to inadequate oxygenation of the pulmonary capillary blood and to pulmonary arterial hypertension, may thus promote extrapulmonary right-to-left shunting and maintenance of an unconstricted ductus, resulting in further hypoxemia and the establishment of a vicious cycle. A return of a transitional (not wholly fetal) circulatory pattern leading to dangerously low and sometimes fatal levels of hypoxemia occurs with most frequency in newborn infants with diaphragmatic hernias, in IDMs, for unknown reasons, in infants with severe endo- or exotoxemia, such as with Group B β-hemolytic streptococcal sepsis, in terminal HMD, and, on rare occasion in infants with no obvious *in utero*, intrapartum, or neonatal cardiopulmonary disease. Persistent pulmonary hypertension, with right-to-left shunting through the foramen ovale in the presence of a closed ductus, has been described in newborn infants following maternal aspirin ingestion, a drug which, like indomethacin, can block prostaglandins synthesis and promote *in utero* ductal closure.

In the presence of severely low levels of arterial oxygen tension, a temporal, right radial or right brachial arterial sample should be compared with a simultaneously drawn aortic or femoral arterial sample for P_{O_2}. A significant O_2 gradient between blood sampled above and below the ductus arteriosus confirms right-to-left ductal shunting. If Pa_{CO_2} is also low or normal and lung fields are clear on x-ray examination, primary pulmonary pathology is an unlikely cause of the pulmonary arterial vasoconstriction and other causes should be sought. Hypovolemia and/or systemic hypotension should be corrected, adequate pulmonary oxygenation and ventilation assured with careful respirator management, and structural factors such as congenital cardiac lesions or pneumothorax ruled out. If dangerous levels of hypoxemia persist, a cautious trial with a vasodilator, such as tolazoline, should be given into a vein draining into the superior vena cava, with careful monitoring of systemic arterial pressure and heart rate because peripheral vasodilitation and systemic hypotension will result if significant amounts of drug reach the systemic vascular bed through the right-to-left ductus shunt. Blood pressure and heart rate monitoring is essential throughout the continued infusion of drug, and dosage must be regulated to prevent pulmonary edema from pulmonary vasodilation with reversal of ductus shunting or severe systemic hypotension.

HYALINE MEMBRANE DISEASE (HMD)

There are many forms of respiratory distress from which newborn infants suffer in their first days of life, the most common of which and the most important worldwide is HMD. This single entity is associated with 30% of all neonatal deaths in the United States and with 50 to 70% of premature deaths. It occurs in infants who are born before term but susceptibility depends more on the stage of lung maturation at the time of delivery than on precise gestational age.

Etiology and Pathogenesis

The presence of adequate amounts of surface-active material to line airspaces is one of the prerequisites for adequate postnatal pulmonary adaptation. This material is capable of maintaining alveolar stability at low pressures so that on end expiration, alveolar collapse does not occur. Surface-active material must not only be present in adequate amounts at birth but also must be regenerated at a rate consonant with its disappearance. This implies functionally intact and viable Type II alveolar cells.

Another prerequisite for extrauterine survival is an adequate surface area for gas exchange across the airspace wall. This implies the development of a sufficient pulmonary capillary bed in contact with an alveolar surface area covered by cells adapted for gas diffusion: Type I epithelial cells.

Surfactant can be present in inadequate amounts after birth from several causes:

1. Extreme immaturity of the alveolar lining cells
2. Diminished or impaired production rate resulting from transient fetal and early neonatal stress
3. Impairment of the release mechanism for surface-active phospholipids from the limiting membrane within the Type II cells
4. Death of many of those cells responsible for surfactant production

Clinical, biochemical, and histologic evidence suggests that the first and third postulates may account for the inability of the very early fetus to survive extrauterine life—regardless of other factors, progressive atelectasis leads to death from pulmonary insufficiency. The natural history and sequential histologic and biophysical events in HMD strongly suggest that the fourth postulate is operative; while more mild and transient types of respiratory distress might be related to the second postulate.

The more immature the lung, the greater the percentage of cuboidal cells lining potential airspaces. Though presumably capable of producing some surfactant under the proper stimulus, this production may not be at a great enough turnover rate for adequate lung stability in the very immature baby. Also the more immature the lung and smaller the pulmonary capillary bed, the greater the ease with which the nutritional blood supply to the developing lung cells can be compromised by fetal hypoxia and hypotension. Those cells which appear to be dividing to allow further budding of the developing airways, and which eventually will produce surfactant, are presumed to have higher metabolic requirements than the Type I cells which eventually line terminal airspaces and have a passive role in gaseous diffusion.

At about 35-weeks' gestation in normally grown infants, abundant numbers of Type II cells are well differentiated and capable of supplying large amounts of surfactant to airways which have a potentially large surface area for gas diffusion, as a consequence of capillary invasion and Type I cell differentiation. Ischemic necrosis of the entire lining of the airway is no longer possible, although profound stress may still affect Type II cells as further maturation occurs. Thus there are thought to be biochemical and anatomic bases for the susceptibility of the immature lung to HMD.

The Role of Stress

The gestational history of infants who present with clinical HMD frequently includes some episode compatible with recent fetal or intrapartum stress, especially vaginal bleeding (in which the fetus may participate), maternal hypotension, difficult resuscitation associated with birth asphyxia or other catastrophic events capable of severely compromising the blood supply to the fetal lung.

This is in contrast to the more insidious, lower grade, and chronic types of stress to which the fetus may be susceptible, such as gradual placental insufficiency brought about by progressive infarction in association with maternal toxemia. This chronic type of stress appears to be associated with a low incidence of HMD, perhaps as a result of prematurely induced lung maturation.

Acute hypoxia is a powerful pulmonary vasoconstrictor in the fetus, potentiated by increased hydrogen ion concentration (low pH). As long as fetal pathways for shunting blood away from the lung are open, pulmonary hypertension, especially in the presence of systemic hypotension, may critically reduce the nutritional blood supply to those pulmonary cells with high metabolic requirements for survival. Maternal (and therefore fetal) oversedation with central respiratory depression, hypovolemia, and hypotension from injudicious handling of the cord circulation before clamping; uncorrected metabolic acidosis which becomes self perpetuating; oxygen lack with persistence of fetal circulatory pathways; or extremes of hypothermia may lead to a progressive loss of lung compliance secondary to Type II alveolar cell death and cessation of surfactant production.

The added risk of HMD ascribed to *elective* cesarean section is a controversial point at the present. Usher's review of the experience at the Royal Victoria Hospital in Montreal suggested strongly that cesarean section *per se* does not influence the incidence of HMD, whereas the risk of death with pulmonary insufficiency was inversely proportional to gestational age up to 38 weeks' gestation.[16]

The role of maternal diabetes is difficult to determine with certainty because these large infants often have an overestimation of gestational age and therefore of their degree of lung maturation. There is some suggestion, however, that infants of diabetic mothers may have a delay of normal lung maturation (see Chap. 16).

Risk of Recurrence

The risk of recurrent HMD in subsequent prematurely born infants of appropriate size for gestational age is 90%, while the risk of occurrence after a small-for-gestational-age infant is less than 5%. This suggests that maternal factors are operative in the delayed maturation of some infants. The secondborn of twins appears to be more often and more severely affected than the firstborn, possibly because of the greater risk of intrapartum asphyxia but possibly also because the firstborn is more frequently smaller than the second twin, suggesting placental insufficiency, chronic stress, and earlier lung maturation.

Clinical Presentation

At the moment of birth, the infant who subsequently presents the full-blown picture of HMD may sometimes appear to be a healthy, pink, normally grown premature infant with a good Apgar score at 1 and 5 minutes. However, many of these infants do have evidence of intrapartum asphyxia or depression and the onset of respiration may be delayed, making resuscitation necessary. Even the infant who initially appears healthy, if carefully observed from the first minutes after birth, exhibits an abnormal pattern of respiration. This may present in the larger premature infant only as tachypnea, and color may be maintained for some time in room air. The asphyxiated or drug-depressed infant, especially the small premature, may have a low respiratory rate and little effective ventilation until central depression is corrected.

Increasing ventilatory effort is evidenced by the forceful intercostal retraction and use of accessory neck muscles for respiration. Such an infant usually begins to have an audible expiratory grunt or cry during the first few hours after birth as a reflection of forcing expired air past the partially closed glottis. This partial Valsalva maneuver initially serves to maintain a positive end-expiratory pressure of 3 to 5 cm of water at the alveolar level. As lung compliance begins to diminish, the percentage of this positive pressure transmitted to the alveolar level declines.

Within hours, oxygen requirements to maintain a satisfactory arterial P_{O_2} increase, and more and more physical effort is required by the baby to maintain open terminal airways as alveolar volume on end-expiration decreases. Increasingly large negative intrapleural pressures are necessary to open alveoli to volumes satisfactory for gas exchange. A characteristic

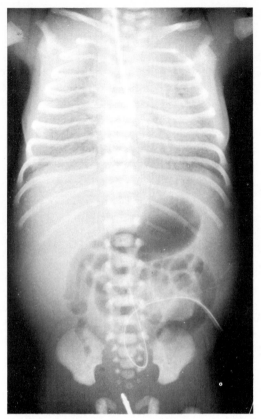

Fig. 20-1. Severe HMD. Note diffuse density of the lung fields compared with intestinal gas, with well-defined air bronchograms. Both lungs are uniformly involved. An umbilical artery catheter lies at the aortic bifurcation (third lumbar vertebra).

"poor air entry" with vigorous ventilatory effort failing to produce audible sounds of normal alveolar filling. Rales are uncommon in the early hours after birth but, as the disease progresses, characteristic dry "sandpaper" breath sounds appear on both inspiration and expiration. Audible cardiac murmurs are uncommon in the first 24 hours of the disease but appear with increasing frequency with time. Tachycardia is frequently present (in the range of 150–160/min), especially if the infant has uncorrected acidosis and hypoxemia, and may be much higher in the presence of hypovolemia. The ECG in the early hours of the disease usually shows a right ventricular preponderance and flattened T-waves but is not characteristic for this disease alone.

X-ray Findings

The early x-ray picture of the chest is usually quite characteristic (Fig. 20-1). Both lung fields show a diffuse, fine reticulogranular pattern with a prominent air bronchogram extending out into the periphery of the lung fields. Central lung markings are not coarse or prominent but the heart border may be fuzzy and obscured. Parenchymal granularity may be more prominent on the right than on the left side early on. A large thymic shadow is almost invariably present (Fig. 20-2). Lower lung field radiolucency may occasionally occur early in the course of the disease but does not persist. The heart often appears enlarged, but its full extent may not be appreciated until serial x-ray films during resolution of the disease show a diminished size. The lateral chest film early on also shows diffuse granularity, prominent air-bronchograms, and, depending on chest cage stability, various degrees of pseudopectus deformity. In the infant with very severe disease, the film of the lungs in the first few hours may already show very heavy, uniform granularity or even a "whiteout," reflecting fluid-filled alveoli, with an air-bronchogram the only visible lung marking. The prognosis in the presence of this lung film, especially if it occurs under 12 hours after birth, is extremely poor.

Clinical Course

The natural history of the disease is one of increasing severity of respiratory symptoms, increasing oxygen dependence and increasingly poor lung function until about 48 to 72 hours after birth when evidence of Type II cell

seesaw type of paradoxical respiration is seen, reflecting poor lung compliance, with protrusion of the abdomen on inspiration as the diaphragm descends forcefully. The less stable the chest cage, the more the anterior chest wall and sternum collapse, producing the appearance of a pseudopectus deformity.

The infant becomes progressively obtunded and flaccid. Marked peripheral vasoconstriction is usually clinically evident with a pale often gray color to the skin, which demonstrates poor capillary filling after compression and often masks severe central cyanosis. Progressive edema develops; shortly after birth it is most apparent in the shiny palms and soles of the infant and in his puffy face. Oliguria in the first 48 hours after birth is common.

On auscultation of the lungs during the first few hours after birth there is usually only

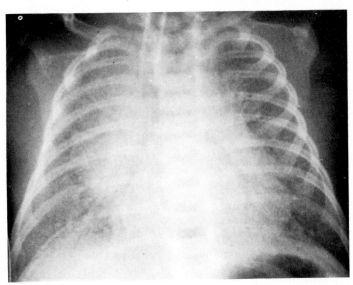

Fig. 20-2. HMD. The Reticulogranular pattern involves both lung fields. A large thymus shadow blends with the right heart border. An endotracheal tube is in place.

regeneration occurs and surfactant production reappears.

Those infants with a good prognosis have a progressive increase in systemic arterial pressure over the first 4 to 5 days after birth as clinical improvement proceeds. Infants who are only moderately ill and who never require assisted ventilation can be managed with an inspired fraction of oxygen $F_{I_{O_2}}$, which rarely needs to be pushed over 60%, and bicarbonate or THAM buffering is seldom needed more than once or twice. By about 48 hours these infants begin to improve clinically, physiologically and biochemically. P_{O_2} begins to rise so that $F_{I_{O_2}}$ can be dropped, often very rapidly, and respiratory rate and effort decrease. This may be associated with some CO_2 retention, but it is rarely severe. The infants become more alert, open their eyes, begin to have diureses, and may tolerate small feedings. Once they have progressed this far, recovery is rapid over the next 3 to 4 days and complications are rare. Closing ductus murmurs may be transiently heard but the persistence of significant shunting is uncommon.

The severely ill infant, however, runs a different course, often modified by the initiation of some sort of ventilatory assistance. The smaller the infant, the earlier after birth his findings of clinical and biochemical deterioration appear. Continuous positive airway pressure (CPAP), continuous negative airway pressure (CNAP), or assisted ventilation may be required, based on unresponsive apnea or very low Pa_{O_2}s in high oxygen concentrations (greater than 60%). This deterioration may be anticipated by careful observation. Respirations become more labored with marked retraction of lower sternum and infracostal area, and the infant uses all of his accessory muscles of respiration. His respiratory frequency may actually begin to decrease, and he lies with eyes closed using all his effort to breathe. Disturbances such as x-ray examinations, which produce bouts of hard crying, may be disastrous. Grunting may actually cease as he worsens still further. Intermittent periods of short apnea may be mixed with other irregular patterns of breathing such as "cogwheel," and, finally, prolonged apnea ensues, which is unresponsive to stimulation. The color changes from pale pink to ashen gray as cardiovascular collapse develops. Arterial pH levels may fall quickly below 7.0 and be difficult to restore to a normal range. Peripheral vasoconstriction is so marked by this time that oxygen unsaturation is very difficult to estimate visually.

Respirator care may stretch out the course of the more severe cases, and a significant proportion can now be salvaged by these techniques. In some, chronic lung disease may follow a prolonged period of high oxygen exposure and assisted ventilation (see Chap. 21).

Other infants deteriorate much more precipitously when, after some hours of uncorrected hypoxia, acidosis, and hypothermia, they are suddenly oxygenated, buffered, and warmed. Sudden pulmonary edema may result with fluid running from the trachea, a whiteout on x-ray of the lungs, and apnea requiring ventilatory assistance. The initiation of low positive end-expiratory pressure, which may be increased as needed, may sometimes prevent such a precipitous outcome.

Pathophysiology

Physiologic measurements in these infants reflect the developing lung pathology and both may depend in part on how the infant has been managed at the time of the measurement. From the initiation of respiration onward, abnormally low compliance measurements may be found, (*i.e.*, a markedly negative intrathoracic pressure necessary to move a normal volume of air). Total ventilation may be greatly increased (in the absence of central depression) and alveolar ventilation thereby maintained at a normal level despite a large functional dead space ventilation, so that Pa_{CO_2} remains normal at first.

In the early hours after birth, pulmonary hypertension relative to systemic pressures may be caused by hypoxia and systemic hypotension. This leads to maintenance of a partial fetal circulatory pattern, with right-to-left shunting through both the ductus arteriosus and the foramen ovale. If the sick infant is not properly resuscitated and enough oxygen is not added to inspired air to maintain arterial P_{O_2} above about 30 to 35 torr, the pulmonary vascular resistance will remain high. A low pH acts synergistically with low Pa_{O_2} on the pulmonary vascular bed contributing to the pulmonary arterial constriction. Early after birth, oxygen unsaturation is principally produced by extrapulmonary shunting through persistent fetal pathways, and the direction and magnitude of these shunts can be changed drastically by changing the relative resistances in aorta and pulmonary artery.

The pathophysiology of the lung at this stage of the disease is dependent upon the dominant shunt pattern into or away from the lung. In the infant with marked hypovolemia from intrapartum blood loss, systemic hypotension results, and, if corrected with whole blood transfusion, the direction of the ductus shunt-

ing may abruptly become left-to-right. If rapid bicarbonate infusion is given for severe metabolic acidosis, pulmonary resistance may fall and the same net effect result. If high oxygen is suddenly added to the inspired gas mixture of a severely hypoxic infant, a rapid dilatation of the pulmonary vascular bed occurs with a lowering of pulmonary arterial pressure and frequently a rise in aortic pressure. This can be shown during the early phase of the disease to reduce drastically the amount of right-to-left shunting through extrapulmonary pathways and often produces a large left-to-right shunt at the ductus level.[17]

If one studies the pathology of twin lambs with induced HMO, one ventilated in 100% oxygen and the other on room air, with Pa_{CO_2} held constant, striking differences in the appearances of the lungs are seen at autopsy.[18] Both animals have severe hypoxia and metabolic acidosis during life, the oxygen-ventilated one being the more severely affected from birth onward. The animal ventilated with room air has tightly constricted small pulmonary arterioles but the capillary bed still contains blood, as do the veins. The alveolar duct epithelium appears vacuolated in places but has not completely sloughed from its basement membrane, and there is no exudation of fluid into the respiratory bronchiole or alveolar duct airspaces, so that no hyaline membranes are formed. However, there is some patchy alveolar exudation fluid which appears to contain protein. The alveoli are fairly well expanded and no atelectasis is present despite very high lung surface tension measurements, even after 10 hours of ventilation (Fig. 20-3).

In contrast, the lung of the twin who has been ventilated from birth with 100% oxygen has considerable loss of alveolar volume with similar high-surface-tension measurements on lung mince. There is extensive sloughing of alveolar duct and respiratory bronchiolar epithelium with massive exudation of protein-containing fluid into these airspaces and typical hyaline membrane formation. The alveoli themselves, though small in size, do not contain excess fluid; capillaries are extraordinarily dilated, sometimes almost appearing as small aneurysms. Veins and arterioles are likewise dilated. The most striking features of these lungs are

1. the difference in alveolar volume despite similar surface tension.

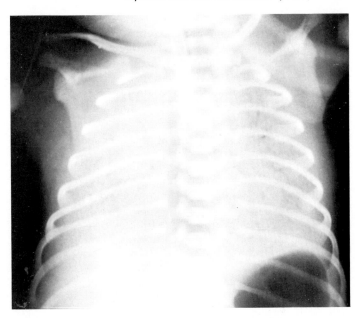

Fig. 20-3. Severe HMD with "white-out" lung fields and very early interstitial emphysema.

2. the massive blood vessel dilatation in the oxygen-treated lung.
3. the absence of slough or exudation forming hyaline membranes in the room-air-treated lung.

If these lungs predict what is happening in the human infant, we can guess that the untreated, acidotic, hypoxic infant in the first hours after birth has "room-air lung" with large right-to-left shunts through extrapulmonary persistent fetal pathways and a relatively clear x-ray picture of the lung. If this abnormal state is abruptly corrected by high oxygen administration, buffering of pH, blood replacement, or the like, in the presence of respiratory bronchiolar and alveolar duct epithelium which has been previously damaged, reversal of the persistent fetal shunting pattern from primarily right-to-left to a large left-to-right shunt, dilatation of the pulmonary vascular bed at all levels and extensive leakage of fluid into alveolar duct and respiratory bronchioles, with a virtual uprooting of cells lining these air spaces, may result. This infant, though temporarily improved with oxygen therapy and buffers, suddenly and rapidly deteriorates with fluid pouring from the trachea. The x-ray film of the lung shows a whiteout and respiration must be supported in some way or the infant will die.

We are thus caught on the horns of a therapeutic dilemma: whether to ignore those abnormalities in physiology and biochemistry from which the infant will die if left untreated, or to knowingly risk massive exudation into the lung. One must try to reach a happy therapeutic medium, correcting hypoxia and acidosis more gradually and in more moderation. It is at this stage of development of the lung pathophysiology in which continuous expiratory pressure (CPAP or CNAP) might best be used, before massive exudation has occurred.[19,20]

Clinical management may be further complicated if hypothermia or hypovolemia are present. As one corrects acidosis and hypothermia, the peripheral vascular bed dilates as well as that of the lung, and any hypovolemia becomes exaggerated by an expanding intravascular volume. Even small blood losses become important because progressive hypotension is common. The judicious use of whole blood transfusion seems proper at this stage if functional or absolute hypovolemia is suspected, again with the risk in mind of further pulmonary exudation.

Early in the course of the disease, severely affected infants may display slightly higher arterial pressures, even when corrected for body size, than the more moderately ill infants, perhaps reflecting the extreme peripheral vasoconstriction which is obvious clinically. Functional hypovolemia can occur as fluid leaks from intravascular to extravascular compartments because of endothelial damage and resultant edema. This extravasation may be promoted by the low serum albumin present in most such infants. Actual hypovolemia can be shown to be present in many of these infants, especially those with a history of maternal vaginal bleeding, placenta abruptio or placenta previa leading to blood loss in which the fetus may participate. It also may be brought about at cesarean section or even at vaginal delivery by positioning the infant above the placental level for some time before cord clamping, so that umbilical arterial perfusion of the placenta continues while umbilical venous return is impeded by hydrostatic pressure. There is some suggestion also that intrapartum asphyxia per se may produce a maldistribution of blood between infant and placenta so that the asphyxiated infant at the time of cord clamping is deprived of an additional volume of blood pooled in the placenta. The prognosis of infants with hypovolemia and HMD is poor. If these infants show systemic hypotension before vasodilatation has been produced with oxygen and buffers, it may be irreversible. However, many infants with initially fairly normal arterial pressure for size may be dangerously hypotensive after vasodilatation, and, if volume replacement is not prompt and quantitative, the prognosis may likewise become grave.

In the more mildly affected infants with respiratory distress, Gluck and coworkers have shown abnormally low levels of phosphatidyl glycerol (PG) and high levels of phosphatidyl inositol (PI) in tracheal effluent similar to patterns found in severe HMD but with intermediate values. Surfactant complex was found in tracheal effluent in the early stages of the disease in about 40% of patients sampled, even with severely affected HMD.[21] These findings are in line with the hypothesis that Type II cell death has occurred, rather than that immaturity alone is responsible for the development of abnormal pulmonary compliance during the height of the disease, and that regeneration of this cell population, as is seen by electron microscopy, is timed with the recovery phase of the disease and the return of normal compliance.

One may speculate that, in mildly and tran-

siently affected infants, cell death has not occurred, but rather that temporary cell malfunction, which may be reversible, is responsible. Those susceptible infants in whom insults go uncorrected for prolonged periods in the neonatal period might reach a critical point of no return, with permanent cell impairment and the typical course of HMD. Early and prompt therapy in such infants who appear to be mildly affected might therefore prevent the development of the full-blown disease in these instances.

Blood Gases and pH (See also Chap. 22)

Arterial blood gases and pH depend both on the stage of the disease and on its severity. In all affected infants, the natural history is one of increasing oxygen requirements for at least 36 to 48 hours, and $F_{I_{O_2}}$s of 50% are often eventually required to maintain Pa_{O_2} at 50 to 70 torr in the aorta. In the more severely affected infants, $F_{I_{O_2}}$ up to 100% may be necessary for adequate blood oxygen levels, even with the use of various types of ventilatory assistance or constant airway pressure. This gradually progressing oxygen requirement is characteristic of HMD and separates it from many of the milder and more transient varieties of neonatal respiratory distress.

Most infants who are not centrally depressed by sedation or birth asphyxia have a normal or even low Pa_{CO_2} (30–40 torr) in the first hours of the disease, when satisfactory ventilation can be achieved by increased respiratory frequency and effort. However, as the disease advances and loss of alveolar volume occurs, ventilatory insufficiency is often reflected by a rising Pa_{CO_2}. The initially depressed infant shows respiratory acidosis of varying degrees from birth onward and may well require early ventilatory assistance.

Arterial pH, even in the vigorous infant, is low (perhaps 7.20–7.30), reflecting metabolic acidosis with normal Pa_{CO_2} and increased base deficit. The latter frequently is in the range of 10 to 15 mmol/liter.* In the depressed infant arterial pH may be lower (between 7.0–7.20 and base deficit 15–20 mmol/liter), but acidosis is of mixed origin, both metabolic and respiratory. In the smallest and sickest infants, usually those suffering from uncorrected se-

---

* 1 mmol = 1 mEq for monovalent ions.

vere birth asphyxia and shock, arterial pH may persist below 7.0 and base deficits reach extremes. These infants rarely survive despite temporarily adequate acid-base correction, and intraventricular hemorrhage is almost always found at autopsy if they are kept alive for over 24 hours.

Other Metabolic Problems

Blood lactic acid levels also reflect the degree of metabolic acidosis. Serum sodium is frequently below 135 mmol/liter initially but may reach high levels if repeated infusions of sodium bicarbonate are used for acid-base correction. Serum calcium is usually 8 to 9 mg/dl initially but falls progressively over the first 72 hours after birth, often to quite low levels. The more immature the infant, the lower the eventual serum calcium level may become. Serum phosphorus may be elevated in the first 3 days, reflecting a catabolic state and poor renal output during this time. Total serum proteins are almost invariably low, even for gestational age, and serum albumin is rarely above 3 g/dl in the severely affected infant. This as well as the frequent occurrence of acidosis may account for the rare incidence of frank tetany. Although jitteriness is common, it is difficult to correlate with serum calcium or glucose levels. Glucose may be low in the first few hours, and in severely asphyxiated infants or infants of diabetic mothers may produce symptoms. Increasing hyperbilirubinemia is common after the first 24 hours and may reach dangerous levels in small premature infants, with low serum albumin and multiple factors such as acidosis, which may change the albumin-binding capacity for bilirubin and indicate need for intervention at a lower level.

Serum potassium is usually normal in the infant who is given acid-base correction and glucose infusion early in the course of the disease but may reach dangerously high levels in those infants in whom persistent acidosis and poor tissue perfusion are allowed to continue, especially in the absence of glucose. Occult hemorrhage into the lung, ventricles or peripheral tissues may account for extremes of hyperkalemia in some infants, as potassium from red cell breakdown enters the intravascular space. Extremes of tissue hypoxia and poor perfusion also may produce hyperkalemia as membrane integrity for maintenance of intracellular potassium is lost. Potassium levels of 7 mmol/liter or above are almost always reflected in ECG changes and associated with a poor prognosis. The electrocardiogram rarely if ever shows the typical peaked T-waves characteristic of hyperkalemia in older patients, but demonstrates an increasing arteriovenous (AV) conduction time. This may progress to very widened conduction complexes and terminate in a sine wave ECG shortly before cardiac arrest. The effects of hyperkalemia noted on the ECG are exaggerated by concomitant hypocalcemia, and are best treated with calcium, glucose, and if necessary, added insulin to facilitate potassium return to the intracellular compartment. After several days of intravenous therapy with glucose, if potassium has not been added, most infants develop low serum potassium levels which may contribute to poor muscle tone, poor ventilatory effort, and ileus. Transient functional ileus is frequently present in these infants, even in the absence of hypokalemia and may temporarily preclude oral feedings. Correction of potassium from either extreme is obviously important for the infant's well-being.

Management (See also Chap. 22)

Successful management of HMD taxes the therapeutic armamentarium of the neonatologist, and many of the necessary procedures are described elsewhere in this book. The infant with HMD is often a desperately ill premature with temporary failure of many vital functions: respiratory exchange, circulation, renal function, alimentation, temperature regulation, and metabolic homeostasis. Table 20-1 serves mainly as a checklist of considerations which should be included in caring for such a baby, and as a cross-reference to other chapters where relevant material is presented.

Complications

Cerebral Hemorrhage. Some infants, especially those of small size (less than 1500 g), who may go through the natural history of severe HMD including the need for CPAP or ventilatory assistance, begin to show clinical pulmonary improvement on the third to fourth day and then suddenly deteriorate. These infants frequently begin to have extensor spasms with eye-rolling, arching of the back, stiffening of the arms and legs, fist-clenching, respiratory arrest, bradycardia, and unresponsiveness. Tremors may occur but frank tonic-clonic

Table 20-1. Management of HMD

1. Verify diagnosis; chest film
2. Stabilize temperature, conserve heat (see Chap. 10)
3. Sample and frequently monitor arterial pH and blood gases
4. Buffer metabolic acidosis with $NaHCO_3$ (see Chap. 29)
5. $F_{I_{O_2}}$ as needed to maintain Pa_{O_2} 60–80 torr
6. Follow blood pressure, hematocrit; transfuse if hematocrit < 45%, falling > 10%, or shocky, hypotensive
7. Special techniques of ventilatory support if $F_{I_{O_2}}$ > 60%, Pa_{O_2} < 50 torr; Pa_{CO_2} > 70; or sustained apnea (see Chap 22) [CPAP, CNAP, IPPB + PEEP, INPB + CNP, etc.]
8. Care of airway, pulmonary toilet (see Chap. 22)
9. Antibiotics (associated pneumonia, catheters, etc.)
10. Nutritional support (see Chap. 42); IV 10% glucose, add electrolytes day 2 or 3
11. Follow serum Na^+, K^+, Cl^-, glucose, and Ca^{++}
12. Observe for complications: pneumothorax, DIC, patent ductus with heart failure, chronic lung disease
13. Other details appropriate to the care of small prematures (see Chap. 14)
14. Exchange transfusion at lower bilirubin levels (high-risk state) (see Chap. 24)

seizures are uncommon. The infant, if ventilation is supported, may survive many days but usually has fixed pupils and semi- or complete coma; signs of peripheral vascular collapse and uncorrectable metabolic acidosis appear progressively. These infants, almost without exception, have large, bilateral intraventricular hemorrhages at autopsy, frequently beginning in the developing vascular bed of the germinal layer lining the posterior portion of the lateral ventricles near the caudate neucleus. Timing of these intraventricular hemorrhages has suggested that they rarely occur in the first 24 hours.[22]

Immaturity of the brain almost surely plays a large role, because such lesions rarely present themselves in premature infants of relatively more advanced gestational age. Episodes of asphyxia *in* or *ex utero,* especially if associated with shock and hypotension, may set the stage for ischemic necrosis of the tissues surrounding the developing vascular bed in the germinal layer. The role of coagulation abnormalities is unclear, although they are common in infants with severe disease.

Smaller hemorrhages into the ventricles may be silent and only picked up on CAT scan of the ventricles, but an increasing number of infants are surviving with diagnosable intraventricular hemorrhage which leads to advancing hydrocephalus, demanding treatment.

Disseminated Intravascular Coagulation (DIC).[23] Most infants with severe HMD have prolonged PT and PTT measurements from birth until clinical improvement is evident. Many also show coagulation factor depression and low platelets characteristic of DIC. However, not all such infants die or show hemorrhagic phenomena, and these coagulation findings are common in severely ill infants with many other types of insults, such as gram-negative or Group B streptococcal sepsis, severe birth asphyxia, hemorrhagic shock, and severe hemolytic disease, resulting primarily from shock and endothelial damage.

Air Leaks and Pneumothorax. The infant whose course has been so severe as to require CPAP with high pressure given by endotracheal tube, assisted ventilation, or both, may suffer from a series of related complications. Dissection of interstitial air following rupture of alveoli may produce large accumulations of multiple compartmented air in the mediastinum. This pneumomediastinum can be so large as to impede venous inflow into the right heart and produce cardiac symptoms. It may rarely dissect into the pericardium and produce tamponade. The most frequent farther dissection is into the pleural space on one or both sides, and this usually causes a rapid deterioration of the infant's status despite assisted ventilation (Figs. 20-4, 20-5).

Pneumothorax is an emergency and requires prompt recognition and localization, and the placement of a large-bore multiple-hole chest tube into the intrapleural space. A small amount of negative pressure is always applied to the chest tube, whose distal end is in an underwater trap. It must also be kept in mind that, with the infant lying supine, pleural air lies anteriorly, where it may be masked by lung thickness. Stiff, fluid-filled lungs, such as those in severe HMD, do not collapse in the

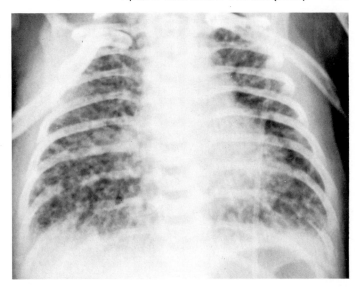

Fig. 20-4. Severe HMD with advanced air dissection (interstitial emphysema). Note bilateral chest tubes which have been placed after pneumothoraces.

same way as a compliant lung does. A cross-table lateral chest film, in addition to an anteroposterior (AP) projection is often helpful in assessing the full extent of pleural versus mediastinal air. The anterior position of the air also is important in the positioning of chest tubes, which frequently have their tips posteriorly and allow air to continue to accumulate anteriorly.

Diffuse collections of interstitial air may collapse alveolar walls containing capillaries, and grossly abnormal ventilation-to-perfusion ratios result. The infant is not only difficult to oxygenate, but Pa_{CO_2} begins to rise. The more pressure is used to ventilate the lung, the more air dissection occurs. This may be lobar in distribution, unilateral or bilateral, or generalized. If diffuse, this is a complication from

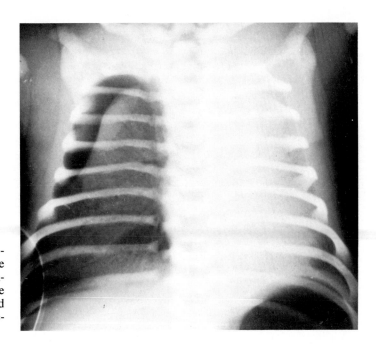

Fig. 20-5. Right tension pneumothorax in a patient with HMD. Note the failure of the stiff and noncompliant lung to collapse despite the tension reflected by widely spaced ribs and bulging interspaces, and mediastinal shift.

which recovery, if it occurs at all, is prolonged and difficult.

Secondary Infection. Another common complication of assisted ventilation or CPAP with endotracheal tube is infection frequently associated with gram-negative organisms such as *Pseudomonas aeruginosa, Aerobactor, Klebsiella,* and *Escherichia coli.* These infections are very difficult to eradicate from a damaged lung and produce a low-grade, chronic pneumonia which further injures an already compromised pulmonary parenchyma. Infection and air dissection, with or without pneumothorax, are responsible for most of the prolonged periods of assisted ventilation, which are necessary in some babies. With these complications, weaning from a respirator or from CPAP becomes protracted, and careful medical and nursing care, including expert pulmonary physical therapy, is essential for survival.

Patent Ductus Arteriosus. One of the common and frequently serious events which complicates the healing stage of HMD is the appearance of heart failure associated with a large left-to-right ductus shunt. By the third day of life most severely ill infants, if carefully observed, have a clearly audible ductus murmur. This does not have the typical diamond-shape sound of a ductus in older children, but is usually low pitched in systole. The higher pitched diastolic component may be difficult to hear until several days have passed. Auscultation of the heart may be made difficult in these infants by the presence of respirators, incubator motors, chest tubes, and ECG leads, but careful daily auscultation is invaluable in picking up these murmurs and anticipating their implications for cardiac and pulmonary function. These infants usually have a gradually increasing basal heart rate and slowly increasing peripheral edema. Descent of the liver is not an early sign. It is at this stage that rapid digitalization and diuresis have their best effect. If therapy is delayed until frank congestive failure has supervened, failure may be irreversible and medically unmanageable. This complication also prolongs the necessity for CPAP or assisted ventilation, and vigorous management is necessary to overcome its adverse effects.

Larger infants (above 1750 g) can usually be conservatively managed with digitalis, diuretics, and fluid restriction, and spontaneous closure will result in a few days. A few ductus will prolong the recovery phase of HMD and a trial of indomethacin may be indicated. Rarely will surgical intervention be indicated. In contrast, many infants of very low birth weight with HMD will have a greatly protracted recovery phase from HMD and may be difficult to extubate or wean from oxygen, despite medical management. It is in this group that early use of indomethacin holds the most promise (see above) and chronic respirator lung disease may be avoided. Surgical closure may also be used if pharmacologic closure does not occur.[24,25]

Pathology

The pathology of the disease is important in understanding its natural history, unmodified by respirator therapy, as well as the healing process and possible sequelae. The initial lesion is one of pulmonary arteriolar vasoconstriction followed by slough of alveolar duct and respiratory bronchiolar lining epithelium. This is followed by an eschar formation in the denuded areas, with fluid containing fibrinogen leaking from adjacent blood vessels, clotting in the presence of tissue thromboplastin and enmeshing the cellular debris in its matrix. With ventilatory effort, this material is deposited around the denuded basement membrane. The replacement of the epithelial lining and the removal of the membrane material are essential for recovery.

The first stage in healing seems to be the migration of new epithelial cells from upper airways still covered with intact epithelium. These cells on electron microscopy have the appearance of rather atypical Type II great alveolar cells, with many lamellar inclusions. The cytoplasm of these cells is often bizarre in shape and crowded with lipid inclusions. It seems likely that a stem cell, capable of mitosis and normally providing the turnover for the population of cells, is stimulated to rapid reproduction and differentiation into Type II cells. Those airways lined with membranes are relined with these cells, which actively invade membrane material and appear to lyse it, possibly by fibrinolytic enzyme release. In some infants, these new Type II cells not only produce large amounts of surface active material but also release it into the airways. In others, the release mechanism may not be operative early in the convalescent course, and cells appear to continue producing many inclusions filled with surfactant, which they are unable to discharge into the alveolar space.

In secondary infection, the effects of chronic high oxygen use, and the mechanical effects of respirators are superimposed on the injured lung, the lung parenchyma appears grossly distorted in its architecture, and many alveoli are obliterated. Capillary obliteration followed by new capillary growth may also appear in the interstitial tissue which becomes filled with proliferating fibroblasts. Dense collagen bands may be laid down around existing open airways, and result in fibrosis. If extra-alveolar dissection of air occurs, false airspaces are created which may be made permanent by epithelialization.

Follow-up

Serious abnormalities in the normal ratio of ventilation-to-perfusion in many areas of the lung result from this sequence of events. Thanks to the growth potential of the newborn lung, even this type of lung pathophysiology may progressively diminish with time because new lung tissue is developed with normal growth. Many infants appearing as pulmonary cripples at discharge from ICNs slowly but progressively improve with time, if they can be kept infection-free. Although clinical episodes resembling bronchiolitis are common in such infants during the first 3 years of life, and although pneumonia is a serious complication on occasion, in most infants symptoms subside progressively with age. What the long-term pulmonary sequelae will be in such infants is unknown at present because intensive care and respirator survival have not been in existence long enough for infants to reach adult life. However, the results thus far are encouraging, even in the seemingly worst survivors, if they live for 1 year. Long-term functional follow-up of this population of infants is mandatory, especially in the face of rapidly changing modes of management which may contribute not only to survival, but to sequelae.

The long-term outlook for the intellectual and neurologic development of these infants is also encouraging, even in those very ill at birth.[26] This may be due in part to the rarity of survival of infants with HMD who also have intraventricular hemorrhage. However, as very immature infants form a greater percentage of the survival population, such as has happened following the introduction of CPAP, more developmental sequelae are becoming apparent in later follow-up. Most infants who have been looked at as long as 4 years approach a normal population. However, perceptual problems do begin to appear in increased frequency as the children reach school age. Genetic and socioeconomic factors seem to play a significant role in the child's eventual developmental achievement, as judged by siblings' development and parental educational and achievement background.

Prevention

The ultimate goal of therapy is prevention. We hope to have eventually at our disposal agents that are safe and capable of prematurely maturing the lung *in utero* to a point at which susceptibility to HMD is markedly reduced. The results of Liggins' controlled trial of glucocorticoid administration to women of less than 37-weeks' gestation in premature labor, in whom labor could be stopped for 48 hours, are encouraging.[9] The use of L/S ratios in amniotic fluid as a guide to the timing of elective cesarean section or induction of labor is also an important preventive. Important, also, is avoidance of situations which compromise the pulmonary circulation in the fetus or newborn, such as maternal hypotension, oversedation, maternal hypoxia or hypercapnia, fetal asphyxia without prompt delivery, delayed resuscitation, uncorrected acidosis or hypoxia, hypothermia and hypovolemia. This requries continued exercise of obstetrical and pediatric judgment, especially in those pregnancies at high risk, good nursing care, and availability of techniques and personnel capable of immediate handling of emergency situations. The regionalization of facilities for the care of high-risk pregnancies, deliveries and newborns is a rational approach toward providing this kind of preventive medicine to many of the patients at risk. Those unanticipated risk deliveries which cannot be carried out in a facility capable of handling a desperately ill infant must have access to an immediate transport system to an intensive care nursery. The further development of this philosophy of prevention, anticipation and prompt management will pay rich dividends in the future.

Table 20-2. Comparison of HMD and Type II RDS

Hyaline Membrane Disease	Type II Respiratory Distress
Premature, AGA	AGA premature near term
Frequent perinatal distress	Maternal oversedation
Decreased surfactant	Aspiration
Widespread atelectasis	Delayed absorption of lung fluid
Tachypnea	Tachypnea
Retractions	Retractions
Grunting	Grunting
Cyanosis	Cyanosis
Chest film: diffuse reticulo- granularity with air-bronchogram	Chest film: hyperaeration with heavy central markings
Progressive O_2 requirement for 2–3 days	Variable O_2 requirement easily hyperoxygenated
Early pulmonary hypoperfusion: shunting common	Significant extrapulmonary shunting uncommon
Hypovolemia common	Hypovolemia rare
Ventilatory assistance often needed	Ventilatory assistance rarely needed
Mortality 20–50%	Most infants survive

TYPE II RESPIRATORY DISTRESS SYNDROME (RDS)

There are many newborn infants with progressive respiratory distress in the first 24 to 48 hours after birth who, by the strict criteria presented in the section on HMD, clearly do not have that disease, but bear many resemblances to it. When critically observed, they have many distinguishing features, a different natural history, and a far more sanguine outlook (Table 20-2). This disorder has been called Type II RDS,[27] aspiration syndrome, and disseminated atelectasis by various authors. Transient tachypnea of the newborn, as originally described, is probably of different etiology.

Predisposed Group

These infants often are large prematures approaching term gestation. The most common feature of the maternal history is heavy medication with analgesics during labor which may or may not be followed by general anesthesia during delivery. Occasionally, there is no such history, but rather some episode which might be associated with intrauterine or intrapartum asphyxia, such as cesarean section, maternal bleeding, prolapsed cord, or maternal diabetes. Most are between 2000 and 3000 g birth weight and show some physical evidence of immaturity. If one excludes IDMs, the infants are appropriately grown for their gestational age. They do not show chronic placental insufficiency as evidenced by being small-for-gestational-age, peeling skin, loss of vernix, or meconium staining of skin, cord, or nails.

Pathogenesis

The most striking historical facts are those of heavy maternal sedation and intrapartum depression in relatively immature infants, resulting in failure to clear the airway of mucus and other accumulated debris. This, combined with the clinical and radiologic findings, strongly suggests lower airway obstruction of a ball-valve type, and overdistention of distal alveoli.

The moderately depressed infant, despite initial suctioning, has depressed gagging, swallowing, and coughing reflexes, and may pool

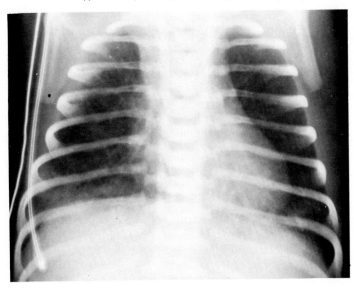

Fig. 20-6. Type II RDS, illustrating hyperaeration of the periphery, with heavy central markings of both lung fields.

secretions in the hypopharynx or tracheo-bronchial tree for many hours after birth. This is especially true if he is assumed to be "normal" at birth and is not carefully nursed until reactive. Added to this, there may be delay in the transitional circulatory pattern for several hours until the infant corrects his birth asphyxia. The removal of the normal intrauterine lung fluid by lymphatics may also be delayed by the same mechanisms.

Clinical Course

Many infants present the typical picture of oversedation: good condition at the moment of birth without evidence of asphyxia, and a good initial Apgar score; cold, tactile, auditory, and, occasionally, painful stimuli keep the infant alert temporarily. When left alone and unstimulated, the infants rapidly become somnolent, may hypoventilate, and have depression of cough, gag, and swallowing reflexes with resulting aspiration.

In the first few hours after birth, frequently by the time they reach the nursery, they can be observed to have abnormal respiratory patterns, and most will begin to grunt promptly. The degree of retraction depends on the extent of the disease and on the maturity of the infant, because the stability of the chest cage increases with gestational age. Flaring of the alae nasae occurs with the onset of the respiratory symp-

toms. Respiratory rates may be normal or even depressed immediately after birth, but, by 6 hours, tachypnea has appeared and may reach extreme rates of 100 to 140/minute. Most infants show visible cyanosis in room air, and supplemental oxygen is required to keep arterial P_{O_2}s within normal limits.

These infants usually have 24 to 96 hours of respiratory distress, during which time oxygen requirements may go as high as 70%. Grunting and retraction may last 24 to 48 hours, and tachypnea is usually the last sign of distress to disappear. Most infants are edematous, relatively oliguric, and have mild functional intestinal ileus, which precludes feeding for 1 to 2 days.

On auscultation, the chest is clear of rales and heart sounds are often distant.

Another striking difference between these infants and those with HMD is their response to hyperoxia. Babies with Type II RDS can be hyperoxygenated in a 100% O_2 environment throughout the course of their disease. Although they may require increasing amounts of oxygen for 1 to 2 days, they usually can be well oxygenated at all times, and oxygen requirements frequently decline rather than increase over the first 48 hours (Fig. 20-6).

Early in the course of their disease, many infants show significant acidosis, which is both metabolic and respiratory in origin. This is reflected by low arterial pH, an elevated base deficit of perhaps 7 to 15 mmol/liter, and a moderately elevated P_{CO_2}. Initial correction of base deficit is usually all that is required for maintenance of normal acid-base balance thereafter. Although respiratory symptoms persist, compensation is usually adequate.

Significant shunting of blood either right-to-left or left-to-right through the ductus arteriosus has not been found, nor do large foramen ovale shunts persist, as in HMD. Systemic hypotension is rare.

X-ray Findings

Initial chest films at less than 6 hours may not be grossly abnormal, except for suggestive increases in bronchovascular markings. By 12 hours after birth, there is usually clear evidence of heavy central markings, exaggerated by a peripheral increased radiolucency. Diffuse overexpansion of the lung fields may also be evidenced by increased AP diameter to the chest as seen on a lateral film of the chest, bulging of intercostal spaces, and, occasionally, flattening of the diaphragm. A prominent thymic shadow is often present. The heavy bronchovascular markings usually persist for 3 to 4 days after birth, but overexpansion may last for a week. Patchy pulmonary infiltrates may be present for several days in some infants. The lobar fissure between right upper and right middle lobes is frequently visualized in early films, and, occasionally, a small amount of fluid is seen in the pleural cavity.

Therapy

In some instances this disease is probably preventable. The excessive use of maternal analgesics, which are depressant to the central nervous system, should be avoided. This is especially important in high-risk pregnancies.

Attention to the details of resuscitation at delivery and careful nursing care thereafter minimize the disease process. The maintenance of adequate oxygenation without risking the dangers of overoxygenation sometimes becomes a therapeutic problem and, in immature infants with persistent respiratory distress, may justify aortic catheterization for monitoring purposes. Many infants, however, can be monitored with radial or temporal sampling once or twice a day and buffered and oxygenated on the basis of these findings. The administration of enough sodium bicarbonate

solution to raise the infant's buffer capacity 5 mmol/liter of body water is usually desirable even in the absence of pH measurements. Repeated buffering is rarely necessary. The parenteral administration of calories and fluid in the form of glucose solution is advisable, especially with very rapid respiratory rates, and in the face of lowered gut motility. Oral feedings may be initiated slowly as symptoms subside.

The primary importance of recognizing infants with Type II RDS as a distinct disease entity is its differentiation from HMD because the prognosis is excellent, and overzealous treatment is unnecessary. The inclusion of these infants in mortality statistics and therapeutic trials of HMD has led to confusion in the past and should be avoided.

INTRAUTERINE ASPIRATION PNEUMONIA (Massive Aspiration Syndrome, Meconium Aspiration Pneumonia)

The presence of meconium in the amniotic fluid is regarded as abnormal, and both the obstetrician and pediatrician must be alerted to possible fetal or neonatal complications. Although many infants whose amniotic fluid has contained meconium at delivery are completely normal at the time of birth, one can be confident that some episode of asphyxia, however brief, has occurred, inducing the passage of meconium. The ease with which meconium is passed *in utero* seems to progress with gestational age, so that a meconium-stained premature or even term infant may well have had a more severe insult than a comparable post-term infant. It is unusual for very immature infants, even under extremes of asphyxia, to have peristalsis and a relaxed anal sphincter. Although the appearance of meconium is regarded by many as normal in breech deliveries, this attitude should not mask the possibility of its induction by asphyxia. Indeed, severe asphyxia is commonly associated with breech deliveries, especially in large babies whose delivery may be mechanically difficult.

The passage of meconium, either *in utero* or intrapartum, always presents the opportunity for its aspiration into the tracheobronchial tree, especially with repeated episodes of severe asphyxia which induce forceful, "terminal-type" gasping. The infant who has chronic placental insufficiency also has lost his vernix, some of which may be floating in the amniotic fluid with his peeling, keratinized skin. The presence in aspirated amniotic fluid of layers of keratinized squamous cells, vernix, and old meconium produces the severest form of massive aspiration syndrome or meconium aspiration pneumonia. This type of infant has surely suffered from chronic *in utero* asphyxia and malnutrition and, if required to deliver from below, may die intrapartum or in the neonatal period. The Apgar score is usually very low, and resuscitation must be prompt, vigorous, and expertly done. The amniotic fluid, which may have the appearance and consistency of pea soup, fills the oropharynx and tracheobronchial tree. Prior to the initiation of air breathing it must be mechanically removed by careful suction, best done under direct vision with an infant laryngoscope. The amniotic content of meconium, vernix and squamous cells may already be packed into terminal airways and impossible to remove, so that, with the introduction of air, it may enter some alveoli, fail to enter others, and have a ball-valve effect on others.

Rupture of alveoli and air dissection into the mediastinum or pleural cavity is common both during and following resuscitation, and must be promptly recognized. Assisted ventilation is frequently needed from the delivery room onward because many not only have severe ventilatory difficulties but are centrally depressed as well.

These infants may appear long and thin, with hanging folds of skin about the knees, buttocks and axillary creases. Little evidence of subcutaneous fat remains, although clearly the infant was fatter at some prior time. The eyes are frequently wide open, and the area between the eyebrows is furrowed longitudinally giving the baby a characteristic worried appearance. The nails, cord, and skin are stained with yellowish pigment. Often the cord has little Wharton's jelly and appears thin. The skin is more keratinized than usual, vernix is absent, and there may be extensive peeling. The chest may appear hyperinflated, and rales and ronchi are common. In such severely affected infants, metabolic as well as respiratory acidosis is present, often extreme, and sodium bicarbonate or THAM is needed for correction. Oxygenation is often poor, with very low Pa_{O_2}s despite 100% oxygen inhala-

tion, as a result of large intrapulmonary shunts and of the persistence of fetal patterns of shunting through the ductus arteriosus and foramen ovale. The chest film shows patchy densities interspersed with radiolucence, which may represent overinflation in some areas (Fig. 20-7).

Treatment

Treatment largely is symptomatic because the infant's pulmonary defenses are mobilized to clear the particulate foreign material by ciliary motion, phagocytosis, enzymatic lysis and, perhaps, eventual fibrosis in some areas. Vigorous pulmonary physical therapy is indicated on a frequent schedule if air dissection has not occurred, and pulmonary lavage has been suggested in extreme instances. Corticosteroid administration has been used with reported good results in uncontrolled series. Steroids may minimize airway inflammation because of presence of foreign material, and may relieve central depression from brain swelling produced by the extreme asphyxia. Antibiotics are indicated to prevent the frequent complication of secondary bacterial pneumonia, especially if steroids are used. Assisted ventilation may be needed for many days and carries a risk of air dissection. Mortality is high in those infants so severely affected as to need a respirator, and in those with seizures. Hypoglycemia, often severe and persistent, is a frequent occurrence in these chronically malnourished infants and may contribute to CNS problems. Careful nursing and the physician's care and attention to detail are necessary for survival. Neurologic sequelae are not uncommon.

OTHER ASPIRATION SYNDROMES

Some infants who have passed meconium intrapartum are severely asphyxiated at birth but have not prolonged *in utero* placental insufficiency. Their meconium staining is dark green rather than yellow. These infants are not malnourished; they may even be preterm, but this is unusual. Some suffer from severe aspiration pneumonia with all the chest findings and complications of the post-term infant. However, many infants who have clearly aspirated meconium at birth are not nearly so severely affected. Although their chest films may look remarkably abnormal, their respi-

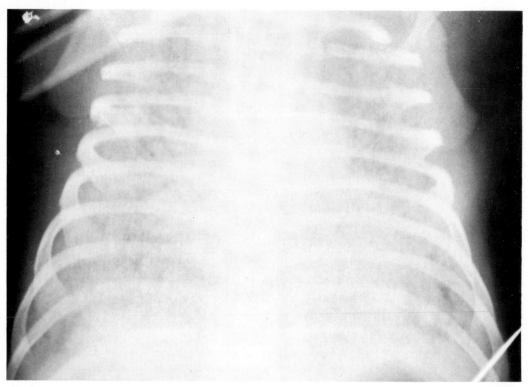

Fig. 20-7. Severe meconium aspiration syndrome, showing shaggy heart border and irregular densities throughout both lungs, and having a wooly quality in this patient.

ratory distress may be mild and transient. Unless complications such as pneumothorax occur, mildly affected infants may need only supportive therapy in the form of supplemental oxygen, fluids, and glucose; initial buffering of pH, and careful nursing care. Their prognoses, if their courses have not been associated with seizures are usually excellent.

Postnatal aspiration of regurgitated feedings is common, especially in small, weak prematures who may be gavage-fed amounts exceeding their capacity. Such aspiration is capable of causing acute apnea with airway obstruction, respiratory distress, and secondary pneumonia. If aspiration, especially of milk curds, is sudden and overwhelming, it may be immediately fatal in the small infant whose cough reflex is poor. Most infants recover if adequately suctioned, although this may require laryngoscopy and direct visualizing of the airway. Those in whom stomach contents have reached the lung may show subsequent signs of respiratory distress with tachypnea, rales, and x-ray evidence of infil-

trates or localized atelectasis. Supportive therapy is usually all that is necessary, and gradual improvement occurs over a 3- or 4-day period.

INFECTIONS OF THE NEWBORN LUNG (See also Chap. 32)

Intrapartum Pneumonia

The introduction of bacteria into the fetal lung may occur *in utero* as the result of infection of the fetal membranes, almost exclusively associated with their rupture more than 12 hours before delivery of the infant. Blood-borne infection across the placenta may also affect the fetal lung secondary to sepsis. On occasion the infant may be unlucky enough to aspirate maternal fecal contents at delivery which may also introduce bacteria into the lung.

Infants with intrauterine pulmonary infection usually show signs of generalized illness from birth onward, often including pneumonia which is widespread and severe. Symptoms of intrapartum infection, however, may be delayed for hours or even 1 or 2 days because aspiration of infected amniotic fluid or fecal contamination may take place during the delivery process, and an incubation period may interpose before overt infection appears. It is therefore reasonable to suspect infants of latent infection for several days when they have been in a possibly contaminated environment. Cultures of skin before bathing (the ear is an untouched area), nasal cavity, and deep oral pharynx may show organisms. Aspiration of the stomach contents for culture and a smear for increased numbers of polymorphonuclear leukocytes and bacteria may support the possibility of bacterial pneumonia in a newborn with respiratory distress. Blood, spinal fluid, and urine may grow organisms in the case of generalized bacterial sepsis with pneumonia, and a smear of the spinal fluid may give early evidence of which organism is involved.

Sepsis and pneumonia are always suspected in the infant whose amniotic fluid is either purulent or foul smelling, or whose mother is febrile either before or after delivery without other demonstrable infection than amnionitis. Prolonged rupture of the membranes alone does not demand immediate treatment. However, neonatal sepsis with pneumonia is a severe and often rapidly fatal illness, and prompt therapy should be given in all reasonably suspect instances. *Pseudomanas, Aerobacteraerogenes,* and *Klebsiella pneumoniae,* along with the *E. coli,* have been, until recently, the most frequent causes of intrauterine or intrapartum sepsis and pneumonia. In recent years, neonatal infection with Group B, β-hemolytic streptococci has assumed a leading role in the morbidity and mortality of infectious origin in the newborn period. These organisms now occur apparently as saprophytes in the vaginal and rectal flora of many parturient women, rarely causing overt symptoms in the mother. The fetus may be infected *in utero,* apparently even with intact membranes, but more commonly with early rupture, and evidence of fetal tachycardia and loss of variability and heart rate pattern during labor may reflect fetal reaction to sepsis. In these cases, systemic symptoms may be present at birth. Often, however, organisms appear to have been acquired by the fetus during the passage through the birth canal, and an interval of a few hours may lapse before symptoms appear.

Often these infants, if preterm, may appear indistinguishable from those with other types of respiratory distress such as HMD. They grunt on expiration, have retraction of sternum and infracostal region, and demonstrate varying degrees of cyanosis, arterial oxygen unsaturation, and CO_2 retention, depending on the stage and severity of the illness. The x-ray in the pre-term infant may present as that of severe HMD, or a white-out, and it is probable that the two conditions coincide in many instances. In infants near term, the x-ray is more likely to show patchy infiltrates more typical of a localized pneumonic process, often with pleural or septal fluid early on, and will only later appear generalized. In those instances of severe generalized pulmonary involvement, sepsis is almost invariably present, and a shock-like syndrome may appear. Recurrent episodes of apnea, followed by cardiovascular collapse, profound hypoxemia, and a persistent transitional circulatory pattern are ominous prognostic signs. A low polymorphonuclear count is common in more severely affected infants, and metabolic acidosis may be profound. The mortality in infants who advance to cardiovascular collapse is high, and a frequent complication is DIC associated with signs of cardiovascular collapse and bleeding. The site of bleeding may be the lung, gastrointestinal tract, skin, vagina, or CNS.

Penicillin is the drug of choice in infants with Group B streptococcal disease, but infants may die in shock after bacterial sterilization has been accomplished. The presence of a specific bacterial toxin has been postulated.

More mildly affected infants may have a much more benign course and lower mortality. Meningitis is a complication in a few newborns with this organism, although it is a more frequent presenting sign in infants past the neonatal period.

Infants with gram-negative sepsis and pneumonia may also have cardiopulmonary symptoms and signs similar to HMD, or present in septic shock. DIC is also a frequent complication, with the possibility of multiple bleeding sites. Specific antibiotic therapy is indicated, depending on the sensitivity of the organism. When septic shock appears from any cause, symptomatic management with plasma expanders, whole blood, ventilatory assistance, IV buffers and other supportive measures are indicated. The mortality remains high in this group of infants.

Nursery-acquired Pneumonia

Nursery-acquired neonatal infection of the lungs is frequently of a different type. Ordinary pathogens such as coagulase-positive staphylococci and group A streptococci are frequently involved, although *E. coli* sepsis and pneumonia also appear as postnatal diseases. These infections are most frequently carried by handlers—from other infants with skin infection such as staphylococcal pustules or impetigo neonatorum caused by β-hemolytic streptococci, or the fulminant "scalded skin" syndrome of highly pathogenic staphylococcal origin. In these cases, pneumonia is usually a secondary phenomenon to primary disease elsewhere and commonly associated with septicemia. The cord stump or circumcision wound are frequent primary sites of purulent infection.

Chest films in staphylococcal pneumonia frequently show consolidation in a lobar distribution and may be extensive, involving parts of one or both lungs. Pleural fluid may accumulate and, if it is in large enough amounts to cause lung compression, may require evacuation. The appearance of pneumatocoeles, often multiple, is common and should not be confused with abscess formation because they are thin-walled and contain only air, and do not present air-fluid levels. They may rupture spontaneously and cause pneumothorax, but otherwise are treated conservatively because they regress completely as the disease process heals. Streptococcal and gram-negative pneumonias are more likely to be widely distributed throughout both lungs, without lobar localization. Their resolution appears complete and without pulmonary sequelae if the infant survives. By contrast, *E. coli* pneumonia is often of insidious onset in an infant of several days of age, with poor feeding, hyper-, or more frequently, hypothermia, jaundice, anemia, and lethargy. Sepsis is the origin of the pulmonary seeding of infection in these cases, the primary site of entry often being the cord stump, circumcision or gastrointestinal tract. Meningitis is common as is secondary hemorrhage, often associated with DIC, and mortality is high.

All of these nursery-acquired infections are best prevented by scrupulous handwashing technique, uncontaminated water, and milk supplies, and individual isolation nursing of each infant. Careful and early observation of minor signs and symptoms may allow early diagnosis, prompt culturing and treatment with specific antibiotics if sensitivities of the organisms are known. Supportive therapy is important, and may include parenteral fluids and buffers, blood transfusion for anemia and exchange transfusions for hyperbilirubinemia, supplemental oxygen, and, in some instances, respirator therapy for apnea. Only with the most vigorous therapeutic approach will these infants survive intact.

Pneumonia Associated with Respiratory Equipment

Another kind of nursery-acquired infection occurs in those infants who are chronically supported by respirators or other techniques, such as CPAP, which utilize prolonged endotracheal intubation. These are secondary, low-grade, chronic pneumonnias from organisms normally considered saprophytic and ubiquitous, such as *Psuedomonas aeruginosa, Alcaligenes,* and *Kelbsiella.* These organisms are frequently water-borne from humidifiers, suction catheters, and other equipment. Endotracheal tube suction material is cultured daily to identify as early as possible the appearance of organisms. Once established, however, their eradication is almost impossible, despite long-term antibiotic therapy with drugs chosen for organism sensitivity. The problems of respiratory care are intensely magnified by this complication because of increased tenacious secretions, with atelectasis or tube occlusion being common occurrences. Vigorous pulmonary physical therapy is mandatory. Much of the chronic respirator lung syndrome, with its high mortality and its long-term pulmonary disability is associated with this disastrous type of secondary infection.

Other Organisms

Viral agents such as the parainfluenza group occasionally have been identified in neonatal pneumonia, but their role even in these instances is somewhat questionable. Pneumonic involvement may also occur with cytomegalic inclusion disease. Spirochetal pneumonia may occur with congenital syphilis, but it is a rare disease in the United States at present. Intrauterine infection with Toxoplasma parasites may also occur, and, rarely, widespread fatal pneumonia results. Other protozoan organisms such as *Pneumocystis carinii,* are occasionally found in chronic pneumonias, but are rare in the United States. Insidious pneumonia caused by chlamydial infection is described in Chapter 32.

PULMONARY HEMORRHAGE IN THE NEWBORN

Pulmonary hemorrhage in the newborn continues to be an enigma. The occurrence of localized extravasations of blood into alveoli is a frequent, almost incidental finding at autopsy, but a massive generalized pulmonary hemorrhage may be a terminal event. Its isolated occurrence without other underlying disease processes is rare, if one looks carefully at intrauterine, intrapartum and neonatal events. Commonly, it is found as a complication of a more generalized disorder, such as bacterial pneumonia, sepsis, hemolytic disease of the newborn, kernicterus, CNS hemorrhage, congenital heart disease with a large left-to-right shunt, or placental insufficiency syndromes associated with intrauterine malnutrition and hypoglycemia. It may appear as a sudden isolated catastrophic hemorrhage, or may, in certain instances, such as infection or kernicterus, be associated with a more generalized bleeding diathesis. In some instances of severe intrapartum asphyxia such as placental abruption, pulmonary hemorrhage may be present at birth. In many of these cases, there are clotting abnormalities, sometimes related to second-stage clotting factors alone, and, in other instances, associated with evidence of DIC.

An infant may present during the course of one of these disorders with sudden and severe respiratory distress, and fresh blood is suctioned from the trachea. Ventilatory assistance is usually mandatory for survival, but the bleeding, if profuse, is rapidly fatal. Fresh whole blood transfusions, or a partial exchange transfusion with fresh whole blood, seems to offer the best approach toward treatment, coupled with vigorous management of the underlying disease. Identification of any abnormalities in clotting mechanisms may be helpful in guiding overall therapy.

The sudden and massive dilatation of the pulmonary capillary bed associated with reversal of fetal ductus shunts and lowering of pulmonary vascular resistance wtih oxygen therapy in a previously vasoconstricted newborn may contribute to the lung being selected as a target organ. A better understanding of the mechanisms involved in control of pulmonary blood vessel tone—arterial, capillary, and venous—as well as an understanding of clotting disorders in the newborn, is essential to any future approach toward prevention.

PNEUMOTHORAX, PNEUMOMEDIASTINUM, AND INTERSTITIAL EMPHYSEMA

Pathophysiology

The dissection of air from the normal alveolar compartments may be one of the most serious complications occurring in the newborn infant. It is seldom a spontaneous occurrence and only rarely appears in an infant without previous underlying pulmonary pathology. When it does occur with a normal lung, it is usually iatrogenic from the use of excessive airway pressures in resuscitation of a depressed infant, at a time when the newborn lung is still fluid-filled. When it occurs spontaneously, it is usually associated with severe underlying pulmonary pathology, either of the obstructive variety, such as with meconium aspiration in which ball-valve air trapping may occur, or with those diseases associated with poor lung compliance. In the latter, such as with HMD, enormous negative intrapleural pressures are created by the infant as he attempts to maintain alveolar ventilation, and grunting produces positive intraalveolar pressures with expiration. Bouts of hard crying with Valsalva maneuvers often precede air dissection in such circumstances.

The most frequent antecedent to air dissection is the use of respirators or continuous positive airway pressure breathing. The creation of sudden high airway pressure gradients across the alveoli, either with positive- or negative-pressure respirators, with very stiff lungs is likely to cause rupture. This is especially true if the infant is struggling against the respirator and breathing or crying out of phase with its cycle. The use of continuous positive- or negative-airway pressure likewise is a hazard for air dissection, especially if the popoff valve is set at a substantially higher pressure than the constant pressure intended, or if kinking of the tubing produces very high pressure inadvertently.

The difficulty of pulmonary toilet in infants with endotracheal tubes in place exaggerates these risks because complete obstruction of some airways and ball-valve obstruction of others may develop secondarily. The most meticulous and experienced physician and nursing care is mandatory in units prepared to assume the responsibilities of respirator or CPAP use if iatrogenic disasters are to be minimized.

Clinical Presentation

The dissection of air from the alveoli frequently follows the tracheobronchial tree and blood vessels retrograde into the loose alveolar tissue in the anterior mediastinum. Here it may be visualized only as a rim of radiolucence around the heart. If the collection is small, it remains asymptomatic. However, large collections of mediastinal air may compress the heart and lungs and venous return to the right heart may be compromised. A typical "sail sign," or visualization of sharp lower edges of the thymus surrounded by air, is diagnostic. The dissection of air, if massive, may reach the pericardium, producing tamponade, and may dissect beneath the parietal pleura, especially well visualized over the diaphragm. A cross-table lateral chest film usually demonstrates the extent of air accumulation better than a lateral with the infant turned on his side. This is especially true if the air dissection breaks out into the pleural space on one or both sides. This occurrence may be unaccompanied by a dramatic change in the clinical status of the baby, if the pneumothorax is not under tension, but usually it is a catastrophic and life-threatening event. One cannot always judge the degree of tension present by mediastinal shift or lung collapse on the film because stiff lungs, such as with severe HMD, may not collapse toward the hilum even under enormous pressure.

The prompt placement of a large bore, multiple-holed chest tube, preferably into the pleural space anterior to the lung rather than posterior, is a medical emergency. This should be accompanied by an underwater trap and about 9 to 10 cm water constant negative pressure because reaccumulation of air in a newborn may readily occur even at low levels of submersion of the chest-tube extension, if suction is not applied. The ease with which the lung can be reexpanded depends to a large extent upon underlying pathology. The absence of normal alveolar surface forces with such entities as HMD promotes collapse. Chest tubes can usually be safely removed once the lung is reexpanded and fluctuation of fluid in the submerged tubing and active bubbling ceases for at least 24 hours. With large pulmonary rents, this may take a number of days, and, on rare occasions, surgical plication is necessary.

Interstitial Emphysema

Another omnious site for widespread air dissection is into the perivascular and peribronchial spaces, which on careful microscopic examination appear to be lymphatic channels. This type of disseminated interstitial air seems limited to those infants on positive-pressure respirators, or consant distending airway pressure, who have extremely poor lung compliance. The distribution is occasionally lobar or even lobular, but is frequently generalized and bilateral. The ability to oxygenate the infant, even with high pressure and high $F_{I_{O_2}}$s, is markedly diminished, and CO_2 retention is common. The outcome is frequently fatal, especially if both lungs are involved. Occasionally, an infant is kept alive for many days or even weeks after x-ray appearance of diffuse interstitial air, and, at autopsy, one can identify large cuboidal cells, occasionally multinucleated, invading these false airspaces and creating a new lining epithelial membrane. On electron microscopy these cells appear to be Type II alveolar cells. If, as seems likely, these false airspaces are lymphatic channels, one can speculate that fluid homeostasis in the lung is grossly distorted by this process because most water absorption from the lung is into lymphatics. If the distribution of air is lobar, eventual lobar emphysema may result and be resectable. But if interstitial emphysema is generalized and severe, no specific therapy seems helpful.

REFERENCES

1. **Arey LB:** Developmental Anatomy, 8th ed. 1965
2. **Farrell PM, Hamosh M:** Clin in Perinatol 5(2): 197, 1978
3. **Epstein MF, Farrell PM:** The choline incorporation pathway: Primary mechanism for *de novo* lecithin synthesis in fetal primate lung. Pediatr Res 9:658, 1975

4. **Wykle RL, Malone B, Synder F:** Biosynthesis of dipalmitoyl-sn-glycero-3-phosphocholine by adenoma alveolar type II cells. Arch Biochem Biophys 181:249, 1977

5. **Engle MJ, Saunders RL, Longmore WS:** Phospholipid composition and acyltransferase activity of lamellar bodies isolated from rat lung. Arch Biochem Biophys 173:586, 1976

6. **Gluck L, Kulovich M, Borer RC, et al:** Diagnosis of the respiratory distress syndrome by amniocentesis. Am J Obstet Gynecol 109:440, 1971

7. **Hallman M, Kulovich M, Kirkpatrick E, Sugarman RG, Gluck L:** Phosphatidylinositol and phosphatidylglycerol in amniotic fluid: Indices of lung maturity. Am J Obstet Gynecol 125:613, 1976

8. **Liggins GC:** Premature parturition after infusion of corticotrophin or cortisol into fetal lambs. J Endocrinol 45:515, 1969

9. **Liggins CG, Howie RN:** A controlled trial of antepartum glucocorticoid treatment for prevention of the respiratory distress syndrome in premature infants. Pediatrics 50:515, 1972

10. **Fargier P, Salle B, Band M, et al:** Prevention du syndrome de detresse respiratoire chez le premature. Nouv Presse Med 3:1595, 1974

11. **Caspi E, Schreyer P, Weintraub Z, et al:** Prevention of the respiratory distress syndrome in premature infants by antepartum glucocorticoid therapy. Br J Obstet Gynecol 83:187, 1976

12. **Horvath I, Mehes K, Fias E, et al:** Prevention of respiratory distress syndrome by antenatal maternal steroid treatment. Acta Paediatr Acad Sci Hung 17:303, 1976

13. **Ballard P, Benson B, Brehier A:** Glucocorticoid effects in the fetal lung. Am Rev Resp Dis 115(Suppl.):29, 1977

14. **Block MF, Kling OR, Crosby WM:** Antenatal glucocorticoid therapy for the prevention of respiratry distress syndrome in the premature infant. Obstet Gynecol 50:186, 1977

15. **Stahlman MT:** Perinatal circulation. Pediatr Clin N Amer 13:753, 1966

16. **Usher RH:** Clinical implications of perinatal mortality statistics. Clin Obstet Gynecol 14:885, 1971

17. **Stahlman MT, Blankenship W, Shepard F, et al:** Circulatory studies in clinical hyaline membrane disease. Biol Neonate 20:300, 1972

18. **Raye J, Gutberlet R, Faxelius G, et al:** Pulmonary pathology in lambs with hyaline membrane disease ventilated with air and 100% oxygen (abstr). Pediatr Res 4:469, 1970

19. **Gregory GH, Kitterman JA, Phibbs RH, et al:** Treatment of the idiopathic respiratory distress syndrome with continuous airway pressure. N Engl J Med 284:1333, 1971

20. **Chernick V, Vidyasogar D:** Continuous negative chest wall pressure in HMD, a 1 yr. experience. Pediatrics 49:753, 1972

21. **Hallman M, Feldman BH, Kirkpatrick E, Gluck L:** Absence of phosphatidylglycerol (PG) in respiratory distress syndrome in the newborn: Study of the minor surfactant phospholipids in newborns. Pediatr Res 11:714, 1977

22. **Tsiantos A, Victorin L, Relier JP, et al:** Intracranial hemorrhage in the prematurely born infant: Timing of clots and evaluation of clinical signs and symptoms. J Pediatr 6:843, 1974

23. **Altstatt L, Dennis L, Sundell H, et al:** The relation of disseminated intravascular coagulation to hyaline membrane disease. Biol Neonate 19:227, 1971

24. **Cotton RB, Stahlman MT, Kover I, Catterton WZ:** Medical management of small pre-term infants with symptomatic patent ductus arteriosus. J Pediatr 92:467, 1978

25. **Cotton RB, Stahlman MT, Bender HW, Graham TP, Catterton WZ, Kovar I:** Randomized trial of early closure of symptomatic patent ductus arteriosus in small preterm infants. J Pediatrics 93:647, 1978

26. **Stahlman M, Hedvall G, Dolanski E, et al:** A six-year follow-up of clinical hyaline membrane disease. Pediatr Clin N Amer 20:433, 1973

27. **Sundell H, Garrott J, Blankenship W, et al:** Studies on infants with type II respiratory distress syndrome. J Pediatr 78:754, 1971

21

Chronic Lung Disorders

Joan E. Hodgman

INTRODUCTION

When use of assisted ventilation for newborn infants became widespread during the decade of 1965 to 1975, chronic pulmonary disease in the nursery population became more common and more severe. Before the use of ventilators, chronic pulmonary disease had been described as of insidious onset in immature infants.[1] Following the introduction of ventilatory assistance, chronic pulmonary disease became primarily limited to infants receiving assisted ventilation.[2] Since 1975, the incidence of chronic pulmonary disease following ventilatory support appears to have decreased in larger infants, but remains significant in very immature infants.[3]

The major problems in this area can be summarized as follows:

1. The accurate definition of BPD and its etiologic relationship to ventilatory therapy
2. The chronic effects of acute pulmonary disease on structure and function in surviving infants
3. The role of the immature lung in producing chronic pulmonary disease of poorly defined etiology such as chronic pulmonary insufficiency of the premature and Wilson–Mikity syndrome

BRONCHOPULMONARY DYSPLASIA (BPD)

This descriptive term was first applied by Northway, Rosan, and Potter to a disease process occurring in infants during respiratory therapy for acute hyaline membrane disease (HMD).[2] Instead of improving rapidly after the initial acute disease, these infants went on to develop chronic pulmonary changes. The pathologic picture was one of alveolar and bronchiolar necrosis and repair with bronchial metaplasia and interstitial fibrosis.

Pathology

In 1972, 147 infants were treated in our nursery on positive-pressure respirators for respiratory failure from all causes. All infants were intubated and treated with positive-pres-

The intensive care of the large number of infants reviewed for this chapter required concentrated and dedicated care from all members of our Newborn Service: faculty, fellows, housestaff nurses. I am particularly indebted to Dr. Robert Cleland, for review of the autopsy material, to Dr. Victory Mikity and Dr. John Richmond for consultation on the radiographs, and to Dr. Annabel Teberg, Dr. Emily Kahlstrom and Dr. Eithne McLaughin for follow-up information on the graduates from our nurseries.

sure respirators of various types. Of these infants, 92 died before discharge from the hospital, and autopsies were obtained on 63. The pulmonary pathology in the 63 autopsied cases was reviewed and classified according to the criteria of Northway, Rosan, and Potter.[2]

Stage I (2 to 3 days) is a period of acute HMD. Twelve infants from our nursery whose age at death ranged from 7 hours to 3 days were classified as Stage I. These cases were indistinguishable from severe HMD without respirator therapy. The bronchiolar epithelium was intact except for early syncytial change.

Stage II (4 to 10 days) is a period of regeneration. Twenty-three of our 63 infants, whose age at death ranged from 8 hours to 18 days were classified as Stage II. Hyaline membrane was present in all the cases but was beginning to break up. Necrosis and repair of alveolar epithelium was evident. Regeneration and proliferation of bronchial epithelium occurred (Fig. 21-1, from a patient who died at 3 days). Ulceration and membrane formation in bronchioles were also present, but fibrosis was not.

Stage III (10 to 20 days) is a period of transition to chronic disease. Eight of our 63 cases whose ages at death varied from 2 to 15 days were classified as Stage III. Extensive repair, with phagocytosis of membrane and advanced alveolar epithelial regeneration, occurred. Bronchiolar metaplasia and interstitial fibrosis were seen in the same sections as residual membrane and cell proliferation (Fig. 21-2 from a patient who died at 5 days).

Stage IV (beyond 1 month) is a period of chronic disease. Five of our 63 cases, whose ages at death ranged from 23 days to 5 months, were considered to demonstrate Stage IV lesions. The most prominent findings in our cases were obliterative bronchiolitis with interstitial fibrosis. Evidence of active epithelial regeneration was still present in the earlier cases. Four of the five infants were 1 month of age or less at the time of death, and none of these could be weaned from the respirator. The youngest infant in this group died at 17 days of age from necrotizing enterocolitis following a very stormy course marked by interstitial emphysema and recurrent pneumothorax. The infant's pulmonary status appeared to be improving at the time of death. The lung shows peribronchial and some interstitial fibrosis with regenerating epithelium (Fig. 21-3). More severe peribronchial fibrosis

with regenerating cuboidal epithelial cells and some residual membrane is seen in an infant dying at 26 days (Fig. 21-4 *Top*). Bronchiolar metaplasia is particularly striking in Figure 21-4 *Bottom* from the same case. This infant was constantly maintained on a respirator from 36 hours until death. Except for brief periods, early in the course, oxygen concentrations of over 60% were required to maintain a P_{O_2} above 40. A patent ductus arteriosus with 80 percent shunt was demonstrated at 7 days, and surgically ligated the same day. Although the infant recovered from the surgical procedure, the course was one of unremitting pulmonary failure, complicated by a pneumothorax at 21 days.

Only one infant in our series died later than 1 month and after being weaned from the respirator. This infant was started on a respirator at 3 hours of age because of severe HMD. After a complicated course, the infant was finally weaned from the respirator at 3 months but remained oxygen-dependent. At 5 months, the infant died of cardiac arrest with cardiac hypertrophy and coronary disease. A section of the lung shows extensive fibrosis with dilated air spaces that are probably regenerated bronchioles, lined by a cuboidal epithelium (Fig. 21-5).

The pathologic changes of BPD represent damage and extensive repair of the alveolar and bronchial epithelium. Bronchiolar metaplasia, peribronchial and interstitial fibrosis appear during the transition to chronic pulmonary disease. Although separation into stages is useful for discussion and classification, the process is obviously continuous. Stage I, describes acute HMD and stage II describes resolution from acute HMD. Stages III and IV represent changes associated with chronic pulmonary disease. It would be less confusing if only these latter two stages were designated BPD. Considerable variability in timing was present in our cases, with some infants showing extensive repair and beginning fibrosis as early as 2 days of age. Fibrosis was more prominent in our infants than reported by Northway, Rosan, and Potter, and was regularly present in all infants who survived longer than 18 days.[2] The early appearance of Stages III and IV changes and the presence of extensive fibrosis in infants dying after 1 to 2 weeks of ventilation have also been reported by others.[4-6]

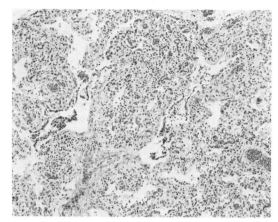

Fig. 21-1. Regeneration and proliferation of bronchiolar epithelium with no fibrosis in an infant who died at 3 days (Stage II of bronchopulmonary dysplasia). (H & E × 125)

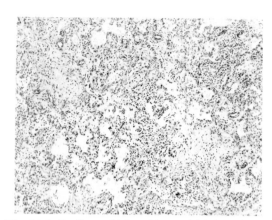

Fig. 21-3. Peribronchial and interstitial fibrosis and regenerative epithelium in an infant who died at 17 days while showing clinical improvement (Stage IV). (H & E × 100)

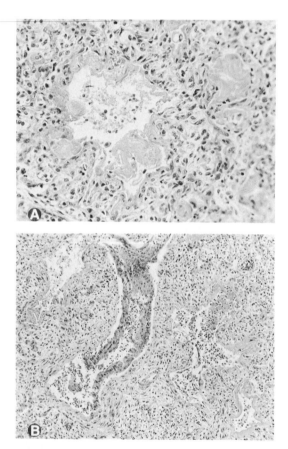

Fig. 21-2. A. Phagocytosis of hyaline membrane with regeneration of alveolar epithelium in an infant who died at 5 days (Stage III). (H & E × 250) **B.** Residual membrane, bronchiolar metaplasia and interstitial fibrosis in the same case. (H & E × 125)

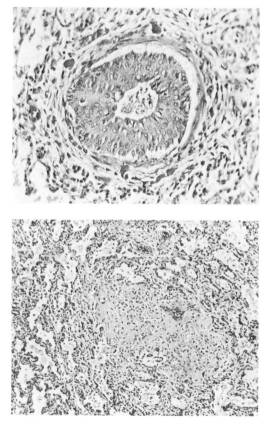

Fig. 21-4. *Top*. More severe peribronchial fibrosis, residual membrane, and regenerating alveolar epithelium in an infant dying at 26 days of progressive pulmonary failure (Stage IV). (H & E × 125) *Bottom*. Metaplasia of bronchiolar epithelium and partial occlusion of the bronchiole. (H & E × 250)

In a recent study of lung biopsies in premature infants requiring prolonged ventilation, proliferation of smooth muscles surrounding the terminal airways was a prominent finding (Fig. 21-6). This change was present in association with evidence of epithelial necrosis and metaplasia in specimens obtained as early as 8 days.[7]

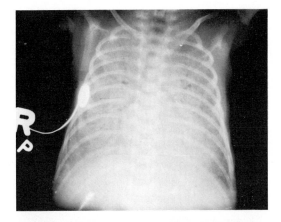

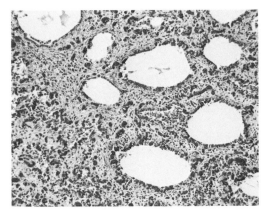

Fig. 21-5. Extensive fibrosis with dilated air spaces probably representing regenerated bronchioles lined by cuboidal epithelium in an infant dying at 5 months after 2 months off the respirator (Stage IV). (H & E × 125)

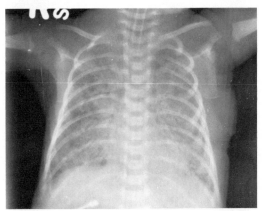

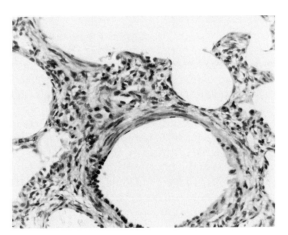

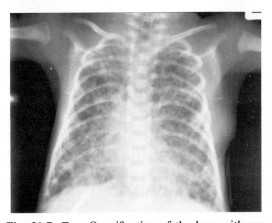

Fig. 21-6. Biopsy at 8 days during surgical ligation for PDA complicating severe HMD. Resolving membrane and early epithelial metaplasia were present. Most striking finding is the smooth muscle lining the terminal airways. (H & E × 250)

Fig. 21-7. *Top.* Opacification of the lung with persistence of air bronchograms at 6 days (Stage II) in the same infant as in Figure 21-3. *Center.* Appearance of small cystic changes characteristic of Stage III in the same infant 1 day later. *Bottom.* Same infant at 14 days showing overexpansion and marked cystic changes throughout all lung fields.

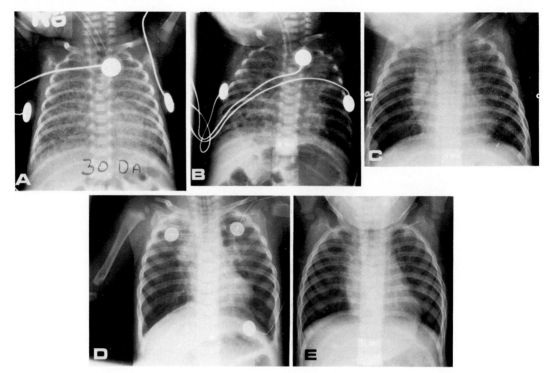

Fig. 21-8. A. Classic cystic changes of Stage III at 1 month of age. **B.** Enlargement of cysts and beginning coalescence at the bases in the same infant at 3 months. **C.** Early Stage IV changes of hyperlucency at the bases and strand-like infiltrates in the apices in the same infant at 4 months. **D.** Accentuated Stage IV changes in the same infant following an episode of severe tachypnea and wheezing at 8 months. **E.** Clearing except for overexpansion by 11 months.

Radiology

The Stage II radiologic picture described by Northway, Rosan, and Potter of complete opacification obscuring the heart borders has been seen occasionally in our infants (Fig. 21-7 *Top*).[2] The earliest radiologic finding of chronic disease consistently seen in our patients has been that described as Stage III, the appearance of small, radiolucent cysts in a generalized pattern, but most prominent in the perihilar areas. These usually appear at about 9 days (Fig. 21-7 *Center*). The cystic areas increase in size and number until they fill the entire lung fields. The lungs become increasingly hyperexpanded during this stage (Fig. 21-7 *Bottom*). The generalized cystic appearance persists until 3 to 4 months with the cystic areas increasing in size and the intervening tissue appearing thicker. Resolution starts with the cystic areas replaced by hyperlucency at the bases and streaky infiltrates at the apices. The hyperlucency and finally the streaky areas in the upper lobes disappear slowly over a period of months. Figure 21-8 A–E demonstrates the progression in one case of the radiologic picture from the generalized cystic appearance at 1 month, through the stage of hyperlucency and apical streaking at 8 months, to resolution, except for persistent hyperinflation, at 11 months. The radiographs from Stage III, through resolution, bear a striking resemblance to those from cases of the Wilson–Mikity syndrome. Differentiation must be made on the basis of pathologic findings or early clinical course (see below).

Late Course and Prognosis

Of the 55 survivors of respirator care in our nursery in 1972, 11, or 20%, had clinical and radiologic evidence of BPD on discharge. All of these infants recovered, although one was oxygen-dependent for 10 months. Six had major recurrent lower respiratory disease characterized by tachypnea and wheezing. One required respirator support during the period of acute illness. Chest radiographs have shown complete clearing by 6 months of age in a few of the infants, but most continued to show mild changes of hyperaeration, peribronchial thickening and streaking in the upper lobes into the second year, with eventual clearing.

Similar radiologic and clinical findings have been reported by others. Johnson and co-workers found that 16 in 55, or 29%, of survivors of positive-pressure ventilation for acute HMD developed BPD before discharge from the nursery.[8] Episodes of recurrent pulmonary infection occurred in many of these infants during infancy, with marked clinical improvement thereafter. At the time of follow-up, 10 of the 16 had coarse stranding and mild peribronchial thickening without overexpansion in the chest film, while the remaining six had completely cleared. Death from cardiopulmonary disease after discharge from the nursery has been reported in about 10% of infants with BPD.[9] In those infants surviving the first year of life, the ultimate prognosis appears good, with no clinical evidence of persistent cardiopulmonary disability.

Pulmonary function studies performed during the first year demonstrated severe maldistribution of ventilation.[10,11] As would be expected from the clinical findings of tachypnea, retractions, and prolonged oxygen dependency, tidal volume was decreased, with a normal minute volume maintained by an increased respiratory rate. Dynamic compliance was decreased and functional residual capacity (FRC) increased, but with a decrease in the amount of FRC occupied by well-ventilated lung. Relative hypoxia and carbon dioxide retention were present with a decrease in pH. In the few infants tested, functional abnormalities persisted beyond infancy in spite of apparent clinical recovery.[12]

Incidence

Accurate figures for the incidence of BPD are difficult to ascertain. The diagnosis can be made with certainty only from cytologic material obtained at autopsy, biopsy, or possibly by tracheal aspiration.[13] Owing to the similarity of radiologic findings in various forms of neonatal chronic pulmonary disease, the relative contributions of immaturity, residual of acute disease, and BPD cannot be easily determined in surviving infants. The problem is further compounded by rapid changes in ventilatory techniques, increasing immaturity in the population of infants ventilated, and increasing rates of survival at all birth weights.

When only autopsied cases are considered, BPD is overwhelmingly, though not exclusively, associated with HMD. Our experience from 1972, reviewed above, is fairly typical. Of the 48 infants dying with HMD, 13, or 27%, had evidence of Stages III to IV BPD. Five of these, or approximately 10%, had chronic Stage IV BPD. Although no infants had evidence of BPD without preceding HMD in this series, diffuse interstitial fibrosis has been reported following ventilation for pneumonia and Wilson–Mikity syndrome.[5]

It is the impression of most neonatologists that BPD is decreasing, but figures to substantiate a significant decrease in the number of cases are not available. Incidence figures must be interpreted cautiously as the population of ventilated infants has changed. In an extensive review of cases from the years 1962 to 1973, Edwards and coworkers reported a constant number of cases yearly, with a decreased incidence in 1973 when changing criteria for ventilatory assistance resulted in a marked increase in the number of infants ventilated.[9] It seems clear that BPD in infants of birth weights greater than 1500 g is uncommon, and that the total number of cases has not increased in spite of increasing survival rates in smaller infants.[14,15] Overall incidence in the most recent reports has been 10% to 15%, with incidences of 20% to 38% in infants of very low birth weight.[3,14] There is no question that chronic lung disease in ventilated infants below 1500 g birth weight contributes significantly to the need for prolonged and costly intensive care.

Etiology

Northway and coworkers, in their original report, made a strong case for the toxic effects of oxygen as the major etiologic factor in BPD. **Oxygen** toxicity received support from the study of de Lemos in which effects of positive-pressure respirators and oxygen were compared in young lambs.[16] Only those animals exposed to high concentrations of oxygen demonstrated acute pulmonary changes. The toxicity of high concentrations of oxygen for pulmonary tissue has been thoroughly demonstrated in both adult humans and animals.[17–19] The early lesions have been consistently described as alveolar thickening and congestion, with an increase in total lung weight ascribed to edema. With longer exposure, capillary proliferation, stromal edema, and, finally, interstitial fibrosis have occurred.

One proposed mechanism for oxygen toxicity involves the ability to form the superoxide anion (O_{2-}), a highly reactive free radical with proven cytotoxic action. Other unstable oxygen metabolites are formed from subsequent intracellular reactions which are capable of various cytotoxic effects, including interaction with DNA and lipid peroxidation of cell membranes. The lung contains a battery of antioxidant enzyme systems, including superoxide dismutase (SOD), which circumvent injury from free oxygen radicals. Tolerance to high oxygen concentrations in immature animals has been related to the ability to rapidly increase pulmonary antioxidant enzyme activity on exposure to hyperoxia.[20] The reaction requires the presence of an as yet unidentified plasma factor. Plasma from infants with HMD and BPD appears to lack this factor when tested in vitro.[21] Small doses of gram-negative bacterial endotoxin have protected lungs of adult rats from oxygen-induced lung injury.[22] The protective effect of endotoxin was associated with an increase in the activity of antioxidant enzyme systems. The effect of oxygen exposure on the protective enzyme systems in the human premature lung has not been tested, but the observations in animals suggest the potential usefulness of this approach.

Boad and coworkers compared human neonatal tracheal epithelium explants exposed to 80% and 20% oxygen concentrations.[23] With high oxygen, loss of ciliary action, early overproduction of mucus followed by later cessation of mucus production, and metaplasia of the epithelium were observed between 24 and 96 hours. The timing of these changes correlates with the earliest changes of Stage II BPD. Changes in tracheal epithelial function, particularly in an infant with an endotracheal tube, might well be important in initiating chronic pulmonary changes.

Oxygen toxicity as the major etiologic factor in BPD has been questioned. BPD has not been found in infants managed with negative-pressure ventilators and without endotracheal tubes, in spite of ambient oxygen concentra-tions up to 100%.[24] No BPD was found in infants given IPPV by mask rather than by endotracheal tube.[25] High peak airway pressures were found to correlate better than ambient oxygen levels with the development of BPD in one study,[26] but there was no relationship to peak airway pressure in another.[27] An increased incidence of BPD associated with pulmonary interstitial emphysema, presumably reflecting an increase in airway pressure, has been reported by some but not all investigators.[10,28] In spite of these confusing reports, in virtually all of the reported cases, four potential contributing factors are present: increased ambient oxygen, positive-pressure ventilation, use of an endotracheal tube, and abnormal or immature lungs. The relative contribution of these factors is impossible to assess from the information currently available.

Increased left-to-right shunting through a **patent ductus arteriosus** (PDA) has been implicated in the etiology of BPD.[29] A potential explanation is suggested by the study of Naulty and coworkers in which ligation of the PDA in symptomatic infants requiring assisted ventilation resulted in a significant increase in lung compliance.[30] Although not a constant finding, the presence of a PDA complicating the course of HMD increases the risk of BPD.[31]

The impact of an added **fluid load** in development of BPD has been retrospectively evaluated by Brown and coworkers.[32] Fluid intake during days 1 through 5 in infants with RDS and PDA without congestive heart failure (CHF) was 105 ml/kg/day. In CHF without BPD, the intake was 118 ml/kg/day, while in CHF with BPD the intake was found to be increased significantly to 150 ml/kg/day. In this study, the principle variable which distinguished infants who developed BPD was the increased fluid intake in the first 5 days of life.

Management

Despite the confusion over specific etiology, sensible management of newborn infants involves attention during assisted ventilation to those factors associated with BPD. Early initiation of ventilatory assistance, control of oxygen levels and pressures, and early weaning from an endotracheal tube can be expected to decrease complications and improve both mortality and long-term outcome. The benefits of restricting fluids during the first few days of life have been confirmed in a prospective study.[33]

Sniderman and coworkers treated infants with chronic lung disease who were ventilator- or oxygen-dependent with 7-day courses of **furosemide** in doses of 1 to 4 mg/kg every 6 hours.[34] Half of the infants with BPD responded to this treatment, while only one-fifth of those considered to have "chronic pulmonary insufficiency of the premature" responded. These results are as expected, considering the differences in the pathologic picture of the two conditions (see below). A trial of furosemide is indicated in infants early in the course of chronic pulmonary disease. Electrolytes must be carefully followed to minimize the complications of hyponatremia, hypokalemia, and metabolic acidosis.

In animals, **vitamin E** deficiency enhances oxygen toxicity, and administration of vitamin E decreases oxygen-induced lung injury.[35] Since premature infants are relatively deficient in vitamin E, a trial of its protective effect was made in infants ventilated for HMD.[36] The initial study showed a decrease in BPD in infants receiving vitamin E. However, in a further study using lower peak inspiratory pressures for ventilation, BPD did not occur in either the treated or control groups.[37] A firm recommendation regarding the administration of vitamin E to premature infants cannot be made at the present time.

Theophylline administered to a limited number of ventilator-dependent infants with BPD resulted in decreased airway resistance, increased compliance, and shortened duration of ventilator weaning in infants less than 30 days.[38] The smooth muscle proliferation around terminal airways reported in Stages II and III BPD may partially explain these beneficial effects, especially the timing. Fibrosis, which increases with duration of ventilation, decreases the response. Dosages used were those recommended for apnea of prematurity. A trial of theophylline seems indicated in infants who are ventilator dependent with BPD.

CHRONIC EFFECT OF PULMONARY DISEASE

Classically, HMD has been considered an acute process with death or complete recovery without sequelae in the newborn period. Reports of follow-up of infants surviving acute HMD have cast doubt on this traditional belief. Lewis reported an increased incidence of acute respiratory disease during the first year of life in nonventilated survivors of acute HMD.[39] Radiographs showed air trapping but no evidence of fibrosis. Outerbridge and coworkers reported that 11 of 53 survivors of acute HMD required hospitalization for subsequent severe lower respiratory infection.[40] Five of the 11 infants were treated with negative-pressure respirators during the newborn period, and six did not require ventilatory assistance. All infants showed clinical and radiologic clearing before discharge from the nursery. Severity of the subsequent disease did not correlate with severity of disease in the nursery, including O_2 administration. Three of the 11 required ventilatory assistance during the subsequent hospitalization. Chest radiographs on follow-up showed varying degrees of peribronchial thickening and pulmonary overdistension.

We have seen a similar process in infants initially treated with assisted ventilation for meconium aspiration without BPD in the nursery. Major recurrent disease, sometimes requiring respirator management, and mild radiographic findings of hyperaeration, peribronchial thickening, and streaking of the upper lobes characterized these patients. Shepard and coworkers reported that 6 of 19 infants who were treated with negative-pressure respirators for acute HMD developed radiograph changes suggestive of pulmonary fibrosis, or overexpansion, or both.[41] Two of these infants had recurrent infections and wheezing. Lung biopsies performed at 18 and 24 months of age in these infants showed peribronchiolar and interstitial fibrosis. Although these findings are similar to those seen during Stage IV BPD, the authors did not find evidence of BPD on radiographs in these infants during their nursery course.

Pulmonary function studies comparing term infants to premature infants with and without HMD suggested an increase in resistance in large airways in premature infants, with an added increase in small airway resistance for survivors of HMD.[42] Because generation of the terminal airways is incomplete in the premature, these findings may represent growth disturbances in lung components related to premature birth, with an additional effect of HMD or its therapy. Stocks and coworkers also reported the appearance of increased airway resistance in prematures at 4 to 10 months of age which was related to the use of IPPV.[43] Finally, Lamarre and coworkers reported follow-up data on 37 infants surviving acute HMD, and found mild persistent abnormalities suggestive of pulmonary fibrosis still present at 8 years of age in patients who had not been treated with respirators.[44] As more survivors of acute disease are studied, the concept of the transient nature of the acute disease, the role of therapy, and the relationship to bronchopulmonary dysplasia require continued evaluation.

CHRONIC PULMONARY DISEASE IN THE IMMATURE LUNG

Functional and structural pulmonary changes have been reported in premature infants without any apparent specific underlying disease. These have been variously called pulmonary insufficiency of prematurity,[45] chronic pulmonary insufficiency of prematurity,[46] and the Wilson–Mikity syndrome.[1] The common denominator appears to be immaturity, with the majority of cases weighing less than 1500 g at birth.

Wilson–Mikity Syndrome

This syndrome of chronic respiratory distress, almost entirely limited to premature infants, was first reported from our center,[47] but subsequently from a wide geographic area.[48–51] From 1957 through 1968, before the use of assisted ventilation in our nursery, we saw a total of 69 cases. Since ventilation of symptomatic premature infants has become routine, the disease as first reported has almost disappeared. The course of the non-ventilated infants will be summarized, not only for historical interest, but also because an appreciation of the problems of these infants is germane to the understanding of current pulmonary problems in the premature.

Clinical Findings

All of our cases, and all but one report in the literature occurred in infants of 36 weeks' or less gestation with normal intrauterine growth.[52] Severity of disease was inversely correlated with length of gestation. Onset symptoms usually appeared at the end of the first week or later, although three infants had both symptoms and diagnostic radiographic findings on the first day of life. Onset symptoms were frequently mild and intermittent. Tran-

sient cyanosis, hyperpnea, and retractions were the most frequent early symptoms. The infant's disease followed a pattern of increasing severity of respiratory symptoms lasting from 2 to 6 weeks after onset. This was followed by a period of severe respiratory symptoms for a few days to several weeks. Systemic symptoms, particularly poor feeding and vomiting, which had been absent during the early course, appeared at this time in the more severe cases.

One-third of the infants died during this acute phase of the disease. Signs and symptoms slowly improved in the survivors. Recurrent lower tract disease requiring hospital admission occurred in several infants. All but two cleared completely by 6 months to 2 years of age. One of the two died at 1 year from heart failure secondary to persistent pulmonary disease. The lungs showed large cystic areas, marked hyperinflation and atelectasis, and some areas of interstitial fibrosis. The second infant was oxygen-dependent for 15 months, but became clinically and radiologically normal by 5½ years.

Radiology

Initial chest films during the first 6 days of life were usually clear, although occasionally early changes of a bilateral, coarse, streaky infiltrate with small cystic areas throughout all lobes of the lung were seen, as in Figure 21-9 *Top,* taken at 4 days. The cystic areas enlarged and became more sharply defined, as seen in Figure 21-9 *Center,* taken of the same infant at 2½ months, following a biopsy. Changes characteristic of improvement occurred between 1 to 5 months. During this second stage, the cystic foci at the bases appeared to enlarge and coalesce. The lower lung fields became hyperlucent and overexpanded, and the upper lobes showed streaky strand-like infiltrates (Fig. 21-9 *Bottom*). The similarity of the radiologic picture to that of Stages III and IV BPD is readily apparent.

Pathology

Ten of the infants seen early in our series of cases had a lung biopsy and all the infants who died were autopsied. The most striking feature of the pathologic material was the absence of structural change in the pulmonary tissue. The earliest biopsy, obtained at 20 days of age in the same infant whose chest radiograph at 4 days is presented in Figure 21-10**A** showed immaturity of the alveolar septa only. A second biopsy was obtained from this infant at 2½ months just before the radiograph shown in Figure 21-9 *Center*. The changes seen in the lung are overexpansion and atelectasis of alveoli without epithelial damage or fibrosis (Fig. 21-10**B**). The infant died of intercurrent diarrhea at 3½ months. At autopsy the lungs showed only hyperaeration (Fig. 21-10**C**). A positive print of a diazo replication of the lung from an infant dying at 29 days of age demonstrates the uneven aeration which is the most striking characteristic of this disorder (Fig. 21-11).

Relation to Chronic Pulmonary Insufficiency of the Premature (CPIP)

Burnard and coworkers surveyed their nursery population of infants less than 1800 g birth weight and reported a spectrum of pulmonary insufficiency ranging from common mild clinical and radiologic manifestations to an occasional infant with the marked findings of Wilson–Mikity Syndrome.[45] Pulmonary function was normal soon after birth but deteriorated in many of the infants during the next 2 to 3 weeks. Almost two-thirds of the infants passed through a phase in which the tests of lung mechanics suggested the presence of overdistension and atelectasis. Abnormal function was not invariably accompanied by radiographic findings.

A syndrome of delayed respiratory distress in small premature infants reported by Krauss and coworkers was designated CPIP.[46] The description fits within the spectrum of findings reported by Burnard and coworkers. These infants were well for the first 3 days, but gradually developed hypoxemia and hypercapnia during the next 2 weeks associated with frequent apneic spells. Chest films during this time were interpreted as normal. During the third and fourth weeks the infants showed a gradual return to normal with complete recovery by 2 months. A mortality of 10% to 20% was attributed to the syndrome.

It seems clear that immature infants have a spectrum of pulmonary insufficiencies, ranging from very mild changes to significant disease requiring ventilatory assistance. Although the severity is related to the degree of immaturity, the relationship is not exact and the reasons why some infants are more affected are not

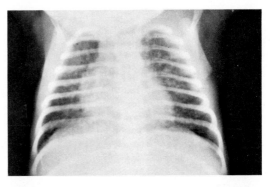

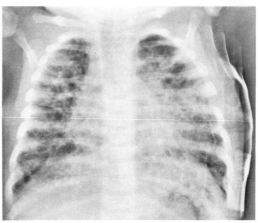

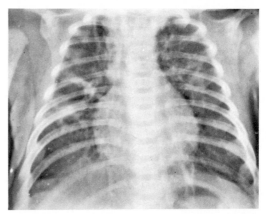

Fig. 21-9. *Top.* Early changes of Wilson–Mikity syndrome at 4 days of age. *Center.* Marked cystic changes in the same case 2½ months. Note the similarity to Stage III bronchopulmonary dysplasia. *Bottom.* Recovery phase of Wilson–Mikity syndrome showing hyperlucency and overexpansion of the bases and streaky infiltrate in the apices. Note the similarity to Stage IV bronchopulmonary dysplasia. (Figs. 21-9–21-11 from Hodgman JE et al: Pediatrics, 44, 179, 1969; Copyright © American Academy of Pediatrics, 1969)[1]

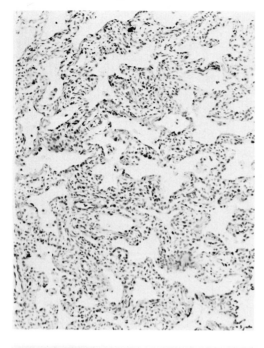

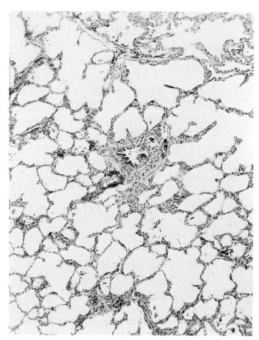

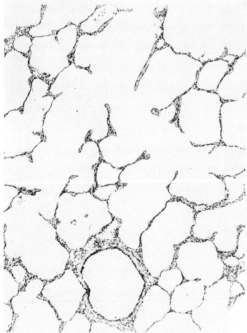

Fig. 21-10. A. First biopsy at 20 days in the same case as Figure 21-9 (*Top, Center and Bottom*) showing immaturity of alveolar septa. (H & E × 125) **B.** Second biopsy taken at 2½ months, 1 day before the radiograph in Figure 21-9 (**B.**) showing hyperaeration. (H & E × 100) **C.** Marked hyperinflation present in the same case at autopsy at 3½ months. (H & E × 125)

clear. All of these infants are demonstrating pulmonary insufficiency of the premature; classifying them by syndromes seems useful only in identifying severity of disease and prognosis.

Etiology

The spectrum of pulmonary insufficiency in the premature infant can best be explained by increasingly abnormal air distribution secondary to characteristics of the premature lung.

In involved infants the FRC decreases, beginning at the end of the first week, accompanied by hypoxia and hypercapnia. As demonstrated by Rigatto and Brady, the premature response to hypoxia is reduction in breathing with resultant apnea and atelectasis.[53] Increased airway resistance and increased compliance in the small airways found in premature infants would lead to alternating areas of hyperaeration and atelectasis.[45] In the most susceptible infants, this maldistribution of air would progress to the degree responsible for the cystic appearance typical of x-ray films of the Wilson–Mikity syndrome after the first month.

Coates and coworkers reported pulmonary function studies in five infants between 8–10 years of age, following clinical and radiologic recovery from Wilson–Mikity syndrome.[54] They found significant differences in airway resistance between these children and normal prematurely born children. The flow rates in the long-term survivors of Wilson–Mikity syndrome also showed an abnormal drop-off, with decreasing lung volumes suggesting persistence of over and under aerated regions of the lung.

There is no evidence for oxygen toxicity in these infants. Biopsy and autopsy material show changes in air pattern, without the necrosis and repair found in oxygen-damaged lungs. A number of our infants had well-developed clinical and radiographic findings before receiving supplemental oxygen.

Current Incidence

Infants with the clinical and blood gas findings characteristic of pulmonary insufficiency are now being ventilated unless the changes are mild. Once the infant is placed on the ventilator, Wilson–Mikity syndrome can not be reliably differentiated from BPD, and the changes of BPD may be superimposed. Support for this opinion comes from a recent study of biopsies from premature infants who required prolonged ventilation.[7] The patchy air pattern characteristic of Wilson–Mikity was found in about 20% of the specimens. In these ventilated infants the pathologic changes of epithelial metaplasia and interstitial fibrosis characteristic of BPD were also present. The report of Philip, who found BPD in very small infants following ventilation for apnea beginning after 48 hours, is consistent with this

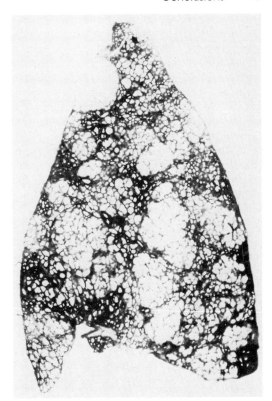

Fig. 21-11. Positive print of diazo replication of the lung of an infant dying at 29 days, showing the characteristic pattern of hyperaeration and atelectasis responsible for the cystic appearance.

view.[55] Some of the chronic lung disease so common in ventilated immature infants of 1000 g birth weight or less is almost certainly caused by pulmonary insufficiency of the premature. Much of the confusion surrounding the etiology of BPD might be clarified if we could better differentiate the various causes of underlying lung disease requiring ventilation in the premature infant.

CONCLUSIONS

The late stages of all the chronic lung disorders discussed are very similar and cannot be differentiated by clinical or radiologic findings. All are characterized by similar radiologic changes (usually mild): hyperaeration, peribronchial thickening or strand-like infiltrates in the apices. Recurrent lower respiratory disease, occasionally severe enough to require ventilatory support, occurs in all. The prognosis is generally good with almost all infants, even those with very protracted disease, showing progressive clearing. Although the general outlook appears favorable, accurate long-term prognosis can be made only on the basis of continued study and follow-up of surviving patients. Some of the chronic pulmonary disease is certainly related to treatment in the neonatal period. Continuing evaluation of the nursery care, especially methods for providing respiratory assistance, should help delineate the etiologic factors involved, leading to further reduction in neonatal mortality and long-term pulmonary morbidity.

REFERENCES

1. **Hodgman JE, Mikity VG, Tatter D, Cleland RS:** Chronic respiratory distress in the premature infant. Pediatrics 44:179, 1969
2. **Northway WH, Rosan RC, Porter DY:** Pulmonary disease following respiratory therapy of hyaline-membrane disease. N Engl J Med 276:357, 1967
3. **Wung JT, Koons A, Driscoll JM Jr, James LS:** Changing incidence of BPD. J Pediatr 95:845, 1979
4. **Anderson WR, Strickland MB:** Pulmonary complications of oxygen therapy in the neonate. Arch Pathol 91:506, 1971
5. **Pusey VA, Macpherson RI, Chernick V:** Pulmonary fibroplasia following prolonged artificial ventilation of newborn infants. Can Med Assoc J 100:451, 1969
6. **Banerjee CK, Girling DJ, Wigglesworth JS:** Pulmonary fibroplasia in newborn babies treated with oxygen and artificial ventilation. Arch Dis Child 47:509, 1972
7. **Light M, Uyemora H, Hodgman JE:** Lung biopsies in premature infants during prolonged assisted ventilation. In preparation
8. **Johnson JD, Malachowski NC, Grobstein R, Welsch RSW, Daily WJR, Sunshine P:** Prognosis of children surviving with the aid of mechanical ventilation in the newborn period. J Pediatr 84:272, 1974
9. **Edwards DK, Dyer W, Northway WH Jr:** Twelve years' experience with BPD. Pediatrics 59:839, 1977
10. **Watts JL, Ariagno RL, Brady JP:** Chronic pulmonary disease in neonates after artificial ventilation: Distribution of ventilation and pulmonary interstitial emphysema. Pediatrics 60:273, 1977
11. **Bryan MH, Hardie MJ, Reilly BJ, Swyer PR:** Pulmonary function studies during the first year of life in infants recovering from the respiratory distress syndrome. Pediatrics 52:169, 1973
12. **Harrod JR, L'Heureux P, Wagenstun OD, Hunt CE:** Long-term follow-up of severe respiratory distress syndrome treated with IPPB. J Pediatr 84:277, 1974
13. **D'Ablang G III, Bernard B, Zaharov I, Barton L, Kaplan B, Schwinn CP:** Neonatal pulmonary cytology and bronchopulmonary dysplasia. Acta Cytol 19:21, 1975
14. **Tooley WH:** Epidemiology of BPD. J Pediatr 95:851, 1979
15. **Hodson WA, Truog WE, Mayock DR, Lyrene R, Woodrum DE:** BPD: The need for epidemiologic studies. J Pediatr 95:848, 1979
16. **deLemos R, Wolfsdorf J, Nachman R, Block AJ, Leiby G, Wilkinson HA, Allen T, Haller JA, Morgan W, Avery ME:** Lung injury from oxygen in lambs: The role of artificial ventilation. Anesthesiology 30:609, 1969
17. **Pratt PC:** Pulmonary capillary proliferation induced by oxygen inhalation. Am J Pathol 34:1033, 1958
18. **Kaplan HP, Robinson FR, Kapanci Y, Weibel ER:** Pathogenesis and reversibility of the pulmonary lesions of oxygen toxicity in monkeys, I. Clinical and light microscopic studies. Lab Invest 20:94, 1969
19. **Cedergren B, Gyllensten L, Wersall J:** Pulmonary damage caused by oxygen poisoning: An electron microscopic study in mice. Acta Paediatr 48:477, 1959
20. **Frank L, Bucher JR, Roberts RJ:** Oxygen toxicity in neonatal and adult animals of various species. J Appl Physiol 45:699, 1979
21. **Frank L, Autor AP, Roberts RJ:** Oxygen therapy and hyaline membrane disease: The effect of hyperoxia on pulmonary superoxide dismutase activity and the mediating role of plasma. J Pediatr 90:105, 1977
22. **Roberts RJ:** Employment of pulmonary superoxide dismutase, catalase, and glutathione peroxidose activity as criteria for assessing suitable animal models for studies of BPD. J Pediatr 95:904, 1979
23. **Boad T, Kleinerman J, Fanaroff A, Matthews L:** Toxic effects of oxygen on culture of human neonatal respiratory epithelium. Pediatr Res 7:607, 1973
24. **Stern L, Ramos A, Outerbridge EW, Beaudry PH:** Negative pressure artificial respiration: Use in treatment of respiratory failure of the newborn. Can Med Assoc J 102:595, 1970
25. **Rhodes PG, Hall RT, Leonidas, JC:** Chronic pulmonary disease in neonates with assisted ventilation. Pediatrics 55:788, 1975
26. **Taghizadeh A, Reynolds EOR:** Pathogenesis of BPD following hyaline membrane disease. Am J Pathol 82:241, 1976

27. **Boros SJ, Orgill AA:** Mortality and morbidity associated with pressure and volume-limited infant ventilators. Am J Dis Child 132:865, 1978

28. **Berg TJ, Pagtakhan RD, Reed MH, Langston E, Chernick V:** BPD and lung rupture in hyaline membrane disease: Influence of continuous distending pressure. Pediatrics 55:51, 1975

29. **Gay JH, Daily WGR, Meyer BHP, Trump DS, Claud DT, Molthan ME:** Ligation of the patent ductus arteriosus in premature infants. J Pediatr Surg 8:677, 1973

30. **Naulty CM, Horn S, Conry J, Avery GB:** Improved lung compliance after ligation of patent ductus arteriosus in hyaline membrane disease. J Pediatr 93:682, 1978

31. **Brown ER:** Increased risk of BPD in infants with patent ductus arteriosus. J Pediatr 95:865, 1979

32. **Brown ER, Stark A, Sosenko I, Lawson EE, Avery MC:** BPD: Possible relationships to pulmonary edema. J Pediatr 92:982, 1978

33. **Bell EF, Warburton D, Stonestreet BS, Oh W:** Randomized trial comparing high- and low-volume maintenance fluid administration in low-birth-weight infants (abstr). Pediatr Res 13:489, 1979

34. **Sniderman S, Chung M, Roth R, Ballard R:** Treatment of chronic lung disease with furosemide (abstr). Clinical Research 26:201, 1978

35. **Poland RL, Bollinger RO, Bozynski, ME, Karna P, Perrin EVD:** Effect of vitamin E deficiency on pulmonary oxygen toxicity (abstr). Pediatr Res 11:577, 1977

36. **Ehrenkrantz RA, Bonta VW, Ablow RC, Warshaw JB:** Amelioration of BPD after vitamin E administration. N Engl J Med 299:564, 1978

37. **Ehrenkrantz RA, Ablow RC, Warshaw JB:** Prevention of BPD with vitamin E administration during the acute stages of respiratory distress syndrome. J Pediatr 92:873, 1979

38. **Rooklin AR, Moonjian AS, Shutack JG, Schwartz JG, Fox WW:** Theophylline therapy in BPD. J Pediatr 95:882, 1979

39. **Lewis S:** A follow-up study of the respiratory distress syndrome. Proc R Soc Med 61:771, 1968

40. **Outerbridge EW, Nogrady MB, Beaudry PH, Stern L:** Idiopathic respiratory distress syndrome. Am J Dis Child 123:99, 1972

41. **Shepard FM, Johnston RB Jr, Klatte EC, Burko H, Stahlman M:** Residual pulmonary findings in clinical hyaline membrane disease. N Engl J Med 279:1063, 1968

42. **Coates AL, Bergsteinsson H, Desmond K, Outerbridge EW, Beaudry PH:** Long-term pulmonary sequelae of premature birth with and without idiopathic respiratory distress syndrome. J Pediat 90:611, 1977

43. **Stocks J, Godfrey S, Reynolds EOR:** Airway resistance in infants after various treatments for hyaline membrane disease: Special emphasis on prolonged high levels of inspired oxygen. Pediatrics 61:178, 1978

44. **Lamarre A, Linsao L, Reilly BJ, Swyer PR, Levison H:** Residual pulmonary abnormalities in survivors of idiopathic respiratory distress syndrome. Am Rev Respir Dis 108:57, 1973

45. **Burnard ED, Grattan-Smith P, Picton-Warlow CG, Grauaug A:** Pulmonary insufficiency in prematurity. Aust Paediatr J 1:12, 1965

46. **Krauss AN, Klain DB, Auld PAM:** Chronic pulmonary insufficiency of prematurity. Pediatrics 55:55, 1975

47. **Wilson MG, and Mikity VG:** A new form of respiratory disease in premature infants. AMA Journal of Diseases of Children 99:489, 1960

48. **Butterfield J, Moscovici C, Berry C, Kempe CH:** Cystic emphysema in premature infants. N Engl J Med 268:18, 1963

49. **Baghdassarian OM, Avery ME, Neuhauser EBD:** A form of pulmonary insufficiency in premature infants. Am J Roentgenol Radium Ther Nucl Med 89:1020, 1963

50. **Swyer PR, Delivoria-Papadopoulos M, Levinson H, Reily BJ, Balis JU:** The pulmonary syndrome of Wilson and Mikity. Pediatrics 36:374, 1965

51. **Sinnette CH, Bradley-Moore AM, Cockshott WP, Edington GM:** Wilson–Mikity respiratory distress syndrome. Arch Dis Child 42:85, 1967

52. **Grossman H, Berdon WE, Mizrahi A, Baker DH:** Neonatal focal hyperaeration of the lungs (Wilson–Mikity syndrome). Radiology 85:409, 1965

53. **Rigatto H, Brady JP:** Periodic breathing and apnea in preterm infants, II. Hypoxia as a primary event. Pediatrics 50:219, 1972

54. **Coates AL, Bersteinsson H, Desmond K, Outerbridge EW, Beaudry PH:** Long-term sequelae of the Wilson–Mikity Syndrome. J Pediatr 92:247, 1978

55. **Philip AGS:** Oxygen plus pressure plus time: The etiology of BPD. Pediatrics 55:44, 1975

22

Special Techniques in Managing Respiratory Problems

W. Alan Hodson and
William E. Truog

INTRODUCTION
(See also Chaps. 20 and 21)

Respiratory diseases in the newborn have unique physiologic, anatomic, and clinical characteristics necessitating special techniques for management. Intensive respiratory care requires a highly skilled team of physicians and nurses, support personnel, unique facilities, equipment, and laboratory services. Promptness and accuracy of diagnosis and subsequent treatment help determine quality of outcome with all neonatal lung disorders. Diagnosis can be made in the majority of cases from clinical and radiographic information alone. Other laboratory aids, particularly blood gas tension determinations, help in assessing the severity of the disease. Knowledge of the pathophysiology of pulmonary disease is essential to the comprehensive management and therefore to the application of special techniques of treatment.

PRINCIPLES OF MANAGEMENT OF RESPIRATORY FAILURE

1. Establish airway
2. Ensure oxygenation
3. Assist ventilation
4. Correct metabolic abnormalities
5. Assess adequacy of ventilation
6. Alleviate cause

Oxygen delivery to the tissues is the goal of management. Patency of the airway is maintained by removal of any obstructing material, such as mucus, and by provision of an artificial airway when necessary. Inspired oxygen is administered in a carefully controlled fashion to provide adequate but not excessive blood oxygen levels. Mechanical assistance to ventilation may be required for hypoxia, CO_2 retention, or apnea. Hypotension, hypovolemia, hypothermia, and severe metabolic acidosis often accompany respiratory failure; correction of these abnormalities is vital to management (see Chaps. 20 and 29). The patient's condition is evaluated continually by clinical and laboratory means and management altered promptly in accordance with the assessment. Finally, the specific cause of the respiratory failure is determined and treated.

ESTABLISHMENT AND MAINTENANCE OF AIRWAY

Physiologic and Anatomic Peculiarities of the Airway

The newborn infant has distinct anatomical and physiologic characteristics of the airways.

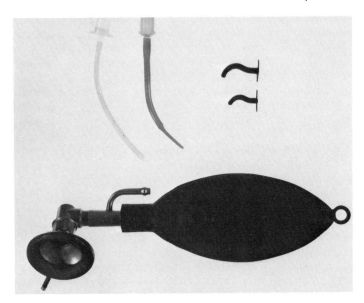

Fig. 22-1. Portex (**top left**) and Cole endotracheal tubes, oropharyngeal airways, sizes 00 (**top right**) and 000. Dräger bag with face mask (**below**).

He is dependent upon nasal breathing for the first few months of life and nasal obstructions due to secretions or congenital abnormalities may produce respiratory distress. The reasons for obligate nose breathing have been the subject of interesting speculation but are not entirely clear.[1] Approximately half of the infant's airway resistance occurs in the nose. However, the narrowness of the lower respiratory tract results in a total airway resistance approximately 15 times greater than that of an adult. Edema and inflammation can produce extremely high resistance in these narrow airways. During expiration, the airways become narrower and resistance increases. Tracheal dimensions as well as lung volumes may differ markedly between large and very small infants.

Techniques for Maintenance of Airway

Suctioning of the oropharynx is required only when there is evidence of accumulation of secretions. A rubber bulb syringe is adequate for this purpose. Nasal suction is seldom necessary unless acute rhinitis occurs. Repeated deep nasal suctioning may cause undue trauma with hemorrhage or edema. Suctioning of the trachea visualized by direct laryngoscopy helps remove meconium which may obstruct the trachea or a major bronchus (see below). A #8 Fr catheter with a single endhole is suitable. Bronchoscopy is rarely indicated in the newborn infant either for therapeutic or

diagnostic purposes because the yield is low and the rate of complications high.

Indications for an Artificial Airway

Artificial airways are needed to relieve airway obstruction, facilitate mechanical ventilation, or avoid insufflation of the gastrointestinal tract. With obstructive lesions, the choice of airways is dictated by the anatomic location of the obstruction. Obstructions of the nose and pharnyx, such as choanal atresia and Pierre Robin syndrome, may be relieved by an oropharyngeal airway. Sizes available for the newborn are 0, 00, 000 (Fig. 22-1). Compromise of the larynx or upper trachea requires endotracheal intubation. Causes of obstruction at this level include laryngeal paralysis, web or stenosis, tracheomalacia, and extrinsic masses such as cystic hygroma, goiter, and hemangioma. Lesions compressing the lower trachea or bronchi require immediate surgical correction if they cause respiratory failure. Endotracheal intubation is also indicated when gastrointestinal distension must be avoided, as in diaphragmatic hernia, duodenal atresia, or perforation of the stomach.

Should mechanical ventilation be necessary, endotracheal tubes and rubber rimmed plastic masks can be used to connect the ventilator to the airway. Endotracheal and nasotracheal tubes currently enjoy the widest acceptance. A round face mask with a rubber or plastic air-filled rim has been used for mechanical ventilation.[2] However, this technique is not usually successful if high inspiratory pressure must be used to ventilate the infant. Marked gastrointestinal distension and pressure necrosis of the face or scalp also may limit the effectiveness of this technique.

Endotracheal Intubation

Route of Intubation. Both orotracheal and nasotracheal intubation are in general use for prolonged mechanical ventilation of term and premature infants. The principal advantage of the nasal route is the stabilization of the tube afforded by the close fit within the naris, but the nasal passages may limit the size of tube which can be used. Necrosis of the nasal septum or the ala nasae can occur if circulation is impaired by a tube that is too large. Orotracheal intubation is more easily and quickly accomplished and is the indicated route for delivery room and other emergency intubations.

Type of Tube. Endotracheal tubes must be flexible, but have sufficient rigidity to prevent kinking and facilitate insertion. They should be of sterile, non-toxic, tissue-implantable material and should be radioopaque to permit localization. Most currently available tubes are made of polyvinyl chloride. There are two shapes: the "shouldered" (Cole) tube and the tube of uniform diameter (Portex) (Fig. 22-1). The Cole tube has a shoulder between the narrow tracheal portion and the wider oropharyngeal portion, designed to prevent passage of the tube too deeply into the trachea; however, the tracheal portion may be too long for very small infants. The Cole tube has about half the resistance to air flow of the uniform-diameter tube. It is simpler to insert and is suitable for emergency resuscitation. The uniform-diameter tube is preferred when intubation is done for prolonged mechanical ventilation because the Cole tube cannot be inserted transnasally and the shoulder may cause dilation of the larynx and damage to the vocal cords.

The endotracheal tube should allow a small air leak between the tube and the glottis. A tube which fits too snugly within the trachea is apt to cause pressure necrosis of the mucosa. If too large a leak is allowed, however, it may be difficult to achieve sufficient pressure for ventilation of noncompliant lungs. As a rough guide, a tube with a 2.5 mm inside diameter will fit infants under 1000 g; a 3.0 mm tube, from 1000 to 1500 g; 3.5 mm, from 1500 to 2500 g; and 4.0 mm, any larger infant.

Technique of Intubation. Orotracheal intubation is a simple procedure and can be accomplished atraumatically within a few seconds. The necessary equipment consists of a straight-bladed laryngoscope, a suction catheter connected to a suction apparatus (or a DeLee mucus trap), an endotracheal tube of the appropriate size with an adapter for the bag or respirator, and an optional flexible (Teflon) introducer, bent so as to prevent its tip from protruding beyond the end of the endotracheal tube. The infant is ventilated with 100% oxygen (40% oxygen if there is no coexisting pulmonary parenchymal disease) by mask for a few breaths. The neck is straightened without hyperextension by placing a small towel under the shoulders, and the head is steadied by an assistant. The laryngoscope is held in the left hand between the thumb and first two fingers. The heel of the hand is placed against the infant's left cheek to provide stability. The blade is introduced into the right side of the mouth, and the tongue is deflected to the left as the blade is advanced into the vallecula, anterior to the epiglottis. The laryngoscope is then tilted in order to elevate the larynx and bring the glottis into view (Fig. 22-2) and the pharynx is suctioned if necessary. A small catheter to provide a low flow of oxygen can be taped to the laryngoscope blade to enhance oxygenation during the intubation process.[3] The endotracheal tube is introduced into the mouth to the right of the laryngoscope, gently guided into the glottis, and the tip positioned 1 to 2 cm below the cords.

Placement of a nasotracheal tube is technically more difficult and often more time-consuming than orotracheal intubation. It is best, particularly in a severely compromised infant, to have an orotracheal tube in place so that the infant can be ventilated while the nasotracheal tube is being positioned. The nasotracheal tube, without an introducer, is inserted through the naris and gently guided along the floor of the nose. The laryngoscope is placed in the mouth to the right of the orotracheal tube, and the tip of the nasotracheal tube is visualized in the posterior pharynx. A Magill forceps is held in the right hand and introduced to the right of the laryngoscope. The nasotracheal tube is grasped a few millimeters back from its tip with the forceps, and the tip of the tube is elevated until it is almost at the glottis. It is helpful to have an assistant grasp the exterior end of the nasotracheal tube to assist in advancing it. The orotracheal tube is left in place until just prior to insertion of the nasotracheal tube in the glottis.

Heart rate should be monitored continuously during any tracheal intubation. If the heart rate falls, intubation should be deferred while the infant is ventilated with a resuscitation bag and face mask.

Positioning of Endotracheal Tube. The length of the trachea from the vocal cords to the carina varies from about 3.6 cm in the smallest premature infants to 6 cm in large, term infants. Optimum positioning for the tip of an endotracheal tube is about the midtrachea, where it is least subject to dislodgment into the pharynx or displacement into a bronchus. The naris-to-midtrachea distance has been shown to be quite predictable from any of several body measurements.[4] The simplest formula is

$$\text{naris–midtrachea distance} = 0.21 \times \text{crown–heel length}$$

which gives ample precision. Nasotracheal tubes should be cut to length before insertion because cutting the tube and reinserting the adapter is both difficult and hazardous once the tube is in place. The length of tube which is left protruding from the naris will depend on the type of fixation to be used. If more than a centimeter of tubing is left unsupported, it may kink. The course of an orotracheal tube through the mouth and pharynx can be variable, making it harder than in the case of a nasotracheal tube to predict the exact length needed.

Immediately upon intubation, position of the tube should be confirmed by inspection and auscultation. Two common errors of tube placement are intubation of the esophagus and intubation of the right mainstem bronchus. The former can be suspected when insufflation through the tube produces abdominal distension with little chest expansion, and when air movement is heard better over the stomach than the chest. Breath sounds that are louder over the right chest than the left suggest that the tube is in the right mainstem bronchus. Auscultation, though helpful, is not reliable because breath sounds are well transmitted in a small chest. Frontal and lateral chest films

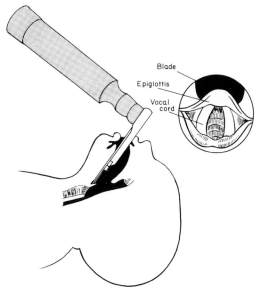

Fig. 22-2. Laryngoscopy for endotracheal intubation.

should be obtained immediately after intubation to confirm tube placement. The lateral view will distinguish between the trachea and the esophagus, and the frontal view will show the position of the tube in relation to the carina.

Fixation of the Tube. Adequate fixation of an endotracheal tube is critical. The lack of a cuff to hold the tube and the leverage exerted by the respirator tubing make the endotracheal tube quite susceptible to dislodgement. Flexion of the infant's neck or even side-to-side movement may cause the tip of the tube to move up and down in the trachea, thereby creating the possibility of the tube slipping back into the posterior oropharynx, or forward into the right main bronchus. Taping the tube to the face and tying it around the head are the most common methods of fixation, but neither is entirely satisfactory. Neither adhesive tape nor umbilical tape adheres well to polyvinyl chloride, particularly after it has become moistened with saliva or nasal secretions. Orotracheal tubes may be sutured to tape or elastoplast on the face, but with some difficulty and hazard. Rigid devices taped or tied to the head which lock to the endotracheal tube may be useful in large active infants, but are probably unnecessary in tiny preterm infants. Mechanical support for the respiratory tubing adds additional safety.

Care of Endotracheal Tubes. The presence of a tube in the trachea interferes with the physiologic mechanisms for clearance of respiratory tract secretions. Meticulous care is needed to prevent accumulation and inspiration of secretions leading to obstruction of the tube. Routine changing of the tube every 24 hours is unnecessary and subjects the infant to repeated risk of trauma to the larynx and interruption of ventilation. The tube need not be changed as long as it remains patent.

Two important aspects of endotracheal tube care are humidification and suctioning. The tube bypasses the nasal and pharyngeal mucosa which normally warms and humidifies inspired gases. If heat and humidity are not provided from an external source, drying of the lower respiratory tract mucosa and secretions as well as hypothermia may result. Inspired gases should be passed through a heated nebulizer so that they are delivered to the airway already warmed and saturated with water vapor. A temperature probe with an audio alarm to detect overheating should be positioned in the inspiratory tubing near the infant. Frequent suctioning of the tracheobronchial tree ensures a patent airway. Hourly suctioning is appropriate for most infants, but volume and quality of secretions vary with the type of pulmonary disease and with the individual patient.

Suctioning is performed with a sterile polyvinyl chloride or polyethylene endhole catheter of a size that will pass easily through the endotracheal tube without fully occluding it. A #5 Fr. catheter is appropriate for a 2.5 or 3.0 mm tube, and a #8 Fr. catheter for a 3.5 or 4.0 mm tube. The suction apparatus should provide at least 75 torr negative pressure; however, higher pressures are sometimes needed.

Immediately before suctioning, $\frac{1}{4}$ to $\frac{1}{3}$ ml of sterile saline is instilled in the endotracheal tube to loosen secretions and the infant is ventilated for 30 to 60 seconds. The respirator or bag is disconnected and the head is turned gently to one side to promote passage of the suction catheter into the contralateral mainstem bronchus. The suction catheter is grasped with a sterile glove and, with the suction eye open, passed as far as it will go with ease through the endotracheal tube. The suction eye is occluded as the catheter is withdrawn over about 5 seconds. The infant is subse-quently ventilated for 30 to 60 seconds with a bag, and the procedure, starting with the instillation of saline, is repeated with the head turned to the opposite side. If a suction catheter can no longer be passed with ease through the endotracheal tube, no force should be applied because this may propel a mucus plug into a lower airway. Rather, the endotracheal tube should be changed promptly.

Removal of the Tube. The problems most likely to be encountered in the immediate postextubation period are inadequate ventilation, manifested by apnea or hypercarbia; obstruction of the larynx by edema; and aspiration caused by incomplete apposition of the vocal cords. The risk of airway obstruction from secretions can be decreased by thorough suctioning of the tracheobronchial tree, the nose, and the mouth before removal of the tube. As a precaution against aspiration, the stomach should be emptied before extubation and feedings should be temporarily withheld. Both systemic corticosteroids and topical racemic epinephrine have been advocated for the management of laryngeal edema associated with endotracheal tubes, although neither therapy has been studied in a controlled fashion.

Long-term Sequelae of Endotracheal Intubation. It is apparent that in all patients endotracheal intubation produces some degree of mucosal injury, usually squamous metaplasia or mucosal necrosis.[5,6] In most infants, there seems to be spontaneous healing without significant sequelae. Hoarseness and stridor are often present following prolonged intubation but usually resolve over a period of days. Persistent lesions may, however, develop in many patients.[7] These complications include laryngomalacia and subglottic stenosis, occasionally requiring tracheostomy. Duration of intubation, pressure from oversized tubes, inadequate humidification, and airway pressure produced by the ventilator all may contribute to the development of laryngotracheal lesions. There may also be an increased risk of otitis media in infants intubated for more than 2 weeks.[8]

Duration of intubation is dictated by the need for continued ventilatory support. In occasional infants requiring very prolonged assisted ventilation (greater than 1 month), tracheostomy tube placement may facilitate development of normal feeding patterns and social interaction, besides bypassing already traumatized areas of the upper airway. However, infant tracheostomy is associated with a significant morbidity and mortality.[9]

OXYGEN THERAPY

Physiologic Considerations of O_2 Administration

The goal of oxygen therapy is to provide adequate tissue oxygenation without undue risk of excessive oxygen administration. Current information indicates that an arterial oxygen tension between 50 and 80 torr is satisfactory. A rational approach to oxygen administration requires understanding of the relationship of the percentage of oxygen inspired to the resultant arterial tension (Pa_{O_2}). The alveolar oxygen tension ($P_{A_{O_2}}$) can be calculated using a simplified version of the alveolar air equation: $P_{A_{O_2}} = P_{I_{O_2}} - P_{A_{CO_2}}$ where $P_{I_{O_2}}$ is the partial pressure of oxygen in the inspired gas and $P_{A_{CO_2}}$ is the partial pressure of carbon dioxide in the alveoli. $P_{I_{O_2}}$ is determined by multiplying the fraction of inspired oxygen ($F_{I_{O_2}}$) by the barometric pressure minus water vapor pressure ($\sim$47 torr), or more simply by multiplying the percentage of oxygen ($F_{I_{O_2}} \times$ 100) by 7 ($Pb - P_{H_2O} = 713$). $P_{A_{CO_2}}$ approximates the arterial P_{CO_2}. The alveolar to arterial oxygen gradient ($AaDO_2$) is normally less than 25 torr while breathing room air. Infants with hyaline membrane disease (HMD) may have an $AaDO_2$ as high as 600 torr while breathing 100% oxygen.[10] This reflects right-to-left shunting of blood most likely caused by perfusion of atelectatic alveoli. Very high inspired oxygen concentrations may be needed to maintain the arterial oxygen, and arbitrary limitations (*e.g.*, 40%) have no physiologic basis. The goal of oxygen therapy is to provide saturated hemoglobin for oxygen tissue delivery. While there may be deleterious effects from a Pa_{O_2} of less than 50 torr, serious brain injury probably does not occur until the oxygen tension is much lower.[11]

Retrolental fibroplasia (RLF) continues to be a serious risk in the smallest premature infants. RLF probably occurs because of retinal arteriolar constriction and secondary hypoxic changes, which may happen when the Pa_{O_2} rises above 80 torr. However, the precise relationship of RLF to Pa_{O_2} and to the presence of adult hemoglobin remains un-

determined.[12,13] The duration and magnitude of the elevation of Pa_{O_2} appear to be important variables; this value should be maintained below 80 torr whenever possible. Most cases occur in infants <1500 g birth weight, with an increasing risk with decreasing birth weight. Although there is usually only a small right-to-left shunt across the ductus arteriosus in neonatal pulmonary disease,[14] the potential exists for large shunts and therefore large discrepancies between right radial (preductal) Pa_{O_2}, reflective of blood perfusing the retinal artery, and postductal aortic Pa_{O_2}, sampled through an umbilical catheter.

Administration of Oxygen

The concentration, humidity, and temperature of inspired oxygen should be precisely controlled. The provision of oxygen between 21% and 100% requires separate line sources of compressed air and oxygen which are connected to a dilutor or mixing chamber. A small error in the setting of the dilutor should be assumed; hence, measurement of the oxygen concentration at the infant's airway is mandatory. This is best accomplished by using an oxygen analyzer. With one such instrument in widespread use, a sensor fuel cell generates a signal proportional to the oxygen concentration passing over its face. This device permits continuous monitoring, rapid calibration, and the use of an alarm to signal undesirable fluctuations.

It is important to ensure that there is no further dilution of the oxygen leaving the mixer before reaching the infant's lungs. An incubator is ineffective in maintaining O_2 concentrations above 30% because opening of the portholes causes considerable dilution. An oxygen hood should be placed around the infant's head (Fig. 22-3). A removable lid allows positioning and suctioning of the infant without lowering the inspired oxygen because oxygen is heavier than ambient air. Small apertures in the head hood provide access for temperatures and oxygen probes and intravenous tubing. Gas flow through the hood should be at least 2 liters/minute to prevent carbon dioxide accumulation. The oxygen-air mixture should be warmed to the same temperature as the incubator air, which should be in the range of the neutral thermal environment for that infant (see Chap. 10).

A simple and effective method for heating

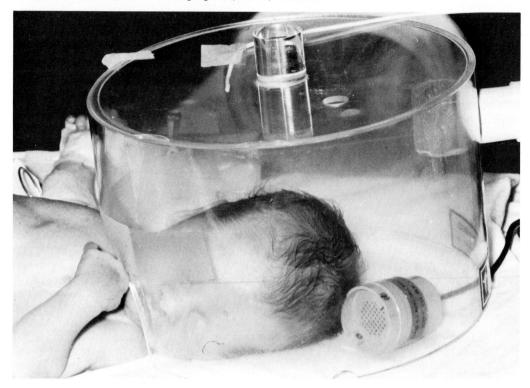

Fig. 22-3. Oxygen hood for administration of controlled oxygen concentration. Note temperature probe passing through the lid, and sensor of oxygen analyzer next to infant's face.

and humidification is to bubble the gas mixture through water containing a heating device. The apparatus and water are replaced every 48 hours to prevent colonization with hydrophilic bacteria. This device needs to be equipped with a warning system to prevent overheating of the inspired air-oxygen mixture which could result in serious injury to the infant.

Assessment of Oxygenation

Until recently, assessment of oxygen tension, the most sensitive measure of oxygenation, has required blood sampling. During the past 5 years, however, a noninvasive device for measuring transcutaneous oxygen tension (Ptc_{O_2}) has been adapted for clinical use. The device consists of a heater to warm the skin to 43 to 45° C, a miniaturized polarographic electrode to measure oxygen tension across the skin in the dilated dermal capillaries, an electronic amplifier, and a recorder (Fig. 22-4).

Arterial P_{O_2} and transcutaneous P_{O_2} are not identical. Differences can be expected to occur because of local O_2 consumption by skin mitochondria and the electrode itself, the effects of heating on O_2-hemoglobin dissociation (which can vary depending on the baseline Pa_{O_2}), and because of O_2 diffusion time and response time of the sensor.[15] In spite of these factors, correlation between Ptc_{O_2} and Pa_{O_2} has been remarkably good over a wide range of infant sizes and postnatal and postconceptional ages (Fig. 22-5).

Use of the transcutaneous oxygen monitor can reduce the number of blood sampling procedures performed on infants who require long-term oxygen therapy. Continuous monitoring for several hours also allows assessment of the effects on oxygenation of infant handling and routine procedures such as airway suctioning, or feeding.

Certain limitations with the device should be noted. Differentiating a decreased skin blood flow from decreased oxygen tension may be difficult, although changes in heater current output may imply an altered skin flow.

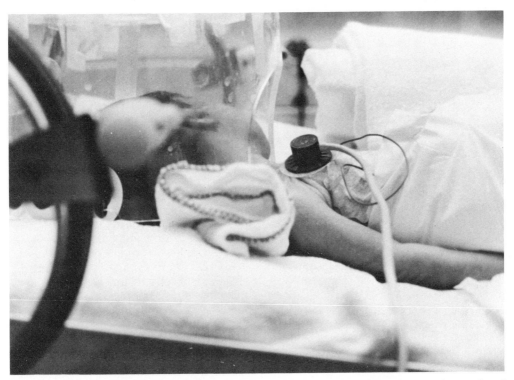

Fig. 22-4. Placement of transcutaneous O_2 electrode on the upper thorax, over the preductal distribution of blood flow.

Ptc_{O_2} and Pa_{O_2} correlations are poorer when the infant is <24 hours old,[16] or is hypotensive or is receiving vasodilator therapy.[17] Frequent instrument calibration at a site distant from potential leaks of oxygen into the ambient air is necessary for proper instrument use. An instrument drift of greater than 10% per hour has been found in 15% of monitored patients indicating the need for frequent comparisons with an arterial sample.[16] Second-degree burns (blistering) may be induced with more than 5 hours of use at a single site on the body. This requires shifting the monitoring site every 3 to 4 hours. For these reasons, the Ptc_{O_2} monitor remains a supplementary tool to other methods of O_2 assessment.

Capillary blood obtained from puncture of a warmed heel can provide useful information about pH and P_{CO_2} in an infant over 24 hours old.[18] The P_{O_2} values, however, are insufficiently accurate at any age to allow their use in optimal patient management. Arterial blood must, therefore, be obtained by catheterization of an umbilical artery or by puncture of the

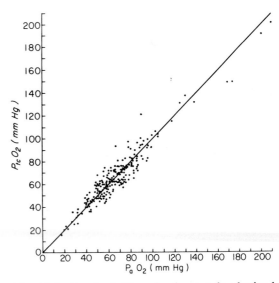

Fig. 22-5. Graph plotting simultaneously obtained arterial P_{O_2} and trancutaneous P_{O_2} in 115 infants >24 hours old (weight range 600–4200 g). (Graham G, Kenny M:unpublished observations)

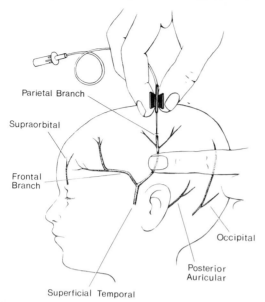

Parietal Branch

Supraorbital

Frontal
Branch

Occipital

Posterior
Auricular

Superficial Temporal

Fig. 22-6. Location of scalp arteries and technique of temporal artery puncture. (Schlueter MA, Johnson BB, Sudman DA et al: Blood sampling from scalp arteries in infants. Pediatrics 51:120, 1973; Copyright American Academy of Pediatrics 1973)

radial or temporal artery. The brachial artery, although larger than the radial, is deeper and less well fixed, making puncture more difficult. Risks of joint infection or of an occlusive hematoma make the aspiration from the femoral artery hazardous.

The techniques of radial or temporal artery puncture are simple, as illustrated in Figure 22-6.[19] A 23- or 25-gauge scalp vein needle is suitable. The radial artery is identified by its location just lateral to the flexor carpi radialis tendon on the palmar surface of the wrist, and its appearance can be highlighted by high-intensity illumination.[20] The superficial temporal artery ascends just anterior to the ear and can be identified by palpation. For arterial puncture, the skin is prepared with an antiseptic solution and the artery is entered against the direction of flow with the bevel of the needle facing upward. Blood should flow spontaneously or with gentle aspiration into the plastic tubing. After removing the needle, continuous pressure is applied to the artery for at least 5 minutes. Repeated punctures can be made at the same site if hematoma formation is prevented. Temporal artery needles have been taped in place and flushed with a heparinized solution for repeated sampling, al-

though the development of cerebral cortical infarction has been associated with long-term temporal artery catheterization.[21]

Umbilical Artery Catheterization

The insertion of a catheter into the umbilical artery is justifiable only if the access it provides to frequent sampling of arterial blood without disturbing the patient will enhance the likelihood of successful treatment of the infant's disease. The necessity for frequent, even half-hourly, sampling of arterial blood for measuring oxygen tension as well as pH and P_{CO_2} has made the umbilical artery catheter the method of choice for obtaining these samples. However, in any individual baby the potentially crippling or fatal complications associated with these catheters, including hemorrhage, ischemic damage to organs, and thrombus formation with distal embolization, must be weighed against the potential benefits to the patient.

The umbilical artery catheter should be non-thrombogenic, transparent, radioopaque, and have markings to indicate length from the tip. It should be nonkinking and have sufficient stiffness to permit easy insertion. Flexibility and a rounded, nonbeveled tip help prevent trauma to the intimal lining. A single endhole permits flushing of the entire catheter. Unfortunately, most umbilical artery catheters are made of polyvinyl chloride, which is not optimally resistant to clotting and may predispose to tissue uptake of plasticizer leached from the catheters.[22] In addition, the radioopaque line on the catheter may contain tiny thrombogenic imperfections.[23]

Technique of Insertion. Placement of the umbilical catheter should be done with aseptic technique, adequate oxygenation, and close monitoring. An open table with an overhead radiant warmer is the most suitable location for the procedure. The infant's arms and legs should be restrained. The umbilical stump and surrounding abdominal skin are cleansed with three applications of an antiseptic solution (usually povidone–iodine), which is allowed to dry and rinsed with water after the catheterization. Caustic skin lesions have resulted from the application of alcohol to small infants. A #5 Fr. catheter is preferable in all infants; however, at times it is necessary to use a #3.5 Fr. catheter on very small babies. The catheter is connected to a three-way stopcock and filled

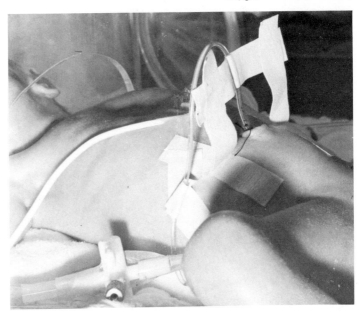

Fig. 22-7. Tape bridge for securing umbilical artery catheter. (Symansky MR, Fox, HA: Umbilical vessel catheterization: Indications, management, and evaluation of the technique. J Pediatr 80:820, 1972)

with sterile heparinized saline. The connection to the stopcock may be made directly or by cutting off the flared end of the catheter and inserting a blunt-needle adapter. The latter technique reduces the "dead space" of the catheter somewhat, but has greater potential for disconnection from the stopcock unless the stopcock has a locking connection. A snug tie of umbilical tape is placed around the base of the cord to be tightened in the event of bleeding. The cord is cut 1 cm from the skin line. If the cord is dry, it may be necessary to cut at the skin line to find soft tissue. Bleeding is usually minimal and can be stopped with sponging. In a fresh cord, the two arteries, which are small, whitish colored, thick-walled, and constricted, are readily differentiated from the larger, thin-walled vein. Selection of the proper vessel may be more difficult when the cord has dried for more than 24 hours. The arterial lumen is gently dilated with an iris forceps. Probing too deeply with a sharp instrument may tear the arterial wall.

The catheter tip is inserted in the lumen and gently advanced with a slight twisting motion with forceps or the fingers. Traction can be applied to the cord with a gauze sponge or with a clamp on Wharton's Jelly. It is common to meet slight resistance to passage of the catheter at 1 to 2 cm, and considerable resistance may be met at the junction of the hypogastric artery at 5 to 6 cm. The resistance may

be caused by spasm of the artery and can usually be overcome by sustained gentle pressure on the catheter for 1 to 2 minutes.

Failure to pass the catheter usually results because of creation of a false tract with subintimal cannulation. If this occurs in both arteries, it may still be possible to cannulate the vessel by performing a subumbilical cutdown procedure.[24] This leaves an almost imperceptible scar at the base of the umbilicus but carries the risk of hemorrhage and accidental entry into the peritoneal cavity.

Once the catheter has been advanced to the desired position (see below) and blood is easily aspirated, the catheter must be secured in place. A purse-string suture through Warton's Jelly will prevent bleeding from the two open vessels. The same suture or a second one should be passed through the skin margin to provide a secure anchor for the catheter. The suture is then tied around the catheter in two places: at the entrance into the vessel and 2 to 3 cm from the cord. A tape bridge incorporating the suture may add some additional security (Fig. 22-7), or the catheter may be taped to the abdominal wall to position it to one side. Tape alone or suture alone is inadequate to secure a catheter.

Location of the Catheter Tip. The tip of an umbilical artery catheter should be at a position in the descending aorta which is not opposite the orifice of any major artery supplying ab-

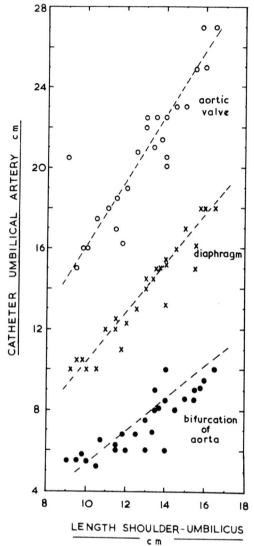

Fig. 22-8. Relationship between the shoulder-to-umbilicus measurement and the length of umbilical artery catheter needed to reach the aortic bifurcation, diaphragm, and aortic valve. (Dunn PM: Localization of the umbilical catheter by post-mortem measurement. Arch Dis Child 41:69, 1966)

artery and the aortic bifurcation. One study has compared the incidence of complications of "high" versus "low" catheter placement.[25] Although there was no difference between groups in the rate of complications requiring catheter removal, there was a higher overall complication rate from the low-position catheters because of more episodes of blanching and cyanosis of the extremities. Thoracic placement allows greater leeway for catheter motion but carries the risk of embolization of clots from the catheter tip or surface into major downstream arteries.

Dunn, on the basis of post-mortem measurements, has constructed graphs which relate the shoulder-to-umbilicus measurement to the length of the catheter required to reach various points in the aorta (Fig. 22-8).[26] This graph is useful as a guide to proper placement and should be displayed near the treatment table. Estimates of catheter position, however, do not obviate the need for confirmation by a

dominal viscera. This placement avoids occlusion of a major artery by the catheter tip and direct injection of hypertonic or highly alkaline solutions into such an artery. The two locations which meet this criterion are the lower thoracic aorta between the ductus arteriosus and the origin of the celic axis, and the lower abdominal aorta between the inferior mesenteric

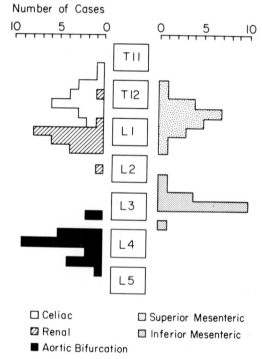

Fig. 22-9. Origins of the major arteries in relation to the vertebral bodies, determined by post-mortem angiography on 27 term and premature infants. (Adapted from Kelly P, Graham CB: Unpublished data)

thoracoabdominal radiograph soon after placement and before medications are infused. The radiographic landmarks are the vertebral body of L4 for low aortic placement and between the body of T4 and T11 for thoracic placement (Fig. 22-9). The catheter tip may enter the pulmonary artery through the ductus arteriosus if positioned above this level. Lateral x-ray films have been recommended for identifying catheter position; however, the nonradiologist will find pertinent landmarks (the 12th rib and the sacrum) easier to identify on a frontal film. Usually the operator can be confident that the catheter has been placed in the artery and not the vein. If there is uncertainty, the frontal film will show the characteristic descent of the arterial catheter into the pelvis and then a cephalad curve toward the aorta. The radiograph will usually be unambiguous if the exterior portion of the catheter does not overlie the pelvis.

Care of Indwelling Catheters. Umbilical artery catheters should be flushed free of blood after each sampling. A continuous fluid infusion is the most satisfactory method for keeping the lumen clear. This is best accomplished with a pump because it is necessary to maintain an infusion pressure greater than aortic pressure. All or part of the infant's fluid requirements can be administered through the catheter, although the administration of medications and blood products may enhance the risk of complications, or shorten the life of the catheter.

Heparin has been advocated as an additive to the fluid infusion or for periodic flushing of the catheter. However, this may induce inadvertent systemic heparinization and increase the infant's risk of a severe hemorrhage. Keeping the catheter free of blood by flushing with any fluid should prevent clotting within the catheter lumen. Evidence for clot formation within the catheter (difficulty in withdrawing blood or a damped blood pressure tracing) is an indication for its removal and possible replacement.

Catheter Removal. Slow withdrawal of an arterial catheter (over 5–10 min) usually permits the artery to constrict and prevents significant bleeding. It is a sensible precaution, however, to have small artery forceps available and to place a purse-string stuture or umbilical tie around the cord stump to be tightened in the event of brisk bleeding.

Complications of Umbilical Catheterization

Limb Ischemia. Blanching or cyanosis of a portion of a lower extremity is a fairly common event, usually occurring shortly after insertion of the catheter. It is probably caused by arterial spasm. The natural history of this condition is not known. No doubt, the safest approach is immediate catheter removal, which has usually been associated with prompt return of the normal circulation. If the other artery is not available, and if maintenance of a catheter is deemed essential, induction of reflex vasodilation may be attempted by warming an extremity other than the ischemic one. Warming the ischemic extremity is undesirable since this will increase local oxygen consumption. The catheter should be removed if there is not improvement in color or pulse in 15 minutes or less.

Thrombosis. Two studies employing angiography report thrombus formation associated with the catheters in 90% of the patients examined.[25,27] These thrombi were all asymptomatic, including thrombi apparently growing retrograde from a low-lying catheter. However, hypertension[28] and infarction of the bowel[29] have been reported following embolization of catheter-related thrombi. The relationship between duration of catheterization and development of arterial thrombosis is unclear. The need for monitoring Pa_{O_2} primarily determines how long the catheter is left in place. Hopefully, the use of the transcutaneous monitor will shorten this time. Development of less thrombogenic materials for catheters may reduce the incidence and severity of thromboembolism.

Infection. Bacterial colonization of umbilical catheters has been reported with frequencies as high as 57%.[30] The source of contamination has not yet been identified. Insertion before 6 hours, removal before 24 hours, and the use of topical antibiotics do not appear to affect the frequency of catheter colonization.[31] Catheter-related bacteremia occurs much less frequently than catheter colonization (in 5% or less of patients), and positive blood cultures drawn through the catheter are of doubtful significance. In controlled studies, catheter-related infection was not prevented by the prophylactic use of ampicillin and kanamycin.[32] No relationship has been established between duration of catheterization and risk of infection.

Other Complications. Significant blood loss is most often a result of accidental disconnection of the infusion tubing, usually at the stopcock. This is less likely to occur with locking connectors. The blood pressure strain gauge connected to the arterial catheter should have an alarm system which will provide immediate warning. Hemorrhage upon removal of the catheter can usually be stopped with pressure, ligation of the cord stump, or suturing.

Vascular perforation by a catheter with a beveled tip may occur. A case of paraplegia has been ascribed to spinal cord ischemia during exchange transfusion through an umbilical artery catheter.[33] Electrocution conducted by the electrolyte solution infused through the catheter is a theoretical possibility. These complications are perhaps preventable and very rare.

A promising innovation in assessment of arterial oxygenation is the use of an indwelling oxygen and carbon dioxide analyzer which provides frequent readout of arterial P_{O_2} and P_{CO_2} without the need for withdrawal of blood samples. At present this device is still in the patient trial stage and not available for routine clinical use.

Oxygen Delivery. It must be remembered that oxygen tension is only one of the critical components in tissue oxygen delivery and emphasis on this measurement must not distract the physician from consideration of the other factors involved. These include cardiac output and its potentially changing distribution, hemoglobin concentration, quantity of red blood cell organophosphates, their interaction with the type(s) of hemoglobin present, and the temperature and pH effects on the patient's oxygen-hemoglobin dissociation curve.

VENTILATORY ASSISTANCE

There has been a marked improvement over the past 5 years in mechanical respirators for newborn infants. Infant respirators are now an essential and common component of neonatal intensive care units. Respirators designed for exclusive use in the newborn permit precise control of the variables affecting the infant's respiratory patterns or frequency. By improving gas exchange and, hence, blood gases, assisted ventilation has made a significant contribution to reducing morbidity and mortality for neonatal respiratory disorders.

Indications

The indications for mechanical intervention in respiratory failure vary slightly from center to center; however, there is general agreement that the Pa_{O_2} should be maintained above 50 torr. There is less agreement on the maximal concentration of oxygen to be used prior to initiating mechanical ventilation. The risk of oxygen damage to the lungs increases with increasing concentration and duration of oxygen exposure. Therefore, the level of inspired oxygen used for initiating mechanical ventilation is arbitrary. All other chemical and laboratory information should be considered and the "critical" inspired oxygen level in making a decision might vary from 60% to 100%. Clinical and radiographic information should permit an estimate of duration and severity of disease, and risk from O_2 toxicity should influence the decision. Because intrapulmonary right-to-left shunting of blood is the major cause of hypoxemia in most infants with respiratory failure, an increase in $F_{I_{O_2}}$ from 0.6 to 1.0 should have very little effect on the Pa_{O_2} if the shunt is greater than 30% (Fig. 22-10).

Carbon dioxide retention is also an important determinant of the need for intervention. Respiratory acidosis has a greater effect on intracellular pH than metabolic acidosis because of the diffusion characteristics of carbon dioxide. Increased cerebral blood flow and enhanced risk of developing intracranial hemorrhage may be additional hazards of hypercapnia. Buffer therapy for respiratory acidosis is not indicated because it is not directed at the cause and its possible benefits are only transient. Most clinicians agree that a Pa_{CO_2} above 70 torr warrants ventilatory support. With an elevated P_{CO_2} less than 70 torr, the decision to provide ventilatory support depends upon other variables such as severity of distress, rate of rise of P_{CO_2}, oxygen requirements and presence, and frequency or duration of apneic episodes. Episodes of prolonged apnea, associated with severe bradycardia or unresponsive to tactile stimulation, require ventilatory support regardless of blood gas values.

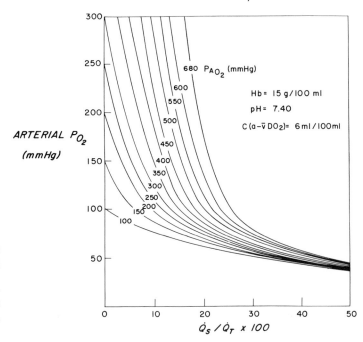

Fig. 22-10. Aterial oxygen tension as a function of shunt fraction for several values of alveolar oxygen tension. (Pontoppidan H, Geffin B, Lowenstein E: Acute respiratory failure in the adult. New Engl J Med 287:743, 1972)

Physiologic Considerations in Mechanical Ventilation

A thorough understanding of the effects of mechanical ventilation on the lungs requires knowledge of respiratory mechanics including pulmonary compliance and airway resistance, respiratory control mechanisms and alveolar gas exchange in the infant.

Lung compliance (change in lung volume/unit pressure change, ml/cm H_2O) depends on the elastic properties of the tissue, which are influenced by the lung volume and abnormalities such as tissue inflammation or edema. Compliance is low if there is either alveolar collapse or overdistension. Expansion from alveolar collapse requires inflation pressures of 12 to 20 cm H_2O. The lungs of infants with HMD will have areas of collapse and over-expansion and there will be nonuniformity of compliance. Other conditions such as pneumothorax, lobar atelectasis, consolidation or pulmonary edema will decrease compliance. The chest wall compliance is usually very high and does not present a problem to mechanical ventilation.

Because the **airway resistance** (cm H_2O/l/sec) is inversely related to the fourth power of the radius, it is high in the infant, increasing at low lung volumes and with obstruction of the airway. High rates of air flow also increase resistance by producing turbulence in the airways.

The rate at which lung areas will inflate is determined by both resistance and compliance. An increase in airway resistance will increase the time required for air to reach the alveoli; a decrease in compliance will result in less airflow required to reach equilibrium. The product of resistance and compliance is a unit of time known as the pulmonary **time constant.** Changes in resistance or compliance, therefore, can alter the pattern or distribution of ventilation.

It is helpful to have an understanding of **lung volumes** when ventilating an infant. The tidal volume (V_T) is approximately 8 ml/kg with one-third consisting of dead space. Mechanical ventilators should permit a tidal volume in the range of 5 to 60 ml, depending upon the size of the infant, with a minimum apparatus dead space.

Air entry into the alveoli depends upon a pressure differential between the upper airway and the alveolus. The pressure differential can be applied through positive pressure at the airway or negative pressure outside the chest; both methods produce similar effects on air movement.

The **circulatory effects** of mechanically applied pressure to the alveoli are important to consider and often overlooked. Normal breathing results in negative intrapleural pressures which enhance venous return and cardiac output, whereas positive pressure breathing or negative pressure around the body impedes venous return and may diminish cardiac output unless the negative pressure is applied around the chest alone. Negative pressure will not impede venous return from the head. The duration of inspiration (the inspiratory:expiratory ratio—I:E) will influence the pulmonary capillary circulation and hence pulmonary blood flow and gas exchange.

Several years ago respirators were designed to permit settings which could mimic the infant's spontaneous respiratory pattern. Efforts were made to allow the infant to trigger each respiration cycle and hence the respirator was adjusted to permit a rapid frequency and a high inspiratory flow rate. Because respiratory control mechanisms are incompletely understood in premature and newborn infants it is unwise to rely on the infant's spontaneous ventilatory response to hypoxia and/or hypercapnia. Improved respirator design has resulted in improved control of several variables including rate, peak airway pressure, mean airway pressure, inspiratory time, inspiratory and expiratory flow rates, I:E ratio, and end-expiratory pressure.

An awareness of all of the physiologic variables affecting gas exchange during different types of lung disease permits comprehensive adjustment of respirator settings.

Bag and Mask Ventilation

Bag and mask ventilation is a short-term substitute for intermittent positive-pressure ventilation with a respirator. It is most commonly employed during resuscitation and may be of help in the management of infants with recurrent apnea before establishing the need for mechanical ventilation. The mask should consist of soft rubber-like material to ensure a tight fit. The bag should be compliant, have a capacity of approximately 500 ml, and permit delivery of 100% oxygen without a cumbersome attachment. A bag similar to the Dräger bag (Fig. 22-1) permits high concentrations of oxygen and is useful in a variety of situations. The incorporation of an additional outlet from the oxygen dilutor allows gas of an appropriate concentration to flow into the bag without

disconnecting the oxygen supply to the incubator, head hood, or respirator. The bag is squeezed with thumb and finger tips, mimicking a natural or spontaneous respiratory pattern. Observation of chest wall movement indicates the adequacy of the tidal volume and guides hand pressure. Auscultation of the chest is advised to determine if air entry sounds adequate and equal bilaterally.

Management of Mechanical Ventilation

Initiation. Several commercially available respirators have been designed specifically for use in infants. The constant pressure generator type with continuous flow is optimal and permits adjustment of a number of variables which influence ventilation. These include rate, peak inspiratory pressure (PIP), mean airway pressure (MAP), positive end-expiratory pressure (PEEP), inspiratory time, air flow, and I:E ratio. It is therefore possible to produce several respiratory patterns.

The appropriate respirator settings should allow the most effective gas exchange with the least risk of lung injury. There is considerable controversy over the relative contribution of high airway pressure (barotrauma) or oxygen toxicity to the pathogenesis of bronchopulmonary dysplasia (BPD). An excess of applied airway pressure or inspired oxygen concentration is certainly undesirable and should be avoided whenever possible. Less certain are the safe or tolerable limits of airway pressure, including the duration of its application during a respiratory cycle. The goal is to maintain an arterial P_{O_2} between 50 and 80 torr and a P_{CO_2} less than 50 torr during the course of acute lung disease. The use of a reversed I:E ratio or an inspiratory plateau may improve gas exchange.[34,35] It has been claimed that reversed I:E ratios and avoidance of high peak airway pressures will result in a decreased incidence of BPD.[35,36] Unfortunately, there are no carefully controlled clinical studies which substantiate this claim, and one study apparently refutes it.[37] Retrospective analysis associating high airway pressure with pathologic changes in the airways at post mortem does not differentiate cause and effect. In other words, abnormal airways may have resulted in the use of high peak airway pressures for satisfactory gas exchange. It would seem wise to avoid the use of high airway pressures (>30 cm H_2O)

unless manipulation of other variables, such as changes in I:E ratio, PEEP, and $F_{I_{O_2}}$, fails to improve gas exchange.[38]

Decreased lung compliance, as in HMD, is the most common physiologic abnormality associated with respiratory failure. A *uniform* decrease in compliance throughout the lung will decrease the time constant; therefore distribution of pressure throughout the lung should be rapid and even. In surfactant-deficient lungs, the terminal air sacules or alveoli will tend to collapse to airlessness, potentially causing local differences in compliance. This will cause uneven distribution and longer equilibration times.

The optimal I:E ratio can only be determined by trial and error, that is, by measurement of improved oxygenation and reduction in the estimated $P_{AaD_{O_2}}$. The use of PEEP will prevent collapse to airlessness of those alveoli already open. Inspiratory pressures of greater than 15 cm H_2O are usually required to open collapsed alveoli. Hence a combination of an increase in the I:E ratio with 2 to 6 cm H_2O PEEP may be optimal during the initial phase of assisted ventilation. With subsequent opening of alveoli, the optimal I:E ratio might need to be decreased. The use of an end-inspiratory pause or plateau should improve the distribution of inspired gas when there are regional differences in airway resistance.[39–41] However, if the alveolar pressure exceeds capillary pressure, there will be tamponading of the pulmonary circulation and some "wasting" of ventilation will occur. Therefore, the settings or adjustment of respiratory variables should be dictated by the type of underlying lung disease; hence, the anticipated aberration in mechanical properties.

Decreased Lung Compliance

If a decreased lung compliance is suspected, it is recommended that the respirator be set with a high flow rate to produce a rapid inspiration with a peak pressure between 25 to 30 cm H_2O. The peak pressure measured in the proximal airway is assumed to be at least 5 cm H_2O higher than in the distal airways. The I:E ratio is set at 1:2, the rate at 30 per minute and the end-expiratory pressure (PEEP) at 3 to 5 cm H_2O. Blood gases should be checked 10 to 15 minutes after the initial settings. If the P_{O_2} is below 50 torr or the

P_{CO_2} is above 50 torr, several adjustments can be made. However, it is recommended to adjust one variable at a time and reassess the change in P_{O_2} and P_{CO_2}. If hypoxemia occurs without hypercapnia, recommended adjustments are (1) increase the I:E ratio, (2) increase peak pressure, (3) increases $F_{I_{O_2}}$, and (4) increase PEEP. The sequencing of these adjustments depends on the existing respirator settings and the degree of hypoxemia. If hypercapnia occurs with a satisfactory P_{O_2}, the sequence might be (1) increase rate, (2) increase peak airway pressure, and (3) decrease PEEP. A marked increase in respiratory rate could have adverse effects on the P_{CO_2} by increasing dead-space ventilation. A moderate degree of hypercapnia (*e.g.*, 50–55 torr) should be well tolerated by the infant and should be accepted by the physician if modest changes in the respirator settings are unsuccessful. Sometimes hypoxemia may persist (*e.g.*, persistent pulmonary hypertension or persistent fetal circulation) in spite of a trial with all combinations of respiratory settings, and attempts at relieving pulmonary vasoconstriction with agents such as tolazoline are indicated. The degree of leaking around the endotracheal tube should always be considered when adjusting pressure and flow rates.

Airway Obstruction

If airway obstruction is present, as may occur with BPD or meconium aspiration, then optimal respirator settings may differ from those used for HMD. Because there is a relatively long time constant, the inspiratory flow rate should not be too rapid. The required peak inspiratory pressure may be below 25 cm H_2O, with an I:E ratio of either 1:2 or 1:3.

Normal Lung Mechanics

Recurrent apneic episodes in the low-birth-weight infant or hypoventilation because of central nervous system depression frequently call for mechanical ventilation. Ventilation of the normal lung requires a low PIP (approximately 10 cm H_2O), a frequency of 20/minute or less, an I:E ratio of 1:3, and a PEEP of 2 cm H_2O (physiologic). Infants with irregular or occasional breathing may be satisfactorily ventilated at a frequency below 10 breaths/minute. If the Pa_{CO_2} is below 35 torr, PIP should be decreased, followed by a reduction in respiratory rate.

Paralysis

Paralysis with pancuronium bromide (Pavulon) may alleviate problems of ventilation in certain infants who do not become synchronized with the respirator or tend to fight or "buck" the respirator.[42] A typical case is a vigorous near-term infant with meconium aspiration and a spontaneous rapid respiratory rate. The vast majority of infants can be ventilated satisfactorily without the use of paralytic drugs.

Weaning

Methods of weaning an infant from the respirator are almost as controversial as those procedures used to establish ventilator settings. The major goal is to minimize complications associated with the treatment of respiratory failure, including barotrauma, air leaks, oxygen toxicity, retention of airway secretions, pulmonary infection, and subglottic stenosis. The reduction of specific respirator settings is influenced by the perceived or relative importance of each of the many variables that contribute to complications. Reduction of the inspired oxygen concentration should be weighed against changes in peak pressure. Generally, attempts to lower PIP should take precedence if the $F_{I_{O_2}}$ is below about 0.6. Lowering of $F_{I_{O_2}}$ to less than 0.4 should precede reductions in rate. A suggested sequence of weaning is (1) reduce PIP to below 30 cm H_2O, (2) reduce $F_{I_{O_2}}$ to below 0.6, (3) further reduce PIP to below 20 cm H_2O, (4) further reduce $F_{I_{O_2}}$ to below 0.4; and (5) reduce frequency. Obviously, not all infants can be weaned in the same manner and the rate and method of weaning will depend on the severity, type, and duration of underlying lung disease. Some infants with chronic pulmonary changes will require assisted ventilation at a low rate, or intermittent mandatory ventilation (IMV) with a PIP above 25 cm H_2O.

Assessment

Generally, the adequacy of ventilation is assessed by observation of chest wall movement, skin and mucous membrane color, estimation of the degree and symmetry of air entry by ausculation, arterial blood gas and pH measurements and transcutaneous P_{O_2} monitoring. The adequacy of cardiac output is judged by continuous measurement of arterial blood pressure, clinical assessment of peripheral perfusion and, when indicated, central venous pressure. A pulmonary-artery catheter (Swanz–Ganz) for measurement of pulmonary artery pressure and the indirect assessment of cardiac output, provides additional, perhaps useful, information; however, placement is a difficult procedure and its use is far from routine at the present time. Alterations in respiratory settings are primarily dictated by the Pa_{CO_2} and Pa_{O_2} as discussed above. The blood gases should be measured within 15 minutes of initiation of mechanical ventilation, change in respirator settings, or change in the infant's clinical condition. The Pa_{CO_2} is the most reliable indication of the adequacy of alveolar ventilation and should be maintained between 35 and 50 torr. Transcutaneous oxygen monitoring has permitted a more rapid assessment of respirator adjustments, reducing the risk for possible hyperoxia and hypoxemia as well as more rapid weaning from the respirator. Respirator adjustments, including $F_{I_{O_2}}$ should be recorded with the pH and blood gas measurement, and kept at the infant's bedside (Fig. 22-11). Computerized methods of tabulating continuous Ptc_{O_2} have been developed and the Ptc_{O_2} records should also be incorporated into the bedside flow sheet. A transcutaneous P_{CO_2} device has been developed recently. Further clinical trials are needed prior to its acceptance for clinical use in the intensive care nursery.

Complications of Mechanical Ventilation (See also Chap. 21)

The incidence of complications arising from the use of mechanical ventilators is difficult to assess. Because of differences in personnel, equipment, and technique, the types and frequency of complications vary from one intensive care unit to another. Pneumothorax, pneumomediastinum, or interstitial emphysema occurs in about 15% of mechanically ventilated infants. Pulmonary air leak may be due to the nature and severity of the disease rather than mechanical ventilation.

Mechanical ventilation may result in hypocapnia or hyperoxia. Hypocapnia resulting in severe respiratory alkalosis may reduce cerebral blood flow, and, because CO_2 freely dif-

DATE AND TIME	RESPIRATORY THERAPY SETTINGS						BLOOD GASES											PHYSICIAN'S ORDERS	INITIALS OF NAMES BELOW		
	FiO$_2$	CONTINUOUS VENTILATOR					pH	PCO$_2$	HCO$_3$ BE	PO$_2$	TYPE	P$_{tc}$O$_2$			BLD QTY	TIME			DOCTOR	NURSE	TECH
		I : E RATIO	RESP RATE	SYS FLOW	PRESS	PEEP						LOW	HIGH	AVG	HCT						

Fig. 22-11. A flow sheet for blood gas values and respiratory therapy orders.

fuses through tissue, the intracellular alkalosis may interfere with cellular metabolism. Hyperoxia increases the risk of RLF in very low-birth-weight infants.

Ventilation with a face mask prohibits nutrition by the oral route and may result in gastric distension.

The most serious hazard is mechanical failure of the ventilator which may be due to accidental extubation, tubing disconnection, or mechanical failure within the respirator itself. Constant attendance by a highly skilled nurse and alarm monitoring of heart rate, blood pressure and respirator pressure should virtually eliminate any compromise to the infant due to mechanical failure.

BPD, first described by Northway and co-workers, is the major pulmonary complication.[43] Histopathologic changes progress in stages and involve airway mucosa, alveolar cells, pulmonary interstitium, lymphatics, overinflation, and fibrosis with characteristic radiographic changes.[43-46] The etiology, and hence the prevention, of BPD is unclear. However, oxygen toxicity and mechanical trauma to the lungs appear to be important contributing factors. Chronic pulmonary changes occur in approximately 12% of infants with HMD.[47] Susceptibility to lung damage is related to a number of variables including immaturity of lungs, severity of HMD, duration and magnitude of oxygen exposure, mechanical injury of positive-pressure ventilation, endotracheal intubation, pulmonary air leak, and patent ductus arteriosus. Many of these variables are simultaneously present during the usual course of respirator management in infants, and every effort should be made to minimize the risks from high airway pressure, oxygen toxicity, and prolonged endotracheal intubation. These risks are often unavoidable and need to be balanced against the risks of inadequate tissue oxygenation.

New patterns of mechanical ventilation, such as the rapid oscillation, low-tidal-volume technique, may help minimize these complications. Such innovations must be tested extensively on experimental animals before being applied to human infants, however.

Continuous Distending Airway Pressure

In 1968, Harrison, Heese, and Klein observed that the expiratory "grunt" associated with HMD could be abolished by endotracheal intubation and that this maneuver was associated with a decrease in arterial P_{O_2}.[48] It was theorized that the partially closed glottis maintained a positive airway pressure during expiration, which prevented alveolar collapse and intrapulmonic shunting. Thibeault, Poblete, and Auld found that some premature infants showed improved oxygenation when FRC was artificially increased by subatmospheric pressure around the thorax.[49] These observations gave rise to the hypothesis that continuous positive transpulmonary pressure might have therapeutic use in HMD. The first report of the clinical application of this technique was by Gregory and coworkers.[50] In 20 infants with HMD, Pa_{O_2} was found to increase following the application of continuous positive airway pressure. Subsequent studies by other investigators have confirmed this finding.

Various terms have been used to describe the imposed positive gradient between airway pressure and intrapleural pressure maintained throughout the respiratory cycle. Continuous positive airway pressure (CPAP) denotes a gas pressure greater than atmospheric continuously applied to the airway during spontaneous breathing. Subatmospheric pressure applied around the thorax during spontaneous breathing is called continuous negative pressure (CNP). Positive airway pressure applied during the expiratory phase of mechanically assisted ventilation is called positive end-expiratory pressure (PEEP).

Equipment. Systems for the application of CPAP are quite simple. The basic components are (1) a source of gas, (2) a device for varying the pressure in the system, (3) a manometer, and (4) a means of connecting the system to the infant's airway. Gas sources are similar to those used in other forms of ventilatory assistance for the newborn. They should be able to supply any selected mixture of air and oxygen with warmth and humidification.

Several devices have been described.[51] The system first reported used an anesthesia reservoir bag with a screw clamp on its open tail piece.[50] This bag, attached to an endotracheal tube, can also be used for periodic manual inflation of the lung, but requires the use of a "pop-off" to prevent high pressures. A length of tubing immersed in a bottle of water can act as a "pop-off" or may itself be used as a pressure regulator. The depth of the tubing end below the surface of the water determines the maximum pressure that can be achieved in the system. Standard orotracheal and nasotracheal tubes and oronasal masks have been used to apply these systems to the airway. Most infant ventilators provide a device which permits various levels of PEEP or CPAP if the infant is breathing spontaneously. CPAP may also be applied through nasal cannulae. The depth of cannulation of the nares should be at least 1 cm, and some have suggested insertion to the nasopharynx beyond the soft palate.[52,53] Because newborn infants breathe preferentially through the nose, it is possible to achieve a pressure of 10 to 12 cm H_2O without taping the mouth.

The components of the CPAP circuits are usually freely interconnected with tubing and T-pieces, without the use of valves. CO_2 rebreathing is prevented by maintaining a gas flow through the system which is at least twice the patient's minute ventilation.

Clinical Indications

The major use of CPAP has been to improve arterial P_{O_2} in order to reduce the $F_{I_{O_2}}$ in infants with HMD who do not require assisted ventilation. The $F_{I_{O_2}}$ at which intervention occurs is arbitrary; 0.6 has been the generally accepted threshold. There is abundant testimony to the resultant improvement in Pa_{O_2}; however, there is no strong evidence that mortality or the incidence of BPD is reduced.[54] Several studies have attempted to determine if early versus delayed application of CPAP is beneficial.[55-57] Guthrie and coworkers, comparing "early" versus "late" application of CPAP in 36 infants with HMD, were unable to demonstrate differences in mortality, or duration of oxygen exposure.[58] The incidence of pneumothorax appears to be increased in those infants treated with CPAP.[54]

At least 2 cm H_2O PEEP are indicated in all infants with an endotracheal tube to provide a physiologic amount of end-expiratory pressure. The use of greater amounts of PEEP will depend on other respirator settings and inspired oxygen concentrations as discussed above.

Physiologic Considerations

Lung Mechanics and Gas Exchange. Owing to the technical difficulties and increased risk inherent in certain invasive procedures on newborn infants, much of the information on the physiology of continuous transpulmonary pressure has been obtained from studies on adults and experimental animals. The limitation of such information is readily apparent: both the physiologic systems and the pathologic processes in these subjects may differ in important respects from HMD in the human neonate.

In most studies on infants with HMD, arterial P_{O_2} increased significantly, and the alveolar–arterial oxygen difference decreased when a transpulmonary pressure between 5 and 10 cm H_2O was applied. No consistent pattern of change has been observed in Pa_{CO_2}, although an increase in P_{CO_2} may occur.[54]

The optimal level of CPAP will vary in the individual patient and the underlying lung disease. Bonta and coworkers have suggested the measurement of esophageal pressure to determine optimal levels of CPAP.[59] In infants with HMD, airway pressure will not be reflected by esophageal pressure until compliance improves, unless high pressures are applied. The pressure at which an increase in esophageal pressure occurs suggests an effective distending pressure has been attained and further increases in CPAP could have deleterious effects on cardiac output.

The exact mechanism responsible for the increase in Pa_{O_2} is still a matter of speculation. Because HMD is characterized by diffuse atelectasis, it would be desirable to have a mode of therapy which prevents collapse of unstable alveoli or even reinflates those already collapsed. On theoretical grounds, it is unlikely that continuous transpulmonary pressure actually accomplishes this. When surfactant is deficient, increments of pressure are more apt to overinflate large alveoli than to expand small or collapsed ones. Lung compliance should increase with alveolar "recruitment" and decrease with overdistension, but attempts to distinguish these two possibilities on the basis of compliance are so far inconclusive. A decrease in dynamic compliance has been reported with the use of both CNP and CPAP in infants with HMD.[60,61] It is also possible that decrease in alveolar or interstitial fluid, or redistribution of blood flow may make a major contribution to the improvement in oxygenation.

An increase in functional residual capacity undoubtedly occurs, enhancing gas exchange in already open alveoli and preventing collapse

to airlessness. An improvement in the ventilation-perfusion ratio in local areas of the lung may also account for some of the increase in Pa_{O_2}.[63]

Airway resistance may increase in some infants[64] while a decrease has been reported in others.[62] A decrease in airway resistance has been reported in infants following operation for congenital heart disease.[65] Nasal prongs result in an increase in the work of breathing by 94%.[66]

Cardiovascular Effects

Cournand and coworkers observed that right-heart filling pressure and cardiac output decreased in response to increasing mean airway pressure.[67] Decreasing cardiac output by inordinate CPAP, in an already compromised infant, is very undesirable. Studies of the effects of CPAP on changes in cardiac output and circulation are lacking in infants. In dogs with normal lungs, the increase in pleural pressure and intravascular pressure within the thorax is about half of the applied airway pressure, and cardiac output falls with each increment in airway pressure.[68] The transmission of applied pressure is much less when there is a general decrease in lung compliance. Studies in animals with normal or abnormal lungs suggest that effects on cardiac output are influenced by the magnitude of applied airway pressure, the extent to which it is transmitted across the lungs (dependent on lung compliance), and blood volume.[69–71] Pulmonary blood flow may also be redistributed with high levels of PEEP.[71] Moderate levels of CPAP or PEEP (less than 10 cm H_2O) probably do not cause important alterations of cardiac output in the majority of patients, but may be hazardous in patients with hypovolemia or compromised myocardial function. A fall in arterial pressure or rise in central venous pressure with clinical evidence of decreased peripheral perfusion may be indicative of adversely high levels of CPAP or PEEP.

OTHER RESPIRATORY PROBLEMS
Apnea (See also Chap. 39)

Recurrent apnea in the premature infant may well account for more patient days in neonatal intensive care units than does any other condition. A major emphasis in the approach to this problem is ascertaining that apnea is in fact idiopathic and is not a secondary sign of some other metabolic or infectious event.

The respiration monitor, utilizing impedance pneumography, and the cardiac monitor are the most commonly used tools for the detection of these episodes. The alarm delay on the apnea monitor should be set long enough to exclude the apneic phases of periodic breathing. These usually last no longer than 12 seconds. Some infants, however, may become cyanotic and bradycardic in less than 12 seconds and therefore the choice of alarm delay should be individualized when possible. Random infant movement during apneic episodes may delay triggering the monitor alarm. Upper-airway obstructive apnea will also not be recorded as long as chest movement occurs.

Most apneic episodes can be aborted by tactile or proprioceptive stimulation. For an infant who is frequently apneic, it is useful to have a device for providing stimulation without entering the incubator. A string tied to the infant's leg and led outside the incubator serves this purpose, as do exterior handles for tilting the mattress tray. More vigorous stimulation, when needed, is accomplished by holding the infant and stroking or patting the trunk.

If the infant does not respond promptly to stimulation, ventilatory assistance with a bag and mask will avert marked cyanosis or profound bradycardia. This equipment should be kept in the incubator of a susceptible infant at all times. Initially, ventilation is with air to avoid excessive oxygen exposure in infants who require such assistance. Oxygen is added only if the color fails to improve.

Recently the methylxanthine class of drugs (caffeine and theophylline) has been shown to be effective in the prevention and treatment of neonatal apnea.[72] Although the exact mechanism of action is unclear, the drugs appear to alter respiratory center output activity and induce a greater sensitivity of the respiratory center to CO_2.[73] An initial dose of 5 mg/kg of aminophylline and subsequent doses of 1 to 2 mg/kg every 6 to 8 hours of either theophylline orally or aminophylline intravenously have been recommended to maintain a blood level of 6 to 12 μg/ml.[74] Both serum theophylline and caffeine levels must be measured in order to properly assess the total effective methylxanthine blood levels.[75] These drugs may have multisystem effects, and signs of overdose include tachycardia, distension, gastrointestinal bleeding, and seizures. There has been only one short-term follow-up study reported to date which indicated no adverse effects in treated infants.[76] However, until more information is known about the drug effects in premature infants, the drugs should be considered for use only as an alternative to long-term mechanical ventilation.

If apnea remains uncontrolled by the above measures, and bag-and-mask ventilation continues to be required for many closely spaced episodes, mechanical ventilation is indicated. Here, as in other applications, the ventilator must be carefully adjusted to maintain physiologic blood gas tensions. Infants who are ventilated for apnea generally require much lower respiratory pressures (sometimes as low as 10 cm H_2O PIP) than do infants with pulmonary disease. Schedules of weaning from the ventilator, in which gradually increasing periods of spontaneous ventilation are alternated with periods of mechanical ventilation, are designed to increase tolerance to the unaccustomed work of breathing. An end-expiratory pressure of 3 to 5 cm H_2O with or without intermittent positive-pressure ventilation may also be useful in the control of apnea.[77]

Meconium Aspiration

Aspiration of meconium or meconium-stained fluid at birth may result in airway obstruction and pneumonitis with sufficiently severe hypoxemia or hypercarbia to require mechanical ventilation. Prevention or amelioration of the disease may be accomplished by sunctioning the oral pharynx of the infant just as the head is delivered, and, following completion of the delivery, by suctioning the trachea of meconium while performing direct laryngoscopy.[78] The physician must balance the time involved in laryngoscopy and suctioning, with its concomitant poor ventilation, with the need to begin effective resuscitative efforts in an infant who is likely to be severely asphyxiated.

For the fully developed syndrome, the care is supportive. Corticosteroids have been shown to have no effect on the course or outcome of the disease.[79] Pulmonary gas exchange has been reported to improve in infants requiring mechanical ventilation when positive end-expiratory pressure was added;[80] however, this form of therapy has not been studied in a controlled manner. Because meconium aspiration syndrome often occurs in term or post-term infants, the effectiveness of mechanical ventilation may be compromised by the infant's struggling and attempting to breathe against the ventilator. Therefore, sedation, with or without respiratory paralysis (pancuronium bromide 0.03–0.06 mg/kg/dose) may be a useful adjunct for acute respiratory care. For those infants with intractible hypoxemia in spite of maximally assisted ventilation, a trial of a pulmonary (and systemic) vasodilator such as tolazoline hydrochloride (1 to 2 mg/kg/hour, continuous infusion), administered into the superior vena caval circulation, has been advocated.[81] However, this agent has multiple effects including systemic hypotension, oliguria, and gastrointestinal hemorrhage,[82] and its overall effect upon an individual patient's course is difficult to predict.

The effects on long-term pulmonary function of neonatal meconium aspiration are presently unknown.

Persistent Fetal Circulation

Persistent fetal circulation (PFC) is a syndrome of several days' to weeks' duration, characterized by hypoxemia and cyanosis, usually without hypercarbia, an anatomically normal heart, and diminished pulmonary blood flow with right-to-left shunts at the foramen ovale and the ductus arteriosus.[83] Treatment involves maintaining adequate tissue oxygenation until the increased pulmonary artery pressure abates. In some infants, the hypoxemia may necessitate mechanical ventilation. PEEP has not been tested in this setting but might pose a theoretical disadvantage because the airway pressure would be transmitted across a normally compliant chest and lung. This positive pressure may impede cardiac output and hence worsen the already diminished pulmonary blood flow. Use of tolazoline hydrochloride to lower the PA pressure has been reported to relieve hypoxemia in some infants.[83] However, as previously noted, this agent has multiple systemic effects.

Again, as in meconium aspiration syndrome, there have been no long-term studies on later pulmonary function in infants with PFC.

Pulmonary Air Leak

Pulmonary air leak may occur as a complication of any of the above-mentioned diseases. The air leak may consist of pulmonary interstitial emphysema, pneumomediastinum, pneumopericardium, and pneumothorax; the latter two usually require immediate treatment by evacuation of the air.

Pneumothorax must be considered whenever there is abrupt worsening of the respiratory or circulatory status of an infant at risk. Unilateral hyperresonance, decreased breath sounds, a shift of the apical cardiac impulse, and skin mottling are useful clinical clues. High-intensity illumination may demonstrate the presence of a pneumothorax if the room can be adequately darkened.[84] Often, however, a definite diagnosis can only be made by radiographic examination. The volume of the extrapulmonary air collection is not always a valid indication of the presence or absence of tension. Interstitial emphysema, often a precursor of pneumothorax,[85] will cause the lung to remain partly expanded even when intrapleural pressure is high. Bilateral pneumothorax may lead rapidly to death and must always be considered in cases of severe deterioration.

Pneumothorax in otherwise asymptomatic infants often resolves without therapy. However, marked mediastinal shift, coexisting pulmonary disease, or use of mechanical ventilation mandate immediate removal of the air. Aspiration with a syringe and needle may be done as an emergency procedure but will rarely be adequate by itself and should be followed with tube thoracostomy.

Thoracostomy tubes should be sterile and of nonreactive rubber or plastic. The wall thickness should be sufficient to prevent kinking and the lumen should be sufficiently large to prevent occlusion by exudate. The presence of at least two holes in the tube reduces the likelihood of occlusion by tissue. Polyvinyl chloride feeding tubes or trochar catheters (Argyle) size 8 or 10 Fr. are suitable for thoracostomy use. Feeding tubes can be inserted by grasping the tip with a clamp and pressing through a previously made incision through the pleura. Trochar catheters can be inserted after a skin incision has been made and can be Z-tracked over a rib for a better seal. However, the latter often require considerable force to insert, and lung puncture has been reported with their use.[86]

It is not usually practical to connect a suction apparatus to the tube before it has been secured, but the pneumothorax should be aspirated with a syringe and the tube occluded with a clamp or stopcock. A purse-string suture is placed in the skin around the tube, which can then be tied securely in place. The tube may become dislodged if care is not taken at this step. Taping alone is inadequate.

The tube is connected to continuous suction at a negative pressure of 10 to 15 cm of water with an underwater seal. A chest film should be obtained soon after thoracostomy. If the pneumothorax has not been evacuated, the infant should be repositioned, the tube stripped, or, if necessary, a second tube inserted.

A thoracostomy tube is left in place until air ceases to bubble from the tube and generally until the risk of recurrent pneumothorax is reduced (*i.e.,* until respiratory distress has subsided or mechanical ventilation is no longer required). The tube is then clamped. If in several hours there is neither clinical nor radiographic evidence of recurrent pneumothorax, the tube is removed and the skin incision promptly closed with a purse-string suture. Antibiotics are not used routinely if the thoracostomy is performed under aseptic conditions.

Pneumopericardium

Another form of air leak, pneumopericardium, characteristically presents with sudden and profound hypotension, distant heart sounds, and rapid death. Emergency treatment is to remove the air by passing a long catheter into the pericardial sac utilizing a subzyphoid approach and constant application of gentle negative pressure on the plunger of the syringe. The tip of the catheter needle should be aimed toward the left midclavicular region and the catheter should travel in a superficial plane towards the pericardial sac, once having penetrated the skin. An 18- or 20-gauge angiocath can be used for this purpose. There will be a gush of air when the pericardial sac is entered, and prompt relief of the hypotension. The needle should be sutured into place and connected to underwater drainage, as the pneumopericardium may recur. Consideration should then be given to replacement or repositioning the tube under direct surgical observation. In spite of these efforts, risk of mortality from pneumopericardium complicating respiratory distress remains very high.

Transient Tachypnea of the Newborn (TTNB)[47]

Unexplained tachypnea or respiratory distress in both full-term and premature infants occurs frequently. Increased perihilar density with fluid in the pleural space or minor fissure is usually seen on the chest film. Delayed absorption of fetal lung fluid has been suggested as an etiologic factor.[87] It is possible that other factors such as aspiration of amniotic fluid or mucus may account for the clinical and radiographic course. In either event, there is no specific treatment and the respiratory distress is self-limited, usually resolving in several days. Management of this illness consists in ruling out other, more treatable, forms of respiratory distress (*e.g.,* pneumonia) and maintaining adequate oxygenation. Usually feedings must be withheld because of the tachypnea. Careful observation is indicated in the first hours of life because TTNB is sometimes difficult to distinguish from early hyaline membrane disease.

INTENSIVE CARE SETTING (See also Chap. 3)

Management of respiratory problems requires specialized personnel and equipment. Nurses must be carefully trained in the techniques of intensive care of infants. Necessary skills include application of ventilatory support equipment, recognition of equipment malfunction, airway management, assessment of ventilation, and use of monitoring equipment. Nurse to patient ratios vary from 1:1 to 1:3, depending on the severity of the illness. Respirator management most often requires a ratio of 1:1.

A physician skilled in neonatal intensive care techniques should be available within the unit at all times and other specialists should be immediately accessible for consultation.

Respiratory therapists are critical to the effective use of respiratory equipment. Maintenance and calibration of all oxygen administration and oxygen-measuring devices require the presence of a respiratory therapist within the hospital around the clock.

Equipment needs for neonatal intensive care include wall sources of compressed air and oxygen, oxygen dilutors, heating and humidification devices, and oxygen-monitoring systems with alarms. Most premature infants need continuous monitoring of temperature, respiratory rate, and heart rate by electrical devices with alarm systems. In the acute phase of illness, or if an umbilical artery catheter is in use, continuous blood pressure monitoring and oscilloscopic ECG display are also advisable. Adequate and safe power sources must be available for all electrical equipment.

A procedure area with a heated table, an operating-room lamp, and surgical supplies facilitates the placement of umbilical catheters, performance of exchange transfusions, and other complex procedures.

The parents of severely ill infants need understanding and support. They experience feelings of anxiety, fear, guilt, and hostility. Many families are ill-equipped for the emotional and financial burden imposed by the hospitalization. A social worker should be available exclusively to the neonatal intensive care unit to provide assistance to parents by delineating parental concerns and helping coordinate communication with the medical and nursing staff and other hospital personnel.

Finally, the physical design of the intensive care unit must facilitate the management of acute respiratory problems. In particular, each patient area should be large enough to accommodate the personnel and enormous amount of equipment, without provoking intolerable crowding. A small number of patients in each room facilitates parental visiting and alleviates the overall level of stress.

Only when adequate attention is paid to these ancillary features of intensive respiratory care of the newborn can the optimal outcome expected for premature infants in this era be approached.

REFERENCES

1. **Polgar G, Kong GP:** The nasal resistance of newborn infants. J Pediatr 67:557, 1965
2. **Helmrath TA, Hodson WA, Oliver TK:** Positive pressure ventilation in the newborn infant: the use of a face mask. J Pediatr 76:202, 1970
3. **Weng JT, Stark FI, Indyk L et al:** Oxygen supplementation during endotracheal intubation of the infant. Pediatrics 59:1042, 1977
4. **Coldiron JS:** Estimation of nasotracheal tube length in neonates. Pediatrics 41:823, 1968
5. **Rasche RFH, Kuhns LR:** Histopathologic changes in airway mucosa of infants after endotracheal intubation. Pediatrics 50:632, 1972
6. **Klainer AS, Turndorf H, Wu WH:** Surface alterations to endotracheal intubation, Am J Med 58:679, 1975
7. **Porkin JL, Stevens MH, Jung AL:** Acquired and congenital subglottic stenosis in the infant. Annals of Otolaryngology 85:573, 1976
8. **Berman SA, Balkany TJ, Simmons MA:** Otitis media in the neonatal intensive care unit. Pediatrics 62:198, 1978
9. **Filston HC, Johnson DG, Crumrire RS:** Infant tracheostomy. Am J Dis Childr 132:1172, 1978
10. **Thibeault DW, Hobel CJ, Kwong MS:** Perinatal factors influencing the arterial oxygen tension in preterm infants with RDS while breathing 100% oxygen. J Pediatr 84:898, 1974
11. **Guthrie RD, Haberkern CM, Woodrum DE et al:** Effects of acute hypoxemia on the EEG of the neonatal primate (abst). Pediatr Res 13:525, 1979
12. **Kinsey VE, Arnold HJ, Kalina RE et al:** PaO_2 levels and retrolental fibroplasia: a report of the Cooperative Study. Pediatrics 60:655, 1977
13. **Lechner D, Kalina RE, Hodson WA:** Retrolental fibroplasia and factors influencing oxygen transport. Pediatrics 59:916, 1977
14. **Murdock AI, Swyer PR:** Contribution to venous admixture through the ductus arteriosus in infants with the respiratory distress syndrome of the newborn. Biol Neonate 13:194, 1968
15. **Indyk L:** PO_2 in the 70's. Pediatrics 55:135, 1975
16. **Graham G, Kenny MA:** Performance of a radiometer transcutaneous oxygen monitor in a neonatal intensive care unit. Clin Chem 26(5):629–632, 1980
17. **Peabody JL, Gregory GA, Willis MM:** Transcutaneous oxygen tension in sick infants. Am Rev Respir Dis 118:83, 1978
18. **Koch G, Wendel H:** Comparison of pH, carbon dioxide, standard bicarbonate, and oxygen tension in capillary blood to arterial blood during the neonatal period. Acta Pediatric Scand 56:10, 1967
19. **Schleuter MA, Johnson BB, Sudman DA et al:** Blood sampling from scalp arteries in infants. Pediatrics 51:120, 1973
20. **Wall PM, Kuhns LT:** Percutaneous arterial sampling using transillumination. Pediatrics 59:1032, 1977
21. **Simons MF, Levine RL, Lubchenco LG et al:** Serious sequelae of temporal artery catheterization. J Pediatr 92:284, 1978
22. **Hillman LS, Goodwin SL, Sherman WR:** Identification and measurement of plasticizer in neonatal tissues after umbilical catheters and blood products. N Engl J Med 292:381, 1975
23. **Clawson CC, Boros SJ:** Surface morphology of polyvinyl chloride and silicone elastomer umbilical artery catheters by scanning electron microscopy. Pediatrics 62:702, 1978
24. **Clark JM, Jung AL:** Umbilical artery catheterization by a cutdown procedure. Pediatrics 59:1036, 1977
25. **Mokrobisky ST, Levine RL, Blumhagen JD et al:** Low positioning of umbilical artery catheters increases associated complications in newborn infants. N Engl J Medicine 299:561, 1978

26. **Dunn PM:** Localization of the umbilical catheter by post-mortem measurement. Arch Dis Child 41:69, 1966

27. **Neal WA, Reynolds JW, Jarvis CW et al:** Umbilical artery catheterization: demonstration of arterial thrombosis by aortagraphy. Pediatrics 50:6, 1972

28. **Plumber LB, Kaplan GW, Mondoza SA:** Hypertension in infants: a complication of umbilical arterial catheterization. J Pediatr 89: 802, 1976

29. **Goetzman BW, Stedalink RC, Bogren HG et al:** Thrombotic complications of umbilical artery catheters: a clinical and radiographic study. Pediatrics 56:374, 1975

30. **Kraus AN, Albert RF, Kannan MM:** Contamination of umbilical catheters in the newborn infant. J Pediatr 77:963, 1970

31. **Powers WF, Tooley WH:** Contamination of umbilical vessel catheters: emergency information. Pediatrics 49:470, 1972

32. **Bard H, Albert G, Teasdale F et al:** Prophylactic antibiotics in chronic umbilical artery catheterization in respiratory distress syndrome. Arch Dis Child 48:63, 1973

33. **Aziz EM, Robertson AF:** Paraplegia: A complication of umbilical artery catheterization. J Pediatr 82:1051, 1973

34. **Smith PC, Schach E, Daily WJR:** Mechanical ventilation of newborn infants: II. effects of independent variation of rate and pressure on arterial oxygenation of infants with respiratory distress syndrome. Anesthesiology 37:498, 1972

35. **Herman S, Reynolds EOR:** Methods for improving oxygenation in infants mechanically ventilated for severe hyaline membrane disease. Arch Dis Child 48:612, 1973

36. **Taghizadeh A, Reynolds EOR:** Pathogenesis of bronchopulmonary dysplasia following hyaline membrane disease. Am J Pathol 82: 241–264, 1976

37. **Boros SJ, Orgill AA:** Mortality and morbidity associated with pressure- and volume-limited infant ventilators. Am J Dis Child 132:865–869, 1978

38. **Boros SJ:** Variations in inspiratory-expiratory ratio and airway pressure wave form during mechanical ventilation: the significance of mean airway pressure. J Pediatr 94:114–117, 1979

39. **Jansson L, Jonson B:** A theoretical study on flow patterns of ventilators. Scand J Respir Dis 53:237–246, 1972

40. **Fuleihan SF, Wilson RS, Pontoppidan H:** Effect of mechanical ventilator with end-inspiratory pause on blood gas exchange. Anesth Analg 55:122–130, 1976

41. **Cheney FW, Burham SC:** Effect of ventilatory pattern on oxygenation in pulmonary edema. J Appl Physiol 31:909–912, 1971

42. **Nugent SK, Laravuso R, Rogers MC:** Pharmacology and use of muscle relaxants in infants and children. J Pediatr 94:481, 1979

43. **Northway WH, Rosan RC, Porter DY:** Pulmonary disease following respiratory therapy of hyaline membrane disease/bronchopulmonary dysplasia, N Eng J Med 276: 357–368, 1967

44. **Edwards DK, Colby TV, Northway WH:** Radiographic-pathologic correlation in bronchopulmonary dysplasia. J Pediatr 95:834–836, 1979

45. **Edwards DK:** Radiographic aspects of bronchopulmonary dysplasia. J Pediatr 95:823–829, 1979

46. **Stahlman MD:** Clinical description of bronchopulmonary dysplasia. J Pediatr 95:829–834, 1979

47. **Hodson WA, Truog WE, Mayock DE et al:** Bronchopulmonary dysplasia: the need for epidemiologic studies. J Pediatr 95:848–851, 1979

48. **Harrison VC, Heese HV, Klein M:** The significance of grunting in hyaline membrane disease. Pediatrics 41:549, 1968

49. **Thibault DW, Poblete E, Auld PAM:** Alveolar-arterial O_2 and CO_2 differences and their relation to lung volume in the newborn. Pediatrics 41:574, 1968

50. **Gregory GA, Kitterman JA, Phibbs RH et al:** Treatment of the idiopathic respiratory distress syndrome with continuous positive airway pressure. N Engl J Med 384:1333, 1971

51. **Gregory GA:** Devices for applying continuous positive airway pressure. In Thibault DW, Gregory GA (ed): Neonatal Pulmonary Care. Menlo Park, Calif, Addison–Wesley, 1979

52. **Novogroder M, MacKuanying N, Eidelman AI et al:** Nasopharyngeal ventilation in respiratory distress syndrome. J Pediatr 82:1059, 1973

53. **Kattwinkel J, Fleming D, Cha CC et al:** A device for administration of continuous positive airway pressure by the nasal route. Pediatrics 52:130, 1973

54. **Belenky DA, Orr RH, Woodrum DE, Hodson WA:** Is continuous transpulmonary pressure better than conventional respiratory management of hyaline membrane disease? a controlled study. Pediatrics 58:800, 1976

55. **Krouskop RW, Brown EG, Sweet AY:** The early use of continuous positive airway pressure in the treatment of idiopathic respiratory distress syndrome. J Pediatr 87:263, 1975

56. **Mockrin LD, Bancalari EH:** Early versus delayed initiation of continuous negative pressure in infants with hyaline membrane disease. J Pediatr 87:596, 1975

57. **Gerard P, Fox WW, Outerbridge EW et al:** Early versus late introduction of continuous negative pressure in the management of the idiopathic respiratory distress syndrome. J Pediatr 87:591, 1975

58. **Rowe JC, Guthrie RD, Hinkes P et al:** Time of initiation of CPAP in HMD. Pediatr Res 12:533A, 1978

59. **Bonta BW, Wekslew L, Warshaw JB et al:** Determination of optimal continuous positive airway pressure for the treatment of IRDS by measurement of esophageal pressure. J Pediatr 91:449, 1977

60. **Bancalari E, Garcia O, Jesse MJ:** Effects on continuous negative pressure on lung mechanics in idiopathic respiratory distress syndrome. Pediatrics 51:485, 1973

61. **Yu VYH, Rolfe P:** Effect of continuous positive airway pressure breathing on cardiac respiratory function in infants with respiratory distress syndrome. Acta Paediatr Scand 66:59, 1977

62. **Saunders RA, Milner AD, Hopkins IE:** The effects of continuous positive airway pressure on lung mechanics and lung volumes in the neonate. Biol Neonate 29:178, 1976

63. **Richardson CP, Jung AL:** Effects of continuous positive airway pressure on pulmanry function and blood gases of infants with respiratory distress syndrome. Pediatr Res 12:771–774, 1978

64. **Gregory GA:** Continuous positive airway pressure (CPAP). In Thibeault DW, Gregory GA: Neonatal Care. Menlo Park, Calif, Wesley, 1979

65. **Cogswell JJ, Hatch DJ, Kerr AA:** Effects of continuous positive airway pressure on lung mechanics of babies after operation for congenital heart disease. Arch Dis Child 50:799, 1975

66. **Goldman SL, Brady JP, Dumpit FM:** Increased work of breathing assocated with nasal prongs. Pediatrics, 64: 1979

67. **Cournand A, Motley HL, Werko I et al:** Physiologic studies of the effects of intermittent positive pressure breathing on cardiac output in man. Am J Physiol 152:162, 1948

68. **Lenfant C, Howell BJ:** Cardiovascular adjustments in dogs during continuous pressure breathing. J Appl Physiol 15:524, 1960

69. **Holzman BH, Scarpelli EM:** Cardiopulmonary consequences of positive end-expiratory pressure. Pediatr Res 13:1112–1120, 1979

70. **Cassidy SS, Robertson CH, Pierce AK et al:** Cardiovascular effects of positive end-expiratory pressure in dogs. J Appl Physiol 44:743–750, 1978

71. **Hedenstierna G, White FC, Mazzone R et al:** Redistribution of pulmonary blood flow in the dog with PEEP ventilation. J Appl Physiol 46:278–287, 1979

72. **Kuzenko JA, Poala J:** Apneic attacks in the newborn treated with amniophylline. Arch Dis Child 48:404, 1973

73. **Davi MJ, Sankaram K, Simons KJ et al:** Physiologic changes induced by theophylline in the treatment of apnea in preterm infants. J Pediatr 92:91, 1978

74. **Aranda JV, Sitar DS, Parsons WD et al:** Pharmacokinetic aspects of theophylline in prematurĕ newborns. N Engl J Med 295:413, 1976

75. **Bory C, Baltassat P, Porthault M et al:** Metabolism of theophylline to caffeine in premature newborn infants. J Pediatr 94:988, 1979

76. **Gunn TR, Metrakos K, Riley P et al:** Sequelae of caffeine treatment in preterm infants with apnea. J Pediatr 94:106, 1979

77. **Kattwinkel J:** Neonatal apnea: pathogenesis and therapy. J Pediatr 90:342, 1977

78. **Carson BS, Losey RW, Bowes WA et al:** Combined obstetric and pediatric approach to prevent meconium aspiration syndrome. Am J Obstet Gynecol 126:712, 1976

79. **Yeh TF, Srinivason G, Harris V et al:** Hydrocortisone therapy in meconium aspiration syndrome: a controlled study. J Pediatr 90:140, 1977

80. **Fox WW, Berman LS, Down JJ et al:** Therapeutic application of end expiratory pressure in the meconium aspiration syndrome. Pediatrics 56:214, 1975

81. **Levin DL, Gregory GA:** The effect of tolazoline on right to left shunting via a patent ductus arteriosus in meconium aspiration syndrome. Crit Care Med 4:304, 1976

82. **Stevenson DK, Kosting DS, Dornall RA et al:** Refractory hypoxemia associated with neonatal pulmonary disease: the use and limitations of tolazoline. J Pediatr 95:595, 1979

83. **Goetzman BW, Sunshine P, Johnson JD et al:** Neonatal hypoxia and pulmonary vasospasm: response to tolazoline. J Pediatr 89:617, 1976

84. **Kuhns LR, Bednorck, FJ, Wyman ML:** Diagnosis of pneumothorax or pneumomediastinum in the neonate by transillumination. Pediatrics 56:355, 1975

85. **Ogata ES, Gregory GA, Kitterman JA et al:** Pneumothorax in the respiratory distress syndrome: incidence and effect on vital signs, blood gas, and pH. Pediatrics 58:177, 1976

86. **Banayale RC, Outerbridge EW, Aranda JV:** Lung perforation: a complication of chest tube insertions in neonatal pneumothorax. J Pediatr 94:973, 1979

87. **Schaffer AJ, Avery ME:** Diseases of the Newborn, 4th ed, p 171. Philadlephia, WB Saunders, 1977

23

Neonatal Heart Disease

*Donald C. Fyler and
Peter Lang*

INTRODUCTION

Since the first edition of this text book, the field of neonatal cardiology has flourished. Notable progress has been made in the physiologic understanding and the pharmacologic manipulation of the ductus arteriosus.[1,2,3,4] Control of the patency of the ductus arteriosus has wide potential value and may be at hand. Noninvasive cardiac diagnosis through the use of two-dimensional echocardiography has proved to be a breakthrough,[5] and, nowadays, it is rare to be without a precise anatomic diagnosis before cardiac catheterization. Primary reparative surgery in early infancy is being increasingly used as the surgical treatment of choice for selected cardiac lesions, and overall surgical mortalities for infant cardiac surgery are improving.[6]

In this chapter, topics considered of interest to the neonatologist are covered; for further detail, standard texts of pediatric cardiology should be consulted.[7,8,9] Much of the statistical data to be presented is derived from the New England Regional Infant Cardiac Program (NERICP), a cooperative venture of all the hospitals in New England providing definitive care to cardiac infants (Table 23-1).

Incidence

The incidence of congenital heart disease has been most reliably estimated to be 7.5 in 1000 live births.[10]

The statistic of most interest in planning services for babies with heart disease is the number who are ill enough to require some intervention. Considering those sick enough to risk the hazard of cardiac catheterization, to require cardiac surgery or to have died with heart disease, there is a maximum of 2.7 sick cardiac infants per 1000 births in New England. Nearly one-half of these babies are first seen before the second week of life.

Mortality

Prior to the philosophy of aggressive intervention, Mitchell found that 2.3 in 1000 live births developed lethal cardiac problems in infancy.[10] New England data covering the period of aggressive palliation indicate that the current infant cardiac fatality rate is more nearly 1.2 in 1000 births. Congential heart disease is a major cause of neonatal death in the Children's Hospital Medical Center, Boston, assounting for one-third of all neonatal deaths.

In a study of perinatal and infant mortality

Table 23-1. New England Regional Infant Cardiac Program (NERICP)* Participating Centers.

Center and Physician	City and State
Hartford Hospital	
Leon Chameides, M.D.	Hartford, CN
St. Francis Hospital	
Ellen Marmer, M.D.	Hartford, CN
Yale–New Haven Hospital	
Norman S. Talner, M.D.	New Haven, CN
Maine Medical Center	
Edward C. Matthews, M.D.	Portland, ME
Boston Floating Hospital	
Marshall B.	Boston, MA
Kreidberg, M.D.	
Children's Hospital	
Medical Center	
Donald C. Fyler, M.D.	Boston, MA
Massachusetts	
General Hospital	
Allan Goldblatt, M.D.	Boston, MA
Dartmouth–Hitchcock	
Medical Center	
Richard J. Waters, M.D.	Hanover, NH
Rhode Island Hospital	
Robert D. Corwin, M.D.	Providence, RI
Medical Center Hospital	
of Vermont	
Mary Fletcher Unit	Burlington, VT
Arthur M. Levy, M.D.	

*The New England Infant Cardiac Program is supported by the Maternal and Child Health Service, Health Service and Mental Health Administration Project #260

in Massachusetts for the years 1967 and 1968, Muirhead and associates found that congenital heart disease accounts for 3% of deaths in the first week of life among live-born, otherwise potentially viable infants.[11] This figure rose to 33% of all deaths in the remainder of the neonatal period. The noncardiac deaths are dominantly related to low birth weight and early gestational age. Because congenital heart disease is primarily a problem of full-term infants, it is easy to conclude that congenital heart disease is a major cause of death of neonates born at term.

In New England, 150 infants die with congenital heart disease each year (Table 23-2; Figs. 23-1, 23-2). Analysis demonstrates the importance of noncardiac anomalies and pre-

maturity in these deaths. Consequently, in estimating the potential for salvage of cardiac infants, it is important to assess the contribution to mortality that is attributable to noncardiac anomalies and to low birth weight. For example, of 31 newborns dead with ventricular septal defect only 10 were not complicated by extracardiac anomalies or low birth weight.

Survival Versus Salvage

It is important to distinguish between survival and salvage. An infant with an uncorrectable cardiac problem may survive because of a palliative operation, but have no expec-

Table 23-2. Mortality of Symptomatic Cardiac Infants Hospitalized in the First 28 Days of Life (1968–1977).

Diagnosis	No.	% Mortality*
D-Transposition of the		
great arteries	289	42
Hypoplastic left ventricle	227	97
Coarctation, complex	181	64
Tetralogy of Fallot	123	35
Heterotaxies	113	61
Pulmonary atresia with		
intact septum	105	74
Ventricular defect		
complex	102	22
simple	99	9
Patent ductus arteriosus	86	21
Endocardial cushion defect	74	50
Single ventricle	69	52
Tricuspid atresia	64	45
Pulmonary atresia with		
ventricular defect	55	46
Total anomalous pulmonary		
venous drainage	55	73
Pulmonary stenosis	50	26
Myocardial disease	38	37
Aortic stenosis	38	63
Truncus arteriosus	35	74
Atrial defect, secundum	32	22
Coarctation, simple	31	39
Others	128	46
Total	2220	50

*Gross mortality through first birthday.

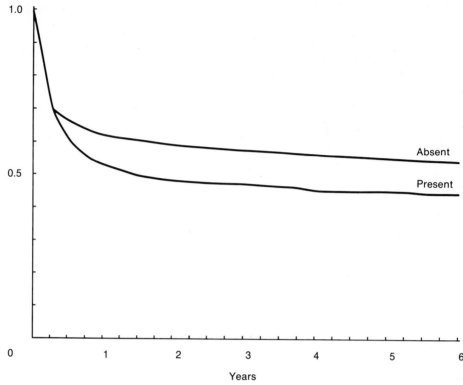

Fig. 23-1. Lifetable for cardiac infants with and without extracardiac anomalies.

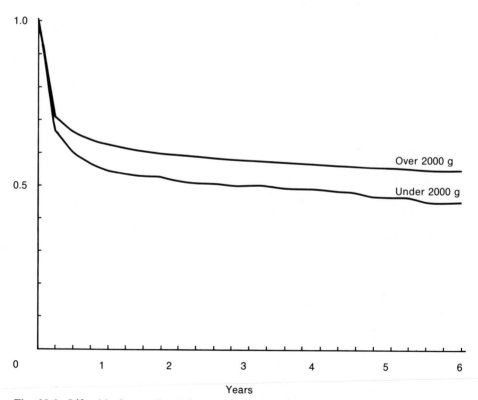

Fig. 23-2. Lifetable for cardiac infants with birth weights under and over 2000 g.

tation of reaching adulthood. Similarly, the cardiac problem may be totally corrected, but in the process the baby may suffer permanent central nervous system damage. Correction of a cardiac defect in a child with major anomalies can scarcely be categorized as a salvaging the baby. Finally, there is little satisfaction in repairing the child's cardiac problem at the price of economic or psychologic devastation of the child and his family.

The New England experience indicates that 50% of newborns symptomatic with heart disease will survive to their fifth birthday. Survival rates beyond 5 years are not established. In 80% of the 5-year survivors, there is no impairment of intellectual or motor development and no limitation of growth. Most of these problems are the result of associated extra-cardiac anomalies and only 3% are acquired during treatment.

With refinement of recognition, transportation, diagnosis, and surgery, it is realistic to suspect that as many as 65% of infants born with potentially lethal heart disease can be successfully salvaged.

Table 23-3. Diagnostic Distribution by 3-Year Periods.* (Percent)

Diagnosis	1969–71 $n = 727$	1972–74 $n = 692$	1975–77 $n = 800$
Transposition of the great arteries	15.7	12.9	10.7
Hypoplastic left-heart syndrome	11.6	10.4	8.7
Coarctation of the aorta, complex	8.7	6.9	8.7
Tetralogy of Fallot	6.5	4.9	5.2
Heterotaxies	5.2	4.8	5.2
Pulmonary atresia with intact septum	5.5	4.6	4.1
Ventricular defect complex	4.4	4.9	4.5
simple	4.0	5.5	4.0
Patent ductus arteriosus	4.1	4.3	3.2
Endocardial cushion defect	2.6	3.8	3.6

* Symptomatic cardiac infants hospitalized in first 28 days of life

Etiologic Considerations

The constancy of the relative diagnostic frequency, year by year, state by state, hospital by hospital, has been notable (Table 23-3). Any etiologic theory must account for this phenomenon as well as the sex differences associated with specific lesions. Thus, males more commonly have coarctation, aortic stenosis, and transposition, while females are prone to have atrial septal defect and patent ductus arteriosus. Maternal diabetes is associated with several cardiac anomalies (see below) while maternal rubella is most often associated with patent ductus arteriosus and narrowed right and left main pulmonary arteries.

Rarely, all children in a family will have the same cardiac defect; and approximately 3.5% of siblings of children with congenital heart disease will also have cardiac anomalies. It is rare for both fraternal twins to have heart disease, yet up to 25% of identical twins will both have cardiac abnormalities. About one-third of patients with congenital heart disease are found to have a positive family history of congenital cardiac abnormalities. Certain chromosomal aberrations are often associated with heart disease; the association of Downs's syndrome and heart anomalies, especially endocardial cushion defect, are common (Table 23-4).

The tendency for various cardiac anomalies to occur together suggests common embryogenesis (*i.e.*, infundibular pulmonary stenosis and ventricular septal defect, or coarctation and patent ductus arteriosus). Similarly, the association of noncardiac anomalies and specific forms of heart disease can be recognized (*e.g.*, asplenia or polysplenia). (See below.)

Certain cardiac lesions are associated with prematurity or low birth weight (Table 23-5). Because closure of the ventricular septum may be recognizably delayed until the first months of life, it is not surprising that among prematures there is a somewhat increased incidence of ventricular septal defect. The increased incidence of patent ductus arteriosus among prematures can be viewed as birth before the programmed time for closure of the ductus; and, at the same time, the effect of hypoxemia of pulmonary origin in promoting ductal patency must be remembered.

Clearly many interdependent factors may play a role in the etiology of congenital heart disease.

Table 23-4. Distribution of Associated Extracardiac Anomalies By System.

System	% of Total
Musculoskeletal	9.4
Central nervous	5.7
Renal–urinary	5.4
Gastrointestinal	4.3
Trisomy 21	4.2
Respiratory	3.7
Maternal rubella	0.9
Trisomy 17–18	0.4
Turner's	0.4
Trisomy 13–15	0.2
Pierre Robin	0.2

Data base 3364 cardiac infants 1968–1977

PHYSIOLOGY

Extensive information concerning the circulatory physiology of fetus and newborn has accumulated. The works of Barcroft,[12] Dawes,[13] Rudolph,[14] and Lind[15] should be consulted for details. Only the central features will be discussed here.

Fetal Circulation

The circulation before birth consists of parallel circuits (Fig. 23-3). Blood in the aorta may follow several channels to a capillary bed, back to the heart, passing through either ventricle, and out again to the aorta. The stream from the ductus venosus by way of the inferior vena cava carries newly oxygenated blood from the placenta. Unlike the circulation after birth, the streams of oxygenated and unoxygenated blood are not separated, although the more oxygenated blood from the inferior vena cava tends to be diverted through the foramen ovale into the left atrium. For this reason, blood entering the ascending aorta from the left ventricle is somewhat higher in oxygen than that entering the descending aorta from the right ventricle by way of the ductus arteriosus.

Because of the parallel arrangement of the ventricles, the potential of each ventricle for pumping different amounts of blood exists. Normally, the volume pumped by the right ventricle is thought to exceed that pumped by the left by a ratio of 125/75. Because both ventricles pump against the systemic resist-ance, the level of pressure in the two ventricles is comparable. The resistance to blood flow through the lungs is great; consequently, only minimal caretaker flow through the lungs occurs *in utero*.

The parallel arrangement of the ventricles allows fetal survival despite a wide variety of cardiac lesions. With total obstruction of either ventricle, the other ventricle assumes the entire cardiac output with surprising success. Reversal of the pulmonary arterial and aortic streams of blood, as occurs in transposition of the great arteries, produces no deleterious effect on the fetus. Indeed the birth weights of these babies are at least normal and possibly greater than normal. Even lesions that cause increased fetal cardiac work, such as central nervous system arteriovenous fistulas, are tolerated surprisingly well. The ability to withstand gross intrauterine circulatory abnormal-

Table 23-5. Incidence of Low Birth Weight (<2500 g) Among Infants Admitted with Heart Disease in First Months of Life.

Diagnosis	Total Patients	No. Low Birth Weight	Percent Low Birth Weight
D-Transposition of great arteries	289	9	3
Hypoplastic left ventricle	226	21	9
Coarctation, complex	181	33	18
Tetralogy of Fallot	123	24	20
Heterotaxies	113	15	13
Pulmonary atresia with intact septum	105	16	12
Ventricular defect			
complex	102	31	30
simple	99	27	27
Patent ductus ateriosus	86	35	41
Endocardial cushion defect	74	20	27
Other heart disease	1192	93	8
Lung disease	206	98	48
Total	2220	422	19

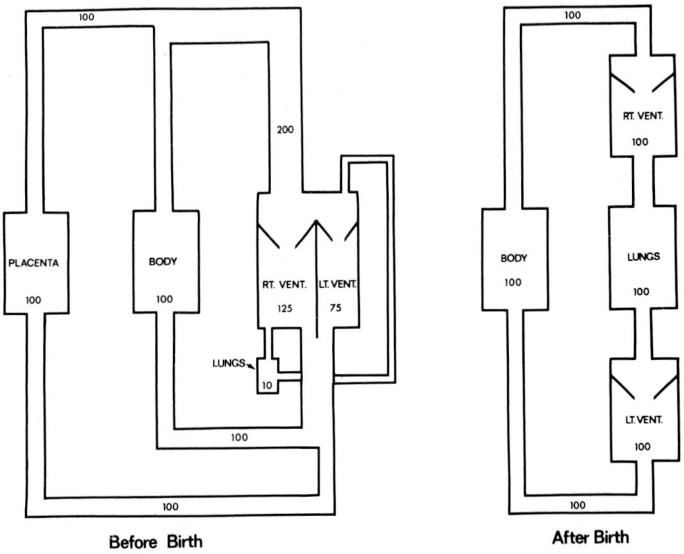

Fig. 23-3. Numbers refer to relative blood flow. Note that the right and left ventricles share in providing systemic blood flow before birth. After birth each ventricle pumps the entire systemic blood flow consecutively with the result that each ventricle pumps approximately the same amount before and after birth. After birth the amount carried by the aorta, is, nonetheless, reduced by 50% because the placenta is removed. Note that the small amount recirculated through the lungs before birth is ignored in these estimations.

ity is in part a result of simultaneous development of the anomaly and adaptation to it. Despite the remarkable ability to adapt, to grow, and to survive, it is apparent that any important limitation in ability to pump (*e.g.,* any limitation in myocardial contractility) will affect the fetus in direct proportion to its severity. Because of the virtual exclusion of the lungs from the circulation, fetal congestive heart failure is a matter of generalized edema. Thus, a newborn with myocardial disease may be born with anasarca. The interplay between the metabolic effects of congestion in the fetus and the possible compensatory role of the placenta is not understood. Because lesions that should cause gross intrauterine difficulty are tolerated surprisingly well, the postulate that the placenta helps to compensate for the metabolic abnormalities resulting from congestive heart failure is tenable.

Circulatory Adjustments at Birth

With the first breath, the resistance to pulmonary blood flow drops sharply. The oxygen content of the left heart and systemic circulation rapidly reaches levels well above that of the fetal circulation. The oxygen saturation in the ascending fetal aorta is 65% while immediately after birth it rises to 93%. The ductus venosus functionally closes, establishing the portal circulation as an independent loop between two capillary beds. With removal of the low resistance placenta, systemic resistance stabilizes at a higher level. The relative fall in the pulmonary resistance and rise in the systemic resistance results in a transitory left-to-right shunt through the ductus arteriosus. The ductus becomes functionally closed toward the end of the first day of life, becoming anatomically obliterated at about 10 days of age. The closure of the ductus is partly the result of direct exposure to highly oxygenated blood; yet, among profoundly cyanotic newborns the ductus may inexorably close, often severing the infant's only source of pulmonary blood flow (*e.g.,* pulmonary atresia). The mechanisms causing closure of the ductus are not completely understood but involve the prostaglandins system, blood oxygen, carbon dioxide, and pH. At birth the left ventricle abruptly becomes the sole supplier of systemic blood flow. The volume it pumps is thereby fractionally increased; the left-to-right shunt through the ductus adds further volume work and the elevated systemic resistance must be overcome. While this is a stressful time for the left ventricle, the magnitude of these suddenly acquired burdens is not so great that detectable left ventricular difficulties are seen normally. Yet, any impairment of myocardial function is likely to be magnified as a consequence. Myocardial disease as a cause of symptoms is more common in the first days of life than at any other time (21 of a total of 81 infants with myocardial disease presented in the first week of life). Recovery from severe left ventricular failure is often surprising.

At birth, the volume of blood to be pumped by the right ventricle decreases to the level of the systemic blood flow; right ventricular pressure falls in porportion to the decrease in pulmonary resistance. Thus, while left ventricular work increases, right ventricular work decreases.

While before birth the two ventricles share in supplying systemic blood flow and placental flow, after birth the two ventricles independently handle the entire cardiac output. Each ventricle effectively pumps blood in amounts comparable to that pumped *in utero*, despite a reduction by 50% in the amount of blood pumped through the aorta because of removal of the placenta (Fig. 23-3). While this arrangement results in pumping comparable amounts of blood by each ventricle before and after birth, it is apparent that a central nervous system arteriovenous fistula will for the same reason—the shift from parallel to serial ventricular pumping—result in an acutely increased volume of work for each ventricle, despite a constant flow through the fistula. Thus, these babies often die immediately after birth, despite normal growth *in utero*.

Closure of the foramen ovale functionally occurs soon after birth, largely as a result of increased left atrial volume and pressure secondary to the ductal left-to-right shunt and the developing differences in diastolic pressure of the two ventricles. Anatomic closure normally is delayed for months or years. Among infants with cardiac defects, factors favoring increased right atrial pressure will favor indefinite patency of the foramen ovale (*e.g.*, pulmonary stenosis), while abnormally increased left atrial pressure promotes early anatomic closure (*e.g.*, ventricular septal defect).

Prior to birth, the pulmonary arterioles are relatively muscular and constricted. With the first breath, total pulmonary resistance falls rapidly, in large part because of unkinking of the vessels with expansion of the lungs. The vasodilatory effect of inspired oxygen also plays a significant role. The muscular constriction relaxes, and, gradually over the subsequent days and weeks, thinning of the muscular wall of the pulmonary arterioles can be demonstrated. During the first weeks of life, the muscular arterioles retain a significant capacity for constriction. Pulmonary alveolar hypoxia normally produces an increase in pulmonary artery pressure at all ages, but, in the young infant, the response is more profound and occurs more rapidly. Thus, the discovery of pulmonary hypertension equal to or greater than systemic pressure is a familiar observation in a sick baby.

Prematurity

The events at birth and in the neonatal period are modified in direct relation to the degree of prematurity. The muscular coat of the pulmonary arterioles develops late in gestation; the more premature the infant the less muscular are his pulmonary arterioles at birth. The most notable consequence of this is that the difference between systemic and pulmonary resistance after birth is greater among prematures than among normals. Consequently, shunting through a ductus arteriosus is often audible. Furthermore, the hypoxia, so common among prematures may be one of the factors that delays closure of the ductus, and, as a result, ductal murmurs are more common. The propensity of the ductus to close at around 41 weeks after conception is clinically recognized. Among infants with persistently patent ductus, the incidence of prematurity is greater than expected.

The prolonged ductal shunting in the premature would probably be of no consequence except that ductal shunting is often promoted by and associated with respiratory distress. How much additional difficulty the ductus shunt causes through increased pulmonary blood volume in an infant already severely ill with respiratory distress is a matter of debate. Sometimes, patency of the ductus arteriosus causes left ventricular failure. Whether medical or surgical interruption of these ductus will have an appreciable effect on survival is undetermined. It is our view that the ductus is rarely a major problem by itself; rather, it is an added problem in an already serious situation. These ductus are found equally among males and females and are considered to be persistent patency of the normal ductus. By contrast, patent ductus unassociated with prematurity is dominantly encountered among females (2:1).

Recognition

Only a small number of infants are born in hospitals equipped for all eventualities. To allow time for transfer to a specially equipped and staffed cardiac center, recognition that the baby has heart disease must be early, or he may not survive transportation, cardiac catheterization and surgery.

Age of Discovery. In recent years, 49 percent of all critically ill cardiac infants born in New England have been admitted to a treatment center within the first week of life. Increased salvage is demonstrable, yet, at the same time, many infants who would formerly have died before transfer are now discovered to have insurmountable problems. In effect, development of an early referral system not only allows greater salvage but also accumulates the most difficult problems.

Murmurs. Hearing a murmur is the commonest means of recognizing infant heart disease. In the recent past, workup consisted of a chest film and an ECG. Nowadays, a two-dimensional echocardiogram is also obtained. This technique demonstrates the anatomic basis for the murmur, occasionally uncovering a potentially lethal lesion in advance of symptoms. Because the transition from fetal to extrauterine circulation continues during the first weeks of life, the earlier the baby is discovered to have heart disease the greater the potential for sudden deterioration. Consequently, safety dictates more frequent initial follow-up.

Cyanosis. Much more threatening than a murmur is the presence of cyanosis. Cyanosis without pulmonary disease is almost invariably the result of a serious cardiac abnormality. Especially in the first week of life cyanosis may be the sole evidence of an important cardiac lesion. Fully one-third of infants with potentially lethal congenital heart disease have cyanosis as their major symptom; another one-third have cyanosis in association with respiratory symptoms. All cyanotic babies should undergo prompt cardiac evaluation in the hope of finding a lesion amenable to surgery.

Cyanosis due to hypoglycemia or methemoglobinemia is rare. Methemoglobinemia should be suspected if the arterial P_{O_2} and arterial oxygen saturation are discordant, the P_{O_2} being normal while the saturation is low.

The clinical recognition of cyanosis is influenced by the baby's hemoglobin. An anemic infant may have severe arterial oxygen unsaturation without obvious cyanosis, while infants with polycythemia may appear cyanotic with normal arterial oxygen levels. A hypothermic infant may seem blue; a baby viewed in fluorescent lighting may appear blue; and blue-colored surroundings may confuse the estimation of cyanosis.

Respiratory Symptoms. Before cardiac surgery was available for small infants, pediatric cardiologists ignored the statements of grandmothers and multiparas that the baby had always breathed too fast as maternal, retrospective aberrations. There is now no doubt that repeated respiratory rates of 60 per minute or greater, not only commonly precede the first detection of a murmur, but, more important may presage deterioration to gross dyspnea and congestive heart failure. Recognition that tachypnea is present prompts discovery that the underlying cause is either heart disease or lung disease. A chest film may provide the answer.

Diagnosis

Number of Diagnostic Entities. The number of cardiac lesions that cause serious disability among newborns is great (Table 23-6). Considering the possible anatomic combinations of lesions, it can be estimated that approximately 100 different physiologic entities are encountered. The commonest general category is D-transposition of the great arteries and includes several different physiologic problems. The combinations of presence or absence of ventricular defects, patent ductus arteriosus, pulmonary stenosis, and coarctation with D-transposition of the great arteries are all included under the rubric D-transposition. It is worth noting that an apparently simple ventricular defect may be a complex surgical problem because the defect is multiple (Swiss-cheese defect) or is associated with an unsuspected additional defect. Significant physiologic problems, such as pulmonary stenosis, may develop with growth of the baby. Comparable comments are applicable to most of the major diagnostic categories. The wastebasket term "heterotaxy" contains the entire gamut of congenital heart disease superimposed on abnormal or discordant sidedness.

Diagnosis Versus Age of Presentation. It is clinically useful to keep in mind the usual time of presentation of infants with various cardiac anomalies (Table 23-7). While ventricular septal defect is far the commonest congenital heart lesion, transposition of the great arteries and the hypoplastic left-heart syndromes are the most common anomalies presenting in the first week of life. Among those whose problem

Table 23-6. Diagnostic Distribution of Symptomatic Cardiac Newborns* Admitted in the First Month of Life (0−28 Days; NERICP 1968−1977)

Diagnosis	Total No.	Percent
D-Transposition of the great arteries	289	13.0
Hypoplastic left-heart syndrome	227	10.2
Coarctation of the aorta		
simple 31 } complex 181	212	9.5
Ventricular septal defect		
simple 99 } complex 102	201	9.1
Tetralogy of Fallot 123 } Pulmonary atresia and ventricular 55 defect	178	8.0
Heterotaxies	113	5.1
Pulmonary atresia with intact septum	105	4.7
Patent ductus arteriosus	86	3.9
Endocardial cushion defects	`74	3.3
Single ventricle	69	3.1
Tricuspid atresia	64	2.9
Total anomalous pulmonary venous connection	55	2.5
Aortic stenosis	38	1.7
Truncus arteriosus	38	1.7
Myocardial disease	38	1.7
Atrial septal defect, secundum	32	1.4
Double outlet right ventricle	28	1.3
L-Transposition of great arteries	14	0.6
Lung disease	226	10.2
Total	2220	100.0

* All infants were born in New England and underwent cardiac catheterization, cardiac surgery or died with heart disease

is cyanosis, transposition of the great arteries is the leading cause for admission through the third week of life; subsequent to that time, tetralogy of Fallot becomes the dominant cause of cyanosis for the rest of childhood. Among cardiac babies admitted because of respiratory symptoms, the hypoplastic left-heart syndromes are the leading cause in the first week, complex coarctations lead in the second week, and thereafter, ventricular septal defect becomes the main cause for symptomatic admission.

Noncardiac Anomalies and Low Birth Weight. Similarly, it is useful to remember the diagnostic possibilities among low-birth-weight babies (Table 23-5) and among those who in addition have other anomalies (Table 23-8). Among prematures, patent ductus arteriosus, coarctation of the aorta, and ventricular septal defect are more commonly encountered. Transposition of the great arteries is rarely associated with low birth weight. Endocardial cushion defects are often associated with Down's syndrome, while transposition of the great arteries is rarely found in association

Table 23-7. Top Five Diagnoses Presenting at Different Ages

Age On Admission: 0–6 Days (n = 1603)	
Diagnosis	*Percent*
D-Transposition of great arteries	15
Hypoplastic left ventricle	12
Tetralogy of Fallot	8
Coarctation of aorta	7
Ventricular septal defect	6
Others	52
Total	100

Age On Admission: 7–13 Days (n = 311)	
Diagnosis	*Percent*
Coarctation of aorta	20
Ventricular septal defect	14
Hypoplastic left ventricle	9
D-Transposition of great arteries	8
Tetralogy of Fallot	7
Others	42
Total	100

Age On Admission: 14–28 Days (n = 306)	
Diagnosis	*Percent*
Ventricular septal defect	18
Tetralogy of Fallot	17
Coarctation of aorta	12
D-Transposition of great arteries	10
Patent ductus arteriosus	5
Others	38
Total	100

with other anomalies if there is no heterotaxy. Cardiac anomalies associated with various syndromes are presented in Tables 23-8 and 23-9.

Maternal Diabetes. Maternal diabetes is associated with an increased incidence of congenital heart disease in the fetus. The lesions encountered include transposition of the great arteries, ventricular septal defect, coarctation and hypoplastic left heart syndrome. Some babies of diabetic mothers have cardiomegaly without other evidence of heart disease. At times this is marked (Fig. 23-4) and occasionally cardiac catheterization is a source of comfort to physician and family, proving that, despite marked cardiomegaly, no cardic dysfunction is measurable. Diabetic cardiomyopathy is usually treated expectantly.

Diagnostic Tools. It is beyond the scope of this chapter to discuss in detail the many noninvasive tools useful in the diagnosis of congenital heart disease. The clinical diagnosis of congenital heart disease implies the routine use of ECGs and chest films. The transcutaneous measurement of partial pressure of oxygen is useful, particularly after the umbilical artery is no longer an accessible source of arterial blood. The phonocardiogram can be used to document the qualities and timing of murmurs and heart sounds. The vectorcardiogram, a three-dimensional ECG technique, has occasional value. External pulse tracing and apexcardiograms have not been systematically used in neonates but perhaps should be. A variety of instruments useful in measuring blood pressure are available. M-mode echocardiography identifies the cardiac chambers, estimates their volume, and allows an inferential diagnosis which is often very helpful. Two-dimensional echocardiography provides a view of the intracardiac anatomy which is comparable to angiography. It is realistic to hope that combinations of the available noninvasive tools, in conjunction with the history and physical examination, will allow precise diagnosis without resorting to cardiac catheterization.

Lung Disease Versus Heart Disease

Even though the gestational age of the baby, maternal diabetes, or delivery by cesarean section are helpful facts, the differential diagnosis between primary lung disease and heart disease causing pulmonary edema is difficult.

A chest film may unequivocally suggest lung disease, but in the presence of diffuse pulmonary changes, possibly compatible with pulmonary edema, caution is necessary. Treatment as a pulmonary problem, even with some initial improvement, may confuse the picture. Recognition that heart disease is the underlying problem is delayed until the physician becomes concerned by the poor response to therapy. It is for this reason that neonatal cardiologists view with reservation such overworked diagnoses as transient tachypnea of the newborn or hyaline membrane disease in the full-term baby.

The issue is most pressing when the infant is dyspneic and cyanotic. While carbon dioxide retention is usually notable among babies with primary lung disease, unfortunately, some severely cyanotic infants with pulmonary parenchymal disease have a normal P_{CO_2}. A time-honored test has been the response of the cyanosis to administration of 100% oxygen; cyanosis from cardiac causes is not changed, while cyanosis with a pulmonary basis may disappear. Refinements of this test, through measurement of umbilical artery oxygen measurements while breathing 100% oxygen versus air, have been used in recent years. Difficulties arise when the situation is not pure. The baby with lung disease and heart disease or the baby with heart disease causing pulmonary venous hypertension and pulmonary edema may give confusing results. Further, an umbilical artery catheter positioned in the descending aorta may detect right-to-left shunting through a ductus arteriosus caused by lung disease, while administration of oxygen may decrease pulmonary resistance and increase pulmonary flow, providing higher oxygen levels in a child with a large pulmonary flow and congestive heart failure. Comparison of the right radial artery or temporal artery may eliminate this source of confusion. With these provisos, the infant who responds to breathing pure oxygen with a marked rise in arterial P_{O_2} to 250 torr or more has lung disease, while the infant who does not raise his preductal arterial P_{O_2} above 100 torr has heart disease. When doubt persists, the diagnosis can be made by two-dimensional echocardiography, by establishing that the cardiac anatomy is normal or sufficiently abnormal to account for a critically ill baby.

In summary, apparent diffuse pulmonary

Table 23-8. Incidence of Severe Associated Noncardiac Anomalies Among Selected Infants with Heart Disease

Diagnosis	Total Patients	Infants with Severe Noncardiac Anomalies	
		No.	*Percent*
Endocardial cushion defect	74	34	43
Patent ductus arteriosus	86	27	31
Ventricular septal defect	201	48	24
Heterotaxies	113	15	13
Tetralogy of Fallot	178	17	10
Coarctation of the aorta	212	19	9
Pulmonary atresia with intact septum	105	1	1
Transposition of the great arteries	289	3	1
Total	2220	271	12

Table 23.9. Infant Pediatric Syndromes Commonly Associated with Cardiovascular Abnormalities

Syndrome	% With Cardiovascular Abnormalities	Common Malformation or Abnoramility
Trisomy 21	40%–50%	Atrioventricular canal, ventricular septal defect, patent ductus arteriosus, ostium primum atrial defect
Trisomy 18	90%	Ventricular septal defect, patent ductus arteriosis, double outlet right ventricle
Trisomies 13–15	80%–85%	Ventricular septal defect
Turner (45:XO)	45%	Coarctation of aorta
Cat's eye (Schachenmann–Schmid–Fraccaro)	40%	Total anomalous pulmonary venous return, tetralogy of Fallot
Ellis–Van Creveld	>50%	Single atrium, ventricular septal defect
Mucopolysaccharidoses		Myocardial hypertrophy, congestive heart failure, valvar regurgitation
Pompe (glycogen storage)	100%	Myocardial hypertrophy, congestive heart failure, endocardial fibroelastosis
Congenital rubella	60%–80%	Patent ductus arteriosus (60%–75%), pulmonary valvar and arterial stenosis, ventricular septal defect (18%)
Williams syndrome		Supravalvar aortic stenosis, localized systemic or pulmonary arterial stenosis
Noonan syndrome	35%–50%	Pulmonary stenosis, atrial septal defect secundum
Holt–Oram syndrome		Atrial septal defect
Di George syndrome	80%	Aortic arch anomalies, tetralogy of Fallot, truncus arteriosus, aortic atresia
Tuberous sclerosis		Rhabdomyomas
Goldenhar syndrome	15%	Tetralogy of Fallot

disease in a full-term baby, particularly if the chest film is compatible with pulmonary edema, should be viewed with caution. With continued concern over the diagnosis, two-dimensional echocardiography will often solve the dilemma.

Management

An infant in difficulty because of heart disease in the first days of life has the potential for very rapid deterioration. Too often, the baby looks as though he will survive, only to be near death hours later. The earlier symptoms appear, the faster deterioration can take place. By the time the infant has reached a month or two of age, concern about sudden shifts in status is less warranted. As a consequence, the earlier an infant develops symptoms, the more rapidly the physician must respond. Cyanosis is a clear indication for immediate catheterization. Delay in order to supply anticongestive medication is rarely fruitful. Surgery offers the only real hope.

The cardiac infant whose symptoms are dominantly respiratory has congestive heart failure. A vigorous trial of oxygen, diuretics, and digoxin may be rewarding. Generally, the younger the baby, the shorter the persistence of improvement. Consequently, these babies are treated and, if only a few days old, are subjected to cardiac catheterization about 6 to 12 hours later, at the peak of improvement. Often the response is so gratifying that the temptation to persist in conservative management is overpowering. This is a dangerous course of action because reappearance of congestive symptoms and a rapid downhill course may be the result.

The rare baby with anasarca because of right-sided congestive heart failure should be managed with diuretics and digoxin, sometimes with surprisingly good results.

Cardiac Catheterization

The miniaturization of standard catheterization and angiographic techniques for the study of infants has been accomplished in the past ten years. Infant cardiac catheterization has become a specific technical art demanding specific training and experience. The neonate undergoing study is ill, often critically ill, and may have a widely fluctuating physiologic state. The combinations of lesions encountered in this age group are large; the natural mortality

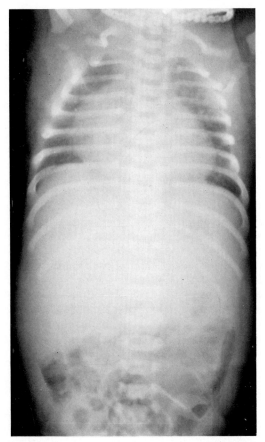

Fig. 23-4. X-ray film of an asymptomatic infant born to a diabetic mother. Gross visceromegaly and cardiomegaly are apparent.

is high. To extract the vital diagnostic information with the least danger to the patient requires vigilance against a multitude of treacherous pitfalls and a finely honed sense of the cost versus benefit relationship of each maneuver contemplated.

Indications. Not long ago, the indication for cardiac catheterization was the presence of cyanosis or tachypnea or both in an infant who had evidence of heart disease. The purpose of the study was to establish the diagnosis. The indications are now becoming more specific, and decisons about cardiac catheterization and its timing are based on the presumptive cardiac anatomy. Rarely is catheterization needed for anatomic reasons. Rather, it is used to provide specific data useful in planning for surgery. What is the pulmonary artery pressure? What is the coronary anatomy? Is there a pressure gradient? While some of this change has been the result of a substantial backlog of experience, in large part it is the result of routine use of two-dimensional echocardiograms.

In general, catheterization for an acyanotic infant in congestive heart failure is better delayed until the full effect of medications has been appreciated. Cyanotic infants who are suffering from a closing ductus arteriosus are best managed with an infusion of prostaglandins E-1, begun before and continued throughout the catheterization.

Risks. Death following cardiac catheterization is rare (0.1%) among children after the first months of life. Early in infancy, the risk is difficult to estimate because of the high natural mortality of the lesions encountered and the frequent temporal association of cardiac catheterization and cardiac surgery. In the first week of life, death within 48 hours of catheterization is 15 times greater than in the fourth week of life. The conclusion that this mortality parallels the natural mortality of the lesions being studied is inescapable. While this provides a universal excuse for a lamentable outcome, the potential for procedural error is undeniably greater in the sick newborn.[16]

If only unequivocally demonstrable damage to the infant is counted, the risk is quite small. We estimate that the mortality directly attributable to cardiac catheterization to be 1% to 2% in the neonatal period. Still, morbidity, such as blood loss, electrolyte imbalance, angiographic myocardial stains, hypothermia, and acidosis, occurs during these studies and influences the outcome of immediately subsequent cardiac surgery.

It is our conviction that the sick infant undergoing cardiac catheterization should be viewed as a treatment problem as well as a diagnostic one. Body temperature should be monitored and maintained with an external source of heat. Oxygen and suction should be available and used as needed. Blood pH and P_{CO_2} should be monitored; sodium bicarbonate solution should be used as indicated and ventilation instituted if carbon dioxide accumulation is identified. The softest and smallest diameter catheter compatible with the purposes of the study should be used and the possibility of perforation of the heart considered whenever a peculiar catheter position develops which is not readily explainable. Arterial pressure measurements and arterial blood samples are obtained from umbilical artery catheters in the first days of life. Later, the femoral artery is used but with some permanent compromise of the artery possible. In recent years, there has been a significant reduction of this complication associated with use of heparin during the procedure. Permanent occlusion of the inferior vena cava or the iliac vein is sometimes observed following newborn cardiac catheterizations. The amount of osmotically active contrast agent should be kept to the minimum needed for diagnosis. In this regard, biplane angiography, preferably cineangiography, should be used in small babies: first, to reduce the total dose of contrast agent; second, to reduce the number of pressure injections; and third, because angiographic monitoring and video replay are possible. No angiography should be done without careful attention to monitoring of the catheter's position and no pressure injections should be made until after a test injection of a small amount of contrast agent.

It is our impression that demonstrable injury to the baby can be held to less than 1% and that deleterious effects of cardiac catheterization that might influence the outcome of cardiac surgery can be held to a minimum by these measures.

Surgery

No neonatal cardiac unit can function safely without 24-hour thoracic surgical back-up. It is often necessary to move the baby directly from the catheterization laboratory to the operating room. Surgical success is a direct reflection of experience. The timing of surgical intervention is related entirely to the anatomic diagnosis and to the degree that survival without surgery is likely. Only neonates who are in danger of death are candidates for cardiac surgery.

At the present time, there are two schools of thought concerning surgical management of infants critically ill with heart disease. The older, conservative view is that a life saving, palliative operation should be done in infancy, followed some months or years later with a reparative operation. The newer view is that, whenever possible, single-stage repair should be carried out, in part to avoid the double jeopardy of two cardiac operations, but more important, to allow the family to live without a surgical sword of Damocles over their heads.

Table 23-10. Cardiac Surgery in the First Months of Life (% First Year Mortality)

Diagnosis	Years					
	1968–1971		1971–1974		1974–1977	
	NO.	% MORTALITY	NO.	% MORTALITY	NO.	% MORTALITY
D-Transposition of great arteries	51	57	36	44	24	54
Coarctation of aorta	28	64	35	54	54	56
Pulmonary atresia with intact septum	32	78	25	68	28	71
Tetralogy of Fallot	24	33	17	41	22	45
Other	94	62	117	62	150	38
Total	229	60	230	57	278	47

The resolution of this difference of opinion will depend primarily on survival statistics with the two surgical philosophies and will likely be different for each type of cardiac defect. In New England, about 40% of operations in the first year of life are reparative procedures. Of 737 infants undergoing cardiac surgery in the first months of life between 1968 and 1977, 337 (46%) survived to the first birthday. Over the years this figure has gradually improved and is most recently 53% (Table 23-10). These are pooled data of several hospitals and several surgeons. If the best results are selected, the figures are considerably better.

The postoperative care of cardiac infants requires fine adjustment of blood volume, body temperature, fluid, and electrolyte balance, and blood pH, P_{O_2} and P_{CO_2}. Close cooperation between the cardiologists and surgeons responsible for the care of these infants is required for optimal management.

VENTRICULAR SEPTAL DEFECT

Interventricular septal defects may be small or large, single or multiple, occur as isolated lesions or in association with other cardiovascular malformations. They are an integral part of complex congenital heart disease lesions such as tetralogy of Fallot, truncus arteriosus, double outlet right ventricle, atrioventricular canal, and have been associated with virtually every other known congenital cardiac malformation. The defect occurs most commonly in the membranous septum and less often in the low portion of the muscular septum. Ventricular septal defects are by far the commonest

of the congenital cardiac lesions and even though only 10% of ventricular septal defects ever cause symptoms, they are still the commonest cause of congestive heart failure after the second week of life (Table 23-7). Extracardiac malformations are also common (24%).

Pathophysiology

The very common small ventricular septal defect does not produce symptoms in infancy. By contrast moderate or large defects cause significant hemodynamic alterations. The decreasing pulmonary resistance after birth results in an increasing left-to-right shunt through a ventricular defect. If the defect is large, there is equilibration of right and left ventricular pressure and pulmonary hypertension. It is interesting to note that the normal regression of pulmonary resistance in the first week of life is delayed in these babies. Nonetheless, sufficient reduction in pulmonary resistance occurs by the second week of life to cause symptoms in many patients. Others, however, presumably with either smaller defects or further delay in the reduction of pulmonary vascular resistance, will develop symptoms as late as 3 to 4 months of age. Symptoms are the result of congestive heart failure or superimposed pulmonary problems such as pneumonia or atelectasis. Congestive heart failure is the result of recirculating an increasingly large amount of blood through the lungs while simultaneously attempting to meet the demand for systemic flow. Mechanical pressure by enlarged structures, particularly the left pulmonary artery and atrium, frequently results in bronchial obstruction and pulmonary atelectasis. The added effect of pulmonary congestion, which produces decreased lung compliance, makes the infants with such a large left-to-right shunt susceptible to recurrent respiratory airway obstruction and infections. Because pulmonary vascular resistance is lower in premature infants at birth, the development of symptoms from a ventricular septal defect occurs earlier. In severe failure, the pulmonary congestion, airway obstruction, or bronchospasm lead to respiratory acidosis. Pa_{CO_2} is increased and pH and Pa_{O_2} are slightly diminished.

Gradual improvement and diminution in pulmonary blood flow in an infant with a moderate to large ventricular defect may occur when there is an anatomic decrease in the size of the defect or the development of right ventricular infundibular stenosis. During childhood, but rarely in infancy, there may be progressive and irreversible increase in pulmonary vascular resistance through the development of anatomic obstructive changes in the pulmonary arterioles. None of these events plays a significant role in the first month of life, though knowledge of these phenomena influences therapy.

Clinical Findings

A small ventricular septal defect is characterized by a regurgitant systolic murmur, harsh or blowing in nature, loudest at the lower left sternal border. Many of these defects close spontaneously. Infants with large septal defects develop congestive failure in the first few months of life with symptoms of tachypnea, fatigue on feeding, decreased oral intake, excessive diaphoresis, and recurrent respiratory infections. Gross dyspnea is a late manifestation. Weight gain lags considerably behind height maturation. The infant often presents with a respiratory infection which may precipitate or mask underlying congestive failure. On examination, the infant is found to be undernourished, usually acyanotic and tachypneic. Pulse is rapid and may be slightly bounding. Cardiac impulse is hyperdynamic. If pulmonary artery hypertension is present, the second heart sound may be single with an accentuated pulmonary closure or, in the absence of pulmonary artery hypertension widely split, occasionally fixed, and with normal intensity of P_2. A gallop sound may be heard. The regurgitant systolic murmur is heard best

at the lower left sternal border but is usually transmitted well to the entire precordium. An apical mid-diastolic flow rumble is usually difficult to appreciate in the neonatal period, particularly when the heart rate is rapid. There is hepatomegaly and frequently pulmonary wheezing and rales. Peripheral edema is rare.

A chest film shows considerable cardiac enlargement, increased pulmonary blood flow, and sometimes pulmonary edema. The main pulmonary artery segment and left atrium are often enlarged. Atelectasis and parenchymal infiltrates are common. The ECG usually reveals left ventricular hypertrophy, and, if the lesion is associated with pulmonary artery hypertension, right ventricular hypertrophy as well. M-mode echocardiography will show evidence of left-ventricular volume overload with large left-atrial and left-ventricular dimensions and hyperdynamic left-ventricular function. The defect may be directly visualized by two-dimensional echocardiography.

Treatment

An infant with a small ventricular septal defect requires no specific treatment, but he should be followed closely with appropriate diagnositc tests at monthly intervals in the first 6 months of life, and at progressively longer intervals thereafter. The infant who develops congestive failure, or who has evidence of pulmonary artery hypertension, should undergo cardiac catheterization to confirm the diagnosis and determine the possible coexistence of other cardiac lesions. Intensive medical therapy with the administration of digitalis and diuretics may result in considerable improvement. Antibiotics, decongestants, and pulmonary physiotherapy should be employed if there are any pulmonary complications. The use of low-sodium formulas may be helpful, but total intake should not be restricted. Palliative or corrective surgery is indicated if the infant (1) does not improve with intensive medical therapy after a reasonable period of observation, (2) requires repeated hospitalizations for respiratory infections, or (3) persists in having significant pulmonary artery hypertension by 9 to 12 months of age. Of infants born with isolated, large defects, 15% succumb in the first year of life, usually as a consequence of associated severe extracardiac congenital anomalies or prematurity (see Table

23-2). Spontaneous closure or decrease in size of the ventricular defect may be anticipated in approximately 20% to 50% of the infants.

Differential Diagnosis

In the neonate, the murmur of a small ventricular septal defect may be difficult to distinguish from that caused by an obstructive lesion or atrioventricular valve regurgitation (mitral or tricuspid regurgitation). Other malformations resulting in a large left-to-right shunt and congestive failure are often difficult to distinguish clinically and should be excluded by echocardiography or if necessary cardiac catheterization. A patent ductus arteriosus is usually associated with bounding pulses and a wide pulse pressure. Endocardial cushion defect is accompanied by a superior QRS axis in the frontal plane, mild systemic arterial oxygen unsaturation, and cardiac enlargement that is out of proportion to the pulmonary plethora. In total anomalous pulmonary venous return with large pulmonary flow (nonobstructed), the ECG shows evidence of isolated right ventricular hypertrophy. Other lesions frequently confused with interventricular septal defects include transposition of the great arteries with a ventricular septal defect, single ventricle, and complex coarctation.

PATENT DUCTUS ARTERIOSUS

The ductus arteriosus, arising from the distal dorsal sixth aortic arch, is well developed by the sixth week of gestation and forms a bridge between the left pulmonary artery and the dorsal aorta, inserting at the aortic isthmus. At term, it is a muscular contractile structure. In the full-term infant, functional closure occurs in the first day of life and anatomic closure by several months of age. Persistence of the ductus arteriosus as an isolated structure, or in association with other cardiovascular lesions, may produce no symptoms or severe hemodynamic changes, depending on its size.

Isolated patent ductus arteriosus, without hyaline membrane disease, is common, accounting for 3.9% of all newborns symptomatic with heart disease (Table 23-6). (Patent ductus arteriosus is also a frequent complication of hyaline membrane disease in the premature infant [see Chap. 20].) It is more prevalent in females, in prematures, in infants born at high altitude, and in those surviving respiratory distress syndrome. It is common in combination with other congenital heart lesions (*e.g.*, coarctation of the aorta, ventricular septal defect, vascular ring). It is the commonest heart disease in congenital rubella, occurring in 60% to 70% of the cases.

Pathophysiology

Ductal constriction and presumably, therefore, functional closure are caused by multiple factors, the most important of which appear to be oxygen tension, the levels of circulating prostaglandins, and available muscle mass. *In vitro* experiments have also implicated constrictive effects by catecholamines, low pH, bradykinin, and acetylcholine. Atropine may delay while acetylcholine, or oxygen administration may promote ductal closure under certain circumstances. Prostaglandin E_1 has been successfully used to dilate a closing ductus in many forms of congenital heart disease in which patency of the ductus arteriosus is necessary to support either pulmonary or systemic blood flow. Delayed closure or persistence of the ductus arteriosus frequently occurs in premature infants with respiratory distress syndrome. Indomethocin, an inhibitor of prostaglandin synthesis, has been used with mixed results to promote closure of the ductus in this situation.

Following birth with a fall in pulmonary vascular resistance and a rise in systemic resistance, a left-to-right shunt may develop through the ductus arteriosus. This may normally occur up to several days after birth. A small right-to-left or bidirectional shunt may occur within the first hour after birth. In the newborn, ductal tone may also regulte flow. If spontaneous closure does not occur and the communication is small, the left-to-right shunt remains small and does not result in any hemodynamic consequences. A moderate-sized patent ductus arteriosus will usually be associated with a significant left-to-right shunt, left-ventricular volume overload, increased left-ventricular end-diastolic volume and pressure, elevation of left atrial pressure, and the development of congestive heart failure. Increased pulmonary blood flow results in increased left-ventricular stroke volume, elevated systolic pressure, wide pulse pressure, and bounding peripheral pulsations.

In the premature infant, failure may appear earlier. The pulmonary vascular resistance is lower because of incomplete development of the medial musculature in the small pulmonary arterioles. Compensatory mechanisms to the increased volume load may also be incompletely developed. In the premature infant with respiratory distress syndrome, there may be an initial period of improvement as the pulmonary status improves, followed by clinical deterioration as left-to-right shunting through the ductus arteriosus increases.

A large patent ductus arteriosus will result in pulmonary artery hypertension because the pressure is transmitted directly from the aorta to the pulmonary artery through the large defect. Both moderate and large ducts are prone to the development of pulmonary vascular obstructive disease at a later age.

Clinical Findings

In the neonate with a patent ductus arteriosus, as in all left-to-right shunts, the normal presence of elevated but decreasing pulmonary vascular resistance determines the clinical manifestations. For this reason, the classical continuous (Gibson) murmur is heard infrequently except in small prematures. Usually there is a crescendo systolic murmur with clicks, sometimes detectably spilling into diastole. S_2 is often not clearly audible. A small ductus may close spontaneously during infancy. The infant with a large patent ductus arteriosus has bounding peripheral pulses, a wide pulse pressure, and a hyperactive cardiac impulse at the apex. The systolic murmur at the base may be accompanied by an apical diastolic rumble. Symptoms and signs of congestive heart failure, growth retardation, poor weight gain, and recurrent pulmonary infections may be present. In a full-term infant with a large patent ductus arteriosus, overt failure usually does not develop until 3 to 6 weeks of age, while in prematures it occurs much earlier. Unlike infants with ventricular septal defects, full-term infants with a patent ductus arteriosus in failure rarely improve spontaneously.

The chest film shows cardiac enlargement, pulmonary plethora, prominent main pulmonary artery, and left-atrial enlargement. The ECG reveals left ventricular hypertrophy, occasionally left atrial hypertrophy, and, in severe failure, ST-T wave changes. Echocardiography shows evidence of a left-ventricular volume overload with a large left atrium, a large left ventricle, and an increase in the ratio of the left atrial to aortic root dimensions.

If pulmonary vascular resistance is high, reversal of the shunt may result in differential cyanosis and the absence of any murmur. The ECG will show right-axis deviation and right-ventricular hypertrophy.

Treatment

The full-term and premature infant with a patent ductus arteriosus and no evidence of cardiovascular embarrassment should be followed and surgical division of the ductus performed between 6 months and 1 year of age. Infants with congestive heart failure should be digitalized and, if necessary, diuretics added. In the sick neonate, clinical differentiation from other lesions may be impossible and cardiac catheterization indicated. Transfusion of packed red cells in the anemic premature may hasten ductal closure by increasing the arterial oxygen content. Interruption of the ductus arteriosus is indicated regardless of age or weight in any infant with a persistent hemodynamically significant left-to-right shunt through a patent ductus arteriosus, particularly if pulmonary artery hypertension is present. Surgical mortality is very low and dramatic improvement often occurs. Complications of surgery include Horner's syndrome, injury to the recurrent laryngeal nerve or lymphatic duct, transient hypertension and atrial fibrillation. Ligation rather than division of the ductus may also result in recanalization and the reappearance of a continuous murmur.

Recent experience indicates that indomethacin may be effective in inducing constriction and closure of the ductus arteriosus in a substantial number of premature infants with hemodynamically significant patent ductus. Success may be related to gestational and post-natal age. Complications of this treatment include transient renal failure related to decreased renal blood flow, necrotizing enterocolitis related to decreased blood flow to the gastrointestinal tract, and intracranial hemorrhage related to decreased platelet function.

Differential Diagnosis

The infant with congestive failure and a large left-to-right shunt caused by a ventricular septal defect, may be clinically indistinguishable from the one having a large patent ductus arteriosus. Other lesions that may result in a large aortic runoff and mimic a patent ductus arteriosus include truncus arteriosus, hemitruncus (right pulmonary artery from the ascending aorta), aortopulmonary window, aneurysm of the sinus of Valsalva, and a large systemic arteriovenous fistula (usually intracranial or hepatic). Truncus arteriosus usually presents in the first week of life, and a large systemic arteriovenous fistula within the first few days after birth.

ENDOCARDIAL CUSHION DEFECT

Defects of endocardial cushion development may be partial, resulting in an ostium primum atrial defect, or complete, resulting in additional significant deficiency of the interventricular septum, producing a common atrioventricular canal. The atrioventricular valves, particularly the anterior mitral valve leaflet, are usually malformed, deficient, or abnormally attached to the ventricular septum. With ostium primum defect, there is a cleft in the mitral valve that is frequently incompetent (50%). In complete atrioventricular canal, the primitive atrioventricular valve may "span" like a sail over both ventricles. This malformation results in a large communication between the right and left atria and the right and left ventricles and occasionally mitral incompetence or tricuspid incompetence. Endocardial cushion defects, as the primary lesions, account for 3.3% of all newborns hospitalized with serious heart disease (Table 23-6). It may occur as an isolated abnormality but is often associated with other malformations such as single ventricle, asplenia syndrome, and Down syndrome.

Pathophysiology

The hemodynamic consequences of ostium primum defect are volume overload caused by a large left-to-right shunt (left atrium to right atrium, or left ventricle to right atrium through the cleft mitral valve) and mitral regurgitation. In complete canal, there is an additional left-to-right shunt through a ventricular septal defect and right ventricular and pulmonary artery hypertension at systemic level. The large volume load, particularly when aggravated by an additional overload caused by mitral regurgitation, results in congestive heart failure which is often severe. Streaming of inferior vena cava blood across the large low-lying defect and cleft common valve leads to mild systemic arterial oxygen unsaturation. Infants with pulmonary artery hypertension are particularly susceptible to the development of pulmonary vascular obstructive disease and its complications in later childhood.

Clinical Findings

Infants with ostium primum atrial septal defects presenting in the neonatal period usually have severe mitral regurgitation, and, like those with complete canal, develop symptoms and signs of congestive failure. Growth retardation may be marked and weight lags considerably behind height maturation. Recurrent pulmonary infections are common. With atrioventricular canal, there is frequently mild cyanosis. Cardiac impulse is hyperdynamic and first heart sound is obscured by a loud pansystolic murmur audible at the apex or left sternal border. S_2 is widely split and fixed. If pulmonary hypertension is present P_2 may be accentuated and S_2 normally split. A loud S_3 and an apical mid-diastolic rumble are present. The chest film shows marked cardiac enlargement, usually out of proportion to the increased pulmonary vasculature, attributable to the large atria. Main pulmonary artery segment is prominent and there is pulmonary vascular engorgement. The ECG is characteristic, showing a superior axis in the frontal plane (commonly $0°$ to $-60°$ in primum defects and $-60°$ to $-100°$ in complete canal). There is often delayed atrioventricular conduction, biatrial, right ventricular, or biventricular hypertrophy. Significant right ventricular hypertrophy is usually indicative of right ventricular hypertension. The vectorcardiogram shows a counterclockwise loop in the frontal plane that becomes superior by 30 milliseconds. Selective left ventriculography shows the pathognomonic "goose-neck sign" that results from the anterior movement of the superior segment of the anterior mitral valve leaflet in diastole, producing an elongated and horizontal left ventricular outflow tract. An echocardiogram may demonstrate the abnormal plane and attachment of the mitral valve as well as the deficiency in the interventricular septum.

Treatment

Treatment with digitalis and diuretics may result in sufficient clinical improvement to delay operative repair into early childhood. In many, however, palliative or corrective surgery has to be performed in infancy. In atrioventricular canal, pulmonary artery banding may be helpful, but, if severe mitral regurgitation is present, primary repair may be necessary. In primum defects with severe mitral regurgitation, closure of the atrial defect with valvuloplasty may result in clinical improvement, but residual mitral regurgitation may later require valve replacement. The prognosis is poor. Only 50% of patients with endocranial cushion defects who become symptomatic in the first month of life survive beyond a year of age and many of these have considerable delay in height and weight maturation.

Differential Diagnosis

Other lesions producing congestive heart failure and pulmonary artery hypertension in early infancy, which may simulate endocardial cushion defects, include ventricular septal defect, single ventricle, double-outlet right ventricle without pulmonary stenosis, D-transposition of the great arteries with a ventricular septal defect, nonobstructive total anomalous pulmonary venous return, corrected transposition of the great arteries with mitral regurgitation, or, more rarely, isolated mitral regurgitation. The characteristic ECG, vectorcardiogram, and echocardiogram in infants with endocardial cushion defect are useful in separating this lesion, but cardiac catheterization is essential for assessing the severity and operability.

TOTAL ANOMALOUS PULMONARY VENOUS DRAINAGE

In the absence of fusion of the common pulmonary vein to the left atrium, communications are established with available systemic venous channels which then drain the pulmonary veins. Anatomically abnormal drainage may be supracardiac (into the right or left superior vena cava), intracardiac (into the coronary sinus, right atrium), or subdiaphrag-

matic (inferior vena cava or porta hepatis). Mixed sites of drainage occur in approximately 10% of the cases. A patent foramen ovale or atrial septal defect is invariably present. Anomalous pulmonary venous return may be associated with the heterotaxy syndrome or the cat's eye syndrome (see below).

Although total anomalous venous return accounts for only 2% of newborns with serious cardiac disease (see Table 23-6), it is an important lesion because it is potentially curable and often misdiagnosed as pulmonary disease.

Pathophysiology

Infants with anomalous pulmonary venous drainage may be divided into two major categories on the basis of the hemodynamic changes produced: nonobstructed and obstructed veins. Nonobstructed pulmonary veins entering the systemic venous circulation or directly into the right heart, result in a large left-to-right shunt, congestive heart failure, and, often, hyperkinetic pulmonary artery hypertension. Systemic output is maintained through an interatrial communication. Despite the obligatory right-to-left shunt through the atrium, the large pulmonary blood flow mixing with the systemic venous return at the right atrium allows a reasonable peripheral oxygen tension and therefore mild cyanosis.

Somewhat different and more acute circulatory changes occur when pulmonary venous return is obstructed. This is true for most subdiaphragmatic drainage and some supracardiac pulmonary venous drainage. The obstruction may take the form of increased resistance to flow produced by a long, common, pulmonary venous channel or localized intrinsic or extrinsic obstruction. Subdiaphragmatic anomalous pulmonary venous return is usually obstructed in the porta hepatis when constriction of the ductus venosus occurs, obstructing flow into the inferior vena cava. (Fig. 23-5**A**, **B**). Obstruction to supracardiac pulmonary venous return may occur because of compression of the common pulmonary venous channel between the left main stem bronchus and left pulmonary artery or because of narrowing at the entry of the common pulmonary vein into the right superior vena cava. Obstruction at the foramen ovale is uncommon but may be seen when pulmonary venous return is to the coronary sinus. Significant resistance to flow through the pulmonary veins results in pul-

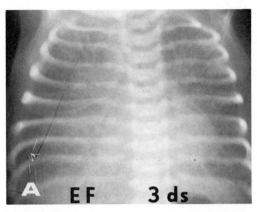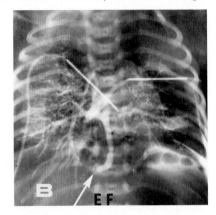

Fig. 23-5. A. Chest film of a 3-day-old infant with obstructed total anomalous pulmonary venous drainage. Note the ground-glass appearance of the lungs and normal heart size. A similar picture may be seen in RDS. **B.** Postmortem angiography showing obstruction of the common pulmonary venous channel below the diaphragm (**arrow**).

monary venous hypertension, pulmonary edema, marked pulmonary artery hypertension, and severe cyanosis. There is respiratory acidosis, and arterial oxygen tension is very low because of the obligatory right-to-left shunt at the atrial level, which is now associated with diminished pulmonary blood flow.

Clinical Findings

Infants with total anomalous pulmonary venous return without significant obstruction usually present after the neonatal period, when the pulmonary vascular resistance decreases and a large left-to-right shunt and congestive heart failure develop. Infants with severely obstructed pulmonary venous return usually present within the first week of life with tachypnea and severe cyanosis. There are symptoms and signs of congestive heart failure and poor peripheral perfusion. A soft continuous murmur may be heard at the site of obstruction. Heart size, as seen on the chest film, is often normal and there is evidence of pulmonary edema. The clinical and the radiographic pictures resemble hyaline membrane disease. The ECG shows right axis deviation, right-atrial hypertrophy and right-ventricular hypertrophy. The infant is critically ill and cardiac catheterization should be performed without delay to confirm the diagnosis and determine the site of the obstruction and drainage. The triad of severe cyanosis and a roentgenographic picture of a normal heart size, associated with pulmonary edema is characteristic (Fig. 23-5A). The prognosis is related to age

of onset of symptoms and severity of the pulmonary hypertension or vascular obstruction. It is most favorable for infants with intracardiac drainage and worst for those with obstructed veins.

Treatment

Primary treatment is surgical. Continuity or redirection of the pulmonary venous drainage into the left atrium is established. The administration of digitalis, diuretics, and supportive medical treatment should be started and cardiac catheterization performed as soon as the presumptive diagnosis is made. Infants with severely obstructed anomalous venous return require immediate surgical intervention; those with congestive heart failure and relatively normal pulmonary artery pressure may improve considerably on medical treatment and corrective surgery can be delayed.

Differential Diagnosis

Respiratory distress syndrome may be clinically indistinguishable from obstructed total anomalous pulmonary venous return. The former, however, is uncommon in full-term infants and the latter rare in prematures. Recently, echocardiography has been very helpful in identifying infants with total anomalous pulmonary venous return. M-mode echocardiograms show a small left atrium and evidence of right-ventricular volume overload, while two-dimensional echocardiograms show the anomalous common venous pathway. Cor triatriatum, stenosis of the pulmonary veins, premature closure of the foramen ovale, and other obstructive left-heart lesions usually do not have severe cyanosis and can be excluded by echocardiography or cardiac catheterization. Nonobstructive pulmonary venous return with large pulmonary blood flow and mild cyanosis should be distinguished from an endocardial cushion defect and other lesions with large left-to-right shunts.

COARCTATION OF THE AORTA

For clinical, prognostic, and probably etiologic reasons coarctation of the aorta is best considered in two separate categories: simple and complex. Simple coarctation, sometimes referred to as "adult coarctation," is usually a discrete constriction at the aortic isthmic area, occasionally associated with a patent ductus arteriosus inserting just at or above it. The complex malformation, which includes "preductal" or "infantile" coarctation, involves tubular hypoplasia of the aortic arch with or without discrete aortic narrowing, a patent ductus arteriosus, and one or more of the following lesions: ventricular septal defect, aortic stenosis, mitral stenosis or regurgitation, hypoplasia of the left ventricle and ascending aorta, and endocardial fibroelastosis. This amalgam of left-sided involvement may be secondary to intrauterine low flow through the left heart with consequent underdevelopment and hypoplasia extending from the left atrium to the aortic isthmus. The right-sided structures are enlarged and hypertrophied, and the patent ductus arteriosus largely or totally supplies the systemic circulation. In both simple and complex coarctation there are great variations possible in the extent and location of the coarctation.

Coarctation occurs in 9.5% of newborns with serious heart disease (Table 23-6). It is one of the common causes of congestive failure in the neonate (Table 23-7). It is more common in males and prematures. Ninety percent of the symptomatic infants have complex coarctation and most of these present within the first 6 weeks of life. Severe extracardiac anomalies, usually renal or gastrointestinal, occur in 6% of these patients.

Pathophysiology

The isthmus is normally smaller than the ascending or descending aorta in newborn infants because only 25% of fetal combined ventricular output passes through the isthmus into the descending aorta, while approximately 60% passes through the ductus arteriosus to the descending aorta. In normal infants, the isthmus gradually grows, but in simple coarctation it remains narrow because of a curtain-like constricting band. The coarctation may become more severe in the neonatal period as ductal closure occurs or during childhood with progressive hypertrophy and endothelial thickening engendered by high blood velocity at the narrow passage. Collateral circulation may be present at birth. In simple coarctation, the increased resistance to flow results in a pressure overload on the left ventricle to which a volume load may be added if there is a patent ductus arteriosus. With a gradual fall in pulmonary vascular resistance following birth, there is a reversal of flow through the ductus arteriosus from the aorta to the pulmonary artery, and a considerable left-to-right shunt may exist. If the heart is unable to compensate for the increased pressure and volume by hypertrophy or dilatation, congestive failure with diminution of systemic output ensues. Left ventricular end-diastolic pressure is elevated with consequent increase in left-atrial filling pressure, pulmonary venous pressure, and the development of pulmonary edema. The increased pulmonary venous pressure also results in pulmonary artery hypertension and right heart failure.

Complex coarctation is characterized by pulmonary artery hypertension with a ductus arteriosus supplying the descending aorta, usually a large intracardiac left-to-right shunt, and increased pulmonary flow. There is a pressure and volume overload on both ventricles with congestive heart failure. In the presence of a large ventricular septal defect and patent ductus arteriosus, the systolic pressure in the pulmonary artery, descending aorta, ascending aorta, and right ventricle is identical. Peripheral pulse pressure is normal and pulses equal throughout. With ductal closure or constriction, the femoral pulsations will diminish. If the coarctation is very severe, perfusion to the lower half of the body, previously supplied by the open ductus, is reduced and manifestations of shock and metabolic acidosis develop.

Clinical Findings

Infants with simple coarctation may be asymptomatic or present with congestive heart failure, usually over the age of 1 month. The femoral pulses are absent or diminished and significantly delayed on comparison to brachial pulses. Left brachial pulses may be decreased if the left subclavian arises at or below the coarctation. Systolic blood pressure in the upper extremities is higher than in the lower extremities, but marked hypertension is uncommon. Pulse pressure in the lower extremities is narrow, often 10 to 15 torr. With patience and a proper soft blood pressure cuff, Korotkoff sounds can be obtained in most infants. An ultrasound flow probe may be helpful. Blood pressure measurement by flush technique, which corresponds to mean systemic pressure, is less reliable. Cardiac impulse is prominent at the apex, xiphoid area, or both. S_3 is often prominent and there may be an apical systolic ejection click. A systolic ejection murmur is usually heard best at the left interscapular area over the back, but it may also be audible at the left-upper sternal border. A continuous murmur may be caused by the presence of a patent ductus arteriosus. Manifestations of congestive heart failure, when present, are those of combined left- and right-heart failure. Peripheral edema is relatively common. The chest film shows cardiac enlargement and pulmonary venous congestion. Rib notching is not seen in the newborn, but the location of the coarctation may be demonstrated by fluoroscopy. The electrocardiogram usually reveals left ventricular hypertrophy or biventricular hypertrophy and right-atrial hypertrophy. Echocardiography shows normal intracardiac structures. Complications such as bacterial endocarditis, subarachnoid hemorrhage, and rupture of the aorta are extremely rare in infancy.

Infants with complex coarctation almost always present with congestive heart failure in the early neonatal period. Generally, the younger the infant the more severe and complex are the associated malformations. Growth and weight gain are inadequate. In addition to the findings described for simple coarctation, there is evidence of a large left-to-right shunt and pulmonary artery hypertension. Femoral pulsations may wax and wane depending on ductal patency. This in itself is a useful diagnostic sign. A pansystolic murmur of a septal defect or mitral regurgitation may be present. The chest film shows considerable cardiac enlargement, pulmonary plethora and edema (Fig. 23-6). The ECG shows right axis devia-

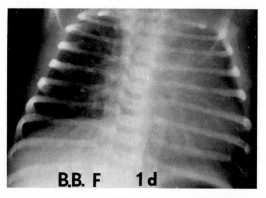

Fig. 23-6. The chest film of a 1-day-old infant with complex coarctation of the aorta. There is marked cardiac enlargement and pulmonary vascular engorgement.

tion, right-atrial hypertrophy, right ventricular hypertrophy, and, often, diminished left ventricular forces. M-mode echocardiography may reveal the intracardiac anatomy. The site of coarctation is often seen by two-dimensional echocardiography.

Treatment

Infants with congestive heart failure should be promptly hospitalized, treated with digitalis, and diuretics added if necessary. In all neonates cardiac catheterization should be performed within 24 to 48 hours after initiation of therapy because the lesion at this age is usually a complicated coarctation and survival without surgery is uncommon. Many infants with complex coarctation become symptomatic because of constriction of the ductus arteriosus. Prostaglandin E_1 infusion can dilate the ductus, restore systemic perfusion, and improve metabolic abnormalities. After an initial period of clinical improvement, rapid deterioration may occur and surgery should therefore not be unduly delayed. The surgical procedures employed depend on the severity of the lesion and include (1) resection of the coarctation with primary anastomosis, subclavian patch-plasty, or construction of a conduit from the ascending to descending aorta; (2) division of the patent ductus arteriosus; and (3) banding of the pulmonary artery if a large ventricular septal defect is present. In infants with simple coarctation who respond well to medical therapy, surgery may be delayed into childhood. Over 95% of infants with simple coarctation survive past 1 year of age. In the presence of a significant patent ductus arteriosus prognosis is poorer. The mortality of infants with complicated coarctation is 85% without surgery. Surgery increases the survival rate to 50%. Regardless of the type of coarctation, the mortality is directly related to age of presentation and is higher in those with pulmonary artery hypertension. The survivors need close medical supervision throughout childhood and may require other operations for the various associated abnormalities at a later time.

Recent reports indicate that patients with coarctation of the aorta, even with excellent surgery, have a significant risk for the development of hypertension as adults. There is suggestive evidence that this risk may be reduced by early surgical intervention.

Differential Diagnosis

A thorough examination, including careful palpation of all peripheral pulses and blood pressure measurement, should lead to the correct diagnosis. Infants presenting under 1 month of age usually have complex coarctation. Complete interruption of the aortic arch is almost always associated with a ventricular septal defect and a systemic patent ductus arteriosus, and is clinically indistinguishable from complicated coarctation. The presence of a ductus arteriosus supplying the descending aorta may be demonstrated by the finding of a higher arterial P_{O_2} in the arms than in the legs. Lesions of the hypoplastic left-heart syndrome may also present with a similar "shock-like" picture or in congestive failure in the first week of life as the ductus arteriosus closes. In these patients, peripheral pulses are frequently diminished throughout and the ECG shows marked diminution in left-ventricular forces. Aortic stenosis and cortriatriatum are rare and may present with pulmonary edema and congestive failure in early infancy.

HYPOPLASTIC LEFT HEART SYNDROME

The syndrome of hypoplastic left heart encompasses a variety of specific cardiovascular malformations producing similar hemodynamic and clinical manifestations. The malformations included in the syndrome are aortic atresia, mitral atresia, premature closure of the foramen ovale, hypoplastic left ventricle with critical mitral stenosis, and/or aortic stenosis. Some cases of severe complex coarc-

tation also fall into this category. The left-heart chamber is usually very small and endocardial fibroelastosis is common. Hypoplastic left-heart syndrome occurs in 10.2% of newborns with serious heart disease and is one of the commonest lesions presenting in the first week of life (Table 23-6 and 23-7). It is less common in very premature (under 4 lb) infants. Familial occurrence is known. It usually occurs as an isolated lesion, although it has been described in association with autosomal trisomy syndromes and in infants of diabetic mothers.

Pathophysiology

Severe obstruction or atresia of the mitral or aortic valve results in reduction or elimination of flow through the left heart. Systemic venous return enters the right heart and is ejected into the pulmonary artery. The systemic circulation is largely or totally supplied by a ductus arteriosus. Blood traversing the lung enters the left atrium and flows through an interatrial defect or patent foramen ovale and returns to the right atrium to join the incoming systemic venous return. Complete mixing, therefore, takes place in the right atrium, with similar oxygen saturation in the right ventricle, pulmonary artery, and aorta. With little or no egress by way of the left heart, pulmonary flow must pass through an interatrial communication. Any limitation of flow through the atrial septum will result in pulmonary venous hypertension. The maintenance of adequate systemic circulation requires patency of the ductus arteriosus. In aortic atresia, the ascending aorta, brachiocephalic vessels, and coronary arteries are perfused in a retrograde fashion from the patent ductus arteriosus. Spontaneous constriction of the ductus results in low systemic blood flow, poor coronary perfusion, congestive failure, and shock with simultaneous flooding of the pulmonary circulation. Closure of the ductus leads to immediate death. Because of poor perfusion, lactacidemia, metabolic acidosis, electrolyte imbalance, and coagulation abnormalities are common.

Clinical Findings

The infants become symptomatic within the first week of life. Congestive failure and a shock-like picture may develop rather precipitously. The baby becomes ashen gray with poor peripheral perfusion and vasoconstriction. The pulses are weak and thready throughout. Ductal constriction may be intermittent and femoral pulses, therefore, intermittently palpable. Symptoms and signs of congestive failure are associated with hypotension and, terminally, with bradycardia. S_2 is usually single and a gallop is present. The chest film shows cardiac enlargement and pulmonary plethora, and the ECG reveals right axis deviation, right-atrial hypertrophy, right-ventricular hypertrophy, and markedly diminished or absent left-ventricular forces. An echocardiogram may be diagnostic in demonstrating a very small or unrecognizable left ventricle or atresia of the mitral or aortic valves. Definite diagnosis of the specific lesion can be made by selective angiography at cardiac catheterization.

Treatment

No adequate treatment is currently available for most lesions grouped under hypoplastic left-heart syndrome. A variety of experimental surgical approaches have been tried without much success. Mortality is 98% by 1 year of age regardless of the type of therapy. Aortic atresia is uniformly fatal, whereas there are a few survivors with mitral atresia or hypoplasia of the left ventricle with severe aortic or mitral stenosis.

Differential Diagnosis

The clinical picture of the hypoplastic left-heart syndrome may be simulated by respiratory distress syndrome, interrupted aortic arch, severe complex coarctation, early neonatal myocarditis, or isolated critical valvar aortic stenosis.

AORTIC STENOSIS

Symptomatic pure aortic stenosis in infancy is rare but important to consider because it is amenable to surgery. The stenosis is invariably valvar rather than supravalvar or subvalvar. Only the most severe aortic valve obstruction results in symptoms in early infancy. The symptoms are those of congestive heart failure, pulmonary edema and sometimes peripheral vascular collapse. The baby may appear ashen and cyanotic, when the pulmonary edema is severe. The cardinal features are tachypnea, cardiac enlargement, and pulmonary venous congestion on chest film, left-ventricular hypertrophy on the ECG, a deformed immobile aortic valve on the echocardiogram, and a stenotic murmur at the upper-right sternal border. In severe left-ventricular failure, the systolic murmur is of low intensity.

Treatment consists in prompt administration of anticongestive medication and oxygen followed as soon as feasible by cardiac catheterization and surgical valvotomy. While most infants with critical aortic stenosis survive surgery, some have associated endocardial fibroelastosis which limits their survival. The asymptomatic infant with auscultatory findings of aortic stenosis and a normal ECG requires continued follow-up because valvar aortic stenosis is frequently a progressive lesion.

D-TRANSPOSITION OF THE GREAT ARTERIES

In transposition of the great arteries, the aorta arises from and above the right ventricle and the pulmonary artery from the left ventricle. In the commonest form, D-(dextro) transposition, also called complete transposition, the aorta is situated anteriorly to and to the right of the pulmonary artery in contrast to its normal rightward and posterior position.

Transposition of the great arteries is the commonest congenital heart lesion presenting in the newborn period (Table 23-6) as well as being a very frequent cause of death among congenital heart disease patients during this period (Table 23-2). The male to female ratio is 1.8:1, and the average birth weight is greater than that for other patients with congenital heart disease, although not greater than that for the general population. Transposition is frequently associated with other cardiac abnormalities including ventricular septal defect, patent ductus arteriosus, hypoplastic right ventricle and coarctation.

Pathophysiology

Normally, the systemic and pulmonary circulations are in series with each other, whereas in complete transposition the circulations are in parallel. Systemic venous blood returns to the right atrium, enters the right ventricle, and exits through the aorta. Pulmonary venous blood, returning from the lung, enters the left atrium and the left ventricle, then goes through the pulmonary arteries and returns to the lung. Without some communication between the pulmonary and systemic circulations, survival is impossible; oxygenated blood cannot be delivered to the systemic circulation, nor can systemic venous blood pick up oxygen in the lung. An atrial communication, ventricular defect, or patent ductus arteriosus, singly or in combination, may provide for mixing between the circulations. The foramen ovale and ductus arteriosus, both normally patent in the fetus, usually close soon after birth. Infants with transposition and intact ventricular septum, therefore, become extremely cyanotic within the first few hours or days after delivery, as closure of the foramen ovale and ductus arteriosus occurs and mixing between the circulations diminishes. The severe hypoxemia also leads to metabolic acidosis. Survival therefore depends on prompt supportive medical or surgical procedures that improve mixing and oxygenation.

Infants born with transposition and a large ventricular septal defect are less cyanotic because the defect allows for adequate mixing. They are often not recognized in the newborn period, but present in subsequent months with congestive failure, which develops as a consequence of both a large volume and pressure load on the left ventricle (supplying the pulmonary circulation). The combination of a large pulmonary flow, pulmonary hypertension, and elevation of left atrial pressure leads to the development of pulmonary vascular obstructive disease within the first 2 years of life.

Anatomic changes during the first few months of life may result in important hemodynamic changes. A large ventricular septal defect may spontaneously diminish in size or close, reducing mixing and increasing hypoxemia. Pulmonary stenosis may develop and result in a decrease in pulmonary flow, and therefore improvement in congestive failure. Atrial defect creation by balloon septostomy, and, occasionally, those performed by surgical septectomy, may spontaneously diminish in size or close. Closure of a patent ductus or foramen ovale may diminish pulmonary blood flow and mixing sufficiently to result in severe hypoxemia.

Clinical Findings

In infants with an intact ventricular septum, severe cyanosis accompanied by mild tachypnea develops soon after birth. Cardiac examination, chest film, and ECG may be nor-

mal. S_2 is normally split and there may be no murmur or there may be a nondescript low-intensity systolic murmur at the upper-left sternal border. If the infant is older than a few days, there may be evidence of congestive heart failure, and the ECG may show some excessive right-ventricular forces.

On a plain chest film, the heart and pulmonary vascularity are initially normal, although at a few weeks of age, cardiac enlargement and pulmonary plethora are noted (Fig. 23-7). M-mode echocardiography may be misleading because the diagnosis is based in part on the subjective right-to-left orientation of the great vessels. Two-dimensional echocardiography has proven to be an extremely valuable diagnostic tool. One of the most important diagnostic tests is the determination of Pa_{O_2} in room air (often less than 30 torr) and then after the inhalation of 100% oxygen for a 10-minute period. Failure of the Pa_{O_2} to rise significantly is strong presumptive evidence for complete transposition and an indication for an immediate cardiac catheterization. The failure to significantly raise systemic arterial O_2 tension is due to inadequate mixing between the pulmonary and systemic circulations.

An infant with transposition and a large ventricular septal defect usually presents with congestive failure and mild cyanosis between 3 to 6 weeks of age. Poor weight gain, tachypnea, and excessive diaphoresis are evident and wheezing is not uncommon. Gallop rhythm may occur due to a loud S_3. S_2 is physiologically split and there is a loud systolic murmur at the lower-left sternal border often associated with a mid-diastolic flow rumble. Rales may be audible in the lungs. The ECG reveals right axis deviation, right-atrial and ventricular hypertrophy, and, frequently, left-ventricular hypertrophy. If the right ventricle is hypoplastic, right-ventricular forces may be absent or reduced. The chest film characteristically shows considerable cardiomegaly and pulmonary plethora. M-mode echocardiography provides strong suggestive evidence for the diagnosis, and two-dimensional studies may be definitive.

The clinical picture in infants with transposition, ventricular septal defect, and pulmonary stenosis or atresia, is virtually indistinguishable from that of tetralogy of Fallot or pulmonary atresia with a ventricular septal defect. The additional presence of a coarctation and a ductus arteriosus in a patient with

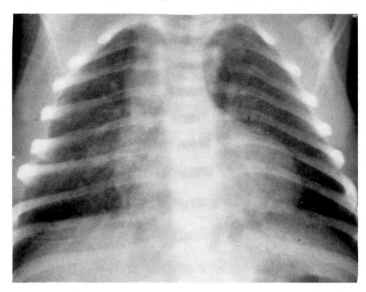

Fig. 23-7. Essentially normal chest film in an infant with transposition of the great arteries with an intact ventricular septum. The chest film in this condition is usually normal in the first few days of life.

transportation and a ventricular septal defect may result in reversed differential cyanosis (pink lower extremities and cyanotic head and upper extremities). Pulmonary artery hypertension is invariably present and the shunt through the patent ductus arteriosus is from the pulmonary artery, containing highly saturated blood, to the descending aorta. Blood entering the ascending aorta and brachiocephalic vessels from the right ventricle is unsaturated. Congestive failure is present and the femoral pulses may be normal because the descending aorta is supplied by a patent ductus arteriosus at systemic pressures.

Treatment

Once the diagnosis of transposition and intact ventricular septum is suspected, cardiac catheterization should be performed. The procedure will establish the diagnosis, and balloon atrial septostomy usually results in considerable clinical improvement. The increase in systemic arterial saturation following balloon septostomy may be satisfactory until definitive repair can be undertaken between 6 months and a year of age. Failure of balloon septostomy may require a second attempt: surgical palliation (by creating an atrial defect) or earlier repair by a Mustard procedure. The type of surgical procedure employed depends on the infant's size, clinical condition, associated malformations, and the available surgical experience. Supportive medical therapy

consists of the administration of oxygen and decongestive medications, and correction of acidosis and anemia. Without therapy, 95% of infants born with transposition die within 1 year. With more aggressive medical and surgical treatment mortality has been reduced to 50% and should continue to decline.

Diagnosis and Differential Diagnosis

Respiratory distress syndrome can be distinguished from transposition by the considerable respiratory effort and characteristic chest film in the former. If intense cyanosis cannot be explained by pulmonary disease and if echocardiography is equivocal, selective right ventricular injection of contrast material will confirm the origin of the aorta from the right ventricle. Depending on the type and severity of the associated cardiac malformations, the clinical symptoms and findings in infants with transposition of the great arteries may closely resemble those of almost any other congenital heart lesion. A single S_2 in a very cyanotic infant, especially when associated with diminished pulmonary vasculature and normal heart size, suggests severe pulmonary stenosis or pulmonary atresia with a ventricular septal defect. The presence of a systolic murmur makes pulmonary stenosis more likely than pulmonary atresia. Infants with critical pulmonary stenosis and intact ventricular septa usually have considerable cardiomegaly. Infants with tricuspid atresia and those with pulmonary atresia and intact ventricular septa can usually be distinguished by the echocardiogram. When D-transposition of the great arteries is associated with a large ventricular septal defect, it is frequently mistaken for other lesions with a large left-to-right shunt, such as a ventricular septal defect with normal aortic root or total anomalous pulmonary venous return without obstruction. Atrioventricular canal defect can usually be differentiated by an ECG showing a superior QRS axis in the frontal plane.

TETRALOGY OF FALLOT

Anatomically, tetralogy of Fallot is characterized by a large, ventricular septal defect and infundibular pulmonary stenosis or atresia. The right ventricular infundibulum is hypoplastic and narrow, and right-ventricular hypertrophy is present. There is often considerable valvar pulmonary stenosis, hypoplasia of the pulmonary arteries, a relatively large ascending aorta, and a right aortic arch (25%). In infants with pulmonary atresia, pulmonary perfusion is by way of a patent ductus arteriosus or aortopulmonary collateral vessels. Tetralogy is one of the most common cyanotic congenital heart lesions presenting in the newborn period (see Table 23-6), and is not uncommonly associated with severe extracardiac malformations (10%).

Pathophysiology

The combination of severe right-ventricular outflow stenosis or atresia and a ventricular septal defect results in decreased pulmonary perfusion, intracardiac right-to-left shunt, and hypoxemia. There is equalization of pressures between the right and left ventricles through the large septal defect. Pulmonary blood flow largely depends on (1) the resistance to flow into the pulmonary circuit (severity of right-ventricular outflow obstruction), (2) the systemic vascular resistance, (3) presence of a ductus arteriosus, and (4) the patency or development of aortopulmonary collateral supply to the lung. The extent of systemic venous admixture (right-to-left shunt by way of the septal defect) is directly related to the severity of the pulmonary stenosis and inversely related to the systemic vascular resistance. The peripheral arterial oxygen saturation will depend on both the amount of venous admixture and the absolute pulmonary flow. For example, in pulmonary atresia with a ventricular septal defect, there is an obligatory large right-to-left shunt through the defect, and pulmonary flow is usually diminished (supplied by a small ductus arteriosus or collateral vessels). Severe cyanosis therefore results. If the newborn has large aortopulmonary collateral vessels perfusing the lung, pulmonary blood flow may be large and the infant may be barely cyanotic, and actually in severe congestive heart failure.

Infundibular hypoplasia and stenosis may be progressive and with time become completely atretic. A patent ductus arteriosus not infrequently closes within the first week of life, resulting in severe and often sudden hypoxemia or cyanotic spells.

Hypoxemia, particularly of rapid onset (as for example during a hyperpneic spell secondary to infundibular spasm or constriction of a ductus arteriosus), may initiate a vicious cycle producing a fall in systemic vascular resistance, acidosis, and increased pulmonary vascular resistance. This results in further reduction of pulmonary flow and an increase in right-to-left shunt by way of the septal defect with more severe hypoxemia, lactacidemia, and metabolic acidosis. The combination of hypoxemia and acidosis (particularly with pH less than 7.1) act synergistically and may result in decreased myocardial contractility, hypotension, and bradycardia. Because of diminished pulmonary perfusion, respiratory compensation for the metabolic acidosis is ineffective despite the hyperventilation induced by acidosis.

Clinical Findings

Cyanosis of varying severity and mild tachypnea are usually present soon after delivery. If hypoxemia is severe, the infant may be hypotonic and hypotensive with a slow heart rate. Hyperpneic spells may develop. These are characterized by a sudden onset of irritability, hyperpnea, and increasing cyanosis. They may be accompanied by loss of consciousness and seizure activity or lead to hemiparesis and death. The spells are due to hypoxemia which may be induced by infundibular spasm or functional closure of a patent ductus. The disappearance of a previously heard right-ventricular outflow systolic murmur or a continuous murmur of a patent ductus arteriosus are pathognomonic features of a "spell," and constitute an indication for immediate therapy. Physical examination of the infant with tetralogy of Fallot reveals a single second heart sound and systolic murmur at the left-sternal border. A continuous murmur of a patent ductus arteriosus or aortopulmonary collaterals may be audible at the base or over the back. In the newborn with pulmonary atresia the systolic murmur is absent and an apical constant systolic ejection click, presumably caused by a dilated aorta, is not infrequently present. Congestive heart failure does not occur except in the infant with pulmonary atresia and very large aortopulmonary collaterals. Delay in height, weight, and skeletal maturation is common, but some infants flourish despite evidently severe hypoxemia. Although subacute bacterial endocarditis and brain abscess are common in older children with tetralogy of Fallot, these complications are extremely rare in infancy. Spontaneous cerebrovascular accidents however are common, particularly in infants with severe hypoxia and relative anemia.

The chest film shows a normal-size heart with right-ventricular enlargement, an absent or diminished main pulmonary artery segment, and diminution of the pulmonary vasculature. The ECG reveals right axis deviation, right-atrial hypertrophy, and right-ventricular hypertrophy. The echocardiogram shows a large aortic root overriding the interventricular septum. Arterial blood gases show a metabolic acidosis with low P_{O_2}, and normal P_{CO_2}.

Treatment

Treatment depends on the severity of the lesion. The newborn with tetralogy of Fallot and mild cyanosis should be carefully observed and repeated measurements of systemic oxygen saturation made until a stable level is apparent. Hyperpneic spells should be treated with oxygen, intramuscular or subcutaneous morphine sulfate (0.1 mg/kg), and the intravenous administration of sodium bicarbonate (approximately 1 mmol/kg). Prostaglandin E_1 may temporarily keep a ductus arteriosus open in the newborn infant and improve pulmonary perfusion. Intravenous propranolol may be of some value in the infant with adequate pulmonary flow, mild hypoxemia, and a very reactive infundibulum. It is important that hemoglobin concentration be maintained at an appropriate level to permit an adequate oxygen content. The presence of severe hypoxemia and the occurrence of a single hyperpneic spell are indications for emergency surgery.

In the past, critically ill infants who required surgery underwent palliative procedures, usually a systemic-to-pulmonary artery shunt (ascending aorta to right pulmonary artery [Waterson shunt]; descending aorta to left pulmonary artery [Potts shunt]; or subclavian artery to branch pulmonary artery [Blalock–Taussig shunt]). These infants would then undergo a reparative operation at an older age. Recently, infants requiring surgery have had one-stage reparative procedures with excellent results. Cardiac catheterization is essential to determine the precise anatomy in these infants. Of particular concern is the presence of multiple ventricular septal defects, the size of pulmonary arteries, and the coronary artery distribution.

In general, the earlier severe hypoxemia develops, the more severe the tetralogy of Fallot and the poorer is the prognosis. The overall mortality is approximately 35% by one year of age (Table 23-2).

Diagnosis and Differential Diagnosis

The tetrad of cyanosis, diminished pulmonary vasculature, a normal-sized heart on the chest film and ECG evidence of right-ventricular hypertrophy are characteristic of tetralogy of Fallot. Pulmonary stenosis with an intact ventricular septum may be difficult to distinguish clinically from tetralogy of Fallot, although it is usually accompanied by cardiac enlargement. Pulmonary atresia with an intact ventricular septum and tricuspid atresia are both characterized by ECG evidence of left-ventricular hypertrophy and an abnormal QRS axis. Double-outlet right ventricle, transposition, or malposition with severe pulmonary stenosis may be suspected from echocardiography, but often can be distinguished with certainty only by cardiac catheterization. The infant with tetralogy of Fallot and absent pulmonary valve usually presents with severe respiratory distress caused by bronchial or tracheal compression by aneurysmally dilated pulmonary arteries.

PULMONARY ATRESIA WITH AN INTACT VENTRICULAR SEPTUM

When the pulmonary valve is atretic and there is no ventricular septal defect, blood cannot pass through the right ventricle in the fetus, and, consequently, the right ventricle is underdeveloped or hypoplastic. The right ven-

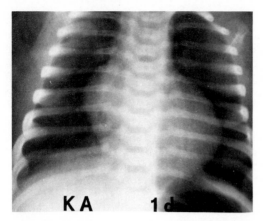

Fig. 23-8. Chest film showing decreased pulmonary vascularity and mild cardiomegaly in a 1-day-old infant with pulmonary atresia and an intact ventricular septum.

tricular cavity is frequently "prune pit" in size and some potential space is filled by heavy, coarse trabeculation. There is membranous pulmonary valvar atresia and, in approximately one-third of the cases, associated infundibular stenosis, hypoplasia, or atresia. The tricuspid valve annulus is small and may be stenotic or incompetent. There is often myocardial fibrosis, segmental coronary artery stenosis, or fistulous tracts draining blood from the right-ventricular sinus into the ascending aorta. The pulmonary arteries are of adequate size and are perfused through a patent ductus arteriosus and rarely through aortopulmonary collaterals. An interatrial communication is essential for survival. Pulmonary atresia with an intact ventricular septum is rarely associated with other cardiovascular or somatic malformations.

Pathophysiology

The major hemodynamic consequences of pulmonary atresia with intact septum are an obligatory right-to-left shunt through an interatrial communication with total systemic venous return entering the left atrium. A patent ductus arteriosus provides the only entrance to the pulmonary circulation. As it closes, and it usually does, pulmonary perfusion is greatly reduced and results in severe hypoxemia, the development of metabolic acidosis, and death. The right ventricle, despite its severe hypoplasia and poor compliance, is capable of generating suprasystemic pressures. This is

probably true *in utero* as well and explains the frequent tricuspid incompetence with right atrial enlargement and the development of coronary artery fistulas that drain blood from the right ventricle into the ascending aorta. The reversal of coronary artery flow ultimately results in myocardial ischemia and fibrosis.

Clinical Findings

The majority of infants are critically ill within the first week of life because of severe hypoxemia. With ductal constriction or closure severe cyanosis, hypotension, bradycardia, hypotonia, and marked acidosis occur. Signs of right-sided failure may develop but are usually absent. The precordium is quiet and there is no thrill. S_2 is single and there is often a pansystolic murmur of tricuspid incompetence. Disappearance of the continuous murmur at the base is indicative of ductal closure. On the chest film, the heart may appear mildly enlarged, the lung fields are ischemic, and the aortic arch is on the left (Fig. 23-8). The ECG usually reveals a QRS axis in the frontal plane between 0° and 90°, absent or diminished right-ventricular forces, and a pattern of left-ventricular hypertrophy.

An M-mode echocardiogram will show normal or somewhat enlarged left-sided structures, a small tricuspid valve and right ventricle, and no visualization of the pulmonary valve. Occasionally, if there is membranous atresia of the pulmonary valve, the membrane will move in a fashion similar to a true valve and the diagnosis cannot be made with certainty. Once the presumptive diagnosis is made, prostaglandins may be given to dilate the ductus arteriosus and increase pulmonary blood flow. There should be rapid improvement in oxygenation and relief of acidosis. Cardiac catheterization is indicated as soon as the presumptive diagnosis is made. Selective right-ventricular angiography is essential for adequate surgical management.

Treatment

Following stabilization with prostaglandins, the treatment of choice is surgical and is indicated as soon as feasible after the diagnosis is established at catheterization. In infants with adequate-sized right ventricle, a pulmonary valvotomy with the additional removal of valve tissue is performed. Some infants may require placement of a pericardial patch across

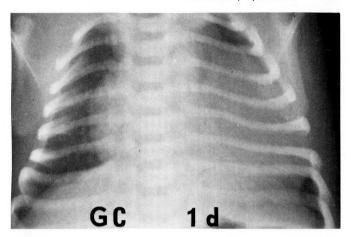

Fig. 23-9. Chest film of a 1-day-old cyanotic infant with Ebstein anomaly of the tricuspid valve. There is marked cardiomegaly.

the right-ventricular outflow tract and valve annulus in order to adequately relieve obstruction. Complete patency or relief of right-ventricular hypertension with maintenance of an adequate cardiac output however, may not be achieved. In infants with severe right-ventricular hypoplasia, and a noncompliant right ventricle, a systemic-to-pulmonary shunt may be necessary to relieve hypoxemia. After a period of time (as the right-ventricular compliance improves and the pulmonary vascular resistance falls), these infants may no longer require shunts to maintain adequate pulmonary blood flow. Without therapy, the malformation is almost uniformly fatal and, with current surgical treatment, about 25% of these newborns survive to 1 year of age (Table 23-2).

Differential Diagnosis

The lesion needs to be distinguished from others causing severe cyanosis in the first week of life. Tetralogy of Fallot or pulmonary atresia with a ventricular septal defect and transposition of the great arteries with an intact ventricular septum are associated with ECG evidence of right-ventricular hypertrophy. Infants with tricuspid atresia or endocardial cushion defect and pulmonary stenosis have a superior frontal plane axis on the ECG. Critical valvar pulmonary stenosis is accompanied by a systolic ejection murmur, congestive heart failure, moderate to marked cardiac enlargement, and right ventricular hypertrophy. Critical pulmonary stenosis with a diminutive right ventricle can be distinguished with certainty only at cardiac catheterization. In Ebstein's anomaly of the tricuspid valve, the

precordium is quiet and cardiac enlargement severe (Fig. 23-9).

HETEROTAXY SYNDROME

The heterotaxy syndrome consist of an anomalous arrangement and malformations of the viscera and/or heart. Visceral heterotaxy should alert the neonatologist to the possibility of associated congenital heart disease, venous anomalies, and splenic abnormalities. Polysplenia may occur without associated heart disease but asplenia is almost invariably accompanied by severe cardiac malformations. Although similar cardiac abnormalities may occur in patients with asplenia and polysplenia, a distinct pattern of cardiac and visceral lesions is usually present in each, enabling clinical differentiation between these entities (Table 23-11). Careful inspection of the chest film will often demonstrate the correct abdominal situs and location of the stomach and liver (Fig. 23-10). Fluoroscopy with barium ingestion and the demonstration of Howell–Jolly bodies on peripheral blood smear may be useful. Polysplenia, asplenia, and venous anomalies (absent inferior vena cava, left inferior vena cava, left superior vena cava) may be demontrated by radionuclide scintigraphy and venography. Recognition of the venous abnormalities is useful in selecting the site for cardiac catheterization. The symptoms, signs and treatment of patients with heterotaxy syndrome depend on the type and severity of the cardiovascular malformation or associated extracardiac abnormalities. Asplenia usually presents with severe cyanosis in the neonatal

Table 23-11. Common Abnormalities in the Asplenia and
Polysplenia Syndrome

Asplenia	Polysplenia
Isolated levocardia or dextrocardia	Dextrocardia or levocardia
Visceral isomerism (midline liver and stomach)	Absent inferior vena cava (renal to hepatic segment)
Transposition of the great arteries	Endocardial cushion defect
Double-outlet right ventricle	Total anomalous pulmonary venous return
Total anomalous pulmonary venous return	Coronary sinus rhythm
Endocardial cushion defect	Bilateral hyparterial bronchi
Pulmonary atresia or pulmonary stenosis	
Single ventricle	
Bilateral superior vena cava	
Absent coronary sinus	
Ipsilateral inferior vena cava and abdominal aorta	
P-wave axis of atrial inversion	
Bilateral eparterial bronchi	
Bilateral trilobed lung	

period. Many of the infants are amenable to palliative surgery. With current management 40% survive to 1 year of age (see Table 23-2).

DEXTROCARDIA

Congenital dextrocardia or a right-sided heart may occur with visceral situs solitus (normal or usual abdominal situs), visceral situs inversus (inversion of viscera), and visceral situs ambiguous (abdominal heterotaxy; asplenia or polysplenia syndrome). Congenital isolated dextrocardia with situs solitus may be (1) secondary to pulmonary hypoplasia or aplasia, the heart and great arteries being structurally normal but the displacement of the heart to the right possibly resulting in tracheal compression and obstruction by the aorta; or (2) associated with ventricular inversion (morphologic left ventricle is right-sided and slightly anterior, and morphologic right ventricle is left-sided and slightly posterior), L-transposition of the great arteries, and other intracardiac malformations.

Mirror-image dextrocardia (i.e., dextrocardia with situs inversus, and ventricular inversion) is usually associated with L-transposition of the great arteries and other intracardiac malformations. It may also occur with normally related great arteries with or without cardiac malformations. D-transposition of the great arteries with situs inversus of the viscera is rare.

Complex cardiac malformations are common in patients with congenital dextrocardia and are virtually always present in those with isolated levocardia (situs inversus of the viscera and a left-sided heart). Accurate diagnosis is best achieved by a segmental approach considering in each case (1) the visceral situs, (2) ventricular loop (i.e., normal or inverted ventricle), and (3) relationship of the great arteries to the ventricles. Situs of the atria almost always corresponds to the situs of the viscera. In situs solitus the suprahepatic segment of inferior vena cava is right sided and empties into a right-sided morphologic right atrium. There are virtually no exceptions to this relationship between the inferior vena cava and localization of the atria. The relationship of the great arteries may be predicted if the type of the ventricular loop present is known. D-loop (right ventricle on the right and anterior and left ventricle to the left and posterior) is usually associated with normally related great arteries or with D-transposition of the great arteries. An L-loop or ventricular inversion is usually associated with L-transposition of the great arteries. Localization of the bulboventricular loop may be determined by visualization of the ventricular morphology on selective angiography or by the ECG. In ventricular inversion, the ECG may show Q-waves in the right chest leads with absent Q-waves in the left precordial leads.

L-TRANSPOSITION OF THE GREAT ARTERIES

In L-transposition of the great arteries with situs solitus, also called corrected transposition, the circulation is physiologically "corrected" and in series. The systemic venous blood enters the right atrium and flows into a right-sided morphologic left ventricule and out into the pulmonary artery. Pulmonary venous blood returns to the left atrium, and by way of the tricuspid valve into the left-sided morphologic right ventricle and out the aorta. The aorta is anterior and to the left of the pulmonary artery. The hemodynamic changes in patients with L-transposition of the great arteries are caused by the commonly associated cardiac abnormalities that include ventricular septal defect (50%), single ventricle (42%), pulmonary stenosis or atresia (45%), and left-atrioventricular valve regurgitation (23%). Conduction disturbances and arrhythmias, particularly complete heart block, are common. Medical and surgical management are directed toward correction or palliation of the associated cardiovascular malformations.

PRIMARY MYOCARDIAL DISEASE

A number of rare diseases of different etiology, but with common clinical manifestations and pathophysiology and affecting the myocardium in the neonate, may be conveniently grouped together. These include myocarditis, endocardial fibroelastosis, glycogen storage disease (Pompe's), neuromuscular diseases, and nonobstructive and obstructive cardiomyopathies. There are no documented cases of rheumatic fever within the first few months of life. Myocarditis is usually the result of a viral infection which may be acquired by the infant *in utero* or after birth. Coxsackie, particularly type B, ECHO, rubella, and other viruses have been shown to cause myocarditis. Damage to the left-ventricular pump results

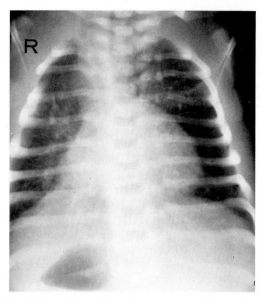

Fig. 23-10. Chest film of a neonate with asplenia syndrome, tricuspid atresia, transportation of the great arteries and a right aortic arch. The liver and stomach are on the right side.

in cardiac dilatation, diminished contractility, and congestive failure. Pulmonary edema may develop and cardiac output is often diminished. Both fibroelastosis and myocarditis are characterized by congestive heart failure, the frequent occurrence of arrythmias, development of left ventricular mural thrombi with occasional embolization and susceptibility to sudden death. The entities are often clinically indistinguishable, although onset of symptoms with fibroelastosis is usually at a few months of age, whereas myocarditis often presents within the first few days of life. A positive family history and mitral regurgitation are common in fibroelastosis and rare in myocarditis. The ECG in acute myocarditis often reveals low QRS voltages, flat or inverted T-waves, and S-T segment depression. If there is an ECG pattern of anterolateral myocardial infarction, the diagnosis of anomalous origin of the left coronary artery from the pulmonary artery should be considered. On chest film, cardiomegaly and pulmonary venous congestion are present, although in the early course of myocarditis, the heart may be normal in size. Pericardial effusion may result in tamponade.

Therapy is supportive and aimed at the congestive heart failure and arrhythmias. Digitalization should be carried out with caution in infants with myocarditis, because they may be unduly susceptible to the drug, and therapy should be maintained until cardiac enlargement subsides. Steroids are indicated in acute myocarditis with a fulminating shock-like picture and when a severe arrhythmia, particularly atrioventricular block, is present.

RHYTHM DISTURBANCES

While any rhythm disturbance may occur in early infancy, those more commonly encountered include sinus tachycardia and bradycardia, premature atrial contractions, paroxysmal artial tachycardia, atrial flutter, and complete heart block. Atrial arrythmias are common, but those of ventricular origin are rare. Acute life-threatening rhythm disturbances such as ventricular fibrillation, ventriclular tachycardia, sinus arrest, or extreme bradycardia usually occur as a terminal event in a systemic illness or in association with severe hypoxemia, acidosis, electrolyte disturbance or drug toxicity (*e.g.*, digitalis). Ectopic atrial beats, atrial bigeminy, and nodal escape beats are of no serious consequence.

Paroxysmal Atrial Tachycardia

Recurrent atrial tachycardia is a common rhythm disturbance in early infancy. It is usually of idiopathic origin but may be associated with the Wolff–Parkinson–White syndrome, cardiac malformation in which there is atrial enlargement (*e.g.*, Ebstein's disease, corrected transposition of the great arteries, tricuspid atresia), or myocarditis. Paroxysmal atrial tachycardia in a female infant is more likely to be associated with congenital heart disease. Onset of the tachycardia in a male less than 4 months of age carries a better prognosis and recurrence is unlikely after a year of age.

Electrocardiographically, the arrythmia is characterized by a rate of over 220 per minute, abnormal or nonidentifiable P-waves (they may be superimposed on the T-waves), and normal QRS morphology with equal R–R interval. The arrhythmia starts and ceases abruptly. The infant may be asymptomatic initially but then becomes irritable, fussy, and refuses feeding. Congestive heart failure develops in approximately 20% after 36 hours and in 50% after 48 hours. Digoxin, preferably by the parenteral route if the infant is acutely ill, usually abolishes the arrhythmia within 6 to 12 hours. It also has the advantage of improving myocardial contractility. (For dosage, see Appendix.) Vagal stimulation maneuvers (unilateral carotid pressure or gagging) should be done with great caution, if at all in a sick infant, and rarely work. Cardioversion with a DC defibrillator (starting with 5 to 10 watt-seconds) may be necessary in some infants. The administration of digitalis should be continued for approximately 1 year after the last episode of arrythmia.

Infants with paroxysmal atrial tachycardia may be recognized *in utero* by a rapid fetal heart rate. If the arrythmia has been present for some time, these infants may develop hydrops. *In utero,* treatment may be effected by administration of digoxin to the mother.

Atrial Flutter

Atrial flutter is less common than paroxysmal auricular tachycardia and may be of idiopathic etiology or associated with the same congenital heart lesions as those producing paroxysmal auricular tachycardia. Congestive heart failure is rare because some degree of atrioventricular block is present. The atrial rate may be 200 to 380 per minute. With a 2:1 block, the ventricular rate at the highest atrial rate would be 190 per minute, a rate insufficient to produce congestive failure in infancy. The ECG tracing reveals flutter waves often seen best in leads II of rV_1. The R–R interval is constant unless the atrioventricular block changes. The treatment of choice is digoxin or cardioversion by DC countershock (initial dose is 5 to 10 watt-seconds). Maintenance therapy with digoxin should probably be continued for 1 year. The addition of quinidine or propranolol may be necessary.

Complete Atrioventricular Block

In complete heart block, the ventricular rate is slower than and independent of the atrial rate. The arrhythmia is not infrequently recognized *in utero*. In approximately 50% of infants with congenital heart block there is an associated cardiovascular malformation (corrected transposition of the great arteries, ventricular septal defect, atrial septal defect). Myocarditis and fibrosis of the atrioventricular node or His bundle have been implicated as etiologic factors. Recent reports note an as-

Table 23-12. Drugs Commonly Used in the Treatment of Cardiovascular Disease in the Newborn

Drug				Side Effects or Toxic Manifestations	Comments
Generic Name	Proprietary Name	Form	Dose and Route		
Digoxin	Lanoxin	Elixer 0.05 mg/ml [bottle, 60 ml] Injection, 0.1 mg/ml [ampule, 1 ml]	*Digitalizing Dose:* Premature—0.04 mg/kg PO,IM,IV Full Term—0.05 mg/kg PO,IM,IV *Initial:* ½ Dig. dose, in 6 hr.—¼ Dig. dose in 12 hr.—¼ Dig. dose	Arrhythmias	ECG monitoring during digitalization Reduce dose with renal disease Check serum potassium and digitalis blood level
Atropine sulfate		0.4 mg/ml(ampule)	0.01 mg/kg/dose SC repeat every 2–4 hr	Hyperthermia Urinary retention Nodal tachycardia	
Ethacrynic acid	Edecrin	50 mg/vial 25 mg/tab	0.5–1.0 mg/kg IV over 5 min 1 mg/kg/dose PO BID	Electrolyte imbalance	
Furosemide	Lasix	10 mg/ml	0.5–1.0 mg/kg IV 1 mg/kg/dose PO BID	Electrolyte imbalance	
Chlorothiazide	Diuril	Suspension 50 mg/ml	20–25 mg/kg/24 hr in divided doses PO	Electrolyte imbalance	
Spironolactone	Aldactone	25 mg/tab	1.5–3.0 mg/kg/24 hr PO in divided doses		Add spironolactone and/or potassium supplement
Potassium	Potassium Triplex	Solution 3 mmol/ml	2 mmol/kg/24 hr PO in divided doses		
Morphine sulfate		2 mg/ml [ampule, 10 ml]	0.05–0.2 mg/kg/dose every 6 hrs IM or SC as needed	Respiratory depression	Antidote 0.01 mg/kg naloxone (Narcan)

THE FOLLOWING DRUGS ARE USED RARELY IN THE NEWBORN PERIOD:
Epinephrine (Adrenalin) and isoproterenol (Isuprel) have been used in the management of refractory congestive heart failure.
Lidocaine, quinidine, procaine amide, and propranolol may be used to control specific rhythm disturbances. Consultation with someone experienced in the ECG diagnosis and treatment of rhythm disturbances is recommended.

sociation between maternal systemic lupus erythematosus and congenital complete heart block. Complete heart block may occur as a complication of cardiac surgery, particularly in the correction of endocardial cushion defects, tetralogy of Fallot, and ventricular septal defects. Most infants with congenital heart block are asymptomatic and require no therapy. The presence of symptoms is usually related to the severity of the associated cardiovascular malformation and the degree of bradycardia. Infants without hemodynamically significant cardiac malformation tolerate bradycardia well, grow, and develop normally. Examination usually reveals cardiac enlargement due to an increased left ventricular end-diastolic volume and the large stroke volume. A systolic ejection murmur and apical mid-diastolic rumble are common. Strokes–Adam episodes may occur, but the initial episode is rarely fatal. The ventricular rate tends to decrease with increasing age. The ECG is usually characterized by normal atrial rate and P-wave configuration, independent ventricular rate with long but equal R–R intervals, and a normal or wide QRS complex. Some patients may respond to medical therapy with isoproterenol HCl (Isuprel) or atropine, but those in congestive heart failure needing digitalization, and infants with postsurgical block, should be electrically paced with epicardial wires. A transvenous pacemaker catheter is helpful as a temporary measure in the acute situation or in preparation for surgery.

REFERENCES

1. Olley PM, Coceani F, Bodach E: E-type prostaglandins: A new emergency therapy for certain cyanotic congenital heart malformations. Circulation 53:728–731, 1976
2. Lang P, Freed MD, Rosenthal A, Castaneda AR, Nadas AS: The use of prostaglandin E₁ in an infant with interruption of the aortic arch. J Pediatr 91:805–807, 1977
3. Friedman WF, Hirschklau MJ, Previtz MP, Pitlick PT, Kirkpatrick SE: Pharmacologic closure of patent ductus arteriosus in the premature infant. N Engl J Med 295:526–529, 1976
4. Heymann MA, Rudolph AM, Silverman NH: Closure of the ductus arteriosus in premature infants by inhibition of prostaglandin synthesis. N Engl J Med 295:530–533, 1976
5. Bierman FZ, Williams RG: Subxyphoid imaging of the interatrial septum in infants and neonates with congenital heart disease. Circulation 60:89–90, 1979
6. Fyler DC: Non-pump cardiac surgery in the New England Regional Infant Cardiac Program. Proceedings of the First Clinical Conference on Congenital Heart Disease. Eds. Tucker BL and Lindesmith GG, Grune and Stratton Inc., San Francisco, CA (accepted for publication, 1979)
7. Nadas AS, Fyler DC: Pediatric Cardiology, 3rd ed Philadelphia, W. B. Saunders, 1972
8. Keith JD, Rowe RD, Vlad P: Heart Disease in Infancy and Childhood, 3rd ed. New York, Macmillan, 1978
9. Moss AJ, Adams FH, Emmanouilides GC: Heart Disease In Infants, Children and Adolescents, 2nd ed. Baltimore, Williams & Wilkins, 1977
10. Mitchell SC, Korones SB, Berendes HW: Congenital heart disease in 56,109 births. Circulation 43:323, 1971
11. Muirhead DM: Report on perinatal and infant mortality in Massachusetts 1967 and 1968. Committee on Perinatal Welfare, Massachusetts Medical Society, Dec., 1971
12. Barcroft J: Researches of Pre-natal Life. Oxford, Blackwell and Mott Ltd., 1944
13. Dawes GS: Foetal and Neonatal Physiology: A Comparative Study of the Changes at Birth. Chicago, Year Book Medical Publishers, 1969
14. Rudolph AM: The changes in the circulation after birth. Circulation 41:343, 1970
15. Lind J, Stern L, Wegelius C: Human and Foetal Neonatal Circulation. Sringfield, Ill, Charles C Thomas, 1964
16. Braunwald E, Swan HJC: Cooperative study on cardiac catheterization. American Heart Association Monograph No. 20. Circulation 37:1 (Suppl III), 1968.

24

Neonatal Jaundice*

M. Jeffrey Maisels

INTRODUCTION

The problem of the jaundiced newborn infant confronts pediatricians daily. Not only is the newborn infant unique because of his limited ability to clear bilirubin from the plasma, but also because (with rare exceptions) the newborn period remains the only time at which an elevated plasma bilirubin concentration *per se* represents a threat to the well-being of the organism.

Chemical Structure and Properties of Bilirubin

A remarkable resurgence of interest in bile pigments on the part of organic chemists has occurred in the last few years and has provided new insights into the chemical and biologic properties of bilirubin. Several recent observations that have been reviewed in-depth,[1-4] may have important implications for our understanding of the potential neurotoxicity of bilirubin as well as the mechanism of phototherapy.[1,2,5-7] Bilirubin is the end product of the catabolism of heme, of which the major source is circulating hemoglobin. The formation of bilirubin from hemoglobin involves an oxidative process in which the alpha-methene

bridge of the heme porphyrin ring is opened, and carbon monoxide and biliverdin are formed (Fig. 24-1). This oxidation is catalyzed by the enzyme microsomal heme oxygenase. The biliverdin is then reduced to bilirubin by NADPH-dependent biliverdin reductase. Because it is derived from cleavage at the alpha position of the heme ring of ferroprotoporphyrin IX, the product thus formed is known as bilirubin $IX\alpha$ (Fig. 24-1). The predominant isomer, bilirubin $IX\alpha$ (ZZ) exists as a charged molecule (dianion) and is thought to be the main component of natural bilirubin found both free and bound to albumin in the human.[2] This form of bilirubin has hydrophilic (polar) properties in eight locations, while the hydrophobic moieties are small. The anion combines with two protons and forms bilirubin acid. Using x-ray crystallography, Bonnett and coworkers have shown that the bilirubin molecule folds up, establishing intramolecular hydrogen bonds to form bilirubin $IX\alpha$ (ZZ) acid (Fig. 24-2).[5] These bonds saturate the hydrophilic (polar) groups of the molecule leaving no affinities for the attachment of water. The molecule therefore becomes hydrophobic and insoluble in water. It is no longer able to bind to albumin but has a pronounced tendency for aggregation and binding to tissues. Under these circumstances, it may be potentially toxic.[2]

* I gratefully acknowledge the helpful advice and criticism of Drs. Rodney Levine and James Kendig.

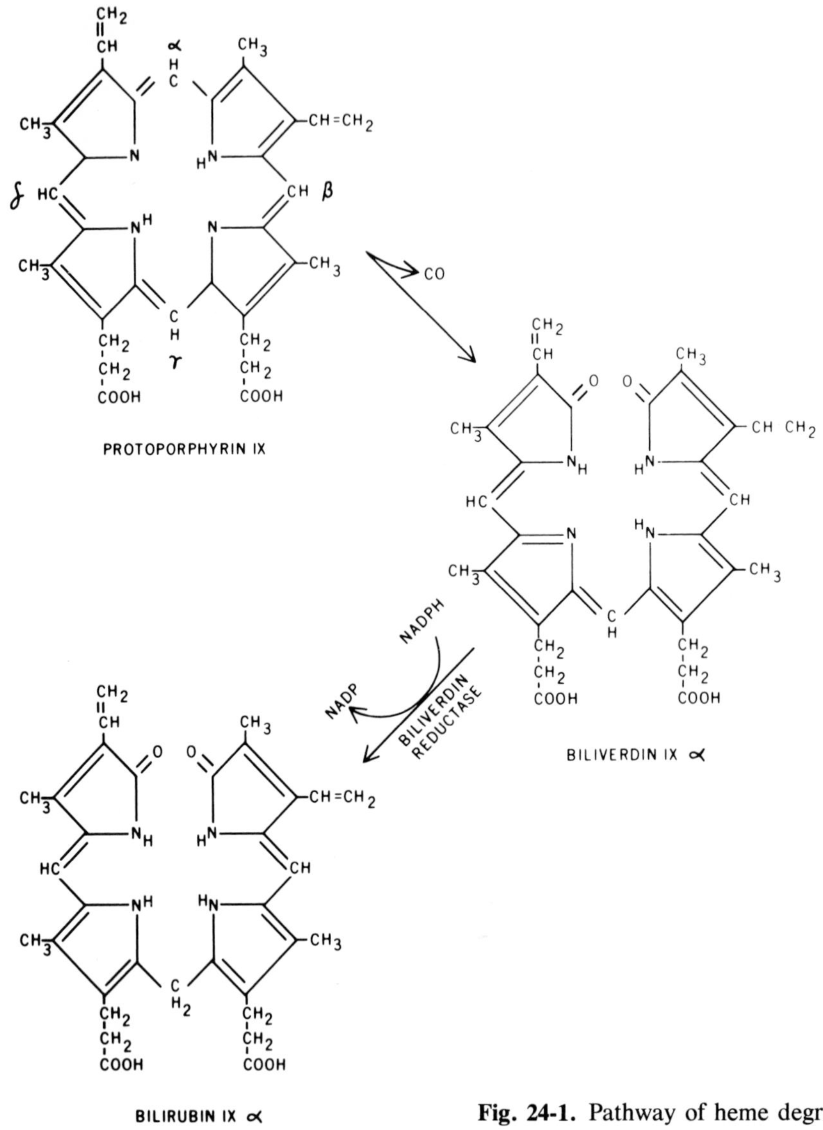
PROTOPORPHYRIN IX
CO
BILIVERDIN IX α
NADPH
NADP
BILIVERDIN REDUCTASE
BILIRUBIN IX α

Fig. 24-1. Pathway of heme degradation.

The presence of such a hydrogen-bonded structure may also explain some of the other biologic properties of bilirubin such as the van den Bergh reaction. For the reaction with the diazo reagent to occur, the hydrogen bonds must be broken (which can be accomplished by the addition of alcohol) and the difference between the indirect and direct diazo reactions may be the presence or absence of intramolecular hydrogen bonding.[3]

Other isomers of bilirubin (IXβ, IXγ, and IXδ) are also found in bile, but only in trace amounts.[2] Additional IXα isomers (EZ, ZE, and EE) result from phototherapy of bilirubin (see above).

Recently, Brodersen has shown that, contrary to what has been accepted almost universally, bilirubin is not a lipophilic substance, and its neurotoxicity is not likely to be caused by its affinity for lipids in the central nervous system.[6] Rather, it appears to be polar with little solubility in triglycerides and increasing solubility in polar solvents.

NEONATAL BILIRUBIN METABOLISM

Bilirubin Production

The normal destruction of circulating red cells accounts for about 75% of the daily bilirubin production in the newborn infant, the

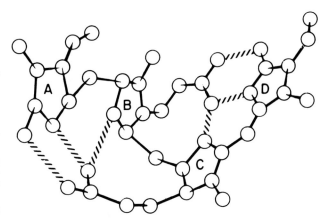

Fig. 24-2. Top. The chemical structure of bilirubin IXα as it is conventionally written. Bilirubin IXα consists of two dipyrroles connected by a central methylene bridge. Two propionic acid side groups are attached to the central pyrrole rings **B** and **C. Bottom.** Involuted hydrogen-bonded structure in which the proprionic acid groups of rings **B** and **C** are linked to the nitrogens of the opposite pyrrole rings (**broken lines**). (Schmid R: Gastroenterology 74:1307, 1978)

senescent erythrocytes being removed from the circulation and destroyed in the reticulo-endothelial system, where the hemoglobin is catabolized and converted to bilirubin. (1 g of hemoglobin, when catabolized, yields 35 mg of bilirubin.)

A significant contribution (25% or more) to the daily production of bilirubin in the neonate, comes from sources other than effete red blood cells (Fig. 24-3). These sources are collectively known as the "early-labeled peak" of bile pigment, from the observation of an early peak of radioactivity which appears as labeled stercobilin in the stool within minutes, to days after the administration of labeled glycine or δ-aminolevulinic acid.[8] This early bilirubin consists of 2 major components: a noneryth-ropoietic component resulting from the turn-over of (nonhemoglobin) heme-protein and free heme, primarily in the liver; and an eryth-ropoietic component primarily arising from ineffective erythropoiesis, the destruction of immature red cell precursors, either in the bone marrow or soon after release into the circulation. There may also be a small contri-bution from bilirubin not arising from heme: the so-called "shunt" bilirubin.

Transport and Hepatic Uptake of Bilirubin

Once bilirubin leaves the reticuloendothelial system, it is transported in the plasma, bound tightly to albumin (the binding affinity is 10^7 to 10^8 mol^{-1}). Binding to albumin is essential because, at pH 7.4, the solubility of unbound bilirubin is extremely low: about 7 nmol/l (0.4 μg/dl).[6] The tightness of this albumin-bilirubin bond may be important in determining the potential toxicity of bilirubin (see below).

The parenchymal cells of the liver have a selective and highly efficient capacity for re-moving unconjugated bilirubin from the plasma, but exactly how this is achieved is unknown. When the bilirubin-albumin com-plex reaches the plasma membrane of the hepatocyte, a proportion of the bilirubin, but not the albumin, is transferred across the cell membrane into the hepatocyte where it is bound to soluble proteins. The transfer of bilirubin from plasma into the liver cell is probably carrier-mediated.[9] Intracellularly, bil-irubin binds primarily to ligandin (Y protein, glutathione S-transferase B) and, to a lesser extent, to other glutathione S-transferases and Z protein.[10]

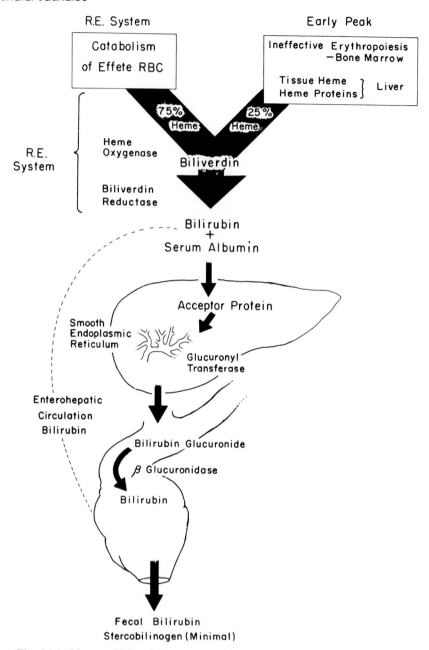

Fig. 24-3. Neonatal bile pigment metabolism.

Bilirubin flux across the hepatocyte membrane is bidirectional, influx and efflux being related to the concentrations and binding affinities of albumin and ligandin in the plasma and hepatocyte respectively. Because the sequestration coefficient is larger than the efflux coefficient, most of the bilirubin entering the liver cell is conjugated and excreted in bile. This is related to the fact that, in the presence of liver cytosol, ligandin binds bilirubin, whereas albumin does not.[11] The administration of phenobarbital increases the concentration of ligandin and provides more intracellular binding sites for bilirubin.[10]

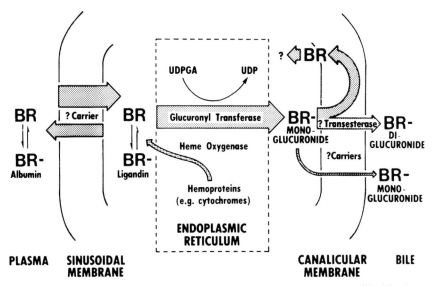

Fig. 24-4. Bilirubin transport and conjugation in the hepatocyte. Bilirubin that has been transferred across the sinusoidal membrane into the hepatocyte is converted by microsomal glucuronyltransferase to bilirubin monoglucuronide. The monoconjugate either is excreted in the bile or converted to diglucuronide by a transesterase believed to be located in the canalicular membrane. (Schmid R: Gastroenterology 74:1307, 1978)

Conjugation and Excretion

Unconjugated (indirect-reacting) bilirubin, which is largely insoluble in aqueous solutions at pH 7.4, must generally be converted to its water-soluble conjugate (direct-reacting bilirubin) before it can be excreted (Fig. 24-4). Under certain circumstances (*e.g.,* phototherapy), direct excretion of unconjugated bilirubin into the bile may occur.

The use of newly developed analytic techniques has established that, in the human adult, the major product of conjugations is bilirubin diglucuronide with monoglucuronides forming a minor fraction. In addition, trace amounts of glucose and xylose conjugates are demonstrable.[3] Most recently, preliminary data from full-term and premature infants revealed the presence of monoconjugates only in the first 24 to 48 hours of life, diconjugates appearing after 48 hours.[12] In both types of the Crigler–Najjar syndrome (see below), the monoglucuronide represents the major pigment fraction of bile.[3] This finding is difficult to interpret, because hepatic bilirubin glucuronyl transferase, which catalyzes the conversion of bilirubin to the monoglucuronide form (Fig. 24-4), is absent or reduced in these syndromes.[3] The fact that these patients ap-

pear to excrete bilirubin monoglucuronide preferentially, suggests that it may be necessary to reassess the previously described enzyme defects in the Crigler–Najjar syndromes.

Two separate enzymes are probably involved in the synthesis of bilirubin diglucuronide. The first is bilirubin uridine diphosphate glucuronyl transferase (UDPG-T), a membrane-bound enzyme associated with the endoplasmic reticulum that catalyzes the formation of bilirubin monoglucuronide. Some of the monoglucuronide formed is stored,[10] some is excreted directly into bile, and some is converted to the diglucuronide (Fig. 24-4). It has been postulated that this latter step is catalyzed by an enzyme functioning as a transesterase, which is located in the plasma membrane of the hepatocytes.[13] Recently, it has been shown that significant quantities of bilirubin monoglucuronide accumulate in the hepatocyte, bound to the intracellular glutathione S-transferases. There is no similar accumulation of the diglucuronide, which is consistent with the hypothesis that synthesis and excretion of diglucuronide occurs in the canalicular membrane (Fig. 24-3).[10]

In the light of better understanding of the structural properties of bilirubin and its conjugation, Schmid concludes that " . . . perhaps the most remarkable aspect of the complex conjugating mechanism of the liver cell is that it seems to serve the sole purpose of altering the involuted hydrogen-bonded conformation of bilirubin IXα . . . ."[3] It is only the bilirubin isomers, that can form intramolecular hydrogen bonds (such as natural bilirubin IXα), that require conjugation for excretion. Other isomers, including those produced by phototherapy, can be excreted directly in bile.

Transfer of Bilirubin into Bile and Intestinal Transport

After conjugation, bilirubin is excreted rapidly into the bile by the liver cell, a process which requires metabolic work for the active transport of bilirubin across a large concentration gradient.

Once in the small gut, conjugated bilirubin is not reabsorbed. In the adult, it is largely reduced to stercobilin by bacteria and an insignificant amount is hydrolyzed to unconjugated bilirubin and reabsorbed by way of the enterohepatic circulation. In the newborn, however, this enterohepatic circulation of bilirubin may be significant (see physiologic jaundice). In conditions with high plasma bilirubin levels and poor hepatic excretion, a gradient for unconjugated bilirubin will exist from the plasma to the intestinal lumen and significant amounts of unconjugated bilirubin may be cleared by diffusion across the itnestinal wall. Figure 24-3 summarizes bile pigment metabolism in the newborn.

FETAL BILIRUBIN METABOLISM
Bilirubin in Amniotic Fluid

Bilirubin can be detected in normal amniotic fluid after about the 12th week of gestation. It subsequently disappears by 36 to 37 weeks. Increased levels of bilirubin in the amniotic fluid are observed in the presence of fetal hyperbilirubinemia (unconjugated) and can be used to predict the severity of Rh hemolytic disease (see below). Increased amniotic fluid bilirubin levels may also be found in the presence of fetal intestinal obstruction.[14]

It is not known precisely how bilirubin gets into the amniotic fluid. Suggested routes include tracheobronchial secretions, excretion by way of the mucosa of the upper gastrointestinal tract, fetal urine and meconium, dif-

fusion across the umbilical cord and fetal skin, or transfer from the maternal circulation.

The most likely of these mechanisms appears to be the first. Studies in rabbits have demonstrated a correlation between increased serum unconjugated bilirubin concentrations and increased tracheal fluid bilirubin concentrations.[15]

Fetal Bilirubin Production, Hepatic Function, and Placental Transfer

The rate of bilirubin production in the fetus has not been determined, but it is reasonable to assume that it is at least as great as that in the newborn (see below). However, the ability of the primate fetal liver to remove bilirubin from the circulation and to conjugate it is severely limited. Lathe and Walker found almost no UDPG-T activity in the livers of three premature infants (25–32 weeks' gestation) who died shortly after birth.[16] Felsher, in studies of electively aborted 8 to 19-week-old fetuses, found markedly reduced activity of hepatic UDPG-T and uridine diphosphate glucose dehydrogenase (UDPG-D), the enzyme which catalyzes the formation of UDPGA.[17] The rate of hepatic bilirubin glucuronidation depends upon the availability of UDPGA as well as the activity of UDPG-T.[17] As virtually all of the fetal bilirubin remains in the unconjugated form, it is readily transferred across the placenta to the maternal circulation, there to be excreted by the maternal liver. Thus, the newborn is rarely born jaundiced except, when in the presence of severe hemolytic disease there is an accumulation of unconjugated bilirubin in the fetus. Because conjugated bilirubin is not transferred across the placenta, it may accumulate in the fetal plasma and other tissues.

PHYSIOLOGIC JAUNDICE OF THE NEWBORN

Almost every newborn infant will develop a serum unconjugated bilirubin concentration of greater than 2 mg/dl (34 μmol/l) during the first week of life, and this transient hyperbilirubinemia in the newborn has, therefore, been called "physiologic jaundice." Gartner and coworkers have conducted an extensive series of studies in the newborn rhesus monkey, a subhuman primate species which develops physiologic jaundice.[18] They found that both

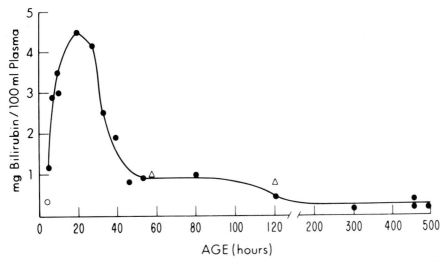

Fig. 24-5. Total bilirubin concentrations in plasma of term (•), premature (Δ), and postmature (○) untreated newborn Macaca mulatta prior to infusion of bilirubin. (Gartner LM, Lee K-S, Vaisman S et al: J Pediatr 90:513, 1977)

the newborn human and monkey develop a strikingly similar biphasic pattern of physiologic jaundice (Figs. 24-5 and 24-6). In the monkey, phase I is characterized by a rapid increase in serum bilirubin levels to 4.5 mg/dl (77 μmol/l) by 19 hours followed by a decline to 1 mg/dl (17 μmol/l) by 48 hours. In phase II, bilirubin levels remain elevated at 1 mg/dl (17 μmol/l) until about 4 days of age when they decline to normal adult values. The term hu-

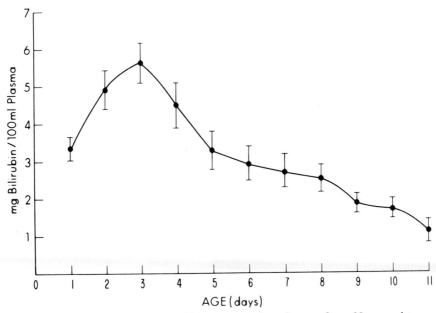

Fig. 24-6. Mean total daily bilirubin concentrations in sera from 29 normal-term human infants. Vertical bars are one standard error of the mean. Phase I lasts until day 5 when phase II begins. (Gartner LM, Lee K-S, Vaisman S et al: J Pediatr 90:513, 1977

Table 24-1. Possible Mechanisms Involved in Physiologic Jaundice.

Increased Bilirubin Load on the Liver Cell

↑ Red blood cell volume
↓ Red blood cell survival
↑ Early-labeled bilirubin
↑ Enterohepatic circulation of bilirubin

Defective Hepatic Uptake of Bilirubin from the Plasma

↓ Ligandin (Y protein)
   Binding of Y and Z proteins by other anions
↓ Relative hepatic uptake deficieny (phase II)

Defective Bilirubin Conjugation

↓ UDP glucuronyl transferase activity
↓ UDP glucose dehydrogenase activity

Defective Bilirubin Excretion

Excretion impaired but not rate limiting

Hepatic Circulation

↓ Oxygen supply to the liver when umbilical cord
   clamped
   Portal blood flow bypassing liver sinusoids if
   ductus venosus patent

man neonate manifests a similar pattern with the duration of each phase approximately three times longer than that in the moneky (Fig. 24-6). In phase I, the serum bilirubin rises to about 6 mg/dl (103 μmol/l) by day 3 and then falls to 3 mg/dl (51 μmol/l) by day 5. In phase II, serum bilirubin concentrations remain between 2 and 3 mg/dl (34–51 μmol/l) for about 3 days and then decline slowly until normal levels are reached by 11 to 12 days of life. Low-birth-weight infants have exaggerated and prolonged hyperbilirubinemia with peak serum bilirubin levels of 10 to 15 mg/dl (171–257 μmol/l) on days 5 to 6 (phase I), and then lower concentrations, which may persist for up to 4 weeks.

Jaundice may result from (1) an increased load of bilirubin on the liver cell, including that contributed by the enterohepatic circulation; and (2) a decrease in the ability of the liver to clear the bilirubin from the plasma as a result of defective uptake, conjugation, or excretion (singly or in any combination). It is likely that physiologic jaundice is the result of a complex interaction of a number of these factors (Table 24-1).

Increased Bilirubin Load on the Liver Cell

Bilirubin Production. Measurements of the production of carbon monoxide (which is produced in equimolar quantities with bilirubin) show that the normal newborn infant produces an average of 8 to 10 mg/kg of bilirubin per day.[19,20] Similar rates of bilirubin production have been found in low-birth-weight infants.[19] This is more than twice the rate of normal daily production of bilirubin in the adult (per kg body weight) and is explained by the fact that the neonate has a higher circulating-red-cell volume (per kg), a shorter mean-red-cell life span and a larger early-labeled bilirubin peak. Bilirubin production decreases with increasing postnatal age but is still about twice the adult rate after age 2 weeks.[19]

Enterohepatic Circulation. The newborn probably reabsorbs significantly larger quantities of unconjugated bilirubin, by way of the enterohepatic circulation, than does the adult. This may result from the absence of bacterial flora and the increased activity of the deconjugating enzyme, β-glucuronidase.[21] As a result, conjugated bilirubin (which is not reab-

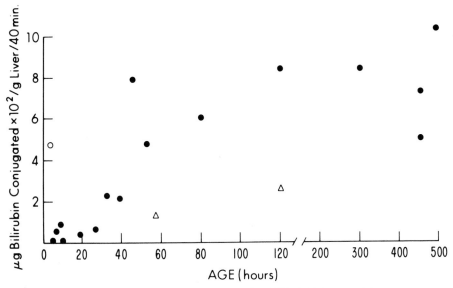

Fig. 24-7 Hepatic glucuronyl transferase activity (bilirubin) in term (•), premature (Δ) and postmature (o) untreated newborn rhesus monkey. (Gartner LM, Lee K-S, Vaisman S: J Pediatr 90:513, 1977)

sorbed) is not converted to urobilin, but is hydrolyzed to unconjugated bilirubin, which is then reabsorbed, thus increasing the bilirubin load on an already stressed liver. Studies in newborn humans and monkeys suggest that the enterohepatic circulation of bilirubin is a significant contributor to physiologic jaundice.[18,22]

Decreased Clearance of Bilirubin from the Plasma

Uptake. Ligandin, which is the predominant bilirubin-binding protein in the liver cell, is deficient in the liver of newborn monkeys. It reaches adult levels by 5 days of life, coinciding with a fall in bilirubin levels and a normal hepatic uptake of sulfobromophthalein (BSP).[23] Furthermore, the administration of phenobarbital will enhance hepatic uptake of BSP and simultaneously increase the concentration of ligandin.[9] Although this suggests that impaired uptake may contribute to the pathogenesis of physiologic jaundice, it does not appear to be rate limiting during phase I (see above).[18] It may be important during phase II, the low grade but more persistent stage of physiologic jaundice.

Conjugation. Deficient glucuronyl transferase activity, (and the resultant impairment of bilirubin conjugation) has long been considered

a major cause of physiologic jaundice. Studies of this sytem have used a variety of substrates and have been restricted largely to non-primates, in which significant species differences may exist in the pattern of development of glucuronyl transferase. Using bilirubin as the substrate, studies in term newborn rhesus monkeys revealed virtually no hepatic glucuronyl transferase activity in the first 24 hours (Fig. 24-7).[18] Activity increased over the next 48 hours coincident with a decline in serum bilirubin levels (descending curve of phase I; Fig. 24-5). By 48 hours, activity levels were close to those of the adult but enzyme maturation in two premature infants was markedly delayed. In a single postmature monkey, activity at 4 hours of life was tenfold greater than term animals of comparable age.

The administration of phenobarbital (5 mg/kg daily for 6 weeks) to pregnant monkeys and in similar dosage to the infants (if not studied within 12 hours of birth) increased hepatic glucuronyl transferase activity by almost threefold: sufficient to abolish, completely, phase I physiologic jaundice (Fig. 24-8). These observations are consistent with the pivotal role of deficient glucuronyl transferase activity (and bilirubin conjugation) in the first phase of neonatal jaundice.

Excretion. The absence of an elevated serum

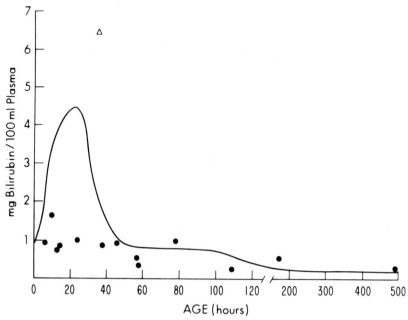

Fig. 24-8 Total bilirubin concentrations in plasma of term (•) and premature (Δ) phenobarbital treated newborn Mucaca mulatta prior to infusion of bilirubin. Solid line represents best fit for the same measurement in untreated newborn monkeys. (Gartner LM, Lee K-S Vaisman S: J Pediatr 90:513, 1977)

level of conjugated bilirubin in physiologic jaundice suggests that, under normal circumstances, the neonatal liver cell is capable of excreting the bilirubin which it has just conjugated. Nevertheless, the ability of the newborn liver to excrete conjugated bilirubin and other anions (drugs, hormones, and so on) is less than in the older child or adult and may become rate limiting when the bilirubin load is significantly increased. Thus, in severe hemolytic disease of the newborn, it is not uncommon to find an elevated serum level of direct-reacting (conjugated) bilirubin.

Hepatic Circulation. It is likely that the liver's capacity for uptake, conjugation, and excretion of bilirubin is also related to its blood supply. While in fetal life this comes from the relatively well-oxygenated blood of the umbilical vein, at birth it is abruptly terminated by the accouchier's clamp on the umbilical cord, and the liver must henceforth rely mainly on the poorly oxygenated portal venous blood. The effect of this apparent "hemodynamic shock" and hypoxia has not been measured in terms of bilirubin clearance, but it may produce temporary impairment until appro-

priate adjustments can take place. If the ductus venosus does not close soon after birth (as may occur in the premature infant), portal blood flow effectively bypasses the sinusoidal circulation of the liver, thus preventing normal bilirubin clearance from the plasma.[24]

Thus, physiologic jaundice appears to result from a decreased ability of the hepatocyte to conjugate bilirubin (phase I hyperbilirubinemia) and to take up bilirubin (phase II hyperbilirubinemia) in the face of a *persistent increase in bilirubin load*. In the absence of this large load of bilirubin, physiologic jaundice probably would not occur.

APPROACH TO THE JAUNDICED INFANT

Because clinical jaundice becomes apparent at serum bilirubin levels of approximately 5 to 7 mg/dl (85–120 μmol/1), between 25% and 50% of all normal newborn infants and a considerably higher percentage of premature infants demonstrate clinical jaundice during the first week of life. It is therefore important for the physician caring for newborn infants to develop a relatively consistent approach to the investigation and management of the jaundiced newborn. Such an approach is suggested by the following questions:

1. Is the jaundice "physiologic" or "pathologic"?
2. If not physiologic jaundice, what are the possible causes?
3. Which infants require further investigation, and what investigations are needed?
4. Is the jaundice a threat to the infant?
    a. What investigations are required to assess the potential danger?
    b. If danger exists, what treatment is appropriate?

Serum Bilirubin Concentration

The first step in assessing any form of jaundice is to measure the total and direct serum bilirubin concentration. While it is true that there is a correlation between the serum bilirubin concentration and the cephalopedal progression of dermal icterus, the clinical estimation of serum bilirubin is not sufficiently reliable to permit omission of laboratory analysis.[25]

Interest has been rekindled in the use of skin reflectance as a screening technique in jaundiced infants. This technique utilizes the fact that skin color can be quantified by measuring the color as a function of wavelength over the visible portion of the spectrum. Utilizing computer-aided reflectometry, Hannemann, DeWitt, and Wiechel found that the serum bilirubin concentration could be predicted within ±2 mg/dl in normal infants, a highly acceptable error for a screening technique.[26] Unfortunately, this method requires complex instrumentation and computer analysis. Yamanouchi and coworkers have now described a method of measuring "transcutaneous" bilirubin levels which appears to offer considerable promise as a screening technique.[27] The instrument, produced by the Minolta Camera Co., is small, hand-held, rechargeable, and simple to operate. Readings are taken from the skin over the forehead. A strobe light passes through a fiberoptic filament and penetrates the blanched skin, transilluminating the subcutaneous tissue. The scattered light comes back through second fiberoptic filaments and is carried to the spectrophotometric module where the in-

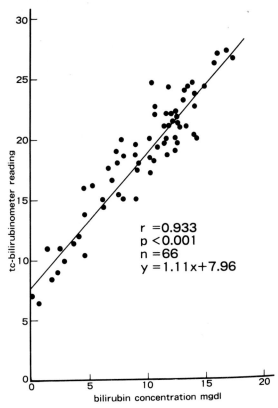

Fig. 24-9. Correlation between transcutaneous (tc) bilirubinometry and serum total bilirubin concentration measured by alkali azobilirubin method. (Yamanouchi I, Yamauchi Y, Ikuko I: Pediatrics 48: 195, 1980; Copyright © American Academy of Pediatrics, 1980)

sity of yellow color (corrected for hemoglobin) is measured. In term and preterm infants, a highly significant linear relationship was found between transcutaneous and serum bilirubin determinations (Fig. 24-9).

When this instrument becomes commercially available, it should find wide application for the screening of newborn infants in hospital nurseries and physicians' offices.

Physiologic versus Pathologic Jaundice

The first step in evaluating jaundice is to decide whether or not it is likely to be "physiologic" or "pathologic". This may not always be easy, because the existence of a serum bilirubin concentration in the so-called physiologic range does not, of course, exclude the possibility that it represents a pathologic process. Indeed, under certain conditions (small, sick premature infants), bilirubin levels well within the physiologic range (<10 mg/dl, 171 μmol/1) may cause kernicterus. On the other hand, in the term infant, there is a tendency to dismiss elevated serum bilirubin concentrations as "physiologic," and it is therefore important to have a fairly clear definition of what physiologic jaundice is not. The conditions under which jaundice cannot be considered to be physiologic are listed below.

Criteria Which Rule Out the Diagnosis of Physiologic Jaundice.*

1. Clinical jaundice in the first 24 hours of life
2. Total serum bilirubin concentrations increasing by more than 5 mg/dl (85 μmol/1) per day
3. Total serum bilirubin concentration exceeding 12.9 mg/dl (221 μmol/1) in a full-term infant or 15 mg/dl (257 μmol/1) in a premature infant
4. Direct serum bilirubin concentration exceeding 1.5 to 2 mg/dl (26–34 μmol/1)
5. Clinical jaundice persisting for more than 1 week in a full-term infant or 2 weeks in a premature infant.

---

* The absence of these criteria does not imply that the jaundice *is* physiologic. In the presence of any of these criteria, the jaundice must be investigated.

Should any of these criteria apply, the jaundice must be investigated. The danger of dismissing any jaundice as "physiologic" without considerable thought, careful review of the maternal and infant history, thorough examination of the infant and, if necessary, further laboratory investigations, is that potentially life-threatening causes of jaundice such as sepsis, hemolysis, galactosemia, and even intestinal obstruction may be missed. It is distinctly unusual, however, for such infants to be otherwise asymptomatic.[28] While there is no doubt that a certain number of infants develop hyperbilirubinemia outside of the physiologic range for which no obvious cause is found, nevertheless this does not permit us to dismiss these instances of jaundice as "physiologic."

Simply stated, the "jaundice equation" is:

Plasma Bilirubin Concentration =
    Bilirubin Load/Bilirubin Excretion

Thus, an increase in load (which may include a significant enterohepatic circulation) or a decrease in excretion, or both, may produce jaundice. On the other hand, a modest increase in load may be accompanied by an increased clearance, leaving the serum bilirubin levels relatively unaffected. In the absence of overt laboratory indications of hemolysis (*e.g.*, abnormalities of red cell morphology, reticulocytosis, positive Coombs' test), more subtle increases in red cell turnover are not detectable by the usual laboratory methods. Furthermore, no clinical method exists for the measurement of enterohepatic circulation or bilirubin clearance. We are, thus, effectively prevented from more clearly defining the cause of hyperbilirubinemia in about 50% of such infants.[29] It should be remembered that the normal newborn's mechanisms for bilirubin clearance from the plasma are already operating at maximal output, so that a relatively slight increase in load, or decrease in clearance, may cause a significant elevation in serum bilirubin.

The differential diagnosis and a practical diagnostic approach to jaundice are outlined in Figure 24-10. Note that a serum bilirubin concentration of 13.0 mg/dl (222 μmol/1) or greater in any infant (term or premature), or the presence of any of the criteria listed previously demand the following basic investigations:

1. Serum bilirubin concentration—direct and total
2. Peripheral blood smear for red cell morphology and reticulocyte count
3. Blood type, Rh, on mother and infant; and direct Coombs' test on infant
4. Hematocrit or hemoglobin

These studies, which can be performed in any hospital laboratory, will define or suggest the cause of jaundice in about 50% of cases[29] and eliminate the need for further investigations. Should this not be the case, the clinical condition, height, duration, and type of bilirubin elevation (direct, indirect, or both) will determine what pathologic conditions should be considered and thus what further diagnostic studies should be performed. Thaler has provided useful algorithms for diagnosing the cause of neonatal jaundice,[30] and McMillan has provided guidelines for obtaining and using clinical and laboratory information in the jaundiced infant (Table 24-2).

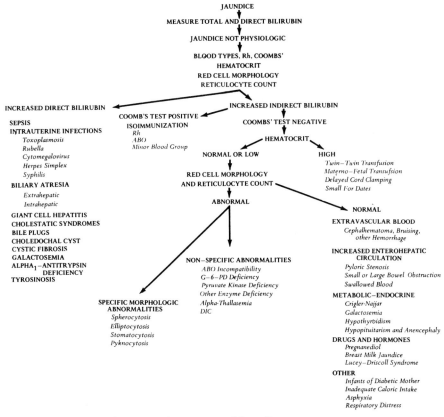

JAUNDICE

MEASURE TOTAL AND DIRECT BILIRUBIN

JAUNDICE NOT PHYSIOLOGIC

BLOOD TYPES, Rh, COOMBS'
HEMATOCRIT
RED CELL MORPHOLOGY
RETICULOCYTE COUNT

INCREASED DIRECT BILIRUBIN

SEPSIS
INTRAUTERINE INFECTIONS
Toxoplasmosis
Rubella
Cytomegalovirus
Herpes Simplex
Syphilis
BILIARY ATRESIA
Extrahepatic
Intrahepatic
GIANT CELL HEPATITIS
CHOLESTATIC SYNDROMES
BILE PLUGS
CHOLEDOCHAL CYST
CYSTIC FIBROSIS
GALACTOSEMIA
ALPHA$_1$—ANTITRYPSIN
    DEFICIENCY
TYROSINOSIS

INCREASED INDIRECT BILIRUBIN

COOMB'S TEST POSITIVE
ISOIMMUNIZATION
Rh
ABO
Minor Blood Group

COOMBS' TEST NEGATIVE

HEMATOCRIT

NORMAL OR LOW

HIGH
Twin—Twin Transfusion
Materno—Fetal Transfusion
Delayed Cord Clamping
Small For Dates

RED CELL MORPHOLOGY
AND RETICULOCYTE COUNT

ABNORMAL

NORMAL

EXTRAVASCULAR BLOOD
Cephalhematoma, Bruising,
other Hemorrhage

INCREASED ENTEROHEPATIC
    CIRCULATION
Pyloric Stenosis
Small or Large Bowel Obstruction
Swallowed Blood

NON—SPECIFIC ABNORMALITIES
ABO Incompatibility
G–6–PD Deficiency
Pyruvate Kinase Deficiency
Other Enzyme Deficiency
Alpha-Thallasemia
DIC

SPECIFIC MORPHOLOGIC
ABNORMALITIES
Spherocytosis
Elliptocytosis
Stomatocytosis
Pyknocytosis

METABOLIC—ENDOCRINE
Crigler-Najjar
Galactosemia
Hypothyroidism
Hypopituitarism and Anencephaly
DRUGS AND HORMONES
Pregnanediol
Breast Milk Jaundice
Lucey—Driscoll Syndrome
OTHER
Infants of Diabetic Mother
Inadequate Caloric Intake
Asphyxia
Respiratory Distress

Fig. 24-10. Diagnostic approach to neonatal jaundice.

NORMAL SERUM BILIRUBIN LEVELS

In the National Collaborative Perinatal Project, conducted from 1959 to 1966, serum bilirubin concentrations were obtained prospectively on more than 35,000 infants (Tables 24-3 and 24-4).[31] The serum bilirubin level was routinely measured at about 48 hours of age and then repeated daily if the initial reading was 10 mg/dl (171 μmol/1) or greater until the value decreased below 10 mg/dl (171 μmol/1). Additional serum bilirubin determinations were obtained when clinically indicated. (Thus, some babies, with a late-rising bilirubin may have been missed). The maximum bilirubin levels measured are shown in Tables 24-3 and 24-4, and indicate that, of infants weighing more than 2500 g at birth, only 6.2% of white infants and 4.5% of black infants had serum bilirubin levels in excess of 12.9 mg/dl (221 μmol/1). Although this population included sick infants and those with hemolytic disease, approximately 95% of all infants had serum bilirubin concentrations which did not exceed 12.9 mg/dl.

Table 24-5 summarizes the data for 11 recent studies of serum bilirubin levels in healthy term infants. Although most of these studies were designed primarily to identify some of the factors which may affect neonatal jaundice (route of delivery, amniotomy, use of oxytocics, feedings, and so on) infants with any neonatal complications were excluded. Furthermore, in each study, serum bilirubin levels were obtained *prospectively in all infants*. This is of considerable importance because retrospective studies have been reported in which serum bilirubin determinations were obtained only on identification of clinical jaundice. This may result in errors in both directions: infants with significant hyperbilirubinemia can be missed;[25] and variations in awareness of jaundice, by different staff at different times, may lead to serious bias in sampling. A review of the data in Table 24-5 reveals that the mean serum bilirubin levels on the third day of life

Table 24-2. The Use of Clinical Data in the Diagnosis of Neonatal Jaundice

Information	Clinical Data	Significance
Family History	Parent or sibling with history of jaundice or anemia	Suggests hereditary hemolytic anemia, such as hereditary spherocytosis
	Previous sibling with neonatal jaundice	Suggests hemolytic disease caused by ABO or Rh isoimmunization or breast milk jaundice
Maternal History	History of liver disease in siblings or disorders such as cystic fibrosis, galactosemia, tyrosinemia, hypermethioninemia, Crigler–Najjar syndrome, or alpha$_1$-antitrypsin deficiency	All associated with neonatal hyperbilirubinemia
	Unexplained illness during pregnancy	Consider congenital infections such as rubella, cytomegalovirus, toxoplasmosis, herpes, syphilis, or hepatitis
	Diabetes mellitus	Increased incidence of jaundice among infants of diabetic mothers
	Drug ingestion during pregnancy	Ingestion of sulfonamides, nitrofurantoins, or antimalarials may initiate hemolysis in G-6-PD deficient infant.
History of Labor and Delivery	Vacuum extraction	Increased incidence of cephalohematoma and jaundice
	Oxytocin-induced labor	(?)Increased incidence of hyperbilirubinemia
	Delayed cord clamping	Increased incidence of hyperbilirubinemia among polycythemic infants
	Apgar score	Increased incidence of jaundice in asphyxiated infants
	Delayed passage of meconium or infrequent stools	Increased enterohepatic circulation of bilirubin; consider intestinal atresia, annular pancreas, Hirschsprung's disease, meconium plug, drug-induced ileus (hexamethonium)
Infant's History	Caloric intake	Inadequate caloric intake results in delay in bilirubin conjugation.
	Vomiting	Suspect sepsis, galactosemia, or pyloric stenosis; all associated with hyperbilirubinemia
	Small for gestational age	Infants frequently polycythemic and jaundiced; consider intrauterine infection
	Head size	Microcephaly seen with intrauterine infections associated with jaundice
	Cephalohematoma	Entrapped hemorrhage associated with hyperbilirubinemia

Infant's Physical Examination	Pallor	Suspect hemolytic anemia
	Petechiae	Suspect congenital infection, overwhelming sepsis, or severe hemolytic disease as cause of jaundice
	Appearance of umbilical stump	Omphalitis and sepsis may produce jaundice
	Hepatosplenomegaly	Suspect hemolytic anemia or congenital infection
	Optic fundi	Chorioretinitis suggests congenital infection as cause of jaundice
	Umbilical hernia	Consider hypothyroidism
	Congenital anomalies	Jaundice occurs with increased frequency among infants with trisomic conditions

Laboratory Data

Maternal	Blood group and indirect Coombs' test	Necessary for evaluation of possible ABO or Rh incompatibility
	Serology	Rule out congenital syphilis
Infant	Hemoglobin	Anemia suggests hemolytic disease or large entrapped hemorrhage. Hemoglobin above 22 gm/dl associated with increased incidence of jaundice
	Reticulocyte count	Elevation suggests hemolytic disease
	Red cell morphology	Spherocytes suggest ABO incompatibility or hereditary spherocytosis. Red cell fragmentation seen in disseminated intravascular coagulation
	Platelet count	Thrombocytopenia suggests infection
	White cell count	Total white cell count less than 5000/mm^3 or increase in band forms to greater than 2000/mm^3 suggests infection.
	Sedimentation rate	Values in excess of 5 during the first 48 hours indicate infection or ABO incompatibility.
	Direct bilirubin	Elevation suggests infection or severe Rh incompatibility.
	Immunoglobulin M	Elevation indicates infection.
	Blood group and direct and indirect Coombs' test	Required to rule out hemolytic disease as a result of isoimmunization
	Carboxyhemoglobin	Elevated in infants with hemolytic disease or entrapped hemorrhage
	Urinalysis	Presence of reducing substance suggests diagnosis of galactosemia

McMillan JA, Nieburg PI, Oski FA: The Whole Pediatrician Catalog; p. 126. Philadelphia, W.B. Saunders Co., 1977

Table 24-3. Highest Total Serum Bilirubin of Newborn by Birth Weight—White.

mg/dl	Under 2501 g			Over 2500 g			Total		
	Live births	Percent	Cumulative Percent	Live births	Percent	Cumulative Percent	Live births	Percent	Cumulative Percent
0–7	488	42.73	100.00	11908	73.73	100.00	12396	71.69	100.00
8–12	336	29.42	57.27	3243	20.08	26.27	3579	20.70	28.31
13–15	128	11.21	27.85	531	3.29	6.19	659	3.81	7.62
16–19	114	9.98	16.64	315	1.95	2.90	429	2.48	3.81
20+	76	6.65	6.65	153	0.95	0.95	229	1.32	1.32
Total	1142	100.00		16150	100.00		17292	100.00	
Unknown	177	13.42		1012	5.90		1189	6.43	
Grand total	1319	100.00		17162	100.00		18481	100.00	

Table 24-4. Highest Total Serum Bilirubin of Newborn by Birth Weight—Black.

mg/dl	Under 2501 g			Over 2500 g			Total		
	Live births	Percent	Cumulative Percent	Live births	Percent	Cumulative Percent	Live births	Percent	Cumulative Percent
0–7	1137	50.29	100.00	11734	74.48	100.00	12871	71.45	100.00
8–12	719	31.80	49.71	3309	21.00	25.52	4028	22.36	28.55
13–15	225	9.95	17.91	412	2.62	4.51	637	3.54	6.19
16–19	113	5.00	7.96	202	1.28	1.90	315	1.75	2.66
20+	67	2.96	2.96	97	0.62	0.62	164	0.91	0.91
Total	2261	100.00		15754	100.00		18015	100.00	
Unknown	356	13.60		1133	6.71		1489	7.63	
Grand total	2617	100.00		16887	100.00		19504	100.00	

(Tables 24-3, 4. Hardy JB, Drage JS, Jackson EC: The First Year of Life. The Collaborative Perinatal Project of The National Institutes of Neurological and Communicative Disorders and Stroke, p. 104. The Johns Hopkins University Press, Baltimore, 1979)

Table 24-5. Serum Bilirubin Levels and Incidence of Hyperbilirubinemia in Normal Full Term Infants; Prospective Studies Since 1973.

| Author | No. of Infants | Age at Time of Measure-ment | Serum Bilirubin mg/dl* | | Hyperbiliru-binemia |
			Mean	+2SD†	
Dahms and coworkers, 1973[56]	199	48 hrs	6.0	11.6	5% ≥ 12.5 mg/dl
	199	72 hrs	6.4	13.5	
Davies and coworkers 1973[46]	78	2 days	5.7	11.0	
	45	5 days	4.7	12.4	
Calder and coworkers,[43]	129	5 days	8.3	16.8	33% > 10 mg/dl
Beazley and Alderman, 1975[41]	1353	3 days	6.8	13.4	8% ≥ 12 mg/dl
	878	6 days	6.6	13.4	
Maisels and Gifford, 1975[29]	246	3 days	6.7	13.5	3.2% > 12 mg/dl
Weakes and Beazley, 1975[42]	447	3 days	6.0	12.3	13% ≥ 10 mg/dl
	343	6 days	4.7	11.4	
Boylan, 1976[47]	197	4 days	4.8		9% > 10.0 mg/dl
Drew and Kitchen, 1976[49]	1107	48 hrs	7.2		8% ≥ 12 mg/dl
	1092	72 hrs	8.2		19% ≥ 12 mg/dl
Chew, 1977[44]	135	3 days	6.5	10.8	7% ≥ 12.0 mg/dl
	135	6 days	5.8	10.2	
Chew and Swann, 1977[45]	196	3 days	6.6	12.5	10% > 12 mg/dl
	196	6 days	5.2	11.2	
Wool and coworkers, 1979 [25]	690	6 days	7.6		20% ≥ 12.0 mg/dl

	Age	n	Mean	+2SD	Median
Composite Data	2 days	1384	6.3	11.3	6.0
	3 days	3668	6.7	12.7	6.6
	4–6 days	2604	6.0	12.6	5.5

* 1 mg/dl ≅ 17.0 μmol/liter
† 2 standard deviations above the mean

in 3668 healthy term infants was 6 to 7 mg/dl (103–115 μmol/1) and that 12.7 mg/dl (217 μmol/1) is 2 standard deviations above the mean. This implies that approximately 97% of all normal infants have serum bilirubin concentrations which do not exceed 12.7 mg/dl, a finding entirely consistent with the data from the Collaborative Perinatal Project (see above and Tables 24-3 and 24-4). In the light of these well-documented observations, the suggestion that significant neonatal jaundice is increasing in frequency must be considered unproven.[32,33]

Factors Influencing Serum Bilirubin Levels

Genetic and Ethnic Influences. Serum bilirubin levels vary considerably among some ethnic groups and in certain geographic locations. For example, Chinese, Japanese, Korean,[34] and American Indian[35] infants have mean maximal serum bilirubin concentrations which are approximately double those of non-Oriental populations.[34] In Hong Kong, 9% of a series of jaundiced infants had already developed kernicterus by the time of admission to the hospital, and 40% required exchange transfusions.[36]

In certain areas of Greece, there is a remarkably high incidence of "idiopathic" hyperbilirubinemia and an increased incidence of kernicterus.[37] Although glucose-6-phosphate dehydrogenase (G-6-PD) deficiency is more common in Oriental and Greek infants, it does not account for these startling differences in the incidence and severity of hyperbilirubinemia.[38] Japanese infants living in the United States have a much higher incidence of hyperbilirubinemia than do their American coun-

Table 24-6. Effect of Induction of Labor With Oxytocin on Mean Serum Bilirubin Levels.

| Author | Age Days | Labor Induced With Oxytocin | | Spontaneous Labor | | p |
		n	Serum Bilirubin mg/dl	n	Serum Bilirubin mg/dl	
Beazley and Alderman[41]	3	149	7.13 ± 3.59	538	6.5 ± 3.2	NS
Chew[44]	3	45	8.5 ± 2.7	45	5.5 ± 2.0	<0.01
Davies and coworkers[46]	2	36	6.8 ± 2.3	28	4.8 ± 2.8	<0.05
Chew and Swann[45]	3	99	7.5 ± 3.3	54	6.1 ± 2.7	<0.05
Calder and coworkers[43]	5	30	9.6 ± 3.9	30	6.4 ± 3.9	<0.005
Wood and coworkers[25]	6	290	7.9	407	7.8	NS
Mean values and totals		*649*	*7.91*	*1102*	*6.18*	

terparts,[39] which suggests that geographic factors alone do not account for these differences. On the other hand, infants born in Australia of parents who have emigrated from Greece do not have higher bilirubin levels than Australian infants.[40] Environmental, rather than genetic factors appear to be important in this population.

Perinatal Factors. Certain antepartum, intrapartum, and postpartum factors have been identified as possibly contributing to an increase in mean serum bilirubin levels in the newborn. Studies by a number of authors have suggested that the method of delivery, use of forceps, use of oxytocic drugs and other drugs taken by the mother, epidural anesthesia, and breastfeeding may be associated with exaggerated serum bilirubin concentrations. Some of these studies are retrospective analyses of large infant populations, in which bilirubin determinations were performed on only those infants noted to be clinically jaundiced.[32] There are inherent weaknesses in this type of study which preclude the drawing of reliable conclusions (see above).

Oxytocin (Table 24-6). Wood and coworkers conducted a prospective study of 690 term infants and found that mean serum bilirubin levels on the sixth day of life were significantly higher when labor was induced for reasons other than postmaturity.[25] However, these authors also noted that infants of <39 weeks' gestation had higher bilirubin levels (9.3 mg/dl = 159 μmol/1) than infants of 39 to 41 weeks'

gestational age (7.3 mg/dl = 125 μmol/1). It is likely that induction of labor produced more infants of <39 weeks' gestation than in the groups which delivered spontaneously, and this alone may account for the differences in serum bilirubin levels found. No effect of oxytocic drug administration on serum bilirubin levels was identified. Beazley and Alderman in a prospective study of 1353 infants, found no difference in mean serum bilirubin levels or the incidence of hyperbilirubinemia (serum bilirubin 12 mg/dl = 205 μmol/1 or greater) following spontaneous labor or after labor which was induced or accelerated by oxytocin.[41] This applied as well when each weight group category was analyzed. However, they observed a significant association (p < 0.001) between the *mean total dose of oxytocin* used for induction and the incidence of hyperbilirubinemia. No similar dose-dependent effect was found when labor was induced or accelerated by prostaglandin E_2,[42] although Calder and coworkers found an increase in mean bilirubin levels following prostaglandin E_2 and oxytocin induction.[43] Other authors have found an increase in mean serum bilirubin levels when labor is induced by amniotomy plus oxytocin[44–46] but not when labor is merely accelerated by oxytocin.[44–47]

The cumulative data (Table 24-6) provide suggestive, but not conclusive, evidence that when labor is *induced* with the aid of oxytocin, mean serum bilirubin levels and the incidence of hyperbilirubinemia (≥12 mg/dl = 205 μmol/

1) are increased. In the two largest studies, however, this effect was not observed.[41,25] Furthermore, in spite of the statistical significance, the magnitude of the increase in mean serum bilirubin levels is *small* and does not suggest the necessity for a change in obstetric practices. Caution must be exercised in interpreting these results because of the distinct possibility that the oxytocin-induction groups contained a greater number of less mature infants. All but one of the studies compared the groups and found no differences in the mean weight or gestational age. However, the findings that full-term infants of <39 weeks' gestation have significantly higher bilirubins (p < 0.001) than those at 40 to 41 weeks emphasizes the possible effect of small (but apparently important) differences in gestational age.[25] Postmature infants are the only infants who do not, invariably, develop physiologic jaundice and it is difficult, if not impossible, to assess gestational age without a potential error of at least two weeks. Because maturity, rather than birth weight, is the dominant factor in determining the ability of the liver to clear bilirubin from the plasma, a skeptical, if not a jaundiced, eye should be cast on the available data. The fact that *not one study* found a significant increase in mean serum bilirubin concentrations when oxytocin was given to *expedite existing labor* is further reason to suspect that this group of infants may have been more mature than those in which labor was induced by oxytocin.

The mechanism for the putative increase in serum bilirubin in association with oxytocin administration is unknown. Using cord blood samples, Buchan found that infants delivered following oxytocin induction had evidence of hemolysis: lower hematocrits, increased plasma bilirubin concentrations, descreased plasma haptoglobin, and increased plasma LDH activity, compared with those born following spontaneous labor.[48] In addition, the oxytocin group had significantly decreased erythrocyte deformability which was shown *in vitro* to be dose dependent. The author suggests that the vasopressin-like action of oxytocin causes activation of electrolyte and water transport across the erythrocyte membrane with consequent osmotic swelling and reduced deformability of the red cells.[48]

Drugs Administered to the Mother. Drew and Kitchen investigated the effect of the administration of various pharmacologic agents to the mothers of 1107 consecutively born infants.[49] Serum bilirubin concentrations were measured at 48 and 72 hours. Administration of narcotic agents, barbiturates, aspirin, chloral hydrate, reserpine, and phenytoin-sodium were associated with lower serum bilirubin concentrations; whereas the use of diazepam (which raised mean bilirubin levels by <1 mg/dl = 17 μmol/l) and oxytocin (significant only at 48 hours) appeared to result in higher bilirubin levels although the magnitude of these changes is clearly unimportant from a clinical standpoint. It should be borne in mind, as well, that the finding of a *lower* bilirubin concentration in association with the administration of a drug could imply an adverse effect of the drug on bilirubin-albumin binding, with potentially disastrous results.[50,51]

Breast-feeding. Many pediatricians have had the impression that breast-fed infants have higher serum bilirubin levels during the first week of life than bottle-fed infants. This concept of "jaundice associated with breast-feeding" must be distinguished from "true breast milk jaundice" (see below) and rests, for the moment, on a body of data which is by no means secure. Table 24-7 summarizes the available data on mean serum bilirubin concentrations obtained in prospective studies of breast- and bottle-fed infants.

In none of the studies listed in Table 24-7 was the serum bilirubin on days 3 or 4 significantly higher in the breast-fed than in the bottle-fed infants. However, in their study of 887 infants of Greek parentage born in Australia and 220 infants of Australian parents, Drew and coworkers found that there was a statistically significant association between serum bilirubin levels at 48 and 72 hours and breast-feeding, but they did not provide the actual bilirubin levels obtained.[40] In a large prospective study, Wood and coworkers found significantly higher bilirubin levels on day 6 in 312 breast-fed infants than in 268 bottle-fed infants. They also found a higher incidence of bilirubin concentrations of 12 mg/dl (205 μmol/l) or greater in the breast-fed group.[25]

Composite data from 680 infants at age 3 to 4 days and 924 infants at 5 to 6 days reveals small differences between breast-fed and bottle-fed infants. It is possible that very large studies of infants 4 to 6 days old might produce unequivocal data supporting the contention

Table 24-7. Effect of Breast-Feeding on Serum Bilirubin Levels in the First 6 Days of Life

Author	Age at Sampling	Mean Serum Bilirubin (mg/dl)				
		n	Breast	n	Bottle	p
McConnel and coworkers[330]	Day 3	50	5.8 ± 3.4	50	4.7 ± 2.2	NS
	Day 5	40	5.6 ± 3.7	43	3.0 ± 2.0	< 0.001
Dahms and coworkers[56]	72 hrs	113	6.9 ± 3.7	86	5.9 ± 3.4	NS
	≥ 12.5 mg/dl		7.9%		2.4%	NS
Gould and coworkers[331]	Day 6	82	3.2 ± 1.65	99	3.2 ± 1.6	NS
Calder and coworkers[43]	Day 5	35	7.7 ± 3.9	45	8.4 ± 4.5	*
Maisels and Gifford[29]	Day 3	115	6.9 ± 3.6	129	6.5 ± 3.2	NS
	≥ 12.0 mg/dl		3.5%		3.1%	NS
Drew[332]	72 hrs	1004				
	> 12 mg/dl		24.0%		19.0%	< 0.02
Boylan[47]	Day 4	60	5.2	137	4.5	*
Wood and coworkers[25]	Day 6	312	8.4	268	6.4	< 0.001
	≥ 12.0 mg/dl		25.3%		12.3%	< 0.001
Composite data	3–4 days	278	6.2 ± 0.84	402	5.4 ± 0.96	
	5–6 days	469	6.2 ± 2.34	455	5.3 ± 2.61	

*Statistical data not given by author and could not be calculated from available information.
NS = not significant

that breast-fed babies of this age have higher mean serum bilirubin levels and/or a greater incidence of hyperbilirubinemia than their formula-fed peers.[52] This remains to be proven and, even if it were so, the differences would be small and of questionable clinical significance. Furthermore, an *association* between breast-feeding and increased levels of serum bilirubin does not, by itself, imply a *causal* relationship.

Other Factors
Early Feeding. The introduction of early feeding as opposed to a 48-hour fast after birth results in a lowering of serum bilirubin levels.[53] The mechanism for this is not known but may be a decrease (following feeding) in entero-hepatic circulation of bilirubin. Gartner and Lee have recently demonstrated that rats who are starved for 48 hours have a significant increase in enteric bilirubin absorption when compared with those who are fed.[54] The serum bilirubin in adults rises after fasting because of a decreased uptake of bilirubin from the plasma.[55]

Weight Loss. Weight loss, by itself, does not appear to be a factor that affects bilirubin levels.[53] Wood and coworkers found an association between poor recovery of birth weight

and neonatal jaundice in breast-fed infants, but this was not found in the bottle-fed group.[25] No such association was found by Dahms and coworkers,[56] and, in a study of 100 breast-fed infants, we found no relationship at all between weight loss and serum bilirubin levels on the third day of life.*

Cord Clamping. A delay of 5 minutes in clamping the umbilical cord produces a 50% increase in red cell volume and blood volume (compared with immediate clamping), and an increase in bilirubin levels at 72 hours in preterm and term infants.[57]

Infants of diabetic mothers and infants who are asphyxiated or hypoxic[58] have an increased incidence and severity of neonatal jaundice. The precise mechanisms involved are not known, although hypoxia has a deleterious effect on liver function.

Vitamin E. Preterm infants, at birth, are deficient in vitamin E, which is important for the prevention of lipid peroxidation of the red cell membrane and subsequent hemolysis. The administration of vitamin E (50 mg/kg intramuscularly) for the first 3 days of life to infants who are <1500 g results in a significant decrease in serum bilirubin levels during the first

* Unpublished data.

weeks.[59] Further studies are needed before this can be recommended as a standard procedure.

Phenolic Detergents. The use of excessive concentrations of a phenolic disinfectant detergent was associated with an epidemic of neonatal hyperbilirubinemia in two hospitals.[60] These epidemics coincided with the time that the nursing staff increased the concentrations of the detergent used for cleaning bassinets and mattresses. Peak bilirubin concentrations as high as 42 mg/dl were recorded and several babies required exchange transfusion. There was no evidence for hemolysis and the pathogenesis of the hyperbilirubinemia is not known. However, *in vitro* studies using liver homogenates have demonstrated that dilutions of the disinfectant compound up to 1:128 significantly inhibited glucuronyl transferase activity, although this could not be confirmed *in vivo* using the Gunn rat.[61] In a subsequent study, use of the disinfectant *at the manufacturer's recommended concentrations* was associated with higher bilirubin levels than those obtained from infants in a nursery where a nonphenolic (quaternary ammonium) disinfectant was used. In view of these observations, it is recommended that phenolic detergents not be used in the nursery.

CAUSES OF INDIRECT HYPERBILIRUBINEMIA

Increased Bilirubin Load

Hemolytic Disease. These conditions are dealt with fully in Chapter 25. Fetomaternal blood group incompatibility, particularly Rh and ABO disease, are the commonest causes of significant hyperbilirubinemia in the newborn, although the introduction of immune globulin prophylaxis and smaller family size have reduced dramatically the incidence of Rh erythroblastosis. Other hemolytic processes include spherocytosis and other morphologic abnormalities of the red cell in addition to red cell enzyme deficiencies (Fig. 24-10 and Chap. 25).

Extravascular Blood. Cephalohematomas, cerebral or pulmonary hemorrhage, or any occult bleeding may lead to an elevated serum bilirubin from breakdown of the extravascular red cells.

Polycythemia. Twin–twin transfusion, maternofetal transfusion, or anything which will produce an elevated hemoglobin level or an increase in the red cell mass, will increase the bilirubin load presented to the liver.

Increased Enterohepatic Circulation. Presumably, this may occur with any form of intestinal obstruction or delay in bowel transit time, allowing more time for bilirubin deconjugation and reabsorption. Thus, jaundice is common in infants with small bowel obstruction and occurs in pyloric stenosis as well.[62,63] Surgical or other correction of the obstruction produces a prompt decline in bilirubin levels.

Decreased Bilirubin Clearance

Inherited Disorders of Bilirubin Metabolism— Nonhemolytic Unconjugated Hyperbilirubinemia. These have been reviewed recently in depth by Valaes.[64] Three degrees of defect are recognized: (1) **marked**—characterized by absolute failure of bilirubin biotransformation through the normal pathway; (2) **moderate**—a marked to moderate decrease in the activity of the pathway with response to inducing agents such as phenobarbital; and (3) **mild**—a mild decrease in the activity of the pathway reaching clinical significance only under special circumstances. The principal characteristics of these three types are listed in Table 24-8.

Transient Familial Neonatal Hyperbilirubinemia (Lucey–Driscoll Syndrome). The serum of pregnant women normally inhibits bilirubin conjugation. In certain women this inhibitory factor (possibly a progestational steroid) appears to be markedly increased, resulting in marked unconjugated hyperbilirubinemia in their offspring.[65] These infants may require exchange transfusion and may have a history of previous siblings with severe jaundice and possibly kernicterus.

Others. See the section on factors influencing serum bilirubin levels (above).

Prolonged Unconjugated Hyperbilirubinemia

Causes of Prolonged Indirect Hyperbilirubinemia

Breast milk jaundice
Hemolytic disease
Hypothyroidism
Pyloric stenosis
Crigler–Najjar syndrome

Breast Milk Jaundice. A small percentage of breast-fed babies develop the syndrome of true

Table 24-8. Congenital Nonhemolytic Unconjugated Hyperbilirubinemia — Clinical Syndromes

Characteristics	Marked (Crigler–Najjar Syndrome) (Arias Type I)	Moderate (Arias Type II)	Mild (Gilbert Syndrome)
Steady state serum bilirubin	> 20 mg/dl	< 20 mg/dl	< 5 mg/dl
Range of bilirubin values	14–50 mg/dl	5.3–37.6 mg/dl	0.8–10 mg/dl
Bilirubin in bile: Total	< 10 mg/dl (increased with phototherapy)	50–100 mg/dl	Normal
Conjugated	Absent	Present (only monoglucuronide)	Present (50% monoglucuronide)
Bilirubin-UDPGT activity *in vitro*	None detected	None detected	20–30% of normal
Bilirubin clearance	Extremely decreased	Markedly decreased	20–30% of normal
Hepatic bilirubin uptake	Normal	Normal	Reduced
Glucuronide formation with other substrates	Reduced	Reduced	Reduced?
Response to phenobarbital			
Plasma bilirubin	Unchanged	Decreased but remains above normal range	Within normal range
Bilirubin-UDPGT activity	None detected	None detected	Within normal range
Glucuronidation of other substrates	Increased from previous subnormal levels	Increased from previous subnormal levels	Increased
Smooth endoplasmic reticulum	Hypertrophy	Hypertrophy	Hypertrophy
Bilirubin encephalopathy	Usually present	Uncommon. May occur only in the neonatal period.	Not present
Genetics	Autosomal recessive Parents often related, both demonstrate impairment of glucuronidation but have normal bilirubin levels.	Heterogeneity of defect distinctly possible. Autosomal dominant? Double heterozygotes? No parental consanguinity. Abnormal glucuronidation or Gilbert's defect in one of the parents.	Autosomal dominant (heterozygotes) Usually one of the parents demonstrates similar abnormality

Valaes T: Clin Perinatol 3:177, 1976

breast milk jaundice. These infants have significant unconjugated hyperbilirubinemia. The serum bilirubin concentration rises progressively from about the fourth day of life and reaches a maximum level of unconjugated bilirubin of 10 to 30 mg/dl (171–513 μmol/l) by 10 to 15 days of life. If breast feeding continues, elevated levels may persist for 4 to 10 days and then decline slowly, reaching normal values by 3 to 12 weeks of age. However, if breast feeding is interrupted at any stage, there is a prompt decline in serum bilirubin levels within 48 hours. With the resumption of nursing, the bilirubin concentration may rise 1 to 3 mg/dl (17–51 μmol/l) but does not reach the previous level. There is no evidence of hemolysis, and liver function studies are normal. The original observations of Gartner and Arias[65a] suggested that a progestational steroid, 3-α-20-β-pregnanediol, present in the milk of certain mothers, was responsible for inhibiting bilirubin conjugation in vitro and could also cause hyperbilirubinemia when administered to full-term infants. Others, while confirming the inhibitory properties of breast milk from certain mothers, have not found this particular steroid to be the offending compound.[66,67] In addition, its inhibitory effect on bilirubin conjugation in vitro has not been confirmed.[35,68,69]

Recent studies have shown that unsaturated fatty acids inhibit bilirubin conjugation.[70,71,73,74] It appears that the inhibitory milks (from mothers of jaundiced infants) have unusually high lipoprotein-lipase activity and can liberate large amounts of fatty acids. When ingested, they lead to release of free fatty acid in the bowel and, since conditions exist in newborn gut which favor transport of free fatty acids into the portal blood, an influx of free fatty acids into the hepatocyte and subsequent inhibition of bilirubin conjugation occurs. A possible mechanism for this inhibition is the competitive binding of hepatic Z protein by fatty acids, although a quantitative role for this protein is poorly defined.[74] This binding results in a decreased level of the bilirubin Z protein complex which may reduce the available substrate for the conjugation reaction. An interesting finding is that the concentration of free fatty acids and inhibitory activity of these milks increases when the milk is frozen and stored at 4°C for 3 to 5 days. This does not occur if the milk is preheated to 56°C for 15 minutes and then frozen.[71] This fact may have important implications for the storage of breast milk and the administration of such milk to low-birth-weight infants.

Additional supporting evidence for the relationship between the inhibitory effect of free fatty acids and prolonged neonatal jaundice is suggested by the observation of Luzeau and coworkers.[75] Three infants who were diagnosed as having breast milk jaundice were given their mother's milk after it had been preheated at 56°C for 15 minutes. This led to the disappearance of the hyperbilirubinemia within 3 to 4 days in all infants.

However, Odievre and Luzeau obtained milk from 50 mothers of infants who had no evidence of prolonged neonatal jaundice.[76] The milk was collected on the 3rd, 6th, 20th and 30th postpartum days and FFA concentration was measured in the fresh samples and in aliquots stored at 4°C for 3 to 5 days. Lipoprotein-lipase activity in fresh milk samples in several mothers was found to equal that of mothers of infants presenting with breast milk jaundice. The activity appeared progressively over the first 30 days and the relative percentage of milk samples containing a large amount of free fatty acids after storage also increased with the time of collection after birth. These findings suggest the presence of some other mechanism for the development of breast milk jaundice in addition to inhibitory activity in the milk, a conclusion which is supported by the observations of Cole and Hargreaves, who found no relationship between the amount of inhibitory substance in breast milk and the degree of neonatal hyperbilirubinemia.[71] It seems likely that the degree of inhibition found in inhibitory milks varies considerably as, one must presume, does the ability of each infant's liver to cope with the inhibition of conjugation. One should not be surprised, therefore, to find a similarly wide spectrum of the clinical presentation of breast milk jaundice, or perhaps varieties thereof.

Recent preliminary observations suggest that the administration of normal human and cow milk to adult rats inhibits enteric bilirubin absorption, while milk from mothers of infants with the breast milk jaundice syndrome does not.[54] This suggests yet another possible mechanism for breast milk jaundice: some factor in the milk which increases absorption of bilirubin in the duodenum and therefore the enterohepatic circulation.

An interesting pattern of neonatal hyperbilirubinemia in the first week of life has been observed in American Indians.[35] Navajo infants have a high incidence of unconjugated hyperbilirubinemia which is exaggerated in those who are breast fed. These investigators identified an inhibitor of glucuronyl transferase activity in colostrum and breast milk in the first three days of life. The degree of inhibition observed was related to the elevation of serum bilirubin. This appears to be a form of breast milk jaundice with a much earlier onset than that seen in Caucasian populations.

It is difficult to find data on the incidence of breast milk jaundice although it has been estimated as 0.5% of breast-fed infants.[34] Winfield and MacFaul found prolonged jaundice in 2.4% of 491 breast-fed infants,[77] and, in a study of 115 totally breast-fed infants, we found 3 (2.6%) with breast milk jaundice.[29]

Approach to the Infant with Breast Milk Jaundice. Although no cases of overt bilirubin encephalopathy related to breast milk jaundice have been reported to date, no prospective studies on either term or preterm neonates with this condition have been done. However, breast-fed infants have higher serum levels of free fatty acids (FFAS) than bottle fed infants,[78] and FFAs have been shown to compete with albumin for bilirubin binding at the primary binding site (see below). There is, therefore, absolutely no reason to believe that significant elevations of serum bilirubin in the breast-fed baby represent less of a threat than to the bottle-fed baby. In this situation, *discretion is by far the better part of valor,* and when the serum bilirubin concentration approaches 16 to 17 mg/dl, we suggest interrupting nursing for 48 hours. In our experience, this is almost invariably followed by a prompt decline in bilirubin levels and nursing can then be resumed. We always provide positive and enthusiastic support to these nursing mothers, making sure that they maintain lactation using a breast pump or manual expression during the period of interrupted nursing, and we strongly reassure them that there is nothing "wrong" with them or their milk. In our experience, this has never led to permanent cessation of nursing nor has it had any serious effect on the mother's subsequent ability to nurse her infant. In fact, the usual rapid decline of bilirubin which occurs with the interruption of nursing is reassuring and allows the mother to resume her nursing without having to be concerned about bilirubin levels and further blood tests.

Pyloric Stenosis. Pyloric stenosis is associated with prolonged indirect hyperbilirubinemia, sometimes of remarkable severity.[62,63] The mechanism for this is not clear, but an absolute decrease in glucuronyl transferase activity has been documented in children with pyloric ste-

nosis.[63] An increased enterohepatic circulation, secondary to the delayed gastrointestinal transit time, may also play a role in the development of jaundice.

Congenital Hypothyroidism. These infants may develop prolonged unconjugated hyperbilirubinemia. There is no hemolysis and it is assumed that hepatic uptake and/or conjugation are affected. The jaundice of hypopituitarism and anencephaly may result from the secondary hypothyroidism that occurs.

Other Causes. See the list of causes (above).

Mixed Forms of Jaundice

In certain conditions, hyperbilirubinemia occurs that is the result of a combination of an increased bilirubin load and decreased bilirubin clearance, so that the jaundice is usually (but not always) characterized by an elevated direct- as well as indirect-reacting bilirubin. An important cause, because of the high mortality with which it is associated, is bacterial sepsis. Jaundice may be a presenting sign of bacterial sepsis and, in particular, urinary tract infection.[79] However, these infants are usually more than 2 weeks old and have other, accompanying symptoms. In the first week of life, sepsis may present with jaundice, but it is not a common cause of unexplained hyperbilirubinemia,[28] and the bilirubin elevation may be **predominantly indirect.** The appearance of a raised direct bilirubin level or any unexplained bilirubinemia outside of the physiologic range demands careful consideration of sepsis as a cause, and, if indicated, cultures of blood, urine, and spinal fluid.

Congenital syphilis, the TORCH group of chronic intrauterine infections (toxoplasmosis, rubella, cytomegalovirus, and herpes simplex), and coxsackie B infection are the other important causes of mixed jaundice. The clinical features and diagnoses of these conditions are described in Chapter 33. Jaundice, thrombocytopenia, hepatosplenomegaly, and intrauterine growth retardation occur in the severe TORCH infections which may, on the other hand, be asymptomatic.

In galactosemia, mixed jaundice occurs because of a combination of hemolytic anemia and liver damage produced by the ingestion of galactose. A positive urine test for reducing substances (nonglucose) will suggest the diagnosis.

BILIRUBIN TOXICITY

The Association Between Hyperbilirubinemia and Kernicterus

The direct association between severe unconjugated hyperbilirubinemia and neurologic damage (kernicterus) was first demonstrated convincingly in 1952 by the studies of Hsia and coworkers[80] and Mollison and Cutbush (Table 24-9).[81] If an infant with kernicterus dies in the neonatal period, coronal sectioning of the brain may reveal a yellow discoloration of the basal ganglia and hippocampus. Numerous animal and human studies have confirmed that bilirubin itself is responsible for the central nervous system damage, although the precise biochemical mechanisms are not known.[4,82]

The clinical manifestations of kernicterus in the term infant are usually seen by the third to fourth day of life and include lethargy, poor feeding, high pitched cry, vomiting and hypotonia. Later, irritability, hypotonia, opisthotonus, and seizures may occur. Survivors usually manifest serious neurologic sequelae, particularly the athetoid form of cerebral palsy, hearing loss, paralysis of upward gaze, and dental dysplasia.[83]

Experiments Versus Surveys

A vast literature exists describing the relationship between brain damage and hyperbilirubinemia.* Unfortunately, the overwhelming majority of these reports are simply retrospective (usually) or prospective (occasionally) *surveys* of a population of infants in whom clinical or pathologic findings are associated with serum bilirubin concentrations. When a follow-up study is performed on a group whose bilirubin concentrations as infants were below 20 mg/dl, and this outcome is compared with another group whose serum bilirubin levels exceeded 20 mg/dl, this is a **survey**—or a report of the author's experience—but it is not an experiment. An **experiment** is performed when the investigator "manipulates the environment by randomly assigning to the test subjects or objects the factors to be investigated." For example, an **experiment** to determine the possible effect of hyperbilirubinemia on the development of ker-

---

* Unless otherwise indicated, bilirubin refers to the unconjugated form.

Table 24-9. Relation Between Maximum Bilirubin Concentration in the Plasma and Kernicterus in Hemolytic Disease of Newborn.

Maximum Bilirubin Concentration (mg/dl)	Total Number of Cases	Number with Kernicterus
30–40	11	8
25–29	12	4
19–24	13	1
10–18	24	0

(From the data of Mollison PL, Cutbush M: In Recent Advances in Pediatrics. New York, Blakiston, 1954)

nicterus requires the **random** assignment of infants, to different treatment regimens (*e.g.,* exchange transfusion at 10 mg/dl versus 20 mg/dl).

Previous Studies

In March 1952, Mollison and Walker reported a prospective randomized, controlled trial on the effect of exchange transfusion versus simple transfusion in the first 9 hours of life on infants with erythroblastosis fetalis.[84] The **mortality** in the "exchanged" group was 13% (8/62) versus 37% (21/57) in the "transfused" group (p = 0.002). Eighteen of the 21 deaths (86%) in the group receiving simple transfusion were caused by kernicterus, versus 4 of the 8 deaths in the group treated with exchange transfusion. Thus, fatal **kernicterus** occurred in 4 of 62 infants who received an exchange transfusion and in 18 of 57 infants who did not (p < 0.001—calculated from author's data). Three of the four kernicteric infants in the exchange transfusion group were premature. The design of this study could not answer the question regarding a critical level of bilirubin and its relationship to kernicterus. However, the study demonstrated beyond reasonable doubt, that exchange transfusion in these infants improved their chance of survival and decreased the risk of fatal kernicterus. In October 1952, Hsia and coworkers reported their findings,[80] which together with those of Mollison and Cutbush,[81] suggested that kernicterus was very unlikely to occur if serum bilirubin concentrations were kept below 20 mg/dl (342 μmol/l). These findings, which resulted from **surveys** (not experiments) could only document an **association** between hyperbilirubinemia and kernicterus and could not establish a critical level for serum bilirubin. Furthermore, important as they are, they have probably been responsible for preventing the appropriate randomized trials from being undertaken.

Wishingrad and coworkers conducted a prospective randomized study of 187 preterm infants with nonhemolytic hyperbilirubinemia, most of whom weighed more than 1500 g.[85] One hundred infants whose serum bilirubin levels exceeded 18 mg/dl (308 μmol/l) after 36 hours of age were randomly assigned to receive or not to receive an exchange transfusion. Thus, 50 infants received exchange transfusions and 50 did not. An additional 87 infants whose serum bilirubin concentrations did not exceed 15 mg/100 dl (257 μmol/l) were selected as a control group. There was no difference in the mortality among the three groups. In the exchange transfusion group, there was no evidence of kernicterus at one year of age in spite of the fact that 7 of the 50 infants had levels of indirect bilirubin exceeding 24 mg/dl (410 μmol/l). In the no-exchange group, ten of the infants had bilirubin levels exceeding 24 mg/dl (410 μmol/l) and one developed fatal kernicterus. Neurologic assessment of the remaining infants at 1 year of life revealed no evidence of kernicterus. It could be concluded from this study that in premature infants weighing more than 1500 g with nonhemolytic hyperbilirubinemia, the risk of kernicterus is extremely low if serum bilirubin concentrations are maintained below 24 mg/dl (410 μmol/l). Other studies have also found that the risk of kernicterus is low in the premature infant if exchange transfusion is performed at bilirubin levels of 20 mg/dl (342 μmol/l).[86,86a] Nevertheless, there are reports of kernicterus occurring in premature infants whose serum bilirubin levels did not exceed 20 mg/dl (342 μmol/l),[87] and, in some small, sick infants, at bilirubin levels of <10 mg/dl (171 μmol/l).[88] However, these, and other reports, are retrospective case reports which do not permit conclusions regarding critical bilirubin levels. Shiller and Silverman, in their study of hyperbilirubinemia in premature infants, found no association between bilirubin levels and neurologic deficit or mental retardation.[86] However, the authors went on to criticize their own (retrospective) follow-up study:

It should be emphasized that the evidence . . . did not result from experiment but rather from experience. The infants were found to have high or to have low concentrations of bilirubin in the serum; they were not allocated to these categories according to an experimental plan. *Data from this and other similar observational studies can be used only to seek hypotheses. Proof of these hypotheses can be obtained only by carefully designed clinical trials* [italics added].

Similar critical analysis must be applied to other follow-up studies *including those in which various tests of bilirubin binding are performed* (see below). The performance of these tests can in no way compensate for fundamental errors in experimental design.

Several studies have suggested, but have not proven, that bilirubin encephalopathy (the clinical equivalent of nonfatal kernicterus) may be asymptomatic in the newborn period and may only manifest itself as subtle changes in neurologic, psychological, or intellectual development months to years later.[89-92] In all of these studies, in which infants were followed for periods of up to 7 years, there appeared to be a significant association between an increased incidence of neurodevelopmental defects and serum bilirubin concentrations which did not exceed 20 mg/dl (342 μmol/l). This association was also reported in *nonasphyxiated full-term infants* whose serum bilirubin levels exceeded 15 mg/dl (257 μmol/l).[89]

Two studies utilized data from the collaborative perinatal project of the National Institute of Neurological and Communicative Disease and Stroke. In this project, serum bilirubin was routinely measured in all infants at approximately 48 hours of age and then repeated daily if the initial reading was 10 mg/dl (171 μmol/l) or greater until the value decreased below 10 mg/dl. When the birth weight was 2250 g or less, the bilirubin level was measured at 4 to 5 days of age. Additional bilirubin determinations were obtained when clinically indicated. The highest serum bilirubin concentration recorded in the neonatal period was the level used in these studies. Scheidt and coworkers studied about 25,000 infants and found an *association* between impaired motor performance at 8 and 12 months of age and serum bilirubin levels between 10 and 14 mg/dl (171–239 μmol/l).[92] This finding was not limited to low-birth-weight infants. Naeye analyzed the outcome of 41,444 children who were followed for as long as 7 years.[90] IQs were measured at 4 years of age and detailed neurologic examinations done at age 7. Patients with physical or laboratory findings known to be associated with mental or motor impairment were excluded from the analysis. Thus multiple births, infants with congenital malformations, birth trauma, hypothyroidism, neonatal hypoglycemia, CNS infection, intrauterine viral infections, and so on, were all excluded, as were infants whose mothers had severe hypotension during labor or delivery or were known alcoholics or drug addicts. In addition, this study examined the effect of amniotic fluid infection (diagnosed by acute inflammation in the plate of the placenta) on mental and motor development. IQs measured at 4 years of age showed an increased frequency of mental impairment in subjects with peak neonatal bilirubin levels of 7 mg/dl (120 μmol/l) and above.

The presence of amniotic fluid infection appeared to potentiate the neurotoxicity of neonatal hyperbilirubinemia and this potentiation increased with the severity of the amniotic fluid infection. Neurologic examination at age 7 years revealed an increase in the frequency of abnormalities when bilirubin levels exceeded 13 to 14 mg/dl (222–239 μmol/l). The frequency of these abnormalities decreased with age but always remained greater in the children who had neonatal hyperbilirubinemia than in those who had normal bilirubin levels. The suggestion that infection may potentiate bilirubin encephalopathy is supported by the findings of Pearlman and coworkers, who found kernicterus at autopsy in four infants, all of whom weighed >2200 g and all of whom had documented sepsis.[93] Again, it must be emphasized that these studies identify an *association* between certain bilirubin levels and intellectual outcome. They *cannot* establish causation.

Conflicting observations have been made by others. Rubin and coworkers prospectively followed 77 infants who had bilirubin levels ranging from 16 to 23 mg/dl (274–393 μmol/l; high bilirubin group) and compared them with 164 infants whose serum bilirubin levels ranged from 11 to 15 mg/dl (188–257 μmol/l; moderately elevated group) and a control group of 125 subjects whose serum bilirubin levels did not exceed 10 mg/dl (171 μmol/l; low bilirubin group).[94] With differences in birth weight and in length of gestation statistically controlled,

high bilirubin levels were found to be significantly associated with poor motor development at 8 months of age and with an increased incidence of neurologic abnormalities at 1 year. However, the high bilirubin group did not differ significantly from the other groups in intellectual performance or neurologic examination at 4 to 7 years of life. These data suggest that the early developmental defects associated with neonatal hyperbilirubinemia may not be apparent subsequently, and that elevated serum bilirubin levels are not predictive of long-term cognitive impairment.

Crichton and coworkers prospectively studied three matched groups of 30 infants with birth weights of 2183 g or less.[95] Maximal serum bilirubin concentrations were 20 mg/dl (342 μmol/l) or greater, 11 to 19.9 mg/dl (188–340 μmol/l), and <11 mg/dl (188 μmol/l) respectively. No significant differences in mean IQ scores or in neurological status were found in the three groups at ages four to 11 years. Nevertheless, the group with the highest bilirubin levels had a significant excess of mentally retarded children. Culley and coworkers studied 371 infants with varying degrees of jaundice and assessed their neurodevelopmental outcome in the sixth year.[96] Neurologic handicap was concentrated among the infants of low birth weight and was not related to jaundice, apart from one case of athetoid cerebral palsy with deafness.

Pearlman and coworkers analyzed the incidence of kernicterus in one hospital in infants weighing 2250 g or less who died on the third to seventh days of life.[97] Between 1971 and 1976, kernicterus was found in 9 of 14 infants, whereas in 1976 and 1977, no kernicterus was found in 34 infants. The only apparent difference between these two populations was a lower mean peak serum bilirubin concentration (8.7 ± 3.4 mg/dl) in the second study (versus 11.1 ± 4 mg/dl in the first). Six infants received exchange transfusions, eleven phototherapy, and four both exchange transfusion and phototherapy in the latter series, whereas no infants received either of these treatments in the first study. The authors suggest that their failure to find kernicterus in recent years may be the result of a more aggressive policy of exchange transfusion and phototherapy, which prevents excessive hyperbilirubinemia, together with the development of more sophisticated intensive care and attention to the maintenance of an optimal physical and bio-chemical milieu. This conclusion (again, based on a survey and not an experiment), may not be warranted. It is possible that the numerous changes in care which occurred over a span of 8 years were the critical factors, and not the bilirubin levels. To illustrate, Cashore and Oh studied 13 infants with birth weights of <1500 g who died.[98] Autopsy revealed kernic-terus in five infants (a remarkably high inci-dence) and no kernicterus in eight. The mean maximum serum bilirubin levels were 8.6 ± 2.4 mg/dl (147 ± 47 μmol/l) in the infants with kernicterus and 8.0 ± 3.8 mg/dl (137 ± 65 μmol/l) in the infants without kernicterus. These differences are not significant. Thus, despite an approach to the treatment of hy-perbilirubinemia which was, apparently, as aggressive as that of Pearlman and coworkers, kernicterus nevertheless occurred in these in-fants.

The studies reviewed above underscore the extreme complexity of attempting to correlate levels of serum bilirubin and subsequent neu-rologic status. The unfortunate fact remains that no prospective randomized studies have been performed that permit the identification of a critical level of serum bilirubin in either full-term or premature infants. Furthermore, it must be reemphasized that *the finding of an association between poor intellectual outcome and certain bilirubin levels in a large group of infants,[90,92] although suggestive, does not by itself provide incontrovertible evidence of cause and effect.* In addition, minor differences in outcome may become statistically signifi-cant when very large population groups are studied, but how this information can be ap-plied, rationally, to the management of the individual infant with jaundice is, as yet, un-answered. Studies which test the hypothesis that a critical level of bilirubin exists have yet to be performed. They could be done by assigning treatment to groups of infants at varying levels of bilirubin, although in the current milieu of newborn care this would be difficult to achieve.

The Chemical Structure, Solubility, and Neurotoxicity of Bilirubin

As discussed above (see section on **Chemical Structure and Properties of Bilirubin**), the acid form of bilirubin IX-α (ZZ) is capable of forming intramolecular hydrogen bonds which

saturate the hydrophilic groups of the mole-cule, leaving no affinities for the attachment of water (Fig. 24-2) and rendering it nearly insoluble in water at pH 7.4. In an alkaline medium, the hydrogen bonds are opened to form the divalent anion which has several hydrophilic groups, resulting in a molecule with much greater (yet still markedly limited) solubility.[1] Other isomers of bilirubin (IX-β, IX-γ and IX-δ) are also found in bile but only in trace amounts, and additional isomers, IX-α (EZ) result from the phototherapy of bilirubin. These additional isomers do not form the intramolecular hydrogen bonds which are present in the acid form of bilirubin IX-α (ZZ), and are therefore soluble in water and in neutral or acid media.[1] Because of its pro-nounced tendency for aggregation, it has been suggested that bilirubin IX-α (ZZ) acid is the neurotoxic form of bilirubin.[6,99] Problems re-main, however, with the application of phys-iochemical observations to the situation *in vivo*. For example, Brodersen has found that the solubility of bilirubin at pH 7.4 is only 7 nmol/l, whereas measurements of free bilirubin in jaundiced infants may be several-fold greater than this (see below).[6] Under these circum-stances, bilirubin would precipitate out of solution. Alternatively, measurements of free bilirubin may include substances other than true free bilirubin. The theoretical possibilities need to be tested *in vivo*.

Recently Broderson has shown that, con-trary to what has been accepted almost uni-versally, bilirubin is not a lipophilic substance and its neurotoxicity is not likely to be due to its affinity for lipids in the central nervous system.[6] Rather, it appears to be polar with little solubility in triglycerides and increasing solubility in polar solvents such as chloroform and dichloromethane. These studies also sug-gest that bilirubin forms a complex with phos-phatidylcholine and that the formation of this complex leads to an accelerated aggregation of bilirubin.

The pH of the plasma has a profound effect on the solubility of bilirubin and its binding to tissue sites (rather than its binding to serum albumin; see below). At a pH of 7.4, the limit of bilirubin solubility is reached with 0.5 moles of bilirubin per mole of albumin, but at a pH of 7.0 this limit is less than 0.1 mole of bilirubin per mole of albumin.[6] Thus, when the concen-tration of bilirubin acid exceeds its solubility,

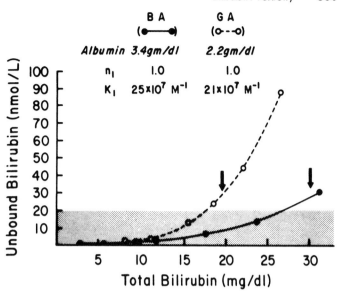

Fig. 24-11. Effects of albumin concentration on the unbound bilirubin concentration. Serum binding in a healthy preterm infant (**GA**) is compared with that in a normal term infant (**BA**). Arrows represent a bilirubin/albumin molar ratio of 1. The arbitrary concentration of 20 nmol/1 unbound bilirubin (**shaded area**) is achieved at a total unconjugated bilirubin concentration of 27.0 mg/dl in the term infant and 17.5 mg/dl in the premature infant, who had a lower serum albumin concentration. (Wennberg RP, Ahlfors CE, Rasmussen LF: Early Hum Dev 3/4:353, 1979)

bilirubin may gradually aggregate and come out of solution.

Albumin Binding and the Concept of Free Bilirubin. Bilirubin is transported in the plasma tightly bound to albumin and the relationship between bound and unbound bilirubin obeys the laws of mass action.[4]

$$\text{Albumin} \qquad\qquad (1)$$
$$+ \ \text{Bilirubin}^{2-} \ \rightleftharpoons \ \text{Albumin-bilirubin complex}$$

The binding can be expressed as follows:[4]

$$Ka_1 \qquad\qquad\qquad\qquad (2)$$
$$= \frac{(\text{albumin-bound bilirubin})}{[\text{unbound bilirubin}] \times (n_1 \ [\text{total albumin}] - \text{albumin-bound bilirubin}])}$$

where Ka_1 is the association constant describing the *affinity* of the primary albumin-binding sites for bilirubin, and n_1 represents the number of sites with affinity Ka_1 per albumin molecule (or the *capacity*); n_1 normally equals one. Because more than 99.9% of the bilirubin is bound, the concentration of unbound bilirubin can be expressed as follows:

$$[\text{unbound bilirubin}]$$
$$\simeq \frac{[\text{total bilirubin}]}{Ka_1 \ (n_1 \ [\text{total albumin}] - [\text{total bilirubin}])} \qquad (3)$$

The unbound bilirubin concentration is therefore a function of four variables: the total bilirubin concentration, the total albumin concentration, the binding capacity (n_1), and the binding affinity (Ka_1). The effect of these variables on unbound bilirubin concentrations is illustrated in Figures 24-11, 24-12, and 24-13.*

In vitro studies and animal studies are consistent with the hypothesis that it is the free or unbound bilirubin that is able to move across the blood–brain barrier, to bind to tissues, and to damage the cells of the central nervous system.[2,6,91,100–103] However Levine, in a sprightly polemic points out that, in fact, no reported experiments have critically tested the free bilirubin theory.[104] In the classic study of Diamond and Schmid, concentrations of bilirubin well in excess of those found in most clinical circumstances were used in order to achieve entry of this pigment into the brain of newborn guinea pigs.[105] In addition, lack of appropriate techniques prevented these authors from measuring the free bilirubin present in the plasma. Furthermore, a poor correlation has been found between the serum free bilirubin level and the level of brain bilirubin in homozygous (jj) Gunn rats,[106,107] although the free bilirubin level correlated directly with the total serum bilirubin level.[107] In these rats, the brain bilirubin level shortly after birth was high, despite the low serum free bilirubin level, and it decreased progressively over the first few weeks of life. Because this decline was

* These figures are based on data obtained in Dr. Wennberg's laboratory using the peroxidase method. They are used for illustrative purposes only and do not define the range of variation to be expected in clinical practice.

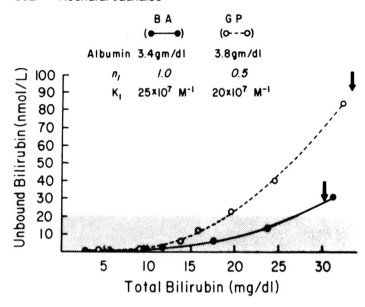

Fig. 24-12. Effect of binding capacity (n_1) on the unbound bilirubin concentration. Similar levels of serum bilirubin produce higher unbound bilirubin concentrations in infant GP whose binding capacity is 50% of BA. (Wennberg RP, Ahlfors, CE, Rasmussen LF: Early Hum Dev 3/4:353, 1979)

unrelated to serum free bilirubin levels, it probably reflected changes in the blood–brain barrier permeability to bilirubin.

It is possible that bilirubin that is tightly bound to albumin could enter cells, as is apparently the case during the transport of vitamin B_{12}.[104] As there must be a relationship between the concentration of free bilirubin and the concentration of bound bilirubin (see equation 1 above), there must also be a *relationship* between the concentration of free bilirubin and its total transport into cells. However, in spite of the suggestive evidence, the finding of such a correlation does not *prove* that the underlying transport mechanism involves the passage of free bilirubin across the cell membranes.[104]

Measurement of Bilirubin Binding

Over the last decade, considerable effort has gone into developing techniques for measuring the binding capacity and affinity of albumin for bilirubin and for understanding the kinetics and physical determinants of such binding. This subject has been reviewed recently in great detail. [104,108–110] Approximately 20 methods have been described for the measurement of bilirubin binding by albumin, although the validity and interpretation of many of these tests remains questionable.[104,109,110] Both the **capacity** and the **affinity** have been measured (see equation 2 above).

Capacity refers to the number of primary binding sites available. Human albumin has a single high-affinity binding site for bilirubin and one or more weaker sites.[111–113] When the primary (tight) binding site on albumin is saturated, there is a rapid rise in the amount of loosely bound or free bilirubin in the plasma. The point at which saturation occurs varies widely. Measurements in a large number of infant sera using different methods indicate that the ability of albumin to bind bilirubin tightly at the primary binding site varies from approximately 0.5 to 1 mole of bilirubin per mole of albumin.[104,112–115] Full-term newborns have binding capacities of the order of 0.6 to 1.0, whereas sick and low-birth-weight infants may have a lower binding capacity, affinity, or both.[112,116] A bilirubin/albumin molar ratio of 1 represents about 8.5 mg of bilirubin per gram of albumin. Thus, a low-birth-weight infant with a serum albumin concentration of 2 gm/dl and an albumin binding capacity of 0.5 mole bilirubin per mole of albumin could only bind, tightly, 8.5 mg/dl (145 μmol/l) of bilirubin. Another infant with the identical serum albumin concentration but a binding capacity of 1 mole bilirubin per mole of albumin would be able to bind 17 mg/dl (291 μmol/l) of bilirubin (Fig. 24-12).

Reserve binding capacity has been used to describe the additional number of tight, or of total, binding sites available in a serum already containing some bound bilirubin.[108] In clinical usage, a formula sometimes employed is:

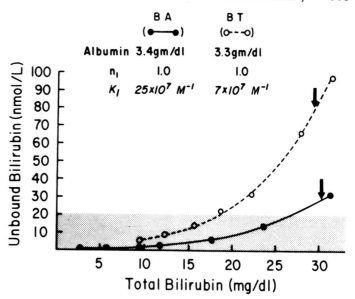

Fig. 24-13. Effect of binding affinity on unbound bilirubin concentration. Binding in a sick infant (BT) is compared with that of a normal infant (BA). Although albumin concentration and binding capacity in BT are normal, unbound bilirubin concentration reaches 20 nmol/1 at a total bilirubin of only 18 mg/dl and is higher throughout the bilirubin range. At any given serum bilirubin level, more bilirubin would tend to be present in the sick infant's tissues. (Wennberg RP, Ahlfors, CE, Rasmussen LF: Early Hum Dev 3/4:353, 1979)

Total binding capacity (mg/dl)
= indirect bilirubin present
+ reserve binding capacity.

The **binding affinity** describes the strength of the bilirubin-albumin bond; that is, it is an expression of the tightness with which bilirubin is bound to the primary binding site. The association constant, Ka_1, is derived from the equilibrium concentrations of bound and free bilirubin (see equation 2 above) and is of the order of 10^7 to 10^8 mol^{-1}.[50,111,112] The affinity can vary, so that even if the same number of binding sites for bilirubin were available on the albumin molecules of two comparable infants, the affinity of the albumin for bilirubin may differ. (Fig. 24-13).

Bilirubin Binding Tests

The tests which have been most widely used in clinical studies are the 2(4'-hydroxybenzeneazo) benzoic acid (HBABA) binding, the salicylate saturation index, peroxidase oxidation, and Sephadex G-25 column chromatography.

The HBABA dye binding method is based on the competitive binding of the dye for the available bilirubin binding sites on albumin. This test measures the theoretical number of albumin sites not occupied by bilirubin and therefore available for binding the dye. However, this method appears to measure not only reserve albumin binding capacity for bilirubin but also non-bilirubin binding sites on albumin.[110]

The salicylate saturation index is based on the observation of a reduction in optical density at 460 nm in icteric sera following the addition of excess sodium salicylate. Odell and coworkers performed a follow-up study on 32 children between the ages of 4 and 7 years of age who were jaundiced in the neonatal period.[91] The salicylate saturation index had been performed on these, as well as about 60 other infants (lost to follow-up), while they were in the nursery. Analysis of the data revealed that if a value of 8 was chosen for the saturation index, 16 of 18 infants with abnormal cognitive function and 5 of 14 normal infants had a saturation index ≥ 8.0 (p < 0.01). However, no correlation was found between IQ and the saturation index. Two-thirds of the infants originally examined did not return to follow-up and those that did had a remarkably high incidence of cognitive dysfunction (56%). The group with abnormal psychometric test results had a high incidence of perinatal complications (in addition to jaundice) which may have contributed to their poor outcome. This study did not test the hypothesis that treatment based on an elevated saturation index would lead to a better outcome. Thus, although a correlation may have been demonstrated between the saturation index and developmental outcome, this can only suggest a hypothesis which needs to be tested by a prospective randomized study.

Bratlid has reported two babies with kernicterus in whom the saturation index was normal,[117] and several theoretical and methodological objections to this method have been identified.[118] This method is technically demanding and requires a degree of precision that is not obtainable in the clinical laboratory. Even in expert hands under carefully controlled conditions, a mean random variation of more than 25% can occur.[119] In a comparison of the HBABA, Sephadex, salicylate saturation index, and the fluorescent dye (DY-7) methods, no correlation was found between the saturation index and the three other methods, nor was any relationship found between the saturation index and the bilirubin-albumin molar ratio.[117–119]

Peroxidase. The peroxidase method is based on the oxidation of bilirubin by hydrogen peroxide in the presence of a peroxidase enzyme (horseradish peroxidase). Because the rate of this reaction is proportional to the enzyme concentration and the equilibrium concentration of free bilirubin in the sample, free bilirubin can be calculated from the rate of oxidation of bilirubin at a standard enzyme concentration. The use of serial additions of bilirubin allows an estimate of bilirubin binding capacity and of the association constant (binding affinity) of bilirubin for albumin in the serum. Measurements of unbound bilirubin concentrations in 117 normal or sick infants with serum bilirubin concentrations of 1.5 to 31 mg/dl (26–530 μmol/l) revealed levels of 0.00006 to 0.0065 mg/dl (1–111 nmol/liter).[112] In two infants with kernicterus, unbound bilirubin was 0.0017 and 0.0013 mg/dl (29 and 23 nmol/liter) and in six infants whose bilirubin exceeded 20 mg/dl, the unbound concentration was 0.0024 $\pm$ 0.00197 mg/dl (41 $\pm$ 34 nmol/liter). No infants with kernicterus were observed when the unbound bilirubin concentration was <.0012 mg/dl (20 nmol/liter).[112,120] However, because only two cases of kernicterus were observed in this population, no critical level of free bilirubin can be inferred from these studies. Cashore and Oh observed kernicterus at autopsy in five low-birth-weight infants.[98] The mean unbound bilirubin concentration, as measured by the peroxidase method in these 5 infants was 0.0016 $\pm$ 0.0005 mg/dl (27 $\pm$ 9 nmol/liter) versus 0.0085 $\pm$ 0.0006 mg/dl (13 $\pm$ 10 nmol/liter, p <0.05) in eight infants without kernicterus. The mean total serum bilirubin concentrations in the two groups, 8.6 mg/dl (kernicterus) and 8.0 mg/dl (no kernicterus), were not significantly different. There were no significant differences in weight, gestational age, highest indirect bilirubin level, albumin concentration, severity of acidosis, or other clinical features between the groups. Although these findings suggested an association between increased unbound bilirubin levels and kernicterus, individual values overlapped considerably, preventing any definition of a level of unbound bilirubin which can be considered toxic (or nontoxic).

An automated method of performing the peroxidase measurement has been described.[121] A disadvantage of the peroxidase method is its extreme sensitivity, which introduces considerable variation within a single day and 11% in day-to-day variations.[112]

Sephadex G-25. This technique has been used extensively in the last few years. A Sephadex column consists of tiny beads of a hydrated polymeric material packed into a tube. Sephadex adsorbs bilirubin actively, the amount of bilirubin adsorbed by the column reflecting the relative affinity of bilirubin for albumin and Sephadex. In other words, the Sephadex appears to compete with albumin for bilirubin binding. A commercial Sephadex test kit, Kernlute*, is available and provides a semiquantitative measurement of the bilirubin binding capacity of albumin. A quantitative assessment of loosely bound bilirubin can be obtained using the Sephadex method to elute the bilirubin from the column and measuring its concentration in the eluate. The Sephadex test is simple to perform but subject to variation as a result of changes in specimen or buffer volume, speed of flow, different batches of Sephadex, tightness of packing, column length and diameter, and so on.[110] The Sephadex method correlates well with the DY-7 fluorescent dye binding method,[119] and with the peroxidase technique in assessing the bilirubin binding capacity. Cashore measured the bilirubin binding capacity of 35 neonatal sera using the Sephadex and peroxidase techniques and found an excellent correlation between the methods (r = 0.961).[114] He found, however,

---

* Specialty Systems Department, Ames Company, Division of Miles Laboratory, Inc., Elkhart, Indiana 46514

that actual measurements of free bilirubin using these methods were strikingly different. Specifically, the free bilirubin concentrations as measured by the Sephadex technique exceeded the values obtained with the peroxidase method by approximately 100fold. It is possible that this difference results from the fact that the Sephadex method measures both unbound and loosely bound bilirubin, whereas the peroxidase method measures only unbound bilirubin. Nevertheless, both methods agree well in their prediction of the point at which the primary sites on albumin will be saturated with bilirubin and the binding capacity exceeded.[114]

A number of studies have been published in which the development of kernicterus has been associated with yellow staining of the Sephadex G-25 column.[116,122-125] These observations suggest that kernicterus is unlikely to occur in the absence of strongly positive staining of the column or when loosely bound bilirubin, as measured by this method, is absent or less than 0.1 mg/dl.

Red Blood Cell Binding. Bratlid measured bilirubin binding by erythrocytes in 105 samples from 72 infants with hyperbilirubinemia, mostly resulting from hemolytic disease.[117] Two infants with clinical signs of kernicterus (one confirmed on postmortem examination) had greatly elevated amounts of erythrocyte-bound bilirubin (4.4 and 6.2 mg/dl) compared with other infants (all less than 2.5 mg/dl).

Front Face Reflectance Fluorometry. Recently, this method has been used for the measurement of total bilirubin and bilirubin binding capacity in whole blood.[126] This method measures the fluorescence of bilirubin itself when bound to albumin and identifies as its endpoint a "flattening" of the fluorescence curve when the high affinity binding sites are saturated. A semiautomated instrument which permits the rapid determination of albumin-bound bilirubin, total bilirubin, and reserve binding capacity on a few drops of whole blood has been produced by Bell Laboratories,* but is not yet commercially available. The presence in serum of certain drugs which fluoresce has not been studied, but could be a source of potential error.[108]

Brodersen has recently described a technique for determining the number of vacant

* Bell Laboratories, Murray Hill, New Jersey 07974

high-affinity bilirubin sites on human serum albumin.[127] This technique uses monoacetyl-4,4'-diaminodiphenylsulphone (MADDS) which is bound selectively to the high-affinity site for bilirubin.

Technical Problems Associated with the Measurements of Bilirubin Binding. There are numerous technical problems associated with all of the above methods for the measurement of free bilirubin and bilirubin binding to albumin.[104,110] The measurement of free bilirubin itself is difficult because of the extremely tight binding of bilirubin to albumin. An affinity constant of 10^8 mol^{-1} means that bilirubin is bound to albumin 10,000 to 100,000 times more tightly than most drugs, making its separation and measurement difficult. A potential problem with the peroxidase technique is that serum contains many components which could act as effectors—substances that could inhibit or stimulate peroxidase independent of the free bilirubin concentration. Vitamin C is known to be a peroxidase substrate, and the presence of vitamin C in serum could introduce significant errors in the peroxidase results, giving falsely low values for the free bilirubin concentrations.[104] Other compounds stimulate the activity of peroxidase and produce falsely elevated values of serum free bilirubin.[104] The free bilirubin concentration is measured by comparing the rate of the peroxidase reaction in the serum to the rate from a standard curve. But, peroxidase is an enzyme which can be affected by the milieu of the serum, so that the rate of reaction in serum may be different from that in the standard, even though the free bilirubin concentration is the same in both serum and standard.[104]

Currently, the binding tests available are not performed in a uniform fashion between institutions nor are there uniform laboratory standards for them, which make comparisons difficult. Elevated levels of direct (conjugated) bilirubin in the range of 2 to 3 mg/dl (34–51 μmol/liter) or greater, interfere with the interpretation of the results of virtually all of the above methods. Many of the tests require dilution of the serum; this acts as a potential source of error by changing the solubility or ionic strength of serum components or perhaps by reducing the effects of weakly bound competitors for bilirubin binding sites.

Clinical Use of Binding Tests. No long-term prospective study of unselected patients using any of these techniques has been performed. Nor have there been any studies which tested the value of these measurements in deciding when to institute treatment for hyperbilirubinemia, and no specific level of free bilirubin has been defined that indicates the necessity for exchange transfusion using these or any other methods. Although there is an association between the finding of kernicterus (or its clinical equivalent) and high levels of free or "loosely bound" bilirubin, [89,91,112,115,116,120,125] individual values overlap so that no clear limits of "safe" nor "toxic" unbound bilirubin levels can be assumed. Despite the circumstantial evidence that a decrease in albumin binding, together with an increase of plasma unbound bilirubin, plays a role in the pathogenesis of "low bilirubin" kernicterus, this mechanism may not, in fact, be the specific cause of kernicterus in such infants.[98]

There is presently no evidence to suggest that treating neonatal hyperbilirubinemia based on tests of bilirubin-albumin binding, will lead to a better outcome than treatment based on the infants' indirect bilirubin concentration. No studies have been designed to test this hypothesis and, therefore, the use of these tests in the making of clinical decisions cannot be recommended currently.

The Effect of Fatty Acids. Studies in animal and human newborns have demonstrated a relation between serum concentrations of unbound bilirubin and levels of FFAs.[128-130] These and several *in vitro* studies suggest that plasma FFAs may competitively inhibit bilirubin binding to albumin, leading to the displacement of bilirubin from its primary binding site. *In vitro* studies indicate that no interference with bilirubin binding occurs as long as the molar ratio of fatty acid to albumin is less than 4:1 or 5:1.[131] However, Odell and co-workers observed competition of FFAs with bilirubin for binding at the high affinity site on albumin at molar ratios of FFAs to albumin of 2:1 to 4:1.[129] They also studied the effect of caloric supplementation on FFA concentrations and bilirubin binding in 16 jaundiced infants. In every case, additional calories produced a simultaneous reduction in FFA and the amount of bilirubin subject to displacement by salicylate. On the other hand, studies with the DY-7 fluorescent dye-binding method show that the effect of certain FFAs is not caused by a competitive binding between FFA and

bilirubin for albumin, but rather to the provision of alternative binding sites for bilirubin on the FFAs, which are themselves either albumin-bound or free in the plasma water in a colloidal state.[132] Brodersen has observed that the addition of 2M laurate to solutions of albumin and bilirubin *increased* the binding of bilirubin to albumin and *reduced* the concentration of free bilirubin to 50% of its previous level.[2] Higher concentrations of laurate were found to displace bilirubin. Elevated levels of serum FFAs occur in response to shock, hypoglycemia, infection, and anoxia and may play a crucial role in the development of bilirubin encephalopathy in infants who are already at risk for kernicterus. Brodersen has derived a theoretical equation for estimating the free bilirubin level in the presence of elevated FFAs.[1] He estimates that at a ratio of FFAs to albumin of 6, the free bilirubin concentration would increase by a factor of 2.6. This suggestion must be confirmed in an appropriate clinical study before it can be applied to clinical practice.

Intravenous Nutrition. The effects of emulsified lipid solutions (Intralipid) on bilirubin binding and transport were studied. [128,133,133a] Intralipid was shown to be capable of binding bilirubin, but it did not compete with bilirubin bound to the high affinity sites on albumin. In fact, once the molar ratio of bilirubin to albumin exceeded 1:1, lower unbound bilirubins were observed in the presence of Intralipid, suggesting that some of the unbound bilirubin was bound to the Intralipid itself. Furthermore, in tissue culture experiments, Intralipid appeared to protect the cells from bilirubin toxicity. Intralipid was also administered to congenitally jaundiced (Gunn) rats in whom the total body bilirubin pool was uniformly labeled with radioactive bilirubin.[133] Intralipid was found to have no effect on the kinetics of bilirubin formation, transport, tissue distribution, or clearance. Thus, the only established, potentially harmful effect of Intralipid resides in its ability to elevate serum FFA concentrations, which, if very high, may interfere with the binding of bilirubin to albumin.

The infusion of synthetic amino acid solutions does not appear to interfere with binding of bilirubin to albumin.[134]

The Effect of pH. Observations in sick low-birth-weight infants suggest that acidosis may have a role in the development of kernicterus.[88,135] Experimentally induced respiratory acidosis increased bilirubin-^{14}C uptake in the brains of newborn guinea pigs[101] and produced an increase in cerebrospinal fluid bilirubin concentrations with gross evidence of kernicterus in newborn puppies.[136] The effect of lowering the pH on the binding of bilirubin to albumin has been measured by a number of techniques. When measured by the Sephadex technique[137] or the fluorescent dye (DY-7) method,[113] a lower pH produces a decrease in albumin binding capacity. However, similar studies using the fluorescence-quenching method[138] or the peroxidase technique[102,139] have not demonstrated any change in bilirubin-albumin binding with changes in pH. The reasons for these differences have been discussed in detail.[1,2,99,140]

However, the correction of neonatal acidosis in 11 sick newborn infants was associated with a significant decrease in the serum free bilirubin concentration as measured by the peroxidase technique.[140] It is possible that acidosis is associated with the presence of other (as yet unidentified) endogenous anions capable of displacing bilirubin from its albumin binding sites, and thereby increasing plasma free bilirubin. With correction of the acidosis, a concomitant improvement in the circulatory and metabolic status of the infants may reduce the effects of these displacers by enhanced clearance, reduction in their formation, or changes in the affinity of anions other than bilirubin for albumin binding sites.[140]

There is evidence that the binding of bilirubin to red cells,[103,141] mitochondria,[142] fibroblasts,[102] and cerebellum tissue[143] in cultures increases when pH is decreased. Wennberg and Rasmussen demonstrated that the uptake of bilirubin by red cells was influenced by pH, whereas albumin binding of bilirubin was not affected.[103] The cellular content of bilirubin was a function of the unbound bilirubin concentration and not the total bilirubin concentration or the bilirubin-albumin molar ratio. The presence of a metabolic acidosis in hyperbilirubinemic adult rats was associated with a significant increase in uptake of bilirubin by the brain, although the acidosis was not associated with an increase in serum levels of free bilirubin.[144] Thus, although the finding of increased deposition of bilirubin in the brain (see above) has been attributed, frequently, to displacement of bilirubin from its albumin

binding site, it seems more likely that these results can be explained by an increase in the binding of bilirubin to the target tissue.[4] These findings are consistent with the hypothesis that the cellular uptake of bilirubin is a function of the concentration of free bilirubin acid. Brodersen[1] points out that the binding of bilirubin to erythrocytes[141] is approximately proportional to the square of the hydrogen ion concentration and it is likely that binding to tissue elements depends on an acidic environment.[2] At physiologic pH, bilirubin exists predominantly as a dianion with only a small fraction present as bilirubin acid. The binding of bilirubin to albumin occurs as a result of attachment of the divalent bilirubin anion to the high-affinity site without involvement of hydrogen ions.[2] Thus, the affinity is constant with varying pH. On the other hand, it has been suggested that the acid, the monovalent anion or both are involved in tissue binding which is likely to be increased in the presence of acidosis.[2,103] A decrease in pH also reduces, markedly, the solubility of bilirubin in plasma, encouraging precipitation of the insoluble acid form.[6] It thus appears that a decrease in pH tends to shift bilirubin away from its specific site on albumin toward tissues, whereas binding to albumin rather than tissues is favored by an increase in pH.

Bilirubin in aqueous solution occurs almost totally as a dinegative carboxylate ion throughout the range of pH from 7 to 11. This ion is in equilibrium with a minute concentration of the electrically neutral acid.[99] The solubility of the acid is extremely low and is exceeded at pH values below 7 to 8, depending upon the bilirubin concentration, and aggregation of the acid takes place.[6] The solubility of bilirubin in aqueous buffers is inversely proportional to the square of the hydrogen ion concentration, a finding which has been verified within the range of pH 7.35 to 8.65.[99]

A decrease in pH of 0.3 produces a fourfold increase in the concentration of bilirubin acid. Because the acid is insoluble in water, Brodersen has suggested that deposition of this substance in the tissues is likely in the presence of acidosis.[6] An alternative possibility is that tissue receptors have an increased affinity for bilirubin in an acid medium.

Cells. The susceptibility of brain cells themselves to damage must be important in determining the risk of bilirubin toxicity. Unfortu-

Table 24-10. Drugs Capable of Interfering with Bilirubin-Albumin
            Binding When Measured with Various Methods.

Sephadex G-25 column chromatography

Sulfisoxazole	Caffeine sodium benzoate
Sulfadimethoxine	Valium injectable
Sulfamethoxypyridazine	Tolbutamide
Sulfamoxole	Furosemide
Sulfafurazine	Ethacrynic acid
Oxacillin	Sodium meralluride
Carbenicillin	Chlorothiazide
Cephalothin	Hydrocortisol
Digoxin	Sodium salicylate

HBABA dye-binding method

Novobiocin	Kanamycin
Sulfisoxazole	Tetracycline
Oxacillin	Erythromycin
Cephalothin	Penicillin
Rifamycin	Ampicillin
Sodium salicylate	Sodium oleate

Bilirubin binding by erythrocytes method

Bile acids	Sodium salicylate
Ethacrynic acid	Sulfisoxazole
Furosemide	Novobiocin
Chlorothiazide	Cloxacillin
Hematin	

Peroxidase (bilirubin oxidation) method*

Sodium salicylate
Sulfisoxazole
Sulfamethoxazole
Other sulfonamides
   (but not sulfadiazine)

*Based on Brodersen's measurements of the binding constants of the drug to the high-affinity site for bilirubin on albumin, the assumed plasma concentration, and the calculated maximal displacement factor. Drugs listed are those which may be used during the neonatal period and in which displacing effect is thought to be significant. Note that the peroxidase method is the only one listed which measures free bilirubin. For further details see Brodersen[2] and Gartner and Lee.[34]

nately, very little is known about what influences this although the effect of pH (see above) and anoxia[145] seem to be important. If unbound bilirubin is the toxic fraction, the cells may be viewed as competing with albumin for the body's miscible bilirubin pool to form bilirubin-cell complexes.[4] Certain cell types and neurons are more likely to be damaged by bilirubin. The distribution of susceptible brain nuclei is similar to the distribution of target nuclei in carbon monoxide poisoning and acute asphyxia suggesting that oxidative metabolism and/or energy reserves are unusually vulnerable in bilirubin-sensitive neurons.[4] The yellow staining of kernicterus may be a relatively late

phenomenon which coincides with the loss of cell membrane integrity, permitting indiscriminate passage of large molecules.[4]

Drugs. The effects of numerous drugs on bilirubin-albumin binding have been tested *in vitro* using different methods. The measured effect varies with the method used, some systems requiring much greater concentrations of the drug than others to demonstrate an increase in unbound bilirubin. Some of the drugs capable of interfering with bilirubin-albumin binding when tested *in vitro* are listed in Table 24-10. Brodersen has provided a list of 150 drugs and their bilirubin displacing effects as measured by the peroxidase method.[2] Nevertheless, the only drug which has been demonstrated to increase the risk of kernicterus in the human newborn is sulfisoxazole.[51]

Other Competing Anions. The effect of exchange transfusion on the albumin binding capacity of infant's serum has been studied using the Sephadex and peroxidase methods.[146,147] Despite the fact that exchange transfusion removes a considerable amount of bilirubin from the infant, replaces much of the infant's serum albumin with bilirubin-free albumin and lowers the free bilirubin level, a single exchange transfusion has no significant effect on the ability of the infant's plasma to bind bilirubin.[146,147] The possibility exists that certain anions are present which interfere with the albumin binding of bilirubin and which are not removed to any great extent by exchange transfusion. The competitors for bilirubin binding to albumin maintain their effectiveness after an exchange transfusion has been performed, and no change in albumin binding capacity is detectable. It has been suggested that a similar mechanism may be operative in the case of acidosis, in which associated endogenous anions may displace bilirubin from its albumin binding sites and increase plasma free bilirubin.[140]

Clinical Status of the Infant. The clinical condition and gestational age of the infant are important and affect the measured bilirubin binding capacity. Infants with respiratory distress, acidosis, asphyxia, hypothermia, hypoglycemia, and sepsis are able to bind less bilirubin per mole of albumin than are well infants.[148] Total binding capacity increases with gestational age but so does serum albumin concentration which, in turn, correlates with binding capacity.

The role of *infection* may be important. Pearlman and coworkers reported three infants with birth weights greater than 2250 g and the pathologic diagnosis of kernicterus who had documented sepsis.[93] One infant was never jaundiced and the other two had maximum serum bilirubin concentrations of 8.6 and 15.6 mg/dl, respectively. Naeye has observed that the presence of amniotic fluid infection is associated with an increase in the damaging effects of bilirubin.[90] The mechanism for this possible effect remains obscure.

Blood-Brain Barrier. A blood-brain barrier exists which limits the entry of certain substances into the central nervous system, but the role of this barrier in the development of kernicterus is unknown. Bilirubin is present in the cerebrospinal fluid in normal newborn infants at a mean concentration of 0.24 ± 0.098 mg/dl in full-term infants and 0.61 ± 0.15 mg/dl in preterm infants.[149] In this study of 100 newborn infants, the ratio of serum bilirubin to spinal fluid bilirubin was 28 ± 24.9 for all infants. However, the ratio was much lower in low-birth-weight infants and increased progressively with age and birth weight. In a group of older children and adults with jaundice, the serum bilirubin-spinal fluid bilirubin ratio was 152.5 ± 175. A significant correlation was found between serum bilirubin and spinal fluid bilirubin levels in the newborn infants ($p < 0.01$). In a study of 23 full-term infants with Rh erythroblastosis, CSF bilirubin concentrations of similar magnitude were found.[150] There are, however, no good data supporting the concept that the blood-brain barrier of newborn infants is "immature."[104] Evidence that increasing age is not necessarily a barrier to the entry of bilirubin into the central nervous system is provided by the documentation of kernicterus in a 16-year-old boy with the Crigler–Najjar syndrome.[151]

Although the blood-brain barrier is ordinarily impermeable to protein-bound material,[100] under certain circumstances (*e.g.*, the infusion of hyperosmolar solutions) serum albumin readily enters the brain.[152] When this occurs, the pattern of uptake into the brain is similar to the distribution seen in kernicterus.[48,61] Studies of newborn and adult rabbits indicate that the newborn animals do not have an immature blood-brain barrier. On the contrary, a sophisticated and selective blood-brain barrier is operative at birth.[153] Although it has been suggested that it is only unbound (free) bilirubin that is capable of crossing the blood-brain barrier, studies of cerebellar bilirubin content in newborn Gunn rats showed an inverse relationship between plasma unbound bilirubin and cerebellar bilirubin.[106,107] Furthermore, the brain will take up endogenously administered enzymes when the barrier is reversibly opened,[154] and incorporate them into brain cells. It is possible that kernicterus may result if the blood-brain barrier was similarly opened in the presence of hyperbilirubinemia. The blood-brain barrier can also be opened by anoxic, ischemic stress.[155] This is

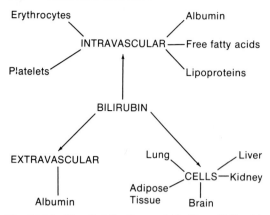

Fig. 24-14. The distribution and binding of bilirubin in the body compartments.

consistent with previous observations in newborn animals in whom kernicterus could not be produced unless the animals were asphyxiated.[145] Indeed, the time of the barrier opening following anoxia-ischemia varies with the length of the insult, which may explain why infants who are asphyxiated at birth display symptoms of kernicterus several days after the asphyxia. It is possible that delayed opening of the blood-brain barrier, coincident with elevations of serum bilirubin could explain this clinical observation.[104,156]

Clinical Management of the Jaundiced Infant. Clearly, there are no simple answers to the problem of the management of the jaundiced infant. When carefully reviewed (see above), the data from numerous studies of bilirubin toxicity are so confusing that they permit almost no rational conclusions regarding a therapeutic approach to the jaundiced infant. In general, high bilirubin levels are bad, but studies documenting the usefulness of measuring loosely bound or free bilirubin have yet to be performed. Furthermore, albumin binding capacity and affinity are not the only factors involved. There is virtually no understanding of the potential for variation in the blood-brain barrier or individual susceptibility to bilirubin damage of cells in the central nervous system. Other factors such as acidosis, asphyxia, hypoxia, and infection may play an important role in "priming" the cells for damage, possibly increasing their affinity for bilirubin, or altering the permeability of the blood-brain barrier.

A review of all the published data on albumin

binding leads one to the conclusion that, at this point, *no single test of the albumin binding of bilirubin is sufficiently reliable to be recommended for routine clinical use.* Currently, the use of such tests should be restricted to properly designed studies. Bilirubin is widely distributed in different body compartments and its particular effect on the cells of the central nervous system may depend on competing affinities of intravascular and extravascular albumin, free fatty acids, lipoproteins, and other tissue and cellular elements (Fig. 24-14). Thus, measurement of the binding of bilirubin to albumin in the intravascular compartment alone may not provide sufficient information to assess the risk of bilirubin toxicity.[110]

Numerous guidelines have been published over the years for the management of jaundiced infants; however, none of them can be regarded as adequately validated nor can any be relied upon in all circumstances. At this time, the most reasonable approach (however imperfect) appears to be the use of the serum bilirubin concentration as an index for exchange transfusion. Tables 24-11 and 24-12 give two schemes for identifying the necessity for treatment in different groups of infants. Table 24-11 is based on the indications for exchange transfusion used at the Albert Einstein College of Medicine. They appear to have been successful in that institution (but not in others) in preventing pathologic kernicterus, at least in low-birth-weight infants.[97] Table 24-12 represents an attempt to provide guidelines for the management of hyperbilirubinemia based on birth weight, the rate of rise in the serum bilirubin, and the presence of potential complicating factors. It cannot be emphasized too strongly that, at the moment, no satisfactory method exists for identifying a critical level of bilirubin. In all cases, a complete assessment of the infant's clinical condition, supported by relevant laboratory tests, is mandatory.

Summary

Bilirubin is toxic to cells, and when the serum concentration of indirect bilirubin is elevated, the pathologic entity of kernicterus may occur. The mode of entry of bilirubin into cells of the central nervous system is unknown. Bilirubin binds reversibly to albumin as well as to cellular membranes and the evidence is

Table 24-11. Guidelines for the Management of Hyperbilirubinemia.

Serum Bilirubin mg/100 ml	Birth weight	<24 hrs	24-48 hrs	49-72 hrs	>72 hrs
<5	ALL				
5-9	ALL	PHOTO-THERAPY IF HEMOLYSIS			
10-14	<2500Gm	EXCHANGE IF HEMOLYSIS	PHOTOTHERAPY		
	>2500Gm		INVESTIGATE IF BILIRUBIN >12 mg		
15-19	<2500Gm	EXCHANGE		CONSIDER EXCHANGE	
	>2500Gm			PHOTOTHERAPY	
20 and+	ALL	EXCHANGE			

□ Observe   ▨ Investigate Jaundice

Use phototherapy after any exchange

In presence of:
1. Perinatal asphyxia
2. Respiratory distress
3. Metabolic acidosis (pH 7.25 or below)
4. Hypothermia (temp below 35° C)
5. Low serum protein (5g/100 ml or less)
6. Birth weight <1500 Gm
7. Signs of clinical or CNS deterioration

} Treat as in next higher bilirubin category

(Modified from Brown, A.K., and Klaus, M.H., and Fanaroff, A.A.)

suggestive, but hardly conclusive, that it is the unbound bilirubin concentration which determines albumin and tissue binding. If this is so, serum albumin and tissues appear to compete with each other for the miscible bilirubin pool. Albumin binding is probably determined by the concentration of free bilirubin anion, which is unaffected by physiologic pH changes. However, bilirubin probably binds to cell membranes, and tissue binding, which may be determined by the concentration of free bilirubin acid, is profoundly influenced by pH.

The measurement of free bilirubin in serum is difficult, and there are insufficient data to justify using such tests in the management of jaundice. At the moment, it appears unlikely that binding tests will provide the necessary information, in individual infants, to predict when the risk of kernicterus will exceed the risk of treatment by exchange transfusion. The accumulated evidence is suggestive, but not conclusive, that hyperbilirubinemia is capable of causing a neurodevelopmental handicap less severe than classical kernicterus. However, there is nothing, at present, to suggest that treating mild jaundice will prevent such a handicap.

MANAGEMENT OF HYPERBILIRUBINEMIA

When the serum bilirubin concentration approaches a level at which kernicterus is likely to occur, hyperbilirubinemia must be treated. This can be done by three methods:

1. Mechanical removal of bilirubin by means of exchange transfusion

Table 24-12. Recommended Maximal Total Serum Bilirubin Concentrations (mg/dl).*

Birth weight (g)†	Uncomplicated course	Complicated course‡
Less than 1,250	13	10
1,250–1,499	15	13
1,500–1,999	17	15
2,000–2,499	18	17
2,500 and up	20	18

*Direct-reacting bilirubin concentrations are not subtracted unless they amount to more than 50% of the total serum bilirubin concentration. Applicable during the first 28 days of life.
†Equivalent gestational age categories may be used in lieu of birth weight for small-for-gestational age (SGA) infants.
‡Complications include perinatal asphyxia and acidosis, postnatal hypoxia and acidosis, significant and persistent hypothermia, hypoalbuminemia, meningitis and other significant infection, hemolysis, and hypoglycemia.
(Lee KS, Gartner LM, Eidelman AI, Ezhuthachan S. Clin Perinatol 4:305, 1977)

2. Use of alternative pathways, that normally play only a minor role, for bilirubin excretion (phototherapy)

3. Acceleration of normal metabolic pathways for bilirubin excretion by pharmacologic means (*e.g.*, phenobarbital)

The action of phenobarbital in lowering serum bilirubin is too slow for the already jaundiced infant and, if there is any role for this drug, it may be in the prevention of hyperbilirubinemia (see below). Suggested guidelines for the use of phototherapy and exchange transfusion based on serum bilirubin levels are outlined in Tables 24-11 and 24-12. It must be recognized that there is no way of applying these guidelines to every jaundiced infant. *Each case must be judged on its own merits* and every effort must be made to diagnose the cause of hyperbilirubinemia before treatment.

Exchange Transfusion

Exchange transfusions are indicated in two situations: (1) to correct anemia rapidly in infants severely affected with erythroblastosis, and (2) to treat potential or actual hyperbilirubinemia. In hemolytic anemia, both of these conditions may exist. The guidelines in Table 24-11 take into consideration the serum bilirubin level, the age of the infant (reflecting the rate of rise of the serum bilirubin), birth weight, and other factors known to affect the risk of

kernicterus (acidosis, hypoxia, hypothermia, hypoalbuminemia, and so on).

Hemolytic Disease. In the past, various criteria for early or immediate exchange transfusion have been proposed based on cord blood levels of hemoglobin and bilirubin. However, recent data suggest that these measurements do not predict the severity of hyperbilirubinemia with sufficient accuracy to warrant their use as therapeutic guidelines.[157,158] On the other hand, the natural history of this disease has been well studied so that plotting the rate of rise of serum bilirubin on a graph allows one to predict whether or not it will reach 20 mg/dl.[159, 160] A useful "rule of thumb" for indicating the need for exchange transfusion in hemolytic disease is a serum bilirubin level of 10 mg/dl (171 μmol/l) by 24 hours, 15 mg/dl (257 μmol/l) by 48 hours, or 20 mg/dl (342 μmol/l) at any age.[160] The use of phototherapy may modify some of these criteria, but by and large they are still applicable.

The presence of anemia that is not immediately life-threatening or of a serum bilirubin rising by more than 0.5 mg/dl/hour suggests that there is a relatively brisk hemolytic process which will require exchange transfusion within the first 12 hours of life. Even though the serum bilirubin has not reached dangerous levels, an early exchange transfusion in this situation is advisable because it will correct anemia and remove a significant proportion of the sensitized red cells, thus aborting the hemolytic process. It also removes some bilirubin before large amounts are distributed in the extravascular space.*

Repeat Exchange Transfusions. When the necessity for the previous exchange is based on the level of serum bilirubin (not the rate of rise of bilirubin), then the indications for repeat exchange transfusion are based on the same serum bilirubin level. Exchange transfusion *per se*, does not appear to improve the bilirubin binding capacity of the patient's serum (see section on Bilirubin Binding, interfering anions).[146, 147]

Severe Hemolytic Disease and Hydrops Fetalis. The determination of amniotic fluid bilirubin levels, and lecithin/sphingomyelin ratios, and

---

* The total bilirubin space is about twice the plasma volume. Thus, at least as much and, in some cases, much more bilirubin will be found outside of the circulation as in it.[151]

ultrasound visualization of the fetus in Rh-sensitized women have allowed optimal obstetric management of the fetus, including intrauterine transfusion and appropriate elective premature delivery. The pediatrician can therefore anticipate with considerable accuracy the likely condition of the infant at delivery. Hydropic infants, or those who are obviously pale and asphyxiated, demand immediate treatment. Otherwise, therapy is based on serial hemoglobin and bilirubin determinations.

The pathogenesis of hydrops fetalis, with its attendant edema and serous effusions, has never been clear. Most authors have suggested that these infants die from congestive heart failure secondary to the severe anemia and that the edema is secondary to the heart failure. However, recent studies of premature infants with moderate-to-severe erythroblastosis show that chronic congestive heart failure is rare at birth in hydropic infants.[161,162] Central venous pressures as measured in the thoracic inferior vena cava do not reflect blood volume alone but also venous tone, pulmonary vascular resistance and right ventricular dynamics.[163,164] Elevated pressures probably result from acute intrapartum asphyxia and may decline to normal or subnormal levels after correction of acidosis, hypoxia, hypercarbia, and anemia.[164] The severely affected infants die from progressive cardiorespiratory failure in which asphyxia and hyaline membrane disease play a major role. Acute intrapartum asphyxia, possibly superimposed upon chronic mild asphyxia in a premature and anemic fetus, leads to delivery of an asphyxiated infant with hypoxemia, hypercarbia, and mixed respiratory/metabolic acidosis. A high incidence of hyaline membrane disease can be expected in such infants.

A linear relationship was found between the umbilical cord hematocrit and the red cell volume,[162] and (in nonhydropic infants) between the hematocrit and the blood volume.[163] No correlation was observed between the severity of hydrops fetalis and the infants' blood volumes (Fig. 24-15).[162]

Specifically, the blood volumes of almost all were within the normal range for infants of similar gestational age (70–90 ml/kg) and only one infant (severely hydropic) had a significantly elevated blood volume (113 ml/kg), while in another, the blood volume was very

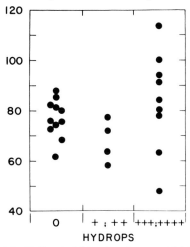

ESTIMATED BLOOD VOLUME at BIRTH
(ml/Kg non-edematous body wt.)

HYDROPS

Fig. 24-15. Estimated blood volumes at birth in 24 infants with varying degrees of hydrops. Note lack of correlation between severity of hydrops fetalis and infants' blood volumes. (Phibbs RH, Johnson P, Tooley WH: Pediatrics 53:13, 1974; Copyright © American Academy of Pediatrics, 1974)

low (48 ml/kg). Not all of the hydropic infants were severely anemic, but most were hypoalbuminemic. These data suggest that low plasma colloid osmotic pressure as a result of hypoalbuminemia is an important mechanism in the pathogenesis of hydrops.

These observations also have important therapeutic implications. In the past, these infants have received immediate exchange transfusions, with little attention to their cardiorespiratory status. It is obvious that their management demands a *comprehensive approach* which includes intensive monitoring and vigorous treatment of asphyxia, acidosis, hypoglycemia, and hypothermia. Assisted ventilation is frequently required and the use of end-expiratory pressure is of value in the presence of pulmonary edema. Attention must be given to thrombocytopenia and possible coagulation disorders, and paracentesis performed if there is significant ascites. In the presence of severe anemia (hematocrit 35% or less), an exchange transfusion of 25 to 80 ml/kg of packed red cells is given within 30 minutes of birth to raise the hematocrit to about 40%.[161] *Phlebotomy should not be routinely performed on these infants* because they are usually normovolemic and may be hypovolemic. In fact, *no manipulations of blood volume should be performed without appropriate measurements of central venous and aortic blood pressures*. Furthermore, in order to monitor accurately the central venous pressure, *the umbilical venous catheter must enter the inferior vena cava* (by way of the ductus venosus). If the catheter is in a portal vein or the umbilical vein, the pressures so measured are meaningless in the interpretation of the infant's circulatory status. Thus the practice of measuring "central venous" pressure using the umbilical vein catheter may lead to serious therapeutic error, unless the position of the catheter tip is confirmed by x-ray or pressure tracing. Note that before making therapeutic decisions based on measurements of central venous pressure, it is necessary to correct acidosis, hypercarbia, hypoxia, and anemia.

Pressures should also be monitored during subsequent exchange transfusions with whole blood. Because the plasma colloid osmotic pressure is low, the infusion of plasma with a normal albumin concentration will draw extravascular fluid into the vascular compartment. This may be of benefit to infants with pulmonary edema or hypovolemia, but could conceivably cause circulatory overload in those with a normal blood volume.[162]

Type of Blood Used for Exchange Transfusion. Blood preserved with one of three types of anticoagulant solutions—heparin, acid-citrate-dextrose (ACD) and citrate-phosphate-dextrose (CPD)—has been used for exchange transfusions. CPD has largely replaced ACD as the standard solution in current use. The anticoagulant preservative solutions and the effects of blood storage produce certain metabolic changes during and after exchange transfusions.[165] Most recently, previously frozen red cells resuspended in plasma or albumin-saline solution have been used for exchange transfusions.[166,167]

ACD and CPD Blood: Metabolic Complications. In CPD, the ratio of citric acid to its sodium salt is reduced, resulting in a higher pH. Total citrate ion of CPD is 15% less than ACD, and the pH of blood at drawing is 7.20 in CPD versus 7.00 for ACD. The dextrose levels are similar, but inorganic phosphate is added to CPD. The CPD solution permits longer maintenance of normal red cell 2,3 diphosphoglycerate (2,3 DPG) levels, enhancing oxygen delivery from the transfused red blood cells to the tissues.[168] Exchange transfusion with 5-day-old ACD blood on the other hand, transiently impairs oxygen delivery to tissues.[169] These changes may be critical when exchange transfusions are performed on sick, hypoxic infants.

The citrate in ACD and CPD blood will bind ionic **calcium** and **magnesium** and produce significant depression in these divalent cations. The temporary hypomagnesemia has not been associated with clinically recognizable problems, but the depression of the calcium ion may produce deleterious hemodynamic and cardiac effects (not caused by "toxicity" of the citrate).[170]

It is common practice to administer calcium gluconate during exchange transfusions to counteract the citrate binding. Measurements during exchange transfusions have not demonstrated any significant effect of calcium gluconate administration on the serum ionized calcium,[171,172] although there is a temporary increase directly after the calcium is given (Fig. 24-16). In some centers, supplemental calcium has never been administered and this has been without apparent ill effects.[173] Calcium chloride (or calcium gluconate) plus heparin can be added to the ACD or CPD blood immediately before the transfusion. The addition of 0.1 g $CaCl_2$ to 1 unit of (heparinized) CPD blood prevented a fall in ionized calcium in term but not in preterm infants.[174] In larger, relatively well infants, it is probably unnecessary to administer additional calcium. Clinical tetany is rarely seen during exchange transfusion, which is remarkable considering the very low levels of ionized calcium that occur. It is also of interest to note that clinical signs such as jitteriness, crying, and irritability occurring during exchange transfusion cannot be correlated with levels of ionized calcium.[171] Parathormone levels rise initially, but then decline during the exchange.[172]

Both ACD and CPD blood have a high glucose content (300–350 mg/dl) that stimulates insulin secretion in the infant and may lead to **rebound hypoglycemia** following the exchange. It is therefore important to monitor blood sugar levels closely in the first few hours after the exchange.

ACD blood contains about 20 mmol/liter of titratable acid; 90% of this results from the added citric acid and the remaining 10% from

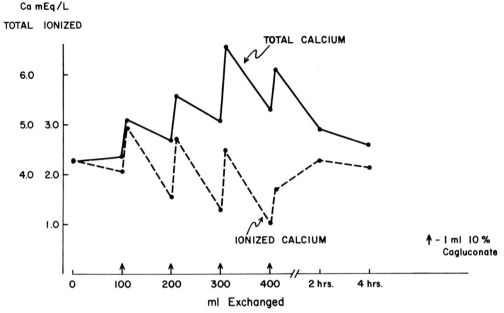

Fig. 24-16. Effect of added calcium gluconate on total and ionized calcium during exchange transfusion with ACD blood. (Maisels, MJ et al: Pediatrics, 53:683, 1974; Copyright © American Academy of Pediatrics, 1974)

the production of acid by the continued metabolism of red blood cells.[165] CPD blood has less than half of the acid load of ACD at the time of drawing,[175] and the pH remains about 7.00 for 7 days (in 2–3 days, ACD blood has a pH of about 6.7.) Some authors have recommended that donor ACD blood be buffered with bicarbonate or THAM prior to exchange transfusion (10mmol to 1.0 M THAM/unit of blood).[176] Others have not done this and with CPD blood that is less than 72 hours old, this may be unnecessary. It is important to understand that it is the *acid load* and not the pH* of the blood which produces acidosis.

Because the citric acid in ACD and CPD blood is readily metabolized in the liver to bicarbonate, most infants should have no difficulty in coping with the infused acid during the exchange (provided it is not performed too rapidly). In fact, most develop a significant *alkalosis after the exchange* that may persist for up to 72 hours.[165]

Nevertheless, because exchange transfu-

sions are usually performed by way of the umbilical vein, the heart is intermittently perfused with blood that is acidemic. This may affect the myocardium directly and could possibly account for the occasional (and apparently unexplained) cardiac arrest that occurs. Therefore, in managing hydropic infants immediately after birth or low-birth-weight infants in shock or marked metabolic acidosis, it may be advisable to buffer the blood.

However, it should be recognized that adding THAM or sodium bicarbonate will elevate the already high osmolarity (>300 mosm/liter) and sodium content (165–170 mmol/liter) of the donor blood.[176,178] Removal of 60 ml of plasma from the donor blood prior to the exchange will reduce the acid and the citrate load and restore the hematocrit toward normal.

Heparinized Blood. This is the safest for exchange transfusions and its use produces no changes in ionized calcium, electrolytes, acid-base balance, or blood sugar levels. There is, however, in response to the administered heparin, a marked rise in nonesterified fatty acids (NEFA) that has caused some concern because of the potential competition between NEFA and bilirubin for albumin binding sites.[179] However, NEFA levels return to normal within 3

---

* Five percent dextrose water, an unbuffered solution with a small amount of dissolved CO_2, has a pH of 4.55 but an acid load of only 0.28 mmol/liter. Its infusion does not, therefore, produce acidosis.[177]

Table 24-13. Size of Exchange Transfusion and Replacement of Infant's Blood.

Donor Volume as Fraction of Infant's Blood Volume	Percent of Blood Volume Removed and Replaced by Exchange
0.5	40
1.0	63
2.0	87
3.0	95

The fraction of blood removed from the infant follows the theoretical equation for the dilution of a closed volume

$$y = 1 - e^{-x}$$

where y = fraction of original fluid removed, x = number of volumes exchanged and e = 2.71828.[179]

hours of the exchange transfusion, and the rise in NEFA occurs while bilirubin is being removed, so that this should not be considered a contraindication to the use of heparinized blood.

Heparinized blood will also affect the coagulation status of the infant although, in most infants, this returns to normal within 4 to 6 hours after the exchange, indicating that the heparin has been metabolized. Protamine sulfate has been used to neutralize the heparin at the end of the exchange. Because some heparin is removed and some metabolized during the exchange, enough protamine is administered to neutralize about half of the heparin in the blood exchanged. This works out to be about 1 mg of protamine for every 100 ml of blood exchanged.[165] It is probably not necessary to use protamine routinely, but it may be indicated in very sick infants, or in those with severe erythroblastosis in whom metabolism of heparin may be impaired as a result of compromised liver function.

On the other hand, in infants with disseminated intravascular coagulation, which is frequently associated with hypoxemia, acidosis, shock, or sepsis, exchange transfusion with fresh heparinized blood may be the ideal therapy, because it heparinizes the infant while simultaneously providing platelets and other clotting factors.

The major disadvantage of heparinized blood is that it must be used within 24 hours of collection, which strains the facilities of most blood banks.

Bilirubin Rebound After Exchange Transfu-

sion. During the exchange, bilirubin from the extravascular space is drawn into the plasma. Partial equilibration between extravascular and plasma bilirubin occurs almost instantaneously,[180] so that by the end of an exchange in which only 13% of the circulating red cells remain, the serum bilirubin is still 45% of the preexchange level. Immediately after the exchange, further equilibration takes place, which is complete within 30 minutes, and which produces the early rebound of plasma bilirubin to 60% of the preexchange level. Despite exchange transfusion, rapid heme breakdown may continue, producing a further increase in serum bilirubin which may necessitate repeat exchange transfusion. This hemolysis may result from catabolism of sensitized red cells that exist as pools previously sequestered in the bone marrow or spleen (and therefore not removed by exchange transfusion), or from production of early labeled bilirubin, or from the hemolysis of transfused red cells.

Efficiency of Exchange Transfusion. The mass of bilirubin removed is related to the plasma bilirubin level[181] and the size of the exchange transfusion, the most critical factor being the amount of plasma removed (Table 24–13).[182]

On the other hand, because of the rapid equilibration between extravascular and plasma bilirubin, the rate of the exchange has little effect on the amount of bilirubin removed. (The extravascular bilirubin concentration decreases at the same rate as the plasma bilirubin concentration, and thus cannot be influenced by the rate of the exchange.) For practical purposes, the size of the blood aliquots exchanged also has no significant effect on the efficiency.[183] Therefore, exchanging in increments of 5 or 10 ml is as efficient as using 20-ml aliquots. Withdrawing 20 ml of blood from a 3000 g infant represents an acute depletion of his total blood volume that will cause a decrease in cardiac return, cardiac output, and blood pressure, particularly if done rapidly.[184] As the cardiovascular system is adapting to these changes an equal volume of blood is rapidly reinfused which reverses the adaption.[183] This is repeated 25 to 30 times during a two-volume exchange. The use of smaller aliquots places less stress on the infant's cardiovascular adaptive mechanisms.

Albumin Administration. The administration of albumin before or during an exchange transfusion has produced conflicting results with regard to its effect on the efficiency of the exchange. Some authors have reported that 1g/kg of 25% salt-poor albumin, given 1 hour prior to the exchange, will increase the amount of bilirubin removed by the exchange, whereas others have not found this to be the case.[181]

Exchange Transfusion Technique. This is described in Allen and Diamond's classic monograph[159] and by Bowman.[185] A few points will be discussed below.

Equipment. The most commonly used technique is the ''push-pull'' method using a single syringe and special four-way stopcock. Various other techniques have been described which include the use of syringe pumps that mechanically infuse and withdraw blood. Simultaneous withdrawal from the umbilical artery and infusion by way of the umbilical vein (using gravity) have also been used.[186] This method adds the hazard of an additional catheter, but may be of considerable value when dealing with very sick infants because it will eliminate swings in blood volume and pressure that occur with the push-pull method. A technique of performing exchange transfusion using peripheral veins has also been described.[187]

Age of Blood. Potassium levels in CPD blood increase rapidly with storage and by 7 days, mean plasma potassium concentration is 11.9 ± 1.5 mmol/liter.[177] Thus, it is recommended that blood used for exchange transfusion should always be no more than 4 days old. However, a recent survey of CPD bank blood, 1 to 4 days old, revealed a mean plasma potassium concentration of 8.5 ± 6.36 mmol/liter.[188] Thirty percent of the units analyzed had potassium concentrations in excess of 9 mmol/liter and 21% had levels greater than 11 mmol/liter. The reasons for this are not clear and these values are surprising particularly in view of the rarity of arrhythmias during exchange transfusion. The problem can be corrected by washing the red cells and resuspending them in fresh plasma.[188] Alternatively the potassium concentration of the blood can be determined prior to the exchange transfusion and the unit rejected if the plasma level exceeds 6 mmol/liter.

Packed Cells Versus Whole Blood. Packed cells are used for partial exchange transfusion when it is necessary to treat severe anemia at birth (see above); otherwise, whole blood is used. This provides plasma with its bilirubin-free adult albumin, immunoglobulins, and opsonic activity. Because of the volumes of anticoagulant solutions added to the donor blood (63 ml CPD or 75 ml ACD), the relatively low (adult) hematocrit of the donor blood is further lowered. Removal of 60 to 70 ml of plasma before the exchange will correct this.

Rate. There is no advantage and considerable risk in performing an exchange transfusion rapidly. A rapid exchange aggravates the cardiovascular changes,[184] may affect cerebral blood flow and intracranial pressure,[189] and does not allow time for the liver to metabolize the infused acid and citrate. With adequate monitoring and good temperature control, there does not seem to be any indication for hurrying with the procedure. Generally, exchange of twice the blood volume should take about an hour in any baby. This means a slower rate for the smaller and sicker infants.

Complications. Careful attention to detail will avoid most of the described hazards of exchange transfusions,[190] although complications related to the placement of the catheter and the procedure itself can never be eliminated completely.[191] This is particularly so because this procedure is now performed on the smallest and sickest infants and may be responsible for problems not previously considered.[189] For example, the high sodium content of CPD blood (165–170 mmol/liter),[178] while of little consequence for the vigorous full-term infant, may not be benign in infants under 1500 g.[192] Unexpected cardiac arrest still occurs in about 1% of infants,[173] but with attention to potassium levels (see above), careful monitoring, and adequate resuscitation, this should be avoidable and immediate mortality from the procedure itself should approach zero.[173]

There have been several reports of necrotizing enterocolitis with intestinal perforation following exchange transfusion. This occurs in term as well as premature infants, and after either single or multiple exchanges. The etiology remains obscure, but it seems possible that positioning the umbilical venous catheter in the portal system, with its close relationship to the mesenteric veins, may well produce retrograde obstructive hemodynamic changes, with hemorrhage and thrombosis at the microcirculatory level. Studies in piglets demonstrated a significant increase in portal venous pressure during the injection phase of the exchange.[193] In some infants, exchange trans-

Table 24-14. Spectral Emission Characteristics of Fluorescent Lamps Used in Phototherapy

Lamp	Range (nm)	Principal Peak (nm)
Daylight	380–700	550–600
Cool white	380–700	550–600
Blue	335–600	425–475
Special blue	420–480	420–480

fusion may be the primary etiologic event, while in others it represents an additional insult to a bowel compromised by infection or hypoxia.[194]

Graft-versus-host disease has been described in infants who received intrauterine transfusions and then exchange transfusions following delivery.[195] These infants apparently did not reject the donor lymphocytes after birth, because the previous introduction of viable lymphocytes during intrauterine life had rendered them relatively immunologically tolerant. The use of exchange transfusion blood deficient in viable lymphocytes was suggested as a means of preventing this in infants who have had intrauterine transfusions.

The unwitting use of hemoglobin SC blood produced massive intravascular sickling and death in one infant, suggesting the advisability of screening donor blood for sickle cell trait or disease.[196]

Phototherapy

In 1958, Cremer and coworkers observed that the exposure of premature infants to sunlight or blue fluorescent light produced a fall in serum bilirubin concentration.[197] Since then, visible light for the treatment of hyperbilirubinemia has been used extensively in Europe, as well as in North and South America.[165] In the United States, it has been estimated that about 90,000 infants annually will be "put under the lights."[198]

Clinical Use of Phototherapy. Effectiveness. There are several well-controlled studies that leave no doubt concerning the effectiveness of phototherapy as a means of preventing or treating moderate hyperbilirubinemia.[198,199] It appears to be more effective than exchange transfusion in achieving prolonged reduction of bilirubin levels in infants with nonhemolytic

jaundice.[200] Phototherapy will modify the course of hyperbilirubinemia in ABO- and Rh-hemolytic disease and will reduce, but not eliminate, the need for exchange transfusion.[199,201]

Characteristics of Light Source and the Dose: Response Relationship. Various types of fluorescent light have been used: broad spectrum, daylight, cool white, and blue or relatively monochromatic "special blue." A quartz halide white light with tungsten filament that has a significant output in the blue spectrum has also been used,[202] although there are no published data regarding its efficiency. These lights have different spectral distributions (the range of wavelength over which the bulb emits) and different peaks of maximal emission (Table 24-14). The lights which are most effective in photooxidizing bilirubin are those having a high-energy output near the maximum absorption peak of bilirubin (450–460 nm). In considering the energy output of various lamps, the relevant unit of measure is the **irradiance or flux**—the quantity of radiant power or energy w*/cm^2—over a particular wavelength interval. The **illuminance** is expressed in foot-candles: standard units of illumination (1 lumen/ft^2) and can be measured by the familiar photographic light meter. This light meter is designed to respond in a manner similar to the human eye and function with a maximum sensitivity between 500 and 600 nm. The measurement (illuminance) is thus a reflection of the sensation of brightness produced by the light (and perceived by the eye or light meter), whereas the irradiance, or flux, in the blue range (425–475 nm) has been demonstrated *in vivo* and *in vitro* to be directly related to the rate of bilirubin degradation.[203–205] A minimum flux of 4μw/cm^2/nm appears to be necessary for effective phototherapy,[206] and the response increases with increasing dose until a saturation point is reached beyond which no further response can be demonstrated.[205] Comparison of reported values by different authors is difficult owing to the fact that measurements are made over different spectral intervals and reported as **irradiance** (the radiant flux impinging on a unit area: w/cm^2) or as **spectal irradiance** (the irradiance over a given spectral interval divided by the width of the interval: w/cm^2/nm). Anderson points out that this latter quantity is only

* w = watts

defined for very narrow wavelength intervals and is not applicable to phototherapy-monitoring instruments currently in use, which use filters that pass relatively broad spectral bands.[207]

Type of Light and Dosage. Although blue light is more effective than white (see above), less is known about the possible side effects of monochromatic light, because most of the experience in phototherapy over the last 20 years has been with broad-spectrum light. Furthermore, blue light obscures the appearance of cyanosis, a sign most physicians are unwilling to do without. The rate of decline in serum bilirubin is related to the amount of energy output in the blue spectrum. There is no information, however, on what the optimal, or the maximum "safe" dose is and for how long it can be applied. Therefore, the lowest dose necessary to achieve the desired result should be used.

The energy output in the blue (425–475 nm) range of phototherapy lights can be monitored clinically using relatively simple instrumentation. Therefore, reporting results of phototherapy in terms of dose, time, and response will allow a more rational approach to its investigation and use. The use of a dosimeter badge which measures the total light dose received by an infant over a period has also been recommended. These devices are not currently available for clinical use and earlier testing revealed problems in uniformity and reproducibility.[208]

Indications for Phototherapy. The major use of phototherapy has been in the prevention and treatment of hyperbilirubinemia in premature infants. Phototherapy should not be used prophylactically in all infants because this will result in 95% of infants being unnecessarily treated. However, its use for 12 to 24 hours in low-birth-weight infants without hemolytic disease when the serum bilirubin concentration reaches 10 mg/dl will prevent it from rising to 15 mg/dl (257 μmol/l) in 80% or more of these infants.[209] In certain low-birth-weight infants who are at particular risk for kernicterus, there may be good reason to start phototherapy well before the serum bilirubin levels reach 10 mg/dl (171 μmol/l),[88,89] and some authors recommend its prophylactic use in this population.[210] However, there are no published data demonstrating that this has reduced the incidence of pathologic kernic-

terus or subsequent neurodevelopmental impairment. In hemolytic disease, phototherapy is indicated as an adjunct to exchange transfusion. It should not be used instead of exchange transfusion when the indications for exchange transfusion already exist. Suggested indications for the use of phototherapy are given in Table 24-11.

Intermittent Versus Continuous Phototherapy. Clinical studies comparing intermittent versus continuous phototherapy have produced conflicting results:[211–214] some studies have found continuous phototherapy to be more effective than the intermittent use of light,[211,212,215] whereas others have not.[213,214] In Vogl's study, 15 minutes of illumination followed by 60 minutes with the lights off was found to be as effective as continuous illumination.[213] In all of the previous studies of intermittent phototherapy, the light-on and light-off periods used were hours in length. Indyk has suggested a model of action of phototherapy which involves a two-step process.[216] He suggests that the time constant for the interaction of a photon of appropriate energy with a bilirubin molecule at a skin binding site is probably of the order of nanoseconds. The products of this reaction then migrate from the skin to the serum, while an unactivated bilirubin molecule assumes the skin site. The migration of bilirubin to the skin takes 1 to 3 hours and is probably the rate-limiting step.[217] Thus, the use of 6 to 12 hour on-off schedules would not be expected to be more effective than continuous illumination. However, intermittent light, timed to match the migration time of bilirubin, should be effective in reducing serum bilirubin while minimizing the total light dosage. The total dose of light can be considered equal to the total number of photons in the blue spectrum that strike the infant during a specified time interval. Based on this assumption, an infant receiving a flux of 60 photons per second, administered continuously for 24 hours, would receive the same total irradiation as an infant receiving a flux of 3600 photons per flash administered by a strobe light that flashes once per minute for 24 hours.[218] However, the observation that intermittent phototherapy is more deleterious than continuous phototherapy to the genetic material of human cells in tissue culture has raised questions regarding intermittent phototherapy regimes,[219] although

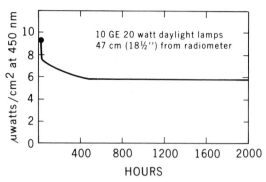

Fig. 24-17. Decay in energy output at 450 nm of phototherapy lamps.

no such adverse effects have been documented in newborn infants and the relevance of such *in vitro* observations to the human newborn is unknown.

Cholestyramine. The administration of cholestyramine to infants undergoing phototherapy appears to accelerate the reduction of serum bilirubin, presumably by decreasing the enterohepatic circulation.[220] However, the complications associated with the administration of cholestyramine make it unsuitable for routine use.

Effective Lamp Life. Wide ranges in decay of energy output have been reported with phototherapy lamps. Overheating in the light chamber produces deterioration of the phosphors and shortens the lamp life, but with adequate cooling effective lamp life is probably several thousand hours.[203] Figure 24-17 shows the change in blue light energy over 2000 hours with continuous usage of a phototherapy lamp. However, irregular decay of the phosphors can occur, so that the use of suitable instrumentation for monitoring energy output in the blue spectrum is extremely helpful in identifying phototherapy lamps that are producing insufficient energy output. Certainly, whenever a "clinical failure" is identified, the output of the lamps should be checked.

Effect of Light on Bilirubin Metabolism. The ability of bile pigments to absorb light depends upon their molecular structure and results in the photodecomposition of bilirubin. Light of wavelengths between 440 and 470 nanometers is the most effective in reducing serum bilirubin levels; wavelengths outside of this spectrum have little effect.[221] Upon exposure to light, the skin of a jaundiced infant loses its yellow color, and this is generally followed by a fall in serum bilirubin concentration. There appear to be two distinct processes which are responsible for these effects: (1) the bilirubin is broken down to more polar, diazo-negative, water-soluble products that are readily excreted in bile and feces and, to a lesser extent, in the urine;[222,223] and (2) the excretion of unconjugated bilirubin is enhanced.[222–224] Thus, the bile and urine of Gunn rats and humans with unconjugated hyperbilirubinemia contain compounds derived from bilirubin,[222,223] as well as intact unconjugated bilirubin itself.[223,224]

Until recently, the predominant mechanism for the formation of the bilirubin-derived compounds was thought to be the photooxidation of bilirubin resulting from a self-sensitized reaction involving singlet oxygen,[225] and there was no ready explanation for the enhancement of excretion of unconjugated bilirubin. Furthermore, the major bilirubin photoderivative excreted in the bile of Gunn rats has not been found among the photooxidative derivatives of bilirubin formed *in vitro*.[7] Most recently, Lightner and coworkers have demonstrated that bilirubin IX-α undergoes geometric photoisomerization in visible light to form what they have termed **photobilirubin** (Fig. 24-18).[226,227] This process does not require oxygen, is much faster than the aerobic photooxidation of bilirubin, and requires much less light. Bilirubin IX-α undergoes rapid and reversible photoisomerization to form ZE, EZ, and EE isomers. These isomers do not form the intramolecular hydrogen bonds which are present in the acid form of bilirubin IX-α (ZZ), and are more polar, less lipophilic, and more acidic than the natural ZZ pigments.[226,227] McDonagh has demonstrated almost instantaneous changes in bile composition in Gunn rats exposed to phototherapy,[228] and has identified the presence of geometric isomers of bilirubin IX-α in the serum of irradiated rats (Fig. 24-19).[229] In addition, when serum from the irradiated rats was injected into homozygous Gunn rats (kept in the dark) there was a prompt transient increase in hepatic bilirubin excretion by the recipient rats. Serum from control rats had no effect.[229]

Thus, it appears that photobilirubin is formed photochemically from bilirubin near the surface of the skin and is then transported in plasma to the liver, where it is excreted in

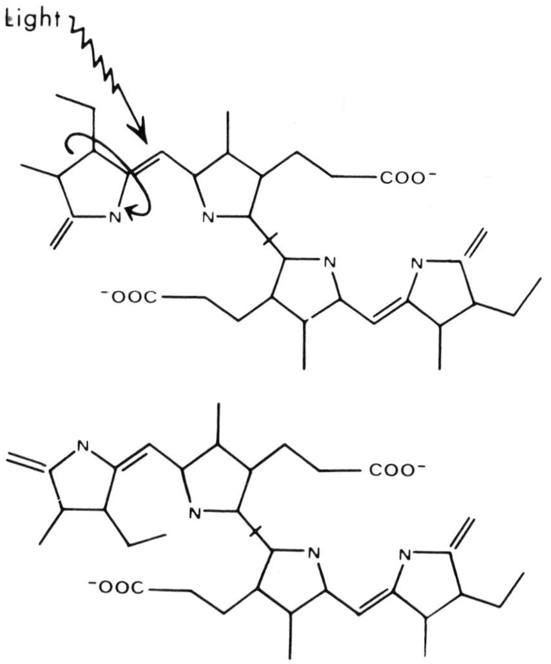

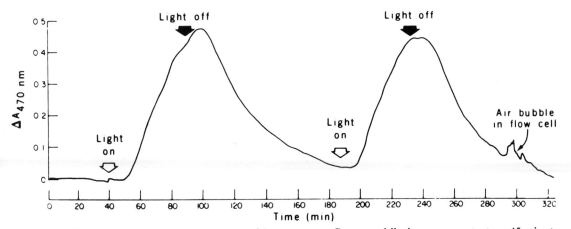

Light

Fig. 24-18. The effect of light (photography) on bilirubin IX-α (Z,Z). The outer ring is turned 180°, and bilirubin IX-α (E,Z) is formed. The product is bound less firmly to albumin, is presumably non-toxic, and is probably excreted in the bile without conjugation. (Brodersen R: In Stern L, Oh W, Frii-Hansen B [eds]: Intensive Care of the Newborn II. New York, Masson Publishing, USA, Inc., 1978)

bile. The formation of these geometric isomers (photobilirubin) that circulate in blood appears to play a role in the enhanced excretion of bilirubin during phototherapy.[229] The formation of photobilirubin appears to be a highly efficient process in which the photobilirubin is continuously removed from the skin by the plasma and is constantly excreted and replenished by newly formed photobilirubin.[226]

The principal site of action of phototherapy appears to be the skin and possibly the cutaneous capillary bed at a depth of no greater than 2 mm.[217] Vogl applied very small patches (4 cm²) of opaque material to the skin and showed that distinct color differences occurred: the covered areas remained yellow while the exposed skin was bleached. Although serum bilirubin concentrations declined, the bilirubin in the areas of skin not exposed to light remained elevated for at least 3 hours.[217] This suggests that bilirubin is rather firmly bound in the skin and subcutaneous tissue and that diffusion from these tissues into the vascular space occurs rather slowly. The skin and subcutaneous tissue thus appear to represent a slowly equilibrating bilirubin space, much slower, for example, than the rest of the extravascular space. The mammalian epidermis will pick up bilirubin either in its free or bound form, although the major uptake is in the form of free (unbound) bilirubin.[230] The liver may be an additional site of photochemical action. Invisible light has been shown to penetrate the abdominal wall in rats,[231] and

Fig. 24-19. Changes in absorbance (470 nm) of homozygous Gunn rat bile in response to two 45-minute periods of irradiation. Note the almost instantaneous changes in bile comosition which occur in response to phototherapy. (McDonagh AF, Ramonas LM: Science 20:829, 1978)

shielding the hepatic area in infants was associated with a decrease in the efficiency of phototherapy.[212]

Biologic Effects and Possible Complications of Phototherapy. The extensive use of light has stimulated considerable interest and research into its possible effects on the human organism. For many years photobiologists have been aware of the numerous effects of light on man and other mammals. These include effects on several biologic rhythms, the pineal gland, gonadal function, and vitamin D synthesis. It is possible to speculate on the potentially harmful effects of various types of light, such as those which may occur in the presence of photochemical sensitizers and cause damage to cell growth and structure.[232] None of these effects have been noted, so far, in human infants in the 20 years that phototherapy has been in clinical use.

Toxicity of Phototherapy Products. Human experience[233] as well as *in vitro*[234,235] and animal studies[105] strongly suggest that the products of photodecomposition have no **neurotoxic effects.** A child with Crigler–Najjar syndrome has been receiving phototherapy for 12 hours a night for 11½ years. Growth and development, bone age, IQ, visual testing, psychological testing, and blood amino acids have all remained normal.*

Red Blood Cells and Platelets. Although very high levels of illumination can produce **hemolysis of red blood cells** *in vitro,*[236] no adverse effects on the survival of normal red cells have been demonstrated with the clinical use of phototherapy.[237] Although there are reports which suggest that increased hemolysis may result from phototherapy in infants with glucose-6-phosphate dehydrogenase (G-6-PD) deficiency,[202,238] in two controlled studies no differences in hemoglobin or hematocrit levels were observed in G-6-PD deficient infants in whom phototherapy was or was not used. Furthermore, phototherapy was effective in reducing serum bilirubin levels in these infants.[239,240] Phototherapy appears to increase the rate of **platelet turnover** resulting in lower mean platelet counts.[72] The lowest platelet count in the group of infants receiving phototherapy was 52,000/mm³ and no bleeding was noted in these infants. The mechanism of action of light on platelets *in vivo* is unknown

* Land VJ: personal communication.

but may be the result of photochemical reactions occurring in the platelet membrane. It is speculated that the shortened platelet lifespan may be the result of sequestration of damaged platelets in the spleen.[72]

Photodynamic Damage. Because bilirubin is a photosensitizer, it has been suggested that it may act as a photodynamic agent in the presence of light and produce damage. However, bilirubin is a weak photosensitizer and no evidence for photodynamic damage (redness, itching, edema, hair loss) exists in jaundiced people exposed to sunlight. In addition, albumin, to which bilirubin is bound, competes with bilirubin for singlet oxygen (which is necessary for the photodynamic response), and thus exerts a protective effect by shielding neighboring molecules from bilirubin-sensitized attack.[241] Oxyhemoglobin also absorbs light and therefore reduces the intensity of photodynamically active light (approximately 415 nm) reaching the bilirubin.

Cell Damage. In a series of studies, Speck and coworkers have demonstrated that phototherapy is capable of damaging DNA of cells growing in culture.[242–244] In addition, they demonstrated that intermittent illumination produced more DNA damage than a similar light dosage administered continuosuly.[219] They also studied the effects of phototherapy on fertilization and embryogenesis using the American sea urchin. Illumination of sperm and oocytes produced abnormal embryos and cleavage patterns.[245] Because it is likely that light penetrates the thin scrotal skin and perhaps even reaches ovaries, it has been suggested that shielding of the gonads with diapers may be indicated during phototherapy.[245]

Oxygen Dissociation. Although phototherapy has been shown to cause hemolysis of fetal red cells and a shift to the right in the neonatal oxygen dissociation curve *in vitro,*[236] these effects were not found in a group of icteric infants receiving phototherapy.[246]

Riboflavin. Riboflavin enhances the photodecomposition of bilirubin *in vitro* and *in vivo.*[247,248] Because riboflavin is a light-sensitive vitamin and has a maximum absorption spectrum at a wavelength similar to that at which the degradation of bilirubin occurs, this vitamin may undergo photodegradation in infants receiving phototherapy. A depletion of riboflavin has been demonstrated in such infants,[249] and this effect may be more pronounced in infants receiving human milk that is relatively poor in riboflavin.[250] However, a daily oral intake of 0.3 mg of riboflavin is adequate to prevent riboflavin deficiency.[251] No clinical consequences of transient riboflavin deficiency have been identified, and the demonstration that the photodynamic action of riboflavin may induce alterations in intracellular DNA should temper enthusiasm for excessive riboflavin supplementation in an effort to enhance the bilirubin-lowering effect of phototherapy.[242]

Intravenous Alimentation. The exposure of amino acid solutions used for intravenous alimentation to light in the blue spectrum produced a significant reduction in tryptophan. In addition, when a multivitamin solution was added to the amino acids, a significant reduction in methionine (40%) and histidine (22%) also occurred. The decrease in methionine was accompanied by an increase in methionine sulfoxide.[252] This raises a question regarding the addition of multivitamin preparations to amino acid solutions and suggests that perhaps multivitamins be delivered separately to infants and shielded from light.

Retinal Damage. Studies of several animal species have demonstrated the potential toxic effects of light on the retina. However, most of these studies were performed in animals whose pupils had been pharmacologically dilated and whose retinas were unusually sensitive to phototoxicity. Messner has studied the effects of clinical levels of phototherapy on the retina of newborn stump-tail monkeys.[253,254] These animals were maintained in standard nursery incubators and were restrained in the supine position facing the light source. However, no mydriatic drops were used and the monkeys could open and close their eyes as desired. One of the eyes was sutured closed and covered with a patch to act as a control. Exposure of the eyes to the phototherapy lights for 12 hours to 7 days produced severe and progressive damage to the retina.[254] In a subsequent study, monkeys were exposed to light for 3 to 10 days and then returned to normal environments for 10 months before being sacrificed.[253] Substantial recovery in retinal cytoarchitecture was evident if the original exposure was for less than 3 days. However, there was some loss of rod and cone cells in all the exposed retinas when compared to the controls. This loss is similar to the normal attrition of photoreceptor cells which occurs in the aging process in the mammalian retina. These changes, therfore, represent a form of **premature aging.** Thus, if an infant suffered phototoxic retinal damage (as a result of a slipped eye patch) visual acuity, electroretinography, and ophthalmic examination may well be normal in childhood although considerable tissue has been lost. It seems prudent to continue to patch the eyes of infants receiving phototherapy. However, displaced patches can obstruct the nares and cause respiratory distress,[255] and the use of patches has also been associated with transient abdominal distension.[256]

Follow-up studies of infants whose eyes have been adequately shielded have yielded normal visual function as assessed clinically and by means of electroretinography.[257-259]

Skin Changes. The skin becomes bleached during phototherapy and skin color therefore cannot be used as a means of assessing serum bilirubin levels; they must be measured at regular intervals. Black infants may show a **tanning effect** from phototherapy.[260] This is the result of exposure to some long wave ultraviolet and short-wave visible light (300–600 nm). This produces pigmentation without an initial erythema and is apparently caused by reoxidation of preformed melanin, a process known as **immediate pigment darkening (IPD).** If this light exposure continues, the initial IPD reaction fades after 1 to 24 hours and is followed within 48 to 72 hours by hyperpigmentation, secondary to increased melanosome synthesis. This occurs in black infants presumably because of the presence of some preformed melanin in their skin.[260] Measurements of irradiance in and out of incubators and the effect of plexiglass interposed between the lights and the baby are shown in Table 24-15. Plexiglass essentially eliminates the passage of short (200–280 nm) and middle wave (280–320 nm) ultraviolet light, but allows a significant portion of the long (320–400 nm) to pass through. Exposure to energies in the 360 to 400 nm wave band may cause an increase in peripheral blood flow and has caused erythema in adults.[261] At wavelengths greater than 650 nm (which includes infrared energy), it can be seen (Table 24-15) that most of this energy is absorbed by the plexiglass. This can lead to a rise in temperature of the plexiglass itself, and, therefore, the incubator. However,

Table 24-15. Irradiance at the Infant Level Inside a C-86 Isolette Incubator with and without Plexiglas Cover

Waveband width (nm)	Available energy (mw/cm²)	Experimental measurement: Energy through 1 layer of ¼ inch Plexiglas G (mw/cm²)	Extrapolated value: Energy through 2 layers Plexiglas G (mw/cm²)
Less than 300	0.00	0.00	0.00
300–360	0.12	0.001	0.0001
360–420	0.15	0.115	0.087
420–460	0.27	0.245	0.223
460–500	0.25	0.227	0.207
500–650	0.53	0.484	0.442
Greater than 650	4.18	0.35	0.17
Total	5.50	1.42	1.15

mw. = milliwatts

Note that the plexiglass essentially eliminates the passage of short (200–280 nm) and middle wave (280–320 nm) ultraviolet light but allows a significant portion of the long (320–400 nm) to pass through. Exposure to energies in the 360–400 nm wave band may cause an increase in peripheral blood flow and has caused erythema in adults.

(Wu PYK , Berdahl M: J Pediatr 84:754, 1974)

if two layers of plexiglass are interposed, the outer layer (such as the shield of the lamp itself) will absorb, largely, the infrared energy and transfer it to the room air by means of air currents.

The "Bronze Baby" Syndrome. The use of phototherapy in infants who have an associated cholestatic jaundice may lead to the development of a dark gray-brown discoloration of the skin, serum, and urine. This has been called the "bronze baby" syndrome.[262] Because the bronzing effect occurs almost exclusively in infants with some degree of cholestasis, it seems reasonable to assume that it is the retention of some product of phototherapy that is producing the color change. During phototherapy, the duodenal bile changes from its normal color to a brownish black.[224] These dark pigments appear to be water-soluble breakdown products of photooxidation, and the retention of these pigments in infants with obstruction to bile flow could explain the bronze color. Most infants with this syndrome have not appeared to suffer any deleterious consequences. However, kernicterus has been described in a full-term infant with the bronze baby syndrome who died.[263] The maximum total serum bilirubin in this infant was 18.0 mg/dl (308 μmol/liter) with a direct-reacting bilirubin of 4.1 mg/dl (70 μmol/liter). At autopsy, the bronze-color stain was noted in abdominal organs, ascitic fluid, and skin, but was absent from the brain and cerebrospinal fluid. In this particular case, however, spectroscopic analysis of serum and ascitic fluid revealed a "shoulder" at 500 nm. Gartner and Lee suggest that this may represent bilirubin in an aggregated or precipitable macromolecular form after critical quantities of unbound bilirubin exist in an aqueous medium.[264] The 500 nm shoulder may represent a specific physical state in which bilirubin gains entrance into the neuronal cell membrane, either alone or in association with FFAs. Discontinuing phototherapy generally results in the disappearance of the bronze pigments.

Gastrointestinal Tract. Some authors have described the development of loose green stools in infants receiving phototherapy,[265] although others did not confirm this.[266] However, Rubaltelli and Largajolli have demonstrated that in jaundiced infants receiving phototherapy the passage of materials through the gut is considerably accelerated.[267] Others have demonstrated a 50% reduction in intestinal transit time and a two- to threefold increase in stool water losses during phototherapy.[268,269] Bakken studied intestinal lactase activity in

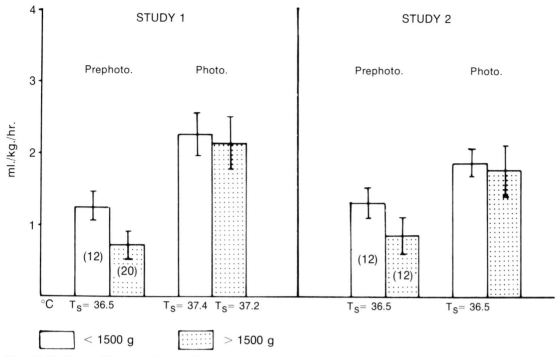

Fig. 24-20. Insensible water loss in infants under phototherapy. Study 1 was performed in Isolette C-86 incubator without servocontrol of skin temperature. Study 2 was performed in Isolette C-86 incubator with servocontrol to maintain skin temperature at 36.5 C. Figures in parentheses denote the number of infants in each group. (Wu PYK, Hodgman JE: Pediatrics 54:704, 1974; Copyright © American Academy of Pediatrics, 1974)

jaundiced, light-treated infants and found significant impairment of their ability to hydrolize lactose.[269a] No intestinal lactase activity was found in the intestinal brush border, and diarrhea stools reverted to normal when these infants were placed on a lactose-free diet. Thus, there seems to be no question that infants receiving phototherapy have increased stool water losses. Lactose intolerance can be documented by the simple demonstration of reducing substances in the stool of such infants and can be treated readily by providing a lactose free formula until the situation has resolved or phototherapy is discontinued. Phototherapy has no effect on the activity of β-glucuronidase in duodenal bile of jaundiced infants.[270]

Fluid Losses, Thermoregulation, and Blood Flow. Significant increases in insensible water loss (IWL) occur during phototherapy (Fig. 24-20), particularly if used in infants who are already under radiant warmers.[271] In full-term infants, IWL increases by 40%,[268] whereas in low-birth-weight infants, IWL may increase by as much as 80% to 190% in nonservocontrolled incubators. This effect can be partially mitigated by the use of servocontrolled incubators.[272] In addition to the previously noted increases in stool water loss, there is an increased fetal excretion of nitrogen, sodium, and potassium.[269] The mechanisms for these changes are not understood, but they do emphasize the need for careful attention to fluid and caloric supplementation during phototherapy.

During phototherapy, there is a marked increase in skin blood flow (228%) and, to a lesser extent, muscle blood flow.[273] When servocontrolled devices are not used, there is also a significant increase in skin temperature from the phototherapy lamps and an increase in incubator temperature, heart rate, and respiration. The use of a servocontrolled device prevents a rise in skin temperature and the previously noted changes in muscle blood flow, respiration, and heart rate, although there remains a significant, but less dramatic, increase in skin blood flow (52%).[273]

Growth. Infants receiving phototherapy gain less weight in the first week of life but show catch-up growth in the next 2 weeks. In a study of 120 infants receiving phototherapy from the second to sixth days of life, 44% of those receiving continuous therapy had regained their birth weights by the seventh day, as compared to 57.6% of those receiving intermittent phototherapy (12 hours on, 12 hours off) and 80% of control infants.[215] Similar, but less marked, changes were seen in length and head circumference. The phototherapy groups had greater increases in weight and length during the second and third postnatal weeks. These growth effects may be caused by the increases in fluid and caloric losses mentioned above. A 2-year follow-up of these infants revealed no differences in weight, length, or head circumference.[274] On the other hand, a 2-year follow-up of another group of infants (studied earlier) revealed significantly smaller head circumferences in those infants who had received phototherapy. Nevertheless, there was no difference in developmental and neurologic performance in the phototherapy infants when compared to the controls.[274] The reason for the difference in growth in this group of infants is not explained. In both of these studies, only 50% of the infants who entered the study were available for follow-up measurements at the age of 2 years. Other studies that have followed the growth of infants receiving phototherapy for 2 to 6 years have found no effect on weight, length, or head circumference.[199,275,276]

Gonadotropins. Changes have been observed in **serum gonadotropins** during and after phototherapy. Values for luteinizing hormone (LH) declined within 24 to 48 hours after commencing phototherapy but increased significantly 6 to 9 days after phototherapy was discontinued.[277] Increases in LH and follicle-stimulating hormone (FSH) were observed 3 to 4 weeks after phototherapy was administered to preterm female infants. In the males, LH increased but FSH did not.[278] These observations suggest that light may affect pituitary-gonadal function in the human neonate, although the mechanism for these changes is not clear.

Physician Management Effects. Certain physician management effects can be characterized as potential complications of phototherapy. Probably the most common "physi-cian effect" of phototherapy is the tendency to treat infants with light without investigating the cause of the jaundice. This may lead to a failure to recognize some life-threatening condition. The bleaching of the skin prevents the clinical assessment of jaundice so that serum bilirubins must be measured. In hemolytic disease, phototherapy, while reducing serum bilirubin levels, cannot of course remove sensitized red cells. In these circumstances, hemolysis continues and the hematocrit must therefore be followed closely.

Electrical. All lamps must be checked for electrical leakage and must be properly grounded.

Effect on the Mother. Seeing an infant under phototherapy may be extremely disturbing to the mother.[279] In particular, the presence of eye patches may interfere with the attachment process between mother and infant and the use of blue lights (which imparts a distressingly cyanotic hue to the infant) may be very frightening.

Exposure of Infants to Radiant Energy in Nurseries. Newborn infants are, of course, constantly exposed to the ambient environmental nursery lighting, as well as light through windows, which varies with the amount of sunlight on any particular day. Lucey has calculated that an infant in an incubator near a window, who is exposed to 6 hours of summer sunlight, receives more radiant energy exposure in the 440 to 470 nm range than does the infant receiving 24 hours of phototherapy (daylight bulbs).[280] Thus, phototherapy may be a less important source of radiant energy than sunlight in some nurseries, and it is certainly a minute portion of the radiant energy exposure an infant will receive in his lifetime.[281]

Other Effects. Phototherapy has been associated with an increased incidence of **hypocalcemia** in preterm infants. The mechanism for this is not apparent.[282] No effect of phototherapy was found on serum **FFA levels** or **leucine amino peptidase values.**[280]

Light penetration has been measured through the **newborn scalp and skull bones,**[280] something which would be expected in view of the common clinical experience with transillumination of the head.

The sera of infants receiving phototherapy have not demonstrated any decrease in the **bilirubin binding capacity of albumin.**[283,284]

Measurements of **urine 17-ketosteroids**[285] and **serotonin** metabolism[286] in infants undergoing phototherapy are normal. Guidelines for the clinical use of phototherapy are given below.

Guidelines for Clinical Use of Phototherapy

1. Perform diagnostic studies to identify the cause of jaundice *before* instituting phototherapy.
2. Measure the energy output of the lamps in the blue spectrum (425–475 nm).
3. Monitor the temperature of infants frequently.
4. Servocontrolled incubator should be used whenever possible and the thermistor probe should be shielded from the light.
5. Monitor fluid balance (twice daily weights, urine output and specific gravity, hematocrit) and provide increased fluid intake if necessary.
6. Shield the eyes and gonads.
7. Measure serum bilirubin levels every 12 hours or more often if indicated. Do not rely on skin color to assess the degree of jaundice.
8. Follow hematocrit, particularly in hemolytic disease.
9. Discontinue phototherapy whenever parents are visiting their infant and always remove eye patches when parents visit.
10. Whether continuous or intermittent phototherapy is used, there is no reason for a mother to be denied contact with her infant during the time that the infant is receiving phototherapy.
11. Use a lactose-free formula if loose stools occur which contain increased amounts of reducing substances.
12. Consider the possibility that phototherapy may be responsible for a decreased platelet count.
13. Check all lamps for electrical leakage and make sure that they are properly grounded.

Pharmacologic Treatment

Numerous pharmacologic agents are capable of stimulating the hepatic glucuronide-conjugating system in animals and some have been used in an attempt to reduce serum bilirubin concentrations in newborn infants.[210] The drug that has been most widely used in human studies is phenobarbital, known to be a potent inducer of microsomal enzymes and which has been shown to increase bilirubin conjugation and excretion and to abolish phase I physiologic jaundice in the newborn.[18] The administration of phenobarbital will also reduce serum bilirubin levels in patients with the Type II Crigler–Najjar syndrome.[287] In addition, phenobarbital will enhance uptake and excretion of certain compounds and will increase bile flow. It thus appears to act on the whole hepatic transport system for organic anions. Administration of phenobarbital to children with intrahepatic cholestasis lowers the serum bilirubin levels by stimulating bile secretion.[288]

Numerous studies have demonstrated that phenobarbital, when given in sufficient doses to the mother, to the baby, or to both, is effective in lowering serum bilirubin levels in the first week of life.[165] When given to mothers of erythroblastotic infants before delivery, phenobarbital-treated infants had a slower postnatal rise of indirect bilirubin than did nontreated controls, and significantly fewer of the phenobarbital-treated group required exchange transfusions.[158] There is no justification for the prophylactic administration of phenobarbital to all pregnant women because the vast majority of their infants will not develop significant hyperbilirubinemia, and because of the many other effects phenobarbital may have on the newborn infant.[165] Combining phenobarbital with phototherapy does not reduce serum bilirubin levels more rapidly than does phototherapy alone.[289]

The use of pharmacologic agents has been suggested in an attempt to reduce the enterohepatic circulation of bilirubin. These include activated charcoal, polyvinylpyrrolidone, and agar,[22,210] which bind bilirubin in the intestinal lumen. None of these substances has been shown to be effective consistently in the treatment of hyperbilirubinemia, and their routine use cannot be recommended.

PREVENTION OF HYPERBILIRUBINEMIA

Both phototherapy and phenobarbital can be used to prevent hyperbilirubinemia. Except under certain circumstances (see above), their prophylactic use in the normal population is not recommended because 95% of infants would be unnecessarily treated. **Early feeding**, however, has been shown to reduce serum bilirubin levels.[53] This may work by decreasing

Table 24-16. Differential Diagnosis of Conjugated Hyperbilirubinemia in Early Infancy.

1. Hepatitis of infectious origin	**4. Hemolytic disease**
Giant-cell hepatitis of presumed viral origin	Erythroblastosis fetalis
Rubella, cytomegalovirus	**5. Heredofamilial and metabolic disease**
Coxsackievirus, echovirus, "massive hepatic	Familial giant cell hepatitis and biliary atresia
necrosis"	Trisomy E
Herpesvirus, varicella	Down's syndrome, leprechaunism
Toxoplasmosis	Zellweger's syndrome ("biliary dysgenesis")
Lues, listeriosis, tuberculosis	Dubin–Johnson disease, Rotor's syndrome
Hepatitis-associated antigen	Wilson's disease
2. Biliary obstruction	Alpha$_1$-antitrypsin deficiency
Extrahepatic atresia	"Idiopathic neonatal hemochromatosis"
Extrahepatic stenosis and choledochal cyst	Fibrocystic disease
Bile plug syndrome	Indian childhood cirrhosis
Tumors (hepatoma, bile duct sarcoma)	Galactosemia, fructosemia, tyrpsinemia
Fibrocystic disease and meconium ileus	Niemann–Pick disease, Gaucher's disease
3. "Toxic" hepatitis	Wolman's disease, glycogenosis IV
Sepsis and coliform pyelonephritis	Cholestatic syndromes, Paucity of intrahepatic
Diarrhea	biliary ducts
Intestinal obstruction (ileum)	Bile salt disorder?
Therapeutic hyperalimentation	Familial hepatosteatosis

Reproduced with permission from Brough and Bernstein: Conjugated hyperbilirubinemia in early infancy. Human Path 5:507–516, 1974

the enterohepatic circulation. It has also been shown that fasting in rats increases the concentration of hepatic microsomal heme oxygenase, thus stimulating the conversion of heme to bilirubin in the liver.[290] The serum bilirubin in adults rises after fasting because of a decreased uptake of bilirubin from the plasma.[55] Early feeding thus appears to be advisable, whenever possible, in the newborn.

CHOLESTATIC JAUNDICE

Cholestatic jaundice is defined as jaundice resulting from failure of excretion of conjugated bilirubin from the hepatocyte into the duodenum, and it is characterized by elevated direct-reacting bilirubin concentrations. Cholestasis in infancy has been reviewed recently and may be the result of a number of conditions frequently posing a difficult diagnostic problem.[291] It is difficult to readily organize the neonatal cholestatic syndromes on a clinical, anatomic, or functional basis because so much overlap exists in the clinical presentations, biochemical abnormalities, and morphologic features of the major disorders.

Thaler has termed the two major categories of hepatobiliary disease **type I and type II cryptogenic infantile cholestasis.**[292] Type I cho-

lestasis refers to hepatocellular disease, generally termed **neonatal hepatitis** or **giant-cell hepatitis,** in which there is no "permanent distortion of the intrahepatic or extrahepatic biliary system" and which is usually self-limiting and has a good prognosis.[292] This diagnosis is applied to unexplained cholestasis in infants.

Type II cholestasis results from various malformations of the biliary system which may or may not be accompanied by parenchymal changes. These are structural abnormalities of the extrahepatic, the major intrahepatic, or both bile ducts, such as atresia, hypoplasia, stenosis, choledochal cyst, or a reduction in the number or size of functional bile ducts and ductules (atresia, hypoplasia, paucity, and cystic dilatation).

For clinical purposes, it is clearly of paramount importance to be able to distinguish between type I cholestasis and a potentially correctable biliary malformation so that, if a correctable lesion is present, surgical correction can be attempted before irreversible changes occur.

Cholestatic Syndromes

Table 24-16 lists the differential diagnosis of conjugated hyperbilirubinemia in early in-

Table 24-17. Etiologic and Structural Classification of Infants and Conjugated Hyperbilirubinemia in the First 4 Months of Life

		Patients
Extrahepatic biliary atresia		32
Hepatitis group		103
Alpha-1-antitrypsin defi-ciency	24	
Galactosemia	1	
Tyrosinosis	1	
Hepatitis B	2	
Rubella	2	
Toxoplasmosis	1	
Cytomogalovirus	1	
Idiopathic hepatitis	71	
Choledochal cyst		2
Total		137

Reproduced with permission from Mowat, Psacharopoulos, Williams: Extrahepatic biliary atersia versus neonatal hepatitis. Review of 137 prospectively investigated infants. Arch Dis Child 51:763–768, 1976

fancy. In the immediate neonatal period, however, perhaps the commonest cholestatic syndrome seen is that associated with the use of **intravenous alimentation** in intensive care nurseries. Measurements of bile acids in low-birth-weight infants show that there is a substantial hepatic excretory defect when compared with older children and adults.[293] This excretory defect appears to be most marked in very low-birth-weight infants. In addition, these infants are particularly susceptible to the development of cholestasis while receiving long-term parenteral alimentation. In infants weighing <2000 g, no evidence of cholestasis was observed when intravenous alimentation was administered for less than 2 weeks. However, seven of eight infants weighing <2000 g, who received alimentation for more than 2 weeks, demonstrated evidence of cholestasis. The effect was not seen in infants who weighed >2000 g. Manginello and Javitt observed a close relationship between sepsis, parenteral nutrition, and the elevation of serum bile acids.[294] Bernstein and coworkers described the histopathology of five infants who developed conjugated hyperbilirubinemia during intravenous alimentation.[295] In none of these infants was sepsis documented. Liver biopsies showed cholestasis and hepatocellular damage including giant-cell transformation.

The pathogenesis of the cholestasis associated with intravenous alimentation solutions is unclear, although it has been suggested that amino acids may inhibit bile flow. Withdrawal of the intravenous alimentation solution generally results in a resolution of the cholestatic jaundice. However, evidence of hepatocellular damage and even fibrosis are cause for concern.[296,297] Thus, all infants receiving intravenous amino acid solutions should have frequent measurements of direct bilirubin and, if possible, serum bile acids.

When cholestasis associated with intravenous alimentation is excluded, 75% of conjugated hyperbilirubinemia during the first years of life is accounted for by two conditions: idiopathic neonatal hepatitis (really a diagnosis of exclusion) and structural abnormalities of the biliary system (Table 24-17).

NEONATAL HEPATITIS AND EXTRAHEPATIC BILIARY ATRESIA (EHBA)

Etiology

The etiologies of biliary atresia and neonatal hepatitis are unknown. Although there are several well-documented causes of hepatitis in the newborn (Table 24-16), the majority are idiopathic. Furthermore, the morphologic, physiologic, and biochemical similarities between hepatitis and atresia have led some workers to suggest that these entities may be expressions of different phases of a similar disease process and that EHBA is frequently, if not always, a consequence of neonatal hepatitis.[298,299] Other features which support this argument are

1. In biliary atresia, clinical jaundice may not be seen for the first time 2 to 3 weeks after birth,[300] which suggests that, in some cases at least, it is not a congenital but rather an acquired malformation. Infants have been described who developed biliary atresia following documented patency of the extrahepatic bile ducts.[301] Others have developed intrahepatic atresia postnatally.[298,302]

2. Biliary atresia is essentially unknown as an incidental finding in infants who die in the neonatal period of other causes and is rarely associated with other congenital anomalies.[303]

3. Bile ducts have been known to open after a surgical finding of atresia.[304,305]

4. Hepatitis and atresia (both intra- and extrahepatic) have occurred in siblings.[303,306]
5. Both hepatitis and atresia have a high incidence in infants with the trisomy 17–18 syndrome, suggesting the possibility of a common prenatal (viral?) insult which produced the chromosomal and hepatobiliary damage.[307]
6. Giant cells are present in both conditions.[292]
7. The bile acid patterns are similar, and infants with extrahepatic biliary atresia frequently show very high levels of chenodeoxycholate early in the course of the disease (before cirrhosis has occurred), which suggests that an underlying hepatitis may be present. It has therefore been suggested that progressive cholestasis itself leads to apposition and then fibrosis of the biliary epithelium. The study of Heathcote and coworkers supported this hypothesis.[298] Seventeen children who developed cholestasis in the neonatal period were followed for a period ranging from 5 months to 22 years. In 11 children, serial liver biopsies showed a progression of the initial lesion from an appearance of giant-cell hepatitis, atresia, cholestasis, or fibrosis to progressive hypoplasia of the intrahepatic bile ducts, portal fibrosis, and, in some, cirrhosis. If it is accepted that EHBA is an acquired disease that follows hepatitis (which may be anicteric), then early detection of cholestasis by the measurement of serum bile acids might suggest the use of hydrocholeretics, such as phenobarbital and cholecystikinin, in an attempt to prevent progression of the disease.[299]

Nevertheless, Thaler points out that it is rare to find extensive hepatocellular disease together with biliary disease in the neonatal period and that the intrauterine viral, protozoal, and bacterial infections producing hepatocellular disease in the newborn do not normally produce bile duct malformations.[308] He further notes that the simultaneous occurrence of atresia in the major bile ducts and terminal intrahepatic ductules is rare and "the manner in which extrahepatic ducts are destroyed by a parenchymal disease process generally leaving the intrahepatic structures intact is difficult to visualize." The pathogenesis and management of neonatal hepatitis and biliary atresia have been discussed in detail at a recent international workshop.[309]

Clinical Features

The clinical picture includes conjugated hyperbilirubinemia which develops at any time from birth to more than 1 month of age. The jaundice persists and hepatomegaly is present early and is frequently accompanied by splenomegaly. Stools are pale and urine is dark. Bilirubin, and not urobilin (virtually none is formed in the bowel in the first 6 weeks of life), is found in the urine.

Neonatal hepatitis and biliary atresia may follow a clinical course so similar that it is frequently impossible clinically to distinguish one from the other, unless spontaneous remission of the cholestatic jaundice occurs, indicating hepatitis.

Javitt has reviewed the reported sex incidence of hepatitis and atresia.[299] When viewed separately, hepatitis occurs more frequently in males (69%) and EHBA somewhat more often in females (60%). If one combines the male and female incidence data for both diseases (on the assumption that atresia is a consequence of hepatitis), it appears that a female infant with cholestatic jaundice stands a considerably greater chance (69%) of developing EHBA than does a male (31%).

Diagnosis

Certain physical findings such as microcephaly, purpura, or radiographic evidence of intracranial calcification will suggest an intrauterine infection. In most cases, however, the history, physical examination, and even the course are of little help in making the diagnosis.

Laboratory Diagnosis. The usual liver function studies—serum transaminases, alkaline phosphatase, lactic dehydrogenase—are rarely, if ever, helpful. A consistently declining conjugated bilirubin level is against EHBA, but the reverse does not rule out hepatitis. During the obstructive phase of the disease, infants with hepatitis may appear to have almost no bile flow.

A number of biochemical and other special tests have been suggested which may help to distinguish neonatal hepatitis from biliary atresia.[310] A problem common to the majority of these tests is that they are, basically, **indirect measurements of bile flow.** Thus, if used during the phase of hepatitis when bile flow is minimal or absent, they may not distinguish between hepatitis and atresia.

The ^{131}I-Rose Bengal Test. The only direct, quantitative measure of the liver's ability to excrete bile is the ^{131}I-rose bengal fecal excretion test. Its major drawback is the necessity for an accurate, 72-hour, urine-free stool collection. All infants with extrahepatic biliary atresia and about 20% of those with hepatitis (at the initial investigation) excrete less than 10% of the administered radioactivity in 72 hours.[311] If the ^{131}I-rose bengal test is equivocal, clarification may be achieved by administering cholestyramine at 4 g/day for 2 to 3 weeks and repeating the test.[312] Alternatively, phenobarbital at 5 to 10 mg/kg/day can be given for 3 to 5 days beginning 1 to 2 days after completing the initial stool collection for ^{131}I-rose bengal. The phenobarbital course is followed by another 72-hour stool collection. It is not necessary to administer additional isotope because less than 10% has been excreted. As phenobarbital stimulates bile flow, infants who have patent extrahepatic ducts will demonstrate a three- to seven-fold increase in fecal radioactivity, whereas no change will occur in infants with extrahepatic biliary atresia.[292] In infants with intact extrahepatic ducts, the administration of phenobarbital may also produce a decline in serum bilirubin and bile acid levels.[288]

The use of ^{131}I-rose bengal for scanning the abdomen with a scintillation camera and performing surface counting over the liver has also been tried.[313] However, these methods are relatively insensitive and frequently do not distinguish between atresia and the obstructive phase of hepatitis.

Analysis of Duodenal Fluid. A simple test of biliary patency has recently been described which consists of visual inspection of a 24-hour sample of duodenal fluid.[314] A #8 radioopaque feeding tube is positioned fluoroscopically between the second and the third portions of the duodenum and two hourly aliquots of the fluid are collected and examined visually. If no bile pigment is observed after a 24-hour collection, surgical exploration is undertaken. All of six infants, who did not have bile pigment present in the duodenal fluid during the 24-hour collection, had exterohepatic biliary atresia. Sixteen infants had bile pigment present in one or more of the duodenal samples and none of these patients had exterohepatic biliary atresia. This is a remarkably simple test

to perform and we have found it to be very useful.

Liver Biopsy. Percutaneous needle biopsy is a safe procedure and in experienced hands should have an accuracy of about 85% to 90%. The single most reliable diagnostic finding is portal ductal proliferation found in EHBA and choledochal cyst. This is typically seen in all portal areas. A focal or irregular distribution suggests that extrahepatic obstruction might not be present. Portal zones are prominent because of periportal fibrosis and proliferation of interlobular ducts. Most (about 80%) infants with intrahepatic cholestasis (Thaler's type I) show extensive giant-cell transformation and portal zones that are inconspicuous or almost normal.[292]

Laparoscopy. Hirsig and Rickham have performed laparoscopy in infants with cholestatic jaundice. They use this technique for obtaining a liver biopsy and for doing choleangiography.[315]

Diagnostic Approach. Without exception, all investigators involved in the management of infants with possible biliary atresia emphasize the necessity for early treatment.[316–318] Because the early operative correction by portoenterostomy has improved significantly, the prognosis for these infants, an aggressive approach to their investigation is necessary. Infants with direct hyperbilirubinemia should be admitted to a hospital immediately and undergo tests for bacterial and viral infection (TORCH screen) and a serum assay for alpha$_1$-antitrypsin deficiency. Urine should be analyzed for glucose, reducing substances, and an amino acid screen. A 24-hour collection of duodenal fluid with visual observation for bile pigment is then performed. (This fluid can be used to measure trypsin activity to detect an infant who might have cystic fibrosis.) If no bile pigment is present in the duodenal drainage, an exploratory laparotomy with operative cholangiogram and liver biopsy should be performed. Current anesthesia and operative techniques pose minimal risk and the possibility of a successful surgical correction outweighs the anesthetic risks which may be associated with the procedure.[315]

Operative Correction

Until recently, the outlook for infants with EHBA was universally poor. Of more than 150 infants treated by Koop, only five had surgically "correctable" lesions and four of these survived.[319] The development by Kasai and Suzuki of the hepatic portoenterostomy procedure to achieve bile drainage, has altered somewhat the prognosis in this condition,[320] although the results are still far from satisfying.

EHBA is generally divided into the surgically correctable and noncorrectable types. The correctable type exists in those infants in whom a patent segment of extrahepatic bile duct is present which is continuous with the portahepatis and thus available for direct anastomosis to the intestine. In the noncorrectable type, there are no extrahepatic bile ducts, although a gall bladder or choledochal duct may be present.

Carcassone and Bensoussan reviewed the data (by questionnaire) from 11 major pediatric surgical centers regarding the anatomic lesions and outcome for infants with EHBA.[321] Of 674 cases in which the anatomy was adequately described, 121 (26%) were correctable and 363 (74%) noncorrectable. In the opinion of Koop, if any patent, even microscopic, bile ducts are found in the portahepatis, the condition should not be described as atresia.[319]

Indeed, the term "correctable" is also a misnomer.[322] In spite of being able to anastomose the bile duct to bowel (usually by means of a modified Roux-en-Y procedure), bile flow is obtained in only 35% of patients, with 32% of all correctable cases surviving 3 to 10 years after treatment.[321] Kasai and Suzuki developed the procedure of removing the extrahepatic bile ducts and anastomosing a loop of bowel to the area of the portahepatis, and showed that bile drainage could be achieved.[320] Following operation on 53 noncorrectable cases, bile drainage occurred in 19.[323] Subsequent results of this procedure were less encouraging. Campbell and coworkers operated on 12 infants and did not achieve sustained bile excretion in any case.[324]

Kobayashi, Utsunomiya, Kawai, and Ohbe treated 97 cases (3 correctable and 94 noncorrectable) with portoenterostomy and achieved bile drainage in 37 infants (38%).[325] Of these, 9 died, 16 developed ascending cholangitis and 11 esophageal varices (5 of which ruptured). Only 14 patients of the total group of 97 had an uneventful course. Odievre and colleagues achieved bile flow in 31 of 49 patients with noncorrectable EHBA, but 30 developed ascending cholangitis, bile peritonitis, or portal hypertension and 26 died.[326] Only one infant (age 21 months) was entirely free of abnormal findings. An overall "cure" rate of 27% can be expected in correctable lesions 1 to 17 years after birth.[321] Of the 68 infants considered "cured," 31 have cirrhosis.

In view of the natural history of this disorder, the timing of operation is crucial in order to prevent progressive cirrhosis. Between 1965 and 1975, survival in 147 patients operated on before 2 months of age was 22%, versus 7% in those operated on after 3 months.[321] Most recently, Kasai has reported bile drainage in 88% of infants with noncorrectable EHBA operated on before 60 days of age and 20% for those treated after 90 days.[318] Alagille reported the results of 91 infants with noncorrectable EHBA who were operated on from September 1969 to December 1976. Thirty-three of these patients have survived with bile flow restoration. Twenty-two of these patients are completely free of jaundice and appear to have a good long-term prognosis.[316]

Gautier, Jehan, and Odievre have classified the histopathologic changes found in the fibrous remnants of the extrahepatic bile ducts at a level just below the portahepatis.[327] They describe three types: type 1, connective tissue with no glands or other epithelial structures and a few inflammatory cells; type 2, abundant connective tissue containing some small glands lined with epithelium, with the additional finding of many mononuclear and polymorphonuclear inflammatory cells; and type 3, connective tissue with central bile ducts lined by columnar epithelium. Glands were found peripherally and many inflammatory cells were present. Following operation, bile flow was restored in 13 of 15 cases of type 2, and 12 of 15 in type 3. Despite the absence of any identifiable biliary structures, bile drainage occurred in 6 of the 13 type-1 patients.

The presence of abundant inflammatory cells in types 2 and 3 but few in type 1 again suggests a dynamic process in which inflammation of well-preserved bile ducts (type 3) may occur, followed by progressive obstruction, disappearance of inflammatory cells, and finally obliteration of ductular lumens.

Chandra and Altman analyzed the results of portoenterostomy based on the size of the atretic ducts.[328] When the duct lumen was 150 μ or greater, (type I) bile drainage occurred in all five patients. When single to multiple ductal structures were present measuring less than 150 μ (type II), drainage occurred in 18 of 21 patients; whereas in those patients with no identifiable epithelial-lined structures in fibrous connective tissue (type III), only one of eight demonstrated bile drainage.

The major complications of portoenterostomy are recurrent cholangitis (in 50%–71% of cases), increased intrahepatic fibrosis and portal hypertension (50%–60% of cases). Altman, Chandra, and Lilly found progressive hepatic fibrosis in 8 of 11 surviving infants after bile flow had been successfully restored.[329] Nevertheless, Kasai has reported 20 of his patients who are well 5 to 22 years after surgery.[318]

Although the outcome for many infants with EHBA remains discouraging, the chances for long-term survival have clearly improved, particularly when operative correction is achieved in the first 2 months of life.

REFERENCES

1. **Brodersen R:** Prevention of kernicterus based on recent progress in bilirubin chemistry. Acta Paediatr Scand 66:625–634, 1977
2. **Brodersen R:** Free bilirubin in blood plasma of the newborn: Effects of albumin, fatty acids, pH, displacing drugs, and phototherapy. In Stern L, Oh W, Friis-Hansen B (eds): Intensive Care of the Newborn, II, pp 331–345. New York, Masson Publishing, 1978
3. **Schmid R:** Bilirubin metabolism: State of the art. Gastroenterology 74:1307–1312, 1978
4. **Wennberg RP, Ahlfors CE, Rasmussen LF:** The pathochemistry of kernicterus. Early Human Development 3/4:353, 1979
5. **Bonnett R, Davies JE, Hursthouse MB, Sheldrick GM:** The structure of bilirubin. Proc R Soc Lond [Biol] 202:249, 1978
6. **Brodersen R:** Bilirubin, solubility and interaction with albumin and phospholipid. J Biol Chem 254:2364–2369, 1979
7. **Stoll MS, Zenone EA, Ostrow JD, Zarembo JE:** Preparation and properties of bilirubin photoisomers. Biochem J 183:139–146, 1979
8. **Robinson SH:** The origins of bilirubin. New Engl J Med 279:143, 1968
9. **Wolkoff AW, Goresky CA, Sellin J, Gratmaitan ZA, Arias IM:** Role of ligandin in transfer of bilirubin from plasma into liver. Am J Physiol 236:E638, 1979
10. **Wolkoff AW, Ketley JN, Waggoner JG, Berk PD, Jakoby WB:** Hepatic accumulation and intracellular binding of conjugated bilirubin. J Clin Invest 61:142–149, 1978
11. **Listowsky I, Gatmaitan Z, Arias IM:** Ligandin retains and albumin loses bilirubin binding capacity in liver cytosol. Proc Natl Acad Sci USA 75:1213, 1978
12. **Rosenthal P, Blanckaert N, Kabra PM, Thaler MM:** Formation and clearance of bilirubin conjugates in human newborns. Gastroenterology 77:A35, 1979 (abstract).
13. **Jansen PLM, Chowdlaury JR, Fischberg EG et al:** Enzymatic conversion of bilirubin monoglocuronide to diglucuronide by rat liver plasma membranes. J Biol Chem 252:2710–2716, 1977
14. **Wynn RJ, Schreiner RL:** Spurious elevation of amniotic fluid bilirubin in acute hydramnios with fetal intestinal obstruction. Am J Obstet Gynecol 134:105, 1979
15. **Goodlin R, Lloyd D:** Fetal tracheal excretion of bilirubin. Biol Neonate 12:1, 1968
16. **Lathe GH, Walker M:** The synthesis of bilirubin glucuronide in animal and human liver. Biochem J 70:705, 1958
17. **Felsher BF, Maidman JE, Carpio NM, VanCouvering K, Woolley MM:** Reduced hepatic bilirubin uridine diphosphate glucuronyl transferase and uridine diphosphate glucose dehydrogenase activity in the human fetus. Pediatr Res 12:838, 1978
18. **Gartner LM, Lee K-S, Vaisman S, Lane D, Zarafu I:** Development of bilirubin transport and metabolism in the newborn rhesus monkey. J Pediatr 90:513, 1977
19. **Bartoletti AL, Stevenson DK, Ostrander CR, Johnson JD:** Pulmonary excretion of carbon monoxide in the human infant as an index of bilirubin production, I, Effects of gestational age and postnatal age and some common neonatal abnormalities. J Pediatr 94:952, 1979
20. **Maisels MJ, Pathak A, Nelson NM, Nathan DG, Smith CA:** Endogenous production of carbon monoxide in normal and erythroblastotic newborn infants. J Clin Invest 50:1, 1971
21. **Brodersen R, Herman LS:** Intestinal reabsorption of unconjugated bilirubin: A possible contributing factor in neonatal jaundice. Lancet 1:1242, 1963
22. **Poland RD, Odell GB:** Physiologic jaundice: The enterohepatic circulation of bilirubin. New Eng J Med 284:1, 1971
23. **Levi AJ, Gatmaitan Z, Adias I:** Deficiency of hepatic organic onion-binding protein, impaired organic anion uptake by liver and "physiologic jaundice" in newborn monkeys. New Engl J Med 283:1136, 1970
24. **Zink J, van Patten GR:** Time course of closure of the ductus venosus in the newborn lamb. Pediatr Res 14:1, 1980
25. **Wood B, Culley P, Roginski C, Powell J, Waterhouse J:** Factors affecting neonatal jaundice. Arch Dis Child 54:111–115, 1979
26. **Hannemann RE, DeWitt DP, Wiechel JF:** Neonatal serum bilirubin from skin reflectance. Pediatr Res 12:207, 1978

27. Yamanouchi I, Yamauchi Y, Ikuko I: Transcutaneous bilirubinometry: Preliminary studies of noninvasive transcutaneous bilirubin meter in the Okayama National Hospital. Pediatrics 65:195, 1980

28. Chavalitdhamrong P-O, Escobedo MB, Barton LL, Zarkowsky H, Marshall RE: Hyperbilirubinemia and bacterial infection in the newborn. Arch Dis Child 50:652, 1975

29. Maisels MJ, Gifford K: Neonatal jaundice and breastfeeding. Pediatr Res 9:308, 1975

30. Thaler MM: Algorithmic diagnosis of conjugated and unconjugated hyperbilirubinemia. JAMA 237:58, 1977

31. Hardy JB, Drage JS, Jackson EC: The first year of life, p 104. The Collaborative Perinatal Project of the National Institutes of Neurological and Communicative Disorders and Stroke. Baltimore, The Johns Hopkins University Press, 1979

32. Campbell N, Harvey D, Norman AP: Increased frequency of neonatal jaundice in a maternity hospital. Br Med J 2:548–552, 1975

33. Sims DG, Neligan GA: Factors affecting the increasing incidence of severe non-haemolytic neonatal jaundice. Br. J. Obstet. Gynecol. 82:863–867, 1975

34. Gartner LM, Lee K-S: Jaundice and liver disease. In Behrman RE (ed): Neonatal Perinatal Medicine, p 394. St Louis, CV Mosby, 1977

35. Saland J, McNamara H, Cohen MI: Navajo jaundice: A variant of neonatal hyperbilirubinemia associated with breast feeding. J Pediatr 85:271, 1974

36. Yeung CY, Tam LS, Chan A, Lee KH: Phenobarbitone prophylaxis for neonatal hyperbilirubinemia. Pediatrics 48:372, 1971

37. Valaes T, Petmezaki S, Doxiadis SE: Effect on neonatal hyperbilirubinemia of phenobarbital during pregnancy or after birth: Practical value of the treatment in a population with high risk of unexplained severe neonatal jaundice. In Bergsma D (ed.), Bilirubin Metabolism in the Newborn. Birth Defects. Original Article Series 6:46, 1970

38. Fessas PH, Doxiadis SA, Valaes T: Neonatal jaundice in glucose-6-phosphate dehydrogenase deficient infants. Br Med J 11:1359, 1962

39. Horiguchi T, Bauer C: Ethnic differences in neonatal jaundice: Comparison of Japanese and Caucasian newborn infants. Am J Obstet Gynec 121:71, 1975

40. Drew JH, Kitchen WH: Jaundice in infants of Greek parentage: The unknown factor may be environmental. J Pediatr 89:284, 1976

41. Beazley JM, Alderman B: Neonatal hyperbilirubinaemia following the use of oxytocin in labour. Br J Obstet Gynecol 82:265–271, 1975

42. Weakes ARL, Beazley JM: Neonatal serum bilirubin levels following the use of prostaglandin E_2 in labour. Prostaglandins 10: 699–714, 1975

43. Calder AA, Ounsted MK, Moar VA, Turnbull AC: Increased bilirubin levels in neonates after induction of labour by intravenous prostaglandin E_2 or oxytocin. Lancet 2: 1339–1342, 1974

44. Chew WC: Neonatal hyperbilirubinaemia: A comparison between prostaglandin E_2 and oxytocin inductions. Br Med J 3:679–680, 1977

45. Chew WC, Swann IL: Influence of simultaneous low amniotomy and oxytocin infusion and other maternal factors on neonatal jaundice: A prospective study. Br Med J 1:72–73, 1977

46. Davies DP, Gomersall R, Robertson R, Gray OP, Turnbull AC: Neonatal jaundice and maternal oxytocin infusion. Br Med J 3: 476–477, 1973

47. Boylan P: Oxytocin and neonatal jaundice Br Med J 3:564–565, 1976

48. Buchan PC: Pathogenesis of neonatal hyperbilirubinemia after induction of labour with oxytocin. Br Med J 2:1255, 1979

49. Drew JH, Kitchen WH: The effect of maternally administered drugs on bilirubin concentrations in the newborn infant. J Pediatr 89:657–661, 1976

50. Levine RL: Perinatal influence on the hyperbilirubinemia of the newborn infant. J Pediatr 90:859, 1977

51. Silverman WA, Andersen DH, Blanc WA, Crozier DN: A difference in mortality rate in incidence of kernicterus among premature infants allotted to two prophylactic antibacterial regimens. Pediatrics 18:614, 1956

52. Krauss AN, Dahms BB, Gartner LM, Auld PAM: Serum bilirubin values in first 4 postnatal days of breast fed and bottle fed infants (letter). J Pediatr 85:285, 1974

53. Wennberg RP, Schwartz R, Sweet AY: Early versus delayed feeding of low birth weight infants: Effects on physiologic jaundice. J Pediatr 68:800, 1966

54. Gartner LM, Lee K-S: Effect of starvation and milk feeding on intestinal bilirubin absorption (abstr). Gastroenterology 77:A13, 1979

55. Bloomer JR, Barrett PV, Rodkey FL, Berlin NI: Studies of the mechanisms of fasting hyperbilirubinemia. Gastroenterology 61: 479, 1971

56. Dahms BB, Krauss AN, Gartner LM, Klain DB, Soodalter J, Auld PAM: Breast feeding

and serum bilirubin values during the first 4 days of life. J Pediatr 83:1049–1054, 1973

57. **Saigal S, O'Neill A, Surainder Y, Chua L-B, Usher R:** Placental transfusion and hyperbilirubinemia in the premature. Pediatrics 49: 406–419, 1972

58. **Drew JH, Barrie J, Horacek I, Kitchen WH:** Factors influencing jaundice in immigrant Greek infants. Arch Dis Child 53:49–52, 1978

59. **Gross SJ:** Vitamin E and neonatal bilirubinemia. Pediatrics 64:321, 1979

60. **Wysowski DK, Flynt JW, Goldfield M, Altman R, Davis AT:** Epidemic neonatal hyperbilirubinemia and use of a phenolic disinfectant detergent. Pediatrics 61:165, 1978

61. **Daum F, Cohen MI, McNamara H:** Experimental toxicologic studies on a phenol detergent associated with neonatal hyperbilirubinemia. J Pediatr 89:853, 1976

62. **Bleicher MA, Reiner MA, Rapaport SA, Track NS:** Extraordinary hyperbilirubinemia in a neonate with idiopathic hypertrophic pyloric stenosis. J Pediatr Surg 14:527, 1979

63. **Wooley MM, Felsher BF, Asch MJ et al:** Jaundice, hypertrophic pyloric stenosis, and glucuronyl transferase. J Pediatr Surg 9:359, 1974

64. **Valaes T:** Bilirubin metabolism: Review and discussion of inborn errors. Clin Perinatol 3: 177, 1976

65. **Lucey JF, Arias I, McKay R:** Transient familial neonatal hyperbilirubinemia. Am J Dis Child 100:787, 1960

65a. **Gartner LM, Arias I:** Studies of prolonged neonatal jaundice in the breast-fed infant. J Pediatr 68:54, 1966

66. **Ramos A, Silverberg M, Stern L:** Pregnanediols and neonatal hyperbilirubinemia. Amer J Dis Child 111:353, 1966

67. **Severi F, Rondine G, Zaverio S and Vegni M:** Prolonged neonatal hyperbilirubinemia and pregnane (3 alpha, 20 beta) diol in maternal milk. Helv Paediat Acta 25:517, 1970

68. **Adlard BPF, Lath GH:** Specificity of the effects of steroids on bilirubin glucuronide transport by liver slice. Biochim Biophys Acta 237:132, 1971

69. **Bevan BR, Holten JB, Lathe GH:** The effect of pregnanediol and pregnanediol glucuronide on bilirubin conjugation by rat liver slices. Clin Sci 29:253, 1965

70. **Bevan BR, Holten JB:** Inhibition of bilirubin conjugation in rat liver slices by free fatty acids, with relevance to the problem of breast-milk jaundice. Clin Chim Acta 41:101, 1972

71. **Cole AP, Hargreaves T:** Conjugation inhibitors in early neonatal hyperbilirubinemia. Arch Dis Child 47:451, 1972

72. **Maurer HM, Fratkin M, McWilliams NB, Kirkpatrick B, Draper D, Haggins JC, Hunter CR:** Effects of phototherapy on platelet counts in low birthweight infants and on platelet production and lifespan in rabbits. Pediatrics 57:506, 1976

73. **Hargreaves T:** Effect of fatty acids on bilirubin conjugation. Arch Dis Child 48:446, 1973

74. **Foliot TA, Ploussard JP, Housset E, Christoforov B, Luzeau R, Odievre M:** Breast milk jaundice: In vitro inhibition of rat liver bilirubinuridine diphosphate glucuronyl transferase activity and Z protein-bromosulfophthalein binding by human breast milk. Pediatr Res 10:594, 1976

75. **Luzeau R, Levillain P, Odievre M, Lemonnier A:** Demonstration of a lipolytic activity in human milk that inhibits the glucuro-conjugation of bilirubin. Biomedicine 21:258, 1974

76. **Odievre M, Luzeau R:** Lipolytic activity in milk from mothers of unjaundiced infants. Acta Paediatr Scand 67:49, 1978

77. **Winfield CR, MacFaul R:** Clinical study of prolonged jaundice in breast- and bottle-fed babies. Arch Dis Child 53:506, 1978

78. **Jesurun CA, Ostrea EM Jr:** Elevated serum bilirubin and albumin saturation in breast fed infants: Role of supplemental feedings. Pediatr Res 13:497, 1979 (abstract)

79. **Seeler RA, Hahn K:** Jaundice and urinary tract infection in infancy. Am J Dis Child 118:553, 1969

80. **Hsia D Y-Y, Allen FH, Gellis SS, Diamond LK:** Erythroblastosis fetalis. VIII. Studies of serum bilirubin in relation to kernicterus. New Engl J Med 247:668, 1952

81. **Mollison PL, Cutbush M:** Haemolytic disease of the newborn. In Gairdner D (ed.): Recent Advances in Pediatrics, p 110. New York, The Blakiston Co., Inc., 1954

82. **Karp WB:** Biochemical alterations in neonatal hyperbilirubinemia and bilirubin encephalopathy: A review. Pediatrics 64:361, 1979

83. **Perlstein MA:** The late clinical syndrome of post-icteric encephalopathy. Pediatr Clin N Amer 7:665, 1960

84. **Mollison PL, Walker W:** Controlled trials of the treatment of hemolytic disease of the newborn. Lancet 1:429, 1952

85. **Wishingrad L, Cornblath M, Takakuwa P, Rozenfeld IM, Elegant LD, Kauffman A, Lassers E, Klein RI:** Studies of non-hemolytic hyperbilirubinemia in premature infants. Prospective randomized selection for exchange transfusion with observations on the levels of serum bilirubin with and without exchange transfusion and neurologic evalu-

ations one year after birth. Pediatrics 36:162, 1965

86. Shiller JG, Silverman WA: "Uncomplicated" hyperbilirubinemia of prematurity. Am J Dis Child 101:587, 1961

86a. Hugh-Jones K, Slack J, Simpson K, Grossman A, Hsia DY-Y: Clinical course of hyperbilirubinemia in premature infants. New Engl J Med 263:1223, 1960

87. Stern L, Denton RL: Kernicterus in small premature infants. Pediatrics 35:483, 1965

88. Gartner LM, Snyder RN, Chabon RS, Bernstein J: Kernicterus: High incidence in premature infants with low serum bilirubin concentrations. Pediatrics 45:906, 1970

89. Johnson L, Boggs TR: Bilirubin-dependent brain damage: Incidence and indications for treatment. In Odell GB, Schaffer R, Simopoulous AP (eds): Phototherapy in the Newborn: An Overview, pp 122–149. Washington, D.C., National Academy of Sciences, 1974

90. Naeye RL: The role of congenital bacterial infections in low serum bilirubin brain damage. Pediatrics 62:497, 1978

91. Odell GB, Storey GNB, Rosenberg LA: Studies in kernicterus. III. The saturation of serum proteins with bilirubin during neonatal life and its relationship to brain damage at five years. J Pediatr 76:12, 1970

92. Scheidt PC, Mellits ED, Hardy JB, Drage JS, Boggs TR: Toxicity to bilirubin in neonates. Infant development during first year in relation to maximum neonatal serum bilirubin concentration. J Pediatr 91:292, 1977

93. Pearlman MA, Gartner LM, Lee K-S, Eidehman AI, Morecki R, Horoupian DS: The association of kernicterus with bacterial infection in the newborn. Pediatrics 65:26, 1980

94. Rubin RA, Balow B, Fisch RO: Neonatal serum bilirubin levels related to cognitive development at ages 4 through 7 years. J Pediatr 94:601, 1979

95. Crichton JU, Dunn HG, McBurney AK, Robertson A, Tredger E: Long-term effects of neonatal jaundice on brain function in children of very low birth weight. Pediatrics 49:656, 1972

96. Culley P, Powell J, Waterhouse J, Wood B: Sequelae of neonatal jaundice. Br Med J II:383, 1970

97. Pearlman MA, Gartner LM, Lee K-S, Morecki R, Horoupian DS: Absence of kernicterus in low birth weight infants from 1971 through 1976: Comparison with findings in 1966 and 1967. Pediatrics 62:460, 1978

98. Cashore WJ, Oh W: Unbound bilirubin and kernicterus in low birth weight infants. Pediatrics, in press

99. Hansen PE, Thiessen H, Brodersen R: Bilirubin acidity. Titrimetric and ^{13}C NMR studies. Acta Chem Scand [B] 33:289, 1979

100. Diamond I: Bilirubin binding and kernicterus. In Schulman I (ed): Advances in Pediatrics, vol 16, p 99. Chicago, Year Book Medical Publishers, 1969

101. Diamond I, Schmid R: Experimental bilirubin encephalopathy. The mode of entry of bilirubin-^{14}C into the central nervous system. J Clin Invest 45:678, 1966

102. Nelson P, Jacobsen J, Wennberg RP: Effect of pH on the interaction of bilirubin with albumin and tissue culture cells. Pediatr Res 8:963, 1974

103. Wennberg RP, Rasmussen LF: Factors determining the cellular uptake of bilirubin. Pediatr Res 12:536, 1978 (abstract)

104. Levine RL: Bilirubin: Worked out years ago? Pediatrics 64:380, 1979

105. Diamond I, Schmid R: Neonatal hyperbilirubinemia and kernicterus. Experimental support for treatment by exposure to visible light. Arch Neurol 18:699, 1968

106. Sato H, Semba R: Relationship between plasma unbound bilirubin concentrations and cerebellar bilirubin content in homozygous Gunn rat sucklings. Experientia 34:221, 1978

107. Sawasaki Y, Yamada N, Nakajima H: Developmental features of cerebellar, hypoplasia and brain bilirubin levels in a mutant (Gunn) rat with hereditary hyperbilirubinemia. J Neurochem 27:577, 1976

108. Cashore WJ, Gartner LM, Oh W, Stern L: Clinical application of neonatal bilirubin-binding determinations: Current status. J Pediatr 93:827, 1978

109. Gitzelmann-Cumarasamy N, Kuenzle CC: Bilirubin binding tests: Living up to expectations? Pediatrics 64:375, 1979

110. Lee K-S, Gartner LM: Bilirubin binding by plasma proteins: A critical evaluation of methods and clinical implications. In Scarpelli EM, Cosmi EV (eds): Reviews in Perinatal Medicine 2:319, 1978

111. Jacobsen J: Binding of bilirubin to human serum albumin: Determination of the dissociation constants. FEBS lett 5:112, 1969

112. Jacobsen J, Wennberg RP: Determination of unbound bilirubin in the serum of newborns. Clin Chem 20:783, 1974

113. Lee K-S, Gartner LM, Zarafu I: Fluorescent dye method for the determination of the bilirubin binding capacity of serum albumin. J Pediatr 86:280, 1975

114. Cashore WJ, Monin PJP, Oh W: Serum bilirubin binding capacity and free bilirubin concentrations: A comparison between Sephadex G-25 filtration and peroxidation techniques. Pediatr Res 12:195, 1978

115. **Schiff D, Chan G, Stern L:** Sephadex G-25 quantitative estimation of free bilirubin potential in jaundiced newborn infant's sera: A guide to the prevention of kernicterus. J Lab Clin Med 80:455, 1972

116. **Kapitulnik J, Valaes T, Kaufman NA, Blondheim SH:** Clinical evaluation of Sephadex gel filtration in estimation of bilirubin binding in serum in neonatal jaundice. Arch Dis Child 49:886, 1974

117. **Bratlid D:** Reserve albumin binding capacity, salicylate index, and red cell binding of bilirubin and neonatal jaundice. Arch Dis Child 48:393, 1973

118. **Seem E, Wille L:** Salicylate saturation index in neonatal jaundice. Biol Neonate 26:67, 1975

119. **Lee K-S, Gartner LM, Vaisman SL:** Measurement of bilirubin-albumin binding, I. Comparative analysis of four methods and four human serum albumin preparations. Pediatr Res 12:301, 1978

120. **Wennberg RP, Lau M, Rasmussen LF:** Clinical significance of unbound bilirubin. Pediatr Res 10:434, 1976 (abstract)

121. **Wennberg RP, Rasmussen LF, Ahlfors CE, Valaes T:** Mechanized determination of the apparent unbound unconjugated bilirubin concentration in serum. Clin Chem 25:1444, 1979

122. **Priolisi A:** Clinical experience with Sephadex gel filtration for the estimation of non-albumin bound bilirubin in sera of jaundiced infants. *In* Bilirubin Metabolism in the Newborn. Vol. 2, Bergsma D and Blondheim SH (eds.), pp. 243–254, American Elsevier, New York, 1976

123. **Valaes T, Kapitulnik J, Kauffmann NA, Blondheim SH:** Experience with Sephadex gel filtration in assessing the risk of bilirubin encephalopathy in neonatal jaundice. *In* Bilirubin Metabolism in the Newborn. Vol. 2, Bergsma D and Blondheim SH (eds.), pp. 215–228, American Elsevier, New York, 1976

124. **Zamet P, Nakamura H, Perez-Robles S, Larroche JC:** Determination of unbound bilirubin and the prevention of kernicterus. *In* Bilirubin Metabolism in the Newborn. Vol. 2, Bergsma D and Blondheim SH (eds.), pp. 236–244, American Elsevier, New York, 1976

125. **Zamet P, Nakamura H, Perez-Robles S, Larroche JC, Minkowski A:** The use of critical levels of birth weight and "free bilirubin" as an approach for prevention of kernicterus. Biol Neonate 26:274, 1975

126. **Lamola AA, Eisinger J, Blumberg WE, Patel SC, Flores J:** Fluorometric study of the partition of bilirubin among blood components: Basis for rapid microassays of bilirubin and bilirubin binding capacity in whole blood. Anal Biochem 101:25, 1979

127. **Brodersen R:** Determination of the vacant amount of high-affinity bilirubin binding site on serum albumin. Acta Pharmacol Toxicol 42:153, 1978

128. **Andrew G, Chan G, Schiff D:** Lipid metabolism in the neonate, II, The effect of intralipid of bilirubin binding in vitro and in vivo. J Pediatr 88:279, 1976

129. **Odell GB, Cukier JO, Ostrea EM Jr, Maglalang AC, Poland RL:** The influence of fatty acids on the binding of bilirubin to albumin. J Lab Clin Med 89:295, 1977

130. **Sato H, Semba R:** Effect of milk on plasma unbound-bilirubin concentration in homozygous Gunn rat sucklings. Experientia 33:59, 1977

131. **Thiessen H, Jacobsen J, Brodersen R:** Displacement of albumin-bound bilirubin by fatty acids. Acta Paediatr Scand 61:285, 1972

132. **Gartner LM, Lee KS:** Bilirubin binding, free fatty acids and a new concept for the pathogenesis of kernicterus. Birth Defects Original Article Series 12:264, 1976

133. **Thaler MM, Pelger A:** Influence of intravenous nutrients on bilirubin transport. III. Emulsified fat infusion. Pediatr Res 11:171, 1977

133a. **Thaler MM, Wennberg RP:** Influence of intravenous nutrients on bilirubin transport II. Emulsified lipid solutions. Pediatr Res 11:167, 1977

134. **Wennberg RP, Thaler MM:** Influence of intravenous nutrients on bilirubin transport. I. Amino acid solutions. Peditar Res 11:163, 1977

135. **Stern L, Doray B, Chan G, Schiff D:** Bilirubin metabolism and the induction of kernicterus. *In* Bergsma D and Blondheim SH (eds.), Bilirubin Metabolism in the Newborn (II) Birth Defects: Original Articles Series, Vol. 12, p. 255, 1976

136. **Lending M, Slobody LB, Meston J:** The relationship of hypercapnea to the production of kernicterus. Dev Med Child Neurol 9:145, 1966

137. **Chunga F, Lardinois R:** Separation by gel filtration and microdetermination of unbound bilirubin, I. In vitro albumin and acidosis effects on albumin-bilirubin binding. Acta Pediatr Scand 60:27, 1971

138. **Levine RL:** Fluorescence-quenching studies of the binding of bilirubin to albumin. Clin Chem 23:2292, 1972

139. **Jacobsen J, Brodersen R:** The effect of ph on albumin-bilirubin binding affinity. Birth Defects Original Article Series 12:175, 1976

140. **Kozuki K, Oh W, Widness J, Cashore W:**

Increase in bilirubin binding to albumin with correction of neonatal acidosis. Acta Paediatr Scand 68:213, 1979

141. **Bratlid D:** The effect of pH on bilirubin binding to human erythrocytes. Scand J Clin Lab Invest 29:453, 1972

142. **Odell GB:** The influence of pH on distribution of bilirubin between albumin and mitochondria. Proc Soc Exp Biol Med 120:352, 1965

143. **Silberberg DH, Johnson L, Ritter L:** Factors influencing toxicity of bilirubin in cerebellum tissue culture. J Pediatr 77:386, 1970

144. **Cashore WJ, Oh W:** Effect of acidosis on bilirubin uptake by rat brain in vivo (abstr). Pediatr Res 13:523, 1979

145. **Lucey JF, Hibbard E, Behrman RE, Esquivel de Gallardo FO, Windle WF:** Kernicterus in asphyxiated newborn rhesus monkeys. Exp Neurol 9:43, 1964

146. **Arkans HD, Cassady G:** Estimation of unbound serum bilirubin by the peroxidase assay method: Effect of exchange transfusion on unbound bilirubin and serum binding. J Pediatr 92:1001, 1978

147. **Valaes T, Hyte M:** Effect of exchange transfusion on bilirubin binding. Pediatrics 59:881, 1977

148. **Cashore WJ, Horwich A, Karotkin EH, Oh W:** Influence of gestational age and clinical status on bilirubin-binding capacity in newborn infants. Am J Dis Child 131:898, 1977

149. **Nasralla M, Gawronska E, Hsia D-Y:** Studies on the relation between serum and spinal fluid bilirubin during early infancy. J Clin Invest 37:1403, 1958

150. **Stempfel R, Zetterstrom R:** Concentration of bilirubin cerebrospinal fluid and hemolytic disease of the newborn. Pediatrics 16:184, 1955

151. **Blumenschein SD, Kallen RJ, Storey B, Natzschka C, Odell GB, Childs B:** Familial nonhemolytic jaundice with late onset of neurological damage. Pediatrics 42:786, 1968

152. **Chiueh CC, Sun CL, Kopin IJ, Fredericks WR, Rapoport SI:** Entry of [³H]norepinephrine, [¹²⁵I]albumin and Evans blue from blood into brain following unilateral osmotic opening of the blood-brain barrier. Brain Res 145:291, 1978

153. **Braun LD, Cornford EM, Oldendorf WH:** Newborn rabbit blood-brain barrier is selectively permeable and differs substantially from the adult. J Neurochem 34:147, 1980

154. **Barranger JA, Rapoport SI, Fredericks WR, Pentchev PG, MacDermot KD, Steusing JK, Brady RO:** Modification of the blood-brain barrier: Increased concentration and fate of enzymes entering the brain. Proc Natl Acad Sci USA 76:481, 1979

155. **Rapoport SI:** Blood-brain barrier in physiology and medicine. New York, Raven Press, 1976

156. **Ito U, Go KG, Walker JT Jr et al:** Experimental cerebral ischemia in mongolian gerbils, III. Behavior of the blood-brain barrier. Acta Neuropathol (Berl) 34:1, 1976

157. **Haque KN:** Value of measuring cord blood bilirubin concentration in ABO incompatibility. Brit Med J 2:1604, 1978

158. **Wennberg RP, Depp R, Heinrichs WL:** Indications for early exchange transfusion in patients with erythroblastosis fetalis. J Pediatr 92:789, 1978

159. **Allen FH, Diamond LK:** Erythroblastosis Fetalis Including Exchange Transfusion Technique. Boston, Little, Brown and Co, 1958

160. **Zuelzer WW, Cohen I:** ABO hemolytic disease and heterospecific pregnancy. Pediatr Clin North Amer 4:405, 1957

161. **Phibbs RH, Johnson P, Kitterman JA, Gregory GA, Tooley WH:** Cardiorespiratory status of erythroblastotic infants: Relationship of gestational age, severity of hemolytic disease, and birth asphyxia to idiopathic respiratory distress syndrome and survival. Pediatrics 49:5, 1972

162. **Phibbs RH, Johnson P, Tooley WH:** Cardiorespiratory status of erythroblastotic newborn infants. II. Blood volume, hematocrit, and serum albumin concentration in relation to hydrops fetalis. Pediatrics 53:13, 1974

163. **Brans YW, Milstead RR, Bailey PE, Cassady G:** Blood volume estimates in Coombs-test-positive infants. N Engl J Med 290:1450, 1974

164. **Phibbs RH, Johnson P, Kitterman JA, Gregory GA, Tooley WH, Schlueter M:** Cardiorespiratory status of erythroblastotic newborn infants. III. Intravascular pressures during the first hours of life. Pediatrics 58:484, 1976

165. **Maisels MJ:** Bilirubin. On understanding and influencing its metabolism in the newborn infant. Pediatr Clin North Am 19:447, 1972

166. **Grawjer LA, Pildes R, Zarif M, Ainis H, Agrawal BL, Patel A:** Exchange transfusion in the neonate: A controlled study using frozen-stored erythrocytes resuspended in plasma. Am J Clin pathol 66:117, 1976

167. **Kreuger A, Blomback M:** Exchange transfusions with frozen blood. Hemostasis 3:329, 1974

168. **Bursaux E, Freminet A, Brossard Y, Poyart CF:** Exchange transfusion in the neonate with ACD or CPD stored blood. Biol Neonate 23:123, 1973

169. **Delivoria-Papadoupoulos M, Morrow G, Oski**

FA: Exchange transfusion in the newborn infant with fresh and ''old'' blood: The role of storage on 2,3-diphosphoglycerate, hemoglobin-oxygen affinity and oxygen release. J Pediatr 79:898, 1971

170. **Bunker JP, Bendixen HH, Murphy AJ:** Hemodynamic effects of intravenously administered sodium citrate. N Engl J Med 266:372, 1962

171. **Maisels MJ, Li TK, Piechocki JT, Wertham MW:** The effect of exchange transfusion on serum ionized calcium. Pediatrics 53:683, 1974

172. **Wieland P, Duc G, Binswanger U, Fischer JA:** Parathyroid hormone response in newborn infants during exchange transfusion with blood supplemented with citrate and phosphate: Effect of IV calcium. Pediatr Res 13:963, 1979

173. **Ellis MI, Hey EN, Walker W:** Neonatal death in babies with rhesus isoimmunization. Q J Med 48:211, 1979

174. **Maisels MJ, Friedman Z, Marks KH, Uhrmann S, Lee C, Denlinger JK:** Calcium homeostasis in exchange transfusion. Pediatr Res 11:537, 1977 (abstract)

175. **Gibson JG II:** International forum. Vox Sang 19:546, 1970

176. **Pierson WE, Barrett CT, Oliver TK Jr:** The effect of buffered and non-buffered ACD blood on electrolyte and acid base homeostasis during exchange transfusion. Pediatrics 41:802, 1968

177. **Walker WF, Griffiths PD:** pH of infusion fluids. Lancet 1:1010, 1967

178. **Bailey DN, Bove JR:** Chemical and hematological changes in stored CPD blood. Transfusion 15:244, 1975

179. **Schiff D, Aranda JV, Chan G, Colle E, Stern L:** Metabolic effects of exchange transfusions. I. Effect of citrated and of heparinized blood on glucose, non-esterified fatty acids, 2-(4 hydroxybenzeneazo) benzoic acid binding and insulin. J Pediatr 78:603, 1971

180. **Sproul A, Smith I:** Bilirubin equilibration during exchange tranfusion in hemolytic disease of the newborn. J Pediatr 65:12, 1964

181. **Chan G, Schiff D:** Variance in albumin loading in exchange transfusions. J Pediatr 88:609, 1976

182. **Valaes T:** Bilirubin distribution and dynamics of bilirubin removal by exchange transfusion. Acta Paediatr 52 (Suppl. 149), 1963

183. **Phibbs RH:** Advances in the theory and practice of exchange transfusions. Calif Med 105:442, 1966

184. **Aranda JV, Sweet AY:** Alterations in blood pressure during exchange transfusion. Arch Dis Child 52:545, 1977

185. **Bowman JM:** Hemolytic disease of the newborn (erythroblastosis fetalis). In Gellis SS, Kagan BM (eds): Current Pediatric Therapy p 262. Philadelphia, WB Saunders, 1971

186. **Martin JR:** A double catheter technique for exchange transfusion in the newborn infant. NZ Med J 77:167, 1973

187. **Campbell N, Stewart I:** Exchange transfusion in ill newborn infants using peripheral arteries and veins. J Pediatr 94:820, 1979

188. **Scanlon JW, Krakaur R:** Hyperkalemia following exchange transfusion. J Pediatr 96:108, 1980

189. **Bada HS, Chau C, Salmon JH, Hajjar W:** Changes in intracranial pressure during exchange transfusion. J Pediatr 94:129, 1979

190. **Odell GB, Bryan WB, Richmond MD:** Exchange transfusion. Pediatr Clin North Amer 9:605, 1962

191. **Simmons PB, Harris LE, Bianco AJ Jr:** Complications of exchange transfusion. Report of two cases of septic arthritis and osteomyelitis. Mayo Clin Proc 48:190, 1973

192. **Doyle PE, Eidelman AI, Lee K-S, Daum C, Gartner LM:** Exchange transfusion and hypernatremia: Possible role in intracranial hemorrhage in very-low-birth-weight infants. J Pediatr 92:848, 1978

193. **Touloukian RJ, Kadar A, Spencer RP:** The gastrointestinal complications of neonatal umbilical venous exchange transfusion. A clinical and experimental study. Pediatrics 51:36, 1973

194. **Shapiro N, Stein H, Olinsky A:** Necrotizing enterocolitis and exchange transfusion. S Afr Med J 47:1236, 1973

195. **Parkman R, Mosier D, Umanski I, Cochran W, Carpenter C, Rosen FS:** Graft versus host disease after intrauterine and exchange transfusions for hemolytic disease of the newborn. New Engl J Med 290:359, 1974

196. **Murphy RJC, Malhotra C, Sweet AY:** Death following an exchange transfusion with hemoglobin SC blood. J Pediatr 96:110, 1980

197. **Cremer RJ, Perryman PW, Richards DH:** Influence of light on the hyperbilirubinemia of infants. Lancet 1:1094, 1958

198. **Maisels MJ:** Phototherapy. In Iatrogenic Problems in Neonatal Intensive Care, p 54. Report of the 69th Ross Conference on Pediatric Research. Ross Laboratories, Columbus, Ohio, 1976

199. **Lucey JF:** Neonatal jaundice and phototherapy. Pediatr Clin North Am 19:827, 1972

200. **Tan KL:** Comparison of the effectiveness of phototherapy and exchange transfusion in the management of nonhemolytic neonatal hyperbilirubinemia. J Pediatr 87:609, 1975

201. **Moller J, Ebbesen F:** Phototherapy in new-

born infants with severe rhesus hemolytic disease. J Pediatr 86:135, 1975

202. **Sisson TRC, Slaven B, Hamilton PB:** Effect of broad and narrow spectrum fluorescent light on blood constituents. *In* Bergsma D and Blondheim S (eds.) Bilirubin Metabolism in the Newborn, II., New York, American Elsevier Publishing Co., Inc., 1976, p. 122

203. **Ente G, Lanning EW, Cukor P, Klein RM:** Chemical variables and new lamps in phototherapy. Pediatr Res 6:246, 1972

204. **Sisson TRC, Kendall N, Shaw E, Kechavarz-Oliai L:** Phototherapy of jaundice in the newborn infant. II. Effect of various light intensities. J Pediatr 81:35, 1972

205. **Tan KL:** The nature of the dose-response relationship of phototherapy for neonatal hyperbilirubinemia. J Pediatr 90:448, 1977

206. **Bonta BW, Warshaw JB:** Importance of radiant flux in the treatment of hyperbilirubinemia: Failure of overhead phototherapy units in intensive care units. Pediatrics 57:502, 1976

207. **Anderson RJ:** Radiometry and dosimetry as applied to phototherapy. US Dept Health, Education, and Welfare, Publication No (NIH) 76–1075, 1977

208. **Hegyi T, Hiatt IM, Vogl TP, Indyke L:** Use of the Beckman film badge for monitoring during phototherapy. J Pediatr 89:473, 1976

209. **Tab PA, Inglis J, Savage DCL, Walker CHM:** Controlled trial of phototherapy of limited duration in the treatment of physiologic hyperbilirubinemia in low-birth-weight infants. Lancet 2:1211, 1972

210. **Lee K-S, Gartner LM, Eidelman AI, Ezhuthachan S:** Unconjugated hyperbilirubinemia in very low birth weight infants. Clin Perinatol 4:305, 1977

211. **Maurer HM, Shumway CN, Draper DA, Hossaini AA:** Control trial comparing agar, intermittent phototherapy and continuous phototherapy for reducing neonatal hyperbilirubinemia. J Pediatr 82:73, 1973

212. **Rubaltelli FF, Zanardo V, Granati B:** Effect of various phototherapy regimens on bilirubin decrement. Pediatrics 61:838, 1978

213. **Vogl TP, Hegy IT, Hiatt IM, Polin RA, Indyk L:** Intermittent phototherapy in the treatment of jaundice in the premature infant. J. Pediatr. 92:627, 1978.

214. **Zachman RD:** Alternate phototherapy in neonatal hyperbilirubinemia. Biol. Neonate 25:283, 1974.

215. **Wu PYK, Lim RC, Hodgman JE, Kokosky MJ, Teberg AM:** Effect of phototherapy in preterm infants on growth in the neonatal period. J. Pediatr. 85:563, 1974.

216. **Indyk L:** Physical aspects of phototherapy.

In Bergsma D, Blondheim SH (eds): Bilirubin Metabolism in the Newborn, II, p 23. New York, American Elsevier Publishing Co., Inc., 1976

217. **Vogl TP:** Phototherapy of neonatal hyperbilirubinemia: Bilirubin in unexposed areas of the skin. J. Pediatr. 85:707, 1974

218. **Indyk L:** The physics of phototherapy. In Brown AK, Showacker J (eds): Phototherapy for Neonatal Hyperbilirubinemia: Long Term Implications, p 207. Washington, D.C., U.S. Department of Health, Education, and Welfare, Publication No. (NIH) 76-1075, 1977

219. **Santella RG, Rosenkranz HS, Speck WT:** Intracellular deoxyribonucleic acid-modifying activity of intermittent phototherapy. J. Pediatr. 93:106, 1978.

220. **Nicolopoulos D, Hadjigeorgiou E, Malamitsi A, Kalpoyannis N, Karli I and Papadakis D:** Combined treatment of neonatal jaundice with cholestyramine and phototherapy. J. Pediatr. 93:684, 1978.

221. **Hewitt JR, Klein RM, Lucey JF:** Photodegradation of serum bilirubin in the Gunn rat. Biol Neonate 21:112, 1972

222. **Callahan EW Jr, Thaler MM, Karon M, Bauer K, Schmid R:** Phototherapy of severe unconjugated hyperbilirubinemia: Formation and removal of labelled bilirubin derivatives. Pediatrics 46:841, 1970

223. **Ostrow JD:** Photocatabolism of labeled bilirubin in the congenitally jaundiced (Gunn) rat. J. Clin. Invest. 50:707, 1971.

224. **Lund HT, Jacobsen J:** Influence of phototherapy on the biliary bilirubin excretion pattern in newborn infants with hyperbilirubinemia. J Pediatr 85:262, 1974

225. **McDonagh AF:** Photochemistry and photometabolism of bilirubin. In Brown AK, Showacre, J (eds): Phototherapy for Neonatal Hyperbilirubinemia: Long Term Implications, p. 171. Publication No. (NIH) 76-1075, U.S. Department of Health, Education, and Welfare, 1977

226. **Lightner DA, Wooldridge TA, McDonagh AF:** Configurational isomerization of bilirubin and the mechanism of jaundice phototherapy. Biochem Biophys Res Commun 86:235–243, 1979

227. **Lightner DA, Woodridge TA, McDonagh AF:** Photobilirubin: An early bilirubin photoproduct detected by absorbance difference spectroscopy. Proc Natl Acad Sci USA 76:29, 1979

228. **McDonagh AF and Ramonas LM: Jaundice phototherapy:** Microflow cell photometry reveals rapid biliary response of Gunn rats to light. Science 20:829, 1978

229. **McDonagh AF, Palma LA, Schmid R:** Geo-

metric isomerization of bilirubin in vivo: An important reaction in phototherapy of neonatal jaundice. Gastroenterology 77:A27, 1979 (abstract).

230. **Kapoor CL, Kirshna Murti CR:** Uptake and release of bilirubin by the skin. Biochem J 136:35, 1973

231. **Sisson TRC, Wickler M:** Transmission of light through living tissue. Pediatr. Res. 7:316, 1973

232. **Wurtman RJ, Cardinali DP:** The effects of light on man. *In* Bergsma D and Blondheim SH (eds.), Bilirubin Metabolism in the Newborn, (II), New York, American Elsevier Publishing Co., Inc., 1976, p. 100.

233. **Karon M, Imach D, Schwartz A:** Effective phototherapy in congenital nonobstructive, nonhemolytic jaundice. New Engl J Med 282:377, 1970

234. **Haddock JH, Nadler HL:** Bilirubin toxicity in human cultivated fibroblasts and its modification by light treatment (34724). Proc Soc Exp Biol Med 134:45, 1970

235. **Silberberg DH, Johnson L, Schutta H, Ritter L:** Effects of photodegradation products of bilirubin on myelinating cerebellum cultures. J. Pediatr. 77:613, 1970.

236. **Ostrea EM, Odell GB:** Photosensitized shift in the O_2 dissociation curve of fetal blood. Acta Pediatr. Scand. 63:341, 1974.

237. **Blackburn MG, Orzalesi MM, Pigram P:** Effect of light on fetal red blood cells in vivo. J Pediatr 80:641, 1972

238. **Kopelman AE, Ey JL, Lee H:** Phototherapy in newborn infants with glucose-6-phosphate dehydrogenase deficiency. J Pediatr 93:497, 1978

239. **Meloni T, Costa S, Dore A, Cutillo S:** Phototherapy for neonatal hyperbilirubinemia in mature infants with erythrocyte G-6-PD deficiency. J. Pediatr. 85:560, 1974

240. **Tan KL:** Photerapy for neonatal jaundice in erythrocyte glucose-6-phosphate dehydrogenase deficient infants. Pediatrics 59:1023, 1977

241. **McDonagh AF:** The Photochemistry and photometabolism of bilirubin. In Odell CB, Schaffer R, Simopoulos AP (eds): Phototherapy in the Newborn: An Overview, p 56. Washington, D.C., National Academy of Sciences, 1974

242. **Speck WT, Chen CC, Rosenkranz HS:** In vitro studies of effects of light and riboflavin on DNA and HeLa cells. Pediatr. Res. 9:115, 1975

243. **Speck WT, Rosenkranz HS:** The bilirubin-induced photodegradation of deoxyribonucleic acid. Pediatr. Res. 9:703, 1975.

244. **Speck WT, Rosenkranz HS:** Intracellular deoxyribonucleic acid-modifying activity of phototherapy lights. Pediatr. Res. 10:553, 1976

245. **Speck WT:** Effect of phototherapy on fertilization and embryonic development. Pediatr. Res. 13:506, 1979

246. **Chandler BD, Cashore WJ, Monin PJP, Oh W:** The lack of effects of phototherapy on neonatal oxygen dissociation curves and hemoglobin concentration in vivo. Pediatrics 59:1027, 1977

247. **Kostenbauder HB, Sanvordeker DR:** Riboflavin enhancement of bilirubin photocatabolism in vivo. Experientia 29:282, 1973

248. **Sanvordeker DR, Kostenbander HB:** Mechanism of riboflavin enhancement of bilirubin photodecomposition in vitro. J. Pharm. Sci. 63:404, 1974

249. **Gromisch DS, Lopes R, Cole HS, Cooperman JM:** Light (phototherapy)-induced riboflavin deficiency in the neonate. J Pediatr 19:118, 1977

250. **Hovi L, Hekali R, Siimes MA:** Evidence of riboflavin depletion in breast-fed newborns and its further exceleration during treatment of hyperbilirubinemia by phototherapy. Acta Paediatr Scand 68:567, 1979

251. **Tan KL, Chow MT, Karim SMM:** Effect of phototherapy on neonatal riboflavin status. J. Pediatr. 93:494, 1978

252. **Bhatia J, Mims LC, Roesel RA:** The effect of phototherapy on amino acid solutions containing multivitamins. J Pediatr 96:284, 1980

253. **Messner KH:** Light toxicity to newborn retina. Pediatr. Res. 12:530, 1978

254. **Messner KH, Maisels MJ, Leure duPree AE:** Phototoxicity to the newborn primate retina. Invest. Ophthalmol. 17:178, 1978

255. **Al–Salihi FL, Curran JP:** Airway obstruction by displaced eye mask during phototherapy. Am J Dis Child 129:1362, 1975

256. **Preis O, Rudolph N:** Abdominal distention in newborn infants on phototherapy—the role of eye occlusion. J. Pediatr. 94:816, 1979

257. **Bhupathy K, Sethupathy R, Pildes RS, Constantaras AA, Fournier JH:** Electroretinography in neonates treated with phototherapy. Pediatrics 61:189, 1978

258. **Dobson V, Corvett RM, Riggs LA:** Long-term effect of phototherapy on visual function. J Pediatr 86:555, 1975

259. **Dobson V, Riggs LA, Signeland ER:** Electroretinographic determination of dark adaptation functions of children exposed to phototherapy as infants. J Pediatr 85:25, 1974

260. **Woody NC, Brodkey MJ:** Tanning from phototherapy for neonatal jaundice. J. Pediatr. 82:1042, 1973

261. **Wu PYK, Berdahl M:** Irradiance in incuba-

tors under phototherapy lamps. J. Pediatr. 84:754, 1974

262. **Kopelman AE, Brown RS, Odell GB:** The "bronze" baby syndrome: A complication of phototherapy. J Pediatr 81:466, 1972

263. **Clark CF, Torii S, Hamamoto Y, Kaito H:** The "bronze" baby syndrome: Post mortem data. J Pediatr 88:461, 1976

264. **Gartner LM, Lee KS:** Commentary: The bronze baby syndrome. J Pediatr 88:465, 1976

265. **Brown RJK, Valman HB, Daganah EG:** Diarrhea and light therapy in neonates. Lancet I:498, 1970

266. **Washington JL, Brown AW Jr, Starrett AL:** The question of diarrhea and phototherapy. Pediatrics 49:279, 1972

267. **Rubaltelli FF, Largajolli G:** Effect of light exposure on gut transit time in jaundiced newborns. Acta Paediatr. Scand. 62:146, 1973

268. **Oh W, Karecki H:** Phototherapy and insensible water loss in the newborn infant. Amer. J. Dis. Child. 124:230, 1972

269. **Wu PYK, Moosa A:** Effect of phototherapy on nitrogen and electrolyte levels and water balance in jaundiced preterm infants. Pediatrics 61:193, 1978

269a. **Bakken AF:** Temporary intestinal lactase deficiency in light-treated jaundiced infants. Acta Pediatr Scand 66:91, 1977

270. **Lund HT, Petersen I:** Beta glucuronidase in duodenal bile of jaundiced newborn infants treated with phototherapy. J Pediatr 85:268, 1974

271. **Bell EF, Neidich GA, Cashore WJ, Oh W:** Combined effect of radiant warmer and phototherapy on insensible water loss in low birth weight infants. J Pediatr 94:810, May 1979

272. **Wu PYK, Hodgman JE:** Insensible water loss in preterm infants: Changes with postnatal development and nonionizing radiant energy. Pediatrics 54:704, 1974

273. **Wu PYK, Wong WH, Hodgman JE, Levan N:** Changes in blood flow in the skin and muscle with phototherapy. Pediatr Res 8:257, 1974

274. **Teberg AJ, Hodgman JE, Wu PYK:** Effect of phototherapy on growth of low birthweight infants—two year follow-up. J Pediatr 91:92, 1977

275. **Drew JH, Marriage KJ, Bayle VV, Bajraszewski E, McNamara JM:** Phototherapy—short and long term complications. Arch Dis Child 51:454, 1976

276. **Ogawa J, Ogawa Y, Onishi S, Shibata T, Saito H:** Five years experience in phototherapy. In Phototherapy for Neonatal Hyperbiliru-binemia: Long Term Implications, Brown AK and Showacre J (eds), U.S. Dept. Health, Education, and Welfare, Publication No. (NIH) 76-1075, 1977, p 49

277. **Dacou-Voutetakis C, Anagnostakis D, Matsaniotis N:** Effect of prolonged illumination (phototherapy) on concentrations of luteinizing hormone in human infants. Science 199:1229, 1978

278. **Lemaitre B, Toubas PL, Guillo TM, Drew XC, Relier JP:** Changes of serum gonadotropin concentrations in premature babies submitted to phototherapy. Biol Neonate 32:113, 1977

279. **Klaus MH:** Important considerations in the clinical management of infants with hyperbilirubinemia. In Odell GB, Schaffer R, Simopoulos AP (eds): Phototherapy in the Newborn: An Overview, p 185. Washington, D.C. National Academy of Sciences, 1974

280. **Lucey JF, Hewitt J:** Recent observations on light in neonatal jaundice, p 123. Publication No. (NIH) 76-1075, Washington, D.C., U.S. Department of Health, Education, and Welfare, 1977

281. **Lucey JF:** Another view of phototherapy. J Pediatr 84:145, 1974

282. **Ramagnoli G, Polidori G, Catalbi L, Tortorolo G, Segni G:** Phototherapy-induced hypocalcemia. J. Pediatr. 94:815, 1979

283. **Cashore WJ, Karotkin EH, Stern L, Oh W:** The lack of effect of phototherapy on serum bilirubin binding capacity in newborn infants. J Pediatr 87:977, 1975

284. **Porto SO, Pildes RS, Goodman H:** Studies on the effect of phototherapy on neonatal hyperbilirubinemia among low-birth-weight infants. II. Protein binding capacity. J Pediatr 75:1048, 1969

285. **Onishi S, Yamakawa T, Ogawa J:** Photochemical and photobiologic studies on the light-treated newborn infant. Perinatology 1:373, 1971

286. **Spennati G, Girotti F, Orzalesi MM:** Urinary excretion of 5-hydroxyindolacetic acid in low-birth-weight infants with and without phototherapy. J Pediatr 82:286, 1973

287. **Yaffe SJ, Levy G, Matsuzawa T, Baliah T:** Enhancement of glucuronide conjugating capacity in a hyperbilirubinemic infant due to apparent enzyme induction by phenobarbital. New Engl. J. Med. 275:1461, 1966

288. **Steihl A, Thaler MM, Admirand WH:** The effects of phenobarbital on bile salts and bilirubin in patients with intrahepatic and extrahepatic cholestasis. New Engl J Med 286:858–861, 1972

289. **Valdes OS, Maurer HM, Shumway CN, Draper DA, Hossaini AA:** Controlled clinical trial of

phenobarbital and/or light in reducing neonatal hyperbilirubinemia in a predominantly Negro population. J Pediatr 79:1015, 1971

290. **Thaler MM, Gemes DI, Bakken AF:** Enzymatic conversion of heme to bilirubin in normal and starved fetuses and newborn rats. Pediatr Res 6:197, 1972

291. **Mathis RK, Andres JM, Walker WA:** Liver disease in infants, II. Hepatic disease states. J Pediatr 90:864, 1977

292. **Thaler MM:** Cryptogenic liver disease in young infants. Prog. Liver Dis. 5:476–493, 1976

293. **Sondheimer JM, Bryan H, Andrews W, Forstner GG:** Cholestatic tendencies in premature infants on and off parenteral nutrition. Pediatrics 62:984, 1978

294. **Manginello FP, Javitt NB:** Parenteral nutrition and neonatal cholestasis. J Pediatr 94:296, 1979

295. **Bernstein J, Chang C–H, Brough AJ, Heidelberger KP:** Conjugated hyperbilirubinemia in infants associated with parenteral alimentation. J Pediatr 90:361, 1977

296. **Rodgers BM, Hollenbeck JI, Donnelly WH, Talbert JL:** Intrahepatic cholestasis with parenteral alimentation. Am J Surg 131:149, 1976.

297. **Touloukian RJ, Downing SE:** Cholestasis associated with long term parenteral hyperalimentation. Arch Surg 106:58, 1973

298. **Heathcote J, Deodhar KP, Scheuer PJ, Sherlock S:** Intrahepatic cholestasis in childhood. N Engl J Med 295:801–805, 1975

299. **Javitt NB:** Cholestasis in infancy: Status report and conceptual approach. Gastroenterology 70:1172–1181, 1976

300. **Mowat AP, Psacharopoulos HT, Williams R:** Extrahepatic biliary atresia versus neonatal hepatitis. Review of 137 prospectively investigated infants. Arch Dis Child 51:763–768, 1976

301. **Holder TH:** Atresia of the extrahepatic bile duct. Am J Surg 107:458–462, 1964

302. **Brent RL:** Persistent jaundice in infancy. J Pediatr 61:111–144, 1962

303. **Hays DM:** Biliary atresia: The current state of confusion. Surg Clin North Am 53:1257–1273, 1973

304. **Gourevitch A:** The surgery of jaundice in the newborn, with special reference to congenital atresia of the bile ducts. Ann R Coll Surg Engl 32:334–357, 1963

305. **Krovetz LJ:** Congenital biliary atresia II. Analysis of the therapeutic problem. Surgery 47:468–489, 1960

306. **Alagille D:** Clinical aspects of neonatal hepatitis Am J Dis Child 123:287–291, 1972

307. **Alpert LI, Strauss L, Hirschhorn K:** Neonatal hepatitis and biliary atresia associated with trisomy 17–18 syndrome. N Eng J Med 280:16–20, 1969

308. **Thaler MM:** Biliary disease in infancy and children. In Gastrointestinal Disease, Sleisinger MH and Fordtran JS (eds), p 1087, Philadelphia, WB Saunders, 1973

309. **Javitt NB (ed):** Neonatal Hepatitis and Biliary Atresia. Washington, D.C., DHEW Publication No. (NIH) 79-1296

310. **Maisels MJ:** Neonatal Liver Disease. In Demers LM, Shaw LM (eds): Evaluation of Liver Function, p 157. Baltimore, Urban and Schwartzenberg, 1978

311. **Thaler MM, Gellis SS:** Studies in neonatal hepatitis and biliary atresia. IV. Diagnosis. Amer J Dis Child 116:280–284, 1968

312. **Poley JR, Smith EI, Boon DJ, Bhatia M, Smith CW, Thompson JB:** Lipoprotein X and the double ^{131}I-Rose Bengal Test in the diagnosis of prolonged infantile jaundice. J Pediatr Surg 7:660–669, 1972

313. **Kimura S:** The early diagnosis of biliary atresia. Prog Pediatr Surg 6:91–112, 1974

314. **Green HL, Helinek GL, Moran R, O'Neill J:** A diagnostic approach to prolonged obstructive jaundice by 24 hour collection of duodenal fluid. J Pediatr 95:412, 1979

315. **Hirsig J, Rickham PP:** Early differential diagnosis between neonatal hepatitis and biliary atresia. J Pediatr Surg 15–13, 1980

316. **Alagille D:** Long term results of hepatic portoenterostomy. In Javitt NB (ed): Neonatal Hepatitis and Biliary Atresia, p 411. DHEW Publication No (NIH) 79-1296

317. **Altman RP:** Biliary Atresia: A surgical–histopathologic correlation. In Javitt NB (ed): Neonatal Hepatitis and Biliary Atresia, p 391 DHEW Publication No (NIH) 79-1296

318. **Kasai M:** Results of surgery for biliary atresia. In Javitt NB (ed): Neonatal Hepatitis and Biliary Atresia, p 417. Washington, D.C., DHEW Publication No. (NIH) 79-1296

319. **Koop CE:** Biliary obstruction in the newborn. Surg Clin N Am 56:373–377, 1976

320. **Kasai M, Suzuki S:** A new operation for "noncorrectable" biliary atresia: Hepatic portoenterostomy. Shujutsu 13:733–739, 1959

321. **Carcassone M, Bensoussan A:** Long-term results in treatment of biliary atresia. In Rickham PP, Hecker W, Prevot J (eds): Long-Term Surgical Results in Children: Progress in Pediatric Surgery, vol 10, pp 151–160 Baltimore, Urban and Schwarzenberg, 1977

322. **Howard ER, Mowat AP:** Extrahepatic biliary atresia. Arch Dis Child 52:825–827, 1977

323. **Kasai M, Kimura S, Asakura Y, Suzuki H, Taira Y, Ohashi E:** Surgical treatment of biliary atresia. J Pediatr Surg 3:665–675, 1968

324. **Campbell DP, Smith EI, Bhatia M, Poley JR, Williams GR:** Hepatic portoenterostomy: An assessment of its value in the treatment of biliary atresia. Ann Surg 181:591–595, 1975

325. **Kobayashi A, Utsunomiya T, Kawai S, Ohbe Y:** Congenital biliary atresia. Analysis of 97 cases with reference to prognosis after hepatic portoenterostomy. Am J Dis Child 130: 830–833, 1976

326. **Odievre M, Valayer J, Razemon-Pinta M, Habib EC, Alagille D:** Hepatic portoenterostomy of cholecystostomy in the treatment of extrahepatic biliary atresia. J Pediatr 88: 774–779, 1976

327. **Gautier M, Jehan P, Odievre M:** Histologic study of biliary fibrous remnants in 48 cases of extrahepatic biliary atresia: Correlation with post-operative bile flow restoration. J Pediatr 89:704–709, 1976

328. **Chandra RS, Altman RP:** Ductal remnants in exterohepatic biliary atresia: A histopathologic study with clinical correlation. J Pediatr 93:196, 1978

329. **Altman RP, Chandra R, Lilly JR:** Ongoing cirrhosis after successful porticoenterostomy in infants with biliary atresia J Pediatr Surg 10:685–691, 1975

330. **McConnell JB, Glasgow JFT, McNair R:** Effect on neonatal jaundice of oestrogens and progestogens taken before and after conception. Br Med J 3:605–607, 1973

331. **Gould SR, Mountrose U, Brown DJ, Whitehouse WL, Barnardo DE:** Influence of previous oral contraception and maternal oxytocin infusion on neonatal jaundice. Br Med J 3:228–230, 1974

332. **Drew JH:** Breastfeeding and jaundice. Keeping Abreast, Journal of Human Nuturing Jan–March: 53, 1978

25

Hematologic Problems

Frank A. Oski

During the neonatal period, the clinician is confronted with a variety of life-threatening hematologic problems. Some of these disturbances are primary while others merely reflect the presence of other diseases. These hematologic problems can be broadly classified into those of anemia and polycythemia, coagulation disturbances, and disorders of leukocyte production and function. Interpretation of laboratory findings and institution of appropriate therapy require an understanding of basic hematologic principles as well as an appreciation of the normal physiologic variations of the formed blood elements and coagulation factors that accompany this period of life.

ANEMIA

Normal Values in the Newborn Period

The definition of normal in the immediate newborn period is influenced by the gestational age of the infant, the site of sampling, and the method by which the umbilical vessels were treated at the time of delivery.

During gestation, the red cell count, the hemoglobin, and hematocrit rise gradually from the 12th to the 34th week (Table 25-1). This rise in hemoglobin is associated with a fall in the mean corpuscular volume of the

erythrocytes, and a decrease in the numbers of circulating immature red cells.

After the 34th to the 35th week of gestation, the mean cord blood hemoglobin is approximately 16.8 g/dl. Values obtained from capillary samples during the first 48 hours of life tend to average 2 to 3 g/dl higher, although differences of 6 to 8 g/dl have been frequently observed.[1]

During the first hours of life, the hemoglobin and hematocrit may rise by 10 to 20% of their initial value. This rise is confined to those infants whose cords were not clamped immediately at the time of delivery.[2]

The blood volume in the term infant at approximately one-half hour of age ranges from a mean of 78.0 ml/kg in an infant whose cord was clamped immediately to a mean of 98.6 ml/kg in the infant with delayed cord clamping. By the third day of life the blood volume in these 2 groups averages 82.3 and 92.6 ml/kg respectively. In the premature infant the blood volume tends to be higher, with mean values ranging from 89 ml/kg to 105 ml/kg.[3,4] This increased blood volume is primarily the result of an increased plasma volume, with the total red cell volume per kilogram body weight being quite similar to that of the term infant. Cassady has shown that the plasma volume decreases with increasing gestational

Table 25-1. Mean Red Cell Values During Gestation.

Gestational Age (in weeks)	Hb (g/dl)	Hemato-crit (%)	RBC (10⁶/mm³)	Mean Corpusc. Vol. (μ³)	Mean Corpusc. Hb (γγ)	Mean Corpusc. Hb conc. (%)	Nuc. RBC (% of RBC's)	Retic. (%)	Diam. (μ)
12	8.0–10.0	33	1.5	180	60	34	5.0–8.0	40	10.5
16	10.0	35	2.0	140	45	33	2.0–4.0	10–25	9.5
20	11.0	37	2.5	135	44	33	1.0	10–20	9.0
24	14.0	40	3.5	123	38	31	1.0	5–10	8.8
28	14.5	45	4.0	120	40	31	0.5	5–10	8.7
34	15.0	47	4.4	118	38	32	0.2	3–10	8.5

Table 25-2. Normal Hematologic Values During the First Twelve Weeks of Life in the Term Infant as Determined by an Electronic Cell Counter.

Age	No. of Cases	Hb g/dl ± S.D.	RBC × 10^6 ± S.D.	Hct % ± S.D.	MCV μ^3 ± S.D.	MCHC % ± S.D.	Retic % ± S.D.
Days							
1	19	19.0±2.2	5.14±0.7	61±7.4	119±9.4	31.6±1.9	3.2±1.4
2	19	19.0±1.9	5.15±0.8	60±6.4	115±7.0	31.6±1.4	3.2±1.3
3	19	18.7±3.4	5.11±0.7	62±9.3	116±5.3	31.1±2.8	2.8±1.7
4	10	18.6±2.1	5.00±0.6	57±8.1	114±7.5	32.6±1.5	1.8±1.1
5	12	17.6±1.1	4.97±0.4	57±7.3	114±8.9	30.9±2.2	1.2±0.2
6	15	17.4±2.2	5.00±0.7	54±7.2	113±10.0	32.2±1.6	0.6±0.2
7	12	17.9±2.5	4.86±0.6	56±9.4	118±11.2	32.0±1.6	0.5±0.4
Weeks							
1–2	32	17.3±2.3	4.80±0.8	54±8.3	112±19.0	32.1±2.9	0.5±0.3
2–3	11	15.6±2.6	4.20±0.6	46±7.3	111±8.2	33.9±1.9	0.8±0.6
3–4	17	14.2±2.1	4.00±0.6	43±5.7	105±7.5	33.5±1.6	0.6±0.3
4–5	15	12.7±1.6	3.60±0.4	36±4.8	101±8.1	34.9±1.6	0.9±0.8
5–6	10	11.9±1.5	3.55±0.2	36±6.2	102±10.2	34.1±2.9	1.0±0.7
6–7	10	12.0±1.5	3.40±0.4	36±4.8	105±12.0	33.8±2.3	1.2±0.7
7–8	17	11.1±1.1	3.40±0.4	33±3.7	100±13.0	33.7±2.6	1.5±0.7
8–9	13	10.7±0.9	3.40±0.5	31±2.5	93±12.0	34.1±2.2	1.8±1.0
9–10	12	11.2±0.9	3.60±0.3	32±2.7	91±9.3	34.3±2.9	1.2±0.6
10–11	11	11.4±0.9	3.70±0.4	34±2.1	91±7.7	33.2±2.4	1.2±0.7
11–12	13	11.3±0.9	3.70±0.3	33±3.3	88±7.9	34.8±2.2	0.7±0.3

(Matoth Y et al: Acta Paediatr Scand 60:317, 1971)[6]

age, although infants with intrauterine growth retardation tend to have greater plasma volumes than those expected for infants of comparable weight.[5]

During the first week of life, in both the normal term and premature infant, there is very little change in the mean hemoglobin concentration, and values at 7 days of age are very similar to the values present at birth (Tables 25-2 and 25-3). After the first week of life the hemoglobin values fall more rapidly in the infants of lowest birth weight. During the first week of life, in an infant of 34 to 35 weeks of gestation or older, a venous hemoglobin sample of 13.0 g/dl or less should be regarded as evidence of anemia. Similarly, a capillary sample of less than 14.5 g/dl indicates the presence of anemia.

Table 25-3. Serial Hemoglobin Values (g/dl) in Low-Birth-Weight Infants.

Birth Weight (g)	Age (in Weeks)				
	2	*4*	*6*	*8*	*10*
800–1000	16.0±0.6	10.2±3.2	8.7±1.5	8.0±0.9	8.0±1.1
1001–1200	16.4±2.3	12.8±2.5	10.5±1.8	9.1±1.3	8.5±1.5
1201–1400	16.2±1.3	13.4±2.8	10.9±1.2	9.9±1.9	—
1401–1500	15.6±2.2	11.7±1.0	10.5±0.7	9.8±1.4	—

(Oski FA, Williams ML: Unpublished data)

Table 25-4. Types of Hemorrhage in the Newborn.

Occult hemorrhage prior to birth
FETOMATERNAL
Traumatic amniocentesis
Spontaneous
Following external cephalic version
TWIN TO TWIN

Obstetric accidents, malformations of the placenta and cord
RUPTURE OF A NORMAL UMBILICAL CORD
Precipitous delivery
Entanglement
HEMATOMA OF THE CORD OR PLACENTA
RUPTURE OF AN ABNORMAL UMBILICAL CORD
Varices
Aneurysm
RUPTURE OF ANOMALOUS VESSELS
Aberrant vessel
Velamentous insertion
Communicating vessels in multilobed
placenta
INCISION OF PLACENTA DURING CESAREAN
SECTION
PLACENTA PREVIA
ABRUPTIO PLACENTAE

Internal hemorrhage
INTRACRANIAL
GIANT CEPHALOHEMATOMA, CAPUT
SUCCEDANEUM
RETROPERITONEAL
RUPTURED LIVER
RUPTURED SPLEEN

Etiologic Factors in Neonatal Anemia

Anemia present at birth or appearing during the first week of life can be broadly categorized into three major groups. The anemia may be a result of (1) blood loss, (2) hemolysis, or (3) underproduction of erythrocytes.

Blood Loss as a Cause of Anemia. Blood loss resulting in anemia may occur prenatally, at the time of delivery, or in the first few days of life. Blood loss may be a result of occult hemorrhage prior to birth, obstetric accidents, internal hemorrhages, or excessive blood sampling on the part of physicians for diagnostic studies (Table 25-4).

Faxelius and associates estimated the red cell volume in 259 infants admitted to a high-risk nursery in an attempt to determine which clinical events were frequently associated with a reduction in red cell mass.[7] A low red cell volume was frequently associated with a maternal history of late third trimester vaginal bleeding; placenta previa or abruptio placenta; nonelective cesarian section; deliveries associated with cord compression; Apgar scores of less than 6; an early central venous hematocrit of less than 45% and a mean arterial blood pressure of less than 30 torr.

Occult Hemorrhage Prior to Birth. Occult hemorrhage prior to birth may be caused by bleeding of the fetus into the maternal circulation or by bleeding of one fetus into another when multiple pregnancies are present.

In approximately 50% of all pregnancies, some fetal cells can be demonstrated in the maternal circulation.[8] In about 8% of pregnancies, from 0.5 to 40.0 ml of blood is transferred from fetus to mother at birth, while in 1% of pregnancies, the blood loss exceeds 40 ml. Fetal to maternal hemorrhages are more common following traumatic diagnostic amniocentesis or external cephalic version prior to delivery.

The clinical manifestations of **fetomaternal hemorrhages** depend on the volume of the hemorrhage and the rapidity with which it has occurred. If the hemorrhage has been prolonged or repeated during the course of the pregnancy, anemia develops slowly, giving the fetus an opportunity to develop hemodynamic compensation. Such infants may only manifest pallor at birth. Following acute hemorrhage, just before delivery, the infant may be pale and sluggish, with gasping respirations and signs of circulatory shock. The typical physical findings and laboratory data that are useful in distinguishing these two forms of fetal to maternal blood loss are described in Table 25-5.

The degree of anemia is quite variable. Usually the hemoglobin is less than 12 g/dl before signs and symptoms of anemia are recognized by the physician. Hemoglobin values as low as 3 to 4 g/dl have been recorded in infants who were born alive and survived. If the hemorrhage has been acute, and particularly when hypovolemic shock is present, the hemoglobin value may not reflect the magnitude of the blood loss. In such instances, several hours may elapse before hemodilution occurs and the magnitude of the hemorrhage is appreciated. In general, a loss of 20% of the blood volume acutely is sufficient to produce signs of shock and will be reflected in a fall in hemoglobin within 3 hours of the event.

Examination of peripheral blood smear provides useful diagnostic information. In acute hemorrhage, the red cells appear normochromic and normocytic, while in chronic hemorrhage, the cells are generally hypochromic and microcytic.

In anemia that is a direct result of a fetal to maternal hemorrhage, the Coombs' test is negative and the infants are not jaundiced. Infants with anemia secondary to blood loss generally have much lower bilirubin values throughout the neonatal period as a consequence of their reduced red cell mass.

The diagnosis of a fetomaternal hemorrhage of sufficient magnitude to result in anemia at birth can be made with certainty only by demonstrating the presence of fetal cells in the maternal circulation. Techniques for demonstrating these cells include the use of differential agglutination, mixed agglutination, fluorescent antibody techniques, and the acid-elution method of staining for cells containing fetal hemoglobin. The Kleihauer technique of acid elution is the simplest of these methods

and the most commonly employed for the detection of fetal cells.[9] The test is based on the property of fetal hemoglobin to resist elution from the intact cell in an acid medium. The acid-elution technique can be relied on with certainty for diagnosis only when other conditions capable of producing elevations in maternal fetal hemoglobin levels are absent. These include maternal thalassemia minor, sickle-cell anemia, hereditary persistence of fetal hemoglobin, and some normal women who show a pregnancy-induced rise in fetal hemoglobin production.[10] In the presence of these conditions, other techniques based on differential agglutination should be employed.

Diagnosis of a fetomaternal hemorrhage may be missed in situations in which the mother and infant are incompatible in the ABO blood group system. In such instances, the infant's A or B cells are rapidly cleared from the maternal circulation by the maternal anti-A or anti-B and are not available for staining. The staining technique therefore must be carried out within several hours of birth in such instances to diagnose the presence of hemorrhage. A presumptive diagnosis may be made

Table 25-5. The Characteristics of Acute and Chronic Blood Loss in the Newborn.

Characteristic	Acute Blood Loss	Chronic Blood Loss
Clinical	Acute distress; pallor; shallow, rapid, and often irregular respiration; tachycardia; weak or absent peripheral pulses; low or absent blood pressure; no hepatosplenomegaly.	Marked pallor disproportionate to evidence of distress; on occasion signs of congestive heart failure may be present, including hepatomegaly
Venous pressure	Low	Normal or elevated
Laboratory hemoglobin concentration	May be normal initially; then drops quickly during first 24 hours of life.	Low at birth
Red cell morphology	Normochromic and macrocytic	Hypochromic and microcytic; anisocytosis and poikilocytosis
Serum iron	Normal at birth	Low at birth
Course	Prompt treatment of anemia and shock necessary to prevent death.	Generally uneventful
Treatment	Intravenous fluids and whole blood. Iron therapy later.	Iron therapy; packed red cells may be necessary on occasion

by demonstrating either marked erythrophag-ocytosis in smears of the maternal buffy coat or a rise in maternal immune anti-A or anti-B titers in the weeks following delivery.

Fetal-to-fetal transfusion is only observed in monozygotic multiple births with mono-chorial placentas. In approximately 70% of monozygotic twin pregnancies, a monochorial placenta exists. It has been estimated that from 13 to 33% of all twin pregnancies in which a monochorial placenta is present will be associated with a twin-to-twin transfu-sion.[11,12] This blood exchange can produce anemia in the donor and polycythemia in the recipient. When a significant hemorrhage has occurred, the difference in hemoglobin be-tween the twins exceeds 5.0 g/dl. This is in contrast to a maximum discrepancy of 3.3 g/dl in cord blood hemoglobin concentration in dizygotic twins.[11]

The anemic infant may develop congestive heart failure, while the plethoric twin may manifest symptoms and signs of the hypervis-cosity syndrome, disseminated intravascular coagulation (DIC), and hyperbilirubinemia.

The hemorrhage may be acute or chronic. Tan and associates, on the basis of a review of 482 twin pairs in which 35 were found to have the syndrome, pointed out how the dif-ference in weight of the twins could be utilized to establish the timing of the hemorrhage.[12] When the weight difference exceeded 20% of the weight of the larger twin, the transfusion was chronic and the smaller infant was invar-iably the donor. The anemic, smaller twin displayed reticulocytosis. When the difference in the weight of the twins did not exceed 20% of the weight of the larger twin, the larger twin was the donor in almost one-half of all in-stances. In these presumably acute transfu-sions, significant reticulocytosis was not ob-served in the anemic donor.

When a twin-to-twin transfusion is sus-pected, attempts to confirm it by placental examination should be made. The placentas of all multiple pregnancies should be routinely examined for purposes of genetic counseling. When hematologic evidence has not been ob-tained and death of the infants has occurred, other findings may suggest the diagnosis. These include hydramnios of one of the am-niotic sacs (the recipient), and oligohydram-nios of the other (the donor), and marked differences in the size and organ weights of the twins.

Obstetric Accidents and Complications. Obstetric accidents and malformations of the placenta and cord may be responsible for major blood loss at the time of delivery. All too frequently, these accidents are unreported to the pediatrician and may result in diagnostic confusion as to the cause of shock in the early hours of life or the presence of pallor and unexplained anemia during the second or third day of life.

Table 25-4 lists the obstetric conditions that can produce neonatal hemorrhage. It should be noted that a severe, and often fatal, fetal hemorrhage may accompany placenta previa, abruptio placentae, or accidental incision of the placenta or umbilical cord during a cesar-ean section.

In women with late third trimester bleeding, Clayton and associates were able to anticipate the birth of a possibly anemic infant by ex-amining the vaginal blood for the presence of fetal erythrocytes by employing the acid-elu-tion technique of Kleihauer.[13]

It is good pediatric practice to routinely obtain a hemoglobin at the time of delivery on all babies born of women with late third trimes-ter bleeding or babies born after a cesarean section. This determination should be repeated in 6 to 12 hours in order to observe the expected fall in hemoglobin owing to the he-modilution that accompanies recent blood loss.

Severe bleeding as a result of an obstetric accident or complication of delivery often results in the birth of a pale, limp infant. Respirations, which usually commence spon-taneously, are often irregular and gasping. They are not associated with retraction as in conditions accompanied by primary pulmo-nary disease. Cyanosis is minimal and the infant's pale color is not improved by oxygen administration. The peripheral pulses are weak or absent and the blood pressure is reduced. The venous pressure measured after the in-sertion of an umbilical catheter will be found to be extremely low.

Internal Hemorrhage. Anemia that appears in the first 24 to 72 hours of life and is not associated with jaundice is commonly caused by hemorrhage at the time of birth or to a postnatal internal hemorrhage. Traumatic de-liveries may result in subdural or subarachnoid hemorrhages of sufficient magnitude to result in anemia. Similarly, cephalohematomas may also be of sufficient size to produce anemia. Breech deliveries may be associated with hemorrhage into the adrenals, kidney, spleen, or retroperitoneal area. Rupture of the liver or subcapsular hemorrhages into the liver occur far more commonly than are clinically recognized. In stillbirths and neonatal deaths, the incidence of hepatic hemorrhages has been found to range from 1.2 to 5.6%.[14-16] An infant with a ruptured liver generally appears well for the first 24 to 48 hours of life and then suddenly goes into shock. The abdomen may appear distended and a mass contiguous with the liver is often palpable. Shifting dullness can often be demonstrated.

Splenic rupture may also occur after a difficult delivery or as a result of the extreme distention of this organ that is often seen in babies with severe erythroblastosis fetalis. The physician should always suspect a rupture of the spleen when an anemic, and often hydropic, infant with erythroblastosis is found to have a low venous pressure at the time of exchange transfusion.

Bleeding into the ventricles and subarachnoid space can also produce significant decreases in hemoglobin concentration. This is more common in infants with birth weights of less than 1500 g.

Iatrogenic Anemia. More and more frequently today, as a consequence of frequent monitoring of critically ill infants, anemia appearing during the third to seventh day of life is caused by excessive blood removal for diagnostic studies. Anemia can generally be produced by removal of more than 20% of a subject's blood volume over a period of 24 to 48 hours. In an infant of 1500 g, this represents a blood loss of 30 ml. When frequent blood sampling is necessary, a flow sheet should be attached to the infant's incubator and the amount removed at any given time recorded. This simple technique will often convert idiopathic anemia to iatrogenic anemia.

Treatment of Anemia Due to Blood Loss. The treatment of the infant depends on the degree of anemia and the acuteness of the hemorrhage. The following guidelines may be employed:

1. If the infant is pale and limp at birth, clear the airway, administer oxygen, and intubate if necessary.
2. Insert a catheter into the umbilical vein. Measure pressure and obtain blood specimens for hematologic determinations and for crossmatch purposes.

3. As soon as it is apparent that pallor is a result of hypovolemic shock or profound anemia and not a consequence of asphyxia, administer 20 ml/kg of available solution. In order of preference these are: Group O, Rh negative blood; plasma; 5% albumin; and isotonic saline. Infants with acute blood loss generally demonstrate dramatic improvement after such a procedure. Infants with massive internal hemorrhages show less evidence of response.
4. A repeat injection of 10 to 20 ml/kg of whole blood may be given after the first transfusion, particularly if whole blood was not administered initially and the venous pressure and arterial blood pressure have not returned to normal.

After resuscitating the infant, make efforts to determine the cause of blood loss. Examine the placenta and cord for evidence of abnormalities. Obtain a blood sample from the mother for the detection of a fetomaternal hemorrhage.

The infant who is mildly anemic at birth as a consequence of chronic blood loss and who is in no distress does not require transfusions. These infants should be treated with ferrous sulfate in a dose of 2 mg of elemental iron per kg of body weight, administered three times daily for 3 months.

HEMOLYTIC ANEMIAS

Anemia as a consequence of a hemolytic process is common in the newborn period and has multiple etiologies (Table 25-6). Unlike the anemias produced by hemorrhage or by failure of red cell production, a hemolytic anemia in the newborn period is almost always associated with elevations in the serum bilirubin values to levels of 10 mg/dl or greater. In general, a hemolytic process is first detected during the investigation of jaundice occurring during the first week of life.

Hemolytic disease in the newborn can be broadly grouped into three large categories: isoimmunization, congenital defects of the red cell, and acquired defects of the red cell.

Isoimmunization

Hemolytic disease in the newborn as a consequence of isoimmunization of the mother is caused by the passage of fetal red cells, possessing an antigen lacking in the cells of

**Table 25-6 Causes of a Hemolytic Process
in the Neonatal Period.**

Immune
1. Rh incompatibility
2. ABO incompatibility
3. Minor blood group incompatibility
4. Maternal autoimmune hemolytic anemia
5. Drug induced hemolytic anemia

Infection
1. Bacterial sepsis
2. Congenital infections
    Syphilis
    Malaria
    Cytomegalovirus
    Rubella
    Toxoplasmosis
    Disseminated Herpes

Disseminated Intravascular Coagulation
Macro and Microangiopathic Hemolytic Anemias
1. Cavernous hemangioma
2. Large vessel thrombi
3. Renal artery stenosis
4. Severe coarctation of the aorta

Galactosemia
**Prolonged or Recurrent Acidosis of a Metabolic or
   Respiratory Nature**
Hereditary Disorders of the Red Cell Membrane
1. Hereditary spherocytosis
2. Hereditary elliptocytosis
3. Hereditary stomatocytosis
4. Other rare membrane disorders

Pyknocytosis
Red Cell Enzyme Deficiencies
   The most common of these are G-6-PD
    deficiency, pyruvate kinase deficiency, 5'
    nucleotidase deficiency, and glucose
    phosphate isomerase deficiency.

Alpha Thalassemia Syndromes
Alpha Chain Structural Abnormalities
Gamma Thalassemia Syndromes
Gamma Chain Structural Abnormalities

the mother, into the maternal circulation where they stimulate the production of antibody. These antibodies, of the IgG class, then return to the fetal circulation, attach to antigenic sites on the surface of the red cell, and lead to its rapid removal and destruction. The incidence and clinical manifestations of isoimmunization depend on the type of blood group incompatibility between mother and fetus. This topic has been the subject of many excellent and comprehensive reviews.[17-20]

The incidence of Rh incompatibility in a population depends in large part, on the prevalence of the Rh-negative antigens. The prevalence of the Rh-negative genotype ranges from approximately zero in Japanese, Chinese, and North American Indian populations, to 5.5% among American Blacks, to about 15.0% among Caucasians living in the United States. Among Caucasian women, it has been estimated that, in approximately 9% of all pregnancies, an Rh-negative woman will carry an Rh-positive fetus. The incidence of hemolytic disease due to Rh incompatibility is in the range of 0.06% with approximately one-half of the infants requiring therapy. Thus, only 1 in 15 pregnancies at risk will result in the birth of an infant with clinical disease. By comparison, 20% of all pregnancies are accompanied by ABO blood group incompatibility between mother and fetus. The hemolytic disease is limited to those situations in which the mother is blood group O and the baby is blood group A or B. This association occurs in 15% of all pregnancies, yet evidence of disease is found in only 3% of all pregnancies and only 1:30 to 1:120 of these infants require exchange transfusions. Thus, although hemolytic disease caused by ABO incompatibility is approximately five times as common as hemolytic disease caused by Rh incompatibility, the number of exchange transfusions performed for this condition is far less. It is estimated that two out of every three exchange transfusions performed for the treatment of isoimmunization are in infants with Rh incompatibility.

Rh Incompatibility. The severity of this disease varies greatly from infant to infant. At present, it has been estimated by Zipursky that the perinatal mortality in this disease is approximately 17.5%, with about 14.0% of deaths as a result of stillbirths.[19] Although hemolytic disease tends to be more severe in a second than a first pregnancy in which sensitization has occurred, the severity of disease in subsequent pregnancies tends to be uniform.

• Pathogenesis of RH Immunization: The entry of fetal cells into the maternal circulation is the cause of Rh isoimmunization. As little as 0.05 to 0.1 ml cells, particularly if given repeatedly, are sufficient to produce immunization. Rh immunization tends to occur more frequently in pregnancies that have been complicated by toxemia, cesarian section, or manual removal of the placenta, because transplacental hemorrhages occur with greater frequency and in greater volume under these circumstances. It has been estimated that 1% of Rh-negative women will develop antibodies as a consequence of these transplacental hemorrhages before the delivery of their first child. An additional 7.5% will manifest evidence of sensitization within 6 months of the delivery of their first child, and an additional 7.5% will show no evidence of immunization 6 months after delivery, but will develop antibodies during their next pregnancy if their fetus is Rh positive, presumably as a consequence of an initial sensitization during their first pregnancy.

• Destruction of Fetal Erythrocytes by Anti-D: The transfer of antibody from the mother into the fetal circulation is responsible for the clinical manifestations of the hemolytic process. The red cell, coated with an antibody of the IgG class, will be removed primarily in the spleen of the fetus. The rate of destruction is proportional to the amount of antibody on the cell. At very high levels of antibody, the cell may exhibit intravascular hemolysis as well as splenic sequestration.

While *in utero,* the chief danger of excess red cell destruction is profound anemia. After birth, the infant is primarily at risk from the toxic products of red cell breakdown such as bilirubin. While *in utero* the infant responds to the increased breakdown of cells by increasing the rate of red cell production. This is reflected by an elevation in reticulocyte count and the presence of nucleated red blood cells in the peripheral circulation. This accelerated demand for red cells results in active erythropoiesis in nonmarrow sites such as the liver, spleen, and lung. A major portion of the hepatosplenomegaly observed in infants with hemolytic disease is a result of this extramedullary erythropoiesis.

In infants with severe Rh incompatibility, the liver and pancreas also exhibit pathologic changes. Islet cell hyperplasia can be observed in the pancreas and focal cellular necrosis with cholestasis may be seen in the liver.

The most severely affected infants will manifest hydrops fetalis. This massive edema with pleural effusions and ascites is not strictly related to the hemoglobin level of the infant. It is believed that other factors play a role in the development of hydrops. These include intrauterine hypoxia, hypoproteinemia, and a lowering of the nonprotein oncotic pressure of the plasma. Hydrops fetalis has been observed in a variety of other conditions (Table 25-7).

• Clinical Manifestations: The main signs of hemolytic disease in the newborn are jaundice, pallor, and enlargement of the liver and spleen.

Jaundice usually becomes evident during the

Table 25-7. Causes of Hydrops Fetalis.

Severe chronic anemia *in utero*
1. Erythroblastosis fetalis
2. Homozygous alpha-thalassemia
3. Chronic fetomaternal transfusion or twin-to-twin transfusion
4. Glucose-6-phosphate dehydrogenase deficiency (rare)

Cardiac failure
1. Severe congenital heart disease
2. Premature closure of foramen ovale
3. Large A-V malformation (hemangioma)[22]
4. Intrauterine arrhythmias

Hypoproteinemia
1. Renal disease
   a. Congenital nephrosis
   b. Renal vein thrombosis
2. Congenital hepatitis

Infections (intrauterine)
1. Syphilis
2. Toxoplasmosis
3. Cytomegalovirus

Miscellaneous
1. Maternal diabetes mellitus
2. Parabiotic syndrome (multiple pregnancy)
3. Sublethal umbilical or chorionic vein thrombosis
4. Fetal neuroblastomatosis
5. Chagas' disease
6. Achondroplasia
7. Cystic adenomatoid malformation of the lung
8. Pulmonary lymphangiectasia
9. Dysmaturity
10. Cardiopulmonary hypoplasia with bilateral hydrothorax
11. Gaucher's disease
12. Choriocarcinoma *in situ*

first 24 hours of life, frequently within the first 4 to 5 hours of life, and becomes maximal by the third or fourth day. The mechanisms of jaundice and the metabolism of bilirubin are extensively discussed in Chapter 24.

The degree of anemia reflects both the severity of the hemolytic process and the infant's capacity to respond to it with increased red cell production. "Late" anemia may develop in infants with Rh isoimmunization. This is observed in two clinical settings. In one, the infant does not become sufficiently jaundiced in the initial newborn period to require exchange transfusion. Continued red cell destruction occurs and the infant can develop severe, often fatal anemia between 7 and 21 days of life. The other, more common, situation occurs in infants who have had exchange transfusions. In these infants, a gradual fall in hemoglobin may be observed with hemoglobin values of 5 to 6 g/dl being reached by 4 to 6 weeks of life. These infants tolerate the anemia very well and spontaneous correction can be expected by 6 to 8 weeks of age. In general, if the hemoglobin is above 12 g/dl at 7 days of age in an infant who has had an exchange transfusion, no further transfusions will be necessary.

Petechiae and purpura may be observed in infants with severe anemia as a result of both thrombocytopenia and a disturbance in the intrinsic system of coagulation. This disturbance may be a result of DIC[21] or a result of hepatic dysfunction with consequent inability to synthesize the vitamin K-dependent factors.[22]

• Laboratory Findings: Decreased hemoglobin concentration, increased reticulocyte count, and increased numbers of nucleated red blood cells in the peripheral blood reflect the presence of the hemolytic process. Hemoglobin determinations performed on venous samples most accurately reflect the severity of the hemolytic process. Values of less than 14 g/dl in the cord blood should be regarded as abnormal. The reticulocyte count is generally greater than 6% and may reach 30 to 40%. In the peripheral blood, nucleated red blood cells may be observed in addition to some degree of polychromasia and anisocytosis. Spherocytes are not present in patients with hemolytic disease as a result of Rh sensitization.

Except when maternal antibodies are present in low titer, the red blood cells of Rh-positive infants will give a positive direct Coombs' test, indicating the presence of maternal IgG on the red cell surface. Occasionally, this coating is sufficiently heavy to block the Rh antigenic sites, causing a false negative result for Rh typing in an infant who is Coombs'-test positive.

• Treatment: At present the management of this problem focuses primarily on prevention of the disease by the administration of anti-Rh immunoglobulin to the mother following the delivery or abortion of an Rh-positive, ABO-compatible infant and on the prevention of intrauterine death of the infant at risk.

The early proposals for the use of anti-Rh immunoglobulin were based on the observation that ABO incompatibility offered protection against the development or Rh sensitization, probably by allowing destruction of the fetal red cells in the mother before they can stimulate Rh antibody formation. Because most, but certainly not all, major transfers of fetal red cells occur at the time of delivery, efforts to destroy such cells were undertaken soon after delivery. The development of a gamma globulin concentrate of anti-D [Rhogam, $Rh_0(D)$ immune globulin (human)] (Ortho Diagnostics) greatly facilitated application of this means of prevention. Prevention of Rh sensitization is now about 90% effective with the use of Rhogam at the time of delivery. Failures appear to be caused by hemorrhages that occur before term and massive hemorrhages that occur at the time of delivery in which the amount of Rhogam administered is inadequate to destroy the large numbers of cells that have entered the circulation. The subject is reviewed in detail in other sources.[24]

Amniotic fluid examination facilitates the decisions of management of patients during pregnancy. Amniotic fluid is normally clear and colorless. It acquires a yellow pigmentation in cases of severe hemolytic disease because of the passage of bilirubin into it. The amount of bile pigment in the amniotic fluid more accurately reflects the degree of fetal involvement than does the maternal antibody titer. The concentration of bilirubin pigments is generally measured by spectrophotometry of amniotic fluid over the range from about 350 to 700 nm. Normal amniotic fluid, when plotted on a logarithmic scale, describes a straight line, but when a pigment is present a bulge appears around 450 nm. This can be

Table 25-8. Antenatal Management of the Rh-Sensitized Mother.

On the basis of	Decide—one of three courses of action

1. History
   Previous blood transfusions or injections
   Previous pregnancies and outcome
	1. Favorable; wait until 38 weeks, then induce labor

2. Serologic tests
   Father's Rh zygosity
   Maternal antibody titer at approximately 16 weeks, 28 weeks, etc.
	2. Risk of hydrops fetalis or stillbirth: early induction of labor between 34 and 38 weeks

3. Amniocentesis
   In first sensitized pregnancy (Coombs' titer >1:32), at 28–29 weeks
   If previously severely affected infant—as early as 20–23 weeks
   Trend of repeat values important
	3. Risk of hydrops fetalis or stillbirth before 34 weeks: intrauterine intraperitoneal transfusion(s), and induce labor at 34–35 weeks

measured and this optical density (OD), as a function of gestational age, can be employed to gauge the severity of the hemolytic process.[25]

The prevention of stillbirths is accomplished by intrauterine transfusions and by the early termination of pregnancy. These aspects of the management of the problem will not be reviewed here but are summarized in Table 25-8.

Newborns with Rh hemolytic disease are at risk of death or damage primarily from anemia or hyperbilirubinemia. As soon as the infant has been delivered and respirations have been established, the infant should be evaluated in an attempt to judge the severity of the hemolytic process. Note should be made of the presence or absence of pallor, organomegaly, petechiae, edema, ascites, and the respirations, pulse, and blood pressure. Cord blood samples should be analyzed for hemoglobin concentration, reticulocyte count, nucleated red blood cell count, blood type, direct Coombs' reaction, and serum bilirubin concentration, both direct-reacting and total.

In the infant with a positive reacting Coombs' test, the major initial decision is whether to perform an immediate exchange transfusion or to observe the infant's clinical status. In many instances, the outcome of previous pregnancies, and the results of amniocentesis during the current pregnancy will provide valuable information as to what to anticipate in the way of severity. Except for the obviously pale or edematous child, the decision to perform an immediate exchange transfusion is based on laboratory findings. Useful guidelines for facilitating such a decision are presented in Table 25-9.

When immediate transfusion is not indicated, serial observations of total serum bilirubin must be made at intervals of 6 to 12 hours during the first several days of life. Decisions concerning exchange transfusion after birth should be based on the trend of serum bilirubin levels plotted on a graph against the infant's age. All infants should have such graphs placed in their charts to facilitate clinical judgements. In general, a trend projecting a bilirubin level of 20 mg/dl in a full-term infant within 72 to 96 hours of age is an indication for exchange transfusion. If the clinical course is complicated by hypoxia, acidosis, or hypoproteinemia, a decision to perform an exchange transfusion at a lower level of unconjugated bilirubin may be made. In infants born prior to term, a convenient guide for the necessity of exchange transfusion can be made employing the infant's birth weight. Infants weighing 1000 g should be exchanged at 10 mg/dl, infants weighing 1500 g at 15 mg/dl, and infants weighing 2000 g or more at 20 mg/dl. Graphs specifically designed for the management of low-birth-weight infants with hyperbilirubinemia are also available.[27]

Table 25-9. Need for Exchange Transfusion in Infants with a Positive Coombs' Test.

	Observe	Consider Exchange	Exchange
At Birth			
History of previous offspring	No need for exchange transfusion	Exchange transfusion necessary or kernicterus	Death or near death from erythroblastosis
Maternal Rh antibody titer	<1:64	>1:64	
Clinical situation	Apparently normal	Induced or spontaneous delivery of premature infant	Jaundice, fetal hydrops
Cord hemoglobin	>14 g/dl	12–14 g/dl	< 12 g/dl
Cord bilirubin	<4 mg/dl	4–5 mg/dl	
After Birth			
Capillary blood hemoglobin	>12 g/dl	<12 g/dl	<12 g/dl and falling in first 24 hours
Serum bilirubin	<18 mg/gl	18–20 mg/dl	20 mg/dl in first 48 hours or 22 mg/dl on 2 successive determinations at 6–8hr intervals after 48 hr
			Clinical signs suggesting kernicterus at any time or any bilirubin level

(McKay RJ: Pediatrics 33:763, 1964; Copyright © American Academy of Pediatrics, 1964)

The procedure for performing exchange transfusions has been described in detail elsewhere.[28] Certain potential hazards of umbilical vein catheterization and exchange transfusion are listed in Table 25-10. (See also Chap. 24.)

ABO Incompatibility. Hemolytic disease in this condition results from the action of maternal anti-A or anti-B antibodies upon fetal erythrocytes of the corresponding blood group. As discussed, although approximately 20% of all pregnancies are associated with ABO incompatibility between mother and fetus, the incidence of severe hemolytic disease is very low. Anti-A and anti-B antibodies are found in IgA, IgM, and IgG fractions of plasma. Only the IgG antibodies cross the placenta and are responsible for the production of disease. These naturally occurring antibodies result from continuous immune stimulation by A and B substances that are present in foods and gram-negative bacteria. It is not understood why some women develop high anti-A or anti-B titers. They may be the result of repeated, asymptomatic bacterial infections. ABO hemolytic disease tends to occur in the newborns of mothers with the high levels of antibody.

Fewer A or B antigenic sites are present on the erythrocytes of the newborn. This fact appears responsible for the weakly reactive Coombs' test in infants with ABO hemolytic disease. The sparse distribution of A and B sites on the red cells of the newborn also serves to explain why the erythrocyte life span in ABO hemolytic disease is only slightly shortened. That this phenomenon is caused by the fetal erythrocyte, and not the nature of the antibody, is supported by the fact that when adult Group A erythrocytes are transfused into a baby with maternally acquired anti-A antibody they are rapidly destroyed and may in fact produce intravascular hemolysis.

The diagnosis of ABO hemolytic disease

depends largely on the clinical, serologic, and hematologic findings in the newborn. These features include (1) the presence of unexplained hyperbilirubinemia in an infant of Group A or B born of a mother of Group O; (2) the presence of mild anemia, reticulocytosis, and spherocytosis; (3) the presence of a weakly positive direct Coombs' test and the elution of anti-A or anti-B antibodies from the red cells of the affected infant; (4) the presence of free anti-A or anti-B antibody in the serum of the newborn; and (5) the presence of relatively high titers of anti-A or anti-B of the IgG type in the serum of the mother.

Some of the features that are useful in distinguishing ABO from Rh incompatibility are listed in Table 25-11.

Treatment of this disease is primarily directed against the prevention of hyperbilirubinemia. Phototherapy will reduce the need for exchange transfusion in this disorder.[29]

Congenital Defects of the Red Cell. Inherited defects of red cell metabolism, membrane function, and hemoglobin synthesis may all manifest themselves in the newborn period.

Enzymatic Deficiencies of the Red Cell. For many years, these defects were grouped together as "congenital nonspherocytic hemolytic anemias." With increased understanding of red cell metabolism, many of these disorders have been identified as resulting from specific, distinct enzyme deficiencies. As yet, not all the defects capable of producing a congenital nonspherocytic hemolytic anemia have been identified, but some order has been imparted to this once large heterogeneous group of disturbances.

The congenital nonspherocytic hemolytic anemias can be most easily classified into three large groups based on the site of the primary metabolic abnormality. These three groups are (1) defects of the Embden–Meyerhof pathway; (2) defects of the pentose phosphate pathway and disorders of the glutathione metabolism; and (3) a miscellaneous group which includes disorders of adenosine triphosphate metabolism.

These disorders are characterized by normal osmotic fragility of unincubated blood, few or no spherocytes, normal hemoglobin type, and the failure of splenectomy to correct the hemolytic process.

Although all these disorders are potentially capable of manifesting themselves in the neo-

Table 25-10. Potential Hazards of Exchange Transfusion.

Type of Hazard	Problems Encountered
Vascular	Embolization with air or clots
	Thrombosis
	Hemorrhagic infarction of the colon
Cardiac	Arrhythmias
	Volume overload
	Arrest
Metabolic	Hyperkalemia
	Hypernatremia
	Hypocalcemia
	Hpomagnesemia
	Acidosis
	Hypoglycemia
Clotting	Overheparinization
	Thrombocytopenia
Infections	Bacteremia
	Hepatitis A or B, or non-AB
	Malaria
	Cytomegalovirus
Miscellaneous	Mechanical injury to donor cells
	Perforation
	Hypothermia

natal period with jaundice and anemia, the hemolytic process may be so mild as to escape detection until later life. With the exception of red cell glucose-6-phosphate dehydrogenase (G-6-PD) deficiency, a defect of the pentose phosphate pathway that is estimated to affect nearly 100 million individuals throughout the world, these red cell disorders are very uncommon and generally unsuspected, and they are rarely diagnosed during the first weeks of life.

• Glucose-6-Phosphate Dehydrogenase Deficiency: In 1960, Panizon called attention to the risks of G-6-PD deficiency during the newborn period, when he described 11 cases of severe jaundice in infants from Sardinia.[30] During the same year, Smith and Vella reported from Singapore on 13 Chinese infants with kernicterus associated with G-6-PD deficiency.[31] In Greece, it has been noted that isoimmunization cannot be demonstrated in one-third of the infants requiring exchange transfusions for hyperbilirubinemia, and in most cases, G-6-PD deficiency is responsible.

Table 25-11. Comparison of Rh and ABO Incompatibility.

	Rh	**ABO**
Blood Group Set-up		
Mother	Negative	0
Infant	Positive	A or B
Type of Antibody	Incomplete (7S)	Immune (7S)
Clinical Aspects		
Occurrence in firstborn	5%	40–50%
Predictable severity in subsequent pregnancies	Usually	No
Stillbirth and/or hydrops	Frequent	Rare
Severe anemia	Frequent	Rare
Degree of jaundice	+++	+
Hepatosplenomegaly	+++	+
Laboratory Findings		
Direct Commbs' test (infant)	+	+ or 0
Maternal antibodies	Always present	Not clear-cut
Spherocytes	0	+
Treatment		
Need for antenatal measures	Yes	No
Exchange transfusion		
Frequency	Approx. ⅔	Approx. $^{1}/_{10}$
Donor blood type	Rh-negative Group-specific, when possible	Rh—same as infant Group 0 only
Incidence of late anemia	Common	Rare

Unlike observations of the increased incidence of jaundice among Greek, Italian, Chinese, Thai, and Hawaiian infants with G-6-PD deficiency, there does not appear to be an increased incidence of jaundice among Negro or Israeli term infants with the same deficiency, unless the infant is either infected or he or his mother received an oxidant compound. Among Black premature infants, however, the incidence and severity of jaundice are greater in those that are deficient in G-6-PD.

Although the increased incidence of jaundice in the newborn infant deficient in G-6-PD is apparently the result of hemolysis, in many instances no offending drug or toxin can be incriminated as the precipitating agent. In these cases, the precise factor or factors responsible for initiating the hemolytic process remain to be explained.

In infants with hemolytic disease caused by G-6-PD deficiency, jaundice, pallor, or signs of kernicterus are the chief physical findings. Hepatosplenomegaly is uncommon and, if present, a second disease such as isoimmunization or infection should be suspected.

In contrast to the jaundice caused by blood group incompatibilities, jaundice usually does not appear during the first 24 hours of life in infants with G-6-PD deficiency. Bilirubin concentration generally peaks between the third and fifth days of life. Jaundice may not manifest itself until late in the first week of life, with peak levels of bilirubin occurring during the second week. It is in this relatively late jaundice that drugs or mothballs are often found to be responsible for the hemolytic anemia.

Hyperbilirubinemia, variable degrees of anemia, and morphologic alterations of the red cell are the chief laboratory findings in infants with hemolytic disease caused by G-6-PD deficiency. Bilirubin levels frequently exceed 20 mg/dl on the third to fifth day of life, and values in excess of 50 mg/dl have been observed. Levels in excess of 20 mg/dl can occur during the second week of life, with resultant kernicterus.

Hemoglobin values may range from normal to as low as 7 or 8 g/dl during the first week of life. Anemia tends to be more profound in those infants in whom hemolysis is triggered by an exogenous agent. However, in some cases, both the hemoglobin level and reticulocyte count may be normal, emphasizing the fact that only a small proportion of the red cell population need be destroyed in order to produce hyperbilirubinemia in the presence of the physiologically immature bilirubin conjugating and excreting mechanisms of the newborn.

In general, the reticulocyte count is elevated. Morphologic abnormalities in a peripheral blood smear consist of a varying number of nucleated red cells, spherocytes, poikilocytes and crenated and fragmented cells—all findings consistent with hemolytic anemia caused by a metabolic derangement of the cells. With supravital staining techniques, red cells containing Heinz bodies are frequently observed during the early phase of the hemolytic episode. Eventually, these cells are cleared by the spleen, and thus may not be found. All of these morphologic abnormalities disappear when the hemolytic episode has abated.

Although normal newborn infants have higher levels of red cell G-6-PD than do adults, this difference does not make it difficult to diagnose G-6-PD deficiency during the neonatal period. Glutathione levels are low and glutathione instability is present, but these tests are not as reliable or as meaningful as studies of enzyme activity. Newborn infants deficient in G-6-PD have markedly reduced levels of enzyme activity that can be detected by screening tests. These screening tests have been proved to be reliable in detecting the hemizygous male or the homozygous female. Direct assay of the enzyme by spectrophotometric techniques is often necessary to identify precisely the heterozygous female.

The basis for treatment of this condition is simple, but often its application may be difficult. Proper care consists in recognition of the deficient patient who is potentially in danger, avoidance of hemolytic compounds in the care of these infants, careful observation for jaundice, and the treatment of hyperbilirubinemia with exchange transfusions.

In nurseries in which a large percentage of the patients are from ethnic groups susceptible to spontaneous hemolysis during the neonatal period, screening procedures should be introduced to identify the infants at risk. Potential hemolytic agents should not be given to the newborn infant deficient in G-6-PD, and should also be withheld from the mother if the child is to be breast fed. Hemolytic anemias have occurred in breast-fed infants of mothers who have ingested fava beans or have been exposed to mothballs.

In the Black infant, there is no apparent danger from the use of naturally occurring vitamin K_1 (Aquamephyton, Konakion), even in doses far in excess of 1.0 mg. Large doses of water-soluble vitamin K analogs (Synkyvite, Hykinone) can produce hemolysis, but in doses of 1.0 mg, they also appeared to have no jaundice-producing effects in the deficient Black. The safe dose for vitamin K analogs has not been determined for the deficient Caucasian infant. Until more information is available, it is advisable to adhere to the recommendations of the American Academy of Pediatrics (1961) and give the minimum dose (1 mg intramuscularly to the premature or full-term infant) of the least toxic preparation: vitamin K_1.

After the deficient infant is discharged from the nursery, careful instructions must be given to the parents with respect to exposure to naphthalene. These infants must not be exposed to blankets, bedclothes, or diapers that have been recently removed from storage in mothballs or in flakes that contain naphthalene. The parents should also be instructed to bring the child immediately to the hospital if pallor, jaundice, or dark urine is noted.

When hyperbilirubinemia occurs, exchange transfusions should be performed for indirect bilirubin levels in excess of 20 mg/dl, even after the first week of life. When an infant deficient in G-6-PD is recognized, family studies should be carried out to detect other individuals who may be at risk from the hemolytic consequences of drug therapy. If hyperbilirubinemia has not resulted in kernicterus, the prognosis for infants deficient in G-6-PD is good. Although these deficient patients will always have red cells with a shorter life span, they will not develop anemia or reticulocytosis unless stressed by drugs, infections, or acidosis.

• Other Metabolic Abnormalities of the Red Cell: are far less common than G-6-PD deficiency and, thus, are unusual causes of a hemolytic process with anemia and jaundice during the newborn period. Virtually all the recognized defects, however, have been described in association with jaundice and anemia during the first week of life. Of this group, red cell pyruvate kinase deficiency appears to be most commonly responsible for a severe hemolytic process during the first week of life. These disorders are generally characterized by the presence of a normal osmotic fragility of unincubated blood, few or no spherocytes in the periperhal blood smear, and the failure of splenectomy in later life to correct the hemolytic process. It is most practical to defer diagnosis of these infants until approximately 3 months of life, after it has been established that the hemolytic process observed in the immediate neonatal period is of a chronic nature, and the more common reasons for such an event have been excluded.

Hereditary Abnormalities of the Red Cell Membrane. • Hereditary Spherocytosis, Elliptocytosis and Stomatocytosis: In approximately 50% of patients with **hereditary spherocytosis,** a history of neonatal jaundice can be obtained. Hyperbilirubinemia may be of sufficient magnitude to require exchange transfusions. Untreated hyperbilirubinemia has resulted in kernicterus in infants with hereditary spherocytosis.

The degree of anemia, reticulocytosis and hyperbilirubinemia are quite variable in these patients, although most patients are mildly to markedly anemic. The hemoglobin tends to fall rapidly during the first several weeks of life, reaching values of 5 to 7 g/dl by 1 month of age. Neither the hematologic values observed during the immediate newborn period nor the values observed during the first several months of life serve as reliable indicators of the eventual severity of the disease. It has been our experience that hemoglobin levels in many infants with values in the range of 4 to 7 g/dl during the first several months of life, subsequently stabilize in the range of 7 to 10 g/dl. Repeated transfusions are rarely needed to maintain adequate hemoglobin levels, except during the course of infections or aplastic crises. It is our opinion that splenectomy

should be deferred until 3 or 4 years of age to minimize the risk of post-splenectomy infections.

Hereditary spherocytosis can be diagnosed during the newborn period. Examination of the peripheral blood reveals the presence of characteristic microspherocytes and the osmotic fragility of erythrocytes is increased. Family studies are extremely useful in confirming the diagnosis, although only in approximately 80% of cases will an affected parent be identified.

Hemolytic disease caused by ABO incompatibility, as well as infections in the neonatal period, share many features in common with hereditary spherocytosis. In these conditions, spherocytosis, increased red cell osmotic fragility and mild anemia, reticulocytosis, and minimal splenomegaly may also be present. Both of these diagnostic possibilities must be excluded before an unequivocal diagnosis of hereditary spherocytosis can be made. The eventual course of the illness will also serve to differentiate between transient diseases of the newborn period and the chronic hemolytic process of hereditary spherocytosis.

Hereditary elliptocytosis may also manifest itself in the newborn period as a hemolytic anemia. Although only approximately 12% to 15% of individuals with this morphologic abnormality can be shown to have a shortened red cell life span in later life, it appears that many more of these patients have a hemolytic anemia during the first several weeks or months of life. The diagnosis can only be established by demonstrating large numbers of elliptical cells in the patient's blood film. Occasionally, during the newborn period, very few elliptocytes may be seen. Other morphologic abnormalities, such as pyknocytes, may be more striking initially, and elliptocytes gradually become the predominant cell type during the first 3 to 4 months of life. In this disorder, as in hereditary spherocytosis, demonstrating an affected parent or sibling helps to establish the diagnosis.

Most patients do not require treatment although an exchange transfusion may be required for infants with hyperbilirubinemia. In those patients with persistent hemolytic anemia, splenectomy has proven beneficial but, as in hereditary spherocytosis, it should be deferred until the patient is 3 or 4 years of age.

Hereditary stomatocytosis, a morphologic

abnormality characterized by the presence of red cells with a linear rather than a central area of pallor, is also associated with a hemolytic anemia whose severity varies in the families in which it has been observed. In none of the patients reported to date have sufficient clinical or laboratory abnormalities been detected in the neonatal period to establish a diagnosis. Laboratory findings are variable but include mild to severe anemia, minimal to marked reticulocytosis, alterations in red cell concentrations of sodium and potassium, increased sodium influx and efflux, and the presence of erythrocytes with either a decreased or increased osmotic fragility.

Disorders of Hemoglobin Synthesis. The common hemoglobinopathies can be diagnosed at the time of birth. Defects involving the beta-chain, such as hemoglobins S or C do not generally produce either anemia or jaundice during the first weeks of life. By 1 month of life, infants with sickle-cell anemia have lower hemoglobins than normal infants, and by 3 months of age virtually all such patients will have hemoglobin values of less than 10.0 g/dl.[32]

Two forms of thalassemia may cause anemia in the immediate newborn period. In homozygous alpha-thalassemia, alpha-chain production is deficient and excess gamma-chains combine to form hemoglobin Bart's.[33] This tetramer has a very high affinity for oxygen and the resultant impaired release of oxygen to the tissues results in severe intrauterine distress. The infant with homozygous alpha-thalassemia is usually stillborn or dies shortly after birth with a picture of hydrops fetalis. Although alpha-thalassemia trait is common among Orientals, Blacks, and persons of Mediterranean origin, homozygous alpha-thalassemia has been reported to date only among Orientals.

The heterozygous form of alpha-thalassemia may be associated with mild anemia and jaundice during the neonatal period. This diagnosis may be confirmed by demonstrating the presence of increased quantities of hemoglobin Bart's, decreased quantities of fetal hemoglobin, and the presence of some degree of hypochromia and microcytosis, when compared with newborn values.

The heterozygous form of beta-thalassemia is not associated with anemia and jaundice during the first weeks of life. Infants with homozygous beta-thalassemia may be slightly anemic at the time of birth with evidence of hypochromia and microcytosis.

Two rare hemoglobinopathies have been described in association with neonatal hemolytic anemias: hemoglobin F-Poole,[34] and hemoglobin Hasharon.[35] Hemoglobin F-Poole is a mutant fetal hemoglobin as a result of an amino acid substitution at the 130th residue of the gamma-chain. This substitution produces an unstable hemoglobin characterized by the presence of hemolytic anemia in the neonatal period in which Heinz bodies are present.

Hemoglobin Hasharon is an alpha-chain mutant. Adults heterozygous for this mutant are usually asymptomatic, but the heterozygous state in the newborn period has been reported to be associated with a moderate hemolytic anemia.

Acquired Defects of the Red Cell. Both infections and drugs may produce a hemolytic anemia in the newborn infant who has no underlying inherited defect of red cell metabolism.

Congenital syphilis, toxoplasmosis, cytomegalic inclusion disease, rubella, generalized coxsackie B infections, and *Escherichia coli* septicemia are examples of infections in which anemia and jaundice are common. Some of the nonhematologic manifestations of the diseases such as the presence of a rash, chorioretinitis, purpura, and hepatosplenomegaly are useful in differentiating these disorders from isoimmunization or other primary red cell abnormalities. Elevations in the white count and the serum IgM level may help to establish the presence of infection. It now appears that the hemolytic process in many of these infections may be secondary to the microangiopathic process caused by the associated DIC.

The red cells of the newborn infant are particularly sensitive to the toxic effects of oxidant drugs. The red cells of infants, particularly those born prematurely, demonstrate increased numbers of Heinz bodies, marked glutathione instability, and an increased tendency to develop methemoglobinemia when incubated in the presence of compounds such as acetylphenylhydrazine or menadione. In many respects, the cells of these infants mimic the metabolic abnormalities observed in cells from subjects with G-6-PD deficiency.

Despite these similarities, these infants have normally functioning pentose phosphate pathways, and red cell G-6-PD activity is increased. This vulnerability to oxidant compounds has been ascribed to a relative deficiency of glutathione peroxidase, an enzyme necessary for the detoxification of hydrogen peroxide.[36] Studies in our laboratory suggest that the availability of pyridine nucleotide cofactors and membrane repair processes may also be responsible for the appearance of these cells as phenocopies, in many respects, of the G-6-PD-deficient erythrocyte. Whatever the mechanism, large quantities of water-soluble vitamin K derivatives, sulfonamides, or other agents known to trigger hemolysis in G-6-PD-deficient individuals should not be administered either to the infant or to the mother at term.

Impaired Red Cell Production. This appears to be an unusual cause for anemia in the newborn period. The most common of the disorders in this category is the Diamond–Blackfan syndrome, also known as congenital hypoplastic anemia or pure red cell aplasia. In approximately one-third of infants with this abnormality, anemia is present at birth.[37] The white count and platelet count are normal. Diagnosis may be established by the finding of anemia and reticulocytopenia, and a marked decrease in the bone marrow erythroid to myeloid ratio in an otherwise healthy newborn. Erythroid to myeloid ratios range from 1:6 to greater than 1:200. Low birth weight occurs in approximately 10% of patients, with about one-half being small for gestational age. Physical anomalies are present in about 30% of patients. Anomalies apparent at birth include microcephaly, cleft palate, eye defects, web neck, and abnormalities of the thumb. Early recognition of this disorder appears to enhance the probability of observing a response to steroid therapy. Allen and Diamond recommend an initial dose of prednisone of 30 mg/day for 2 weeks. A response as reflected in a reticulotytosis and rise in hemoglobin generally occurs during this interval. After the hemoglobin has returned to normal, the medication is reduced to the lowest dose necessary to maintain a hemoglobin in the acceptable range. Pure red cell aplasia has also been observed in association with triphalangeal thumbs.[38]

The Differential Diagnosis of Anemia in the Neonate

Although seemingly paradoxical, at no other time than the first week of life does such a myriad of disorders result in anemia. The need for rapid treatment often adds to the diagnostic confusion. It is because of these reasons—multiple causes and the need for prompt therapy—that the fundamentals of diagnosis should be appreciated and practiced with precision and without delay. One approach to the differential diagnosis of anemia in the newborn is offered in Figure 25-1.

Attempts at diagnosis properly begin with a history, when the cause is not immediately apparent. In the family history, attention should be paid to the presence of anemia in other members of the family, or to unexplained episodes of jaundice or cholelithiasis. A positive family history is frequently obtained in cases of infants with hereditary spherocytosis, while a history indicating affected siblings may be encountered in cases of patients with enzymatic defects of the red cell.

In the maternal history, information should be obtained concerning drug ingestion near term. Information concerning drugs known to initiate hemolysis in G-6-PD deficiency should especially be sought, as well as any history of recent exposure to mothballs containing naphthalene.

The obstetric history should provide information on vaginal bleeding during pregnancy, the presence or absence of placenta previa, abruptio placentae, vasa previa, or cesarean section. Additional questions to be answered include (1) Was the birth traumatic? (2) Was the birth attended by a physician? (3) Did the cord rupture? and (4) Was it a multiple birth?

The age at which anemia is first noted is also of diagnostic value. Marked anemia at birth is generally the result of either hemorrhage or severe isoimmunization. Anemia manifesting itself during the first 2 days of life is frequently caused by internal or external hemorrhages, while anemia appearing after the first 48 hours of life is most commonly hemolytic and is generally associated with jaundice.

The basic laboratory studies in the initial investigation of anemia should include hemoglobin determination, reticulocyte count, examination of a peripheral blood smear, a direct Coombs' test of the infant's blood, and examination of the maternal blood smear for fetal erythrocytes. From these few studies and the history, a diagnosis often can be made. If the diagnosis has not been made, at least the list of diagnostic possibilities has been greatly shortened.

The reticulocyte count provides the first

THE ANEMIC NEWBORN

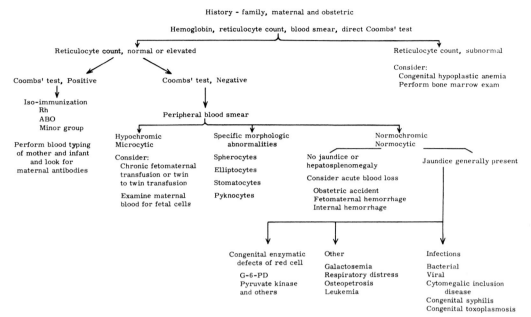

Fig. 25-1. An approach to the differential diagnosis of anemia in the newborn. (Oski F, Naiman J L: In Haematologic Problems of the Newborn. Philadelphia, W. B. Saunders, 1972)[35]

valuable laboratory clue. If the anemia is a result of either hemorrhage or hemolysis, the reticulocyte count usually is elevated. If the anemia is associated with reticulocytopenia, the diagnosis of congenital hypoplastic anemia must be considered as well as processes that might result in bone marrow infiltration, such as congenital leukemia. In reticulocytopenia, a bone marrow examination is necessary to establish the diagnosis.

When the reticulocyte count is elevated, a variety of diagnostic possibilities remains, if obstetric hemorrhage has already been excluded. A positive direct Coombs' test will identify the infants with isoimmunization in the Rh, ABO, or minor blood group systems, after which both infant and mother must be blood typed and a search made for maternal antibodies.

If the Coombs' test is negative, other forms of hemolytic disease as well as occult hemorrhage remain to be excluded. At this point, careful attention must be paid to red cell morphology. While examining the smear, attention should be paid to the numbers of platelets present and to any peculiarities of the leukocytes.

If the peripheral smear reveals the presence of hypochromic microcytic red cells, iron deficiency should be considered as a likely cause of the anemia. Iron-deficiency anemia can result from chronic fetomaternal hemorrhage or twin-to-twin transfusion. If fetomaternal hemorrhage is suspected, the mother's blood should be examined for cells containing fetal hemoglobin.

The presence of morphologic abnormalities such as spherocytes or elliptocytes aids in establishment of a diagnosis of hereditary disorder of red cell morphology. I pyknocytes are present in large numbers, then this poorly understood acquired defect of red cells must be considered as a distinct diagnostic possibility. Pyknoctyes have also been observed in newborns with hemolysis as a consequence of G-6-PD deficiency.

If the red cells are normocytic and normochromic, the anemia may be the result of acute blood loss or a congenital enzymatic defect of the red cell, or secondary to a systemic disease in the infant. In this event, the birth history, the history of the first few days of life, and the physical examination aid in the differential diagnosis.

Anemia as a result of acute hemorrhage is generally not associated with jaundice or hep-

Table 25-12. Neonatal Polycythemia.

Possibly Caused by Placental Hypertransfusion	Possible Association
Twin-to-twin transfusion	Placental insufficiency
Maternofetal transfusion	Small-for-gestational-age infants
Delayed cord clamping	Postmaturity
Intentional	Toxemia of pregnancy
Unassisted home delivery	Placenta previa
	Endocrine and matabolic disorders
	Congenital adrenal hyperplasia
	Neonatal thyrotoxicosis
	Maternal diabetes
	Miscellaneous
	Trisomy 21, 13, 18
	Hyperplastic visceromegaly (Beckwith's syndrome)
	Erythroderma icthyosiforme congenita

atosplenomegaly. Pallor is prominent and the infant may be in shock. Internal hemorrhage must be suspected in infants born after a traumatic delivery.

Pyruvate kinase deficiency, hexokinase deficiency, G-6-PD deficiency, and the other enzymatic defects of the red cell may result in a hemolytic anemia during the first week of life. G-6-PD deficiency should be strongly suspected in Mediterranean and Oriental male infants. The other anemias show no racial predisposition.

A variety of infections may produce a hemolytic anemia characterized by normochromic cells. Red cell fragmentation and spherocytes also may be observed. Cytomegalic inclusion disease, toxoplasmosis, and congenital syphilis are usually accompanied by prominent hepatosplenomegaly, jaundice, and thrombocytopenic purpura. Diagnosis of cytomegalic inclusion disease is supported by finding the characteristic cells in the urinary sediment, and it is confirmed by isolation of the salivary gland virus from the urine. Serologic studies are necessary to establish a diagnosis of congenital syphilis or toxoplasmosis. Other infections also may be accompanied by anemia and jaundice, and appropriate blood and urine cultures should be performed in all infants with obscure hemolytic anemias during the first weeks of life. Measurement of the serum IgM level may provide useful information. The presence of an elevated IgM level in a newborn infant strongly suggests that an antecedent intrauterine infection has occurred.

When a burr cell anemia is present in an infant who is ill with sepsis, acidosis, or hypoxia, laboratory evidence of DIC should be collected and evaluated. Performance of a platelet count, prothrombin time, partial thromboplastin time, thrombin time, Factor V assay, and measurement of fibrin split products are most useful in establishing this diagnosis.

In most newborn infants with anemia, a diligent search is required to reveal the diagnosis. In certain instances, the diagnosis must be deferred until the infant is older; in others the anemia disappears, the cause remains undetermined, and the curiosity unsatisfied.

POLYCYTHEMIA IN THE NEWBORN

A venous hemoglobin of greater than 22.0 g/dl or a venous hematocrit of more than 65% during the first week of life, should be regarded as polycythemia. Table 25-12 gives a list of conditions that may cause or be associated with polycythemia.

The symptoms observed in the polycythemic infant appear to be primarily a consequence of the associated increase in blood viscosity. After the central venous hematocrit reaches 60% to 65%, any further increase will result in an exponential increase in blood viscosity.[40] Some of these infants have inherently rigid red cells that will result in greater than expected viscosity at any given hematocrit reading.[41]

Respiratory distress, cyanosis, congestive heart failure, convulsions, priapism, jaundice, renal vein thrombosis, hypoglycemia, and hypocalcemia all appear to be more common among infants with polycythemia. Many infants with polycythemia are asymptomatic.

It still remains unclear whether efforts should be made to reduce the hematocrit in infants who are asymptomatic. Treatment of infants with symptoms should be designed to reduce the venous hematocrit to less than 60%. This can be readily accomplished by the performance of a partial exchange transfusion, using fresh frozen plasma. The following formula may be employed to approximate the volume of exchange required to reduce the hematocrit to the desired level.

Vol. of exchange (ml)
$$= \frac{\text{Blood vol.} \times (\text{Observed Hct} - \text{Desired Hct})}{\text{Observed Hct}}$$

(Assume a blood volume of 100 ml/kg)

Unless the infant can be demonstrated to be hypervolemic, simple phlebotomy should not be performed to reduce the hematocrit. Most of these infants have a reduced cardiac output as a consequence of their hyperviscosity, and further reduction in blood volume may, in fact, aggravate the symptoms.[42]

FETAL HEMOGLOBIN, THE NEONATAL RED CELL, AND 2, 3-DIPHOSPHOGLYCERATE

Human tissue metabolism critically depends on an adequate supply of oxygen. The oxygen transport system in man is the erythrocyte. The erythrocyte serves this role because it contains the iron-protein conjugate, hemoglobin. The red cell's primary function is to bring oxygen to the tissues in adequate quantities, at a partial pressure sufficient to permit its rapid diffusion from the blood. The ultimate supply of oxygen to the cell is determined by a number of factors including the content of oxygen in the inspired air; the pulmonary and alveolar ventilation; the diffusion of oxygen from the alveolar air to the capillary bed; the cardiac output; the blood volume; the hemoglobin concentration; and the passive diffusion of oxygen from the capillaries to the cells. The initial passive diffusion of oxygen from the

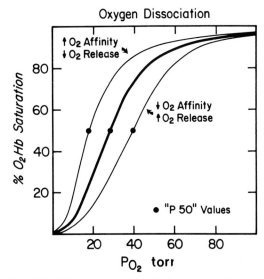

Fig. 25-2. The oxygen dissociation curve of normal adult blood. The P_{50}, the oxygen tension at 50% oxygen saturation, is approximately 27 torr. As the curve shifts to the right, the oxygen affinity of hemoglobin decreases and more oxygen is released at a given oxygen tension. With a shift to the left, the opposite effects are observed. A decrease in pH or an increase in temperature decreases the affinity of hemoglobin for oxygen.

lungs and its final release to the tissues is determined in large part by the affinity of hemoglobin for oxygen.

The oxygen-hemoglobin equilibrium curve reflects the affinity of hemoglobin for oxygen (Fig. 25-2). As blood circulates in the normal lung, arterial oxygen tension rises from 40 torr and reaches approximately 110 torr, sufficient to ensure at least 95% saturation of the arterial blood. The shape of the curve is such that a further increase in the oxygen tension in the lung results in only a very small increase in the degree of saturation of the blood. As blood travels from the lung, the oxygen tension falls as oxygen is released to the tissues from hemoglobin. In the normal adult when the oxygen tension has fallen to approximately 27 torr, at a pH of 7.4 and a temperature of 37°C, 50 percent of the oxygen bound to hemoglobin has been released. The P_{50}, the whole blood oxygen tension at 50% oxygen saturation, is thus stated to be 27 torr. When the affinity of hemoglobin for oxygen is reduced, more oxygen is released to the tissues at a given oxygen tension. In such situations the oxygen-hemoglobin equilibrium curve is shifted to the right of normal. It has long been recognized that increases in blood acidity, carbon dioxide content, ionic concentration, or temperature are capable of decreasing the affinity of hemoglobin for oxygen and thus shifting the curve to the right. When the affinity of hemoglobin for oxygen is increased, such as occurs with alkalosis or a decrease in temperature, the equilibrium curve appears shifted to the left and the tension must drop lower than normal before the hemoglobin releases an equivalent amount of oxygen.

Fetal Hemoglobin and the Organic Phosphates

Benesch and Benesch[43] and Chanutin and Curnish[44] demonstrated that a variety of organic phosphates, when added to adult hemoglobin in solution, has the ability to reduce the affinity of hemoglobin for oxygen. Of the organic phosphates tested, the compound, 2,3-diphosphoglycerate (2,3-DPG) appeared to be the most potent modifier of hemoglobin function. Of the organic phosphates normally found in human erythrocytes, 2,3-DPG is present in highest concentration, averaging approximately 5 μmol/ml of red cells, and thus is quantitatively the most important with respect to modulating hemoglobin's affinity for oxygen.

After the role of 2,3-DPG in altering the affinity of adult hemoglobin for oxygen was recognized, numerous investigators examined its interaction with fetal hemoglobin in an attempt to determine why the fetal erythrocyte demonstrates a higher affinity for oxygen than the adult erythrocyte.

In 1930, Anselmino and Hoffman[45] first observed that the oxygen affinity of human fetal blood was greater than that of maternal blood. Fetal blood had a P_{50} value some 6 to 8 torr lower than that of the normal adult. In 1953, Allen, Wyman, and Smith[46] demonstrated that although intact fetal cells possess a higher affinity for oxygen than do the red cells of adults, when adult and fetal hemoglobin solutions were dialyzed against the same buffer, the resulting oxygen affinities were identical.

This puzzling observation was resolved by the finding that the affinity of fetal hemoglobin for 2,3-DPG is far less than that of adult hemoglobin.[47] When 2,3-DPG is added to solutions of fetal hemoglobin, the decrease in oxygen affinity produced by this compound is much less than that observed with adult hemoglobin.

From these studies it appears that the major reason that the blood of the newborn infant possesses an oxygen-hemoglobin equilibrium curve that is shifted to the left of that of the normal adult is the failure of fetal hemoglobin to bind 2,3-DPG to the same degree as does adult hemoglobin.

The position of the oxygen-hemoglobin equilibrium curve in the neonate is determined by the relative proportions of adult and fetal hemoglobin present and the red cell 2,3-DPG concentration. Infants with similar fetal hemoglobin concentrations can have different P_{50} values if they differ significantly in their red cell 2,3-DPG concentrations; alternatively, infants with similar 2,3-DPG concentrations may have dissimilar P_{50} values if they differ in their percent fetal hemoglobin. The need to consider both the proportion of adult and fetal hemoglobin and the 2,3-DPG content of the cells explains why previous investigators failed to find a direct relationship between fetal hemoglobin values alone and the position of the curve.

The level of red cell 2,3-DPG gradually increases with gestation and, at term, its concentration within the infant's erythrocytes is similar to that of the normal adult. The 2,3-DPG levels fall transiently during the first several days of life and then rise. By the end of the first week of life, in the term infant, the 2,3-DPG levels are considerably higher than they are at birth.

In the term infant, the oxygen-hemoglobin equilibrium curve gradually shifts to the right and the P_{50} value approximates that of the normal adult by approximately 4 to 6 months of age (Table 20-13).[48] A significant increase in P_{50} can be observed during the first week of life. This increase is a result of the rise in the red cell 2,3-DPG level. It is tempting to speculate that it is caused by the transient rise in the serum inorganic phosphate level which so commonly occurs during this period.

In the premature infant, born with lower 2,3-DPG levels and higher fetal hemoglobin values, the shift in the position of the curve is far more gradual.[48] In all infants, the position of the curve appears to be directly correlated with the "functioning" DPG fraction.[48]

Exchange transfusion following birth pro-

Table 25-13. Oxygen Transport in Term Infants.

No. of Infants	Age	Total Hemoglobin (g/dl blood)	O_2 Capacity (ml/dl blood)	P_{50} at pH 7.40 (mm Hg)	2,3-DPG mmol/ml RBC	Fetal Hemoglobin (% of total)
19	1 day	17.8 ± 2.0	24.7 ± 2.8	19.4 ± 1.8	5433 ± 1041	77.0 ± 7.3
18	5 days	16.2 ± 1.2	22.6 ± 2.2	20.6 ± 1.7	6850 ± 996	76.8 ± 5.8
14	3 weeks	12.0 ± 1.3	16.7 ± 1.9	22.7 ± 1.0	5378 ± 732	70.0 ± 7.33
10	6–9 weeks	10.5 ± 1.2	14.7 ± 1.6	24.4 ± 1.4	5560 ± 747	52.1 ± 11.0
14	3–4 months	10.2 ± 0.8	14.3 ± 1.2	26.5 ± 2.0	5819 ± 1240	23.2 ± 16.0
8	6 months	11.3 ± 0.9	14.7 ± 0.6	27.8 ± 1.0	5086 ± 1570	4.7 ± 2.2
8	8–11 months	11.4 ± 0.6	15.9 ± 0.8	30.3 ± 0.7	7381 ± 485	1.6 ± 1.0

duces rapid alterations in the infant's oxygen-hemoglobin equilibrium curve.[49] The early changes produced are a function of the storage characteristics of the blood employed. The use of fresh heparinized blood or blood stored in the anticoagulant citrate-phosphate-dextrose, for periods of up to 1 week, produce a prompt increase in the P^{50} value of the infant to that of the normal adult.

Although the oxygen-carrying capacity of the blood decreases during the first 3 to 4 months of life because of the progressive fall in total hemoglobin concentration, this fall is accompanied by an increase in the oxygen-unloading capacity caused by the gradual shift to the right in the position of the oxygen-hemoglobin equilibrium curve. As a result, at a mixed venous oxygen tension of 40 torr, arbitrarily selected as the normal central venous oxygen tension at rest, the 3-month-old infant is delivering more oxygen to his tissues than the newborn infant, despite the fact that his hemoglobin has fallen from 17.0 g/dl to approximately 11.0 g/dl.[50]

COAGULATION DISTURBANCES

It has been estimated that approximately 1% of all nursery admissions are complicated by problems of hemorrhage or thrombosis.[51] With the prolongation of life in small and desperately ill premature infants, the incidence of clinical coagulation problems appears to be even greater.

The bleeding problems of the newborn can be conveniently divided into the following broad categories:

1. Inherited defects of the coagulation mechanism
2. Accentuation of the normally occurring transitory deficiencies of the coagulation mechanism characteristic of this period of life
3. Transitory disturbances secondary to an associated disease process
4. Quantitative or qualitative abnormalities of the platelets

Normal Blood Coagulation

The standard nomenclature for the coagulation factors is listed in Table 25-14. According to current concepts, 2 major pathways exist to activate the coagulation system. In Figure 25-3, a simplified version of the entire sequence is depicted, based on the formulation of Stormorken and Owren.[52]

In brief, an intrinsic system, occurring within the vessel lumen, and not requiring the presence of tissue factor, is triggered by the activation of Factor XII and Factor XI through surface contact, collagen, antigen-antibody complexes, or negatively charged substances. This complex, in the presence of calcium, activates Factor IX, that, in turn, interacts with Factor VIII, platelet phospholipid, and calcium to form a complex that activates Factor X. In the extrinsic system, tissue thromboplastin, along with Factor VII and calcium, form a complex that also activates Factor X. From this point, both the intrinsic and extrinsic systems proceed in a similar fashion.

Activated Factor X, with Factor V, platelet phospholipid, and calcium activate Factor II to thrombin. Thrombin, next, cleaves fibri-

Table 25-14. The Blood-Clotting Factors.

Factor Number	Synonyms	Definition
I	Fibrinogen	A protein that when modified by thrombin, forms the clot (fibrin).
II	Prothrombin	An alpha-globulin that, when acted on by thromboplastin accelerators and calcium, is converted to thrombin.
III	Thromboplastin	An unidentified substance or substances present in tissues that promote prothrombin conversion to thrombin. In plasma it is formed only by interaction of several factors and is quickly destroyed.
IV	Calcium	Necessary in the first and second stages of coagulation.
V	Proaccelerin, labile factor, Ac globulin	A plasma factor that participates in the first and second stages of coagulation.
VI	Accelerin, serum Ac globulin	Active form of Factor V. Terms no longer employed.
VII	Proconvertin, stable factor, SPCA, autoprothrombin I	A plasma factor required for the conversion of prothrombin to thrombin. Increases 2½ times in the process of clotting.
VIII	Antihemophiliac factor (AHF), antihemophiliac globulin (AHG)	A thromboplastic precursor the deficiency of which is responsible for classic hemophilia. It is found in the beta-globulin fraction.
IX	Plasma thromboplastin component (PTC), Christmas factor, autoprothrombin II	A factor that participates in thromboplastin formation. An alpha-globulin.
X	Stuart–Prower factor, Stuart factor, Prower–Stuart factor	Participates in thromboplastin formation and prothrombin conversion.
XI	Plasma thromboplastin antecedent (PTA)	Reacts with activated Hageman factor and forms thromboplastin substance.
XII	Hageman factor, contact factor	A factor concerned with initiation of clotting in vitro. Becomes activated by contact with rough surface. Deficiency unaccompanied by clinical manifestations.
XIII	Fibrin-stabilizing factor	A serum factor responsible for the stabilization of the fibrin clot.

nogen into fibrinopeptides and fibrin monomers; these polymerize and are stabilized as insoluble fibrin by means of activated Factor XIII.

Once fibrin is deposited on vessel walls or in tissues, it is slowly broken down into soluble fibrin split products by plasmin. Plasmin is a proteolytic enzyme and plasminogen is its inactive precursor. The inactive precursor can be converted to plasmin by a variety of sub-stances normally present in plasma, urine, and tissues. Normal blood also contains substances that inhibit the activators of plasminogen and inhibitors of plasmin as well. Thus, both the coagulation mechanism and also the fibrinolytic system are held in a state of dynamic equilibrium that can be easily upset by a variety of stimuli.

Many of the coagulation factors are not present in normal concentration in the blood

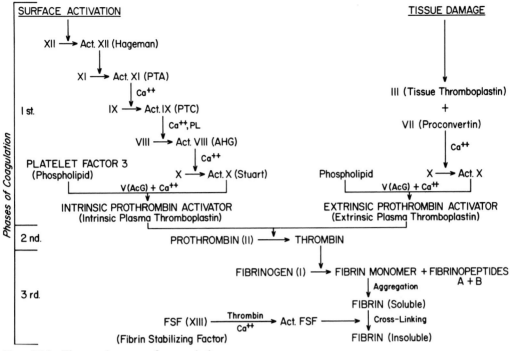

Fig. 25-3. The pathways of coagulation.

of the newborn infant. These deviations from normal adult values are particularly marked in the premature infant. Several recent publications have described these developmental changes.[53,54] The usual values encountered in the term and preterm infant are summarized in Table 25-15. It should be noted that the vitamin K-dependent factors (Factors II, VII, IX, and X) and Factors XI, XII, and XIII are generally decreased while the levels of fibrinogen, Factors V, and VIII and platelets are in, or near, the normal adult range.

Inherited Defects of the Coagulation Mechanism

Although the majority of infants with congenital deficiencies of the coagulation factors do not bleed during the first weeks of life, all of the congenital defects may manifest themselves with hemorrhage in the newborn period.

It is not clear why hemorrhage does not occur more frequently. None of the coagulation factors cross the placenta so that infants with hemophilia can be diagnosed at birth and are presumably at risk from hemorrhage.

From studies of patients with Factor VIII deficiency (classical hemophilia), it would ap-

pear that only the most severely affected persons bled during the newborn period.[55] When bleeding occurs in the newborn, it is most commonly a result of a circumcision. More serious bleeding may take the form of giant cephalohematoma, intracranial hemorrhages, hemarthroses, and intramuscular hematomas. Petechiae and flat ecchymotic areas are uncommon isolated manifestations of hemophilia.

Vitamin K Deficiency

Vitamin K deficiency or true "hemorrhagic disease of the newborn" is caused by an accentuation of the normally occurring transient deficiencies of the coagulation mechanism that characterize this period of life. Bleeding caused by vitamin K deficiency is completely preventable if the recommendations of the American Academy of Pediatrics are followed. The administration of 1 mg of the naturally occurring vitamin K_1 (phytonadione) will correct the deficiency state and has not been reported to produce undesirable side effects.

Bleeding caused by vitamin K deficiency may occur on the first day of life but is more

Table 25-15. Coagulation Factors and Test Values in Term and Premature Infants.

	Normal	Term Infant (cord blood)	Premature Infant (cord blood)
Fibrinogen (mg/dl)	200–400	200–250	200–250
Factor II (%)	50–150	40	25
Factor V (%)	75–125	90	60–75
Factor VII (%)	75–125	50	35
Factor VIII (%)	50–150	100	80–100
Factor IX (%)	50–150	25–40	25–40
Factor X (%)	50–150	50–60	25–40
Factor XI (%)	75–125	30–40	—
Factor XII (%)	75–125	50–100	50–100
Factor XIII (titer)	1:16	1:8	1:8
Partial thromboplastin time (sec)	30–50	70	80–90
Prothrombin time (sec)	10–12	12–18	14–20
Thrombin time (sec)	10–12	12–16	13–20

commonly observed on the second or third day of life. Bleeding from the gastrointestinal tract, umbilical cord, circumcision site, nose, and into the scalp, as well as generalized ecchymosis, are the most frequent external manifestations of the disease. Internal hemorrhages may also occur. Prolonged oozing from capillary punctures may be the first clue to its presence.

The laboratory features of the disease are summarized in Table 25-16 and contrasted with those observed in neonates with DIC. Vitamin K deficiency is characterized by a marked prolongation in the prothrombin time and par-

Table 25-16. Differential Features of Hemorrhage Disease of the Newborn.

Features	Vitamin K Deficiency	DIC
Uniformity of clotting defect	Constant	Variable
Capillary fragility	Normal	Usually abnormal
Bleeding time	Normal	Often prolonged
Clotting time	Prolonged	Variable
One-stage prothrombin	Very prolonged (5% or less)	Moderately prolonged
Partial thromboplastin time	Prolonged	Prolonged
Thrombin time	Normal for age	Usually prolonged
Fibrin degradation products	Not present	Present
Factor V	Normal	Decreased
Fibrinogen	Normal	Often decreased
Platelets	Normal	Often decreased
Red cell fragmentation	Not present	Usually present
Response to vitamin K	Spectacular	Diminished or absent
Associated disease	Usually trivial (trauma may be precipitating factor)	Severe. May include sepsis, hypoxia, acidosis, or obstetric accident
Previous history	No vitamin K given or mother receiving barbiturates or anticonvulsants	Above illnesses. Vitamin K given

Table 25-17. Conditions Associated with Disseminated Intravascular Coagulation in the Newborn.

Obstetric Complications	Neonatal Infections	Miscellaneous Conditions
Abruptio placentae	Bacterial, both gram-negative	Respiratory distress syndrome
Preeclampsia and eclampsia	and gram-positive	Severe erythroblastosis fetalis
Dead twin fetus	Disseminated herpes simplex	Giant hemangioma
Fetal distress during delivery	Cytomegalovirus infections	Renal vein thrombosis
Amniotic fluid embolism	Rubella	Severe acidosis and
Breech delivery	Toxoplasmosis	hypoxemia
	Syphilis	Indwelling catheters

tial thromboplastin time. Slight prolongations of either of these tests should not be used as an explanation for serious hemorrhages.

Treatment of bleeding due to vitamin K deficiency consists of the intravenous administration of 1 mg of vitamin K_1. If this deficiency is responsible for the abnormal test results, dramatic correction may be observed in a period as short as 2 hours. Maximal correction may be observed in 24 hours. It is important to remember that neither the prothrombin time nor the partial thromboplastin time, or the level of Factor II may reach the expected adult normal values for a period of several weeks to months. The response to vitamin K is less marked in the premature infant, but even in these infants, if otherwise well, a therapeutic response can be anticipated.

Disseminated Intravascular Coagulation (DIC)

DIC is an acquired pathophysiologic process characterized by the intravascular consumption of platelets and plasma clotting factors, most notably Factors II, V, VIII, XIII, and fibrinogen. This widespread coagulation within the circulation results in the deposition of fibrin thrombi in small vessels and the production of a hemorrhagic state when the level of platelets and clotting factors drop to values that are insufficient to maintain hemostasis. The accumulation of fibrin in the microcirculation also produces mechanical injury to the red cells, leading to erythrocyte fragmentation and a hemolytic anemia.

DIC occurs in association with a variety of disorders and has been the subject of several excellent reviews.[54,56-58] Clinical conditions in the newborn period which may be accompanied by DIC are summarized in Table 25-17. Gram-negative septicemia, acidosis, hypoxia, and hypotension appear to be the most common initiating events during the first several days of life. Coagulation disturbances characteristic of DIC are seen in many of the sickest infants with the respiratory distress syndrome. The majority of evidence indicates that the disturbance in coagulation reflects the severity of the disease process and in no way is responsible for the idiopathic respiratory distress syndrome. Hemorrhage, however, may be a terminal event in many of these sick infants.

The clinical manifestations are variable, and in part are determined by the associated disease process and in part by the severity of the coagulation disturbance. In a typical case, oozing at puncture sites is noted in a sick infant. Closer examination usually reveals the presence of petechiae and scattered purpura. Clinical manifestations may include pulmonary, cerebral, and intraventricular hemorrhages. Also observed are bleeding from the umbilical stump and body orifices, and thrombosis of peripheral or central vessels with tissue necrosis and gangrene.

Laboratory abnormalities include the presence of a hemolytic anemia with red cell fragmentation visible on the peripheral smear, variable degrees of thrombocytopenia, and a prolongation of the prothrombin, partial thromboplastin, and thrombin time. The levels of Factor V and fibrinogen are most commonly decreased in the sickest infants. This decrease may reflect impaired hepatic synthesis in a very sick, immature infant and does not establish the presence of DIC. The presence of elevated levels of fibrin split products occurs invariably in older infants, children, and adults with DIC, but may not always be present in the neonate. This may be a result of a relative deficiency of plasminogen and plasminogen activators during this period of life. The laboratory features characteristic of DIC are described in Table 25-17. In some pathologic states, thrombocytopenia or hypofibrinogenemia may be present without the laboratory findings of DIC.

Treatment must be directed at both the underlying disease process and the coagulation abnormality. Success, in general, depends on the ability to correct the condition that initiated the process of DIC rather than merely on the management of the hematologic abnormalities. Management of the patient thus may include the administration of appropriate antibiotics, correction of abnormalities of pH and electrolytes, and maintenance of adequate oxygenation and blood pressure. The decision to treat the abnormalities of coagulation must be based on the clinical findings as well as on the laboratory results. If the infant is bleeding or has evidence of thrombotic complications, and laboratory studies support the diagnosis of DIC, then treatment appears indicated.

More controlled experience is necessary before the optimal form of treatment for DIC in the newborn can be established. The two major forms of treatment at present are the use of heparin in conjunction with replacement of plasma and platelets, or the use of exchange transfusion with relatively fresh blood (blood of less than 72 hours of age).

Heparin therapy should be reserved for those clinical conditions in which thrombosis is clearly evident. The aim of heparin therapy is to maintain the whole blood clotting time in the range of 20 to 30 minutes or the partial thromboplastin time (PTT) in the range of 60 to 70 seconds if the normal PTT value is 40 seconds. Heparin should be administered in an initial dose of 100 to 200 units/kg of body weight and then at a maintenance dose of 600 units/kg per day. The maintenance dose may be given continuously or given as 100 units/kg at 4-hour intervals. The dose of heparin should be adjusted in keeping with the results of the monitoring test. Effective treatment should be reflected by a return toward normal of Factors II, V, VIII, fibrinogen, and platelets. It may be necessary to administer fresh frozen plasma, 10 ml/kg, and platelets, 1 unit/5 kg, of body weight to correct existing deficiencies once adequate heparin therapy has been achieved. The use of plasma and platelets alone appears to provide little benefit to the patient.

Heparin therapy should be continued until the process of DIC has been halted.

A 2-volume exchange transfusion with fresh heparinized blood or blood stored less than 72 hours in citrate-phosphate-dextrose (CPD) also may be used to control the bleeding and terminate the consumption process. The exchange transfusion may need to be repeated every 12 hours if coagulation studies have not returned towards normal. Maintenance of the partial thromboplastin time at less than twice the normal value appears to be a convenient guide to management.

Platelet Disturbances

A platelet count of less than 100,000/mm^3 is abnormal in either the term or premature infant. The level of platelets in the blood reflects a balance between their production and their destruction. Thrombocytopenia, therefore, may result from a decreased production of platelets, increased destruction of platelets, or a combination of the two. Platelet production is evaluated chiefly by inspection of the number and appearance of megakaryocytes in a carefully collected sample of bone marrow. This is not always easy to accomplish in a small infant. Platelet destruction may be evaluated by determination of the platelet survival, using platelets labeled with isotopes such as chromium-51 or by merely monitoring the disappearance rate of platelets following a transfusion of unlabeled platelets. An additional clue to the mechanism of thrombocytopenia may be obtained from an evaluation of platelet size. Young platelets are larger than old platelets. The predominance of large platelets in a peripheral smear of blood collected in EDTA, to prevent platelet aggregation, suggests that the thrombocytopenia is a result of peripheral platelet destruction with a compensatory increase in young platelets from the bone marrow.

There are many causes for thrombocytopenia in the newborn. The most common of these disorders are listed in Table 25-18, and have been reviewed in detail elsewhere.[59-61]

Immune Thrombocytopenia. A variety of con-

Table 25-18. Etiologic Classification of Neonatal Thrombocytopenia.

Immune Disorders
Passive (acquired from mother)—ITP, drug-induced thrombocytopenia, systemic lupus erythematosus
Active
  Isoimmune—platlet group incompatibility
  Associated with erythroblastosis fetalis—caused by the disease or exchange transfusion

Infections (? mediated in part by intravascular coagulation)
Bacterial—generalized sepsis, congenital syphilis
Viral—cytomegalic inclusion disease, disseminated herpes simplex, rubella syndrome
Protozoal—congenital toxoplasmosis

Drugs (administered to mother)—nonimmune mechanism (*e.g.,* thiazide diuretics, tolbutamide)

Congenital Megakaryocytic Hypoplasia
Isolated—congenital hypoplastic thrombocytopenia
Associated with absent radii, microcephaly; rubella syndrome; pancytopenia; and congenital anomalies
  (Fanconi's anemia)
Associated with pancytopenia but no congenital anomalies
Associated with trisomy syndromes—D_1 (13), E (18)

Bone Marrow Disease
Congenital leukemia

Disseminated Intravascular Coagulation (DIC)
Sepis
Obstetric complications—abruptio placentae, eclampsia, amniotic fluid embolism, dead twin fetus
Anoxia
Stasis—giant hemangioma (including placental chorangioma), renal vein thrombosis, polycythemia

Inherited (Chronic) Thrombocytopenia
Sex-linked
  Pure
  Aldrich's syndrome
Autosomal
  Pure—dominant or recessive
  May–Hegglin anomaly—dominant

Miscellaneous
Thrombotic thrombocytopenic purpura
Inherited metabolic disorders—glycinemia, methylmalonic acidemia, isovaleric acidemia
Congenital thyrotoxicosis

ditions are associated with the passage of antibody from the mother across the placenta to the infant, resulting in immunologic destruction of the infant's platelets. The antibody may be formed against an antigen on the mother's platelets (autoimmune) or those of the infant (isoimmune).

The maternal disorders in which thrombocytopenia may occur in both the mother and infant include idiopathic thrombocytopenic purpura, drug-induced thrombocytopenia, and systemic lupus erythematosus.

In isoimmune thrombocytopenia, the thrombocytopenia is confined to the infant. In this condition, the infant possesses a platelet antigen lacking in the mother, the infant's platelets cross the placenta into the maternal circulation, and they result in the formation of antibodies by the mother against the foreign platelet antigen. This immunologic mechanism is analogous to that of red cell sensitization that occurs in erythroblastosis fetalis.

Infants born with immune thrombocytopenia show wide variation in their clinical manifestations, although bleeding manifestations appear to be more severe in the isoimmune form of the disease. Infants tend to show maximal signs of bruising and bleeding shortly after birth as a consequence of the mechanical trauma of the birth process. The commonest type of bleeding consists of generalized petechiae and purpuric spots. Bleeding from other sites may be observed such as oozing from the cord, epistaxis, hematuria, melena, and bleeding from needle punctures. Intracranial hemorrhages may also occur.

Jaundice may develop as a consequence of the increased breakdown of red cells within entrapped hemorrhages. Hepatosplenomegaly is absent in these conditions. Bone marrow examination usually reveals the presence of normal to increased numbers of megakaryocytes.

The measurement of platelet counts obtained from fetal scalp samples may assist in the decision to deliver an infant by cesarean section from a mother with autoimmune thrombocytopenia.[61a]

It has been estimated that approximately 10% of infants born to mothers with autoimmune thrombocytopenia die in the neonatal period as a consequence of hemorrhage, while 15% of infants with isoimmune thrombocytopenia succumb.[62] These figures appear excessive. The thrombocytopenia of passively acquired thrombocytopenia may persist for 1 to 4 months, while the course of isoimmune thrombocytopenia is generally only of 1- to 6-weeks' duration.

Treatment is generally reserved for the infant with bleeding. In infants with passive forms of thrombocytopenia, exchange transfusion followed by platelet transfusions appear to be most effective in management. In infants with isoimmune thrombocytopenia, transfusions of platelets obtained from the mother will normalize the platelet count and produce a cessation of bleeding. Neither steroids nor splenectomy has been demonstrated to be of benefit, and splenectomy should never be considered in management of the newborn.

In pregnancies complicated by isoimmune thrombocytopenia, it would appear to be advantageous to reduce the hazards of bleeding in subsequent children by delivering the infant by cesarean section.

Other Forms of Thrombocytopenia. As indicated in Table 25-18, a variety of other disorders may produce a reduction in platelet count. Infections are a leading cause of thrombocytopenia. Inherited defects in platelet production or platelet function may also manifest themselves at this period of life. An approach to the mutliple diagnostic possibilities is outlined in Table 25-19.

In this scheme, it is as important to study the mother as it is to study the infant. Points requiring specific inquiry include (1) a history of previous bleeding in the form of purpura, bruising, or nosebleeds that might suggest a diagnosis of maternal ITP at some time in the past; (2) ingestion of drugs that might cause thrombocytopenia in the mother and infant (for example, quinidine and quinine) or the infant alone (thiazide diuretics, tolbutaminde); (3) previous infants affected with purpura, suggesting either one of the immune or inherited thrombocytopenias; (4) skin rash or exposure to rubella in the first 8 weeks of pregnancy. The results of the routine test for syphilis should be sought and recorded rather than left buried among the other routine laboratory results performed earlier in pregnancy. Finally, an accurate platelet count should be performed on the mother as soon as possible after delivery to separate immune neonatal thrombocytopenia caused by maternal ITP from that due to platelet isoimmunization (in which case the mother's platelet count is normal).

Physical findings of importance in differential diagnosis in the affected newborn include the presence or absence of hepatosplenomegaly and congenital anomalies. Hepatosplenomegaly is often accompanied by jaundice and suggests an infectious process as the most likely cause of thrombocytopenia. In some cases, congenital leukemia may also have to be considered. Among the congenital anomalies associated with neonatal thrombocytopenia, the commonest group recognizable at birth is that occurring in the rubella syndrome (congenital heart defects, cataracts, and microcephaly). Deformity and shortening of the forearms should suggest bilateral absence of the radii with associated megakaryocytic

Table 25-19. Approach to the Diagnosis of the Thrombocytopenic Newborn.

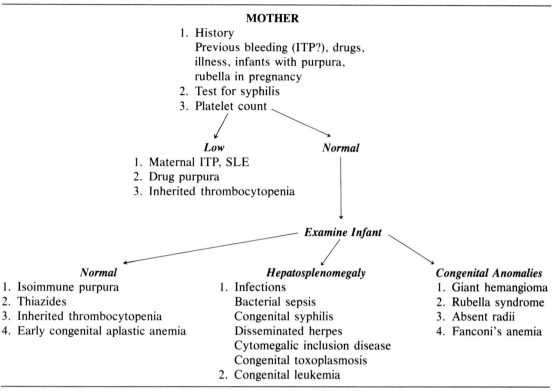

thrombocytopenia. A single large hemangioma or multiple smaller hemangiomas point to these tumors as the problem site of platelet trapping leading to thrombocytopenia.

Complete blood count on the infant should include hemoglobin, white cell count, platelet count, and smear. Associated anemia may be due to blood loss, concurrent hemolysis (as might occur in one of the infectious processes), or marrow infiltration caused by congenital leukemia. Leukocytosis of a mild degree may accompany infection or blood loss, but when this exceeds 40,000 to 50,000/mm³ it should point either to congenital leukemia or to the absent radii syndrome. Bone marrow examination is essential not only for assessment of megakaryocytes, but also to exclude underlying infiltrative disorders such as leukemia. Increased numbers of megakaryocytes suggest either consumption coagulopathy or one of the immune thrombocytopenias, although megakaryocytes may be diminished in number in some infants with these disorders. A decrease in the number of megakaryocytes generally suggests one of the types of congenital me-

gakaryocytic hypoplasia. It is important, however, to exclude the immune disorders, if possible, by serologic tests before arriving at this diagnosis, because of its ominous prognosis. When in doubt, it is wise to defer such a diagnosis until follow-up observations clarify the situation. Repeat bone marrow examination may be necessary.

Serologic tests for platelet antibodies are at present difficult, time-consuming, and available only in a small number of laboratories. Should isoimmune thrombocytopenia be suspected by the finding of an otherwise normal thrombocytopenic newborn of a healthy mother with a normal platelet count, blood should be drawn from the mother soon after delivery and serum frozen and saved until antibody testing can be carried out. Because results of such studies are usually not available for some time, their chief value lies in the management of subsequent pregnancies, much in the manner of maternal Rh antibody tests in predicting the occurrence of erythroblastosis fetalis.

The response to platelet transfusions may

Table 25-20. The White Cell Count and the Differential Count During the First Two Weeks of Life.

Age	Leukocytes	Neutrophils			Eosinophils	Basophils	Lymphocytes	Monocytes
		Total	Seg	Band				
Birth								
Mean	18,100	11,000	9400	1600	400	100	5500	1050
Range	9.0–30.0	6.0–26			20–850	0–640	2.0–11.0	0.4–3.1
Mean %	—	61	52	9	2.2	0.6	31	5.8
7 Days								
Mean	12,200	5500	4700	830	500	50	5000	1100
Range	5.0–21.0	1.5–10.0			70–1100	0–250	2.0–17.0	0.3–2.7
Mean %	—	45	39	6	4.1	0.4	41	9.1
14 Days								
Mean	11,400	4500	3900	630	350	50	5500	1000
Range	5.0–20.0	1.0–9.5			70–1000	0–230	2.0–17.0	0.2–2.4
Mean %	—	40	34	5.5	3.1	0.4	48	8.8

be of both therapeutic and diagnostic aid.[63] Platelet counts following transfusion have been shown to correlate with the known pathogenetic mechanisms in several infants with either increased platelet destruction or impaired platelet production.[64]

LEUKOCYTE DISTURBANCES
The Normal Leukocyte Count

The white cell count at birth may range from 9,000 to 30,000/mm³ with the mean count generally in the range of 15,000/mm³ for the term infant. The total white count gradually falls during the first week of life and reaches a mean value of approximately 12,000/mm³ by the seventh day.

During the first days of life, the differential count reveals a preponderance of polymorphonuclear neutrophils. Neutrophils average 61% of the total cells with 20% to 40% of the neutrophils being band forms. Promyelocytes and myelocytes may also be seen. Immature forms are more frequently observed in premature infants during the first 72 hours of life.

Between the fourth and seventh day of life, in the term infant, the lymphocyte becomes the predominant cell, and remains so until approximately the fourth year of life. Table 25-20 lists the normal white cell findings during the first 2 weeks of life.

Although it has been commonly believed that the measurement of the total white count and the performance of a differential cell count provides little helpful information in the diagnosis of bacterial infections in the neonatal period, recent evidence suggests that the white count and differential can be extremely useful.[65-67]

The following clinical conditions do not appear to have any effect on the total neutrophil count during the first days of life[61]: birth weight or gestational age; route of delivery; maternal diabetes; prolonged rupture of the membranes if mother remains afebrile; uncomplicated hyaline membrane disease; transient tachypnea of the newborn; phototherapy, and nonhemolytic hyperbilirubinemia.

Noninfectious conditions which affect the neutrophil count include maternal hypertension, intraventricular hemorrhage, and hemolytic disease. Elevations in the band to neutrophil ratio, in the absence of infection,

may be observed in infants of diabetic mothers, those with meconium aspiration or hypoglycemia, and infants with Apgar scores at 5 minutes or less than 6. Alterations produced by low Apgar scores, hypoglycemia, and seizures return to normal within 24 hours of the event.

Neutropenia (defined as an absolute neutrophil count of less than 7800/mm³ in the first 60 hours of life and less than 1750/mm³ after 60 hours of life) is the single most useful alteration in white cell count to indicate the presence of infection. When neutropenia is present the infant has approximately a 75% chance of being infected. If the neutropenia is present in an infant with respiratory distress, the chances are about 85% that the infant is infected. The presence of morphologic alterations in the leukocytes is also strongly suggestive evidence of the presence of a bacterial infection. These morphologic alterations include the presence of toxic granulation, Döhle bodies, and vacuolization of the neutrophils.

The neutrophil response to infection includes the processes of adhesion, diapedesis, chemotaxis, immune adherence, phagocytosis, and intracellular killing and ingestion. Studies of these neutrophil functions during the neonatal period suggest that chemotaxis and phagocytosis may be impaired as a consequence of deficiencies of humoral factors. This subject has been well reviewed in recent publications.[68,69] (See also Chap. 31.)

Neutrophil disturbances during the newborn period are primarily of two types and both are apparently uncommon. These two clinical problems are those of neutropenia and neonatal leukemia. The subject of neonatal leukemia is described in Chapter 36.

Neutropenia

Neutropenia, the presence of less than 1000 neutrophils/mm³ can be caused by a variety of pathologic states. The most common is probably overwhelming sepsis. The recognized complications of primary neutropenia include omphalitis, skin infections, septicemia, and meningitis.

The clinical and diagnostic features of these forms of neutropenia are described in Table 25-21.

In addition to neutropenic states that may manifest themselves during the first weeks of

(*Text continues on p. 580.*)

Table 25-21. The Clinical and Laboratory Features of the Neutropenias.

Diagnosis	Clinical Features	Laboratory Findings
Neutropenia secondary to infection	Infant ill with septicemia, pneumonia, meningitis, or profound diarrhea	Total white count is frequently less than $5,000/mm^3$ with neutrophils of less than $1000/mm^3$ E. Coli, Streptococcus, and Shigella recognized causes. Toxic granulation often prominent Blast forms may be present. Thrombocytopenia often present
Neutropenia associated with maternal neutropenia	Infant usually asymptomatic	Neutropenia present in both mother and infant Mother may have lupus erythematosus A leukocyte agglutinin may be present in maternal sera
Neutropenia associated with maternal isoimmunization to fetal leukocytes	Infant generally asymptomatic but serious infections have been described	Bone marrow aspirate generally reveals a paucity of myeloid forms beyond the myelocyte stage of maturation Leukocyte agglutinin present in maternal sera directed against infant's white cells
Genetic agranulocytosis	Infections include otitis media, pneumonia, meningitis, multiple furuncles, deep abscesses, and omphalitis May involve more than one family member	Bone marrow may be hypocellular or of normal cellularity with virtual absence of white cell precursors or maturation arrest at myelocyte stage
Chronic benign granulocytopenia of childhood	Infant usually asymptomatic May have furuncles, paronychia, ulcerations in genital area, or gingivitis	Marrow cellular with all but the most mature myeloid forms present in normal numbers Spontaneous cure may occur in later childhood

Disorder	Clinical Features	Laboratory Features
Neutropenia and pancreatic insufficiency	Infants usually asymptomatic in neonatal period. Steatorrhea and growth failure may be observed early in life	Bone marrow hypocellular. Mild thrombocytopenia may also be present. Absence of pancreatic enzymes with normal sweat electrolytes. Epiphyseal stippling may be observed. More than one family member may be involved
Reticular dysgenesis	Infants profoundly ill with overwhelming septicemia. Total white count 0–600/mm^3	No granulocytes or granulocyte precursors present in bone marrow. Spleen and thymus devoid or virtually devoid of lymphocytes
Drug-induced neutropenia	Cutaneous infections may be present. More severe infections uncommon	Maternal ingestion of thiazides, Dilantin, amidopyrine, thiouracil, propylthiouracil, phenothiazines, trimethadione, sulfonamides, and others. Marrow reveals either a maturation arrest or depletion of myeloid precursors
Cyclic neutropenia	Symptoms not reported in neonatal period. By 6 weeks of age infant may have recurrent attacks of stomatitis, otitis media, furunculosis, and pneumonia	Neutropenia intermittent. Cycles frequently of 21 days. Neutropenia generally associated with maturation arrest of myeloid elements. More than one family member involved
Lazy leukocyte syndrome	Symptoms uncommon in newborn. Clinical features include unexplained fever, stomatitis, otitis media, furunculosis, and pneumonia	Marrow appears normal. Leukocytes have impaired chemotaxis and random mobility
Neutropenia associated with inborn errors of metabolism	Symptoms are those of underlying metabolic error. Lethargy, vomiting, and ketosis common	Neutropenia observed in hyperglycinemia, methylmalonic acidemia, and isovalericacidemia

Table 25-22. Anomalies of the Leukocytes.

Anomaly	Appearance	Associated Findings
Increased numbers of nuclear projections of the neutrophils	15% or more of the neutrophils contain 2 or more nuclear projections	Trisomy for one of the chromosomes of the D group
Pelger–Huet anomaly	Virtual absence of leukocytes containing more than 2 lobes	Autosomal dominant inheritance No associated disease
May–Hegglin anomaly	Leukocytes containing Döhle bodies Giant platelets	Thrombocytopenia may be present Autosomal dominant inheritance
Hereditary hypersegmentation of the neutrophils	Most neutrophilic leukocytes contain 4 or more lobes	Autosomal dominant inheritance (Undritz, 1939) Must be distinguished from the hypersegmentation of the leukocytes observed in pernicious anemia
Chediak–Higashi anomaly	Multiple refractile gray-green inclusions in the leukocytes Large red or blue inclusions in the lymphocytes	Multiple pyogenic infections, albinism, hepatosplenomegaly, mental retardation, increased incidence of lymphoma
Jordans' anomaly	Vacuoles in cytoplasm of granulocytes	One family with muscular dystrophy, another with ichthyosis
Alder's anomaly	Increased numbers of course, dark azurophilic granules in the cytoplasm of the neutrophils	No pathologic significance Must be distinguished from toxic granulation Inherited as an autosomal recessive
Reilly bodies	Same as Adler's anomaly	Observed in patients with gargoylism In these patients lymphocytic inclusions and bone marrow granules of acid mucopolysaccharide may also be seen

life, congenital anomalies of the leukocytes may also be recognized. The characteristic features of these leukocyte anomalies and their associated findings are listed in Table 25-22.

REFERENCES

1. **Moe PJ:** Umbilical cord blood and capillary blood in the evaluation of anemia in erythroblastosis fetalis. Acta Paediatr Scand 56:391, 1967
2. **Usher R, Shepard M, Lind J:** The blood volume of the newborn infant and placental transfusion. Acta Paediatr Scand 52:497, 1963
3. **Usher R, Lind J:** Blood volume of the newborn premature infant. Acta Paediatr Scand 54:419, 1965
4. **Schulman I:** Characteristics of the blood in foetal life. *In* Walker J, Turnbull AC (eds): Oxygen Supply to the Human Fetus, p. 43. Springfield, Ill, Charles C Thomas, 1959
5. **Cassady G:** Plasma volume studies in low birth weight infants. Pediatrics 38:1020, 1966
6. **Matoth Y, Zaizov R, Varsano I:** Postnatal changes in some red cell parameters. Acta Paediatr Scand 60:317, 1971
7. **Faxelius G, Raye J, Gutberlet R, Swanstrom S, Tsiantos A, Dolanski E, Dehan M, Dyer N, Lindstrom D, Brill AB, Stahlman M:** Red cell volume measurements and acute blood loss in high-risk newborn infants. J Pediatr 90:273, 1977
8. **Zipursky A, Hull A, White FD, Israels LG:**

Foetal erythrocytes in the maternal circulation. Lancet 1:451, 1959

9. **Kleihauer E, Hildegard B, Betke K:** Demonstration von fetalem Hamoglobin in den Erythrocyten eines Blutausstrichs. Klin Wochenschr 35:637, 1957

10. **Pembrey ME, Weatherall DJ, Clegg JB:** Maternal synthesis of hemoglobin F in pregnancy. Lancet 1:1350, 1973

11. **Rausen AR, London RD, Mizrahi A, Cooper LQ:** Generalized bone changes and thrombocytopenic purpura in association with intrauterine rubella. Pediatrics 36:264, 1965

12. **Tan KL, Tan R, Tan SH:** The twin transfusion syndrome. Clinical observations on 35 affected pairs. Clin Pediatr 18:111, 1979

13. **Clayton EM, Pryor JA, Wierdsma JG, Whitacre FE:** Fetal and maternal components in third-trimester obstetric hemorrhage. Obstet Gynecol 24:56, 1964

14. **Potter EL:** Fetal and neonatal deaths: a statistical analysis of 2000 autopsies. JAMA 115:996, 1940

15. **Holmberg E:** Rupture of liver in new-born observed at General Lying-In Hospital in Helsingfors from 1924 to 1932. Finska Lak-Sallsk Handl 75:1067, 1933

16. **Henderson JL:** Hepatic haemorrhage in stillborn and newborn infants; clinical and pathological study of 47 cases. J Obst Gynaecol Br Commonw 48:377, 1941

17. **Naiman JL:** Current management of hemolytic disease of the newborn infant. J Pediatr 80:1049, 1972

18. **Queenan JT:** Modern Management of the Rh Problem. New York, Harper and Row, 1967

19. **Zipursky A:** Erythroblastosis fetalis. *In* Nathan DG, Oski FA, (eds): Hematology of Infancy and Childhood, p 46. Philadelphia, WB Saunders, 1974

20. **Liley AW:** Diagnosis and treatment of erythroblastosis in the fetus. Adv Pediatr 15:29, 1968

21. **Chessells, JM, Wigglesworth JS:** Haemostatic failure in babies with Rhesus isoimmunization. Arch Dis Child 46:38, 1971

22. **Hathaway WE:** Coagulation problems in the newborn infant. Pediatr Clin N Amer 17:929, 1970

23. **Cassady G:** Non-immunologic hydrops fetalis associated with large hemangioendothelioma. Pediatrics 42:828, 1968

24. **Queenan JT:** Modern Management of the Rh Problem, 2nd ed. Hagerstown, Harper and Row, 1977

25. **Bowman JM, Pollack JM:** Amniotic fluid spectrophotometry and early delivery in the management of erythroblastosis fetalis. Pediatrics 35:815, 1965

26. **McKay RJ:** Current status of exchange transfusion in newborn infants. Pediatrics 33:763, 1964

27. **Cockington RA:** A guide to the use of phototherapy in the management of neonatal hyperbilirubinemia. J Pediatr 95:281, 1979

28. **Bowman JD, Friesen RF:** Hemolytic disease of the newborn. *In* Gellis SS, Kogan BM (eds): Current Pediatric Therapy, Vol 4, p. 405. Philadelphia, WB Saunders, 1970

29. **Kaplan E, Herz F, Scheye E, Robinson L Jr:** Phototherapy in ABO hemolytic disease of the newborn. J Pediatr 79:911, 1971

30. **Panizon I:** L'ictere grave du nouveau-ne associe a une deficience en glucose-6-phosphate dehydrogenase. Biol Neonate 2:167, 1960

31. **Smith GD, Vella F:** Erythrocyte enzyme deficiency in unexplained kernicterus. Lancet 1:1133, 1960

32. **Van Baelen H, Vandepitte J, Eeckels R:** Observations on sickle-cell anaemia and haemoglobin Bart's in Congolese neonates. Ann Soc Belge Med Trop 49:157, 1969

33. **Hunt JA, Lehmann H:** Haemoglobin Bart's: a foetal haemoglobin without α-chains. Nature 184:872, 1959

34. **Lee-Potter JP, Deacon-Smith RA, Simpkiss H, Kamuzora H, Lehmann H:** A new cause of haemolytic anaemia in the newborn. J Clin Pathol 28:317, 1975

35. **Levine RL, Lincoln DR, Buchholz WM, Gribble J, Schwartz HC:** Hemoglobin Hasharon in a premature infant with hemolytic anemia. Pediatr Res 9:7, 1975

36. **Gross RT, Bracci R, Rudolph M:** Hydrogen peroxide toxicity and detoxification in the erythrocytes of newborn infants. Blood 29:481, 1967

37. **Diamond LK, Wang WC, Alter BP:** Congenital hypoplastic anemia. Adv Pediatr 22:349, 1976

38. **Aase JM, Smith DW:** Congenital anemia and triphalangeal thumbs. A new syndrome. J Pediatr 74:471, 1969

39. **Oski FA, Naiman JL:** *In* Hematologic Problems of the Newborn, 2nd ed, p 33. Philadelphia, WB Saunders, 1972

40. **Stone HO, Thompson HK Jr, Schmidt-Nielsen K:** Influence of erythrocytes on blood viscosity. Amer J Physiol 214:913, 1968

41. **Gross GP, Hathaway WE, McGaughey HR:** Hyperviscosity in the neonate. J Pediatr 82:1004, 1973

42. **Gersony WM:** Persistence of the fetal circulation: A commentary. J Pediatr 82:1103, 1973

43. **Benesch R, Benesch RW:** The effect of organic phosphates from the human erythrocyte on the allosteric properties of hemoglobin. Biochem Biophys Res Commun 26:162, 1967

44. **Chanutin A, Curnish RR:** Effect of organic and inorganic phosphates on the oxygen equi-

librium of human erythrocytes. Arch Biochem 121:96, 1967

45. **Anselmino KT, Hoffman F:** Die Ursachen des Icterus Neonatorum. Arch Gynäk 143:477, 1930

46. **Allen DW, Wyman T, Smith CA:** The oxygen equilibrium of fetal and adult human hemoglobin. J Biol Chem 203:84, 1953

47. **Bauer C, Ludwig I, Ludwig M:** Different effects of 2,3-diphosphoglycerate and adenosine triphosphate on the oxygen affinity of adult and foetal human hemoglobin. Life Sciences 7: 1339, 1968

48. **Delivoria-Papadopoulos M, Rončevíc NP, Oski FA:** Postnatal changes in oxygen transport of term, premature and sick infants: The role of adult hemoglobin and red cell 2,3-diphosphoglycerate. Pediatr Res 5:235, 1971

49. **Delivoria-Papadopoulos M, Morrow G III, Oski FA:** Exchange transfusion in the newborn infant and fresh and "old" blood: The role of storage on 2,3-diphosphoglycerate hemoglobin-oxygen affinity, and oxygen release. J Pediatr 79:898, 1971

50. **Oski FA:** Clinical implications of the oxyhemoglobin dissociation curve in the neonatal period. Crit Care Med 7:412, 1979

51. **Hathaway WE:** Letter: Fibrin split products in serum of newborn. Pediatrics 45:154, 1970

52. **Stormorken H, Owren PA:** Physiopathology of hemostasis. Sem Hemat 8:3, 1971

53. **Buchanan GR:** Neonatal coagulation: Normal physiology and pathophysiology. Clin Haematol 7:85, 1978

54. **Hathaway WE, Bonnar J:** Perinatal Coagulation. New York, Grune and Stratton, 1978

55. **Strauss H:** Clinical pathological conference. J Pediatr 66:443, 1965

56. **Abildgaard CF:** Recognition and treatment of intravascular coagulation. J Pediatr 74:163, 1969

57. **Karpatkin M:** Diagnosis and management of disseminated intravascular coagulation. Pediatr Clin N Amer 18:23, 1971

58. **Lascari AD, Wallace PD:** Disseminated intravascular coagulation in the newborn. Clin Pediatr 10:11, 1971

59. **O'Gorman Hughes DW:** Neonatal thrombocytopenia: assessment of aetiology and prognosis. Aust Paediatr J 3:226, 1967

60. **Pearson HA, McIntosh S:** Neonatal thrombocytopenia. Clin Haematol 7:111, 1978

61. **Pochedly G:** Thrombocytopenic purpura of the newborn. Obstor Gynecol Survey 26:63, 1971

61a. **Scott JR, Cruikshank DP, Kochenour NK, Piikin RM, Warenski JC:** Fetal platelet counts in the obstetric management of immunologic thrombocytopenic purpura. Am J Obstet Gynecol 136:495, 1980

62. **Anthony B, Krivit w;** Neonatal thrombocytopenic purpura. Pediatrics 30:776, 1962

63. **McIntosh S, O'Brien RT, Schwartz AD, Pearson HA:** Neonatal isoimmune purpura: response to platelet infusions. J Pediatr 82:1020, 1973

64. **Gill FM, Schwartz E:** Platelet transfusion as a diagnostic and therapeutic aid in the newborn. Soc Pediatr Res Res, 1971

65. **Manroe BL, Weinberg AG, Rosenfeld CR, Browne R:** The neonatal blood count in health and disease, I. Reference values for neutrophilic cells. J Pediatr 95:89, 1979

66. **Xanthou M:** Leucocyte blood picture in ill newborn babies. Arch Dis Child, 47:741, 1972

67. **Gregory J, Hey E:** Blood neutrophil response to bacterial infection in the first month of life. Arch Dis Child 47:747, 1972

68. **Dosseth JH:** Microbial defenses of the child and man. Pediatr Clin N A 19:355, 1972

69. **Quie PG:** Disorders of phagocyte function. Current Problems in Pediatrics 11, 1972

26

Carbohydrate Homeostasis in the Fetus and Newborn

Richard M. Cowett
Leo Stern

Following a period of primary dependence on the maternal organism for substrate, the fetus is delivered not only with the need of providing itself with glucose for energy and accelerated growth but also with the necessity of maintaining a balance between glucose deficiency and excess. The variable and intermittent nature of exogenous oral intake in the neonate accentuates the potential problem. Maturation of carbohydrate homeostasis results from a balance between substrate availability and coordination of developing hormonal, enzymatic, and neural systems. The number of conditions producing or associated with neonatal hypo- and hyperglycemia, especially in the sick term or low-birth-weight infant, emphasizes the vulnerability of the neonate to carbohydrate disequilibrium.

GLUCOSE HOMEOSTASIS IN THE FETUS

It is apparent that the neonate depends upon substrate previously accumulated *in utero* to support carbohydrate needs in the period immediately following delivery. Until recently, exogenous glucose (from the mother) was thought to be the only substrate utilized in fetal oxidative reactions. This was based on the original work of Bohr and others who estimated the respiratory quotient (R/Q) to be one, as well as the rapid rate of glucose utilization, which was in excess of the utilization rate of other substrates.[1] Subsequent investigations have suggested that R/Q may be close to, but less than, one. Furthermore, carbon balance data support the conclusion that glucose uptake represents only 23% of fetal carbon uptake.[2] Other substrates such as lactate and amino acids have also been considered as important for fetal oxidative reactions, especially in the fasted state.[3]

Maternal glucose delivery to the fetus is controlled by factors influencing blood flow and maternal glucose concentration. While analyses of factors affecting delivery of glucose are limited, a number of hormones are thought to play major roles. Increased cortisol and estrogen in pregnancy result in increased insulin secretion and peripheral insulin resistance. The placenta contains an insulinase-like substance capable of degrading insulin. Human placental lactogen (HPL) also is important because it promotes release of glycerol and free fatty acids. The integration of these effects results in an adequate supply of glucose for the fetus because insulin increases glycogen, fat, and protein synthesis, while HPL decreases maternal glucose utilization.[3]

It has been suggested that the control of glucose in human pregnancy is not as rigid as previously assumed, resulting in wider swings of fetal glucose concentration than anticipated. Figure 26-1 shows the minimal diurnal variations of maternal glucose and insulin, in early and late pregnancy in one series.[4,5]

In studies in late gestation using fetal lambs, glucose turnover rates (analyses of glucose kinetics) have been compared to umbilical glucose uptake rates. These studies suggest that fetal gluconeogenesis and not simply exogenous glucose delivery may be important contributions to fetal glucose homeostasis.[1] These data indicate that the simple dependency relationship of the fetus on the mother for substrate delivery may, in fact, be much more complex.[6]

The role of insulin in fetal glucose homeostasis has received considerable attention, but the results are conflicting. While earlier work suggested that insulin may not control the rate of fetal glucose utilization, other investigations utilizing the lamb fetus as a model suggest that infusion of insulin into the fetal circulation leads to an increase in glucose uptake and utilization. Although this action of insulin requires further corroboration, these findings would correlate with the well-accepted, growth-promoting effect of insulin *in utero*.[7]

GLUCOSE HOMEOSTASIS AT DELIVERY

Heretofore, glucose has been considered to be the major substrate for brain oxidative metabolism, which requires a constant supply of glucose, although ketones, glycerol and lactate can also be used.[8] Glucose is extracted at a given rate per unit time, irrespective of its concentration in the blood, as long as a minimum amount is available.[9] At the time of birth, the plasma glucose concentration is euglycemic, in the range of 70% to 80% of the maternal concentration. The last maternal meal, the length of labor, the mode of delivery, and the type of intravenous fluid administration to the mother all influence the actual concentration.[10]

The adaptation from fetal to neonatal life has been studied in neonatal lambs by analyzing the significance of the plasma glucagon elevation after delivery, known to occur in a number of species including the human. An adrenergic mechanism has been postulated for not only the observed surge in plasma glucagon, but also for the observed maintenance of low plasma insulin levels. Lipolysis, glycogenolysis, and ketogenesis are favored and may be part of the adaptation from the fetal to the neonatal period.[11]

In the immediate neonatal period, the concentration of glucose in the newborn declines to approximately 50 mg/dl by 2 hours of age but equilibrates at approximately 70 mg/dl by 72 hours after birth.[12] The actual concentration may be further influenced by environmental temperature and heat loss sustained by the infant (see below). Cornblath and Reisner have evaluated the blood glucose concentration over time in an analysis of both term and low-birth-weight neonates and have suggested that concentrations below 40 mg/dl or greater than 125 mg/dl are abnormal after 3 days of age (Figure 26-2).

It has been suggested that maternal hormonal/substrate balance regulates fetal glucose concentration, and that delivery causes a readjustment necessary to develop subsequent control.[14] The repetitive occurrence of wide variations in neonatal glucose concentration and the delayed disappearance of an exogenous glucose load in both term and preterm infants indicate that regulation of carbohydrate metabolism is relatively poorly developed in the newborn at birth.[15]

GLUCOSE HOMEOSTASIS IN THE NEWBORN

In the adult, control of glucose homeostasis is precise, and fine control of endogenous hepatic (splanchnic) glucose production is characteristic of the response to either glucose deprivation or exogenous administration. When glucose is infused at a rate equal to or greater than endogenous glucose production, hepatic production of glucose will be diminished.[16–20]

Indirect methodology, incorporating stepwise incremental glucose infusions, was initially employed to determine the rate of basal glucose output in the infant.[21] Studies in the neonatal puppy, utilizing the prime-plus-constant-infusion technique, have shown that basal glucose production is two to three times the adult value, expressed per unit body weight.[22] These studies were dependent upon the assumption that the newborn was as sen-

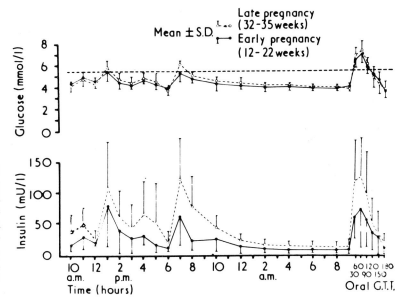

Fig. 26-1. Plasma glucose and insulin concentrations during diurnal evaluation, and an oral glucose tolerance test, in nine normal women evaluated in early and late pregnancy. Conversion 1 mmol/l = 18 mg/dl. (Gillmer MDG, Beard RW, Brooke FM et al: Br Med J 3: 399, 1975)

sitive as the adult to minute changes in glucose concentration. Subsequent investigations in puppies and in the lamb have suggested that precise regulation of glucose homeostasis is not fully developed.[19,20,23] Hepatic suppression of endogenous glucose production does not occur promptly in the neonatal period.

There are a number of studies of glucose production in the human newborn, using stable nonradioactive isotopes such as ^{2}H at the sixth carbon of glucose,[24,25] ^{13}C at the first carbon,[26,27] and uniformly ^{13}C-labelled glucose.[28] The values obtained range from 2.5 to 6.1 mg/kg/minute, depending on the age of the newborn, the label used, and the general medical condition of the infant.

There is data evaluating the autonomic and enzymatic control of neonatal glucose homeostasis suggesting that glycogenolysis is insufficient to maintain glucose production.[29] Other

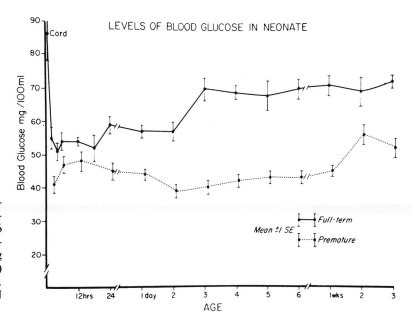

Fig. 26-2. Blood glucose concentrations in 179 full-term infants weighing >2.5 kg (206 determinations) and in 104 low-birth-weight infants weighing <2.5 kg (442 determinations) during the neonatal period. (Cornblath M, Reisner SH: N Engl J Med 273:378, 1965)

studies of glucose kinetics have focused on the developmental maturation of the newborn liver, and have provided quantitative data concerning steady-state hepatic glucose output and peripheral utilization. There is evidence that hepatic unresponsiveness to insulin may be a major factor responsible for the inefficiency in glucose homeostasis noted in the neonatal lamb model.[19,20] To date these findings have not yet been corroborated in the human newborn using stable tracer kinetics. Evaluation of opposing or synergistic hormonal, neural, metabolic, and enzymatic systems is required to understand the maturation of neonatal glucose homeostasis.

HYPOGLYCEMIA IN THE NEWBORN

Hypoglycemia is usually defined as ≤25 mg/dl in plasma in the low-birth-weight infant and ≤35 mg/dl in plasma of the term infant at ≤72 hours of age. After 72 hours, plasma glucose concentration should be ≥45 mg/dl.[12] The main clinical difficulty is the nonspecific nature of the symptoms, which are listed below. These difficulties are compounded by the occurrence of symptoms at different levels of blood glucose in individual infants and the lack of a universal threshold below or above which symptoms can be expected.

Signs and Symptoms of Neonatal Hypoglycemia

Abnormal cry	Hypothermia
Apathy	Hypotonia
Apnea	Jitteryness
Cardiac arrest	Lethargy
Convulsions	Tremors
Cyanosis	Tachypnea

Further difficulties may result from lack of attention to the details of laboratory measurement of glucose. One of the most troublesome problems is the failure to measure the glucose concentration rapidly enough, with subsequent red cell oxidation of glucose resulting in falsely low plasma values. A number of centers use the Dextrostix technique, which is reliable if directions are followed carefully. Abnormally low or high values need to be corroborated with laboratory determination of glucose concentration before correction of the suspected hypoglycemia. It is important also to remember that blood glucose concentration is usually 10% to 15% lower than the corresponding plasma glucose value.

A number of different classifications have been employed for hypoglycemia in the neonatal period. Cornblath and Schwartz[12] and others[30,31] have focused on the clinical course, emphasizing time of presentation, duration, severity, and response to therapy. Another schema considers the biochemical and physiologic parameters, and evaluates the relationship of hepatic production to uptake in contrast to peripheral utilization.[32,33] This system would compare decreased hepatic glucose production caused by enzymatic or substrate deficiencies to that secondary to increased insulin concentration. Inadequate glucose production includes those conditions involving decreased availability of substrate (i.e., glycogen, lactate, glycerol, and amino acids), altered sensitivity to neural or hormonal factors, immature or altered enzymatic pathways (i.e., decreased gluconeogenesis and/or increased peripheral utilization rates) or all of the above. In contrast, hypoglycemia secondary to increased insulin concentration would include all conditions in which there is an absolute or relative increase in insulin concentration.

IMPRECISE/DIMINISHED HEPATIC GLUCOSE PRODUCTION

Neonatal hypoglycemia, except for insulin excess, is caused primarily by diminished hepatic glucose production. Hepatic control of glucose homeostasis and its relationship to disequilibrium in the neonate have only recently been subjected to study.[34] Conditions in the newborn which produce hypoglycemia through either imprecise control of glucose production or diminished substrate availability include: prematurely born infants appropriate for gestational age (AGA), small for gestational age (SGA) infants, perinatally stressed and asphyxiated infants, cold-stressed infants, and neonates with congenital heart disease or sepsis. Infants may also be hypoglycemic because of glucagon deficiency or deficits in intermediary metabolic pathways. Examples are glycogen storage disease type I and fructose 1,6 diphosphatase deficiency, reflecting a series of hereditary metabolic disorders in which hypoglycemia may be the initial or most obvious presenting feature.

Preterm AGA Infants

The AGA infant born before term may develop hypoglycemia. In 1968, Raivio and Hallman reported a frequency of 1.4% in AGA infants.[35] Fluge noted that as many as 14% of AGA prematures showed evidence of neonatal hypoglycemia.[31]

The diminished oral and parenteral intake in the low-birth-weight infant may partially explain the lower plasma glucose seen in these infants and their propensity toward hypoglycemia. Functionally immature gluconeogenic and glycogenolytic enzyme systems present in the neonate potentiate these difficulties. The relatively increased size of the brain (13% of the body mass in the newborn versus 2% in the adult) may be responsible for the greater proportion of glucose consumption during periods of fasting, an effect magnified in the low-birth-weight infant.

SGA Infants

Many centers have reported a relatively high frequency of hypoglycemia in SGA infants ever since Cornblath and coworkers, in 1959, described its occurrence in eight infants born to mothers with toxemia.[36] Lubchenco and Bard,[37] deLeeuw and deVries,[38] and others have all substantiated the commonness of hypoglycemia in these infants. Toxemia has frequently been associated with this occurrence, and the incidence of hypoglycemia was highest (61%) in those infants born to mothers with relatively low urinary estriols, compared to 19% in infants born to mothers with normal estriol levels.[38,39] Reduction in energy reserves manifested as decreased glycogen deposition, combined with increased utilization of substrate, may result in the appearance of hypoglycemia. Furthermore, the occurrence of a reduced muscle mass in the face of normal insulin production (see below) provides for a degree of relative hyperinsulinemia which may contribute to the resultant hypoglycemia.

There have also been a number of studies evaluating intermediary metabolism postnatally. A functional delay in the development of phosphoenolpyruvate carboxykinase (PEPCK), thought to be the rate limiting enzyme of gluconeogenesis, in SGA infants was suggested by Haymond and coworkers.[40] This was substantiated by Williams and coworkers, who studied the effect of oral alanine feeding on glucose homeostasis in the SGA infant, compared to AGA infants.[41] Oral alanine feeding enhanced plasma glucagon in both groups, but only stimulated hepatic glucose output in the AGA infants.

The effect of intravenous glucagon on plasma amino acids has been evaluated in various types of infants, including the SGA infant. SGA infants in the first hours of life had significantly lower total amino acids compared to a comparable group of AGA infants, although the response to glucagon in the SGA infants mimicked the control (AGA) group. It is speculated that the inability of the SGA infant to extract specific gluconeogenic amino acids could account for the susceptibility to hypoglycemia in these stressed infants.[42]

The role of glucagon was also evaluated by Mestyan and coworkers by measuring 17 amino acids before and during glucagon infusion in normoglycemic and hypoglycemic SGA infants.[43] In the normoglycemic group, most amino acid concentrations declined significantly but this did not occur in the SGA infants who were hypoglycemic. Although the effect was transient in nature, these results reinforce the importance of glucagon in acute hepatic glucose homeostasis. In another investigation, neonatal lambs between 1 and 3 days of age were infused with somatostatin alone or in combination with insulin and glucagon during a 2-hour interval. Plasma glucose concentration fell when both insulin and glucagon were suppressed acutely, suggesting that the latter is of importance in maintaining glucose concentration during short-term fasting. It was concluded that the ratio between the two hormones acutely affects glucose homeostasis.[44]

The secretion of glucagon and insulin has been evaluated in SGA infants.[45] Both SGA and AGA infants, after being fed oral glucose and protein (1 g/kg each after a 4-hour fast), had similar secretions of both pancreatic hormones. The authors speculated that the instability of glucose metabolism in the SGA infant resulted from the rapid disappearance rate of glucose and probably also from a transient deficiency of hepatic gluconeogenic enzymes but not from altered secretory patterns of glucagon and insulin.[45]

Infants Experiencing Perinatal Stress/Hypoxia

Infants who develop an increased rate of glucose utilization may be prone to hypoglycemia. An increased rate of anaerobic glycolysis in combination with an increased rate of glycogenolysis is probably the underlying biochemical mechanism. Only two moles of ATP are generated by the Embden–Meyerhof anaerobic pathway. Thus, 18 times more glucose is required to produce the same amount of ATP in contrast to aerobic oxidation, which results in 36 moles of ATP. Because the low-birth-weight infant is subject to hypoxia, the combination of decreased substrate availability and increased rate of utilization may result in hypoglycemia. In addition, increased lactate production may result in an associated acidosis. Beard has emphasized the association between hypoxia and hypoglycemia in the low-birth-weight infant and noted increased metabolic needs out of proportion to substrate availability.[46,47] The difficulties are all accentuated in infants who are clinically compromised and are thus unable to replace substrate from the usual exogenous (oral) sources.

Cold-stressed Infants

Hypoglycemia has been identified in infants who experience cold injury. Mann and Elliott described 14 infants who suffered neonatal cold injury following prolonged exposure to environmental temperatures below 90°F.[48] Marked hypoglycemia was documented in three of six infants in whom it was measured. The hypoglycemia is presumed to be the result of free fatty acid (FFA) elevation secondary to a cold-induced norepinephrine response.[49] Recognition of the potential occurrence of hypoglycemia following cold stress should result in consideration of parenteral treatment in conjunction with warming the infant. In addition, this relationship needs to be considered in the evaluation of blood glucose levels in infants with either temperature instability or who are in a suboptimal thermal environment.

Neonatal Sepsis

Hypoglycemia has been identified with increased frequency in association with neonatal sepsis. Yeung noted hypoglycemia in 20 of 56 infants with signs of sepsis.[50] He suggested that inadequate caloric intake in these infected infants may predispose to hypoglycemia. The possibility of an increased metabolic rate was also suggested because ≥100 kilocalories/kg/day had been infused intravenously in these infants. A decreased rate of gluconeogenesis has also been documented in laboratory animals following gram-negative bacterial infection.[51] The possibility of increased peripheral utilization because of enhanced insulin sensitivity in sepsis has been considered.[52] It is likely that one or more of these factors will operate in specific circumstances to produce the resultant hypoglycemia.

Infants with Congenital Heart Disease/Congestive Heart Failure

An inverse relationship has been noted between the concentration of cardiac glycogen and the level of maturity at birth, with low levels in the offspring of mammals born with relative maturity (i.e., man, monkey, sheep, and so on). These reserves are rapidly depleted during anoxia.[53] Benzing and coworkers reported on a series of 27 patients in whom the simultaneous occurrence of hypoglycemia and acute congestive heart failure was noted in association with congenital heart disease.[54] Reduced dietary intake in association with diminished hepatic glycogen resulted in hypoglycemia. This has been further substantiated by Amatoyakul and coworkers, who noted the association of congestive heart failure with hypoglycemia in infants without significant heart defects.[55] The pathophysiology of hypoglycemia in cyanotic congenital heart disease has been studied by Haymond and coworkers.[56] Six subjects were evaluated between 13 and 67 months of age. Glucose and alanine turnover, using studies of metabolic clearance rates in these infants, were compared to controls. A subtle defect in hepatic extraction of gluconeogenic substrates was suspected, possibly secondary to decreased hepatic perfusion. It is apparent that the presence of either hypoglycemia or congestive heart failure should be considered when one or the other appears.

Infants Manifesting Defective Gluconeogenesis/Glycogenolysis

Hypoglycemia has been noted in infants unable to sustain normal gluconeogenesis. Glucagon is influential in hepatic glucose production since it enhances glycogenolysis and gluconeogenesis. A recent report has documented an infant with isolated glucagon deficiency and neonatal hypoglycemia. The diagnosis was based on low basal glucagon concentration as well as a diminshed response to hypoglycemia and alanine infusion, both potent stimulators of glucagon secretion, in an infant in whom normal insulin secretion was present.[57] Vidnes has also reported on three infants with persistent neonatal hypoglycemia, one of whom evidenced an abnormal subcellular distribution of PEPCK (see above) in the extramitochondrial fraction.[58,59]

The specific enzymatic deficiency that may affect gluconeogenesis in the neonate is type I glycogen storage disease (glucose-6-phosphatase deficiency). The deficiency is an autosomal recessive genetic defect which may occasionally present in the neonatal period with severe hypoglycemia and hepatomegaly.[12]

Galactosemia may present early in infants, with cataract formation, septicemia, and hepatocellular jaundice appearing as clinical manifestations, in addition to hypoglycemic symptoms and a positive reducing test in the urine. Several inborn errors of galactose metabolism are known to occur in man. The most common is a defect in galactose-1-phosphate uridyl transferase, along with the two variants, Duarte and Negro. Other disorders, including galactokinase and uridine diphosphogalactose-4-epimerase deficiency, have been described. The diagnosis involves the demonstration of a low true glucose level in the face of normal total hexoses, together with the determination of the enzymatic defect, which can be analyzed in both red and white blood cells. Exclusion of milk and milk products (lactose) is the treatment of choice. Because early intervention prevents sequellae, routine neonatal screening has been recommended.[60]

Hereditary fructose intolerance has also been documented in the neonatal period, particularly in infants who ingest sweets or fruit juices. The major intolerance is caused by fructose-1-phosphate aldolase deficiency. The hypoglycemia is secondary to an inhibition of hepatic glucose release, and absence of a hyperglycemic response to glucagon following ingestion or parenteral administration of fructose. A second enzymatic defect, fructose-1,6-diphosphatase deficiency, has also been associated with hypoglycemia.

HYPERINSULINISM

Hypoglycemia following increased plasma insulin has now been associated with several discrete disorders of the islets, including the infant of the diabetic mother, infants with hemolytic disease of the newborn, pancreatic nesidioblastosis, discrete or multiple islet cell adenomatosis, and infants undergoing exchange transfusion. The infant with Beckwith–Wiedemann Syndrome should also be considered along with other rare causes of hyperinsulinemic hypoglycemia.

The Infant of the Diabetic Mother (see also Chap. 16)

The infant of the diabetic mother (IDM) may show profound, though often asymptomatic, hypoglycemia immediately at birth. Although there is a tendency for spontaneous recovery in the ensuing 12 to 24 hours, this is by no means certain, and severe and protracted hypoglycemia may persist. It has been suggested that in the IDM, hyperinsulinism secondary to prolonged intrauterine islet cell stimulation occurs as a result of maternal hyperglycemia.[61] Although insulin does not cross the placenta, glucose readily does, and both islet cell hyperplasia and high serum insulin levels have been demonstrated in the newborn IDM. The somatic overgrowth, resulting in the typical overweight-for-gestational-age infant, is evidence of the prime role of insulin as a growth factor in the perinatal period. Of interest in this regard is the work of Susa and coworkers, who studied rhesus monkey fetuses in whom an implanted minipump delivered insulin over a prolonged period. This resulted in a hyperinsulinemic, euglycemic milieu *in utero*. Fetal macrosomia with selective organomegaly of the spleen, heart, liver, and placenta were noted. The brain, kidney, and lung were not enlarged. These studies confirm the selective growth promoting effects of insulin *in vivo*.[62,63]

There is normally an inverse relationship between glucose and plasma FFA's whereby hypoglycemia results in an elevation of the serum FFA levels and vice versa.[64] This response, which may at least in part be mediated by catecholamine-induced activation of the lipase system, provides an alternate source of "fuel" for metabolic functions. This elevation does not occur in the IDM,[65] possibly as a result of a poor catecholamine response to the hypoglycemia.[66] In the infant of the diabetic mother such a finding would suggest a long-standing (intrauterine) hypoglycemic experience with subsequent adrenal medullary exhaustion. Such long-standing experience might also explain the frequent lack of symptoms postnatally, despite extremely low blood levels, as an expression of acclimation to chronic, persistent, low blood glucose levels.

Although pathologically there appear to be more than ample glycogen stores in the liver, their release by the usual doses of glucagon (30 μg/kg/body weight) is often poor.[67] Such infants may respond to much higher doses (300 μg/kg) with a prolonged and sustained glucose release, often resulting in almost paradoxical hyperglycemia.

Another current area of investigation involving the IDM (and his mother) is the evaluation of **Hb A$_{I_c}$**. Glycohemoglobin is a posttranslation modification of normal adult hemoglobin (Hb A), which has been shown to correlate directly with glucose concentration over time. Diabetic therapy has been evaluated in pregnancy by measurement levels of Hb A$_{I_c}$, and the lower levels noted closer to term in the pregnant diabetic have been attributed to closer medical supervision and more rigid glucose control.[68]

Rh Incompatibility

Hyperinsulinism has been implicated as the cause of the hypoglycemia seen in infants with severe Rh isoimmunization.[69–72] These children are invariably severely affected by their disease, with profound anemia and hepatosplenomegaly at birth. The shock and collapse seen on occasion may be caused primarily by the profound hypoglycemia and, under such circumstances, glucose administration in addition to measures taken to correct the anemia may be critical. The IDM and severely Rh-affected infant share several pathologic hallmarks. In addition to the hyperinsulinism and islet cell hyperplasia, both show almost identical edematous placental changes. The IDM, just as his Rh-affected counterpart, has excessive islands of extramedullary hematopoiesis in both liver and spleen. Although this latter finding may be the result of insulin stimulation, the precise cause of the hyperinsulinism itself in the Rh-affected infant is uncertain. It is possible that an increase in glutathione, resulting from massive hemolysis of red blood cells, may act as a stimulus to insulin release.

Metabolic Effects of Exchange Transfusions

Hypoglycemia, although not often considered, may be a real problem following exchange transfusion. In this connection, the exchange blood and its preservatives are more critically important in the newborn, in whom a double volume washout is being undertaken, than in an adult, who is receiving 450 mg of the blood-preservative mixture to be diluted in a total 5 to 6 liter blood volume.

Heparinized blood contains no added glucose. Moreover, the heparin, by raising the FFA levels, contributes to the hypoglycemic potential of the transfusion blood, so that under some circumstances (*e.g.*, severe Rh incompatibility with hyperinsulinism) its use would be contraindicated unless a concomitant IV glucose infusion is administered to prevent and/or treat the hypoglycemia.[73] With citrated blood, acid citrate dextrose (ACD) or citrate phosphate dextrose (CPD), the added dextrose will yield a blood-preservative mixture containing as much as 300 mg/dl glucose. In this situation, although immediate hypoglycemia is not a problem, the high glucose load results in a reactive insulin response. When the glucose "bolus" is suddenly terminated at the end of the exchange procedure, a state of hyperinsulinism ensues. Studies documenting this occurrence have shown a precipitous 2-hour, post-exchange fall in blood glucose to levels below those present before undertaking the exchange procedure.[74] Once again, the severely Rh-affected infant is at greatest risk, but even mildly affected and nonerythroblastotic exchanged infants may respond in such a manner. Recognition of this possibility should lead to its detection and treatment.

Beckwith–Wiedemann Syndrome

In 1964, Beckwith and associates described a syndrome characterized by omphalocele, muscular macroglossia, and visceromegaly.[75] Wiedemann almost simultaneously described a similar clinical picture in three siblings.[76] It was subsequently shown that hypoglycemia may be an associated metabolic component of this syndrome, occurring in approximately

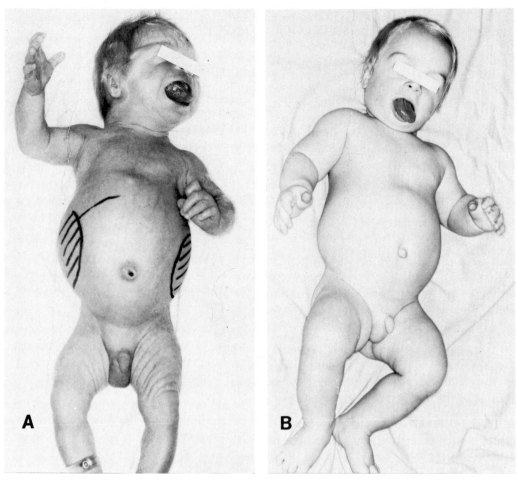

Fig. 26-3. Infant with Beckwith–Wiedemann's Syndrome at birth (**A**) and at six months (**B**), after glucose homeostasis had been achieved. Although liver and spleen have receded in size, the tongue is still large. (Courtesy of Dr. David Schiff, Department of Pediatrics, University of Alberta)

50% of the cases reported. Hyperinsulinism is responsible for both the hypoglycemia and the somatic and visceral growth abnormalities. Pathologically, islet cell hyperplasia of the pancreas has been demonstrated in these infants, although the etiology of the syndrome remains unclear. The hypoglycemia is ultimately self-limiting but may be relatively protracted and difficult to control. In a carefully studied patient, with resistant hypoglycemia and hyperinsulinism, Schiff and coworkers were ultimately able to achieve adequate control of glucose levels with a combination of epinephrine (1:200, acqueous solution; Susphrine) and diazoxide therapy, which suppressed both basal insulin release and that in the post-prandial state.[77] The infant presented at birth with an umbilical hernia, macroglossia, and hepatosplenomegaly as well as hyperinsulinism and profound recalcitrant hypoglycemia. Normal glucose control was achieved by 1 month of age. At 6 months, somatic growth was normal, hepatosplenomegaly had receded, but the macroglossia was still present. At 2 years of age, growth was normal, and the tongue, although still large, could be kept within the mouth without any evidence of malocclusion (Fig. 26-3).

Nesidioblastosis, Islet Cell Adenomas

Although rare at any age in childhood, infants with nesidioblastosis,[78,79] discrete islet cell adenoma,[80,81] or adenomatosis[82] have been reported and successfully treated. Hyperinsulinism, without other apparent cause and resistant hypoglycemia should raise these rare, but nevertheless real, possibilities. Preoperative confirmation may be sought either by means of regular gastrointestinal radiographic studies, peritoneal air insufflation, abdominal angiography, and/or ultrasound examination, but surgical exploration may be necessary as a definitive diagnostic as well as therapeutic measure.

Other Causes of Hyperinsulinism

Isolated instances have also been reported which mimic the problem of insulin excess and resultant hypoglycemia. Zucker and coworkers have reported symptomatic neonatal hypoglycemia in association with maternal administration of chlorpropamide.[83] This resulted in stimulation of both the maternal and the fetal beta cells. Because the teratogenicity of the drug is a concern, its use is limited, especially because control of glucose is insufficient for the management of diabetes in pregnancy. Benzothiadiazide diuretics have also been implicated in the production of insulin secretion.[84] It has been suggested that the drug produces elevated maternal blood glucose levels and results in stimulation of the fetal islets with subsequent neonatal hypoglycemia. There is also a report of an infant in whom hypoglycemia may have been caused by an insulin-releasing substance, possibly from the gut.[85] Neonatal hypoglycemia has also been associated with administration of salicylates,[86] the suggested mechanism being an uncoupling of mitochondrial oxidative phosphorylation. The association of congenital adrenal hyperplasia and hypoglycemia has also been recorded.[87] Hypoglycemia has been noted in individuals who are sensitive to leucine. This amino acid, among others, may cause increased insulin release following ingestion of milk.[88] Finally, a recent report denotes the potential of hypoglycemia after beta-sympathomimetic tocolytic therapy, which is being used increasingly to inhibit premature labor. While the specific mechanism of action is not known, a possible explanation involves increased pancreatic secretion of insulin in response to a specific glucose concentration.[89]

EVALUATION OF NEONATAL HYPOGLYCEMIA

As in other areas of neonatology, a detailed maternal history and a thorough physical examination are important in determining the probability of neonatal hypoglycemia and its etiology when present. Maternal history, which includes family or maternal history of diabetes or other glucose intolerance, drug ingestion (chlorpropamide, benzothiadiazide diuretics, and salicylates), and blood group incompatability (Rh) or preeclampsia should alert the physician to the potential problem of hypoglycemia. Perinatal history, including birth asphyxia and/or trauma and the presence of cold injury, is of further importance in establishing the possibility.

A thorough physical examination will indicate whether an infant is AGA, SGA, or large for gestational age (LGA) and also what the gestational age of the infant is. The appearance of the IDM, from Class A or B (LGA) versus Classes C through F (SGA), is well recognized, as is that of the infant with Beckwith–Wiedemann syndrome. Prolonged jaundice and cataracts suggest galactosemia, while the infant with unexplained hepatomegaly should be considered for the possibility of glycogen storage disease.

Most etiologies of hypoglycemia should be apparent following a detailed maternal history, review of labor and delivery, and physical examination of the infant. However, appropriate laboratory studies may include plasma glucose, insulin, gulcagon, lactate, alanine, ketones, FAAs, and pH, as well as cortisol, growth hormone, and thyroid function studies in some cases. Tolerance tests, such as those for glucose, galactose, fructose, glucagon, insulin, and tolbutamide, are usually reserved for confirmation of suspected diagnoses. In some research laboratories, stable nonradioactive isotopes are being used to analyze glucose kinetics.

HYPERGLYCEMIA IN THE NEWBORN

Hyperglycemia may also be a problem for the newborn because of the potential for an osmotic diuresis and resultant dehydration.[90–92] Originally, Gentz and Cornblath described hyperglycemia in SGA newborns with **transient neonatal diabetes** in the first six weeks of life.[93] Symptoms included failure to thrive and dehydration, despite adequate oral intake. Insulin was used to treat the extreme hyperglycemia, which was without concomitant ketosis or acidosis. Subsequently, others have confirmed the presence of this entity and suggested that deficient insulin secretion or production of a biologically inactive form of insulin was responsible for its appearance.[94,95] The association of hyperglycemia and a chromosome deletion (46,xxDq−) of number 13 has also been reported in an infant who was SGA.[96]

Of current interest, in view of the widespread use of parenteral alimentation to nourish low-birth-weight infants, are the increasing number of reports documenting the occurrence of hyperglycemia. Dweck and Cassady reported that 43 of 50 infants who weighed 1000 g or less showed plasma glucose concentrations of 125 mg/dl or greater during parenteral glucose administration. Thirty six of these infants had plasma glucose levels >300 mg/dl, usually within 24 hours of birth.[90] Diminished tolerance to glucose was inferred in these very low-birth-weight infants who did not manifest the well-known adult Staub–Traugott effect (*i.e.*, lower blood glucose concentration and increasingly rapid disappearance rates of glucose following its repeated administration).[97]

Hyperglycemia was evaluated by Zarif and coworkers by measuring glucose, insulin, and growth hormone during the first 5 days of life prospectively in low-birth-weight infants receiving a parenteral and/or oral glucose load.[98] Hyperglycemia was noted in 32 of 75 infants and an association was seen between death and hyperglycemia. Insulin and growth hormone responses were not felt to be of etiologic significance, but the authors did note that most infants had been stressed, suggesting the possibility of increased secretion of cortisol, catecholamine, or both.

Exogenous insulin as a treatment for hyperglycemia, specifically to increase glucose disposal, was evaluated in eight infants of <1500 g by Pollak and coworkers.[99] A saline placebo was given during infusion of 14 mg/kg/min of exogenous glucose on day one and was followed on day two by 10 mU/kg/min of insulin infused over 50 minutes under similar conditions of glucose administration. Normogly-

cemia resulted from the exogenous administration of the insulin. The authors speculated that hyperglycemia during exogenous infusion of glucose was either the result of persistent endogenous hepatic glucose production or decreased peripheral utilization, but the two entities could not be differentiated. It appeared, however, that an elevated plasma insulin concentration was required to achieve appropriate control of glucose homeostasis.

A second series of studies defined tolerance for glucose in 35 clinically healthy AGA infants weighing 750 to 1500 g and between 3 and 38 days of age.[100] Infants were given graded doses of glucose at either 8, 11, or 14 mg/kg/min for 3 hours by continuous peripheral intravenous infusion. Plasma glucose and insulin concentrations and timed urine volume and glucose concentrations were measured. Nine infants received 8 mg/kg/min and, in these infants, plasma glucose and insulin concentrations were similar in the steady state period of analysis. None of these infants evidenced hyperglycemia. In contrast, 10 infants receiving 14 mg/kg/min of exogenous glucose developed significantly higher plasma glucose and insulin responses in contrast to the infants receiving 8 mg/kg/min of exogenous glucose. Sixteen infants received 11 mg/kg/min and the plasma glucose concentration significantly increased to from 140 to 160 mg/dl in a comparable time period, but the plasma insulin concentrations were not significantly different from baseline. Half of these infants developed hyperglycemia (plasma glucose concentration >150 mg/dl) with concomitant glucosuria. All of these infants had been clinically asymptomatic for at least 48 hours prior to the study but had been clinically ill prior to that time (Table 26-1). These findings parallel the work of others who have also suggested that clinical morbidity could unfavorably affect glucose homeostasis in the newborn.[101] Stable isotope tracer analyses and other techniques will provide differentiation of the characteristics of glucose metabolism in these infants, and should help explain the clinical appearance of hyperglycemia.

TREATMENT

The treatment of neonatal hypo- and hyperglycemia begins with identification of its po-

Table 26-1. Frequency of Different Clinical Morbidities* (N = 35)

Group	Glucose Infusion Rate (mg/kg/min)	No Glycosuria	Glycosuria	Frequency† Low	High	Statistical Significance
1 (n = 9)	8	9	0	4	5	None
2A (n = 9)	11	9	0	9	0	p. <0.05
2B (n = 7)	11	0	7	2	5	None
3 (n = 10)	14	0	10	8	2	None

*Clinical morbidities include the following: Apgar score ≤6 at 1 min; Apgar score ≤6 at 5 min; sepsis or necrotizing enterocolitis, apnea ≥4/24 hr; respiratory distress syndrome requiring use of respirator; hypocalcemia ≤7 mg/100 ml; serum bilirubin ≥10 mg/100 ml at 48 hr; patent ductus arteriosus with congestive heart failure.
†Low frequency = 1 to 2 clinical morbidities; high frequency = 3 to 8 clinical morbidities
(Cowett RM, Oh W, Pollack A et al: Pediatrics 63:389, 1979; Copyright © American Academy of Pediatrics, 1979)

tential in the infant at risk, documentation of its presence by appropriate laboratory measurement (Dextrostix and confirmatory blood or plasma glucose determinations), and corrective measures to either raise or lower blood or plasma glucose concentration.

Feedings generally are advocated as either 5% dextrose or formula but probably should only be used to maintain a glucose concentration already in the euglycemic range. Using 6 mg/kg/min as the concentration of glucose required to maintain homeostasis, it is unreasonable to expect that oral feedings alone will provide for adequate glucose intake in infants who are hypoglycemic. We advocate parenteral (intravenous) treatment of the hypoglycemic condition using a constant infusion pump to avoid fluctuations in the rate of infusion that would result in irregular rates of endogenous insulin release. Oral feedings should be initiated as tolerated. Repeated documentation of blood or plasma glucose concentration should be an integral part of the treatment of any infant. The glucose infusions should be gradually reduced rather than abruptly terminated, to avoid sudden reactive hypoglycemia due to "uncovered" hyperinsulinism. Once oral feedings are initiated, evaluation of the glucose concentration just before a subsequent feeding provides an analysis of the infant's status.

Parenteral therapy should begin with 6 mg/kg/min followed by graded increases to achieve euglycemia with the minimum concentration of glucose required. A peripheral vein rather than an umbilical vessel is the preferred route of infusion. However, other than in an emergency, rates greater than 15 mg/kg/min should be given only when using a central venous approach. Rates greater than 20 mg/kg/min are probably contraindicated by either route. Acute administration of 25% glucose by bolus infusions of up to 4 ml/kg, if required for relief of acute symptoms (*e.g.*, seizures), must be followed by parenteral infusion until the effect of the bolus infusion on acute pancreatic insulin release is no longer apparent.

Calculation of parenteral glucose therapy must include the actual concentration of glucose present in the administered fluids. A hydrated form of glucose (mol. wt. 198) is used by most manufacturers to prepare the parenteral fluid so that the actual amount of sugar available is approximately 10% less.[102] This is of particular concern when very-low-birth-weight or severely hypoglycemic infants are being treated.

Treatment with a number of specific agents is indicated when parenteral therapy above 15 mg/kg/min is not effective in maintaining euglycemia. **Corticosteroids** have been shown to be effective in the therapy of hypoglycemia. Although several glucose-producing reactions are enhanced by the steroids, the major effect is probably that of gluconeogenesis from noncarbohydrate (protein) sources. The alleged "superiority" of ACTH over cortisone was in all likelihood the result of the use of crude hog pituitary extract, from which the patient received the added benefit of "pollutant" growth hormone. Current preparations afford no advantage between the two. Hydrocortisone is given at a dose of 5 mg/kg/day either intravenously or orally every 12 hours or prednisone is used at a dose of 2 mg/kg/day orally. As with all forms of therapy, gradual diminution of the dosage administered, in concert with decreasing parenteral concentrations of glucose and increasing oral intake of nutrients, will successfully allow weaning of the infant.

The use of **glucagon** provides a highly effective method of releasing glycogen from the liver and can indeed be utilized as a therapeutic means of assessing whether or not the liver contains adequate stores. Thus, its failure in some growth-retarded infants is considered to be evidence for a lack of hepatic glycogen stores in these children. In the IDM, there is often a failure to respond to the usual doses (30 μg/kg), despite the presence of more than adequate hepatic glycogen stores. These infants will frequently respond to higher doses (300 μg/kg) with a prolonged and sustained hyperglycemia (see above), so that the higher dose might well be used as initial therapy in the IDM.[12]

Like glucagon, **epinephrine** is capable of promoting glycogen to glucose conversion, but in far smaller quantities. For this effect, therefore, glucagon is the drug of choice. The hyperglycemic potential of epinephrine in blocking glucose uptake by peripheral muscle presupposes an adequate blood level to start with and is, therefore, of little practical benefit in the hypoglycemic state. Epinephrine is, however, a powerful anti-insulin, a fact which explains its success as an effective anti-hypoglycemic agent in IDMs, as well as in other hyperinsulinemic states. The agent most commonly used is a 1:200 epinephrine in aqueous suspension (Sus-phrine), which can be readily administered subcutaneously.[103]

Phenobarbital, commonly used in the treatment of seizures, may have value if these are of hypoglycemic origin, over and above its effect as a sedative agent. Experimentally, phenobarbital appears to increase the amount of glucose in the brain, at a given blood level, in hypoglycemic animals.[104] The effect is not caused by a decrease in metabolic demand by the brain under these conditions, suggesting that glucose transport into the brain may be enhanced by an enzyme system induced by the barbiturate. These observations would explain the frequently seen diminution in severity and intensity of hypoglycemic seizures following phenobarbital therapy in the absence of any effect of the drug on blood glucose levels.

Diazoxide, in a dose of 10 to 15 mg/kg/day, probably exerts its effect by suppressing pancreatic insulin secretion, although some have suggested a direct effect on hepatic glucose production.[105] The drug should be used only when other methods have failed.[106]

Surgical intervention is indicated with nesidioblastosis or when an islet cell adenoma or adenomatosis has been confirmed.

The treatment of hyperglycemia is usually successfully accomplished by lowering the concentration of parenteral glucose administered. The ease with which this can be accomplished may be diminished because of the requirements of at least 60 kcal/kg/day to spare protein for subsequent somatic growth.[107] Before lowering the concentration of parenteral glucose administered on the basis of hyperglycemia alone, measurement of urine concentration and volume is required to confirm the presence of an osmotic diuresis, which may be absent in the very low-birth-weight infant.[100] The absolute level of hyperglycemia at which untoward CNS effects are first manifest has not been documented in the human. However, the presence of intracranial bleeding has been reported in newborn puppies in whom acute hyperglycemia was produced by "standard regimens" of glucose therapy.[108] Caution and further evaluation are necessary to define the effect of acute and chronic hyperglycemia on the central nervous system of the infant at risk.

REFERENCES

1. **Battaglia FC, Meschia G:** Principle substrates of fetal metabolism. Physiological Reviews 58:499–527, 1978
2. **James EJ, Raye JR, Gresham EL et al:** Fetal O_2 consumption, CO_2 production, and glucose uptake in a chronic sheep preparation. Pediatrics 50:361–371, 1972
3. **Hay WW, Jr:** Fetal glucose metabolism. Semin Perinatol 3:157–177, 1979
4. **Gilmer MDG, Beard RW, Brooke FM et al:**

Carbohydrate metabolism in pregnancy. I. Diurnal plasma glucose profile in normal and diabetic women. Br Med J 3:399–402, 1975

5. Gilmer MDG, Beard RW, Brooke FM et al: Carbohydrate metabolism in pregnancy. II. Relation between maternal glucose tolerance and glucose metabolism in the newborn. Br Med J 3:402–404, 1975

6. Hay WW, Jr, Sparks J, Quisell B et al: Comparison of umbilical glucose uptake and fetal glucose turnover rates (abstr). Pediatr Res 12:394, 1978

7. Simmons MA, Jones MD, Jr, Battaglia FC et al: Insulin effect on fetal glucose utilization. Pediatr Res 12:90–92, 1978

8. Schwartz AL: The metabolism of carbohydrate. In Cornblath M, Schwartz R (eds): Disorders of Carbohydrate Metabolism in Infancy, pp 3–23. Philadelphia, WB Saunders, 1976

9. McIlwain H: Biochemistry and the central nervous system. Edinburgh, Churchill-Livingstone, 1971

10. Fisher DA: Perinatal insulin, glucagon, and carbohydrate metabolism. In Bloom RS, Sinclair JC, Warshaw JB (eds): Perinatal endocrinology, pp 30–37. Symposium in perinatal and developmental medicine, No 8, Mead Johnson, 1975

11. Grajwer LA, Sperling MA, Sack J, Fisher D: Possible mechanisms and significance of the neonatal surge in glucagon secretion: Studies in newborn lambs. Pediatr Res 11:833–836, 1977

12. Cornblath M, Schwartz R: Disorders of Carbohydrate Metabolism in Infancy, 2nd ed. Philadelphia, WB Saunders, 1976

13. Cornblath M, Reisner SH: Blood glucose in the neonate and its clinical significance. N Engl J Med 273:378–381, 1965

14. Milner RDG: The growth and development of the endocrine pancreas. In Davis JA, Dobbing J (eds): Scientific Foundations in Pediatrics, pp 507–513. Philadelphia, WB Saunders, 1974

15. Shelley HJ, Bassett JM: Control of carbohydrate metabolism in the fetus and newborn. Br Med Bull 31:37–43, 1975

16. Soskin S, Essex HE, Herrick JF et al: The mechanism of regulation of the blood sugar by the liver. Am J Physiol 124:558–567, 1938

17. Madison LL: Role of insulin in the hepatic handling of glucose. Arch Intern Med 123:284–292, 1969

18. Steele R: Influences of glucose loading and of injected insulin on hepatic glucose output. Ann NY Acad Sci 82:420–430, 1959

19. Cowett RM, Susa JB, Oh W et al: Endogenous glucose production during constant glucose infusion in the newborn lamb. Pediatr Res 12:853–857, 1978

20. Susa JB, Cowett RM, Oh W et al: Suppression of gluconeogenesis and endogenous glucose production by exogenous insulin administration in the newborn lamb. Pediatr Res 13:594–599, 1979

21. Adam PAJ, King KC, Schwartz R: Model for the investigation of intractable hypoglycemia: Insulin-glucose interrelationship during steady state infusions. Pediatrics 41:91–105, 1968

22. Kornhauser D, Adam PAJ, Schwartz R: Glucose production and utilization in the newborn puppy. Pediatr Res 4:120–128, 1974

23. Varma S, Nickerson H, Cowan JS et al: Homeostatic response to glucose loading in newborn and young dogs. Metabolism 22:1367–1375, 1973

24. Bier DM, Arnold KJ, Sherman WR et al: In vivo measurement of glucose and alanine metabolism with stable isotropic tracers. Diabetes 26:1005–1015, 1977

25. Bier DM, Leake RD, Haymond MW et al: Measurement of "true" glucose production rates in infancy and childhood with 6,6 dideuteroglucose. Diabetes 26:1016–1023, 1977

26. Kalhan SC, Savin SM, Adam PAJ: Measurement of glucose turnover in the human newborn with glucose-1-^{13}C. J Clin Endocrinol Metab 43:704–707, 1976

27. Kalhan SC, Savin SM, Adam PAJ: Attenuated glucose production rate in newborn infants of insulin dependent diabetic mothers. N Engl J Med 296:375–376, 1977

28. Cowett RM, Susa JB, Sommer M et al: Kinetic studies with ^{13}C-U-glucose in pregnant women and their offspring (abstr). Pediatr Res 13:357, 1979

29. Chlebowski RT, Adam PAJ: Glucose production in the newborn dog. II. Evaluation of automatic and enzymatic control in the isolated perfused canine liver. Pediatr Res 9:821–828, 1975

30. Gutberlet RL, Cornblath M: Neonatal hypoglycemia revisited, 1975. Pediatrics 58:1–17, 1976

31. Fluge G: Clinical aspects of neonatal hypoglycemia. Acta Paediatr Scand 63:826–832, 1974

32. Senior B: Current concepts. Neonatal hypoglycemia. N Engl J Med 289:790–793, 1973

33. Milner RDG: Annotation: Neonatal hypoglycemia. A critical appraisal. Arch Dis Child 47:679–682, 1972

34. Cowett RM, Schwartz R: The role of hepatic control of glucose homeostasis in the etiology

and neonatal hypo and hyperglycemia. Semin Perinatol 3:327–340, 1979

35. **Raivio KO, Hallman N:** Neonatal hypoglycemia. I. Occurrence of hypoglycemia in patients with various neonatal disorders. Acta Pediatr Scand 57:517–521, 1968

36. **Cornblath M, Odell GB, Levin EY:** Symptomatic neonatal hypoglycemia associated with toxemia of pregnancy. J Pediatr 55:545–562, 1959

37. **Lubchenco LO, Bard H:** Incidence of hypoglycemia in newborn infants classified by birth weight and gestational age. Pediatrics 47:831–838, 1971

38. **deLeeuw R, deVries IJ:** Hypoglycemia in small for dates newborn infants. Pediatrics 58:18–22, 1976

39. **Koivisto M, Jouppila P:** Neonatal hypoglycemia and maternal toxaemia. Acta Paediatr Scand 63:743–749, 1974

40. **Haymond MW, Karl IE, Pagliara AS:** Increased gluconeogenic substrate in the small for gestational age infant. N Engl J Med 291:322–328, 1974

41. **Williams PR, Fisher RH, Jr, Sperling MA et al:** Effects of oral alanine feeding on blood glucose, plasma glucagon, and insulin concentrations in small for gestational age infants. N Engl J Med 292:612–614, 1975

42. **Reisner SH, Aranda JV, Colle E et al:** The effect of intravenous glucagon on plasma amino acids in the newborn. Pediatr Res 7:184–191, 1973

43. **Mestyan MJ, Schultz K, Soltesz G et al:** The metabolic effects of glucagon infusion in normoglycaemic and hypoglycaemic small for gestational age infants. II. Changes in plasma amino acids. Acta Paediatr Acad Sci Hung 17:245–253, 1976

44. **Sperling MA, Grajwer L, Leake RD et al:** Effects of somatostatin (SRIF) infusion on glucose homeostasis in newborn lambs: Evidence for a significant role of glucagon. Pediatr Res 11:962–967, 1977

45. **Salle BL, Ruiton-Ugliengo A:** Effects of oral glucose and protein load on plasma glucagon and insulin concentrations in small for gestational age infants. Pediatr Res 11:108–112, 1977

46. **Beard AG, Panos TC, Marasigan BV et al:** Perinatal stress and the premature neonate. II. Effect of fluid and caloric deprivation on blood glucose. J Pediatr 68:329–343, 1966

47. **Beard AG:** Neonatal hypoglycemia. J Perinat Med 3:219–225, 1975

48. **Mann TP, Elliott RIK:** Neonatal cold injury due to accidental exposure to cold. Lancet 1:229, 1957

49. **Schiff D, Stern L, Leduc J:** Chemical thermogenesis in newborn infants. Catecholamine excretion and the plasma non-esterified fatty acid response to cold exposure. Pediatr 37:577–582, 1966

50. **Yeung CY:** Hypoglycemia in neonatal sepsis. J Pediatr 77:812–817, 1970

51. **LaNoue KF, Mason AD, Jr, Daniels JP:** The impairment of glucogenesis by gram negative infection. Metabolism 17:606–611, 1968

52. **Yeung CY, Lee VWY, Yeung CM:** Glucose disappearance rate in neonatal infection. J Pediatr 83:486–489, 1973

53. **Shelley HJ:** Glycogen reserves and their changes at birth and in anoxia. Br Med Bull 17:137–143, 1961

54. **Benzing G, Schubert W, Hub G et al:** Simultaneous hypoglycemia and acute congestive heart failure. Circulation 40:209–216, 1972

55. **Amatayakul O, Cumming GR, Haworth JC:** Association of hypoglycemia with cardiac enlargement and heart failure in newborn infants. Arch Dis Child 45:717–720, 1970

56. **Haymond MW, Strauss AW, Arnold KJ, Bier DM:** Glucose homeostasis in children with severe cyanotic congenital heart disease. J Pediatr 95:220, 1979

57. **Vidnes J, Ø Yas Æter S:** Glucagon deficiency causing severe neonatal hypoglycemia in a patient with normal insulin secretion. Pediatr Res 11:943–949, 1977

58. **Vidnes J, Søvik O:** Gluconeogenesis in infancy and childhood. II. Studies on the glucose production from alanine in three cases of persistent neonatal hypoglycemia. Acta Paediatr Scand 65:297–305, 1976

59. **Vidnes J, Søvik O:** Gluconeogensis in infancy and childhood. III. Deficiency of the extramitochondrial form of hepatic phosphoenolypyruvate carboxykinase in a case of persistent neonatal hypoglycemia. Acta Paediatr Scand 65:307–312, 1976

60. **Levy HL, Hammersen G:** Newborn screening for galactosemia and other galactose metabolic defects. J Pediatr 92:871–877, 1978

61. **Pedersen J:** The Pregnant Diabetic and Her Newborn: Problems and Management. Baltimore, Williams & Wilkins, 1977

62. **Susa JB, McCormick KL, Widness JA, Singer DB, Oh W, Adamsons K, Schwartz R:** Chronic hyperinsulinemia in the fetal rhesus monkey: Effects on fetal growth and composition. Diabetes 28:1058–1063, 1979

63. **McCormick KL, Susa JB, Widness JA, Singer DB, Adamsons K, Schwartz R:** Chronic hyperinsulinemia in the fetal rhesus monkey: Effects on hepatic enzymes involved in li-

pogenesis and carbohydrate metabolism. Diabetes 28:1064–1068, 1979

64. **Dole VP:** A relation between non-esterified fatty acids in plasma and the metabolism of glucose. J Clin Invest 35:50, 1957

65. **Koldovsky O:** Free fatty acids and glucose in the blood of various groups of newborns. Acta Pediatr Scand 53:343, 1964

66. **Stern L, Ramos AD, Leduc J:** Urinary catecholamine excretion in infants of diabetic mothers. Pediatrics 42:598, 1968

67. **Cornblath M, Nicolopoulos D, Ganzon AF, Levin EY, Gordon MH, Gordon HH:** Studies of carbohydrate metabolism in the newborn infant. IV. The effects of glucagon on the capillary blood sugar in infants of diabetic mothers. Pediatrics 28:592, 1961

68. **Widness JA, Schwartz HC, Schwartz R:** Glycohemoglobin: Its importance in pregnancy and to the newborn of diabetic mothers. In Moss AJ et al (eds): Pediatrics Update: Review for Physicians. Elsevier, New York, 1980

69. **Barrett CT, Oliver TK, Jr:** Hypoglycemia and hyperinsulinism in infants with erythroblastosis fetalis. N Engl J Med 278:1260–1263, 1968

70. **Oh W, Yap LL, D'Amodio MD:** Hypoglycemia in severely affected Rh erythroblastotic infants (abstr). J Pediatr 74:813, 1969

71. **Schiff D, Lowy C:** Hypoglycemia and excretion of insulin in urine in hemolytic disease of the newborn. Pediatr Res 4:280–285, 1970

72. **Mølsted-Pedersen L, Trautner H, Jørgensen KR:** Plasma insulin and K values during intravenous glucose tolerance test in newborn infants with erythroblastosis foetalis. Acta Paediatr Scand 62:11–16, 1973

73. **Schiff D, Aranda JV, Chan G, Colle E, Stern L:** Metabolic effects of exchange transfusions, I. Effect of citrated and of heparinized blood on glucose, non-esterified fatty acids 2-(4 hydroxybenzeneazo) benzoic acid binding and insulin. J Pediatr 78:603, 1971

74. **Schiff D, Aranda JV, Colle E, Stern L:** Metabolic effects of exchange transfusions, II. Delayed hypoglycemia following exchange transfusion with citrated blood. J Pediatr 79:589, 1971

75. **Beckwith JB, Wang CI, Donnel GN, Gwin JL:** Hyperplastic fetal visceromegaly with macroglossia, omphalocele, cytomegaly of adrenal fetal cortex, postnatal somatic gigantism, and other abnormalities: Newly recognized syndrome (abstr 41). Proc Am Pediatr Soc Seattle, June 16–18, 1964

76. **Wiedemann HR:** Complexe malformatif familiale avec hernie ombilicale et macroglossie—un syndrome nouveau? J Genet Hum 13:223, 1964

77. **Schiff D, Colle EC, Wells D, Stern L:** Metabolic aspects of the Beckwith-Wiedemann syndrome. J Pediatr 82:258, 1973

78. **Hertz PU, Koppel G, Hacke WH et al:** Nesidioblastosis: The pathologic basis of persistent hyperinsulinemic hypoglycemia in infants. Diabetes 20:632–642, 1977

79. **Woo D, Scopes JW, Polak JM:** Idiopathic hypoglycemia in sibs with morphological evidence of nesidioblastosis of the pancreas. Arch Dis Child 51:528–531, 1976

80. **Baerentsen H:** Case report: Neonatal hypoglycemia due to an islet cell adenoma. Acta Paediatr Scand 62:207–210, 1973

81. **Burst NRM, Campbell JR, Castro A:** Congenital islet cell adenoma causing hypoglycemia in a newborn. Pediatrics 47:605–610, 1971

82. **Habbick BF, Cram RW, Miller KR:** Neonatal hypoglycemia resulting from islet cell adenomatosis. Am J Dis Child 131:210–212, 1977

83. **Zucker P, Simon G:** Prolonged symptomatic neonatal hypoglycemia associated with maternal chlorpropamide therapy. Pediatrics 42:824–825, 1968

84. **Senior B, Slone D, Shapiro S et al:** Benzothiadiazides and neonatal hypoglycemia. Lancet 2:377, 1976

85. **Stern C:** Idiopathic hypoglycemia. Proc R Soc Med 66:345–346, 1973

86. **Pickering R:** Neonatal hypoglycemia due to salicylate poisoning. Proc R Soc Med 61:1256, 1968

87. **Gemelli M, DeLuca F, Barberio G:** Hypoglycemia and congenital adrenal hyperplasia. Acta Paediatr Scand 68:285–286, 1979

88. **Brown RE, Young RB:** A possible role for the exocrine pancreas in the pathogenesis of neonatal sensitive hypoglycemia. Am J Dig Dis 15:65, 1970

89. **Epstein MF, Nicholls E, Stubblefield PG:** Neonatal hypoglycemia after beta-sympathomimetic tocolytic therapy. J Pediatr 94:449–453, 1979

90. **Dweck HS, Cassady G:** Glucose intolerance in infants of very low birth weight. I. Incidence of hyperglycemia in infants of birth weights 1,100 grams or less. Pediatrics 53:189–195, 1974

91. **LeDune MA:** Intravenous glucose tolerance and plasma insulin studies in small for date infants. Arch Dis Child 47:111–114, 1972

92. **Fox HA, Krasna IH:** Total intravenous nutrition by peripheral vein surgical patients. Pediatrics 52:14–20, 1973

93. **Gentz JCH, Cornblath M:** Transient diabetes

of the newborn. Adv Pediatr 16:345–363, 1969

94. **Sodoyez-Goffant F, Sodoyez JC:** Transient diabetes mellitus in a neonate. J Pediatr 91: 395–399, 1977

95. **LeDune MA:** Insulin studies in temporary neonatal hyperglycemia. Arch Dis Child 16: 393–394, 1971

96. **Leisto J, Raivio K, Krohn K:** Neonatal hyperglycemia and chromosomes deletion (46, xx, Dq–). J Pediatr 88:989–990, 1976

97. **Dweck HS, Brans YW, Sumners JE et al:** Glucose intolerance in infants of very low birth weight. II. Intravenous glucose tolerance tests in infants of birth weights 500–1380 grams. Biol Neonate 30:261–267, 1976

98. **Zarif M, Pildes RS, Vidyasagar D:** Insulin and growth hormone responses in neonatal hyperglycemia. Diabetes 25:428–433, 1976

99. **Pollak A, Cowett RM, Schwartz R et al:** Glucose disposal in low birth weight infants during steady state hyperglycemia: Effects of exogenous insulin administration. Pediatrics 61:546–549, 1978

100. **Cowett RM, Oh W, Pollak A et al:** Glucose disposal of low birth weight infants: Steady state hyperglycemia produced by constant intravenous glucose infusion. Pediatrics 63: 389–396, 1979

101. **Lilien LD, Rosenfield RL, Baccaro MM:** Hyperglycemia in stressed small premature neonates. J Pediatr 94:454, 1979

102. **Cowett RM, Susa JB, Schwartz R, Oh W:** Concentration of parenteral glucose solution. Pediatrics 59:791, 1977

103. **McCann ML, Likly B:** The role of epinephrine prophylactic therapy in infants of diabetic mothers. Proc Soc Pediatr Res 3:5, 1967

104. **Mayman CI:** Carbohydrate metabolism in the brain of experimental animals. In Hildes JA, Naimark A, Ferguson MH (eds): Studies in Physiology, pp 83–92. Winnipeg, University of Manitoba Press, 1969

105. **Victorin LH, Thorell JI:** Plasma insulin and blood glucose during long-term treatment with diazoxide for infant hypoglycemia. Case report. Acta Paediatr Scand 63:302–306, 1974

106. **Altszular N, Hampshire J, Moraru E:** On the mechanism of diazoxide-induced hyperglycemia. Diabetes 26:931–935, 1977

107. **Andersen TL, Muttart CR, Beiber MA, Nicholson JF, Heird WC:** A controlled trial of glucose vs. glucose and amino acids in premature infants. J Pediatr 94:947–951, 1979

108. **Arant BS, Jr, Gooch WM III:** Effects of acute hyperglycemia on brains of neonatal puppies (abstr). Pediatr Res 13:488, 1979

27

Calcium and Magnesium Homeostasis in the Newborn

Reginald C. Tsang and
Jean J. Steichen

CALCIUM

CALCIOTROPIC HORMONES

Physiology[1,2]

Parathyroid hormone (PTH) increases serum Ca through mobilization of calcium from bone, increased renal tubular reabsorption of calcium, and stimulation of 1,25-dihydroxyvitamin D production. Although PTH action on bone results in an increase in serum phosphate, its potent phosphaturic effect overwhelms the bone effect and results in lowered serum phosphate. PTH production is stimulated by decreased serum Ca or acute decrease of serum Mg. Chronic hypomagnesemia appears to decrease secretion of PTH.

Calcitonin lowers serum calcium and phosphate through inhibition of bone resorption and increased renal clearance of calcium and phosphate. Calcitonin production is increased when serum calcium concentrations are elevated.

Vitamin D is produced endogenously (vitamin D_3) in the skin or ingested (vitamin D_3 or D_2). Conversion to 25-hydroxyvitamin D occurs in the liver and subsequent conversion to

1,25-dihydroxyvitamin D occurs in the kidney. The final metabolite, 1,25-dihydroxyvitamin D, is considered the physiologically active vitamin D and its production is facilitated by PTH and decreased phosphate. Hypocalcemia probably stimulates production of 1,25-dihydroxyvitamin D through stimulation of PTH. 1,25-Dihydroxyvitamin D increases the absorption of calcium and phosphate from the intestine and facilitates PTH-induced mobilization of calcium and phosphate from bone[3] (Fig. 27-1).

During pregnancy, calcium is actively transported across the placenta from mother to fetus. During the last trimester, net calcium transport to the fetus may reach 150 mg/kg of fetal weight/day,[4] which is the largest amount of calcium intake a person will achieve in his life. Both total and ionized calcium concentrations are elevated in fetal blood and higher than maternal values. Indeed, the fetal plasma calcium concentrations are the highest concentrations that the baby will have in his life. PTH probably does not cross the placenta,[5] and there appears to be maternofetal autonomy of parathyroid function. Fetal PTH function appears to be relatively suppressed by the high fetal plasma ionized calcium, although the fetal parathyroids are capable of being activated if there is sufficient stimulus.

Supported in part by NIH-NICHD Grant HD11725-02 and the Children's Hospital Research Foundation, Cincinnati, Ohio

CALCIUM - PARATHYROID - VITAMIN D INTERRELATIONSHIPS

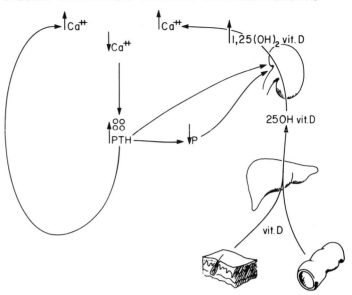

Fig. 27-1. Vitamin D metabolic pathway and its interrelationship with parathyroid hormone (PTH) and calcium. PTH increases in response to hypocalcemia. PTH results in hypophosphatemia and stimulates 1,25-dihydroxyvitamin D (the active metabolite of vitamin D) production from 25-hydroxyvitamin D. Both increased 1,25-dihydroxyvitamin D and increased PTH act to restore serum Ca to normal. Vitamin D (D_3) is synthesized in the skin or ingested (D_2 or D_3). (Tsang RC, Noguchi A, Steichen JJ, Pediatr Clin North Am 26:223, 1978)

Calcitonin probably does not cross the placenta,[6] and, as with PTH, fetal calcitonin function may be autonomous from that of the mother. Relatively high fetal serum concentrations of calcitonin probably reflect the need for protection of the rapidly mineralizing fetal skeleton.

Vitamin D and 25-hydroxyvitamin D may cross the placenta,[7] but 1,25-dihydroxyvitamin D crossover is less certain. Fetal 1,25-dihydroxyvitamin D production may be decreased,[8] probably through hypercalcemia and suppression of parathyroid function, and possible hyperphosphatemia. Because there is presumed to be little need for fetal intestinal calcium and phosphate absorption, dormancy of 1,25-dihydroxyvitamin D function would be expected.

Calciotropic Hormones in the Neonatal Period

Full-term infants increase their serum PTH concentrations after birth.[9–11] The increase is coincident with a fall in plasma total and ionized calcium concentrations, presumably reflecting the abrupt withdrawal of the maternofetal calcium transfer. Apparently the increased PTH concentrations reflect increasing PTH production, in an attempt to rectify the disturbance in serum calcium concentration. The ability of the neonatal parathyroids to respond to a hypocalcemic stress increases with postnatal age[12] and presumably reflects increasing adaption to extrauterine existence.

In premature infants[10,12] and infants of diabetic mothers (IDM),[11] the parathyroid adaptation to a relatively lower extrauterine serum calcium milieu appears to be blunted. However, ultimately these infants seem to be able to increase their PTH production appropriately in response to hypocalcemic stresses. Thus, in preterm infants and IDMs, temporary neonatal hypoparathyroidism may be a problem accentuating and perpetuating the tendency toward decreased serum calcium concentrations after birth (Fig. 27-2).

In newborn rats, calcitonin administration results in decrease of plasma calcium and phosphate concentrations.[13] The sensitivity to calcitonin appears to be greater in newborn versus older rats.[14] Plasma calcitonin concentrations are generally higher in newborn animals than those in adults.[15] Increases in plasma calcitonin concentrations during feeding of newborn rats with milk may be related to the need to prevent hypercalcemia during suckling periods.[16]

In newborn infants, thyroid gland calcitonin content is very high compared to that of adults.[17] Serum calcitonin concentrations are also relatively high at birth, with further increases after birth. The postnatal increase in serum calcitonin concentration occurs in full-

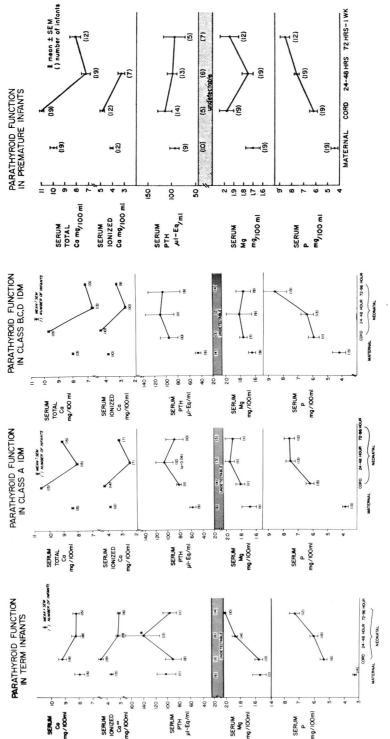

Fig. 27-2. Serum PTH concentrations in term infants, infants of diabetic mothers (class A and classes B, C, or D) and preterm infants. In term infants, decrease in serum calcium (total and ionized) is associated with significant increase in serum PTH at 24 hours of age. In infants of class A diabetic mothers the increase of PTH levels is equivocal. In infants of insulin-dependent diabetic mothers there is no significant increase in serum PTH values in spite of marked decrease in serum calcium. Similarly, in preterm infants there is no significant increase in serum PTH values. (Tsang RC, Chen I-W, Friedman MA, Chen I: J Pediatr 83:728–738, 1973; and Tsang RC, Chen I-W, Friedman MA et al: J Pediatr 86:399–404, 1975)

term infants,[18] low-birth-weight infants,[19] and IDMs.[18] Elevated serum calcitonin concentrations in low-birth-weight infants appears to be correlated with low serum calcium concentrations,[19] supporting the thesis that elevated calcitonin concentrations in the newborn period could aggravate the tendency toward hypocalcemia at this age.

Serum 25-hydroxyvitamin D concentrations in neonates appear to be related to gestational age.[20] Premature infants are apparently less able to increase their serum 25-hydroxyvitamin D concentrations than are full-term infants.[21] Some premature infants with low serum Ca concentrations may have associated low serum 25-hydroxyvitamin D concentrations,[22] although the etiologic relationship is unclear.

Serum 1,25-dihydroxyvitamin D concentrations have recently been measured in cord blood of full-term neonates. 1,25-dihydroxyvitamin D concentrations are decreased, but by 24 hours of age the concentrations have reached normal adult values.[8] Increased postnatal production of 1,25-dihydroxyvitamin D could be related to the decrease in serum calcium with increase of PTH production. The increase coincides with the conversion from an intrauterine existence dependent on the placental "lifeline" for supply of calcium, to an extrauterine existence dependent on intestinal calcium supply. Because 1,25-dihydroxyvitamin D is important in intestinal calcium absorption, its activation would be expected in the postnatal period.

NEONATAL HYPOCALCEMIA (Table 27-1)

Early neonatal hypocalcemia occurs within the first few days of life, with the lowest concentrations of serum calcium being reached at 24 to 48 hours of age. An infant can be considered to be hypocalcemic when serum calcium concentrations are below 7 mg/dl or when ionized calcium concentrations are below 3 to 3.5 mg/dl (depending on the particular ion-selective electrode that is used). Hypocalcemia in the newborn period can be accompanied by hyperphosphatemia (serum phosphate concentrations above 8 mg/dl) or hypomagnesemia (serum magnesium less than 1.5 mg/dl). It can be asymptomatic or there may be signs of neuromuscular hyperactivity, muscle twitching, or even convulsions. The most commonly encountered causes of neo-

Table 27-1. Neonatal Hypocalcemia.

"Early" neonatal hypocalcemia
1. Preterm infants
2. Infants with birth asphyxia
3. Infants of insulin-dependent, diabetic mothers

"Late" neonatal hypocalcemia
1. Intake of high-P containing milks
2. Intake of high-P containing rice cereals
3. Intestinal calcium malabsorption
4. Hypomagnesemia
5. Hypoparathyroidism
6. Rickets

Decreased ionized calcium
1. Exchange blood transfusions (citrated donor blood)
2. Increased free fatty acid (intravenous lipid infusions)
3. Alkalosis

natal hypocalcemia are prematurity (a third of infants <36 weeks' gestational age have hypocalcemia),[23,24] birth asphyxia (a third),[25] and infants of mothers with insulin-dependent diabetes (half).[26] Infants with intrauterine growth retardation (IUGR) may have hypocalcemia if they are also premature or have experienced birth asphyxia; otherwise there does not appear to be an increased incidence of hypocalcemia related to this condition.[27] Early neonatal hypocalcemia appears to be related to decreased calcium intake in association with temporary neonatal hypoparathyroidism, possible hypercalcitonemia, and, in some instances, possible disordered vitamin D metabolism. In rare instances, maternal hyperparathyroidism may be associated with congenital hypoparathyroidism, thought to be related to suppression of the fetal parathyroids through accentuation of fetal hypercalcemia.

"Late" neonatal hypocalcemia occurs towards the end of the first week of life and generally presents as neonatal tetany. The condition is probably related to the ingestion of milks with relatively high phosphate contents, acting through the production of hyperphosphatemia.[28] Maternal disturbance of vitamin D function has been proposed as an additive mechanism, possibly related to poor dietary intake of vitamin D during pregnancy[29] and compounded by seasonal variations in sunlight exposure. Associated factors include increased maternal age and parity, and poor socioeconomic classes.[29] At present, late neonatal hypocalcemia appears to occur infrequently in the United States, probably because of the greater use of "humanized" milk formulas with lower phosphate contents. Other potential causes of late neonatal hypocalcemia include ingestion of high phosphate containing cereals, intestinal malabsorption of calcium, hypomagnesemia (see below), hypoparathyroidism, and rickets.[30]

Decreases in serum ionized calcium can occur without decreases in total calcium concentration. The classic example is the effect of citrate contained in acid citrate dextrose (ACD) or citrate phosphate dextrose (CPD) donor blood, especially during an "exchange" blood transfusion. Citrate complexes calcium and results in decreased ionized calcium. Similarly, increases in long-chain free fatty acids also can complex calcium, and should be watched for during intravenous infusion of lipid-containing solutions.[31] Finally, alkalosis from overtreatment with alkali, or hyperventilation from infant respirators, can result in shifts of calcium from the ionized state to the protein-bound fraction.

Diagnosis of Hypocalcemia

The clinical features of twitching of muscles and extremities, convulsions, high-pitched cry, laryngospasm, Chvostek's sign (facial muscle twitching on tapping), and Trousseau's sign (carpopedal spasm on constriction of limbs) may be present. A family history of calcium-related disorders, or a maternal history suggestive of hyperparathyroidism (nausea, vomiting, polyuria, hypertension, renal stones) may be present although the maternal signs and symptoms may be confused with pregnancy-related complications.

Determination of ionized calcium concentrations is desirable, although ion-selective electrode methodology is still unreliable. Electrocardiographic QT intervals (QT_C, or QT interval corrected for heart rate, >0.04 sec, or Q_0T_C, the beginning of Q to the beginning of T, corrected for rate, > 0.2 sec) are of some value in monitoring the course of the infant's hypocalcemia, but do not predict ionized calcium.

Identification of hyperphosphatemia (serum P $>$ 8 mg/dl) may indicate high phosphate ingestion. Hypomagnesemia (serum Mg $<$ 1.5 mg/dl) should be sought because its treatment may be important (see below). Assays of the calciotropic hormones are still of limited value in view of the heterogenicity of circulatory forms of PTH and calcitonin, and the differences in specificity of available antisera. Serum 25-hydroxyvitamin D concentrations below 10 ng/ml may be indicative of rickets, although there is an overlap of values with those of normal infants. Chest films may identify the absence of the thymus as part of DiGeorge's syndrome (thymic aplasia, hypoparathyroidism, and immunologic disturbance).

Prevention and Therapy of Hypocalcemia

Prevention of early neonatal hypocalcemia in infants at risk for the condition can be achieved through oral calcium supplementation at a dose of 75 mg elemental calcium/kg/day (Fig. 27-3).[32] Short-term use of 1,25-dihydroxyvitamin D_3 at relatively high doses of 0.5 μg/kg/day for 2 days can also prevent neonatal hypocalcemia,[33] but such regimens should still be considered experimental.

Treatment of hypocalcemia can be instituted with oral or continuous intravenous calcium salts. In the authors' experience, 75 mg/kg/day of elemental calcium (for example, as calcium gluconate) given over 48 hours is effective and relatively safe. Daily serum calcium determinations should be performed to verify concentrations within the 8 to 10.5 mg/dl range. Alternatively, calcium can be administered at 75 mg/kg/day for 24 hours followed by half the dose for 24 hours, and a quarter of the dose for an additional 24 hours before discontinuation, accompanied by daily serum calcium determinations.

With oral calcium therapy, hypertonic solutions (such as Neo-calglucon) should probably be avoided in view of the theoretical potential for precipitating necrotizing enterocolitis in infants at risk for this condition.[34] Also, increase in frequency of bowel movements can be expected.[32] Solutions such as 10% calcium gluconate (intravenous preparation) are well tolerated orally by low-birth-weight infants, and the daily dose can be given in 4- or 6-hour intervals.

With the intravenous mode of therapy, continuous infusion is probably more efficacious than intermittent therapy because renal loss of calcium appears to be greater with the latter

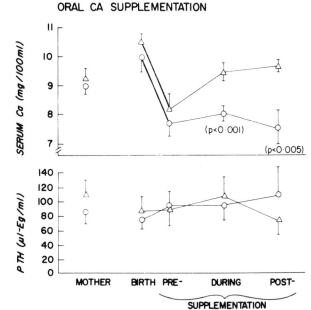

ORAL CA SUPPLEMENTATION

Fig. 27-3. Oral calcium supplementation in premature infants and infants with birth asphyxia. Daily dose of elemental calcium 75 mg/kg/day prevents hypocalcemia without apparent effect on serum PTH concentrations. Treated infants Δ-----Δ, pair matched controls ○-----○. (Adapted from Brown DR, Tsang RC, Chen I-W: J Pediatr 89:973, 1976)

therapy. However, with continuous therapy, constant cardiac monitoring for signs of bradycardia should be performed. Accidental infusion at faster rates than intended (such as when the intravenous tubing is "flushed") may cause bradycardia and cardiac standstill. This mishap is particularly likely to occur with umbilical venous catheters when the catheter tip is close to the heart. For this reason, it is recommended that calcium-containing intravenous tubing should be labeled: "Danger—Calcium Infusion—Do Not Flush."

Intermittent intravenous therapy is useful in situations in which admixture of calcium with other fluids might lead to precipitates forming within the intravenous solutions. When bicarbonate therapy is required, either a separate intravenous calcium infusion is required, or intermittent calcium infusions can be given after temporary cessation of bicarbonate therapy.[35] Boluses of calcium salts should probably not be given at a rate greater than 2 ml (10% calcium gluconate)/kg body weight/10 minutes and cardiac monitoring should be carried out simultaneously.

With either approach to intravenous administration of calcium, skin sloughs can occur if there is extravasation of the salt into subcutaneous tissues. Intraarterial infusion of calcium salts is potentially fraught with many dangers, and should not be done. Anecdotal

cases of massive sloughing of soft tissue in the areas perfused by the artery receiving the infusion have been reported, and inadvertent administration into a mesenteric artery potentially can lead to necrosis of intestinal tissues.[36]

Where hypocalcemia is secondary to specific etiologies, resolution of the primary disease often leads to correction of hypocalcemia. Substitution of low-phosphate formulas (such as Similac PM 60/40) is useful in infants suspected to be suffering from high-phosphate intake. Removal of complexing agents will resolve conditions caused by complexing of calcium.

Rickets

Infantile nutritional rickets remains a problem even in "westernized" countries and countries with apparently abundant sunshine. Predominantly, reports of rickets come from migrant populations with dietary practices adverse to intestinal calcium and phosphate absorption (such as phytate-rich foods), and whose clothing styles might prevent adequate sunlight exposure. Dietary supplementation with vitamin D at 400 IU/day is still recommended for prevention of rickets in all infants.[3]

Premature infants are particularly prone to rickets. Standard infant formulas are fortified with 400 IU vitamin D/liter. However, because premature infants generally do not ingest a

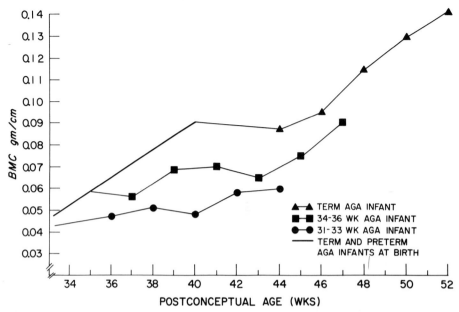

Fig. 27-4. Bone mineral content (BMC) in premature infants fed standard proprietary formula and examined prospectively. Regression line (**solid**) represents *intrauterine* bone mineral increases. Postnatal BMC in term infants, 34- to 36-week gestational age infants, and <33-week infants is shown. Postnatal bone mineral content in preterm infants increases at a much slower rate than that achieved *in utero*. (Adapted from Minton S, Steichen JJ, Tsang RC: J Pediatr 95:1037, 1979)

liter of formula each day, the absolute amount of vitamin D would be low, especially in very small infants. Thus for premature infants, a daily additional supplement of 400 IU vitamin D is recommended.[37] In infants receiving parenteral alimentation, accidental omission of calcium and vitamin D may give rise to rickets. Hepatic cholestasis associated with hyperalimentation may result in impaired 25-hydroxy-vitamin D metabolism and rickets.[38]

Based on recent studies, human breast milk appears to have much higher vitamin D content than previously suspected.[39] In some studies, breast milk also appears to have a significant antirachitic effect. However, the protection afforded by breast milk, especially during prolonged breast feeding, appears to be incomplete, and until there is more information, breast-fed infants should continue to receive vitamin D supplementation.[3]

Osteopenia in Premature Infants

During the last trimester, significant calcium and phosphate is transferred daily from mother to fetus. Using conventional formula feeding, preterm infants receive much less calcium and phosphate in their formulas than they would have received *in utero*. The low calcium and phosphate intake may be the major reason why preterm infants are often described as having "washed out" bones on x-ray films. Less commonly, fractures may develop in very low-birth-weight infants in the intensive care nursery.

Recently, using photon absorptiometric techniques for longitudinal follow-up of bone mineral content, preterm and small-for-dates infants have been demonstrated to have decreased bone mineral content and little postnatal mineralization for 2 months after birth (Fig. 27-4).[40] When preterm infants are given calcium and phosphate supplemented formulas, the bone mineral content appears to approach that expected *in utero*.[41] By standard metabolic balance techniques, calcium retention rates comparable to that achieved *in utero* can also be demonstrated in infants supplemented with calcium.[42]

Thus, it appears that osteopenia of prematurity is predominantly a problem of lack of mineral intake after birth. The safety of mineral supplementation of such infants, however, needs to be further evaluated.

MAGNESIUM

Magnesium homeostasis is intimately related to calcium homeostasis. The effects of magnesium on parathyroid hormone function have been alluded to in the earlier discussion. Hypomagnesemia commonly results in hypocalcemia. The mechanisms for production of hypocalcemia include decreased parathyroid hormone production, decreased end-organ responsiveness to parathyroid hormone, and decreased heteroionic exchange of calcium for magnesium at the bone site.[43]

MAGNESIUM DEFICIENCY AND HYPOMAGNESEMIA (Table 27-2)

Decreased Magnesium Intake

Magnesium depletion in pregnant rats results in fetal mortality, fetal malformations, fetal hypomagnesemia, and decreased skeletal magnesium content. Fetal hemolytic anemia, with extreme alterations in red cell morphology, possibly related to decreased hemoglobin synthesis or membrane abnormalities, has been demonstrated, in association with active fetal erythropoiesis in liver, spleen and adrenals; hypoproteinemia; and edema.[44]

Human fetal magnesium depletion is less well documented. An infant born of a mother with celiac disease and apparent magnesium deficiency had neonatal seizures with hypomagnesemia and hypocalcemia, responsive to magnesium therapy; the authors report felt that the infant's hypomagnesemia might be related to maternal magnesium deficiency.[45]

Hypomagnesemia occurs in IDMs. The severity and incidence of hypomagnesemia is directly related to the severity of maternal diabetes. Hypomagnesemia is also related to maternal hypomagnesemia, younger mothers, and prematurity. Because diabetes mellitus itself can be associated with hypomagnesemia, it is possible that neonatal hypomagnesemia in IDMs reflects maternal magnesium deficiency. Hypomagnesemia in IDMs is associated with neonatal hypocalcemia and decreased parathyroid function.[43]

Hypomagnesemia occurs more frequently in small-for-gestational-age (SGA) infants than in appropriate-for-gestational-age infants. The hypomagnesemia occurs particularly in young primiparous mothers, especially those who have toxemia of pregnancy.[46] The association of neonatal hypomagnesemia with young primiparous mothers has been interpreted as reflecting poor maternal nutritional intake and, possibly, magnesium deficiency. Magnesium deficiency has also been suspected as a factor in toxemia of pregnancy. Thus a possible cause for neonatal hypomagnesemia in SGA infants is maternal magnesium deficiency.

Specific intestinal magnesium malabsorption has been reported in the neonatal period.[47,48] The condition apparently predominates in males.[49] Irritability, eye rolling, muscle twitching, and convulsions occur. Hypocalcemia has occurred in all reported instances.

Intestinal operations that have involved intestinal resection, increased intestinal losses through ileostomy or fecal fistulas, and rapid intestinal transit times may lead to magnesium deficiency. Theoretically, operations affecting proximal jejunal function will particularly affect magnesium balance because the major portion of intestinal magnesium absorption appears to occur at this site.[49]

Clinical assessment of magnesium deficiency is difficult because magnesium is predominantly an intracellular rather than an extracellular cation. Magnesium-loading tests have been suggested. Infants retaining more than 40% of a magnesium load appear to have a higher incidence of neuromuscular signs than do infants excreting less than 40%. It has been proposed that high magnesium retention after a magnesium load may reflect magnesium deficiency.[50]

Table 27-2. Neonatal Hypomagnesemia

Decreased magnesium intake
1. Maternal magnesium deficiency
2. Maternal diabetes
3. Small for gestational age infants
4. Specific intestinal magnesium malabsorption
5. Intestinal surgical operations

Magnesium loss
1. Exchange (citrated) blood transfusion
2. Hepatobiliary disorders

Other causes
1. Increased phosphate intake
2. Maternal hyperparathyroidism

The treatment of choice for acute hypomagnesemic seizures is 50% magnesium sulfate ($MgSO_4$, 0.1–0.3 ml/kg), given intramuscularly or intravenously. Intravenous injections should be monitored with blood pressure measurements for systemic hypotension, and an ECG for prolonged atrioventricular conduction time, or sinoauricular or atrioventricular block should be done. The dose may need to be repeated every 8 to 12 hours.

If oral fluids are tolerated, 50% $MgSO_4$ can be given at a dose of 0.1 ml/kg/day, preferably diluted five fold. In specific magnesium malabsorption, daily oral doses of 1 ml/kg/day may be required because intestinal magnesium absorption may be as low as 10%. Large doses of calcium or vitamin D appear to be detrimental to magnesium status because increased intestinal calcium absorption may decrease intestinal magnesium absorption and increased calcium excretion would also increase magnesium losses.[49]

Hypomagnesemia Due to Magnesium Loss

In the newborn period, "exchange" blood transfusions utilizing citrate as anticoagulant result in complexing of citrate with magnesium. The resultant losses of magnesium can lead to hypomagnesemia, especially with multiple exchanges.[51] Infants with congenital biliary atresia and neonatal hepatitis have significantly lower seum Mg concentrations than do control infants.[52] The mechanism of hypomagnesemia is probably increased aldosterone-related renal losses of magnesium. Other potential causes of hypomagnesemia in neonates include defects in renal tubular reabsorption of magnesium[53] and high doses of the antibiotic gentamicin, which theoretically may cause increased magnesuria.[54]

Other Causes of Hypomagnesemia

Increased phosphate intake may lead to decreased magnesium absorption, and infants on high-phosphate milk preparations have lowered serum Mg concentrations. In infants with uremia, serum Mg concentrations are decreased, which is in contrast to adults with renal failure who have increased serum Mg concentrations. Higher dietary phosphate in infancy may play a role in decreasing Mg concentrations in uremic infants.[55] Elevation of serum phosphate decreases serum magnesium, possibly through transfer of magnesium from extracellular to intracellular sites.

Maternal hyperparathyroidism has been associated with neonatal hypomagnesemia. Negative magnesium balance may occur with hyperparathyroidism. In one infant with hypomagnesemia and hypocalcemia, it was felt that maternal hyperparathyroidism with negative maternal magnesium balance may have accounted for the neonatal hypomagnesemia.[56] Alternatively, neonatal hypoparathyroidism may lead to hypomagnesemia.[57] Because neonatal hypoparathyroidism occurs with maternal hyperparathyroidism (presumably by suppression of the fetal parathyroids by high ionized Ca concentrations *in utero*), it is theoretically possible that neonatal hypomagnesemia resulting from maternal hyperparathyroidism might also be related to neonatal hypoparathyroidism.

HYPERMAGNESEMIA

Neonatal hypermagnesemia most commonly occurs after maternal magnesium sulfate administration for preeclampsia. In mothers given magnesium sulfate, serum Mg concentrations have been reported from 2.6 to 14.0 mg/dl with umbilical cord serum concentrations from 2.0 to 11.5 mg/dl.[58,59] Elevated neonatal serum Mg concentrations can persist beyond 3 days of age. Premature infants appear to have more elevated serum Mg concentrations, presumably because of decreased Mg excretion. Infants with birth asphyxia also appear to have elevated serum Mg concentrations at 2 days of age, possibly also reflecting decreased renal Mg excretion.[60]

Clinical signs of neuromuscular depression may not correlate with serum Mg concentrations, although there appears to be a better correlation with the duration of maternal magnesium sulfate therapy,[58] possibly reflecting tissue magnesium content. A delay in passage of meconium (meconium plug syndrome) has been thought to be related to neonatal hypermagnesemia.[61] However in pregnant and newborn rats and dogs, there is no effect of hypermagnesemia on intestinal motility or consistency of meconium.[62]

In adults with hypermagnesemia, hypotension and urinary retention occur at serum Mg concentrations of 4 to 6 mg/dl, central nervous system depression, hyporeflexia, and ECG abnormalities (increased atrioventricular and ventricular conduction time) at 6 to 12 mg/dl, and respiratory depression, coma, and cardiac arrest above 12 mg/dl.[63] These physical signs are all theoretically possible in the newborn period and should be watched for in infants whose mothers have received magnesium sulfate. However, with judicious use of magnesium sulfate in the mother, signs of magnesium intoxication should be rare in the infant.[59]

Elevation of serum Mg theoretically suppresses parathyroid function. Indeed, neonatal hypermagnesemia has been recently found to be associated with suppressed serum PTH concentrations. However, the total and ionized calcium concentrations are increased in hypermagnesemic neonates when compared with control infants. It is possible that bone exchange of magnesium for calcium may have been the reason for increased serum Ca in these infants.[60]

The most effective treatment of severely depressed hypermagnesemic infants is exchange blood transfusion with citrated blood. Citrated donor blood is particularly useful because the complexing action of citrate would expedite removal of magnesium from the infant. Theoretically, ethacrynic acid diuretics with adequate fluid intake may hasten magnesium excretion.[49] Supportive measures such as respiratory assistance may also be needed. Asymptomatic hypermagnesemia usually is not treated.

REFERENCES

1. Tsang RC, Donovan EF, Steichen JJ: Calcium physiology and pathology in the neonate. Pediatr Clin North Am 23:611, 1976
2. Tsang RC, Steichen JJ, Brown DR: Perinatal calcium homeostasis: Neonatal hypocalcemia and bone demineralization. Clin Perinatol 4:385, 1977
3. Tsang RC, Erenberg A: Calcium homeostasis in the newborn: The calciotropic hormones: parathyroid hormone, calcitonin and vitamin D. In Moss AJ et al (eds): Pediatric Update: Review for Physicians, p 193. Elsevier, New York, 1980
4. Shaw JCL: Evidence for defective skeletal mineralization in low birth weight infants: The absorption of calcium and fat. Pediatrics 57:16, 1976
5. Garel JM, Dumont D: Distribution and inactivation of labelled parathyroid hormone in the rat fetus. Horm Metab Res 4:217, 1972
6. Garel JM, Millhaud G, Sizonenko R: Thyrocalcitonin et barriere placentaire chez le rat. C R Acad Sci [D] (Paris) 269:1785, 1969
7. Haddad JG, Jr, Boisseau V, Aviola L: Placental transfer of vitamin D_3 and 25-hydroxycholecalciferol in the rat. J Lab Clin Med 77:908, 1971
8. Steichen JJ, Gratton TL, Tsang RC, DeLuca HF: Perinatal vitamin D homeostasis: 1,25-$(OH)_2$ D in maternal, cord and neonatal blood. Clin Res 25:567A, 1977
9. David L, Anast CS: Calcium metabolism in newborn infants. The interrelationship of parathyroid function and calcium, magnesium and phosphorus metabolism in normal, "sick" and hypocalcemic newborns. J Clin Invest 54:287, 1974
10. Schedewie HK, Odell WD, Fisher DA, Krutzik SR, Dodge M, Cousins L, Fiser WP: Parathormone and perinatal calcium homeostasis. Pediatr Res 13:1, 1979
11. Tsang RC, Chen I-W, Freidman MA, Gigger M, Steichen J, Koffler H, Fenton L, Brown DR, Pramanik A, Keenan W, Strub R, Joyce T: Parathyroid function in infants of diabetic mothers. J Pediatr 86:399, 1975
12. Tsang RC, Chen I-W, Freidman MA, Chen I: Neonatal parathyroid function: Role of gestational age and postnatal age. J Pediatr 83:728, 1973
13. Garel JM, Barlet JP: The effects of calcitonin and parathormone on plasma Mg levels before and after birth in the rat. J Endocrinol 61:1, 1974
14. Copp DH: Parathormone, calcitonin and calcium homeostasis. In Comar CL, Bronner F (eds): Mineral Metabolism, Vol III, Calcium Physiol. New York, Academic Press, 1969
15. Garel JM, Barlet J-P: Calcium metabolism in newborn animals: The interrelationship of calcium, magnesium and inorganic phosphorus in newborn rats, foals, lambs and calves. Pediatr Res 10:749, 1976
16. Cooper GW, Obe JF, Touverud SU, Munson PL: Elevated serum calcitonin and serum calcium during suckling in the baby rat. Endocrinology 101:1657, 1977
17. Wolfe HJ, DeLellis RA, Voelkel EF, Tashjian AH: Distribution of calcitonin-containing cells in the normal neonatal human thryroid gland: A correlation of morphology with peptide content. J Clin Endocrinol Metab 41:1076, 1975
18. Bergman L, Kjellmer I, Selstam U: Calcitonin and parathyroid hormone—relation to early neonatal hypocalcemia in infants of diabetic mothers. Biol Neonate 24:1, 1974
19. David L, Salle B, Chopard P, Grafmeyer D: Studies on circulating immunoreactive calcitonin in low birth weight infants during the

first 48 hours of life. Helv Paediatr Acta 32: 39, 1977

20. **Chan GM, Tsang RC, Chen I-W, DeLuca HF, Steichen JJ:** The effect of $1,25(OH)_2$ vitamin D_3 supplementation in premature infants. J Pediatr 93:91, 1978

21. **Hillman LS, Haddad JG:** Perinatal vitamin D metabolism, II. Serial 25-hydroxyvitamin D concentrations in sera of term and premature infants. J Pediatr 86:928, 1975

22. **Rosen JF, Roginsky M, Nathenson G, Finberg L:** 25-hydroxyvitamin D. Plasma levels in mothers and their premature infants with neonatal hypocalcemia. Am J Dis Child 127:220, 1974

23. **Tsang RC, Oh W:** Neonatal hypocalcemia in low birth weight infants. Pediatrics 45:773, 1970

24. **Tsang RC, Light IJ, Sutherland JM, Kleinman L:** Possible pathogenetic factors in neonatal hypocalcemia of prematurity. J Pediatr 82:423, 1973

25. **Tsang RC, Chen I, Atkinson W, Hayes W, Atherton H, Edwards N:** Neonatal hypocalcemia in birth asphyxia. J Pediatr 84:428, 1974

26. **Tsang RC, Kleinman L, Sutherland JM et al:** Hypocalcemia in infants of diabetic mothers: Studies in Ca, P, and Mg metabolism and in parathormone responsiveness. J Pediatr 80:384, 1972

27. **Tsang RC, Gigger M, Oh W, Brown DR:** Studies in calcium metabolism in infants with intrauterine growth retardation. J Pediatr 86:936, 1975

28. **Oppe TE, Redstone D:** Calcium and phosphorous levels in healthy newborn infants given various types of milk. Lancet 1:1045, 1968

29. **Purvis RJ, Mackay GS, Cockburn F, Barrie WJMcK, Wilkinson EM, Belton NR, Forfar JO:** Enamel hypoplasia of the teeth associated with neonatal tetany: A manifestation of maternal vitamin D deficiency. Lancet 2:811, 1973

30. **Tsang RC, Steichen JJ, Chan GM:** Neonatal hypocalcemia, mechanism of occurrence and management. Crit Care Med 5:56, 1977

31. **Whitsett JA, Tsang RC:** In vitro effects of fatty acids on serum ionized Ca. J Pediatr 91:233, 1977

32. **Brown DR, Tsang RC, Chen I-W:** Oral calcium supplementation in premature and asphyxiated neonates. J Pediatr 89:973, 1976

33. **Chan GM, Tsang RC, Chen I-W, DeLuca HF, Steichen JJ:** The effect of $1,25-(OH)_2$ vitamin D_3 supplementation in premature infants. J Pediatr 93:91, 1978

34. **Willis DM, Chabot J, Radde IG, Chance GE:** Unsuspected hyperosmolality of oral solutions contributing to necrotising enterocolitis in very-low-birth-weight infants. Pediatrics 60:535, 1977

35. **Nervez CT, Shott RJ, Bergstrom WH, Williams ML:** Prophylaxis against hypocalcemia in low-birth-weight infants requiring bicarbonate infusion. J Pediatr 87:439, 1975

36. **Book LS, Herbst JJ, Stewart D:** Hazards of calcium gluconate therapy in the newborn infant: Intra-uterial injection producing intestinal necrosis in rabbit ileum. J Pediatr 92:793, 1978

37. **Lewin PK, Reid M, Reilly BJ, Swyer PR, Fraser D:** Iatrogenic rickets in low birth weight infants. J Pediatr 78:207, 1971

38. **Farrel MK, Suchy FJ, Tsang RC, Steichen JJ, Whitsett JA, Partin JC, Schubert WK:** Neonatal "hepatic rickets" in premature infants receiving parenteral alimentation (abstr). Pediatr Res 12:434, 1978

39. **Sahashi Y, Suzuki T, Higaki M, Asano T:** Metabolism of vitamin D in animals, V. Isolation of vitamin D sulfate from mammalian milk. J Vitaminol 13:33, 1967

40. **Minton SD, Steichen JJ, Tsang RC:** Bone mineralization in term and preterm appropriate for gestational age infants. J Pediatr (in press)

41. **Steichen JJ, Gratton TL, Tsang RC:** Osteopenia of prematurity: The cause and possible treatment. J Pediatr 75:1037, 1979

42. **Day GM, Chance GW, Radde IC, Reilly BJ, Park E, Sheepers J:** Growth and mineral metabolism in very low birth weight infants. II. Effects of calcium supplementation on growth and divalent cations. Pediatr Res 9:568, 1975

43. **Tsang RC, Strub R, Steichen JJ, Brown DR, Hartman C, Chen I-W:** Hypomagnesemia in infants of diabetic mothers: Perinatal studies. J Pediatr 89:115, 1976

44. **Cosens G, Diamond I, Theriault LL, Hurley LS:** Magnesium deficinecy anemia in the rat fetus. Pediatr Res 11:758, 1977

45. **Davis JA, Harvey DR, Yu JS:** Neonatal fits associated with hypomagnesemia. Arch Dis Child 40:286, 1965

46. **Tsang RC, Oh W:** Serum magnesium levels in low birth weight infants. Am J Dis Child 120:44, 1970

47. **Stromme JH, Nesbakken R, Normann T et al:** Familial hypomagnesemia. Acta Paediat Scand 58:433, 1969

48. **Paunier L, Radde IC, Kooh SW, Conen PE, Fraser D:** Primary hypomagnesemia with secondary hypocalcemia in an infant. Pediatrics 41:385, 1968

49. **Tsang RC:** Neonatal magnesium disturbances. A review. Am J Dis Child 124:282, 1972

50. **Byrne PA, Caddell JL:** The magnesium load test. II. Correlation of clinical and laboratory data in neonates. Clin Pediatr 14:460, 1975

51. **Bajpai PC, Sugden D, Stern L et al:** Serum ionic magnesium in exchange transfusion. J Pediatr 70:193, 1967

52. **Kobayashi A, Shiraki K:** Serum magnesium level in infants and children with hepatic diseases. Arch Dis Child 42:615, 1967

53. **Booth BE, Johanson A:** Hypomagnesemia due to renal tubular defect in reabsorption of magnesium. J Pediatr 84:350, 1974

54. **Bar RS, Wilson HE, Mazzaferri EL:** Hypomagnesemic hypocalcemia secondary to renal magnesium wasting. Ann Intern Med 82:646, 1975

55. **Ghazali S, Hallett RJ, Barratt:** Hypomagnesemia in uremic infants. J Pediatr 81:747, 1972

56. **Monteleone JA, Lee JB, Tashjian AH, Cantor HE:** Transient neonatal hypocalcemia, hypomagnesemia and high serum parathyroid hormone with hyperparathyroidism. Ann Intern Med 82:670, 1975

57. **Taitz LS, Zarate-Salvador C, Schwartz E:** Congenital absence of the parathyroid and thymus glands in an infant. Pediatrics 38:412, 1966

58. **Lipsitz PJ:** The clinical and biochemical effects of excess magnesium in the newborn. Pediatrics 47:501, 1971

59. **Stone SR, Pritchard JA:** Effect of maternally administered magneisum sulfate on the neonate. Obstet Gynecol 35:574, 1970

60. **Donovan EF, Tsang RC, Steichen JJ, Strub RJ, Chen I-W, Chen M:** Neonatal hypermagnesemia: Effect on parathyroid hormone and calcium homeostasis. J Pediatr 96:305, 1980

61. **Sokal MM, Koenigsberger MR, Rose JS, Berdon WE, Santulli TV:** Neonatal hypermagnesemia and the meconium plug syndrome. N Engl J Med 286:823, 1972

62. **Cooney DR, Rosevear W, Grosfeld JL:** Maternal and postnatal hypermagnesemia and the meconium plug syndrome. J Pediatr Surg 11:167, 1976

63. **Randall RE, Cohen MD, Spary CC et al:** Hypermagnesemia in renal failure. Ann Intern Med 61:73, 1964

28

Inherited Metabolic Disorders

Y. Edward Hsia and
Barry Wolf

INTRODUCTION

Genetically determined metabolic diseases affect at least 1 in every 200 infants. Separately, these diseases are rare, but they are important causes of morbidity and mortality in the newborn and will present diagnostic challenges to any active neonatal service. They are important because timely diagnosis and treatment may be lifesaving or may prevent brain damage in many of these conditions. Recognition that a disease is genetic enables families to be forewarned about recurrence risks, often with the offer of antenatal diagnosis as an option for future pregnancies.

Of the various ways that genetic abnormality can cause disease, the expression of abnormal genes can either disrupt the finely tuned fetal developmental schedule to produce physical malformations,[1,2] or it can block or upset a normal physiologic function. Some aberrant functions are nonessential: pentosuria, which is caused by deficiency of the enzyme xylulose dehydrogenase, is completely innocuous. Some genetic diseases, such as the muscular dystrophies, have no identified metabolic cause as yet, although these diseases must be the result of mutant gene expression. This chapter will focus on the inherited abnormalities of metabolic function that are of impor-

tance in the newborn period, generally on those that have a known biochemical lesion. Genetic defects of leukocytes and the immune system, of hemoglobin and the coagulation system, of the endocrine system, and of special organs and tissues are discussed in Chapters 31, 25, and 44, respectively.

Deranged metabolic functions that have a known genetic basis can be grouped functionally into abnormalities of (1) structural proteins, (2) membrane proteins, (3) enzymes of intermediate metabolism, and (4) lysosomal degradation of macromolecules.[3] Abnormal structural proteins undermine cellular integrity or function in disorders of collagen metabolism and the hemoglobinopathies. Many abnormalities of membrane transport affect intestinal intake or renal tubular reabsorption of small molecules such as sugars and amino acids; several of these are benign with little pathologic significance for infants. Deficiencies of enzymes of intermediary metabolism may result in (1) failure to produce a needed metabolic product, (2) accumulation of a toxic metabolic substrate or (3) diversion of metabolites to alternate biochemical pathways with toxic products; any of these may lead to metabolic disease, growth failure, or death.[4] Blocked lysosomal degradation of specific macromolecules results in progressive trapping of undegraded material in lysosomes, and engorging of cells and organs, which impairs their normal function. This type of process causes progressive degeneration, often with organomegaly.

This discussion of the clinical manifestations of the inborn errors of metabolism is concerned primarily with their medical presentations and only secondarily with their biochemical classification. For systematic biochemical approaches, the reader is referred to special texts.[5-10]

Clinical manifestations of inborn errors of metabolism are protean, including gastrointestinal disturbances, cardiorespiratory difficulties, neurologic abnormalities, anemia, jaundice, rashes, and even loss of normal temperature control. Usually, the clinical syndrome is nondiagnostic, and metabolic disturbances must be detected by laboratory investigations. Severe acute metabolic disorders may mimic overwhelming sepsis, birth trauma, or cardiorespiratory failure, which may prove fatal before appropriate diagnostic tests can be conducted. Chronically progressive metabolic disease may cause failure to thrive, developmental retardation, or degeneration, with a course that is so insidious that disease is not suspected for many months. Within this range of presentations, the possibility of an inheritable metabolic disease should be considered when there is (1) a positive family history; (2) a suggestive diet history; (3) otherwise unexplained hypoglycemia, metabolic acidosis, lacticacidosis, ketonuria, or hyperammonemia;[11,12] (4) seizures, neurologic abnormalities, or developmental retardation; (5) other characteristic physical signs; (6) failure to thrive; or (7) an abnormal metabolic screening test in a presymptomatic infant.[9,13] Confirmatory tests and special investigations would then be required to establish a definitive diagnosis.[14] The finding of a rare biochemical abnormality in an ill infant does not necessarily mean that the cause for the illness has been identified because an association could be secondary to a nongenetic cause or could be coincidental, unless this association is found consistently.

In this chapter, diagnostic approaches, initial treatment, and long-term management of a few representative disorders will be described as will the roles of counseling, carrier detection, and antenatal diagnosis in disease prevention.

FAMILY HISTORY

Autosomal dominant single gene disorders already affecting one of the parents rarely present in the newborn period except for some of the chondrodystrophies, osteogenesis imperfecta tarda, and other malformation syndromes (see Chap. 37).[1,2,15,16] A positive family history of dominant conditions (*e.g.,* type II hyperlipoproteinemia) may allow early prophylactic treatment to be offered, and of later onset diseases (*e.g.,* polycystic kidneys, Huntington's chorea, or neurofibromatosis) may alert the physician to families who would benefit from genetic counseling[17] because any child of an affected parent has a 50% risk of being affected.

Sex-linked disorders are mostly recessive and include glucose-6-phosphate dehydrogenase (G-6-PD) deficiency, Menkes disease, Hunter's syndrome, Fabry's disease, Lesch–Nyhan disease, Duchenne type muscular dystrophy, and the two common types of hemophilia. Disorders affecting male siblings or male maternal relatives (see Chap. 37) indicate that a male infant of a carrier mother has a 50% risk of being affected. For conditions which are lethal for the male before he can reproduce, and when no sibling or maternal relative is affected, the likelihood is up to 33% that the patient suffered a fresh mutation, so that the mother need not be a genetic carrier.[18] In this circumstance, a subsequent male infant need not be at risk. In some X-linked recessive disorders, the heterozygous carrier state can be detected, but in others no reliable tests have yet been established. The most noteworthy of the few dominant sex-linked disorders, hypophosphatemic rickets, is of no importance in the newborn period because the characteristic hypophosphatemia may be delayed several months. Ornithine transcarbamylase deficiency, however, is lethal in the newborn male, and of varying severity in the heterozygous female.[11,12] In X-linked dominant inheritance, any child of an affected mother has a 50% risk of being affected, but the condition is more severe in males, and all daughters but no sons of an affected father will be affected.

Autosomal recessive inheritance is the genetic pattern for most inborn errors of metabolism. Both parents of an affected child would be heterozygous genetic carriers, usually with no prior family history outside the siblings, unless there has been consanguinity. Therefore, if a couple has one offspring with a known autosomal recessive disease, the recurrence risk is 25% for any subsequent infant of that couple. The existence of prior siblings affected with any ill-defined or undiagnosed illness, particularly with onset in infancy, alerts the physician to the possibility of a genetic disease (*e.g.,* if prior siblings have had problems such as meconium ileus, growth failure, or chronic respiratory infections, the diagnosis of cystic fibrosis is a strong possibility in families of Western European origins).

Maternal histories of diabetes or thyroid disease are routinely sought (see Chaps. 16 and 44), but diseases such as phenylketonuria or maple syrup urine disease in the mother are also associated with high threat of brain damage and malformations *in utero* to the infant of an affected mother.[1,7] The infant might be protected successfully from intrauterine chemical toxicity by careful control of the maternal diet during pregnancy. Mothers of microcephalic infants should be tested for undiagnosed maternal phenylketonuria, particularly if their own intelligence is subnormal, because treatment might help to protect fetuses in future pregnancies.[6] Medications used for maternal genetic disease may subject an infant to serious hazards too. For instance, D-penicillamine therapy for Wilson's disease or cystinuria might cause grave connective tissue defects in the fetus.[6] The risk of genetic myopathies, chondrodystrophies, certain connective tissue disorders, and other genetic diseases affecting the mother may be dangerous for both the pregnant woman and her fetus.[16]

Fetal loss may be caused by many maternal and fetal factors. In families with inborn errors of metabolism, there is often a history of repeated abortions or stillbirths as well as of neonatal deaths. Hydramnios has been associated with cystic fibrosis and other metabolic diseases, as well as with renal or gastrointestinal malformations.

DIET HISTORY

Diet history is of paramount importance in many inborn errors of metabolism because dietary components may precipitate or aggravate metabolic disturbances in some of these and they may relieve them in others. When an inborn error of metabolism is suspected, a careful diet history should be taken, searching for any relationship between symptoms and the types or times of food intake.

Characteristically, hypoglycemia from most causes is relieved by eating, and the response may be biochemically confirmed by blood glucose levels before and after feeding (see Chap. 26)[6,19] Whether hypoglycemia is symptomatically relieved by glucose alone, by all carbohydrates, or by any food, indicates an infant's capacity to convert carbohydrate, fat, or amino acid precursors to glucose. Exquisite intolerance to fasting is characteristic of hepatic glycogenoses (particularly type I), of von Gierke's disease in which neither gluconeogenesis nor glycogenolysis can sustain blood glucose, and of fructose 1,6-diphosphatase deficiency in which glucogenesis is blocked.[6,8]

Symptoms of vomiting, lethargy, and hypotonia, precipitated by diet, are characteristic of several metabolic diseases (Table 28-1). The type of food causing toxicity and the rapidity with which symptoms are produced help to localize the area of intermediary metabolism involved. Many of these conditions, such as galactosemia, glucose-galactose malabsorption, organic acidemias, and urea cycle enzyme defects, can be rapidly lethal in early infancy.

If acute toxicity from food is possible, all oral feeding should be immediately suspended. For example, severe gastrointestinal symptoms, vomiting, abdominal distension, and frothy or watery diarrhea are induced by intolerance to carbohydrate; explosive diarrhea is especially likely to occur in lactase deficiency or glucose-galactose malabsorption; and accompanying jaundice with liver failure suggests galactosemia, fructose intolerance, hereditary tyrosinemia, and some of the urea cycle enzyme defects.[6] Fulminant neurotoxicity with seizures and coma would suggest amino acid and protein toxicity. Unless the infant is already severely malnourished, when carefully planned parenteral hyperalimentation may be necessary, it should be possible to avoid all exposure to a suspected food until preliminary consulations and tests have indicated that it is safe to reintroduce such foods, with close observation for toxic effects. Other conditions of later onset are included in Table 28-1 because their prompt recognition in affected family members may be the only clues for early detection and treatment of these conditions in presymptomatic infants.

Toxicity caused by allergies to milk proteins

or other allergens is beyond the scope of this chapter.

CLINICAL FEATURES OF METABOLIC ERRORS

Hypoglycemia, acidosis, ketosis, and hyperammonemia are common to many metabolic errors. Because of overlap in the clinical features of many disorders, these metabolic disturbances will be reviewed first.

Hypoglycemia

Hypoglycemia is so frequently encountered in the care of ill infants that its neonatal signs and symptoms should be thoroughly familiar to anyone caring for the newborn (see Chap. 26).[19] Insidious onset of hypoglycemia produces somnolence, lethargy, and refusal to feed. Acute onset produces tremulousness, irritability, incessant weak or high-pitched crying, perspiration, irregularities of respiration, eye-rolling, vomiting, poor feeding, lethargy, convulsions, and coma. Hypoglycemia may be precipitated exogenously by components of the diet, it may be primarily caused by endogenous inability to sustain blood glucose, or it may arise from a combination of both. For inborn errors of metabolism to be differentiated from other causes of hypoglycemia, attention must be paid to unusual patterns of onset or response and to association with other metabolic disturbances. For instance, in fructose intolerance, hypoglycemia presents only after fructose has been introduced into the diet, but, in fructose-1,6-diphosphatase deficiency, the hypoglycemia is accompanied by ketosis and lactic acidosis, is resistant to treatment, and is aggravated by dietary fructose. The hypoglycemia of the hepatic glycogenoses is associated with a voracious appetite, poor tolerance to fasting, and hepatomegaly. Therefore, the possibility that an inborn error of metabolism is responsible must be excluded if hypoglycemia is associated with food intake rather than with fasting, if it is less responsive to administration of glucose than expected, if it is associated with unusually extreme ketoacidosis or other metabolic disturbances, or if it is recurrent despite adequate nutrition. The biochemical relationship of the inborn errors of carbohydrate and organic acid metabolism with glucose are diagrammed in Figure 28-1. The inborn errors of metabo-

lism producing hypoglycemia are listed in Table 28-2.

How hypoglycemia results from defective glycogenolysis or glucogenesis can be readily appreciated. In fructose-1,6-diphosphatase deficiency, glucogenesis is blocked, with persistent hypoglycemia. In fructose intolerance, the primary defect of fructose-1-phosphate aldolase results in fructose-1-phosphate accumulation only after fructose ingestion. This accumulation then secondarily inhibits fructose-1,6-diphosphate aldolase (Fig. 28-1, 14), blocking glucogenesis and producing episodic hypoglycemia after dietary fructose. Hypoglycemia arising in metabolic disorders that are remote from the pathways outlined in Figure 28-1 has no clear explanation, but may be caused by metabolites that inhibit glucose formation or release.

Metabolic Acidosis, Lactic Acidosis and Ketosis

The clinical features of metabolic acidosis, lactic acidosis, and ketosis are nonspecific. These metabolic disturbances are associated with increased depth rather than with higher rate of respiration, and in ketosis enough volatile acetone may be emitted in the expired air to be detectable by its sweetish smell. There may be lethargy, irritability, difficulty with feeding, vomiting, dehydration, crying spells, convulsions, and coma. Correlation of clinical severity with the metabolic disturbance depends on the rate of onset. Acute acidosis can lead to prostration with marked dyspnea that, on occasion, has led to the erroneous diagnosis of pneumonia. Chronic acidosis may show no physical signs except failure to thrive until the metabolic disturbance is extreme. If the acidosis has no obvious exogenous cause, if it is resistant to therapy, or if there are repeated attacks of acidosis, especially if the attacks can be related to diet (Table 28-1), an inborn error of metabolism should be strongly suspected.[4]

The inborn biochemical lesions that are associated with metabolic acidosis, lactic acidosis, and ketosis are listed in Table 28-2, and the biochemical relationships of the inborn errors of carbohydrate metabolism with lactate, acetate, and acetone are diagrammed in Figures 28-1 and 28-2.[6,8,19] Many of the inborn errors of amino acid metabolism producing

(*Text continues on p. 618.*)

Table 28-1. Metabolic Conditions Aggravated by Constituents of Food.

Toxic Constituent	Condition	Location in Figures	Toxic Effects
Carbohydrate			
Galactose	Galactosemia	28-1(9)	Gastrointestinal, liver damage, brain damage, hypoglycemia, cataracts
Galactose	Galactokinase deficiency	28-1(8)	Cataracts
Fructose	Fructose intolerance	28-1(14)	Gastrointestinal, hypoglycemia, liver damage
Fructose	Fructose-1,6-diphosphatase deficiency	28-1(11)	Hypoglycemia, ketosis
Sucrose and lactose	Disaccharidase deficiencies	—	Diarrhea, growth failure
Glucose and galactose	Glucose-galactose malabsorption	—	Gastrointestinal, dehydration
Glycerol	Glycerol intolerance	28-1(19)	Hypoglycemia, ketosis
Protein and Amino Acids			
All nitrogenous foods	Uremia	—	Azotemia
All nitrogenous foods	Disorders of urea cycle	28-4(1)-(5)	Hyperammonemia
All nitrogenous foods	Hyperornithinemia	28-4(6)	Hyperammonemia
All nitrogenous foods	Familial protein intolerance	?	Gastrointestinal
All protein	Trypsinogen deficiency	—	Gastrointestinal, malnutrition
Lysine	Periodic lysinemia	28-2(17)	Hyperammonemia
Lysine	Persistent hyperlysinuria with hyperammonemia	28-2(19)	Hyperammonemia
Lysine	Glutaricacidemia	28-2(14)	Acidosis, posturing, retardation
Tryptophan	Blue diaper syndrome	Tryptophan malabsorption	Retardation, irritability, fevers
Tryptophan	Tryptophanuria	28-2(16)	Severe retardation, ataxia, photosensitivity, hyperpigmentation
All branched-chain amino acids	Maple syrup urine disease	28-3(3)	Metabolic ketoacidosis
Valine	Hypervalinemia	28-3(2)	Hypotonia, nystagmus, coma
Leucine and isoleucine	Hyperleucine-isoleucinemia	28-3(1)	Hyptotonia, seizures, ?deafness, ?retinal degeneration
Leucine	Isovalericacidemia	28-3(4)	Ketoacidosis, ataxia
Leucine	β-Methylcrotonylglycinuria	28-3(5)	Gastrointestinal, hypotonia, ?muscular atrophy

Substance	Disease		Clinical features
Isoleucine	α-Methylacetoacetic aciduria	28-3(6)	Gastrointestinal, ketoacidosis, hyperammonemia
Isoleucine, valine, threonine, and methionine	Propionicacidemias and Methylmalonicacidemias	28-3(7)-(9)	Gastrointestinal, ketoacidosis, hypoglycemia, hyperammonemia
Leucine and other amino acids	Leucine sensitivity	–	Hypoglycemia
All sulfur amino acids	Sulfite oxidase deficiency	28-3(14)	Severe retardation, ectopia lentis
Homocystine, methionine	Homocystinuria	28-3(12)	Ectopia lentis, ?retardation
Methionine	Oasthouse urine disease	Methionine malabsorption	Convulsions, edema, retardation, white hair
Glutamate	Chinese restaurant syndrome	Glutamate sensitivity	Possibility of neurotoxicity in infants
Tyrosine and phenylalanine	Neonatal tyrosinemia	?28-2(7)	?Benign
Tyrosine and phenylalanine	Hereditary tyrosinemia	28-2(7)	Hyperkeratosis, dendritic corneal ulcers
Phenylalanine	Phenylketonuria	28-2(6)	Retardation presenting later
Gluten	Coeliac syndrome	Gluten sensitivity	Steatorrhea, stunted growth

Fats and Fatty Acids

Substance	Disease		Clinical features
Neutral fats	Hyperlipidemia type I	Lipoprotein lipase	Abdominal cramps
Neutral fats	A-β-Lipoproteinemia		Steatorrhea, acanthocytosis, later stunted growth, retinitis, ataxia
Neutral fats (and protein)	Cystic fibrosis	?	Meconium ileus, steatorrhea, chronic respiratory infections
Neutral fats	Cholestatic syndromes	–	Jaundice, itching, diarrhea
Cholesterol	Hyperlipidemia type II	28-1(18)	Xanthomata and early myocardial ischemia in homozygotes; midadult myocardial ischemia in heterozygotes
Chlorophyl (phytanic acid)	Refsum's disease	Phytanic acid oxidase	Late onset of polyneuritis, ataxia, retinitis, with ichthyosis

Minerals

Substance	Disease		Clinical features
Iron	Hemochromatosis	?	Adult onset of bronze diabetes
Copper	Wilson's disease	?	Late onset of liver damage and basal ganglia degeneration

acidosis are diagrammed in Figure 28-2, which shows how these are related to the citric acid cycle.

Metabolic Acidosis. Acidosis results from an imbalanced excess of hydrogen ions in the *milieu interieur*. This could be caused by cellular hypoxia or by energy starvation (hypoglycemia) with accumulation of lactate and other glycolytic by-products. Inborn metabolic errors can lead to abnormal concentrations of metabolites, interfering with normal oxidative catabolism. Newborn infants are particularly vulnerable to an acid load because of their limited renal capacity to excrete hydrogen ions.

Levels of the abnormal organic acid in iso-valeric acidemia, propionic acidemia or methylmalonic acidemia are insufficient *per se* to account for the degree of acidosis, and must produce acidosis by inhibiting other biochemical pathways. For instance, experimental evidence that α-ketoisocaproate inhibits ketoglutarate and pyruvate catabolism offers an explanation for ketogenesis and acidogenesis in maple syrup urine disease (Fig. 28-3,#3).[4] In most inborn errors, the biochemical mechanisms underlying metabolic acidosis are obscure. In pyroglutamic acidemia, however, the amount of pyroglutamate in the blood can be so great that it is equivalent to the base deficit.[4]

Alkalosis occurs in the hyperammonemia syndromes.

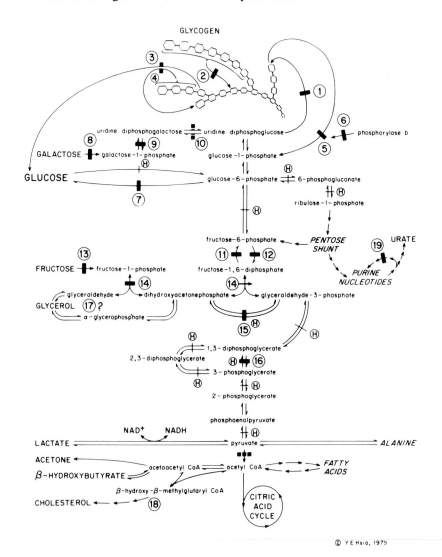

© Y E Hsia, 1979

Lactic acidosis. Whenever anoxia or other factors impair normal oxidative phosyhorylation, the strongly charged pyruvate produced from glycolysis is shuttled to the less reactive lactate by the ubiquitous enzyme lactate dehydrogenase, with conversion of its nicotinamide adenine coenzyme from the reduced NADH form to the oxidized NAD^+ form.[17] Because other NADH oxidation pathways would also be impaired, the equilibrium ratio of pyruvate: lactate (normally 1:15) will be pushed even more toward lactate (Fig. 28-2 #4). Lactic acidosis thus arises both from excess production, by glycolysis in peripheral tissues, and from depressed oxidative phosphorylation in the liver. Lactic acidosis, usu-

ally with corresponding elevations of pyruvate and of alanine (all three are normally in close dynamic equilibrium) has been reported in many families with apparent defects of the pyruvate decarboxylase enzyme system (Fig. 28-2,#1). Some of these patients have had severe metabolic disturbances, with moderate failure to thrive, intermittent ataxia, and retardation; others have had more severe degenerative neurologic disease with optic atrophy or lenticular cataracts, and variable metabolic involvement.[6] Hyperalaninemia with ataxia responsive to thiamine therapy appears to be one such syndrome. Lactic acidosis with hypotonia, cranial nerve lesions, and degenerative brain disease, which characterize the sub-

◀ **Fig. 28-1.** Metabolic map of carbohydrate metabolism indicating sites of enzyme defects. The branched polysaccharide structure of glycogen is represented by the hexagons at the top. The Embden–Meyerhof pathway of glycolysis descends down the center of the figure to the citric acid cycle. Glucose, other hexoses, and glycerol enter this schema from the **left;** lactate, ketone bodies and cholesterol are related to pyruvate and acetyl CoA as shown on the **lower left.** Purine nucleotide synthesis and fatty acid synthesis are related to carbohydrate metabolism as shown on the **right.**

Solid bars indicate the sites of enzyme defects; **interrupted bars** designate postulated blocks. Enzyme deficiencies causing hemolytic anemia are located by a circled **H.**

The following abbreviations are used for coenzymes, which are included only when relevant to the cause or treatment of an inborn error.

Ad-B$_{12}$	5'-Deoxyadenosyl-cobalamin	NAD	Nicotinamide adenine dinucleotide
ATP	Adenosine triphosphate	NAD$^+$	Oxidized form of NAD
CoA	Coenzyme A	NADH	Reduced NAD
CoQ	Coenzyme Q	OH-B$_{12}$	Hydroxocobalamin
FAD	Flavine adenine dinucleotide	Pyr P	Pyridoxal phosphate
FADH	Reduced FAD	ThPP	Thiamine pyrophosphate
Me-B$_{12}$	Methylcobalamin		

Enzyme Reaction	*Deficient in*
1. Glycogen synthetase	Glycogenosis type 0
2. Brancher enzyme	Glycogenosis type IV
3. Debrancher amylo-1,6 glucosidase	Glycogenosis type III
4. Debrancher oligo-1,4→1,6-glucantransferase	Glycogenosis type III
5. Phosphorylase	Glycogenosis type VI (also V—muscle)
6. Phosphorylase kinase	Glycogenosis type VIII
7. Glucose-6-Phosphatase	Glycogenosis type I, von Gierke's
8. Galactokinase	Galactokinase deficiency
9. Galactose-1-phosphate uridylyl transferase	Galactosemia, variants
10. Uridyldiphosphogalactose epimerase	Benign variants
11. Fructose-1,6-diphosphatase	Fructose-1,6-diphosphatase deficiency
12. Phosphofructokinase	Muscle glycogenosis type VII
13. Fructokinase	Benign fructosuria
14. Fructose-1-phosphate aldolase Fructose-1,6-diphosphate aldolase	Fructose intolerance
15. Triosephosphate isomerase	Triosephosphate isomerase deficiency
16. Phosphoglycerate kinase	Phosphoglycerate kinase deficiency
17. Undetermined	Glycerol intolerance
18. 3-hydroxy-3-methylglutaryl CoA reductase	Rate limiting step in cholesterol biosynthesis
19. Hypoxanthine-guanine phosphoribosyltransferase	Hyperuricemia

Table 28-2. Genetically Determined Disease Causing Hypoglycemia or Metabolic Acidosis.

Condition	Location in Figures	Hypoglycemia	Acidosis	Ketosis	Lactic-acidemia
CARBOHYDRATE METABOLISM					
Galactosemia	28-1(9)	+	+	+	
Fructose-1,6-diphosphatase deficiency	28-1(11)	+	+	+	+
Fructose intolerance	28-1(14)	+	+		+
Glycogenosis					
Type O	28-1(1)	+	+	+	−
Type I	28-1(7)	+	+	±	+
Type II	Lysosomal	±		±	
Type III	28-1(3),(4)	+	+	+	+
Type VI	28-1(5)	+	+	+	+
Type VIII	28-1(6)	±	±	±	±
Glycerol intolerance	28-1(17)	+		+	
ORGANIC ACID METABOLISM					
Phosphoenolpyruvate carboxykinase deficiency	28-2(3)	+			+
Pyruvate carboxylase deficiency	28-2(2)	+			+
Leigh's subacute necrotizing encephalopathy	?28-2(1)				+
Pyruvate decarboxylase deficiency	?28-2(1)				+
Hyperalaninemic lactic acidosis	?28-2(1)	+	+		+
Lactic acidosis	?28-2(1)	?			+
BRANCHED-CHAIN AMINO ACID METABOLISM					
(Leucine sensitivity)	−	±			
Maple syrup urine disease	28-3(3)	+	+	+	+
Isovalericacidemia	28-3(4)		+	+	+
α-Methylacetoaceticaciduria	28-3(6)		+	+	
Succinyl CoA:3-ketoacid CoA tranferase deficiency	28-2(5)		+	+	
Propionicacidemia	28-3(7)	+	+	+	+
Methylmalonic acidemia	28-3(8),(9)	+	+	+	+
OTHER AMINO ACIDS AND ORGANIC ACIDS					
Hereditary tyrosinemia	28-2(8)	+			
Pyroglutamic aciduria	?		+		
Glutaricacidemia	28-2(14)		+		
OTHER CONDITIONS					
NADH oxidation deficiency	28-2(4)		+		+
Lysosomal acid phosphatase deficiency	Acid phosphatase		+		
Cystinosis	Lysosomal transport defect	+			
Lowe's syndrome	?		+		
Other causes of uremia	−		+		
Progressive intrahepatic cholestasis	?	+			
Other causes of liver failure	−	+			
Combined immune deficiency disease	Adenine deaminase	+			

acute necrotizing encephalomyelopathy of Leigh, may be another syndrome. (Earlier reports of pyruvate carboxylase deficiency, Fig. 28-2,#2, may prove to be a secondary phenomenon.[6,8]) Other patients may have had lactic acidosis precipitated by disorders such as fructose-1,6-diphosphatase deficiency or propionic acidemia. Excess turnover of the Embden–Meyerhof pathway in glycogenosis type I has been invoked as an explanation for overproduction of lactate (Fig. 28-1,#7); blocked gluconeogenesis would seem to be the mechanism in some disorders (Figs. 28-1, #11, #14); NADH oxidation blocks have been described (Fig. 28-2,#4).[4,6,8] Inhibition of multiple enzyme reactions may explain why α-ketoglutarate is elevated in some cases of lactic acidosis. In propionic acidemia, some lactate may be formed by direct α-hydroxylation of propionate.

Ketosis. The common ketone bodies, acetone, acetoacetate, and β-hydroxybutyrate, are formed when the production of acetyl CoA exceeds the oxidative capacity of the citric acid cycle. Acetyl CoA is condensed and then reduced to form the other ketone bodies (Figs. 28-1, 28-2, and 28-3). Increased ketones in body fluids is rapidly followed by ketonuria. Unbalanced gluconeogenesis from fatty acids or the ketogenic amino acids will lead to ketosis, as will metabolic blocks that either impede normal oxidative energy metabolism or cause overproduction of acetate. Metabolic blocking of α-methylacetoacetyl CoA degradation (Fig. 28-3, #6–#10) leads to production of the unusual long-chain ketone, butanone.

Hyperammonemia

Hyperammonemia can be fulminant in the newborn or subacute in older infants. Characteristic features of hyperammonemia produce a recognizable syndrome that demands urgent blood ammonia determinations.[11,12,20]

Fulminant hyperammonemia starts in the first few days or weeks of life in an infant who is asymptomatic at birth. The attack is often precipitated by the first protein feeding, and successively produces lethargy, somnolence, refusal of feedings, vomiting, alternating hypertonia, hypotonia, grunting respirations, sweating, seizures, coma, and death. The alternating rigidity and flaccidity is occasionally accompanied by unusual posturing of the arms,

reminiscent of the flapping asterixis of hepatic coma in older patients. Subacute hyperammonemia produces similar but less severe neurologic signs. Irritability, screaming attacks, and feeding difficulties are prominent complaints, and episodes of constipation may initiate or aggravate hyperammonemic attacks because of increased ammonia uptake from the stagnant colonic contents. Hyperammonemia should be associated with recent protein intake, although this is often masked by a confusing history of multiple formula changes for postulated food intolerances.

The genetic causes of hyperammonemia are listed in Table 28-3.[4,11] Inborn errors of the urea cycle enzymes generally are associated with mild alkalosis, whereas inborn errors of branched-chain amino acid catabolism are associated with metabolic acidosis.

Nongenetic causes of hyperammonemia in infants are rare, but include severe liver failure from such etiologies as sepsis or hepatitis and from hyperalimentation. Reye syndrome has not been reported in young infants. In addition, severe transient hyperammonemia has recently been described in several preterm newborns with normal urea cycle enzyme activities and normal plasma and urinary organic acids and amino acids. Shortly after birth, these infants developed respiratory distress progressing to coma. Following aggressive treatment they displayed normal uncomplicated clinical courses.[20]

Normally, blood ammonia levels are closely constrained in dynamic equilibrium with aspartate, glutamate, and glutamine. The intimate relationships among these compounds, the urea cycle, and the citric acid cycle, are diagrammed in Figure 28-4, from which it can be seen that excess ammonia is biochemically diverted to aspartate, glutamate, and glutamine, and then, in the liver, to urea biosynthesis.

Many acute metabolic diseases result in liver necrosis (see below); in any of these, hepatocellular damage can produce secondary hyperammonemia. Alzheimer type II astrocyte changes in the brain provide neurohistologic evidence of possible hyperammonemia, although they may also be caused by other metabolic toxins.[4] These changes should be sought in infants dying of suspected hyperammonemia, even if the diagnosis was not confirmed before death.[11,12]

CLINICAL ABNORMALITIES
Neurologic Abnormalities in Inborn Errors

Disturbances of tone, movement, and alertness, and seizures associated with hypoglycemia, acidosis, and hyperammonemia have already been discussed. Any severely ill infant, regardless of the cause, will show hypotonia, lethargy, and somnolence, with or without irritability, and chronic debilitation will retard physical and mental development. Specific neurologic features, however, have been associated with some inborn errors of metabolism (Table 28-4).[4,8]

Seizures in the newborn are most commonly caused by birth trauma, anoxia, infections, or acute systemic metabolic disturbances (see Chap. 39). In addition, seizures appear in some inborn errors of metabolism even in the absence of generalized disturbances.

One rare genetic cause of seizures in the newborn, associated with severely disorganized EEG patterns, responds dramatically to injections of pyridoxine, and can be effectively treated by continual treatment with large doses of pyridoxine. Infants with **pyridoxine-dependent seizures** do not have vitamin deficiency, although pyridoxine deficiency in infants will

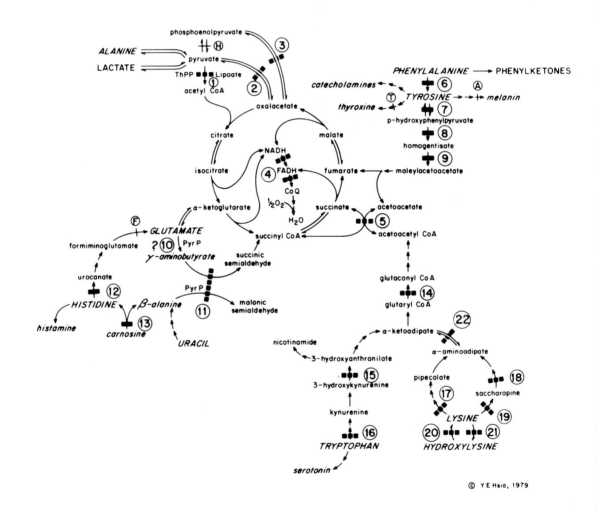

© Y E Hsia, 1979

also produce convulsions.[5,6] It has been postulated that the biochemical lesion may be an abnormality of brain glutamate decarboxylase, correctable by high concentrations of its cofactor, pyridoxal phosphate (Fig. 28-2, #10). Failure of glutamate decarboxylation would interrupt the normally highly active glutamate shunt (Fig. 28-2) in the brain, preventing formation of α-aminobutyrate, a neuroinhibitor, and causing accumulation of glutamate, a neurostimulator.[4] The concept that this is the basis for the seizures is speculative. Other inborn errors of metabolism may also produce seizures by disturbing the balance of neuroactive metabolites in an analogous fashion, with either excess formation of an epileptogenic agent, or suppressed formation of a neuroinhibitor.

Myoclonus, which occurs in a few inborn errors of metabolism, also is of obscure pathogenesis (Table 28-4). α-Ketoglutamate has been found in the cerebrospinal fluid of patients with hepatic coma and caused somnolence or myoclonus in rats (Fig. 28-4). This suggests that a specific toxic metabolite may cause the specific neuromuscular features of some inborn errors of metabolism.[4]

Cerebellar ataxia or choreoathetoid move-

◄ **Fig. 28-2.** Metabolic map of citric acid metabolism and related pathways of catabolism of some amino acids, indicating sites of inborn errors of metabolism causing biochemical disturbances. The conversion of triose phosphates by way of pyruvate to acetyl CoA is at the **top left** leading to the citric acid cycle. The glutamate cycle, with the important biogenic amine, γ-aminobutyric acid, is included, as well as β-alanine and its metabolism. The catabolism of phenylalanine and tyrosine are at the **top right,** indicating pathways of pigment and hormone formation from tyrosine; those of tryptophan and lysine are at the **bottom,** including the relation of serotonin, or 5-hydroxytryptamine, to tryptophan. Within the citric acid cycle is diagrammed the oxidative pathway of energy metabolism by which protons are transferred from NADH to molecular oxygen. Disorders of glycine and proline catabolism have been omitted.

Symbols and abbreviations are the same as for Fig. 28-1. The sites of metabolic blocks causing albinism are labeled **A,** and defects of thyroid hormone synthesis are labeled **T.** The symbol **F** locates the site of action of formiminofolate transferase on histidine catabolism.

Enzyme	*Deficient in*
1. Pyruvate dehydrogenase complex	? Lactic acidosis
	? Thiamine responsive hyperalaninemic hyperpyruvicacidemia
	? Leigh's subacute necrotising encephalopathy
2. Pyruvate carboxylase	Pyruvate carboxylase deficiency
3. Phosphoenolpyruvate carboxykinase	Phosphoenolpyruvate carboxykinase deficiency
4. Undetermined	Enzyme defects of the respiratory chain
5. Succinyl CoA-3-ketoacid CoA transferase	Succinyl CoA-3-ketoacid CoA transferase deficiency
6. Phenylalanine hydroxylase	Phenylketonuria and variants
7. Cytosol tyrosineaminotransferase	Hypertyrosinemia
8. p-Hydroxyphenylpyruvate oxidase	Hereditary tyrosinemia and variants
9. Homogenetisic acid oxidase	Alcaptonuria
10. Glutamate decarboxylase	? Pyridoxine-dependent seizures
11. ? β-Alanine aminotransferase	β-Alaninemia
? γ-Aminobutyric aminotransferase	
12. Histidase	Histidinemia
13. Carnosinase	Carnosinemia
14. ? Glutaryl CoA dehydrogenase	Glutaricacidemia
15. Kynureninase	Xanthurenicaciduria
	3-Hydroxykynureninuria
16. Undetermined	Tryptophanuria
17. Lysine dehydrogenase	Periodic hyperlysinemia
18. Undetermined	Saccharopinuria
19. Lysine α-ketoglutarate reductase	Persistent lysinemia with pipecolatemia
20. Undetermined	Hydroxylysinuria
21. Lysine hydroxylase	Ehlers-Danlos syndrome variant
22. ? δ-aminoadipate transaminase	Aminoadipic aciduria

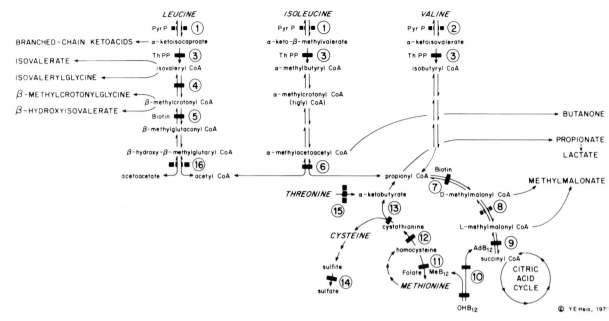

Fig. 28-3. Metabolic map of branched-chain amino acid and sulfur amino acid catabolism, indicating sites of inborn errors of metabolism. The catabolism of leucine, isoleucine, and valine descend to common intermediary metabolites from the **top.** Organic acids and other compounds excreted in these metabolic disorders are indicated on the left or right. The catabolism of threonine and methionine, with the pathways of vitamin B_{12} coenzyme synthesis, are **below.**

Metabolic blocks at six, seven, eight, nine, and ten have all produced the syndrome of ketotic hyperglycinemia.

Enzyme Reaction	*Deficient in*
1. ? Branched-chain amino acid transaminase	Hyperleucine-isoleucinemia
2. ? Valine transaminase	Hypervalinemia
3. Branched-chain ketoacid decarboxylase complex	Maple syrup urine disease and variants
4. Isovaleryl CoA dehydrogenase	Isovalericacidemia
5. β-Methylcrotonyl CoA carboxylase	β-Methylcrotonylglycinuria
	? biotin-responsive variant
6. β-Ketothiolase	β-Ketothiolase deficiency
7. Propionyl CoA carboxylase	Propionicacidemia and variants
8. ? Methylmalonyl CoA racemase	Methylmalonicacidemia
9. Methylmalonyl CoA carbonylmutase	Methylmalonicacidemia and variants
10. Steps in B_{12} coenzyme synthesis	B_{12}-dependent methylmalonicacidemias
11. Homocysteine-methionine methyltransferase and steps in folate coenzyme turnover	Inborn errors of folate metabolism
12. Cystathionine synthase	Homocystinuria
13. Cystathionase	Cystathioninuria
14. Sulfite oxidase	Sulfite oxidase deficiency
15. ? Threonine deaminase	Threoninemia
16. β-Hydroxy-β-Methyl-glutaryl CoA lyase	β-Hydroxy-β-Methyl-glutaryl CoA lyase aciduria deficiency

ments occur in some of the ill-defined lactic acidoses, as well as in several other disorders listed in Table 28-4. There is no clear information on the mechanisms responsible for these neurologic abnormalities, except that

Parkinsonian tremors can be aggravated by phenothiazine derivatives, and sometimes respond to L-dopa therapy, indicating a key role of catecholamines in basal ganglion function.

Retardation in metabolic errors is sometimes

Table 28-3. Genetically Determined Diseases Causing Hyperammonemia.

UREA CYCLE ENZYME DEFICIENCIES	LOCATION IN FIGURES
Carbamyl phosphate synthetase deficiency	28-4(1)
Ornithine transcarbamylase deficiency	28-4(2)
Citrullinemia	28-4(3)
Argininosuccinic acidemia	28-4(4)
Argininemia*	28-4(5)
DISORDERS OF DIBASIC AMINO ACIDS	
Ornithinemia	?
Periodic hyperlysinemia with hyperammonemia	28-2(17)
Persistent hyperlysinuria*	28-2(19)
Familial protein intolerance*	?
DISORDERS OF BRANCHED-CHAIN AMINO ACIDS	
β-Ketothiolase deficiency*	28-3(6)
Propionicacidemias	28-3(7)
Methylmalonicacidemias	28-3(8),(9)

* Only in some patients

associated with failure of postnatal myelination or interconnection of neural tracts, again possibly from neurotoxic metabolites. For instance, α-ketoisocaproate, which accumulates in maple syrup urine disease, inhibits the myelination of cultured fetal rat cerebellar tissue (Fig. 28-3, #3).[4] In many of the lysosomal storage diseases, on the other hand, in which there is arrested degradation of neurolipids, normal central nervous system turnover of these compounds is blocked, with more or less rapid deterioration of brain function, depending on the nature of the enzyme defect and the degree of enzyme impairment in genetic variants.[3,6,8] Table 28-5 lists the clinical features found in the lysosomal storage diseases that may appear in early infancy.

Megencephaly develops in some of the lysosomal storage diseases because of progressive infiltration and engorgement of brain tissue.[3]

Microcephaly is found with reduced brain growth. It can be either apparent at birth or it can become manifest only postnatally. Disorders of folic acid metabolism may have microcephaly as the sole physical abnormality, although with underlying ventricular dilatation and EEG abnormalities.[4]

Other Physical Abnormalities

In the lysosomal storage diseases, accumulation of undegraded macromolecules in tissue cells may give rise exclusively to central nervous system abnormalities, as in Tay–Sachs disease; to both brain and systemic abnormalities, as in GM_1 gangliosidosis and Niemann–Pick disease; or to primarily systemic abnormalities as in Pompe's type II glycogenosis and Wolman's lipid storage disease, in both of which death occurs in midinfancy with little neurologic involvement.[3,6,8]

Systemic abnormalities in the lysosomal storage diseases typically are organomegaly, especially hepatosplenomegaly, and occasionally skeletal dysplasia. Cardiomegaly with cardiomyopathy is a feature of Pompe's glycogenosis. Skin involvement in the lysosomal disorders results in thickening and loss of elasticity, with coarsening of the facial features from thickened skin covering misshapen facial bones. This may be exaggerated by thickening of the tongue and enlargement of the cranium (Table 28-5).[3,16]

Liver enlargement is infiltrative in the lysosomal storage diseases, generally with splenomegaly. In other inborn errors, liver enlargement may be from hepatocellular toxicity. When hepatotoxicity is acute and severe, as in galactosemia, there is necrosis with liver failure. Less acute liver damage leads to liver swelling with scarring and eventually splenomegaly from portal hypertension, as in glycogenosis type IV or in familial cholestasis.[15]

Jaundice appears in the cholestatic syn-

(*Text continues on p. 628.*)

Table 28-4. Neurologic Abnormalities in Inborn Metabolic Diseases.
(Other than those secondary to hypoglycemia, acidosis, hyperammonemia, severe liver involvement, or lysosomal storage)

Condition	Location in Figures	Seizures	Retardation	Other Neurologic Signs
CARBOHYDRATE METABOLISM				
Glycogenosis Type V	28-1(5)			Muscle cramps with
Glycogenosis Type VII	28-1(13)			exercise in older patients
Triosephosphate isomerase deficiency	28-1(15)		+	Spasticity
Phosphoglycerate kinase deficiency	28-1(16)	+	+	Later ataxia, speech problems
AMINO ACID AND ORGANIC ACID METABOLISM				
Albinism	28-2(A)			
Leigh's subacute necrotizing encephalopathy	?28-2(1)	+	+	Ataxia, ocular palsies
Hyperalaninemic lacticacidosis	?28-2(1)	+	+	Intermittent ataxia
Phenylketomuria	28-2(6)	+	+	Manifestations long after neonatal period
Hypertyrosinemia	28-2(7)	+	+	
β-Alaninemia	28-2(11)	+	+	Somnolence, hypotonia
Carnosinemia	28-2(13)	+	+	Myoclonic spasms
Tryptophanuria	28-2(16)		+	Cerebellar ataxia
Oasthouse urine disease	Methionine malabsorption	+	+	
Blue diaper syndrome	Tryptophan malabsorption		+	Irritability
Hydroxykynureninuria	28-2(15)		±	Infantile spasms
Hartnup disease	Neutral amino acid transport defect		?	Transient cerebellar ataxia at later age
Hydroxylysinuria	28-2(20)		+	
Persistent hyperlysinemia	28-2(19)	+	+	Hypotonia
Lysinuria	?		+	
Saccharopinuria	28-2(18)		?+	
Pipecolatemia	?			Cerebellar ataxia
Histidinemia	28-2(12)	±	±	?speech difficulties, ataxia
Hydroxyprolinemia	?		?+	
Hyperleucine-isoleucinemia	28-3(1)	+	+	Nerve deafness
Hypervalinemia	28-3(2)		+	Lethargy, nystagmus
Isovalericacidemia	28-3(4)		+	Drowsiness, cerebellar ataxia
β-Methylcrotonylglycinuria with β-hydroxyisovaleric aciduria	28-3(5)			?Spinal muscular atrophy
Nonketotic hyperglycinemia	?Glycine cleavage enzyme deficiency	+	+	
Hypersarcosinemia	–		?+	?Hypertonia, swallowing difficulties

Condition	Location in Figures	Seizures	Retardation	Other Neurologic Signs
AMINO ACID AND ORGANIC ACID METABOLISM (*continued*)				
Homocystinuria	28-3(12)		?+	
Cystinuria	Transport defect		?	
Argininosuccinicaciduria	28-4(4)			Cerebellar ataxia
Ornithinemia	28-4(6)			Myoclonic spasms
VITAMIN METABOLISM				
Pyridoxine dependent seizures	28-2(10)	+	+	Dramatic response to pyridoxine
Folate malabsorption of infancy	–	+	+	Ataxia, athetosis in an older patient
Formiminotransferase deficiency	28-2(F)		+	Microcephaly
Methyltetrahydrofolate transferase deficiency	28-3(11)		+	Microcephaly
Methylenetetrahydrofolate reductase deficiency	–		+	Microcephaly
Methylmalonicaciduria with homocystinuria	28-3(10)	+	+	?Hypertonia, ?cerebellar ataxia in some older patients
OTHER CONDITIONS				
Hyperuricemia	Hypoxanthine-guanine phosphoribosyltransferase deficiency		+	Choreoathetosis, compulsive automutilation
Oroticaciduria	28-4(7)		+	Lethargy
Glutathionemia	?		+	
Hyperserotoninemia	?	+	+	Cerebellar ataxia
A-β-Lipoproteinemia	–			Spinocerebellar ataxia, later, retinitis
Refsum's disease	Phytanate oxidase deficiency			Polyneuritis, ataxia, retinitis in adult life
Crigler–Najjar disease	Conjugation defect		+	Kernicterus
Menkes' kinky-hair disease	Copper transport defect	+	+	Hypotonia, hypothermia
Lowe's oculocerebrorenal syndrome	?		+	Hypotonia episodic hypertension, hypothermia, indifference to pain, areflexia, dysphagia
Adrenogenital syndrome	Steroid metabolism	+		
α_1-antitrypsin deficiency	–	+		

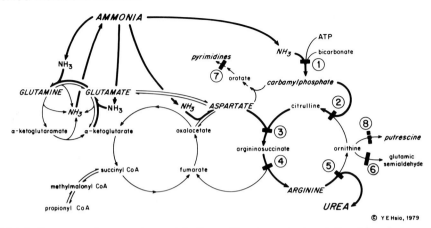

Fig. 28-4. Metabolic map of ammonia metabolism. The important relationships between ammonia, glutamate, and aspartate are emphasized. The purine nucleotide cycle which releases large amounts of ammonia from muscle has been omitted. The relationship of the citric acid cycle to the arginine cycle is shown, as is the synthesis of pyrimidines from aspartate and carbamyl phosphate. How disorders of propionate metabolism produce hyperammonemia is not clear. α-Ketoglutaramate, depicted on the left, has been found in the cerebrospinal fluid of patients with hepatic coma.

Enzyme Reaction	Deficient in
1. Carbamylphosphate synthetase	Carbamylphosphate synthetase deficiency
2. Ornithine transcarbamylase	Ornithine transcarbmylase deficiency
3. Argininosuccinate synthetase	Citrullinemia
4. Argininosuccinase	Argininosuccinicaciduria
5. Arginase	Argininemia
6. Ornithine transaminase	Gyrate atrophy of the retina
	One form of ornithinemia
7. Orotidine-5'-phosphate pyrophosphorylase and orotidine-5'-phosphate decarboxylase	Oroticacidurias
8. Ornithine decarboxylase	Hyperornithinemia

A transport defect of ornithine re-entry into the mitochondrion is the probable cause of hyperornithinemia with homocitrullinemia.

dromes, in Crigler–Najjar syndrome (because of abnormal bilirubin metabolism), in hepatotoxicity, and also in the congenital hemolytic anemias.[21] Other inherited causes of jaundice in the neonatal period and infancy include galactosemia, the G-6-PD deficiencies, fructose intolerance and α_1-antitrypsin deficiency. The differential diagnosis of jaundice and the importance of the time of its onset are discussed in Chapter 24.

Skin abnormalities[22] besides those arising from lysosomal storage or liver disease, include eczematous rashes in phenylketonuria, the immune deficiencies,[23] some complement abnormalities, and the Wiskott–Aldrich syndrome;[15] erythematous acrodermatitic rashes in disorders of zinc or essential fatty acid metabolism and maple syrup urine disease; keratosis palmoplantaris in hypertyrosinemia;

a malar flush in homocystinuria; and blotchiness of the skin in familial dysautonomia.[8] Photosensitivity occurs in the cutaneous albinism syndromes, cystinosis, tryptophanuria, and some of the porphyrias. Xanthomata may be present even at birth in homozygous patients with hyperlipidemia type II. The skin has abnormal thickness and texture not only in inherited abnormalities of collagen and elastic tissue, but also in some of the lysosomal storage diseases[3] and the goitrous cretinism syndromes.[8] Severe pruritus in the cholestatic syndromes results in scratching and keratinization. Among the genetically determined dermatologic diseases are xeroderma pigmentosa caused by deficiency of a DNA repair enzyme, which can present with a photosensitive red scaly rash in infancy; and two of the forms of Ehlers–Danlos syndrome, one resulting from

Table 28-5. Lysosomal Storage Diseases with Clinical Manifestations in Early Infancy.

Condition	Metabolic Defect	Clinical Features
Cytinosis	?Membrane transport	Photophobia, corneal crystals, retinal depigmentation and peripheral degeneration
Pompe's glycogenosis type II	α-Glucosidase	Severe weakness, cardiomegaly, macroglossia
Mucopolysaccharidoses Hurler's type I*		Coarse facies, macroglossia, hepatosplenomegaly, skeletal dystrophy
Mucolipidosis I (Gal + disease)	Undetermined	Coarse facies, hepatosplenomegaly, skeletal dystrophy, some have cherry red spot in eyes; may have corneal clouding
Mucolipidosis II (I-cell disease)	Undetermined	Quiet inactive behavior, retarded development, failure to thrive, coarse facies, skeletal dystrophy, gingival hyperplasia
Mucolipidosis III (pseudo-Hurler)	Undetermined	As for type I
Mucolipidosis IV	Undetermined	Congenital corneal clouding, retardation evident later
Fucosidosis	α-L-Fucosidase	Coarse facies, macroglossia, hepatosplenomegaly, skeletal dystrophy, initial hypotonia, later hypertonia, frequent infections
Mannosidosis	α-Mannosidase	Large head, coarse facies, hepatosplenomegaly, skeletal dystrophy, retardation, frequent infections, later coarsening of facies
GM$_1$ Gangliosodosis	Acid-β-galactosidase	Coarse facies, macroglossia, hepatosplenomegaly, skeletal dystrophy, some have corneal clouding, some have cherry red spot in eyes, initial hypotomia, later hypertonia, spasticity, convulsions
GM$_2$ Gangliosidosis Sandhoff, type O	N-acetyl-β-hexoseaminidase A and B	Large head, some have hepatosplenomegaly, optic atrophy, cherry red spot, hypertonia, myoclonic seizures
Tay–Sachs, type B	N-Acetyl-β-hexoseaminidase B	Hyperacusis, weakness, later amaurosis, retardation, convulsions, most have cherry red spot in eyes
GM$_3$ Gangliosidosis	?"synthetase"	Coarse facies, macroglossia, hepatosplenomegaly, contractures and thick skin
Gaucher's-infantile variant	Glucocerebrosidase	Hepatosplenomegaly, skeletal dystrophy, increased bruisability
Krabbe's	Galactocerebrosidase	Hyperirritability, stiffness, fevers, later hypertoxicity, amaurosis
Niemann-Pick	Sphingomyelinase	Cachexia, hepatosplenomegaly, retardation, some have cherry red spot in eyes
Wolman's disease	Acid lipase	Diarrhea, failure to thrive, hepatosplenomegaly, calcification of adrenals, cachexia
Acid phosphatase deficiency Lysosomal Total	Acid phosphatase	Diarrhea, hepatomegaly, hypotonia, convulsions, perhaps choreoathetosis, lethargy, opisthotonus, increased bleeding, failure to thrive
Farber's disease	Acid ceramidase	Hoarseness, stiffness, subcutaneous nodules, arthropathy, failure to thrive
β-Xylosidase deficiency	β-Xylosidase	Choreoathetosis, blindness, deafness

* None of the other mucopolysaccharidoses has clinical manifestations until > 1 year of age.

lysine hydroxylase deficiency and the other from procollagen peptidase deficiency, which show marked skin hyperelasticity and fragility with joint laxity in the young infant.[15,16] Profuse sweating occurs in some of the hyperammonemia syndromes, in some other metabolic diseases, and in dysautonomia. Absent tearing is characteristic of dysautonomia.[8]

Hair abnormalities are odd findings in a few inborn errors. In oasthouse urine disease, the skin and hair are very fair; in older infants with untreated phenylketonuria, hair is underpigmented. Some patients with agrininosuccinicaciduria have trichorrhexis nodosa with increased hair fragility, but any severe protein-calorie dysnutrition can also cause pigmentary and friability changes in the hair. In Menkes' disease, the twisted hair shafts, pili torti, are an important diagnostic finding although not usually seen in the newborn period.

Bone and joint abnormalities are a systemic manifestation of many of the lysosomal storage diseases.[2,10,16,24] Just as skin is thickened, so in some of these conditions connective tissue is thickened and rendered inelastic with decreased joint mobility. Skeletal malformations, involving distortion of vetebral bodies, ribs, and long bones of the extremities, are of some aid in the radiologic differentiation of some of the lysosomal diseases. These malformations are evident in infancy in only the more severe lysosomal diseases, but radiologic surveys of the skull, vertebrae, ribs, and long bones may provide important diagnostic clues to these diseases.[25–27] The long marfanoid body habitus of homocystinuria may be apparent in infants, but it is not a well-studied or reliable index of that disorder in infancy.

Eye abnormalities are also unusual but important findings in some of the inborn errors of metabolism; a thorough eye examination, preferably by an ophthalmologist, should be done whenever an inborn error of metabolism or a degenerative lysosomal disease is suspected (Table 28-6).[28,29] Congenital corneal cloudiness occurs in mucolipidosis III and IV, and appears in infancy in some of the other lysosomal storage diseases; it can be seen secondary to glaucoma, as in Lowe's syndrome. Corneal deposits of cystine crystals are seen in cystinosis; in older children copper deposits are responsible for the Kayser–Fleischer rings of Wilson's disease. Keratoconjunctivitis is not always infective;

it can be a sign of congenital erythropoietic porphyria, and can arise because of absent tearing in some cases of anhydrosis or in familial dysautonomia. Corneal ulceration appears in dysautonomia, and painful dendritic corneal ulcers are typical of hypertyrosinemia, in which relief can be obtained by diet restriction of tyrosine.

Cataracts are seen in galactosemia and galactokinase deficiencies, although they are very faint initially, opacifying with prolonged exposure to galactose. In Lowe's syndrome, dense nuclear cataracts are present at birth. Cataracts have been reported in some patients with lactic acidosis. Ectopia lentis, presumably caused by pathologic weakness of the suspensory ligament system, is seen in sulfite oxidase deficiency and homocystinuria, disorders of sulfur metabolism (Fig. 28-3, #14, #12), and in hyperlysinemia.

Retinal abnormalities found in metabolic conditions include infiltration in some of the lysosomal diseases,[3,28,29] typically Tay–Sachs disease, leaving a clearer macula that appears as a cherry red spot. Optic atrophy is associated with some lysosomal diseases and some patients with lactic acidosis. Gyrate atrophy of the choroid and retina is pathognomonic of ornithine transaminase deficiency. Retinal depigmentation and dystrophy are important early neonatal findings in cystinosis. Abnormal retinal pigmentation in infants is often indicative of intrauterine infection, but retinitis pigmentosa appears in older patients with a-beta-lipoproteinemia and Refsum's disease, as well as a host of inherited eye diseases.[28]

SCREENING

Presymptomatic screening of all newborns for inborn errors of metabolism is not only possible, it is necessary to detect those disorders that are treatable.[30–36] To date, screening has focused on PKU and hypothyroidism, but multiple entities can be evaluated on a single neonatal blood specimen.

Theoretically, all infants at risk for a condition should be tested by an accurate, reliable, efficient test which must be economical, with minimal hardship for infants. In practice, the specimen tested can be cord blood, capillary blood, urine, sweat, tears, hair, nails, or stools. In pilot projects, there has been analysis of chromosomes, many proteins, enzymes, and metabolites. Microbiologic assays and chromatographic and other techniques, adapted to automated multitest equipment, have all been successfully developed for centralized testing of large numbers of samples. Results have to be monitored, interpreted, and followed up by a responsible comprehensive service program to ensure that identified abnormalities are confirmed and adequately treated.[35-38]

Phenylketonuria (PKU)

PKU is the prototype of conditions for which screening seems justified. The incidence is about 1 per 15,000 in Caucasian populations; it is less common in Oriental, Black and Ashkenazi Jewish populations. The condition is featureless in early infancy, developmental retardation becoming evident only in the second 6 months of life. Dietary restriction, started within the first 2 months of life, has proven effective in preventing most of the brain damage.[5,6,8,9,35-38] The cost of testing programs and effective treatment of affected infants has been demonstrably less than the cost of caring for untreated brain-damaged patients, so there is financial justification for screening programs as well.

Because the protein product of the structural gene, phenylalanine hydroxylase, is found almost exclusively in the liver, the enzyme can be measured reliably only in liver tissue. Screening tests must therefore focus on abnormal concentrations of the enzyme's substrate, phenylalanine, in the peripheral blood. After birth, some infants with PKU have elevated blood phenylalanine levels within one day, but some patients with phenylketonuria will not have high blood phenylalanine until the fifth day. Because of changing obstetric practices in the United States, which include discharging mothers and babies from hospital early, it seems prudent to recommend that all babies have a blood test for phenylalanine on discharge from hospital, but that a repeat test be obtained the first time the baby is seen by a health professional after discharge, preferably during the second week of life.

Hyperphenylalaninemia by itself does not make the diagnosis of phenylketonuria. The upper limit of normal for phenylalanine in the first few days of life falls from 4 to 2 mg/dl. Of infants found to have higher levels, some also have elevated tyrosine, indicating that the metabolic block is beyond phenylalanine hydroxylase (Fig. 28-3); some have modest transitory elevations; others have marked elevations which are either not as severe as in phenylketonuria or are not associated with as much production of the phenylketone by-products. Hence, a group of conditions categorized as benign hyperphenylalaninemias or atypical PKUs have been uncovered by large-scale newborn screening programs. These infants, if proven not to have PKU, may have no danger of brain damage (their management is discussed under Treatment).

Urine phenylketones do not appear until the blood phenylalanine level has exceeded 15 to 20 mg/dl for at least several weeks. Urine testing is therefore unsatisfactory for diagnosis of PKU in the immediate newborn period.

More malignant variants of PKU have recently been discovered that are caused by abnormalities of regeneration or synthesis of the biopterin cofactor. Because this cofactor serves tyrosine and tryptophan hydroxylases as well as phenylalanine hydroxylase, affected patients have grave defects in dopa and serotonin metabolism unbenefited by dietary treatment for PKU. Experimental therapy is being explored for these variants.[39]

Other Inborn Errors of Metabolism

Galactosemia screening can be performed either by assay for blood galactose concentration or for red cell uridyl transferase activity (Fig. 28-1, #9). The disease is rare (about 1 per 75,000), and clinical toxicity may be lethal before the results of a screening test are obtained.[40] **Maple syrup urine disease** is detectable by elevated blood leucine levels; many of the other aminoacidopathies can be detected by abnormal amino acid concentrations or by patterns in the blood or urine. **Cystic fibrosis,** affecting 1 in 2000 infants of Western European ancestry, can be screened by detection of serum proteins in meconium or stool or on a blood spot.[41] **Sickle-cell disease,** affecting 1 in 500 American Black infants, and other hemoglobinopathies have been detected by cord blood tests. A small dried blood specimen can also be used to test for G-6-PD deficiency, angioneurotic edema, or α_1-antitrypsin deficiency.

Hypercholesterolemia in newborn infants is relatively common (1 per 300 births), but it alone is not indicative of type II hyperlipidemia.[6,8] The therapeutic value of early detection

(*Text continues on p. 634.*)

Table 28-6. Physical Abnormalities in Inborn Errors of Metabolism Other than Lysosomal Storage Diseases.

Condition	Location in Figures	Organomegaly	Skin and Appendages	Eyes
Glycogenosis				
von Gierke's type I	28-1(7)	Liver, kidney		
Pompe's type II	Lysosomal	Heart, liver		
Cori's type III	28-1(3),(4)	Liver		
Anderson's type IV	28-1(2)	Liver, spleen		
Hers' type VI	28-1(5)	Liver		
type VII	28-1(6)	Liver		
Galactokinase deficiency	28-1(8)			Cataracts
Galactosemia	28-1(9)	Liver*	Jaundice and petechiae	Cataracts
Fructose intolerance	28-1(14)	Liver*	Jaundice and petechiae	
Lacticacidosis	?28-2(1)	Liver in some	Flushing in some	Some have cataracts
Leigh's encephalopathy	?28-2(1)			Some have optic atrophy
Phenylketonuria	28-2(6)		Eczema later	
Hypertyrosinemia	28-2(7)		Keratosis palmoplantaris	Dendritic corneal ulcers
Hereditary tyrosinemia	28-2(8)	Liver,* spleen	Jaundice and petechiae	
Tryptophanuria	28-2(16)		Photosensitivity, hyperpigmentation	
Hyperleucine-isoleucinemia	28-3(1)		Retinal degeneration	
Maple syrup urine disease	28-3(3)	Liver	Acrodermatitis has been seen	
Propionicacidemia	28-3(7)		Desquamative rash has been seen	
Homocystinuria	28-3(1)		Malar flush in older patients	Ectopia lentis ? age of detectability
Sulfite oxidase deficiency	28-3(4)			Ectopia lentis
Cystinosis	Lysosomal cystine storage			Corneal crystals, retinal depigmentation
Hartnup disease	Tryptophan malabsorption		Pellegra-like rash in older patients	
Oasthouse urine disease	Methionine malabsorption		White hair, edema	
Ornithine transcarbamylase deficiency	28-4(2)	Liver*	Jaundice, bleeding	
Citrullinemia	28-4(3)	Liver*	Jaundice, bleeding	
Argininosuccinic aciduria	28-4(4)	Liver*	Jaundice, bleeding, tri-	

Hyperornithinemia	28-4(6)			Gyrate atrophy of retina
Persistent hyperlysinemia	22-2(19)		Synophrys, (lax joint ligaments)	Ectopia lentis
Pipecolatemia	?	Liver		
Familial protein intolerance	?	Liver, abdominal distension		
Homozygous hyperlipidemia Type II			Xanthomata	
A-β-Lipoproteinemia				Retinitis pigmentosa
Refsum's disease	Phytanate oxidase defect		Ichthyosis	Retinitis pigmentosa
Lowe's oculocerebrorenal syndrome	?			Dense cataracts, glaucoma, bulphthalmos
Familial cholestasis		Liver, spleen	Jaundice, pruritus, clubbing	
Crigler–Najjar's congenital non-hemolytic jaundice	Conjugation defect	Liver, spleen	Jaundice, (kernicterus)	
Gilbert's congenital nonhemolytic jaundice	Mild conjugation defect	Liver	Jaundice	
Dubin-Johnson's chronic idiopathic jaundice	Bile excretory defect	Liver	Mild jaundice	
Congenital erythropoietic porphyria			Photosensitivity, vesicular eruptions with scarring, hypertrichosis	Keratoconjunctivitis
Angioneurotic edemia	C1 esterase inhibitor		Acute circumscribed skin and glottic edema	
?Leiner's infective seborrhea	C5 complement defect		Seborrheic dermatitis (infections, diarrhea)	
Wiskott–Aldrich syndrome			Eczema (infections, thrombocytopenia)	
Familial dysautonomia	?		Blotchiness of skin, absent fungiform papillae on tongue	Absent tearing
Menkes' kinky hair disease	Copper transport defect		Pili torti; fair complexion	Corneal ulcers

* Some patients have acute hepatic necrosis

of hypercholesterolemia depends on whether lowering blood cholesterol can be shown to lower the incidence of occlusive coronary disease in adults and on determining the optimal time in children or infancy for the initiation of treatment.[42] Even if diet treatment need not be started until a much older age, screening of the newborn might be an effective, albeit indirect, way to find young families at risk, in order that prophylactic treatment and genetic counseling can be offered.

If a battery of screening tests is to be run on a small sample of blood, it is particularly desirable to look for abnormalities of **thyroid hormone**.[36,43,44] In fact, an increasing number of states are requiring screening for hypothyroidism because early treatment with thyroxine can prevent mental retardation (see Chap. 44).[44] Incidence has been estimated at 1 per 3000 to 5000. Testing immunoglobulins for evidence of intrauterine infection should also be considered.

DIAGNOSIS

For inborn disorders of metabolism, a complete diagnosis should include (1) a clinical diagnosis of the phenotype, (2) a metabolic diagnosis of the nature and extent of chemical disturbances, (3) a biochemical diagnosis of the enzyme or protein defect primarily responsible for the disease, and (4) a genetic diagnosis of the pattern of inheritance in a particular family.

The **clinical phenotype** need not correspond to the biochemical diagnosis because there is often such heterogeneity of expression of enzyme deficiencies that many enzyme deficiencies may mimic one another or nongenetic disorders, and also a single enzyme deficiency may have varying pleiotropic clinical manifestations. A **metabolic** diagnosis is essential for rational corrective treatment. A precise **biochemical** diagnosis forms the basis for predicting complications and prognosis. A **genetic** diagnosis is required for detecting affected or carrier relatives and estimating risks to future children.

Minimal diagnostic workup for possibly inherited metabolic diseases consists of the following considerations. A **family history** of unexplained illnesses or known problems should be carefully sought, as should a **diet history** of possibly toxic foods in relatives as well as the patient. Growth of body weight, length, and head size should be recorded. Developmental achievements, neurologic function, and clinical symptoms should be thoroughly evaluated with particular attention to skin, eye, or organ abnormalities. **Blood tests** for glucose, electrolytes, lactate and ammonia should be considered, as well as bilirubin, alkaline phosphatase, and serum proteins. Routine urine tests, when metabolic errors are suspected, should include inspection, smell, testing for reducing substances, and at least a simple ferric chloride test for unusual color reactions. Qualitative urine amino acid patterns should also be obtained. Of course, nongenetic causes of disease such as infections should be excluded. To complete a diagnostic workup, technically sophisticated metabolic studies or enzyme assays may be required that are performed only in specialized centers. Particularly with rare disorders, with which clinical experience has been limited, consultation should be sought with investigators in centers experienced with the disorder. A biochemical diagnosis can sometimes be made on plasma or blood cells, but often can be made only on cultured cells from a skin biopsy or from biopsied organ tissue, generally the liver. Both for the sake of the patient and for optimal collection of information, tissue biopsies should be planned carefully with respect to preservation of enzyme viability as well as of histologic detail. A liver biopsy may only yield nondiagnostic changes if a portion is not immediately frozen and sent for appropriate tests. Anesthetic risks are great in some metabolic diseases, and indications must be very carefully weighed before any surgery is planned.

Examination of the Urine

Unusual colors or smells in the urine may be valuable clues to inborn errors of metabolism. Table 28-7 lists conditions in which the smell, color or deposits in the urine are immediate indicators of specific diagnoses. Therefore, the clinician must be alert to the need for sniffing and inspecting the patient and the patient's urine whenever an inborn metabolic error is a possibility. Smells are notoriously difficult to describe or identify, but when the unknown smell can be compared with the smells of known standards, identification of smells is quite accurate. In PKU, the

Table 28-7. Smells, Urine Colors, and Sediments found in Inborn Errors of Metabolism.

Condition	Location in Figures	Smell, Color or Sediment	Substance
Smells			
Any cause of ketosis with acetonuria	—	Sweetish	Acetone
Phenylketonuria	28-2(6)	Musty or mousy	Phenylacetate
Hereditary tyrosinemia	28-2(8)	Stale cabbage (rancid butter)	α-Keto-γ-methiolbutyrate
Maple syrup urine disease	28-3(3)	Maple syrup (burnt sugar)	Branched-chain α-ketoacids
Isovalericacidemia	28-3(4)	Sweaty feet (cheesy)	Isovalerate, butyrate, hexanoate
β-Methylcrotonylglycinuria	28-3(5)	Cat's urine	β-Hydroxyisovalerate
Oasthouse urine disease	Methionine malabsorption	Dried celery	?α-Hydroxybutyrate
Trimethylaminuria	?	Stale fish	Trimethylamine
All intestinal malabsorption syndromes		Foul, fecal	Fatty acids
Urine Color or Sediment			
All choluric jaundice syndromes	—	Yellow	Bile pigments
Alcaptonuria	28-2(9)	Black on standing	Homogentisate
Congenital erythropoietic porphyria (and acute intermittent porphyria in adults)			
Hemoglobinurias		Red	Hemoglobin
Hyperuricemia	Hypoxanthine-guaninephosphoribosyl transferase	Sandy	Uric Acid
Oroticaciduria	28-4(7)		Needle-like crystals of orotic acid
(also in ornithine transcarbamylase deficiency)	28-4(2)		
Blue diaper syndrome	Tryptophan malabsorption	Indigo blue	Indican

penetrating musty odor does not appear until the infant is many weeks of age, whereas in maple syrup urine disease the definitive sweetish smell of maple syrup can be detected in early infancy.

Regardless of smells, colors, or sediments, urine tests for unusual metabolites should start with inspection, microscopy of urinary sediment for crystals, and the standard tests for protein, ketones, glucose, and reducing substances.[13] It is not sufficient to test only for glucose by a specific glucose oxidase test, because detection of nonglucose reducing substances, such as galactose, by nonspecific tests may be lifesaving, as in the case of galectosemia, which can be discovered by this means. The addition of 10% ferric chloride to a sample of urine yields color reactions with many unusual aldehydes and ketones in addition to the phenylpyruvic acid of phenylketonuria and the acetoacetate of any ketonuria, thus providing further diagnostic information.[14,30-32]

Other screening tests have been devised to detect traces of ketoacids, free sulfhydryl groups, excess glycosaminoglycans (mucopolysaccharides), unusual amino acid patterns, and various specific chemicals or enzymes.[9,33]

Amino acid patterns in the urine can be analyzed by several chromatographic or electrophoretic techniques.[5,9] Interpretation is complicated by the fact that renal tubular reabsorption of amino acids is much less complete in the newborn infant than in later infancy. Generalized aminoaciduria can appear normally in prematurity or can be produced by many drugs, heavy metal poisoning, severe systemic illness, particularly liver failure, and any cause of renal tubular damage. A specific pattern of excess amino acids is diagnostic of many membrane transport disorders (e.g., cystinuria) and of many enzyme deficiencies (e.g., phenylketonuria). Interpretation still requires experience, however, because some abnormal amino acid patterns have several possible causes. For example, fructose intolerance can mimic the amino acid pattern of hereditary tyrosinemia. Normal urine amino acid patterns do not exclude all of the aminoacidopathies, because normal renal reabsorptive capacity may not be saturated even by fivefold increases, specifically of plasma ornithine or arginine. Therefore, whenever a persistently abnormal urine amino acid pattern is not easily interpretable, plasma amino acids should be analyzed with careful attention to technical details, such as the specification of fasting or postprandial specimens, and the prompt deproteinizing of plasma to avoid *in vitro* changes in amino acid concentrations.

Organic acids and ketones vary in ease of detection according to their stability, concentration, and reactivity.[34] Acetone is relatively easy to measure but is volatile; methylmalonate is stable and has unique color reactions which are useful for measuring it; other organic acids must be identified and quantitated by gas chromatography.[9,34] In the absence of universal color reactions for the organic acids, as in the amino acids, some of the organic acidemias are only beginning to be recognized and studied. Undoubtedly, many other clinically important organic acidemias will be discovered with increased use of the more readily available gas chromatographic and mass spectrographic techniques.

Stool

Inspection of the stool is just as important in some metabolic diseases as it is in infants with diarrhea or malnutrition. Its consistency and color are altered in malabsorption states. Offensive, greasy stools are characteristic of incomplete fat assimilation. A frothy stool indicates that carbohydrate has passed through undigested to the colon to be fermented by colonic microorganisms. Special tests on the stools, apart from microscopy and tests for pH, blood, fat content, or undigested meat fibers, include an assay for pancreatic enzymes, detection of reducing substances in disaccharidase deficiency, and detection of serum proteins in suspected cystic fibrosis. Analysis of fecal amino acid patterns, which are distinctive in membrane transport disorders such as Hartnup disease, is of research interest but of limited practical value.

Blood and Bone Marrow

Routine peripheral blood counts and smears can also supply clues to various metabolic disorders. For example, intermittent neutropenia and thrombocytopenia may be present in tyrosinemia and in many types of organic acidemia. Vacuolated lymphocytes are seen in a number of glycogen, mucopolysaccharide, and lipid-storage diseases.

The presence of cystine crystals or engorged lysosomes in bone marrow macrophages and histiocytes are diagnostic of several specific lysosomal disorders. Marrow iron in sideroblastic anemias and hemochromatosis are discussed in Chapter 25.

In any ill infant, routine blood tests are obtained for glucose, urea nitrogen, electrolyte, and hydrogen ion concentrations. Liver function tests, when indicated, include at least bilirubin, alkaline phosphatase, and serum proteins. Additionally, when an inherited metabolic disease is suspected, lactate should be determined if there is a large anion gap, as should ammonia if there are suggestive symptoms. Specific tests are best deferred until preliminary blood and urine investigations have narrowed the diagnostic possibilities.

Postmortem Studies

When an infant dies with signs and symptoms suggestive of a metabolic disorder, a full skeletal survey, an autopsy examination, and an assay of a biopsy specimen of skin or rapidly frozen tissues (*e.g.,* liver) might still provide a definitive diagnosis, essential for counseling the parents and relatives about recurrence risks and the possibility of fetal diagnostic tests for future pregnancies.

TREATMENT

As discussed under diet history, exogenous components of the diet are toxic in many inborn errors of metabolism; therefore, one basic principle of treatment is to restrict toxic foods. In the vitamin-responsive diseases, in which the biochemical defects affect a vitamin cofactor,[45] large doses of the vitamin can be dramatically beneficial. Metabolic disturbances require prompt corrective measures. Some of these are discussed under representative genetic disorders. Symptomatic treatment is self-evident and obvious precautions should be undertaken, such as avoidance of dangerous medications in pharmacogenetically susceptible disorders, or overexposure to sunlight in photosensitive states.[36]

The following metabolic disorders are discussed not because they are the most common, but because they represent diverse presentations and illustrate different principles for treating inborn errors of metabolism.[38]

von Gierke's Glycogenosis Type I

In von Gierke's disease, blocked glucose release from the liver results in severe hypoglycemia, secondary lactic acidosis, hyperlipidemia, hyperuricemia and moderate ketonuria (Fig. 28-1). There is hepatomegaly, thrombocytosis with bleeding episodes, and occasionally steatorrhea. The principle of treatment, as in all causes of hypoglycemia, is to restore blood glucose to physiologic levels and sustain it at these levels. Both gluconeogenesis and glycogenolysis produce phosphorylated glucose that cannot cross the cell membrane until dephosphorylated; the debrancher enzyme alone releases free glucose from the branch points of glycogen (Fig. 28-1, 3). In this disease, because of blocked hydrolysis of glucose-6-phosphate, only carbohydrate food that is broken down to glucose in the intestine will contribute to the extracellular glucose pool. To avoid extremes of postprandial hyperglycemia with resultant reactive hyperinsulinemia and eventual obesity, there should be small frequent feedings with small amounts of fat and protein to retard gastric emptying and intestinal absorption. Strict attention to feeding by a rigid timetable may prevent the complication of hypoglycemic seizures; overnight, slow intragastric glucose infusions have proven beneficial;[46] and careful regulation of caloric intake may avoid the complication of exogenous obesity. If dietary management alone does not suffice, measures such as portal vein diversion or even liver transplantation may be required in older patients. To avoid the late complication of hyperuricemia, allopurinal treatment is indicated, but can be started when the child is older. Other hepatic glycogenoses are metabolically milder, and have patent gluconeogenic pathways that render them easier to treat with high-protein diets.[6,8]

Galactosemia

Mild congenital cataracts and minimal intrauterine growth retardation suggest that the fetus with galactosemia is susceptible to galactose toxicity *in utero* (although galactosemic mothers have borne some healthy nongalactosemic infants). Postpartum exposure of the galactosemic infant to galactose, however, can be catastrophic. There is severe vomiting and diarrhea, liver enlargement and jaundice, secondary bleeding, cerebral congestion or edema, exacerbation of the cataracts, and renal tubular damage with generalized aminoaciduria as well as galactosuria. Patients are unduly susceptible to bacterial septicemia or meningitis.[40] Emergency treatment of a suspected case of galactosemia is the immediate cessation of all milk (lactose) intake. Dehydration, sepsis, hypoglycemia, and electrolyte disturbances may require parenteral fluid and antibiotic therapy. Because the diagnosis can be readily confirmed by red cell enzyme tests at any time and because treatment is so simple, there is never any justification for delaying treatment until a diagnosis has been made. If an infant is vomiting, has an enlarged liver with jaundice, and a reducing sugar in the urine which is not glucose, galactosemia should be the working diagnosis until proven otherwise. Oral feedings can be safely reestablished with commercial synthetic galactose-free (lactose-free) milk formulas.[47] In the older child, mixed feeding with natural or processed foods is acceptable, provided no galactose or lactose is in the food. Expert nutritional supervision is needed for the management of these patients. They can do well with prompt diagnosis and optimal treatment: recovery of hepatic function is gratifyingly good in most infants diagnosed in time, brain function may escape damage, lenticular opacities may be negligible, and recovery of renal function recovery is complete.

G-6-PD Deficiency

Persons with X-linked recessive G-6-PD deficiencies usually first manifest hemolytic anemia following exposure to one of a variety of oxidizing chemicals or drugs, such as primaquine, sulfonamides, or aspirins. Mediterranean and Oriental varieties can be severe enough to cause icterus gravis neonatorum. Treatment consists of treating the anemia, any consequent hyperbilirubinemia, and withdrawing the symptom-promoting substances, as well as warning the affected patient against future drug contacts.[6]

PKU

Dietary treatment of PKU is urgent because of the proven risk of progressive brain damage if treatment is not started within the first 2 months of life. When an infant is found to have elevated blood phenylalanine on a screening test, at least one more fasting blood phenylalanine should be obtained to confirm the diagnosis, preferably by an accurate quantitative chemical or chromatographic test. If the blood phenylalanine exceeds 15 mg/dl, and if the blood tyrosine level is <4 mg/dl, a presumptive diagnosis of phenylketonuria can be made, and the infant should be given a restricted phenylalanine diet.[6,47,48]

Phenylalanine is an essential amino acid. Even the infant with PKU must have some for protein synthesis; moreover, because tyrosine is formed from phenylalanine, tyrosine becomes an essential amino acid for these infants.

A commercial synthetic milk formula, Lofenalac, has 12 mg phenylalanine/dl and 120 mg tyrosine/dl in the standard dilution. This formula has insufficient phenylalanine for a rapidly growing young infant. In the first few weeks, a growing infant (with phenylketonuria) requires daily 50 to 150 mg phenylalanine/kg body weight. This intake is best regulated by

mixing Lofenalac with other formulas having known high-phenylalanine content (cow's milk has 150 to 180 mg phenylalanine/dl). Every infant placed on a restricted phenylalanine diet must be monitored regularly for adequate nutrition and growth, as well as for satisfactory phenylalanine concentration.

To avoid malnutrition, these patients must have fasting phenylalanine levels of >3 mg/dl, and probably at any level below 15 mg/dl the patient is safe from brain damage. If all treated infants are carefully followed, those who do not have true PKU will be identified by their better tolerance for phenylalanine, and, if their diet allocation is adjusted according to blood level, no infant on a restricted diet should suffer from malnutrition. Benign hyperphenylalaninemic infants can be withdrawn from the diet when it has been demonstrated that their blood phenylalanine does not rise above 20 mg/dl, even on a normal diet. Most high-grade proteins contain 5% to 7% phenylalanine; when other foods are offered to the growing infant, the diet is best calculated by an experienced dietician or nutritionist. The problem of when the diet can be safely discontinued is beyond the scope of this book.

High neonatal phenylalanine can be secondary to high tyrosine in prematurity, immature development of tyrosine enzymes, liver disease, or rare inherited errors of tyrosine metabolism. Mild hypertyrosinemia can be corrected in immaturity by large doses of vitamin C. When hypertyrosinemia persists, even in the absence of any definable disease, there is concern that mental development might be suppressed.[4,6]

Maple Syrup Urine Disease

The classic variant of this disease is associated with severe metabolic disturbances (Tables 28-2 and 28-3), which may require parenteral fluid and electrolyte therapy.[6-9] The princples of dietary treatment are the same as for PKU.[47,48] A synthetic amino acid mixture, low in the branched-chain amino acids, must be substituted for dietary protein. When an artificial diet is being given, attention must be paid to the intake of vitamins, essential fatty acids, and trace elements, in order to avoid malnutrition. Milder variants of maple syrup urine disease are easier to treat, and there is a thiamine-responsive variant that should be treated with large doses of the vitamin.

Methylmalonic acidemia

Methylmalonic acidemia, a disorder of organic acid metabolism, is characterized by severe metabolic ketoacidosis, hyperglycinemia, and occasionally hyperammonemia, which can be lethal in infants or can cause serious brain damage.[5] Patients with this disorder do not tolerate excesses of the amino acids—isoleucine, valine, threonine, and methionine—whose catabolism is slowed by an enzymatic block causing toxic metabolites to accumulate. Affected individuals should be given restricted protein or synthetic amino acid diets low in branched-chain amino acids. It is critical to adjust the dietary protein between an excess that may disturb metabolism and an inadequate intake that may interfere with nutrition. Also, a synthetic diet must be closely monitored for adequate intake of water, calories, vitamins, essential fatty acids, and trace elements. When hyperammonemia is a complication, therapeutic measures similar to those used in ornithine transcarbamylase deficiency must be followed.

Several variants of methylmalonic acidemic are caused by defective metabolism of vitamin B_{12} cofactors (Fig. 28-3, 9, 10). Patients with some of these variants improve markedly following pharmacologic doses of vitamin B_{12}, even with near normal dietary protein. Various enzyme cofactor treatments are also applicable in about 20 other various enzyme deficiency disorders.[45]

Ornithine Transcarbamylase Deficiency and Other Hyperammonemia Syndromes

Ornithine transcarbamylase deficiency is a sex-linked urea cycle defect which is characterized by severe hyperammonemia in male infants; it is usually a less severe condition in females (Fig. 28-4, 2). These patients have secondary oroticaciduria.[6]

When hyperammonemia of any etiology is extreme, no treatment will be effective. When it is moderately severe, the first approach is to reduce dietary intake of nitrogenous food. A growing infant requires at least 1.5 g protein/kg body weight daily. If this amount is not tolerated, the next measure is to reduce colonic reabsorption of ammonia by avoiding constipation and by acidifying colonic contents with lactulose, or by suppressing bacterial breakdown of urea of the colon with antibiotics or urease inhibitors.[11] Administration of acids may promote greater ammonia excretion in the urine and is worth trying as an adjunct to other procedures. Peritoneal dialysis and exchange transfusions have been tried as desperate measures for hyperammonemia or hepatic necrosis; hepatic transplant has not yet been attempted for this in newborn infants. The amino acid arginine may become growth-limiting in this condition, requiring supplementation as in citrullinemia, argininemia, and lysinuric protein intolerance.

Recent attempts at treating urea cycle enzyme defects with synthetic diets consisting of α-ketoacid or lactoacid analogues of the essential amono acids, aimed at decreasing nitrogenous amino acids while supplying the necessary carbon skeleton substrates, have been encouraging.[8] Greatest success has been achieved when the treatment was initiated presymptomatically in infants of families known to be at risk.

Oroticaciduria

This exceedingly rare disorder is an example of an inborn metabolic disease causing deficiency of an essential metabolite. There are defects in orotidylic pyrophosphorylase and orotidylic decarboxylase activities, blocking *de novo* synthesis of pyrimidines. Affected infants present with severe megaloblastic anemia and developmental retardation. Treatment with uridine dramatically reverses the deficiency, corrects the megaloblastic anemia, and may arrest or prevent brain damage, if started in time.[6]

Other Forms of Treatment

Besides the various modes of therapy described in the above examples, other metabolic disorders have been successfully treated by supplying essential products of altered metabolic steps such as thyroxine in hypothyroidism, cortisol in adrenogenital syndrome, or pancreatic enzymes in cystic fibrosis of the pancreas. Direct supplementation of a deficient enzyme with a highly purified normal enzyme has sometimes produced transient alleviation of biochemical abnormalities but has never altered clinical symptoms or disease progression. Current research efforts have been directed at "genetic engineering" or the introduction of normal genetic information into cells *in vitro,* with the ultimate hope of applying such techniques to cells *in vivo* in patients with enzymatic defects to induce production of normal enzymes.[49] Finally, the most universally applicable prevention for families with inborn errors of metabolism is genetic counseling.[17] This provides the family members with knowledge on their risks of bearing children with the same disorder and allows them to consider alternate family-planning options.

PRENATAL DIAGNOSIS

The reproductive options of many families at risk of having children with genetic or developmental defects has been widened by the possibility of fetal diagnostic tests in midpregnancy.[50] It is possible, by means of diagnostic ultrasound, to detect anencephaly by the end of the first trimester. Amniotic fluid can be safely obtained in the second trimester with negligible maternal risk and small obstetric risk of fetal loss. Amniotic fluid analysis for elevated α-fetoprotein will identify fetuses with major neural-tube malformations for parents who have had a child with spina bifida or anencephaly.[52,53] Other amniotic fluid proteins, blood group antigens or other cellular markers, such as histocompatibility factors (HL-A), can be used for linkage analysis because more and more genes are being localized onto chromosomes and linked to genes causing diseases[54] (*e.g.*, the adrenogenital syndrome, 21-hydroxylase deficiency, has been closely linked to the HL-A locus).[55] Viable fetal cells from the amniotic fluid can be cultured for chromosome karyotyping of the fetus, if advancing maternal age or familial chromosomal anomalies increase the risk of the fetus having chromosomal abnormalities.[56]

Biochemical testing of amniotic cell enzymes has already been used successfully to diagnose or to exclude specific enzyme disorders in families with known risks. For the sex-linked recessive disorders, even if no test is available for detecting an affected fetus, determination of the chromosomal sex allows a family with hemophilia, for instance, to select only female infants. The ability to obtain a few drops of fetal blood has augmented the number of genetic disorders diagnosable *in utero* to include hemophilia;[57] all of those detectable in erythrocytes, such as hemoglobinopathies;[58] and even those manifested in leukocytes.[59] Furthermore, direct analysis of DNA with the aid of restriction enzymes has opened up possibilities for determining the genetic status of the fetus for many more inherited disorders.[60,61]

REFERENCES

1. **Warkany J:** Congenital Malformations: Notes and Comments. Chicago, Year Book, 1971
2. **Smith DW:** Recognizable Patterns of Human Malformation, 2nd ed, Philadelphia, WB Saunders, 1976.
3. **Hers HG, Van Hoof F (eds):** Lysosomes and Storage Diseases. New York, Academic Press, 1973
4. **Hsia YE, Wolf B:** Disorders of amino acid metabolism. In Seigel GJ, Albers RW, Katzman R, Agranoff BW (eds): Basic Neurochemistry, 3rd ed. Boston, Little Brown, 1980
5. **Scriver CR, Rosenberg LE:** Amino Acid Metabolism and Its Disorders. Philadelphia, WB Saunders, 1973
6. **Stanbury JB, Wyngaarden JB, Fredrickson DS (eds):** The Metabolic Basis of Inherited Disease, 4th ed. New York, McGraw-Hill, 1978
7. **Bondy PK, Rosenberg LE (eds):** Duncan's Diseases of Metabolism, 7th ed. Philadelphia, WB Saunders, 1974
8. **Gardner L (ed):** Endocrine and Genetic Diseases of Childhood, 4th ed. Philadelphia, WB Saunders, 1975
9. **Nyhan WL (ed):** Heritable Disorders of Amino Acid Metabolism. New York, J Wiley, 1974
10. **Brock DJH, Mayo O (eds):** The Biochemical Genetics of Man. New York, Academic Press, 1978
11. **Hsia YE:** Inherited hyperammonemic syndromes. Gastroenterology 67:347, 1974
12. **Packman S, Mahoney MJ, Tanaka K, Hsia YE:** Severe hyperammonemia in a newborn with methylmalonyl CoA mutase deficiency. J Pediatr 92:769, 1978
13. **Buist NRM, Shaver BM:** A guide to screening newborn infants for inborn errors of metabolism. J Pediatr 85:511, 1973
14. **Holtzman NA:** Rare diseases, common problems: Recognition and management. Pediatrics 62:1056, 1978
15. **McKusick VA:** Mendelian Inheritance in Man: Catalogs of Autosomal Dominant, Autosomal Recessive, and X-linked Phenotypes, 5th ed. Baltimore, Johns Hopkins, 1978
16. **McKusick VA:** Heritable Disorders of Connective Tissue, 4th ed. St. Louis, CV Mosby, 1972
17. **Hsia YE, Hirschbern K, Silverberg RL, Godmilow L (eds):** Counseling in Genetics. New York, AR Liss, 1979

18. **Murphy EA, Chase GA:** Princples of Genetic Counseling. Chicago, Year Book, 1975
19. **Cornblath M, Schwartz R:** Disorders of Carbohydrate Metabolism in Infancy, 2nd ed. Philadelphia, WB Saunders, 1976
20. **Ballard RA, Vinocur B, Reynolds JW, Wennberg RP, Merritt A, Sweetman L, Nyhan WL:** Transient hyperammonemia of the preterm infant. N Engl J Med 299:920, 1978
21. **Oski FA, Naiman JL:** Hematologic Problems in the Newborn. Philadelphia, WB Saunders, 1972
22. **Moschella S, Pillsbury DM, Hurley H (eds):** Dermatology, 2nd ed. Philadelphia, WB Saunders, 1975
23. **Stiehm ER, Fulginiti VA (eds):** Immunologic Disorders in Infants and Children. Philadelphia, WB Saunders, 1973
24. **Legum CP, Schoor S, Berman ER:** The Genetic Mucopolysaccharidoses and Mucolipidoses: Review and comment. Adv Pediatr 24:305, 1976
25. **Kaufman HJ (ed):** Progress in Pediatric Radiology, Vol 4, Intrinsic Diseases of Bones. Basel, S Karger, 1973
26. **Taybi H:** Radiology of Syndromes. Chicago, Year Book Medical, 1975
27. **Rimoin D (ed):** Skeletal dysplasias. Clin Orthopod Related Res 114:2–179, 1976
28. **Bergsma D, Bron AJ, Cotlier E:** The eye and inborn errors of metabolism. Birth Defects Original Article Series XII: 3, New York, AR Liss, 1976
29. **Goldberg MF (ed):** Genetic and Metabolic Eye Disease. Boston, Little, Brown and Co, 1974
30. **Thomas GH, Howell RR:** Selected Screening Tests for Genetic Metabolic Diseases. Chicago, Year Book, 1973
31. **Hill A, Casey R, Zaleski WA:** Difficulties and pitfalls in the interpretation of screening tests for the detection of inborn errors of metabolism. Clin Chim Acta 72:1, 1976
32. **Burton BK, Nadler HL:** Clinical diagnosis of the inborn errors of metabolism in the neonatal period. Pediatrics 61:398, 1978
33. **Thomas GH, Scott CI:** Laboratory diagnosis of genetic disorders. Pediatr Clin North Am 20: 105, 1973
34. **Tanaka K:** Disorders of organic acid metabolism in biology of brain dysfunction. In Gaull GE (ed): Biology of Brain Dysfunction, vol 3, New York, Plenum, 1975
35. **Task Force on Genetic Screening:** The pediatrician and genetic screening (every pediatrician a geneticist). Pediatrics 58:757, 1976
36. **American Academy of Pediatrics Committee on Genetics:** Screening for congenital metabolic disorders in the newborn infant: congenital deficiency of thyroid hormone and hyperphenylalaninemia. Pediatrics 60:389, 1977
37. **Grover R, Wethess, D, Shahidi S, Gross M, Goldberg D, Davidow B:** Evaluation of the expanded newborn screening program in New York City. Pediatrics 61:740, 1978
38. **Milunsky A (ed):** The Prevention of Genetic Disease and Mental Retardation. Philadelphia, WB Saunders, 1975
39. New varieties of PKU. Lancet 1:304, 1979
40. **Levy HL, Sepe SJ, Shih VE, Vawter GF, Klein JO:** Sepsis due to Escherichia coli in neonates with galactosemia. N Engl J Med 297:825, 1977
41. **Crossley J, Elliott RB, Smith P:** Dried-blood spot screening for cystic fibrosis in the newborn. Lancet 1:472, 1972
42. **Breslow JL:** Pediatric aspects of hyperlipidemia. Pediatrics 62:510, 1978
43. **Fisher DA:** Neonatal Thyroid Screening. Pediatr Clin North Am 25:423, 1978
44. **Fisher DA, Dussault JH, Foley TP, Klein AH, LaFranchy S, Larsen PR, Mitchell MD, Murphey WH, Walfish PG:** Screening for congenital hypothyroidism: Results of screening one million North American infants. J Pediatr 94:700, 1979
45. **Rosenberg LE:** Vitamin-Responsive Inherited Metabolic Disorders. Adv Hum Genet 6:1, 1976
46. **Perlman M, Aker M, Slonim AE:** Successful treatment of severe type I glycogen storage disease with neonatal presentation by nocturnal intragastric feeding. J Pediatr 94:772, 1979
47. **Acosta PB, Elsas LJ:** Dietary Management of Inherited Metabolic Disease: Phenylketonuria, Galactosemia, Tyrosinemia, Homocystinuria, Maple Syrup Urine Disease. Atlanta, ACELMU, 1976
48. **American Academy of Pediatrics Committee on Nutrition:** Special diets for infants with inborn errors of amino acid metabolism. Pediatrics 57:783, 1976
49. **Sinsheimer RL:** Genetic engineering and gene therapy: Some implications. In Cohen BH, Lilienfeld AM, Huang PC (eds): Genetic Issues in Public Health and Medicine, p 439. Springfield, Thomas, 1978
50. **Golbus MS:** The prenatal diagnosis of genetic defects. In Caplan RM, Sweeney WJ (eds): Advances in Obstetrics and Gynecology, p 106. Baltimore, Williams & Wilkins, 1978
51. **Golbus MS, Loughman WD, Epstein CJ, Halbasch G, Stephens JD, Hall BD:** Prenatal genetic diagnosis in 3000 amniocenteses. N Engl J Med 300:157, 1979
52. **Brock DJH:** Biochemical and cytological methods in the diagnosis of neural tube defects. In Steinberg A, Bearn AG, Motulsky AG, Childs B (eds): Progress in Medical Genetics, II, p 1. Philadelphia, WB Saunders, 1977
53. **Crandall BF, Labherz TB, Freihube R:** Neural

Tube Defects: Maternal serum screening and prenatal diagnosis. Pediatr Clin North Am 25: 619, 1978

54. **Bergsma D (ed):** Human Gene Mapping. New York, Intercontinental Medical Book, 1974

55. **Dupont B, Oberfield SE, Smithwick EM, Lee TD, Levine LS:** Close genetic linkage between HLA and congenital adrenal hyperplasia (21-hydroxylase deficiency). Lancet 2:1309, 1977

56. **Yunis JJ (ed):** New Chromosomal Syndromes. New York, Academic Press, 1977

57. **Firshein SI, Hoyer LW, Lazarchick J, Forget BG, Hobbins JC, Clyne LP, Pitlick FA, Muir WR, Merkatz IR, Mahoney MJ:** Prenatal diagnosis of classic hemophilia. N Engl J Med 300:937, 1979

58. **Leonard CO, Kazazian HH:** Prenatal diagnosis of hemoglobinopathies. Pediatr Clin North Am 25:631, 1978

59. **Newburger PE, Cohen HJ, Rothchild SB, Hobbins JC, Malawista SE, Mahoney MJ:** Prenatal diagnosis of chronic granulomatous disease. N Engl J Med 300:178, 1979

60. **Wong V, Ma HK, Todd D, Golbus MS, Dozy AM, Kan YW:** Diagnosis of homozygous α-thalassemia in cultured amniotic-fluid fibroblasts. N Engl J Med 298:669, 1978

61. **Kan YW, Dozy AM:** Antenatal diagnosis of sickle-cell anemia by DNA analysis of amniotic-fluid cells. Lancet 2:910, 1978

29
Fluid and Electrolyte Management
William Oh

Fluid and electrolyte therapy constitutes one of the most commonly encountered clinical problems in the newborn period. In treating the common clinical disorders (*i.e.,* respiratory distress syndrome, sepsis, major surgical conditions, and so on), maintenance of normal fluid and electrolyte balance could influence the outcome of the underlying illness.

The goal of fluid and electrolyte management is to restore fluid and electrolyte losses resulting from an underlying pathology and to maintain that balance by appropriate calculation of parenteral or oral intake during the period of illness. The principle of fluid and electrolyte treatment in the neonatal period is similar to that established for older children, except for some variations and specific features of body composition, physiologic water and electrolyte losses such as insensible water loss, and the neuroendocrine control of fluid and electrolyte balance.

Another major consideration in handling fluid and electrolyte problems in the neonate is the relative limitation of some renal functions, particularly in preterm, low-birth-weight infants, which leaves less room for error in the calculation. Therefore, to appropriately manage the parenteral fluid therapy in the neonate, the clinician should have the funda-mental knowledge of normality in the newborn infant regarding body composition, insensible water loss, neuroendocrine control of water and electrolyte balance, and renal function. In addition, he should develop a system of approach so that the handling of the fluid and electrolyte problem is a combination of mathematical calculation of fluid and electrolyte for replacement of deficit, and provision of intake to balance outgo, along with clinical assessments to monitor the appropriate response to treatment.

BODY COMPOSITION IN THE FETAL AND NEONATAL PERIOD

Changes in Body Fluid During Growth. The total body water (TBW) is conventionally divided into two major compartments: intracellular (ICW) and extracellular (ECW). The ECW is further divided into interstitial fluid compartment and intravascular compartment, which represents plasma volume. Figure 29-1 shows the approximate distribution of body fluid in the various compartments in an infant at term.

In the early stages of fetal development, water constitutes a large portion of the body composition.[1] It has been estimated that TBW is high: 94% of the body weight during the

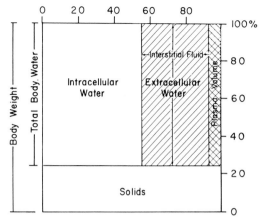

Fig. 29-1. Percentage distribution of body fluid in a term newborn.

third month of fetal life. As the gestational age increases, the TBW gradually declines, so that if a fetus is born prematurely at 32-weeks' gestation, the TBW is approximately 80%, and at term the TBW decreases to about 78% (Fig. 29-2). The changes in extracellular water (ECW) and intracellular water (ICW) during growth also assume certain characteristics. ECW decreases from 60% body weight at the fifth month of fetal life to about 45% at term, and ICW increases from 25% in the fifth month of fetal life to approximately 33% at birth.

A contraction of ECW normally occurs during the first few days of life. In low-birth-weight infants, 32 to 34 weeks of gestation, the ECW declines from 45% to 39% at the end of the first week of life.[2] This reduction of ECW is accompanied by an improvement in renal function.[3] Appropriate fluid and electrolyte intakes should allow for the normal transition of body fluid from fetal to neonatal status; if fluid and/or electrolyte overloading takes place during the first week, ECW may remain expanded and can be associated with certain undesirable clinical complications, such as congestive heart failure secondary to patent ductus arteriosus with left-to-right shunt[4] and necrotizing enterocolitis.[5]

Characteristics of Solute Distribution in Body Fluid. As shown in Figure 29-3, the major cation in the plasma is sodium. Potassium, calcium, and magnesium constitute the balance of the cation fraction. The anion is primarily chloride, with protein, bicarbonate and some undetermined anion constituting the smaller

fraction of the total anions. The interstitial fluid has a similar solute composition to that of the plasma except that its protein content is lower. The ICW contains K^+ and Mg^+ as its primary cations, while organic phosphate and inorganic phosphate are the major anions, with bicarbonate contributing a smaller fraction.

The electrolyte composition in the body fluid of the newborn infant also largely depends on the gestational age. Per unit body weight, a preterm, low-birth-weight infant has a larger extracellular ion content than a term infant simply on the basis of larger ECW. Conversely, the ICW electrolyte content is lower in a preterm infant because of a smaller ICW. These concepts are important considerations when calculating electrolyte losses and replacement and during parenteral fluid therapy.

Because fetal fluid and electrolyte balance *in utero* also depends on the maternal homeostasis and placental exchange, the neonatal fluid and electrolyte status at birth is influenced significantly by the maternal fluid and electrolyte state. For instance, it is well recognized that maternal hyponatremia during labor may result in hyponatremia in the newborn infant as well.[6]

Insensible Water Loss in the Neonatal Period

Data on insensible water loss (IWL) in newborn infants has been well established by several authors. Because of differences in methodology, technique, and study designs,

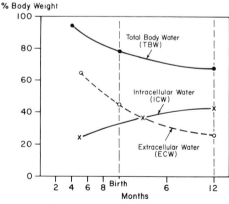

Fig. 29-2. Changes in body fluid during fetal and neonatal life. (Data modified from those of Friis-Hansen B: Pediatrics [Suppl] 47:264, 1971, copyright American Academy of Pediatrics, 1971)

the normal values have ranged from 0.7 to 1.6 ml/kg/hour.[7,10,13,14] There is also a considerable degree of controversy as to the appropriate unit of expressing IWL. Theoretically, caloric expenditure is the ideal reference unit for IWL, because the latter depends entirely on the evaporative heat loss through the skin and respiratory tract. Because heat loss is also closely related to body weight and surface area, most studies in the past have used these two parameters as units of expressing IWL. However, Sinclair and coworkers have recently shown that within the range of 1 to 4 kg body weight, the systematic variations in expressing the metabolic rate on the basis of body weight or surface area are significant and that the least degree of error is achieved when the calculation of metabolic rate is based on body weight minus extracellular fluid.[8] At any rate, for practical purposes, body weight would still be the most desirable parameter for expressing IWL and heat expenditure.

Several factors may increase the IWL in infants while others may reduce it. Recent studies have confirmed that the IWL is inversely proportional to birth weight or gestational age (Fig. 29-4).[9,10] The reasons for the greater IWL in very low-birth-weight infants include increased permeability of the skin epidermis to water, larger body surface area

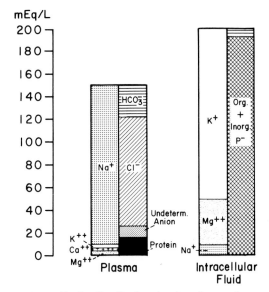

Fig. 29-3. Ionic distribution in the plasma (representing extracellular fluid) and in the intracellular fluid compartment.

per unit of weight, and greater skin blood flow relative to metabolic rate. Although not proven beyond doubt, it has been suggested that the higher respiratory rate in the low-birth-weight infant may partially account for the higher IWL. Hyperthemia increases the IWL by in-

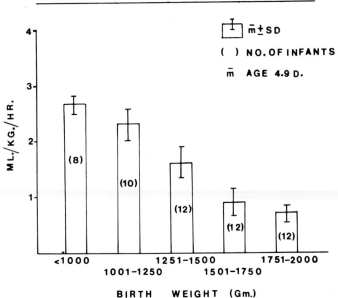

Fig. 29-4. Inverse correlation between insensible water loss and body weight. (Wu PYK et al: Pediatrics 54:704, 1974, copyright American Academy of Pediatrics, 1974)

Table 29-1. Factors Affecting Insensible Water Loss in Newborn Infants.

	Changes in IWL
Level of maturity[10]	Inversely proportional to birth weight and gestation (Fig. 29-4)
Respiratory distress	Probably increased, but no precise data available
Ambient temperature above the neutral thermal zone[7,11]	Increment proportional to the increase in ambient temperature above the neutral zone
Elevated body temperature[7]	Up to three- fourfold increase above 37°C
High relative humidity[7]	Reduction of 30%
Activity[14]	1.7-fold increase above basal value
Use of radiant warmer[10,12]	50% increase
Use of phototherapy[10,13]	50% increase

creasing metabolic rate; more recently it has also been shown that elevation of ambient temperature $\geq 1°C$ above the range of neutral thermal environment will result in a significant increase in IWL. The study by Bell and co-workers has shown that keeping the ambient thermal environment 1°C above the range of thermal neutrality in low-birth-weight infants results in an increment in IWL through an increase in evaporative heat loss. Oxygen consumption (heat production) was unchanged. In contrast, an ambient thermal environment of 1°C below the range of thermal neutrality results in no change of IWL in spite of a significant increase in oxygen consumption. Under a cooler environment, the infant increases his heat production to maintain body temperature, and reduces his heat loss by the evaporative route because the nonevaporative heat loss is accelerated on the basis of a greater thermal gradient between the skin, air, and incubator walls. This series of observations clearly demonstrates the close relationship between ambient thermal environment and fluid and energy balance in infants.

Use of a radiant warmer[12] and phototherapy[13] also increases IWL by about 50% of basal values. The mechanism is simply an increase of heat expenditures (including evaporative heat loss) when radiant energy is absorbed by infants subjected to phototherapy or who are nursed under a radiant warmer. In addition, peripheral blood flow increases during phototherapy,[15,16] and the radiant warmer

may also participate in this mechanism. A recent study showed that infants nursed in a radiant warmer and treated with phototherapy tripled their IWL when compared with the values obtained when they are maintained in an incubator with neutral thermal environment, not receiving phototherapy.[18]

Factors that may reduce IWL include the use of a heat shield, high relative humidity in the ambient environment, and placement of the infant under assisted ventilation with humidified gas. Heat shields reduce IWL by half in low-birth-weight infants but not in large-sized infants.[9,17] High ambient relative humidity reduces IWL by 30%,[7] and in a ventilator, when the inspired air is properly warmed and humidified (which is mandatory for proper respiratory care), the evaporative water loss through the respiratory tract can be completely eliminated, hence reducing the IWL. Table 29-1 summarizes these factors.

It becomes obvious that in calculating maintenance fluid for infants with various clinical conditions and environmental factors, the amount of IWL will vary and should be modified accordingly. This consideration becomes more critical when the infant's fluid intake is solely derived from parenteral route.

Endocrine Control of Fluid and Electrolyte Balance

Pituitary gland (antidiuretic hormone), adrenal cortex (mineralocorticoids), and parathyroid glands are the three major endocrine organs that regulate the water and electrolyte balance in the body fluid. In the human newborn, the pattern of antidiuretic hormone (ADH) secretion and metabolism is not well established. Indirect evidence, based on data obtained by water deprivation and loading, suggest that neonates can regulate water balance by means of ADH control in the same manner as adults do, although within a certain physiologic limitation. For instance, the urinary concentrating mechanism of a newborn infant is limited to the maximum of 800 mosm/l upon water deprivation, while in the adult, urine concentration of 1200 mosm/l can be achieved on the same challenge.[19] On water loading, the newborn infant can attain its maximal diluting mechanism only at 5 days of age or older.[20] It is not clear whether ADH deficiency or inadequate renal tubular function is the primary reason for the lack of appropriate concentrating and diluting response to water deprivation or loading, although it is conceivable that both hormonal and end-organ factors are responsible for such a phenomenon. (See below for further discussion.)

The role of mineralocorticoids such as aldosterone in the regulation of electrolyte balance, particularly sodium, has been reported recently by several workers. Beitins and coworkers demonstrated the high level of serum aldosterone in the neonate;[21] in preterm, low-birth-weight infants, a feedback mechanism between Na intake, Na excretion and serum aldosterone level is intact and appropriate.[22]

Data on serum parathyroid hormone levels in the newborn infant are lacking. However, studies on calcium and phosphate balance suggest that newborn infants may have relative and transient hypoparathyroidism,[23] accounting for the frequent occurrence of hypocalcemia in infants associated with high-risk factors such as diabetic pregnancy, toxemia, and in preterm, low-birth-weight infants with respiratory distress syndrome.[24] (Also see Chap. 27.)

Renal Functions in Relation to Fluid and Electrolyte Therapy

For many years, it has been largely assumed that the renal function of the newborn infant is immature[25] and that this limitation in renal function contributes significantly to the problem in the proper homeostasis of fluid and electrolyte in disease state. Recent work further demonstrates that the renal function in neonates depends on the gestational age, and its efficiency is appropriate for the homeostatic environment it has during intrauterine existence.[25] The overall glomerular and tubular functional status is capable of handling some physiologic variations in fluid and electrolyte load but imbalance may occur when given an overwhelming challenge.

PRINCIPLES OF FLUID AND ELECTROLYTE THERAPY

As in older children, three essential steps should be followed in the treatment of infants with fluid and electrolyte disorders.

1. Estimate the quantity of fluid and electrolyte losses.
2. Calculate fluid and electrolyte for replacement of losses, maintenance, and replacement of current abnormal losses.
3. Institute a system of monitoring the adequacy of therapy.

Estimate of Fluid Loss. Fluid loss is conveniently estimated on the basis of degree of dehydration. If sequential data on body weight are available, a reduction in body weight during a short period of time will generally provide an accurate assessment of the degree of dehydration. In this context, it should be pointed out that during the first week to 10 days of life, a 5% to 10% reduction in body weights should be considered normal because it represents the normal contraction of body fluid and tissue breakdown during a catabolic state. Hence, during the first week of life, dehydration is considered when weight loss exceeds 10% to 15% of the birth weight.

In the absence of body weight data, clinical evaluation of physical signs may provide an approximate estimation of degree of dehydration, particularly in cases of isotonic dehydration. Dry skin, dry mucous membranes, and a slightly sunken fontanel are signs of 5% dehydration; loose abdominal skin turgor, a markedly sunken fontanel and eyeballs, severe oliguria, and signs of circulatory insufficiency (*i.e.*, tachycardia, mottled skin, hypotension) are evidence of 10% dehydration; clinical signs of shock and generally a moribund-looking infant usually indicate 15% dehydration.

Calculation of Fluid Deficit for Replacement. Fluid deficit is calculated on the basis of estimated degree of dehydration. If an accurate weight change has been obtained during the

Table 29-2. Calculation of Total Solute Deficits.

Type of Dehydration	Plasma Na (mmol/l)	Calculation for Solute Deficit*	Solute† (mosm)	Deficit/kg Na⁺ (mmol)	K⁺ (mmol)
Isotonic	140	$(0.7 \times 280) - (0.6 \times 280)$	28	14	14
Hypotonic	127	$(0.7 \times 280) - (0.6 \times 254)$	44	22	22
Hypertonic	153	$(0.7 \times 280) - (0.6 \times 306)$	12	6	6

* Solute deficit = $[TBW_e \text{ (l)} \times solute_e \text{ (mosm/L)}] - [TBW_o \text{ (l)} \times solute_o \text{ (mosm/L)}]$ where subscript $_e$ and $_o$ are *expected* and *observed* respectively. $TBW_e = 0.7$ l/kg, $TBW_o = 10\%$ deficit or $0.7 - 0.1 = 0.6$ l/kg, $solute_e = 140 \times 2 = 280$ mosm/l, assuming total solute = twice the plasma Na concentration, $solute_o$ = observed plasma Na $\times$ 2.
† Total solute deficit is equally divided between Na⁺ and K⁺.

dehydration periods, the difference in weight can be considered as the amount of fluid deficit. If such an observation is unavailable, the use of clinical signs for the estimation of percentage of dehydration will suffice. The rapidity of deficit replacement depends on the severity of the dehydration. As a rule, dehydration of acute onset and of short duration requires a more rapid correction and vice versa. The exception to this rule is found in the case of hypertonic dehydration in which an exceedingly rapid expansion of body fluid may result in convulsions.

Estimate of Electrolyte Loss. The nature and extent of electrolyte disturbances along with fluid disorders can often be determined by a carefully obtained clinical history and physical examination, and by measurement of serum electrolytes. Using serum Na values as the criteria, the type of electrolyte disturbance is divided into isotonic or isonatremic (serum sodium within normal range of 136–143 mmol/l), hypotonic or hyponatremic (serum Na <130 mmol/l) and hypertonic or hypernatremic (serum Na >150 mmol/l). Electrolyte disorders depend on the nature of the underlying causes of fluid and solute abnormalities. For instance, severe diarrhea usually leads to isotonic dehydration; prolonged febrile illness with diarrhea, and inappropriate use of milk formula are common causes of hypertonic dehydration; and inappropriate parenteral fluid administration, central nervous system diseases, and fluid overload to the mother prior to the delivery of the infant are frequently associated with hypotonic dehydration.

In addition, physical signs may provide a lead to the type of dehydration present (*e.g.*, doughy and thickened skin turgor in hypertonic

dehydration), and the diagnosis can be confirmed by serum electrolyte determination. With the current availability of micromethods, electrolyte determinations are feasible even in the infants of smallest size. It also should be stressed that in neonates with severe underlying pathology such as sepsis, respiratory distress syndrome, and so on, the clinical signs, particularly those related to central nervous system manifestations, may not be readily discernible. Therefore, it is of utmost importance that serum electrolytes be determined before initial fluid therapy and be serially monitored during the course of treatment.

Calculation of Electrolyte Deficit for Replacement. Electrolyte deficit is calculated on the basis of the difference in expected total body solute before dehydration and the observed total body solute during the dehydrated state. Examples of such calculations in isotonic, hypotonic, and hypertonic dehydration are listed in Table 29-2. It is a common practice to replace half or two-thirds of the estimated deficit within the first 24-hours of therapy and the balance during the second 24 hours of therapy. It is also important to refrain from adding potassium to the parenteral solution until the infant has established urinary flow.

Fluid and Electrolyte Maintenance. IWL, urinary water loss, stool water loss, and water for tissue growth are the four components to be considered in calculating the daily maintenance fluid requirement. Stool water loss averages approximately 10 ml/kg/day, while water for tissue growth is about 20 ml/kg/day (assuming 70% of 30 g/kg/day new tissue [average weight gain in growth] is water). In the first 10 days of life, stool water loss is minimal and the infant is not in the growth phase.

Therefore, the two main components that need to be accounted for are IWL and urinary water loss.

In a full-term infant under basal conditions, IWL is approximately 20 ml/kg/day.[7] Urinary water loss will depend on the amount of solutes to be excreted through the kidney and the urinary concentration. In most term infants receiving parenteral fluid administration, we provide 10% glucose and 2 to 3 mmol/kg/day of Na and K, which would provide a solute load of approximately 15 mosm/kg/day. Because urinary concentration in the newborn infant generally ranges from 280 to 300 mosm/l, an allowance of approximately 50 ml/kg/day of fluid for the formation of urine would be appropriate. Hence, in a term infant, the initial fluid prescription for maintenance would be 70 ml/kg/day during the first day and increase to 80, 90, and 120 ml/kg/day on days 3, 5, and 7 respectively. The increment is to fulfill the requirement generated by increasing solute load and the amount of water loss by an increasing volume of stool. In older, orally fed infants, the maintenance fluid requirement is between 120 and 150 ml/kg/day because of a larger solute intake and the water requirement for growth.

In low-birth-weight infants, the maintenance fluid requirement is larger because of a higher IWL. The inverse correlation between IWL and birth weight (and gestational age) has been well documented (Fig. 29-4).[10] Therefore, the IWL component of the maintenance fluid should be increased proportionately with decreasing birth weight or gestation.

In infants cared for under a radiant warmer or receiving phototherapy, the allowance for IWL should also be increased by 50% of its basal values. The combination of both increases the IWL by 100%.[18] Elevation of ambient temperature above the range of thermal neutrality,[26] also increases the IWL significantly.[11,27] Therefore, one of the important aspects in maintaining IWL within a normal range is to constantly focus attention on appropriate temperature control, maintaining the incubator temperature within the neutral thermal zone.

It should be pointed out that there are a number of factors that may reduce the IWL: use of a plastic heat shield can reduce IWL by 50% in the low-birth-weight infant,[9] and, if the infant is being artificially ventilated, the warmed and fully humidified inspired air in the respirator will completely eliminate the respiratory component (30%) of the IWL.

In infants with perinatal asphyxia, it is highly desirable to maintain a low fluid intake during the first 24 to 48 hours of life in anticipation of the potential development of acute renal insufficiency as a result of renal injury or inappropriate ADH secretion, the latter as a consequence of central nervous system injury. Both conditions may result in oliguria and anuria—hence the fluid restriction. The fluid prescription can be revised upward when normal urinary flow is established during the second and third day of life.

The electrolyte requirements for maintenance primarily involve Na^+, K^+, and Cl^-, and these represent the amount of loss through the kidney and in the stool. Based on balance study data, this amount is constant and similar to those of older infants at 2 to 3 mmol/kg/24 hours for each of the elements.

Example of Fluid and Electrolyte Calculation. A 3 kg infant is admitted with 10% isotonic dehydration (serum Na = 140 mmol/l). The formula may be used to calculate fluid and electrolyte intake for the first 24 hours of therapy (Table 29-3).

This fluid formula can be given to the infant by adding 48 mmol NaCl into 600 ml of 5% glucose in water, with addition of KCl as soon as the infant voids. The repair of intracellular potassium deficit may be done at a slower rate (over a 48-hour period). If the infant also has a significant metabolic acidosis, the Na^+ can be given in the form of Na lactate or bicarbonate and the chloride can be given in the form of KCl.

Concurrent Abnormal Losses. It is important that current abnormal losses be replaced during the course of parenteral fluid therapy. This usually involves accurate collection and estimation of abnormal fluid losses, such as vomiting, diarrhea, bile, or ileostomy drainage. The fluid replacement should correspond to the estimated amount of fluid loss. Solute replacement should correspond to the estimated solute content of the fluid loss. The approximate electrolyte content of each kind of drainage is listed in Table 29-4.

Monitoring the Effectiveness of Parenteral Fluid Therapy. During the course of parenteral

Table 29-3. Calculation of Fluid and Electrolyte Intake.

	Water (ml)	Na$^+$ (mmol)	K$^+$ (mmol)
Maintenance	300	6	6
	(100 ml/kg × 3 kg)		(2 mmol/kg)
Deficit			
Fluid	300		
	(0.10 × 3 kg)		
Solute		42	42
		3(0.7 × 280) − 3(0.6 × 280) = 84	
		(equally divided between Na$^+$ and K$^+$)	
Concurrent Loss =	0	0	0
(*Assuming none*)			
Totals	600	48	48

fluid therapy, detailed and organized data collection can clearly reflect the effectiveness of treatment. Data to be collected at a designated interval should include intake, output, body weight changes, urinary specific gravity (or osmolarity), serum electrolyte including blood urea nitrogen, and clinical assessment for the presence of edema, dehydration, or evidence of acute water overload. The interrelationships among the various parameters are shown in Figure 29-5. Frequent causes of inadequate fluid administration are underestimation of fluid requirement for maintenance, and neglect in replacing the abnormal concurrent losses during the therapy period. These factors will result in the reduction of urine volume, increase in urine specific gravity and, if these compensatory steps are inadequate, a significant weight loss and clinical signs of dehydration. If an excessive amount of fluid is administered, the urine volume will be high and the urine specific gravity low. If these compensations are tested to the maximum, fluid retention will take place resulting in edema and weight gain. If the rate of overhydration is rapid, pulmonary edema and congestive heart failure may occur, particularly in ill neonates with underlying cardiopulmonary disorders.

Urinary specific gravity is a convenient and accurate approximation of urinary solute excretion. An exception to the rule would be in cases of significant glycosuria in which a high specific gravity may be observed, reflecting the presence of glucose rather than electrolytes. Specific gravity should be determined at 6- to 8-hour intervals with the use of a reflectometer.

Stationary weight or appropriate weight gain when deficit therapy is being instituted, no clinical evidence of fluid overload such as edema or congestive heart failure, and maintenance of urinary specific gravity at 1.008 to 1.012 would indicate success in maintaining fluid balance. Serial daily serum electrolyte determinations would provide evidence of electrolyte balance (or imbalance).

During the first week of life, a 5% to 10% weight loss is considered physiologic and is partly the allowance for the normal contraction of the extracellular fluid. Therefore, in using weight changes as an index for fluid balance, a weight loss of 1% to 2% per day should be considered normal. In fact, a rigid insistence on maintaining a zero weight (or fluid) balance during the first week of life may lead to fluid overload.

Table 29-4. Electrolyte Content of Various Fluids.

Fluid	Na	K (mmol/l)	Cl
Gastric	20–80	5–20	100–150
Small intestine	100–140	5–15	90–120
Bile	120–140	5–15	90–120
Ileostomy	45–135	3–15	20–120
Diarrheal stool	10–90	10–80	10–110

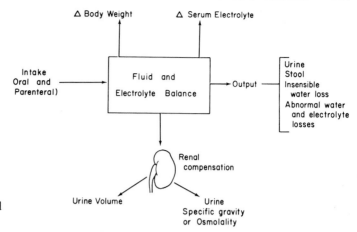

Fig. 29-5. A system of monitoring fluid and electrolyte therapy.

Acid-Base Balance

The buffer system (primarily bicarbonate and its weak acid counterpart, carbonic acid), renal and respiratory compensations, are the three major mechanisms responsible for the maintenance of normal acid base equilibrium in the body fluids. H^+ changes in the body fluid follow the Henderson–Hasselbalch equation:

$$pH = 6.1 + \log \frac{HCO_3^-}{H_2CO_3 \text{ or } (S.P_{CO_2})}$$

where 6.1 is the pK constant of carbonic acid, $S.P_{CO_2}$ the amount of CO_2 dissolved in the body fluid which is nearly equivalent to the amount of total weak acid (H_2CO_3). It can be seen from this formula that any increase or reduction of $^-HCO_3$ fraction in the buffer pair will result in alkalosis or acidosis respectively. Because H_2CO_3 is interchangeably related to P_{CO_2} under the constant influence of a catalyst, carbonic anhydrase, any alteration in P_{CO_2} in the body fluid would also alter the pH values. Hence, hyperventilation with reduction of P_{CO_2} will result in **respiratory alkalosis,** and hypoventilation with hypercarbia will result in **respiratory acidosis.**

A good example of respiratory alkalosis is that of an infant who is hyperventilated by a mechanical ventilator (respirator). In respiratory distress syndrome, the respiratory component of the acidosis is caused by retention of CO_2 in the body fluid as a result of pulmonary insufficiency. **Metabolic acidosis** is also seen in respiratory distress syndrome as a result of significant lactic acidemia, the latter as a result of anaerobic metabolism under hypoxemic conditions. An excellent example of metabolic alkalosis is that of infants with congenital pyloric stenosis. In the latter cases, the abnormal loss of gastric contents by persistent vomiting results in a marked excess of bicarbonate content in the body fluids in amounts exceeding the bicarbonate excreting capacity of the kidney.

In all instances of acid-base disturbance, a compensatory mechanism takes place either by the lung or by the kidney. If the compensatory mechamism is adequate, the pH value may be normalized at the expense of an altered bicarbonate or carbonic acid concentration. In this instance, the acid-base disturbances are termed *compensated*. For instance, if a neonate with respiratory distress syndrome has the following acid base values: pH = 7.38, P_{CO_2} = 32 torr, bicarbonate content = 15 mmol/l, and base deficit = −10 mmol/l, the acid base status would be considered compensated metabolic acidosis. Hyperventilation results in lower P_{CO_2} compensation for the reduced bicarbonate content (base deficit), hence normalizing the pH values.

SPECIFIC CLINICAL CONDITIONS WITH FLUID AND ELECTROLYTE PROBLEMS

Respiratory Distress Syndrome (Hyaline Membrane Disease). Earlier studies by Cort have shown that in respiratory distress syndrome (RDS), the renal functions are markedly reduced and that hyperkalemia and hyperphosphatemia are common occurences.[28] More recent observations, however, seem to indicate

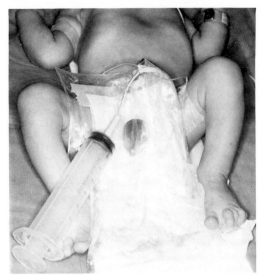

Fig. 29-6. Urine collection in infant using a pediatric urine collector.

that if the cardiorespiratory status is kept within the physiologic range, the renal functions in RDS infants are comparable to non-RDS infants within the same range of gestational age.[29] Also, with appropriate fluid and electrolyte management by the parenteral route, there is less likelihood of hyperkalemia, hyperphosphatemia, and azotemia.

The parenteral solution should include fluid and electrolyte for maintenance, taking into consideration the variable requirement for IWL as a result of the infant's physiologic and pathologic status and environment. Because RDS affects almost exclusively preterm infants, the IWL is high and should be appropriately accounted for.

Because limitation in renal concentration capability is characteristic of preterm infants with or without RDS, it is apparent that adequate fluid intake is essential to maintain an appropriate fluid balance. The precise volumes required will vary from one infant to another depending on the gestation, birth weight, presence or absence of perinatal asphyxia, environmental factors (*e.g.*, radiant warmer versus incubator), and all the factors cited previously that may affect the fluid requirement of preterm infants. In general, an infant weighing 1500 g with RDS, but without perinatal asphyxia, who is being cared for in an incubator would receive a fluid volume of 80 ml/kg during the first day as a 5% to 10% glucose solution. This

will fulfill the requirement for IWL (35–40 ml/kg/day) and urinary water loss (40–45 ml/kg/day for solute load of 10 mosm/kg/day). The amount of fluid administration in the subsequent days should be guided by a careful monitoring of intake, output, body weight changes, urine specific gravity, and serum electrolyte determinations. To assure a reasonably accurate parenteral fluid intake, a calibrated infusion pump should be used. For urine collection, a pediatric urine collector may be used in the larger preterm infant. To avoid skin irritation and excoriation from frequent changing of the urine collector, the urine can be aspirated from the collector from time to time for volume determination through a feeding tube placed within the urine bag (Fig. 29-6). In very small male infants in whom urine collector application is impractical, an appropriate size test tube may be fitted onto the penis for urine collection (Fig. 29-7).

Urine volumes, urine specific gravity, and changes in body weight are the three important guidelines for fluid calculation. During the first week of life, the infant should lose approximately 10 to 20 g/kg/day of weight. If, at the same time, the urine volume and specific gravity are within the normal range (40–50 ml/kg/day and 1.008–1.012, respectively), the fluid intake of the previous 24 hours can be continued for the next 24 hours. Day-to-day adjustment of the fluid intake may be made according to these three parameters.

Moderate to severe forms of RDS are as-

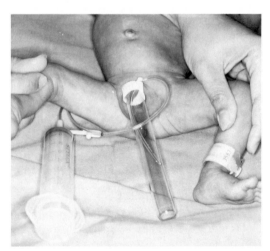

Fig. 29-7. Urine collection in a small preterm male infant using an appropriate size test tube.

sociated with significant incidence of congestive heart failure and pulmonary edema from left-to-right shunt across the patent ductus arteriosus (PDA).[30,31] It has further been shown that fluid overload may enhance the occurrence of this complication.[32] Bell and associates, in a randomized study, showed that a high fluid intake significantly increase the incidence of PDA and left-to-right shunt. This study clearly emphasizes the importance of careful monitoring of fluid and electrolyte intake in high-risk infants to avoid significant cardiopulmonary complications.

During the first 12 to 24 hours of life, it is usually not necessary to add Na to the parenteral fluid, particularly if it is anticipated that Na bicarbonate may be used for the treatment of metabolic acidosis. Potassium supplementation (2 mmol/kg/24 hr) should be added as soon as the infant voids unless serum K^+ is elevated. Sodium (in the form of NaCl) should be added starting on the second day of age at a dose of 1 to 2 mmol/kg/24 hours.

Serial serum electrolyte determinations should be done at 24- to 48-hour intervals. Hyperkalemia may occasionally occur; in such instances, supplemental K in the parenteral fluid should be discontinued until the serum K level returns to normal range. Correction of hypernatremia or hyponatremia (if they occur) has been described below.

RDS is commonly associated with a combined respiratory and metabolic acidosis resulting from hypercarbia and lactic acidemia respectively. In severe RDS, when the acidosis is predominantly respiratory, some form of assisted ventilation should be instituted. On the other hand, if the acidosis is primarily metabolic, Na bicarbonate (0.9M $NaHCO_3$) may be used as a buffer to correct the acidotic state. The dose of $NaHCO_3$ should be calculated on the basis of the following formula:

dose of $NaHCO_3$ (mmol)
    = base deficit (mmol/l) $\times$ body weight $\times$ 0.4.

The common clinical practice is to calculate the base deficit from the pH and Pa_{CO_2} by using an appropriate nomogram.[33] Base deficit may also be derived from a known pH and plasma CO_2 content or bicarbonate concentration. The 0.4 value in the formula represents the bicarbonate space which is confined mostly to the extracellular fluid compartment. It should be noted that there is some disagreement on the true bicarbonate space, the values ranging from 0.3 to 0.6 of body weight.

The calculated $NaHCO_3$ dose may be given intravenously at a rate of 1 mmol/min or by slow infusion over a 2- to 3-hour period. If the bolus infusion is chosen, it is advisable to utilize a half-strength solution by diluting an equal volume of 0.9M $NaHCO_3$ with sterile water. The slow infusion with diluted $NaHCO_3$ may lessen the risk of sudden osmolar changes in the intravascular and extracellular fluid compartment,[34] which have been implicated as causing the increased incidence of intracranial hemorrhage in infants given a large dose of $NaHCO_3$.[35]

The data purporting to show beneficial effects of $NaHCO_3$ in treating infants with RDS is still controversial.[36–39] Table 29-5 compares the four studies that addressed this question; the answer is at best equivocal. Therefore, the current approach is not to treat RDS with aggressive $NaHCO_3$ therapy, but rather to treat significant metabolic acidosis (pH $\leq$ 7.20) with an appropriate dose of $NaHCO_3$, at the rate and by the method of infusion cited above.

Because of its buffering effect on the carbon dioxide, Tris (hydroxymethyl) aminomethane (THAM) has been suggested for treating respiratory acidosis. However, the effect of THAM on reducing plasma CO_2 is at most transient and would require a large continuous dose of THAM to effectively neutralize the CO_2 accumulated as a result of respiratory insufficiency. The dose needed to accomplish this would far exceed the therapeutic safety of THAM. Furthermore, because of its corrosive quality, local tissue sloughing may occur if subcutaneous infiltration takes place. Hence, in treating acidosis of RDS, THAM is generally not used.

Congenital Pyloric Stenosis. The magnitude of fluid and electrolyte disturbance in congenital pyloric stenosis depends entirely on the duration and severity of its main symptomatology, vomiting. In severe and persistent vomiting, the electrolyte abnormality is usually that of hypochloremic alkalosis and hypokalemia. Studies have shown that in infants with severe vomiting caused by congenital pyloric stenosis, intracellular Na is increased and K is decreased.[40] The intracellular K deficiency is frequently reflected in the form of low serum K. An ECG may also show evidence of intracellular hypopotassemia with depressed and

Table 29-5. Comparison of Studies to Evaluate the Effects of Alkali Therapy on Premature Infants with RDS.

Authors	N	Gestation (weeks)	Birth Wt. (g)	Study Design and Mode of Therapy	Beneficial effect on neonatal mortality
Usher R	70	32	1745	All study infants had RDS. Experimental group received intravenous glucose beginning at 3 hr and slow infusion of sodium bicarbonate to maintain pH at 7.3–7.4.	Yes
Sinclair J	20	30	1305	Infants with RDS were randomized into four groups: one group control and each of the other three groups received either unlimited oxygen, alkali, or respirator.	No
Hobel CJ	90	37	1300–2250	Infants with acidosis (pH < 7.25 at 30 min of age) were randomized into early (< 30 min) or late (> 2½ hr) treatment with sodium bicarbonate. Other treatment protocols were comparable.	Improved only in infant weighing between 1000–1500 g
Corbett A	62	30–32	1500	Randomized assignment into liberal and restricted sodium bicarbonate therapy.	No

wide T waves and prolongation of S-T segment. These infants usually appear chronically dehydrated and emaciated; the metabolic alkalosis leads to lethargy, stridor, shallow and slow respiration, and, in some cases, tetany. Serum electrolyte determination reveals in addition to low K, a high pH (>7.50), low chloride (<90 mmol/l), and elevated bicarbonate or CO_2 content; serum Na level may be within normal range.

Parenteral therapy consists of fluid replacement of calculated deficit and maintenance. The chloride deficit should be corrected with the use of NaCl. When the infant's urination is established, KCl should be added to the parenteral fluid. Specific treatment of the metabolic alkalosis with such agents as NH_3Cl is usually not necessary. In most instances, cessation of vomiting by withholding oral intake, correction of dehydration, and replacement of Cl and K deficits by providing NaCl and KCl respectively will restore the blood pH value to within a normal range. Complete correction of intracellular electrolyte abnormalities, particularly the K deficit, may take 7 to 10 days. However, surgical correction of the congenital pyloric stenosis is advisable following 24 to 48 hours of parenteral fluid therapy in order to avoid prolonged starvation.

Diarrhea Dehydration. The principle of parenteral fluid therapy for diarrheal dehydration in the neonate is generally similar to that of older infants and children. Because of lower physiologic reserves, severe dehydration without prompt treatment in the neonate may quickly lead to contraction of intravascular volume, shock, and cardiorespiratory arrest. Therefore, the handling of a moderate to severe dehydration from diarrhea requires exquisite skill in initiating a parenteral fluid line and prompt expansion of the intravascular space.

Following stabilization, an estimate of fluid and electrolyte deficits should be made according to the methods described elsewhere in this chapter. Appropriate fluid and electrolytes are given parenterally to cover deficit, maintenance requirement and concurrent abnormal losses such as persistent diarrhea, during the repair period. Metabolic acidosis is a frequent finding in diarrheal dehydration. However, it frequently does not require specific correction with the use of a buffer, such as sodium bicarbonate or lactate, because correction of the dehydration and maintenance of positive fluid and electrolyte balance will normalize the acid-base status within 24 to 48 hours. Prerenal azotemia is also a common occurrence in diarrhea dehydration and is usually corrected spontaneously within 3 to 4 days following correction of the dehydration state.

Institution of oral fluid intake should be carried out with extreme care. The infant's gastrointestinal tract is frequently in a very precarious state following a diarrheal episode. Introduction of oral intake sooner than indicated frequently leads to recurrence of diarrhea, which may proceed into a protracted diarrheal state. The latter is a serious and difficult problem to handle, particularly in a very young and small infant. A vicious cycle of diarrhea, starvation, malnutrition, and more diarrhea may necessitate a very long period of fasting and the use of intravenous alimentation. (See Chap. 42.)

The appropriate period of fasting depends on the severity of the diarrheal episode. As a rule, a more severe diarrheal state will require a longer period of fasting and vice versa. Also, the number of diarrheal stools following fasting will provide a good guideline for the duration of fasting. It should also be pointed out that in prolonged diarrheal states, a transient lactase deficiency may occur[41] which may require the use of a lactose-free milk formula during the resumption of milk intake.[41a]

Parenteral Alimentation. (See Chap. 42.) The pioneer work by Dudrick and coworkers in experimental animals[42] and subsequently by his colleagues in infants[43] has shown that metabolic needs and normal growth rate can be sustained by parenteral hyperalimentation alone. This is achieved by parenterally feeding infants with hypertonic glucose, protein hydrolysate, trace elements, and vitamins along with fresh plasma transfusion at regular intervals. Detailed discussion of this technique is found in Chapter 42.

The complication rate of parenteral hyperalimentation is high and the possible undesirable effects include thrombosis, embolism, bacterial and fungal infections, hyperammonemia, metabolic acidosis, hyperglycemia, rebound hypoglycemia, glycosuria, and osmotic diuresis. Expert nursing care with daily renewal of parenteral solution, intravenous tubing, filter, and surgical dressing minimize the infection rate.

In low-birth-weight infants, total parenteral alimentation is not routinely used because of high rates of complication and the technical difficulty of placing central venous catheters in a small infant. In these subjects, parenteral nutrition through a peripheral vein is preferred. With this form of parenteral nutrition, the glucose concentration in the infusate is generally limited to 12% because a higher glucose concentration carries the risk of tissue sloughing if infiltration of the intravenous site occurs. Because of the limitation in glucose concentration, the caloric intake of infants receiving nutritional supports solely from this route is often inadequate. This problem is heightened by our axiom of not giving too much fluid,[4,32] and the frequent occurrence of hyperglycemia in these infants when a large dose of glucose is given.[45,46] Under the circumstances, it may be necessary to use intravenous fat emulsion as a supplemental source of calories. The usual precautions and monitoring for toxicity should be observed when intravenous fat emulsion is infused. Giving an intravenous fat emulsion also resolved the problem of essential fatty acid deficiency that occurred when infants received a prolonged period of parenteral nutrition without fat.[47] It has been estimated that supplying 4% of the caloric intake in the form of intravenous fat emulsion is sufficient to prevent the development of biochemical or clinical essential fatty acid deficiency.

Fluid and Electrolyte Management of Neonatal Surgical Patients

If the surgical conditions result in an abnormal loss of fluid and electrolyte, leading to a significant degree of dehydration and electrolyte aberration, the repair of the deficit should be achieved before surgery. For example, in congenital pyloric stenosis with severe dehydration and electrolyte disturbance, the surgical repair of the pyloric stenosis should be postponed over a 48- to 72-hour period while fluid and electrolyte therapy is in progress. Failure to do so may result in a stormy postoperative course.

Table 29-6. Sample of Intake and Output Sheet.

NAME: _____

HOSPITAL NO: _____

DIAGNOSIS: _____

		INTAKE					OUTGO								
			ORAL		URINE			OTHERS			Body	SERUM ELECTROLYTE			
		IV		Type of		Specific	Glucose	Source							
Date	Shift	Type of Fluid	ml	Fluid	ml	Gravity	(0 to ++++)	Stool, gastrostomy, etc.	ml	D	Wt. (kg)	Na	K	Cl	BUN
													mmol/l		mg/dl
	7-3														
	3-11														
	11-7														
24 Hr Total															

656

During surgery, the calculated fluid and electrolyte requirements and rate of administration should be continued. The anesthesiologist and the members of the surgical team should be apprised of the plan for the parenteral fluid therapy in order to avoid unnecessary error in the administration of parenteral fluid resulting from lack of communication. The abnormal fluid loss, blood loss, or both should be recorded and repaired either during surgery or immediately thereafter.

During the first 2 postoperative days, some infants, particularly those who received general anesthesia, may have reduced urine flow as a result of increased secretion of ADH.[48] It has also been shown that for some unknown reason, the IWL in the postoperative neonate is significantly reduced.[49] Therefore, during the immediate postoperative period (24 hr), the parenteral fluid intake should be reduced to avoid overhydration and water intoxication. Again, a system of careful monitoring of fluid and electrolyte balance (Table 29-6) is an important step in the day-to-day calculation of fluid and electrolyte needs.

Neonatal Sepsis

Infants with sepsis will require intravenous fluid therapy to provide a route of administering antibiotics intravenously, and to provide fluid and electrolyte maintenance if the infant cannot tolerate oral feeding as a result of the severe illness. In both instances, accurate intake and output calculation is important in maintaining homeostatic balance.

In sepsis complicated by meningoencephalitis, hyponatremia without dehydration is not an uncommon complication. Symptoms such as hyperreflexia and convulsions may ensue. The treatment of choice in this instance is correction of the hyponatremia with hypertonic NaCl solution.

TECHNICAL ASPECTS OF PARENTERAL FLUID THERAPY

Blood Sampling. Because of their size and often precarious state, blood sampling for electrolyte analysis in newborn infants can impose a serious problem. In most pediatric services, venous blood is obtained from the antecubital vein, femoral vein, external jugular vein, and, at times, even the internal jugular vein. The antecubital vein is by far the safest site for blood sampling; unfortunately, in small infants, it is often difficult to obtain an adequate blood specimen from this site. The femoral vein is a convenient site for blood sampling; however, proximity to the femoral artery and the risk of traumatizing the hip joint and its surrounding bony structures make this method of blood sampling undesirable, particularly in the small neonate. External jugular vein puncture is a good choice if the infant is free of cardiorespiratory symptoms. In general, internal jugular vein puncture should be avoided in newborn infants because of the risk of incurring injury to adjacent structures such as the trachea, carotid artery, or vagus nerve.

It is apparent from the previous discussion that sampling capillary blood by heel puncture is by far the least traumatic method of blood letting in the newborn period. The correlations between capillary and venous blood samples in regard to electrolyte values are satisfactory. The validity of the capillary blood samples can be further enhanced by warming the heel with a warmed, wet towel (40°C) for 5 to 10 minutes. The latter procedure will improve local circulation which, in turn, will partially abolish the capillary-venous difference in various parameters including hematocrit.[50] Because the amount of blood obtained by heel puncture is limited, the neonatal service should be supported by a laboratory capable of performing microanalysis. For infants who require frequent monitoring of arterial acid-base and blood-gas values, an indwelling catheter (size 3.5 or 5.0 F) may be inserted into the umbilical artery and retrogradely passed into the aorta just above the diaphragm. (See Chap. 22) for further details.) For occasional sampling of arterial blood for blood-gas analysis, direct arterial puncture of the temporal, radial, or brachial arteries may be done using a butterfly needle inserted against the arterial inflow. Skill and experience are obviously necessary. Complications such as arteriospasm, bleeding, or infection are rare.

More recently, transcutaneous P_{O_2} monitors have been introduced into the intensive care nursery for clinical application. They have proved to be an excellent method of guiding oxygen therapy with less sampling of arterial blood. When modern instrumentation allows for the measurement of transcutaneous pH and P_{CO_2}, there will be no need of placing umbilical arterial catheters or direct arterial puncture for blood sampling, both of which carry a certain degree of risk for complications.

Intravenous Fluid Infusion. In infants, the branches of the superficial temporal vein and facial vein are the most commonly used sites for the intravenous infusion. With practice and skill, a suitable size scalp vein needle can be inserted into these venous tributaries with ease. The needle can be immobilized by appropriate taping. Infusion of hypertonic parenteral solutions such as THAM, 0.9M $NaHCO_3$, or 50% glucose should be avoided. Infiltration of these hypertonic solutions into the subcutaneous tissue may result in sloughing and necrosis of the adjacent tissue. Veins in the antecubital fossa or dorsa of the hands and feet are also appropriate sites for intravenous infusion. However, subcutaneous infiltration is more common in these sites because of the relative difficulty in the immobilization of the infusion needle.

The umbilical vein has long been a favorite site for intravenous infusion because of the relative ease in placing a catheter in this vessel. However, recent reports have documented the complications arising from umbilical venous catheterization and fluid infusion, including infection, hepatic necrosis, and phlebitis. If the use of umbilical venous infusion is mandatory for lack of other alternative sites, the catheter tip should be placed in the inferior vena cava through the ductus venosus. If the latter cannot be entered, one should avoid placing the catheter in the hepatic portal sinuses, particularly if infusion of hypertonic solution such as $NaHCO_3$ is anticipated. This can be achieved by placing the catheter no more than 8 cm from the skin of the umbilicus. In any case, the position of the catheter should always be determined or confirmed radiologically.

Cutdown or insertion of an intracath (saphenous, basilic, cephalic, or jugular vein) should be used only in infants who may require a prolonged period of intravenous infusion. Infection is the most common complication from this route of parenteral infusion. Meticulous aseptic care of the cutdown sites and frequent dressing change will reduce the incidence of local and systemic infection.

In all cases of parenteral fluid infusion, a constant infusion pump should be employed, along with a volumetric chamber, to assure a constant rate of infusion. A fluctuating infusion rate may result in erratic blood glucose values and overhydration. The latter may significantly alter the cardiorespiratory status of a sick neonate with congestive heart failure and pulmonary edema.

Hypodermoclysis. With the advent of the advanced technique of intravenous fluid infusion, the use of hypodermoclysis as a means of providing fluid and electrolyte to sick infants has largely been abandoned. The theoretic disadvantage of hypodermoclysis lies primarily in the erratic and unpredictable absorption of water and electrolyte in a sick infant with poor peripheral circulation. In some cases, water and sodium from the extracellular fluid may actually be transferred into the hypodermoclysis site, resulting in contraction of the extracellular space and hypovolemia. Furthermore, the risk of infection and cellulitis is high. Therefore, this method of administering fluid to newborn infants should be avoided.

Intake and Output. Fluid and electrolyte balance in an infant can be achieved by keeping an accurate record of intake and outgo. A sample intake and output flow sheet is listed in Table 29-6. Accurate and thorough record keeping should be done by both the medical and nursing personnel. Therefore, the record sheet is best organized around the routine 8-hour nursing rotations.

REFERENCES

1. **Friis–Hansen B:** Body composition during growth. Pediatrics (Suppl) 47:264, 1971
2. **Kagan BM, Stanincova V, Felix NS, Hodgman J, Kalman D:** Body composition of premature infants: Relation to nutrition. Am J Clin Nutr 25:1153, 1972
3. **Oh W, Oh MA, Lind J:** Renal function and blood volume in newborn infant related to placental transfusion. Acta Paediatr Scand 56:197, 1966
4. **Bell EF, Warburton D, Stonestreet BS, Oh W:** Randomized trial comparing high and low volume maintenance fluid administration in low birth weight infants with reference to congestive heart failure secondary to patent ductus arteriosus. N Engl J Med 302:598, 1980
5. **Bell EF, Warburton D, Stonestreet BS, Oh W:** High volume fluid intake predisposes premature infants to necrotizing enterocolitis. Lancet 2:90, 1979
6. **Alstatt LB:** Transplacental hyponatremia in the newborn infant. J Pediatr 66:985, 1965

7. **Hey EN, Katz G:** Evaporative water loss in the newborn baby. J Physiol (London) 200: 605, 1969

8. **Sinclair JC, Scopes JW, Silverman WA:** Metabolic reference standards for the neonate. Pediatrics 39:724, 1967

9. **Fanaroff AA, Wald M, Gruber HS, Klaus MH:** Insensible water loss in low birth weight infants. Pediatrics 50:236, 1972

10. **Wu PYK, Hodgman JE:** Insensible water loss in preterm infants: Changes with postnatal development and non-ionizing radiant energy. Pediatrics 54:704, 1974

11. **Bell EF, Gray JC, Weinstein M, Oh W:** The effects of thermal environment on heat balance and insensible water loss in low birth weight infants. J Pediatr (in press)

12. **Williams PR, Oh W:** The effects of radiant warmer on insensible weight loss in newborn infants. Am J Dis Child. 128:511, 1974

13. **Oh W, Karecki H:** Phototherapy and insensible water loss in the newborn infant. Am J Dis Child 124:230, 1972

14. **Zweymuller E, Preining O:** The insensible water loss in the newborn infant. Acta Paediatr Scand (Suppl) 205, 1970

15. **Oh W, Yao AC, Hanson JS, Lind J:** Peripheral circulatory response to phototherapy in newborn infants. Acta Paediatr Scand 62:49, 1973

16. **Wu PYK, Wong WH, Hodgman JE, Levan NE:** Changes in blood flow in the skin and muscle with phototherapy. Pediatr Res 8:257, 1974

17. **Bell EF, Weinstein MR, Oh W:** Heat balance in premature infants: Comparative effects of convectively heated incubator and radiant warmer, with and without plastic heat shield. J Pediatr (in press).

18. **Bell EF, Neidich GA, Cashore WJ, Oh W:** Combined effect of radiant warmer and phototherapy on insensible water loss in low birth weight infants. J Pediatr 94:810–813, 1979

19. **Calcagno PL, Rubin MI, Weintraub DH:** Studies on the renal concentrating and diluting mechanisms in the premature infant. J Clin Invest 33:91, 1954

20. **McCance RA, Naylor NJ, Widdowson EM:** Response of infants to a large dose of water. Arch Dis Child 29:104, 1954

21. **Beitins IZ, Bayard F, Levitsky L, Ances IG, Kowarski A, Migeon CJ:** Plasma aldosterone concentration at delivery and during the newborn period. J Clin Invest 51:386, 1972

22. **Siegel SR, Fisher DA, Oh W:** Serum aldosterone levels related to sodium balance in the newborn infant. Pediatrics 53:410, 1974

23. **Tsang RC, Light IJ, Sutherland JM, Kleinman LI:** Possible pathogenic factors in neonatal hypocalcemia of prematurity. J Pediatr 82:423, 1973

24. **Tsang R, Oh W:** Neonatal hypocalcemia in low birth weight infants. Pediatrics 45:773, 1970

25. **Edelman CM Jr, Spitzer A:** The maturing kidney. J Pediatr 75:509, 1969

26. **Brück K, Parmelee AH, Brück M:** Neutral temperature range and range of "thermal comfort" in premature infants. Biol Neonate 4:32, 1962

27. **Hey EN, Katz G:** Optimum thermal environment for naked babies. Arch Dis Child 45:328, 1970

28. **Cort RL:** Renal function in the respiratory distress syndrome. Acta Paediatr Scand 51: 343, 1961

29. **Siegel SR, Fisher DA, Oh W:** Renal function and serum aldosterone levels in infants with respiratory distress syndrome. J Pediatr 83: 854, 1973

30. **Kitterman JA, Edmunds LH Jr, Gregory GA, Heyman MN, Tooley WH, Rudolph AM:** Patent ductus arteriosus in premature infants. Incidence relation to pulmonary disease and management. N Engl J Med 287:473, 1972

31. **Thibeault DW, Emmanouilides GC, Dodge ME, Cachman RS:** Early functional closure of the ductus arteriosus associated with decreased severity of respiratory distress syndrome in preterm infants. Am J Dis Child 131:741, 1979

32. **Stevenson JG:** Fluid administration in the association of patent ductus arteriosus complicating respiratory distress syndrome. J Pediatr 90:257, 1977

33. **Siggard–Andersen O:** The pH–log pCO2 blood acid base nomogram revised. Scand J Clin Lab Invest 14:598, 1962

34. **Siegel SR, Phelps DL, Leake RD, Oh W:** The effects of rapid infusion of hypertonic sodium bicarbonate in infants with Respiratory Distress D. Pediatrics 51:651, 1973

35. **Simmons NA, Adcock EW III, Bard H et al:** Hypernatremia and intracranial hemorrhage in neonates. N Engl J Med 291, 1974

36. **Hobel CJ, Oh W, Hyvarinen MA, Emmanouilides GC, Erenberg A:** Early versus late treatment of neonatal acidosis in low birth weight infants: Relation to Respiratory Distress Syndrome. J Pediatr 81:1178, 1972

37. **Usher R:** Reduction in mortality from respiratory distress syndrome and prematurity with early administration of intravenous glucose and sodium bicarbonate. Pediatrics 32:966, 1963

38. **Sinclair JC, Engel K, Silverman WA:** Early correction of hypoxemia and acidemia in infants of low birth weight: A controlled trial of oxygen breathing, rapid alkali and assisted ventilation. Pediatrics 42:565, 1968

39. **Corbet AJS, Adams JM, Kennedy JD et al:**

Controlled trial of bicarbonate therapy in high-risk premature newborn infants. J Pediatr 91:771, 1977

40. **Benson CD, Lloyd JR:** Infantile pyloric stenosis. Am J Surg 107:429, 1964

41. **Sunshine P, Kretchmer N:** Studies of small intestine during development, III. Infantile diarrhea associated with intolerance to disaccharides. Pediatrics 34:38, 1964

41a. **Leake RD, Schroeder KC, Benton DA, Oh W:** The use of soy-based formula in the treatment of infantile diarrhea. Am J Dis Child 127:374, 1974

42. **Dudrick SJ, Wilmore DW, Vars HM:** Long-term total Parenteral nutrition with growth in puppies and positive nitrogen balance in patients. Surg Forum 18:356, 1967

43. **Wilmore DW, Groff DB, Bishop HC, Dudrick SJ:** Total parenteral nutrition in infants with catastrophic gastrointestinal anomalies. J Pediatr Surg 4:181, 1969

44. **Driscoll JM, Heird WC, Schullinger JN, Gon-** gaware RD, Winter RW: Total intravenous alimentation in low birth weight infants: A preliminary report. J Pediatr 81:145, 1972

45. **Dweck HS, Cassady G:** Glucose intolerance in infants of very low birth weights 1,100 grams or less. Pediatrics 53:189, 1974

46. **Cowett RM, Oh W, Pollak A, Schwartz R, Stonestreet BS:** Glucose disposal of low birth weight infants: Steady state hyperglycemia produced by constant intravenous glucose infusion. Pediatrics 63:389, 1979

47. **Friedman Z, Danon A, Stahlman MT, Oates JA:** Rapid onset of essential fatty acid deficiency in the newborn. Pediatrics 58:640, 1976

48. **Bennett EJ, Daughety MJ, Jenkins MT:** Fluid requirements for neonatal anesthesia and operation. Anesthesiology 32:343, 1970

49. **Lester J:** Insensible water loss in infants. J Pediatr Surg 2:483, 1967

50. **Oh W, Lind J:** Venous capillary hematocrit in newborn infants and placental transfusion. Acta Paediatr Scand 55:38, 1966

30
Renal Diseases

Pedro A. José,
Leticia U. Tina,
Zoe L. Papadopoulou,
and Philip L. Calcagno

HUMAN RENAL ANATOMICAL DEVELOPMENT

Fetal Development

The human kidney originates from the nephrogenic cord and develops sequentially: the pronephros (a cervical structure), the mesonephros (a thoracic structure), and the metanephros (an abdominal structure).[1,2] The pronephros, appearing at about the third fetal week, consists of several pairs of nephrotomes (rudimentary nephrons comprised of a vascular glomus; the periglomus space opens into the coelom at one end and into the tubule leading into the pronephric duct at another end). The human pronephros, though nonfunctional and degenerated by the fourth fetal week, forms the pronephric duct, which serves as a conduit for the mesonephric nephrons. The mesonephros commences its development just prior to the complete degeneration of the pronephros. The mesoneprhos consists of 30 to 40 glomerulotubular units. Direct aortic branches form glomeruli which are enclosed by a Bowman's capsule opening into a distinct proximal convoluted tubule and a distal tubular segment. No loop of Henle, macula densa, or juxtaglomerular apparatus (JGA) is found. The urine formed by the mesonephric kidney drains into the mesonephric duct (wolffian duct) and subsequently into the cloaca. The development of the metanephros or definitive kidney occurs before the mesonephros degenerates completely, by the 12th to 14th fetal week.

The metanephros is derived from both mesoderm and ectoderm. The definitive nephron originates from the nephrogenic blastema (mesoderm) caudal to the mesonephros. The collecting ducts, calyces, pelvis, and ureter are derived from the ureteric bud (ectoderm), which originates from the cloacal end of the mesonephric duct. The primary collecting tubule subsequently undergoes repetitive division into several generations of collecting tubules. The ampulla (anterior end of the collecting tubule) growing into the nephrogenic blastema induces nephron formation which continues until 32 to 36 fetal weeks.

The metanephros consists of a glomerulus enclosed by a Bowman's capsule which opens into a proximal convoluted tubule, then to the loop of Henle, and then into a distal convoluted tubule. Urine formed in these nephrons drains into the structures derived from the ureteric bud and thence into the bladder. The process of glomerular development is still obscure; nonetheless, by the 13th fetal week, well-developed arteriole glomerular tufts are found in the juxtamedullary and pelvic connective tissue areas.

The afferent arteriole, after forming the glomerular tuft, emerges as the efferent arteriole. The sites of entrance and exit are in close proximity. Additionally, the afferent arteriole contains the juxtaglomerular cells, which are responsible for renin secretion. These cells, in combination with the contiguous macula densa cells of the distal tubule, form the juxtaglomerular apparatus.

By the end of the fourth month, the arcuate vessels are well developed so that the cortical and medullary portions of the kidney may be differentiated. Maturation of the glomerular tubular units proceeds from the juxtamedullary zone outward to the periphery of the cortex. At 40 to 42 fetal weeks, the juxtamedullary glomeruli are twice the size of the outer cortical glomeruli. By the postnatal age of 1 year, the juxtamedullary glomeruli are only 20% larger than the outer cortical glomeruli, similar to that observed in the adult human.

During the period of metanephronogenesis, the kidneys migrate cranially from the area of fourth lumbar vertebra to the level of the first lumbar or twelfth thoracic vertebra. In addition, during the upward migration, the kidneys rotate a quarter turn medially so that the pelvis is directed medially rather than anteriorly.

Postnatal Development

Nephron development postnatally is accomplished by nonuniform glomerular and tubular growth and a decrease in interstitial tissue. Anatomic glomerular tubular relationships approach adult levels by the sixth postnatal month. The glomerular diameter increases approximately one-and-a-half fold, whereas proximal tubular length increases almost fourfold during this period of time.[3] In the full-term neonate, the thin loops of Henle are limited to the descending limbs and arise primarily from the second to third generation of nephrons. At some undetermined time after birth, the thin portions of the loops of Henle arise from other generations of nephrons and extend to the ascending limb. Thus, in the neonate the thin loops of Henle are primarily associated with those glomeruli in the immediate juxtamedullary area. Cortical volume as compared to the medulla in the neonate is less than 3:1 ratio of adults.

Immediately prior to birth, the intrarenal circulation appears to be mainly medullary through the juxtamedullary and pelvic arteriole glomerular units and arteriole rectae.[4] Following birth, a cortical circulation is then anatomically possible with the functional appearance of postglomerular cortical vessels. The precise chronologic anatomic circulatory development from birth to adulthood is unknown.

HUMAN RENAL PHYSIOLOGY
Fetal

The human pronephros is nonfunctional; however, function has been described for the human mesonephros. In human abortuses, Urografin injection into the abdominal aorta resulted in opacification of the kidneys, thereby indicating a renal filtering capacity.[5] Elaboration of urine has been demonstrated in the mesonephros of a 10- to 12-week-old fetus.[6] Additionally, renal tissue culture studies of 9-week-old human fetuses showed secretory ability of the proximal segment and a reabsorptive capacity of the distal elements.

Fetal metanephric function has been only indirectly studied by examination of urine obtained immediately after birth. Based on morphology and staining characteristics, the loop of Henle and macula could be functional by 13 to 17 fetal weeks.[7,8] *In vitro* proximal tubular tissue cultures of human fetal 14 weeks metanephric tissue showed tubular ability to perform active transport.[9]

The role of the mesonephric and metanephric kidneys in fetal homeostasis is still unclear.

Postnatal

General. Ninety-three percent of preterm and term infants void in the first 24 hours and ninety-nine percent within 48 hours.[10,11] Thereafter, urine flow is normally 1 to 3 ml/kg/hour.[12] The frequency of voiding after the first 72 hours may be up to 20 or more times in 24 hours. Average voiding patterns beyond the neonatal period are presented in Table 30-1.

Glomerular Filtration Rate (GRF). In the first 24 hours of life, the glomerular filtration rate may be as low as 4 ml/min/1.73 m^2 in infants of 25 weeks gestational age.[13] The GFR increases with gestational age, and, by 34 to 36 weeks of gestation, values of 25 ml/min/1.73 m^2 are achieved, similar to those reported for full-term infants.[13-16] The GFRs in newborns who are small for gestational age are similar to those in infants whose birth weights are appropriate for the same gestational age.[15] The rise in GFR in preterm infants after birth is greater than that occurring during intrauterine life.[13,17] The GFR increases two- to threefold after 1 to 13 weeks of postnatal life.[18-20] The rapid increase in GFR relative to body size, kidney weight, or surface area continues during the first three months of life.[21] Thereafter, a slower rise is noted until adult values are reached by 12 to 24 months of life.[22]

A similar developmental pattern of GFR has been noted in experimental animals.[23-27] In addition, it has been shown by Tavani and coworkers and others that the rise in filtration rate during the first days of life is caused primarily by enhanced perfusion of outer cortical nephrons.[25,26,28,29,30] The increase in GFR with age may be caused by increase in glomerular perfusion pressure, increase in surface area available for filtration, and/or an increase in glomerular permeability.[31] A rise in glomerular plasma flow also appears to play a major role.[28,30]

Renal Blood Flow (RBF). Studies of renal plasma flow (RPF) in the newborn using clearance of para-aminohippurate (PAH) are not true determinations of RPF because the extraction ratio of PAH in the newborn is only 60% as compared to over 90% in the adult.[32] Values of 90% are achieved by 3 months of life in the term infant.[32] The relationship between the clearance of PAH and gestational age below 35 weeks has recently been reported.[32a] PAH clearance increased from 20 ml/min/1.73 m^2 at 30 weeks to about 45 ml/min/1.73 m^2 by 35 weeks of age.[36] The clearance of PAH in term newborns under 12 hours of age averages 83 ml/min/1.73 m^2.[16] An increase to 120 ml/min/1.73 m^2 is apparent in the first week of life. As with GFR, a more rapid increase in the clearance of PAH occurs in the first 3 months. As noted above, PAH extraction approaches adult levels at this time. Thereafter, a slower rise is noted until adult values are reached by 12 to 24 months of age.[21,22,37] Renal plasma flow (clearance of PAH divided by the extraction ratio of PAH) is also lower in the newborn as compared to the adult. In the first 12 hours of life, the estimated RPF is 150 ml/min/1.73 m^2 and increases to about 200 ml/min/1.73 m^2 in the first week of life. Based on these calculations, the filtration fraction

Table 30-1. Average Voiding Frequency.

Age	Voids/24 Hours
3–6 mo	20
6–12 mo	16
1–2 yr	12
2–3 yr	10
3–4 yr	9
12–adult	4–6

(GFR/RPF) of 0.20 is similar to that obtained for adults.[38] In some animals, the filtration fraction has been reported to be lower in younger than in older animals.[23,33]

The low RPF in the neonate is related in part to a low perfusion pressure but is mainly due to a higher renal vascular resistance.[24,30,39,40] The renal fraction of cardiac output in the term newborn is calculated as approximately 4% to 6% in the first 12 hours and 8% to 10% in the first week of life compared to the usual adult value of 25%. This calculated figure is in close agreement with data obtained in newborn animals.[41,42]

The renal blood flow distribution in the young is different from that reported in adults.[34,35] When compared to the adult, the newborn kidney shows a greater percentage of blood flow to the inner cortical and medullary areas.[34,35,43,44] The maturational period varies from species to species. Renal blood flow distribution has not been studied in normal human neonates. Gruskin and coworkers have shown that the baby with cyanotic heart disease has an intrarenal blood flow distribution like the normal newborn.[45] The lower extraction ratio of PAH in infants younger than 3 months may be related to a relatively greater perfusion of the juxtamedullary nephrons in infants in comparison to the adult. With maturation, as total renal blood flow reaches adult levels, a greater fraction of the RBF is received by the outer cortical nephrons. The maturational pattern of single nephron filtration distribution also follows a centrifugal pattern.[25,26,28,43] Recent studies from our laboratory indicated that during the immediate neonatal period in the canine, the differential increase in outer versus inner cortical nephron perfusion is paralleled by similar changes in single nephron filtration distribution.[28]

The mechanisms involved in the age-related

increase and redistribution of RBF have been investigated in our laboratory and by others.[24,25,30,40,46] The factors that have been considered include anatomic and hemodynamic events. Anatomic increase in vessel size may not explain the changes in RBF distribution. While glomerulogenesis may persist after birth in preterms under 36 weeks' gestational age,[1] the increase in renal blood flow continues long after nephron formation has ceased. Hemodynamic factors such as low cardiac output or perfusion pressure may account for only part of the low renal blood flow.[43] The increase in RBF with maturation is mainly caused by a drop in afferent and efferent vascular resistances.[30,40]

The drop in renal resistance with age may be caused by myogenic or neural mechanisms. The roles of several vasoactive agents in the regulation of RBF in the young have been studied, especially prostaglandins, bradykinin, angiotensin II, and catecholamines.[47] The low levels of renal prostaglandins of the E series found in the young,[48] caused either by increased degradation[49] or by decreased production, might account for lower RBF. Urine levels of bradykinin, another vasodilator, presumably synthetized in the distal tubule, have also been reported to be decreased in human neonates.[86] The vasodilator properties of prostaglandins may be mediated by bradykinin. However, when prostaglandin synthesis is inhibited by indomethacin in the adult, renal blood flow is unchanged or a redistribution to the outer cortex occurs, so that a deficiency of prostaglandin or bradykinin might be expected to produce the converse pattern to that found in the neonatal kidney.[50] Moreover, increased renal prostaglandin production has been reported in the perinatal period.[51,85] Inhibition of prostaglandin synthesis in the young, however, does not decrease renal blood flow or alter its distribution,[52] and stimulation of endogenous renal kinin production does not result in an increase in the GFR.[53]

It is unlikely that the increased renal vascular resistance of the newborn is caused by the renin-angiotensin system, despite the high renin-angiotensin values, because inhibition of the renal vascular effects of angiotensin II does not result in an increase in neonatal renal blood flow.[54] On the other hand, catecholamines may play an important role in controlling renal blood flow. Studies suggest that the high renal vascular resistance in the newborn may be caused by enhanced responsiveness to the effects of the adrenergic system.[46] This may not be related to catecholamine levels but instead to differences in adrenergic receptor occupancy or affinity.[55] The clinical relevance of these observations remain to be determined.

Renin-Angiotensin System. A very active renin-angiotensin-aldosterone system in the neonatal period is now well established.[56-59] In addition, the levels of peripheral renin activity (PRA), angiotensin II, and probably aldosterone are higher in preterm infants than in term infants.[58-66] The levels of PRA are inversely related to gestational age, decreasing from 60 ng/ml/hour at 28 weeks to about 10 to 20 ng/ml/hour at term.[67] A slight increase occurs at 3 to 6 days of postnatal life. A marked decline in PRA levels occurs in the next 3 to 6 weeks. Thereafter, a gradual decline is noted. By 3 to 5 years of age, PRA levels are similar to those of adults on a normal salt intake.[56]

The high PRA in the neonatal period has been attributed to increased secretory rate and to decreased clearance or lesser volume of distribution.[68,69] PRA increases appropriately following change in position from the recumbent to the upright posture, volume depletion, hemorrhage, aortic constriction, furosemide administration, and hypoxia.[66,69-74] It appears that the increase in PRA after furosemide or tilting may be less in younger infants as compared to older persons.[70]

Volume expansion with normal saline, the administration of propranolol, indomethacin, or antidiuretic hormone (ADH) decrease PRA levels.[75,76] In most instances, however, the decrease is less in younger animals than in adults.[76] The administration of saralasin, a competitive antagonist of angiotensin II, results in an increase in PRA, indicating that the short loop feedback is intact in the newborn.[75-78] Recent studies also suggest that the cryorenin fraction may be greater in younger animals as compared to older animals.[69] The serum angiotensin converting enzyme (ACE) has also been determined in the preterm and term infants.[79] Cord blood ACE levels were found to have a significant negative correlation with birth weight and gestational age. The greatest decrease in ACE levels occurred at about 35 weeks of gestation. ACE activity in peripheral blood of preterm infants was higher than that found in term infants but similar to maternal levels. ACE levels in term infants were significantly lower than adult values. A gradual increase with postnatal age has been described.

The physiologic significance of the high PRA levels in the neonatal period is still unknown. Siegel and coworkers demonstrated a dependence of blood pressure on renin-angiotensin activity in fetal lambs,[77] and a correlation between plasma angiotensin II levels and blood pressure has been reported in infants.[59] However, Jose and coworkers,[54] Moore and coworkers,[80] and Bailie and coworkers[75] were unable to show an effect on blood pressure with the infusion of the angiotensin II antagonist, saralasin, in puppies, lambs, or piglets. Moreover, Godard and coworkers showed no correlation between blood pressure and PRA in 24 healthy term newborns studied from 1 day to 9 weeks of life.[58] Jose and associates also were unable to demonstrate a role of the renin-angiotensin system in the regulation of neonatal renal blood flow.[54] Spitzer and Schoeneman have suggested that the high PRA and aldosterone levels in the newborn may be involved in the limited ability of the newborn kidney to excrete a salt load.[81] In the preterm, however, Sulyok and coworkers have reported that the increased activity of the renin-angiotensin-aldosterone system is closely related to the renal salt wasting and negative salt balance that occurs in the first few weeks of extrauterine life.[65] This is of interest because in fetal lambs the administration of furosemide may increase PRA but not plasma aldosterone levels.[82]

Prostaglandins. The ontogeny of the renal prostaglandin system is not as extensively studied as the renin-angiotensin system. Prezyna reported a gestational age-related appearance of the renomedullary body, a structure presumably concerned with prostaglandin (PG) synthesis.[83] Day and coworkers isolated PGA_2, E_2, and F_2 from fetal kidneys.[84] Friedman and Demers recently reported the ability of the fetal kidney (gestational age greater than 28 weeks) to synthesize PGs.[48] The fetal vascular tissue and fetal pig renal cortical slices have been reported to produce more PGI_2 than PGE_2. The fetal tissues apparently produced more PGI_2 than did the adult tissues.[85] It was suggested that the greater biosynthetic ability of the young may be related to lack of a PG

inhibitor of synthesis in the neonatal period.[85] These studies would suggest that the low renal blood flow in the neonatal period may not be caused by decreased renal PGs. However, the catabolizing enzymes for PG may be greater in the immediate neonatal period in the rat. Thus the role of PGs in neonatal renal homeostasis remains to be defined. Preliminary studies by Robillard and coworkers indicate that fetal renal PGs are not essential in the regulation of blood flow or salt excretion by the fetal kidney.[52]

Kinins. There is only one study of urinary kinins in the newborn human. Prematures have undetectable levels of urinary kinins.[86] Solhaug and coworkers recently reported that the renal kallikrein system in puppies may be stimulated by the infusion of the undecapeptide substance P.[53] Low doses of substance P did not alter glomerular filtration rate while high dosages decreased GFR. The effects were not related to any change in perfusion pressure.

Erythropoitein. See Chapter 25.

Tubular Function.

Sodium Regulation. Normally growing infants remain in balance and maintain normal extracellular composition while on widely varying salt intakes. However, in apparently healthy very low-birth-weight infants, hyponatremia without evidence of water retention has been observed in the first week of life. A negative sodium balance occurs in the healthy preterm infant in the first week of life. Sulyok and coworkers showed that this may amount to 15 to 30 $\mu mol/min/1.73$ m^2.[87] They also showed that the alterations in serum and urinary chloride paralleled the changes in Na metabolism although the chloride changes were less marked and of a shorter duration.[87] Sodium chloride supplementation of 3 mmol/kg/day may prevent the decline in serum levels of sodium and chloride.[88,89] In the sick, low-birth-weight infant, the net loss of sodium was eight to nine times greater than the negative sodium balance of 1 to 2 mmol/kg/day that is normally noted in the first 3 to 5 days of postnatal life.[90] Several studies have demonstrated that the negative Na balance occurring in the preterm infant is mainly caused by a high renal fractional excretion of sodium chloride.[87,89] Fractional Na excretion is inversely correlated with gestational age, with values as high as 5% to 6% at 28 weeks of gestational age.[13,15,17] The effect of postnatal age on fractional sodium excretion in preterm infant was recently reported by Ross and coworkers in 22 infants whose weights were appropriate for gestational age (28–33 weeks).[14] The fractional sodium excretion in these prematures ranged from 1% to 5% in the perinatal period, with the highest levels noted in the first 10 days of life. By 1 month of age, fractional sodium excretion was less than 0.40%.[14] Term newborns have basal fractional sodium excretion similar to adults on a normal salt intake (1%–2%).

In the neonatal rat, before a proximal tubular length of 1500 μ is reached, high fractional sodium excretion is the rule.[91] A similar mechanism may be operative in the very low-birth-weight infant. Tubular hyporesponsiveness to the effects of aldosterone has been suggested as an additional explanation.[65] Higher aldosterone levels are found in preterm than in term infants, and a sharp increase occurs in the first week of life. This high aldosterone level could represent an attempt to compensate for increased proximal tubular rejection and subsequent increased distal tubular load.

Other conditions that may increase fractional sodium excretion include hypoxia, respiratory distress, hyperbilirubinemia,[92] and acute tubular necrosis. Recently the use of theophylline to treat apnea of prematurity has been associated with hyponatremia and increased fractional sodium excretion.[93]

Under ordinary circumstances, the term and preterm newborn can tolerate a varied sodium intake. However, under conditions of sodium loading, the neonatal kidney may not be able to excrete the excess sodium. In term infants, increasing the sodium intake from 1 to 3 mmol/day will result in an appropriate increase in sodium excretion.[94] The tolerance limits, however, are much narrower in the newborn than in the older child. Aperia and coworkers have suggested an upper limit of 12 mmol NaCl/kg/day. Higher sodium diets may result in an increase in extracellular fluid volume.[95,96]

The mechanisms for the limited response to sodium loading by the neonatal kidney have been the subject of extensive investigations.[97–99] The GFR, which increases only slightly and transiently following acute saline loading, may be a major limitation. More importantly, the increase in fractional sodium excretion in the young following an acute saline load may be only 1% to 3% compared to a 5% to 7% increase in the adult.[100] While it seems that the proximal tubule responds to the load appropriately, the distal tubule is limited in its ability to reject the load presented from more proximal parts of the nephron.[100,101] This avidity of the distal tubule for salt has been ascribed to high circulating levels of aldosterone[81] or to a greater load of the more mature juxtamedullary nephrons.[102] Recently, data have been presented which show a decreased ability of the neonate to increase natriuretic factors,[103] including oxytocin and renal kinin release.[53,104] Such findings, if confirmed, would seem to provide a more satisfactory explanation for the limited ability of the neonate, especially the preterm, to excrete a salt load.

The response to salt load in the neonate may be modified by the existing extracellular fluid balance[105] or by the ionic species given with the sodium (i.e., bicarbonate). Prior sodium chloride administration increases the ability of the newborn (like the adult) to excrete an acute sodium load; in addition, sodium as bicarbonate may be excreted faster than sodium chloride.[106] It must be emphasized that, compared to the adult, the ability to excrete sodium bicarbonate is still limited.

It has been suggested that the correction of acidosis by rapid infusions of hypertonic sodium bicarbonate results in an increased incidence of intracranial hemorrhage.[107] Simmons and coworkers reported that when the total daily dose of administered sodium was less than 8 mmol/kg and serum sodium levels were below 150 mmol/liter, the incidence of intracranial hemorrhage decreased significantly.[108] In a controlled trial by Corbet and coworkers, the correction of acidosis by constant infusion did not increase the incidence of intraventricular hemorrhage.[109] However the incidence of death was greater in those infants receiving more than 8 mmol/kg/day of sodium bicarbonate. Thomas suggested that the cause of the intraventricular hemorrhage with sodium bicarbonate administration may be related more to the changes in osmolality than to the sodium concentration.

The ability of the neonate to excrete a sodium load increases linearly with age until adult values are reached by 1 year of life. Preliminary studies in our laboratory have shown a similar age-related phenomenon.[112]

Potassium. In the first 10 days of postnatal

life, serum potassium levels may be as high as 7 mmol/liter. Thereafter, the levels range from 3.5 to 5.5 mmol/liter. The newborn may have a lesser ability than the adult to excrete a potassium load.[113] In contrast to a negative balance of sodium and chloride in the premature infant early in neonatal life, potassium balance is constantly positive in the neonatal period.[87]

Recent studies have suggested that the potassium permeability of the tubular luminal membrane is low in the newborn and increases with age. Similarly, a maturational process has been described for the Na-K-ATPase that may mediate the transport of potassium.[114]

Dilution and Concentration. The basal urine osmolality of the preterm human infant is similar to that achieved by the term newborn.[115] Although the fetus normally elaborates a urine hypotonic to the plasma, the fetal lamb near term can produce a concentrated urine.[116] Following fluid restriction, the mean urine osmolality achieved in prematures was 482 mosm/kg [370–680] and that for term newborns was 528 [210–650].[117,118] By 15 to 30 days in both term and preterm infants, maximal urine osmolality may be as high as 950 with a range from 780 to 1100. The majority of infants are still not able to concentrate as well as adults by 6 to 12 months of life.[21] However, at 2 months, some infants can concentrate their urine up to 1200 mosm. Asphyxia and hyperbilirubinemia may impair the ability of the neonatal kidney to maximally concentrate the urine.[92]

The inability of infant kidneys to maximally concentrate urine may be related to several factors including maturation of the countercurrent multiplication and exchange systems and a diminished response of the distal nephron to the effects of ADH.

In the rat kidney, Trimble[119] and Edwards and Mandel[120] have shown a direct relationship between growth of the loops of Henle, increased corticopapillary gradient, and urinary concentrating ability. The less steep medullary gradient in the young animal may be related to a decreased ability of the loop of Henle to pump sodium against a medullary gradient. While this has been related to the immaturity of the Na-K-ATPase system, Bursch[121] has shown that urine concentrating ability in the rat precedes the major increase in renal Na-K-ATPase. Augmentation of maximum urinary

concentration in the newborn has been demonstrated with urea or protein loading; these data suggested that low urea levels limited the ability of the newborn to concentrate the urine.[122,123] However, in these studies, even after urea or protein loading, the ratio of urine to plasma osmolality did not approach the adult values of 4 nor were adult values of TcH_2O achieved.[122,123] Urea loading in adults also enhances osmolar concentration.[124]

In the rat, urea loading did not increase the urine osmolality in those less than 10 days old, whereas an effect was seen in those older than 20 days.[119] In humans, increasing protein intake had a greater effect in infants at 4 to 6 weeks than it did at 1 to 3 weeks.[115] It has been suggested that the effectiveness of urea in increasing urine osmolality later in the neonatal period may be caused by a more efficient urea recycling by the kidney.[120]

The low levels of circulating ADH may be a cause of the inability to concentrate. It is generally assumed that these lower ADH levels found in infant plasma are not low enough to limit concentrating ability. Recently, the levels of ADH in the newborn have been measured by radioimmunoassay. ADH levels in umbilical artery and vein are elevated in preterms and term infants; by 2 hours of life adult levels are reached.[126] Hoppenstein also showed that the high plasma ADH levels in term infants decrease rapidly in the first 24 hours.[127] ADH levels of 1.3 μU/ml are detected at 22 to 100 days, and 3.6 μU/ml at 100 days to 3 months. Inappropriate ADH secretion is not uncommon in preterm and term newborns.[128,129] This indicates that the ability of the newborn to secrete ADH is not a limiting factor. In addition, studies in animals show that the sensitivity of the osmoreceptor and volume receptor for ADH secretion is similar in the newborn and the adult.[130,131,132] In the fetus, these receptors may in fact be more sensitive than those of the term newborn.

A diminished end-organ responsiveness to ADH in the young has been advanced as a limiting factor in the ability of the newborn to maximally concentrate his urine.[133] Svenningsen and Aronson[115] showed that the response of the term and preterm newborn kidney to exogenous arginine vasopressin (AVP) or 1-Desamino-8-D-arginine vasopressin (DDAVP) was less and of shorter duration at 1 to 3 weeks as compared to that obtained at 4 to 6 weeks.

Failure of earlier studies to show renal hyporesponsiveness may be because the infants (age 8–53 days) were studied as a group.[134] In the neonatal rat, urine osmolality was less than the corresponding papillary osmolality, indicating that complete osmolar equilibration did not occur. The cyclic AMP response to ADH stimulation of neonatal rat kidneys, inner renal medulla, and isolated collecting duct of neonatal rabbits is less than that of the adult.[135] In the rat, specific binding sites for ADH increase with age and slightly precede the onset of adenylate cyclase responsiveness.[136] Although a similar maturational pattern of ADH-stimulated adenylate cyclase has been reported in the piglet and the puppy,[137,137a] studies by Horster did not demonstrate decreased ADH effect on the collecting tubules in the latter species.[23]

Acid Base Regulation (See Chap. 29).

Acid-base balance in the fetus is mainly dependent upon maternal control mechanisms. However, the fetal kidney, at least after the second half of pregnancy, is able to acidify the urine.[138]

In the immediate postnatal period, the ability of the neonatal kidney to create and maintain a maximal hydrogen ion gradient is limited. Rapid postnatal maturity is achieved, however, so that by the end of 2 weeks pH values as low as those in adults (4.5–5.3) are recorded.[139]

In healthy preterm infants, during the first 4 weeks of postnatal life, the anion gap (serum sodium minus serum bicarbonate and chloride) ranges from 15 to 22 mmol/liter as compared to values of 9 to 12 mmol/liter in term newborns and adults.[87] The serum bicarbonate level may be as low as 14 mmol/liter in the preterm infant;[140] full-term values are 21 to 22 mmol/liter.[141] These levels are lower than adult values of 24 to 27 mmol/liter and are accompanied by a slightly higher serum chloride level. The maximal rate of HCO_3 reabsorption in preterm[142] and term[141] infants is about 2.5 mmol/dl of glomerular filtrate, similar to that reported in adults. The low serum HCO_3 levels in the newborn have been ascribed to a lower renal threshold for bicarbonate. The mechanism for the low bicarbonate threshold is unknown but may be a consequence of the expanded extracellular fluid volume in the neonate.[143]

The ability of the newborn kidney to excrete an acid load is limited, probably by the decreased excretion of urinary buffers, including phosphate and ammonium ions. Pretreatment of infants with phosphate, change of formula from breast milk to cow's milk, or increasing protein intake enhances the ability of the newborn to excrete titratable acids and ammonia.[144] Limited substrate availability and limitation of ammonia synthesis may hamper the ability of the newborn to excrete an acid load. Preterm infants excreted 0.44 mmol/acid/100 mg nitrogen, compared to 0.75 mmol/acid/100 mg nitrogen in term infants studied by Sulyok at 1 week of age.[145] This resulted in a positive hydrogen balance in the preterm during the first 3 weeks of extrauterine life. The ability to excrete a maximal acid load is quickly attained by 1 to 2 months in term and preterm infants.[146] This is caused by a more rapid maturation of titratable acid excretion; ammonia production may not reach adult levels until 2 years of life.[147]

Late metabolic acidosis. About 9% of preterm infants gradually develop a partially compensated hyperchloremic metabolic acidosis during the second to third week of life (late metabolic acidosis); spontaneous remission occurs in the next 2 weeks. This occurs at a time when there is an apparent delay in postnatal weight gain.[148] Radde and coworkers studied the effects of sodium bicarbonate treatment of late metabolic acidosis.[149] Strict maintenance of acid-base homeostasis was associated with greater increases in length compared to a control group. However, there were no differences in weight gains in the two groups. Schwartz and coworkers showed no correlation between correction of acidosis and weight gain in preterm infants.[140] They also showed that the values for titratable acids, ammonia excretion, net acid excretion, and minimum urinary pH were similar in preterm infants with bicarbonate levels lower than 18 mmol/liter and in those infants with higher levels of bicarbonate.

Renal Excretion of Calcium, Magnesium and Phosphorus (See Chap. 27). Eighty percent of the infant's skeletal calcium is acquired in the last trimester of pregnancy. Total serum calcium is 5.5 mg/dl in the second trimester and increases to 11.0 mg/dl in the third trimester. During the final weeks of gestation, fetal calcium levels are usually 2 mg/dl greater than corresponding maternal values. In the term newborn, total and ionized calcium decline in the first 4 days of extrauterine life, after which total calcium increases to 10 mg/dl. Thereafter, there is a gradual decrease with age until adult values are reached by 6 to 12 years of age.[150] In the very low-birth-weight infants, calcium levels fall by the second day and may not increase until the 12th week of life. The urinary excretion of calcium varies as a function of body weight (3 mg/kg/24 hours).[151] The ability to excrete a calcium load in the young is limited.[152] Apparently, parathormone (PTH) does not play a major role in the immediate regulation of renal calcium excretion in the newborn dog.[152] PTH levels may also not be entirely regulated by serum calcium levels.[153]

Serum magnesium levels are similar in preterm and term infants. The levels apparently do not change with age. The ability of the newborn kidney to handle magnesium has not been studied.

Serum phosphorus levels are high in the second trimester (14 mg/dl) and decrease to 6.0 mg/dl in the third trimester. In term infants, cord blood levels are 6.17 ± 1.03 and 6.55 ± 1.10 mg/dl at 3 to 24 hours. Thereafter, the levels rise to about 8 mg/dl, a plateau occurs at about 1 to 2 weeks, and subsequently there is a gradual fall. By 1 month, the levels are 5.75 ± 0.91 mg/dl.[154] Similar changes are observed in the preterm infant. Fractional reabsorption of phosphate increases with gestational age from 85% at 28 weeks to 98% at 40 weeks.[13] With the increase in serum phosphate levels after birth, the fractional phosphate reabsorption decreases to about 73%.[13] Acute intravenous phosphate loading fails to produce a significant increase in fractional phosphate excretion, suggesting maximal transport of phosphorus in the basal state. However if the phosphate load is increased by a change in formula from breast milk to cow's milk, the renal clearance of phosphate is increased.[155] The tubular transport maximum for phosphate is less in the young than in adults.[156] Decreased phosphate load may contribute to the limited ability of the young to excrete an acid load.[156]

Serum alkaline phosphatase levels range from 35 to 105 U/liter at birth and 70 to 250 at 1 month to 1 year of life. The isoenzyme patterns are 20% intestine, 15% liver, and 65% bone. After 18 years of life, the liver fraction increases to 65% while bone fraction decreases to 15%.[150]

Hypocalcemia (See Chap. 27). Hypocalcemia is a frequent problem in early postnatal life, especially in infants with gestational ages of less than 38 weeks. In one series, 3.2%

presented with serum calcium levels of less than 7 mg/dl during the first 36–48 hours of life; ⅔ were premature infants.[153] Studies by several investigators have shown that the PTH levels are low in the first 2 days of life in AGA infants. Thereafter PTH levels increase. The PTH rise in infants of diabetic mothers and in preterm infants is delayed until the age of 4 days. The incidence of hypocalcemia in preterm infants, infants of diabetic mothers, and asphyxiated infants is significantly greater than in healthy term newborns.[153] The mechanism of hypocalcemia is not well known. It does not seem related to the aforementioned delayed rise in PTH seen in infants in this category because when clinical hypocalcemia is manifest PTH levels often tend to rise. Nonetheless, the inverse correlation between PTH and serum calcium is not apparent. Thus the hypocalcemia may be caused by end-organ hyporesponsiveness. Other possible mechanisms include increased secretion of cortisol and calcitonin.[153,157-160] Apparently, vitamin D is not a causal factor.[159]

Renal Regulation of Glucose. Studies available on glucose reabsorption show low maximum reabsorption at birth with gradual increase with age.[13,161] The proximal tubular reabsorption of glucose in the young is difficult to assess and compare to adult values because of nephron heterogeneity. Nonetheless, an adult maximum value is obtained after the first year of life when a more homogeneous population of nephrons is obtained.

Renal Regulation of Amino Acids. Generalized aminoaciduria occurs in the neonate and the infant as a result of lowered tubular reabsorption. When correction is made for glomerular filtration rate, however, net tubular reabsorption is the same in infancy as in childhood.[162] It has been suggested that this represents another example of variation in glomerulotubular balance and heterogeneity of the nephron population in the neonate/infant as compared to the older child and adult.

The ontogeny of amino acid reabsorption in human kidney has been recently described.[163]

CLINICAL EVALUATION OF RENAL FUNCTION

History

Oligohydramnios may suggest either renal agenesis, hypoplasia, dysplasia, or an obstructed urinary tract, provided no loss of

Table 30-2. Failure of Urine Formation in the Immediate Newborn Period.

Causes
Postnatal intravascular hypovolemia
Restriction of oral fluid
Bilateral renal agenesis
Tubular necrosis
Bilateral renal vein thrombosis
Congenital nephrotic syndrome
Congenital pyelonephritis
Congenital nephritis

(From Moore ES, Galvez MB: J Pediatr 80:867, 1972)

amniotic fluid is documented.[164] Alternatively, polyhydramnios may be associated with a newborn recipient twin in the transplacental transfusion syndrome. These patients may have dilated renal tubules and enlarged bladders. A discussion of fetal renal structure and its relationship to amniotic fluid disorders is available.[165]

A history of delayed micturition in the first 24 to 48 hours may suggest various etiologies.[166] The most likely cause is inadequate perfusion of functioning kidneys in an otherwise perfectly normal neonate. The other causes may be classified into those that are associated with failure of urine formation (Table 30-2) and those secondary to obstruction to urinary flow (Table 30-3). To the latter should be added posterior urethral valves. Additional history should address conditions conducive to renal vascular problems. Severe asphyxia may be associated with renal tubular

Table 30-3. Obstruction to Urine Flow in the Immediate Newborn Period.

Causes
Imperforate prepuce
Urethral strictures
Urethral diverticulum
Hypertrophy of the verumontanum
Neurogenic bladder
"Megacystic syndrome"
Ureterocele
Renal tumors

(Moore, Galvez)[166]

necrosis or massive medullary hemorrhage, or more commonly a transient microscopic hematuria.

Physical Examination

The presence of single umbilical arteries has been associated with urinary tract anomalies. The classic Potter's facies, with low-set ears, flattened nose, hypertelorism, epicanthal folds, and micrognathia, would indicate bilateral renal agenesis. Small deformed ears may indicate renal anomalies, and, if unilateral, a renal lesion may exist on the ipsilateral side. Trisomy syndromes should be readily recognizable with their expected renal anomalies.

The "prune-belly" syndrome, with absent abdominal musculature, bilateral cryptorchidism, and urinary tract dilatation, is a well-recognized entity. Patients with myelomeningoceles often have neurogenic bladders and may be born with bilateral hydronephrosis.

Abdominal palpation may reveal such renal anomalies as ectopic kidney, horseshoe kidney, and enlarged kidneys (hydronephrotic, polycystic, multicystic, tumor, renal vein thrombosis) as well as an enlarged bladder secondary to outlet obstruction.

Urinalysis

In the neonate, urinary specific gravities are usually low, with osmolalities ranging from 60 to 600 mosm/liter. The urine pH is usually 6.0 to 7.0, but, as noted previously, the term neonatal kidney rapidly achieves the ability to lower the urine pH to 5.0 or less, after the second week of life. Urates, which are excreted in large amounts during the first week of life, may give false-positive tests for proteinuria. The average urinary excretion of protein is reported to be 0.86 mg/m^2/hr at 28 weeks of gestation; it peaks at 2.48 ± 4.0 mg/m^2/hr at 34 weeks and decreases to 1.29 ± 1.84 mg/m^2/hr at 40 weeks.[13] DeLuna and Hullet reported a mean excretion of 45 mg/day in term newborns. Twelve percent of infants studied by Arant had protein excretion rates of greater than 4 mg/m^2/hr.[13] These infants did not manifest any evidence of disease. In this same study, only 3% had greater than 30 mg/dl in a random specimen. Transient proteinuria may normally be observed in the first 3 days of life. Thus, proteinuria greater than 30 mg/dl or persisting beyond 6 days of life is an indication for further study.[168,169]

Transitory glycosuria in the first week of postnatal life has been found in 20% of term and preterm newborns.[13,168] Excretion is greatest in infants less than 34 weeks of gestational age.[13]

Leukocyturia is normally absent in the neonate, but epithelial cells are common and should not be mistaken for leukocytes. These may be either squamous, particularly in females from vaginal sloughing, or tubular epithelial cells. It has been suggested that the presence of epithelial cells in the urine may direct attention to prenatal or postnatal asphyxia.[170,171] Urine collected by chatheterization or suprapubic bladder aspiration may eliminate spurious findings; a careful "clean-catch" voided urine, however, yields comparable results.[172]

Red blood cells are also not normally found in the newborn's urine. Cylinduria does occur, however, but rapidly disappears within the first week.[168]

The urine of newborns is normally sterile.

Serum Urea Nitrogen and Creatinine

The BUN values in the immediate neonate are usually in the range of 5 to 20 mg/dl, even if the infant has bilateral renal agenesis. Low initial values with renal insufficiency reflect placental function. Thereafter, rises in BUN suggest renal dysfunction if the infant is on the usual infant formulas. Levels as high as 30 mg/dl may be achieved in normal infants when fed a formula of high-protein concentrations. The serum creatinine values at birth are at or near the adult level, falling within approximately 2 to 4 weeks to the levels seen at 1 month of age (0.1–0.2 mg/dl). Thus, early serum creatinine values, unless elevated above usual adult values (0.5–1.1 mg/dl), may be of little aid in estimating renal function in the newborn infant.

Renal Clearance Tests

Urea clearances are of little value in estimating glomerular filtration rate; beyond 1 to 2 weeks of age, endogenous creatinine clearance is useful in assessing glomerular function. To obtain accurate measurement of glomerular filtration rate, however, inulin clearances (C_I) may be used, necessitating priming and maintaining doses of inulin IV, collection of blood samples, and urethral catheterization for accurate collection of serial urines. This restricts its general clinical usefulness. Alternatively, single injection techniques with radioactively labeled substances, without need for bladder catheterization, have been used. Currently, these methods without urine collection do not give information better than those achieved with endogenous creatinine clearances.

Renal blood flow may be measured by determining the clearance of para-aminohippurate (C_{PAH}); the technique is similar to the inulin clearance with the same clinical disadvantages. Furthermore, C_{PAH} clearances, as noted previously, do not accurately measure renal blood flow below 6 months of age because of reduced extraction of PAH by the infant kidneys.

Serum Chemistries

Serum sodium values in premature infants and full-term infants are approximately 145 ± 5 mmol/liter. Hypernatremic dehydration in the neonate may, in a male suggest the possibility of nephrogenic diabetes insipidus. Hyponatremia occurs in small-for-gestational age infants, as well as in sodium-wasting states, such as cystic fibrosis or renal and adrenal salt-wasting diseases.

Hyperkalemia is a normal transitory finding.

Hyperchloremia occurs in both premature and full-term infants, although it is more marked in the premature.

Values for pH normally range from 7.24 to 7.38 in the first few hours after birth; thereafter, a mean of 7.42 is observed. Serum bicarbonate levels of 21 to 22 mmol/liter, are observed during the first year of life. Metabolic acidosis in an infant without diarrhea may represent aminoacidemia, organic acidemia, or renal tubular acidosis, either primary or secondary.

Total serum calcium values of 8.6 ± 0.8 mg/dl, ionized calcium values of 4.1 ± 0.6 mg/dl, and phosphorus values of 6.9 ± 1.2 mg/dl are normally found.[173] Magnesium values range from 1.5 to 2.5 mmol/liter.

Urine Specific Gravity/Osmolality

The average maximal urinary concentration is 600 to 700 mosm/liter (specific gravities 1.018–1.021) in the neonate; increases to an average value of 1,000 mosm/liter may be seen at 1 to 2 months. Standardized tests for urinary concentrating ability include the following:

1. Infants and children are given either half-cream milk or full-cream milk (dried milk

dissolved in half the usual amount of water with sugar added) for 24 hours in amounts calculated to provide their usual caloric intake. Urine is collected at intervals of 3 to 4 hours. Maximum osmolality is taken as the highest value obtained in the urine samples. In the series described, the following averages were obtained: third day, 515 mosm/liter; sixth day, 663 mosm/liter; tenth to thirtieth days, 896 mosm/liter; and age 1 to 2 months 1054 mosm/liter.[174,175]

2. Infants and children over 2 months of age may be tested by administering intramuscularly pitressin tannate in oil in a dosage of 0.1 ml (0.5 pressure units)/6 kg of body weight, following which fluid is restricted for 16 hours. All urine specimens voided are collected separately with the highest osmolality or specific gravity achieved considered as the maximal concentrating ability. A median value of 1000 mosm/liter may be achieved by 2 years of age.[176]

There are obvious dangers inherent in performing these tests on children suspected of having diminished urinary concentrating ability. Such patients should be observed for dehydration and, if a weight loss of greater than 4% occurs, the test should be terminated.

Radiologic Investigation of the Kidney

An abdominal flat plate may yield some information regarding renal size, radiopaque nephrolithiasis, or nephrocalcinosis.

Intravenous pyelography may be performed using contrast agents such as diatrizoate sodium (50% Hypaque) or diatrizoate sodium and methylglucamine diatrizoate (37% Renovist) in doses of 3.5 to 4.0 ml/kg of body weight. This test has proven to be of value in suspected renal vein thrombosis. Should no visualization of the kidneys be noted 5 to 10 minutes after injection, a second injection of contrast material may be utilized with films taken at 15- to 20-minute intervals. Rarely, a 24-hour film may be necessary for visualization if extremely slow renal excretion occurs. Most cases of hydronephrosis, multicystic kidneys, polycystic kidneys, and Wilms' tumors may be visualized by the procedure. Unilateral nonvisualization of a kidney requires the use of other diagnostic procedures such as retrograde pyelography.[177] Complications of intravenous pyelography include rare instances of renal cortical ischemia, medullary necrosis, and pulmonary edema.[178] Extreme caution should be exercised in prematures because of the high osmotic load of the dye.

Radionuclide Evaluation of the Kidney

Radionuclides may be helpful in the evaluation of the neonatal kidney when there is no visualization of the kidney by intravenous pyelography or to evaluate flank masses. Differential function of the kidneys may be grossly assessed by these radioactive agents.

[131]I-Hippuran renal scans indicate functioning renal tissue. When renograms are also obtained, the uptake, transit time, and excretion of the agent can be followed. The uptake and transit time reflect renal blood flow and tubular transport; the excretion phase is associated with flow through the pelvis and the ureter. Therefore, a delayed uptake and transit suggests decreased renal perfusion, intrinsic renal disease, or both, whereas a decreased excretion suggests extrarenal obstruction. Delayed excretion caused by obstructive factors may be delineated by comparing the renal scan data with the renogram results.

Intrarenal blood flow distribution studies have not yet been performed in infants; however, the disappearance of intravenously injected ^{133}Xe has been utilized in adults to measure cortical and inner cortical blood flow.

A comprehensive review on renal radionuclide utilization in pediatrics is available.[179]

Ultrasonography. Nephrosonography is a safe and very useful aid in the newborn especially when congenital renal anomalies are suspected or when oliguria or anuria is present. It has been shown to be of value in the localization and study of nonfunctioning kidneys, in distinguishing cystic from solid space-occupying masses in the kidney, and in determining kidney size and the presence of obstruction.[180,181]

We prefer to perform ultrasonography first, then consider radionuclide evaluation, and use intravenous pyelography last.

ACQUIRED RENAL ABNORMALITIES

Acquired neonatal anatomical abnormalities of the kidney or its nephrons may be classified broadly as those associated with circulatory abnormalities and those secondary to infection. Circulatory disorders probably are the most common etiologic group in acquired renal disease in the newborn. Vascular occlusion may occur with either renal artery or renal vein thrombosis.

Renal venous thrombosis is seen in newborn infants in association with asphyxia and hypoxia, vomiting, diarrhea and dehydration, hyperosmolality, intravascular clotting, cyanotic heart disease, and following angiocardiography, and it may occur in infants of diabetic mothers.[185,186] Oppenheimer and Esterly[187] and Avery and coworkers[186] reviewed 4000 neonates who died in the first 14 days of life and noted that 15.8% of those with a history of maternal diabetes had evidence of venous thrombosis at autopsy. Similar lesions were found in only 0.8% of infants of nondiabetic mothers. The authors suggested that the thrombi probably developed *in utero*. Recently Stuart and coworkers presented evidence of platelet hyperfunction and increased synthesis of prostaglandin endoperoxides in infants of diabetic mothers.[188] However, in Arneil's report of 115 cases, no relationship between renal venous thrombosis and diabetes could be found.[190]

Under 1 month of age, the babies affected are preponderately males. The occlusion may be unilateral or bilateral; the kidney is palpably enlarged in 60% of patients. Blood pressure is variable but usually normal. Oliguria may be noted. In more than half of the cases, hematuria is present. Hyperosmolality, microangiopathic hemolytic anemia, low fibrinogen levels, and thrombocytopenia are usually present. In addition, azotemia, metabolic acidosis, and abnormalities in serum sodium concentration may be noted.

Diagnosis. The presence of hematuria, enlarged kidneys, and intravascular clotting suggest renal venous thrombosis. A flat plate of the abdomen may be ordered to determine the size and location of the kidneys and to help locate abnormal calcifications. For more accurate determination of the presence and size of the kidney, a nephrosonography is called for. If the tests are suggestive, (enlarged kidneys) one may perform an inferior vena cavogram and intravenous pyelogram. Differential diagnosis includes hydronephrosis, cystic disease, and tumors of renal and adrenal origin.

Treatment. Oliguric infants should be treated as having acute renal failure. Intravascular coagulation should be corrected. This may necessitate the use of heparin at a dose of 100 U/kg body weight, followed by a continuous intravenous infusion at 25 U/kg/hr.[190] The dose is then adjusted to maintain the clotting time at 2 to 2.5 times control values. Heparin is continued until the platelet count and clotting factors return to normal. Nephrectomy during the acute phase is not indicated. Bilateral thrombosis with anuria may be managed by dialysis. The extent of dialytic intervention is an unresolved issue.

The nephrotic syndrome, usually secondary to slow forming renal venous thrombosis, is uncommon in the newborn period. However, hypertension in infancy may develop.[190]

Renal artery thrombosis has been associated with highly placed umbilical artery catheters,[182] patent ductus arteriosus,[183] sepsis, cardiac arrythmias, hypercoagulable states, and trauma.[184] Physical examination is nonspecific. Hypertension is common, and cardiorespiratory and neurologic symptoms are often seen in hypertensive neonates. Palpably enlarged kidneys are rare. Urinalysis may be normal but more commonly reveals microscopic hematuria, rarely gross hematuria, and proteinuria. Renal function may be diminished and irreversible renal cortical necrosis or infarction may occur. Peripheral renin activity is elevated for age.[182] Diagnosis is made by arteriography. Radionuclide studies may be used for followup.[182] When obstructive uropathy is suspected, ultrasonography and a voiding cystourethrogram may be performed before proceeding towards intravenous urography. Any underlying problem should be corrected. Aggressive treatment of the hypertension is essential. Failure of antihypertensive therapy is an indication for nephrectomy in cases of unilateral renal artery thrombosis. Thrombectomy and anticoagulant therapy remain to be evaluated. Significant mortality occurs. Among survivors, most can be weaned off their medications in 3 to 6 months.

Hypertension in the newborn has been defined as systemic blood pressure greater than 90/60 torr in term infants and greater than 80/45 in preterm infants. Adelman reported an incidence of 2.5% of intensive care nursery admissions.[182] Over 75% may be caused by renal artery thrombosis. The next most common cause is renal artery stenosis (18%). Rare causes include cogenital renal anomalies, adrenal hyperplasia, hypoplastic aorta, and coarctation of the aorta. In some cases, no clear etiology could be found. Signs and symptoms are nonspecific. Heart failure may be present.

Therapy should be directed at identifying and correcting the etiology. In one series, 85% of the infants had an indwelling umbilical artery catheter prior to or at the onset of hypertension. Mild hypertension (10 torr greater than the upper limits of normal) may respond to salt restriction or diuretics. Greater elevations of blood pressure may be treated with hydralazine (5 mg/kg/day) and methyldopa (25 mg/kg/day). When pulmonary and heart disease are not present, propranolol (2-4 mg/kg/day) may be used in lieu of methyldopa. Extreme elevations of blood pressure may be managed with diazoxide (5 mg/kg/dose IV). Nitroprusside may be used starting at a dose of 2 μg/kg/min Thiocyanate levels should be monitored if nitroprusside is used for more than 3 days. Uncontrollable hypertension caused by unilateral renal disease may necessitate nephrectomy.

Renal necrosis. Renal conditions in which vascular occlusion may not be readily demonstrable, but in which ischemic changes occur, include renal cortical, tubular, medullary, and papillary necrosis.

Bilateral renal cortical necrosis is rare, often fatal, and most often associated with circulatory failure and/or disseminated intravascular coagulation.[191-194]

Laboratory findings. Azotemia, metabolic acidosis, albuminuria, and microscopic hematuria may be found. Scan may reveal poorly or nonfunctioning kidneys. However, plain films of the abdomen may demonstrate both kidneys outlined by a rim of calcification extending throughout the outer cortex.[195]

Roentgenology. One can distinguish between renal cortical and renal tubular/medullary necrosis; in the latter, one usually finds renal function sufficient for adequate renal visualization by intravenous pyelography. During the acute phase, a prolonged nephrogram may be seen, whereas at a later date renal scarring and papillary necrosis occur.[196,197] The characteristic finding of cortical rim calcification is noted in renal tubular necrosis, chronic pyelonephritis, tuberculosis, and hyperparathyroidism. Treatment is that of acute renal failure (see below) and of underlying conditions.

Acute tubular necrosis may occur in those same circumstances that give rise to cortical necrosis and, in some instances, the two coexist. As noted previously, renal function is better preserved with acute tubular necrosis than with acute cortical necrosis.

Renal medullary necrosis[198,199] most often is caused by episodes of severe vascular collapse as with neonatal asphyxia, gastroenteritis, or hemorrhage, and occurs more frequently in females. In long-term cases, the heart may show left-ventricular hypertrophy. This is another example of an enlarged kidney with hematuria.

Renal papillary necrosis is rare in neonates and infants. The kidneys may be palpably enlarged, and gross or microscopic hematuria is almost invariably present. Urinary infection may be associated with it. Uremia is the principal cause of death after an illness lasting 1 to 3 weeks. A case report with a review of the literature, and a hypothesis as to etiology, invoking prostaglandin action, is available.[200]

ACUTE RENAL FAILURE

Acute renal failure (ARF) is a clinical syndrome that occurs following a sudden reduction in renal function; its hallmark is progressive azotemia.[201] In the newborn, renal dysfunction may be the first manifestation of renal dysplasia or agenesis. Some degree of ARF may be seen in 25% of all neonatal intensive care admissions, of which a quarter may be caused by acute tubular necrosis.

ARF should be suspected if the BUN is greater than 20 mg/dl, the rise in BUN is greater than 5 mg/dl/day,[202] serum creatinine rises more than 0.2 to 0.5 mg/dl/day, or oliguria occurs, defined as urine output less than 25 ml/kg/24 hours.[203] Renal failure can occur even when urine output is normal (nonoliguric renal failure).

Etiology

ARF may be caused by prerenal, renal, or obstructive uropathy.

Prerenal failure may be caused by underperfusion of the kidney because of inadequate cardiac output or by hypovolemia. The former may be seen in asphyxiation at birth, cardiac failure, hypoxia, or respiratory distress syndrome. Hypovolemia may be caused by blood loss, fluid and electrolyte loss through the skin, gastrointestinal tract or the kidney, or sequestration as seen in sepsis, ascites, or chylothorax. Recent studies have reemphasized the importance of hypoxia and shock as major contributory factors in the development of acute renal failure.[204,205] Depending upon the degree of hypoxia, oliguria with decreased sodium excretion or a diuresis may be observed.[206,207] Intermittent positive pressure ventilation,[208] vasodilators, or vasoconstrictors may decrease renal blood flow and produce renal failure.[209]

Intrinsic Renal Failure

Acute tubular necrosis has been used synonymously with acute renal failure.[201] Intrinsic renal failure may follow prolonged hypoxia, hypovolemia or hypoperfusion, disseminated intravascular coagulation, renal arterial and venous thrombosis, or toxic nephropathy (*i.e.,* drug induced). Congenital renal malformations causing renal failure in the neonatal period are listed below.[210]

Parenchymal Malformations Associated with ARF

1. Renal agenesis
2. Renal hypoplasia
3. Renal dysplasia
4. Renal dysplasia with urinary tract obstruction
5. Infantile polycystic disease

Obstructive Uropathy

This may be caused by intrarenal obstruction (urate nephropathy) or extrarenal obstruction, such as seen in congenital malformations of the lower urinary tract. Anatomic obstructions include posterior urethral valves, Eagle–Barrett syndrome (absent abdominal musculature), congenital urethral stricture, and neuropathic bladder.

Acute renal failure caused by intrinsic kidney damage has been traditionally divided into two categories: nephrotoxic injury and renal ischemia. Oliguria usually follows the initial insult. The mechanism for the initiation or maintenance of the oliguria in acute renal failure remains controversial.[211] Evidence has been presented for tubular factors including abnormal back diffusion of filtrate through damaged tubular epithelium and tubular obstruction. There may also be altered glomerular dynamics. Failure of filtration may be caused by resetting of afferent and efferent arteriolar resistances, alterations in glomerular ultrafiltration coefficient, or both.

Recent studies have shown that prevention of renal ischemia may not prevent the fall in glomerular filtration and development of severe ARF. However, agents that increase renal blood flow and increase osmolar excretion, such as mannitol, furosemide, and prostaglandins, may ameliorate the severity of ARF. In addition, Seigel and coworkers have shown that prior infusion of Mg-ATP may prevent the development of renal failure.[212] Most of the studies on ARF have been done in adult animals. Bidani and coworkers showed that mercuric chloride-induced renal failure was associated with a greater mortality and slower recovery in young rats as compared to older animals.[213]

Diagnosis of the Type of ARF

Adult criteria of ARF, including oliguria and azotemia, may not be applicable to the newborn. The influence of gestational age, postnatal age, concomitant disease, and drug therapy on renal function presents special problems inherent in the preterm and term infants.

Acute renal failure is usually suspected when oliguria or azotemia are noted. Oliguria in the neonate may be defined as urine flow of less than 25 ml/kg/24 hours. Acute renal failure may however occur even with normal urine flow rates. Anderson and associates reported that the incidence of nonoliguric renal failure in adults may be as high as 59%.[214] The incidence of nonoliguric renal failure in the newborn is not known. In our series, three of ten newborns with acute renal failure had normal urine flow rates.[215]

The normal range of BUN in the neonate is 3 to 10 mg/dl.[216] In the preterm with a very high protein intake, the BUN may be greater than 20 mg/dl.[217] Hypercatabolic states, as in sepsis, sequestered bleeding, large areas of tissue necrosis, and hemoconcentration, and inborn errors of urea excretion may result in elevated urea levels despite normal renal function. Although in the adult, severe renal failure is characterized by a daily increase in BUN of from 10 to 30 mg/dl, in the newborn an increase of 5 mg/dl/day may suggest renal failure. The lesser increments in BUN may be related to the higher anabolic states in the newborn as compared to the adult. Catabolic states such as sepsis, hyperpyrexia, and starvation may double the rate of rise in blood urea in any age group.[202]

In the newborn, serum creatinine may not be useful as in older infants and children in the assessment of renal function, without considering the factors that influence its levels. Creatinine is an end product of creatine metabolism, and plasma creatinine in the steady state is related to the muscle mass. In the newborn, serum creatinine is the consequence of maternal plus fetal production so that neonatal levels approximate maternal values. The high levels of creatinine noted at birth usually decrease by 2 weeks of postnatal age.[216,218] Small changes in very low creatinine values allow large potential errors. A sustained rise in serum creatinine (0.2–0.5 mg/day) is indicative of a reduction of glomerular filtration rate. Values of GFR are influenced by gestational age and postnatal age.[13–21] The timing of umbilical cord clamping may also transiently affect the glomerular filtration rate during the first 24 hours of life.[16]

The electrolyte abnormalities that occur in acute renal failure are quantitatively different in the newborn as compared to older children. In the newborn with severe renal failure, serum potassium may rise at a rate of 0.4 to 0.8 mmol/liter/day, whereas in older age groups the increment is usually over 1 mmol/liter/day. Similarly, the rise in serum phosphorus and magnesium and the fall in serum calcium associated with severe reduction in glomerular filtration rate is less rapid in the newborn than in adults.[202]

The diagnosis of acute renal failure caused by tubular necrosis is arrived at after elimination of other diagnostic possibilities. The history, physical examination, urinalysis, and other laboratory tests will usually categorize the cause of the renal failure (*e.g.*, prerenal failure, renal parenchymal disease, tubular necrosis, or uropathic obstruction). The occurrence of azotemia with normal urine flow rates may be seen in nonoliguric renal failure, increased urea production, inborn errors of urea excretion, or prerenal failure following diuretic therapy. Anuria is suggestive of renal agenesis or aplasia, severe renal dysplasia, vascular accidents, cortical necrosis, or obstruction. Oliguria with azotemia may be seen in renal vascular disease, renal parenchymal disease (*i.e.*, interstitial nephritis), oliguric tubular necrosis, or prerenal failure.

Several laboratory aids have been used to help differentiate the entities causing renal failure (Table 30-4). In prerenal failure, the urinary sodium concentration is relatively low while the urine: plasma ratios of urea, creatinine, and osmolality are high, indicating a concentrated urine. In contrast, in acute tubular necrosis, the urinary sodium concentration is high, and the low values are found for the urine: plasma ratios of urea, creatinine, and osmolality. While these values are used mainly to distinguish prerenal failure from acute tubular necrosis, Miller and coworkers have recently reported that urine chemistries in acute obstruction may resemble those of oliguric acute tubular necrosis, while acute parenchymal renal disease (such as glomerulonephritis and interstitial nephritis) produces a urine similar to that found in prerenal failure.[219]

In adults, the ratio of urinary sodium to the urine: plasma creatinine ratio (renal failure index) has been reported to be a more accurate guide in the diagnosis of acute tubular necrosis.[219] A renal failure index of less than 1 was generally found in prerenal failure, and greater than 2 in acute tubular necrosis. In newborns, however, the fractional sodium excretion is not only influenced by intrarenal and extrarenal mechanisms,[220] but also by gestational and postnatal age as well.

The ratio of urine to plasma creatinine is least in the most preterm newborns and increases with postnatal age. Norman and Asadi found that the renal failure index in newborns with acute tubular necrosis was significantly greater (15.9) than those reported in adults.[205] Mathew and coworkers recently reported that the renal failure index was greater than 3 in infants with ARF whose gestational ages were greater than 33 weeks.[220a] Therefore, renal failure index in the newborn needs further evaluation in terms of gestational and postnatal age.

The ratio of urine to plasma osmolality has been reported to be consistently close to one in acute tubular necrosis regardless of age.[221] Norman and Asadi, Gordillo–Panigua, and Velasquez–Jones found that the ratio of urine to plasma osmolality in acute renal failure caused by tubular necrosis in newborns was consistently less than 1.1, similar to that reported in adults.[205,222]

The establishment of urine flow may be used as a diagnostic as well as a therapeutic ma-

Table 30-4. Laboratory Aids in the Differential Diagnosis of
Acute Renal Failure.

	Prerenal oliguria		Low-output acute tubular necrosis	
	Adult	*Infant*	*Adult*	*Infant*
Urine Na, mol/liter	<20	<10	>25	>40
FeNa, %	< 1	< 1.8	> 3	>10
U/P osm	> 2	> 2	< 1.1	< 1.1
U/P urea	>20	>20	<10	< 5
U/P creatinine	>40	>20	<10	< 5
Urine sediment (*casts*)	hyaline and granular		cellular	

U = Urine; P = plasma; FeNa = fractional sodium excretion
(Adapted from Medani et al: Contrib Nephrol 15:47, 1979)

neuver in distinguishing prerenal failure from oliguric acute renal tubular necrosis. The first step is to assure adequate volume repletion. This may require the infusion of electrolyte solutions, dextrose in water, albumin, or blood, depending upon the putative cause of volume contraction. If there is no evidence of circulatory overload and the central venous pressure is not elevated, a fluid challenge of 10% dextrose in water with 30 mmol/liter sodium chloride at 20 ml/kg in 1 to 2 hours may be undertaken. If adequate urine output is not established in 1 to 2 hours, a trial of mannitol, furosemide, or both may be indicated. In the case of prerenal failure, 60 ml/m^2/hour of 12.5% mannitol solution will result in a urine output of at least 12 ml/m^2/hour within 1 hour of the infusion.[222] Of 53 newborns with oliguria, Gordillo–Panigua and Velasquez–Jones found seven newborns who eventually were diagnosed as having acute renal tubular necrosis.[222] All those infants had an inadequate response to mannitol, whereas all of the remaining 46 infants had positive responses.[222] It should be noted that the use of mannitol is contraindicated in the presence of congestive heart failure.

Williams and coworkers found that intravenous furosemide gives results comparable to the mannitol infusion test.[202] However, loop diuretics may increase urine flow in renal parenchymal as well as prerenal oliguria.[223] A dose of 1 to 2 mg/kg can be administered intravenously.[209] There should be an increase in urine flow of 50% or greater within 1 to 2 hours after the injection of furosemide. In a number of adults with normovolemic oliguric renal failure, intravenous furosemide resulted

in an increase in urine flow to nonoliguric rates.[223] Those who responded appeared to have an earlier stage of acute renal failure. Whether the conversion of oliguric to nonoliguric renal failure alters the natural course of the disease in adults, children, or newborns remains to be determined.

In nonoliguric renal failure, fluid and electrolyte losses should be replaced to avoid dehydration.

If oliguria is established, fluid intake should be restricted to that required to replace insensible water loss, urine, and any other extrarenal water and electrolyte loss. Insensible water loss varies greatly depending upon gestational age and environmental conditions. Nutritional status should be monitored carefully to provide a minimal exogenous caloric intake of 40 Kcal/kg/day as carbohydrate and fat. Recent studies in infants and adults suggest that addition of essential amino acids or organic acids may be beneficial.[224]

In the well-managed patient, severe hyperkalemia is rarely a problem. Hyperkalemia is a constant threat to the patient with ARF, especially in the presence of sepsis, necrotic tissue, or blood. In the first 10 days of life, potassium may normally be as high as 7 mmol/liter. Thereafter, the following definitions apply.

Mild hyperkalemia, defined as serum potassium of 6.0 to 6.5 mmol/liter with a normal ECG, may be treated with exchange resins such as sodium polysterene sulfonate (1 g/kg) in sorbitol, given as a retention enema. **Moderate hyperkalemia,** defined as serum potassium 6.5–7.5 mmol/liter, peaked T waves on EKG, needs to be treated immediately. Infusions of hypertonic dextrose with insulin (1 unit/3 g) at 0.5 g/kg/dose or infusion of $NaHCO_3$ may be administered. **Severe hyperkalemia,** defined as serum potassium greater than 7.5 mmol/liter with major ECG abnormalities, should be treated with calcium gluconate at 100 mg/kg with ECG monitoring. Because the effects last for only 5 minutes, this should be followed immediately by intravenous glucose and bicarbonate and preparation of the patient for dialysis.

Other complications include hemorrhage, hypertension, and infection. There are no available data on pharamacokinetics of drugs in renal failure of the newborn. Therefore, blood levels should be obtained whenever possible.

The indications for dialysis in the newborn are not well established. In our institution, we have used the following as guides to the initiation of dialysis therapy: severe hyperkalemia, circulatory overload, pulmonary edema, and uremia. The blood levels of urea and creatinine at which dialysis is indicated are not established. We have found that a BUN greater than 50 mg/dl is associated with the abnormalities listed above.

Course

In oliguric renal failure in adults, urine flow usually decreases within a day of the initiating injury. The duration of the oliguria is quite variable, ranging from hours to weeks, 1 to 2 weeks being the usual period. Oliguria lasting more than 4 weeks is suggestive of cortical necrosis. The diuretic phase of oliguric renal failure may be heralded by an increase in urine volume and improvement in renal function. In approximately two-thirds of the patients, GFR may remain 20% to 40% below normal for a year or more after the episode of oliguria. In addition to the reduction in GFR, a variety of tubular functions may be persistently abnormal.[201] Nonoliguric renal failure tends to have a shorter period of significant azotemia and a lower mortality.[214] The mortality in adults is usually secondary to infections or hemorrhagic complications.[223]

The course of acute renal failure in the newborn is poorly documented. In our series, the etiologies were varied but often included birth asphyxia, hypotension and disseminated intravascular coagulation.[215] Forty percent died, generally of concurrent illness. The ma-

jority of deaths were in the first week. Of the ten patients studied at our hospitals, five died in the first week. The survivors began to recover within a week after the onset of azotemia. Follow-up data from a few weeks to several years suggests that about 50% will have normal renal function and that the rest be abnormal, having decreased GFR, decreased concentrating ability, and decreased ability to acidify the urine.

Extensive prospective data on neonatal renal failure are lacking. There are few ongoing studies relating etiology, diagnosis, course, and prognosis.[205] As the data become available, early diagnosis and appropriate therapy may improve the outlook of the newborn with acute tubular necrosis.

EDEMA OF THE NEWBORN (See also Chap. 29)

Edema of the newborn constitutes a major clinical problem. Consideration of the causes of edema requires knowledge of the mechanisms of edema formation.[225,226] Approximately 75% of the newborn body weight is water and does not approach the adult value of 65% until the end of the first year. Extracellular water in the skin and subcutaneous tissue together account for 16% of the infants total body water, compared with 8% in the adult. The extracellular fluid volume is composed of interstitial and intravascular fluid, in the ratio of 3:1. The Starling forces (hydraulic and colloid osmotic pressures) govern the rate of capillary exchange of fluid with the interstitial space. However, considerable derangements of Starling forces can be present in the vicinity of a normal capillary before edema fluid becomes apparent clinically.[226] This observation suggests that other important homeostatic mechanisms may be available to prevent large accumulations of edema fluid. Recent concepts view **interstitial tissues** as a buffer force between the interstitial space and vascular compartment; the **lymphatics** return to the circulation any positive new flow of fluid appearing at the interstitial space; and a **noncompliant interstitial space** modulates tissue hydrostatic pressure with changes in interstitial fluid volume. Increases in tissue hydrostatic pressure occur with small increases in interstitial fluid volume. Such backpressure lowers the hydrostatic gradient which draws fluid out of the capillary. The interstitial compartment contains collagen, which forms a network of interlacing fibers through a matrix of gel composed of protein, salts, and mucopolysaccharide. Fluid in the interstitial space is in the form of gel with very free-flowing channels of water. The relationship of interstitial fluid pressure to changes in interstitial water content is most significant in defining clinical states of edema. Excessive accumulation of edema fluid can be brought about by

1. increases in capillary hydrostatic pressure.
2. decrease in plasma oncotic pressure.
3. diminished tissue hydrostatic pressure or reduced rates of lymphatic drainage.

With this background, we can discuss the common problems associated with edema in the newborn with the exception of renal failure and congestive heart failure, which are covered elsewhere.

In utero and immediately after birth, the extracellular fluid mass is greater than that of the intracellular fluid. This relationship reverses early in the postnatal period. Weight loss within the first few days after birth of a normal newborn would indicate recovery from **physiologic edema.** MacLaurin has shown that normal newborns have limited ability to concentrate the urine maximally.[227] He suggests that the neonatal decrease in weight was largely a consequence of this, resulting in the transfer of water from the intracellular to the extracellular compartment. However, studies have shown that late edema of the newborn occurs in the presence of a rise in GFR with improvement of concentrating ability and without change in the serum proteins.

The amount of blood received by the newborn from the placenta may vary considerably. This influences water content and compartmentalization. The type of delivery also affects water content of the newborn. During the first twenty-four hours, babies born after elective cesarian section have a higher body water content.[228]

Salt intake. Renal handling of salt during maturation has been described. Newborn infants challenged with large salt intake remain in positive balance and may show edema if salt intake is not curtailed.

Edema of the Preterm infant. Permeability of the capillaries is increased in the preterm infant allowing transcapillary escape of albumin.[229] This may play a role in the physiochemical properties of the interstitial gel in the newborn infant having a large compartment assigned to the skin. It would appear that such factors as asphyxia, hypotension, poor tissue perfusion, and **failure to maintain appropriate body temperature** could very well allow for excessive fluid shifts.

Edema associated with **vitamin E deficiency** would create a disturbance in capillary permeability caused by a deficiency of the antioxident effect of vitamin E.[230]

Rh incompatibility. The data of Baum show an interesting correlation between the colloid osmotic pressure of cord venous blood and gestational age in both hydropic and nonhydropic infants with Rh incompatibility.[231] Hydropic infants could be noted with normal levels of plasma protein and albumin concentration, while in severe cases of Rh incompatibility very low levels of protein may be operative in the formation of edema.

Nephrotic Syndrome. Edema in nephrotic syndrome is related primarily to protein loss. A reduction in the effective arterial blood volume occurs despite expansion of the extracellular fluid compartment. Several entities have been reported with onset during the first year of life. Most of the conditions that cause nephrotic syndrome during the first year of life have been summarized by Kaplan and coworkers (Table 30-5).[232] Such a classification is comprehensive and essential for genetic counseling, management, and prognosis. Measuring levels of alpha fetoprotein in the amniotic fluid has made prenatal diagnosis possible. Intrauterine infections with toxoplasmosis cytomegalovirus have been associated with nephrotic syndrome as well.

Rare causes of edema in the newborn include **hereditary hypoparathyroidism,** the edema perhaps caused by decreased sodium excretion of the kidney.[233] Edema in association with **hypomagnesemia** and **hypocalcemia** may be caused by salt and water retention caused by solute load of cow's milk.[234]

Management should be based on understanding the pathophysiologic events that have led to edema formation. Careful assessment of dietary intake of salt and water is important. Accurate measurements of weight and urine output and blood pressure recordings are essential in management. Diuretics may be ap-

Table 30-5. Classification of the Nephrotic Syndrome in the First Year of Life.

Classification	Etiology	Age at onset	Noteworthy features	Pathology
A. Infantile microcystic disease	Autosomal recessive	Birth to 3 mo	Toxemia of pregnancy Prematurity Placentomegaly	Dilated proximal renal tubules
B. Minimal lesion nephrotic syndrome	Usually idiopathic	>6 mo	Usually responds to corticosteroid therapy	Fusion of foot processes on electron microscopy
C. Focal glomerular sclerosis	idiopathic	>6 mo	Microhematuria and corticosteroid resistance with progressive renal failure may be seen	Focal segmental or diffuse glomerular sclerosis
D. Omniglomerular diffuse mesangial sclerosis	Idiopathic Possible familial	<6 mo	Progressive development of renal failure	Omniglomerular diffuse mesangial sclerosis, interstitial fibrosis
E. Epimembranous glomerulopathy	Congenital syphilis	<6 mo	Clinical features of congenital syphilis	Epimembranous nodules; Epimembranous IgG and fibrin, or IgG, IgA, IgM, and β_1C globulin deposition Epimembranous deposits
F. Conditions which rarely may be associated with the nephrotic syndrome	Idiopathic	<2 yr	1. Genital anomalies	Glomerular sclerosis and interstitial fibrosis
	Familial	<2 yr	2. Nephroblastoma	
		1 case at birth, usually > 3–4 yr	3. Nail-patella syndrome	Focal glomerular sclerosis; by electron microscopy, lucent areas and collections of collagen fibrils in glomerular basement membrane
	Mercury intoxication	<2 yr	4. May have other clinical signs of mercury poisoning	Minimal or no change

(Kaplan et al: J Pediatr 85:615, 1974)

propriate if caution is utilized in infants with low colloid osmotic pressure or hypovolemia. A volume expander like salt-poor albumin 0.5 g/kg, infused within 1 to 2 hours, when combined with a diuretic such as furosemide, is usually effective in mobilizing edema fluid. A clear understanding of the complications following diuretic use is essential.

DIURETICS IN THE DEVELOPING KIDNEY

Very few studies are available dealing with the effects of diuretics in term and preterm infants. Walker and Cumming studied the diuretic response of normal infants, 6–67 days of age, to single doses of mercaptomerin, chlorothiazide, acetazolamide, or triamterene.[235] Peak diuresis occurred in 2 to 4 hours after drug administration. Mercaptomerin increased sodium excretion sevenfold compared to a three- to fourfold increase noted with the other diuretics. In these infants, spironolactone produced an increase in urine flow and sodium excretion. The response was qualitatively similar to that reported in adults. A tendency for GFR to decrease was noted with chlorothiazide. Engle and coworkers showed that the diuretic response of furosemide given at 1 mg/kg parentally or 2 mg/kg orally was unrelated to age.[236] Ross and coworkers reported similar conclusions in low-birth-weight infants.[237] However, Woo and coworkers suggested that the response to furosemide in stressed term infants may be less intense but more prolonged, when compared to adults.[238] Aranda and coworkers showed that, with fluid overload, the plasma clearance of furosemide was lower and volume of distribution greater in the preterm and full-term neonate as compared to adults.[239] They related the latter to decreased protein binding. Wemby and coworkers reported that diuretics did not significantly displace bilirubin.[240] The effect of aminophylline on renal function in preterm newborns with apnea has been published.[241] While the effects are minimal, increases in GFR and fractional sodium excretion have been reported. Noorderwier and coworkers studied the dose response curves to constant infusion of furosemide, ethacrynic acid, hydrochlorothiazide, and amiloride in 5 to 10 day old anesthetized piglets.[242] The diuretic responses in piglets were similar to those noted in adults. In the unexpanded state, in the puppy, amiloride inhibited sodium reabsorption to a greater extent than in adults. Amiloride also had a greater effect on potassium secretion in the newborn dog than in the adult dog during saline expansion.[243]

KIDNEY INFECTIONS

Infections of the kidney in the newborn occur most frequently in males and are usually a consequence of coliform septicemia.

Symptoms and signs include hyperbilirubinemia, irritability, anorexia, vomiting, and failure to thrive.

Diagnosis may be made by blood and urine cultures.

In general, before 12 months of age, the male predominance obtains; further, the male is more likely at any age to have serious disease because boys have a higher incidence of associated structural abnormalities and obstruction. However, if patients with obstructive disease are removed from the sample, there is an equal sex incidence of urinary tract infection in the first postnatal year. Thereafter, the incidence is higher in the female, with ratios ranging from 9:1 to 30:1. Additionally, because minor anomalies of the urogenital tract are reported to occur in 1 of 8 newborns, a potential for urinary tract infections exists.

Neonates of low birth weight or large infants are more at risk to develop urinary tract infection. Usatisfactory weight gain is the most frequent symptom. Bergstrom and coworkers reported that fever was common in infants who became ill after the tenth day of life.[244] Other symptoms included vomiting, lethargy, diarrhea, and jaundice.[245] It is important to note, however, that in a recent study of full-term and premature infants, bacteriuria was found in 0.7% of full-term infants and in 2.9% of premature infants, the majority of whom were asymptomatic.[246] This study suggests that routine screening in the healthy full-term neonate (*e.g.*, urinalysis and cultures) may not be profitable; furthermore, asymptomatic urinary tract infection is more common that symptomatic in the premature. The natural history of asymptomatic bacteriuria is unknown. In infancy, failure to thrive with recurrent episodes of fever are the usual presenting signs. Occasionally, a careful history of micturition may reveal infrequency and/or a poor urinary stream.

The diagnosis of urinary tract infection depends upon the demonstration of "significant bacteriuria." If one utilizes the "clean-catch midstream technique," a culture revealing colony counts of 100,000/ml of a single species is indicative of urinary tract infection. Contaminated urines are more often associated with lesser colony counts and/or multiple organisms. The urine should be cultured immediately or within 24 hours of refrigeration. The clean-catch midstream technique is often difficult to carry out in the nursery; in general, a substitute method has been utilized using sterile urine collectors attached to the perineal area. Should this technique be used, recleaning and reapplication of subsequent sterile collectors are needed if the infant does not void within 45 minutes. In general, this technique too often has yielded contaminated cultures and is unsuitable for diagnosis. Alternative methods of collection include percutaneous, suprapubic bladder aspiration or urethral catheterization. With the latter methods, colony counts of 100/ml or less may be considered significant because the healthy urinary tract should not harbor bacteria. Urine obtained by suprapubic bladder aspiration is sterile.

To perform the **percutaneous suprapubic bladder aspiration**

1. Place the infant in a supine position with the lower extremities in a frog-leg position.
2. Cleanse suprapubic area with alcohol and paint it with iodine.
3. Locate the symphysis pubis with an index finger, with a 20-ml syringe with a 21-gauge, 1.5-inch needle attached; penetrate the abdominal wall and bladder in the midline about 1.5 to 2.0 cm superior to the symphysis pubis with a rapid movement directing the needle toward the bladder fundus at a 30° angle.
4. Aspirate the urine and withdraw the needle. To enhance the likelihood of success, the neonate should not have voided within 1 hour prior to the procedure. Localization of the bladder by sonography may be necessary.

To accomplish **urethral catheterization** in the neonate, a small sterile feeding tube is passed into the urethra. Thoroughly cleanse the urethral area with an antiseptic solution and rinse with sterile water. In patients in whom outlet obstruction is suspected, Renografin may be instilled through the catheter and a voiding cystogram performed to determine the existence of vesicoureteral (V–U) reflux. In infants, the short intramural portion of the ureter in relation to its width (<2.5:1) has been implicated etiologically in the high incidence of recurring urinary tract infections. The V–U reflux may be primary or secondary. The **primary** form may be associated with ectopic ureteral orifices and persistent reflux. The **secondary** variety is found with infection and may disappear with cessation of the infection.

The urinary tract and ureteral structure should also be studied by sonography, radionuclide studies, or intravenous urography in all patients in whom a urinary tract infection is diagnosed.

Pathogenesis

The intestinal tract can serve as a reservoir for pathogenic organisms with perineal urethral spread. Prevention of infection through the ascending route depends upon bladder defense mechanisms including phagocytic activity of the bladder mucosa and mechanical emptying (voiding). Failure of complete bladder emptying because of a fault in the urinary outlet mechanism may provide the basis for bacterial growth in the bladder. Recently, bacterial adherance to epithelial cells and vaginal IgA levels have been implicated.

Uropathogenicity of *Escherichia coli* subgroups has been postulated because nine such subgroups usually account for 50% of the infections. However, this concept is not currently widely accepted.

The renal medulla is the usual site of involvement by the invading organism whether by the hematogenous or ascending (urethra-bladder-ureter-kidney) route. The hematogenous route becomes of major importance in (1) the newborn period; (2) children with renal developmental defects such as hypoplasia, dysplasia, or cystic disease; and (3) congenital obstructive lesions of the urinary tract. Special features of the renal medulla that may be related to its vulnerability include low total blood flow, high osmolality (possible interference with phagocytosis), dependency on anaerobic metabolism, and being the site of ammonia production. Ammonia may interfere with the fourth component of complement and thus may reduce medullary bactericidal antibody activity.

Renal function studies utilizing inulin and para-aminohippurate (PAH) clearances have suggested that changes in renal cortical blood flow may occur early in infants and children with recurrent urinary tract infection.[247] It was suggested that the diminished renal cortical blood flow as measured by C_{PAH} reflected early renal functional derangement which may be reversible with therapy. The effects of infection on subsequent renal development and function are not known, although limited longitudinal studies show a tendency to reversibility of diminished clearances in infants.[247]

Treatment

Surgical therapy will not be discussed here (see Chap. 28); patients with compromised renal function secondary to an anatomic obstruction that is accessible to operative intervention may be helped immeasurably.

The effectiveness of an antimicrobial program may depend upon factors such as urinary pH, presence of obstruction, and the susceptibility of the invading bacteria. In acute episodes of urinary tract infection without obstruction, a recover rate of 70% to 80% may be anticipated; however, recurrences are common and may occur in 30% to 40%. In the neonate, short-term therapy with drugs such as kanamycin (15 mg/kg/day in two divided doses) or tebramycin (3–6 mg/kg/day in two divided doses) is the usual. When these drugs are used, BUN levels should be monitored at 5-day intervals and at the conclusion of therapy. Until the cultures are available, tebramycin is usually given in combination with ampicillin. Further chemotherapy with other drugs will depend on recurrence of the susceptibility of the organism.

Prognosis

In patients with structural abnormality of the urinary tract, the prognosis depends upon the severity and potential reversibility. The natural history of patients with asymptomatic or symptomatic urinary tract infections without associated urinary tract abnormality is unknown. In general, data from patients studied in the Department of Pediatrics, Georgetown University Hospital suggest that such patients followed 1 to 12 years have a good prognosis. Longer follow-up is obviously necessary. Some investigators believe that the patient may be at continual risk for life.

Drugs such as methicillin and gentamicin, endogenous substances such as uric acid, and disease caused by immune complex deposition may produce interstitial nephritis. In one study, acute interstitial nephritis was seen at autopsy in 10% of infants who died in the prepartal, perinatal period, and during infancy.[248]

FUNCTIONAL ABNORMALITIES OF THE KIDNEY

Nephrogenic Diabetes Insipidus (NDI)

The renal origin of this form of diabetes insipidus was described in 1947.[249] The onset is in the neonatal or early infancy period with failure to thrive, vomiting, constipation, recurrent fevers, and recurrent episodes of dehydration with hyposthenuria. Polyuria and polydipsia may not be prominent features. Mental retardation may be a serious sequela.

Renal function is usually normal. Hypernatremia and hyperchloremia are seen with dehydration episodes. In a male patient, hyposthenuria with severe dehydration may suggest this diagnosis. A simple water deprivation test will separate normal subjects or patients with psychogenic polydipsia from children with diabetus insipidus.[250] The lack of response to administration of exogenous antidiuretic hormone differentiates this condition from the pituitary forms of diabetes insipidus.

The bladder is frequently enlarged in these patients, apparently as a consequence of the persistent polyuria.[251] Massive dilatation of the urinary tract, including bilateral hydronephrosis, in the absence of any organic obstructive uropathy may occur.[252]

The renal microscopic findings may reveal normal glomeruli and tubules; however, microdissection has shown a decrease in the length of the proximal tubular convolutions.[253] Short proximal convoluted tubules have been demonstrated in both nephrogenic diabetes insipidus and cystinosis.[254,255]

A male predominance is noted in the disease with a sex-linked recessive mode of transmission originally considered.[249] However, symptomatic females have been reported as an autosomal dominant trait with incomplete penetrance.[251,256]

The basic defect is unknown; end-organ (renal) unresponsiveness to circulating antidiuretic hormone is generally proposed. The lack of tubular-hormone response could be caused by several possible faults: an enzymatic defect in the receptor site, in the receptor-enzyme coupling mechanism, or in the core enzyme. The adenyl cyclase system has been proposed as the site for vasopressin action.[257-259] At least two types of NDI have been described: one in which ADH does not increase urinary cyclic AMP levels and another in which ADH increases cyclic AMP levels but still does not increase renal concentrating abilities.

The mental retardation that may occur in these patients is believed secondary to the bouts of hypertonic dehydration. Hypernatremia of diverse etiology in childhood has been associated with cerebral damage and subsequent mental retardation.[260] In addition, large water intake may present problems in infancy meeting the caloric requirements. Normal growth and social contact occur when an adequate nutritional diet and reasonable water intake are effected.

Differential diagnosis. This includes primarily pituitary diabetes insipidus, NDI secondary to obstructive uropathy, potassium depletion, hypercalcemia, structural medullary cystic disease, and essential hypernatremia.

Prognosis. Early diagnosis and treatment determines the prognosis. Death may occur in early infancy if inadequate attention is paid to fluid management during dehydration episodes. Physical and mental retardation may persist, although early diagnosis and therapy may prevent or partially reverse the developmental abnormalities.

Therapy. The most important therapy for these patients is the provision of water in association with a low-protein diet, thereby sacrificing growth in favor of mental development. As the child grows older he will regulate his own water intake. Diuretics may be a valuable adjunct to therapy: 25 mg/kg per day of chlorothiazide or 5 mg/kg per day of hydrochlorothiazide may be used initially with higher doses needed in occasional patients. Therapy may be prolonged for 12 to 24 months or longer, until spontaneous improvement occurs with age. Some patients may not respond to thiazide therapy. The thiazides cause mild hypovolemia, thus allowing for enhanced proximal sodium reabsorption with volume depletion.[261-263] Periodic peripheral blood studies should be done because of the hematologic side effects of these drugs.[264] Furosemide, orally in doses of 2 mg/kg/day in two divided doses, may be effective in yielding an antidiuretic response when daily sodium intake is limited.

Renal Alkalosis with Hyperplasia of the Juxtaglomerular Apparatus, Hyperaldosteronism, and Normotension (Bartter's Syndrome).

Patients with this syndrome display a hypokalemic, hypochloremic metabolic alkalosis with normal blood pressures despite elevated serum levels of angiotensin and increased urinary aldosterone excretion.[265] Renal biopsy reveals marked hyperplasia of the juxtaglomerular apparatus, macula densa enlargement, and an abnormal PAS-positive membrane between the juxtaglomerular wall and macula densa.[266]

Diagnosis may vary from infancy to 25 years of age.

Symptoms and signs. These may occur shortly after birth. The earliest symptoms and signs are failure to thrive, polyuria, polydipsia, constipation, muscle weakness, salt craving, and occasionally tetany. In the pediatric age group, growth retardation is a frequent feature; in adults it is not. Renal insufficiency and/or renal osteodystrophy are uncommon.

Characteristic biochemical features include hypokalemia, hypochloremia, hyponatremia, and metabolic alkalosis; occasionally, hypercalcemia, hypomagnesemia, and hyperlipidemia occur.

Hyposthenuria occurs with no response to the exogenous vasopressin administration. Urinary acidification responses are diminished and hydrogen ion excretion occurs mainly as ammonium. Urinary wasting of potassium and chloride occurs in the face of lowered serum concentrations. Proteinuria is variable and microscopic hematuria is uncommon. Lowered or normal inulin and PAH clearances may be found.

Plasma renin/angiotensin levels are elevated and variably respond to plasma volume expansion by intravenous dextran, saline, or albumin infusion. Aldosterone secretory rates are increased, although urinary aldosterone excretion may be normal or increased.

Renal morphology reveals atrophic to enlarged glomeruli, as well as immature (fetal-like, primitive) glomeruli. The juxtaglomerular apparatus is hyperplastic with macula densa enlargement and a PAS-positive membrane separating the two structures. Hypokalemic tubular lesions are present.

The syndrome is thought to be transmitted by means of a mutant autosomal recessive gene.

The pathophysiologic mechanism of this disorder is a subject of great controversy. Several postulates have been forwarded, including defective sodium transport in various segments of the renal tubule, defective chloride transport in the ascending limb, defective potassium handling by the kidney, resistance to angiotensin II, generalized defect in cation transport, and abnormalities of prostaglandin and kinin metabolism.[266-276]

Although patients with idiopathic hypokalemic metabolic alkalosis and hyperreninemia have been lumped under the heading of Bartter's syndrome, the clinical picture is not totally uniform. The renal response to salt restriction has been variable.[265,266,276] Recently, Robson and others showed that the ability to conserve salt in Bartter's syndrome may be age related, with younger patients demonstrating greater salt wasting than patients over age 3.[277] The variability of the manifestations may also be noted in the reports of normal levels of urine and plasma aldosterone.[278] Several investigators have suggested that variations in the clinical presentation of patients with idiopathic hyperkalemic alkalosis may indicate a spectrum of a single pathologic entity or represent multiple etiologic conditions.[279]

The differential diagnosis includes pyloric stenosis, Fanconi's syndrome, and renal tubular alkalosis. Primary hyperaldosteronism is characterized by hypertension, sodium retention, and lack of elevated plasma renin/angiotensin levels. Secondary hyperaldosteronism with hypertension or edema should be readily distinguished.

The prognosis is variable with mild disease not diagnosed until adolescence or adult life, whereas severe diseases may terminate in death in infancy or early childhood. The physical and mental growth of these children have been described.[280,281]

Therapy consists of supplemental sodium and potassium chloride administration, combined with spironolactone or triamterene therapy, propanolol to decreases renin secretion, and prostaglandin synthetase inhibitors.[277,279]

Renal Tubular Alkalosis

Metabolic alkalosis as a consequence of possible congenital, familial, or acquired renal tubular defects has been reported.[282-293] In retrospect, many of these have been considered as undocumented patients with Bartter's syndrome,[265] yet some clearly are not because no juxtaglomerular hyperplasia existed. Signs and symptoms are similar: failure to thrive, fever, recurrent bouts of dehydration, polyuria, polydypsia, salt craving, muscle weakness, and bouts of tetany. A hypokalemic, hypochloremic metabolic alkalosis is the main biochemical feature. Glomerular function is normal, but urinary concentrating ability is impaired. Urinary potassium or chloride wasting occurs; urinary aldosterone excretion rates may be normal or elevated. Renal morphologic findings are nonspecific or secondary to potassium depletion. The condition may be familial or acquired. No definitive pathogenic mechanism was outlined for any of these patients. Therapy consists of fluid management for dehydration coupled with supplemental sodium or potassium chloride administration throughout childhood.

Hypochloremic, hypokalemic metabolic alkalosis may also be caused by diarrhea, vomiting, brain disease, abuse of laxatives and diuretics, and recently, to decreased chloride intake from milk formulas with absent or minimal chloride levels.

Renal Tubular Acidosis (RTA)

RTA is a clinical condition caused by impaired renal acidification in which the glomerular function is normal or is comparatively less impaired than the tubular function. Conversely, glomerular acidosis occurs in chronic renal insufficiency as part of the uremic syndrome. Further classification has differentiated two main forms. One is based on a defect in proximal tubular reabsorption of bicarbonate, while the other manifests an inability to establish a hydrogen ion gradient in the distal tubule. Proximal RTA, or Type 2 RTA, is thus distinguished from distal RTA, or Type 1 RTA, also called "classic" RTA. In some patients, the delineation between proximal and distal RTA is difficult to establish because they share features of both. Two patterns of combined RTA have been described:[294] hybrid 1,2 RTA and a second pattern, found in some infants with apparently classic distal RTA but with associated bicarbonate wasting (type 3).[295] In addition, another type of RTA is characterized by acidosis and hyperkalemia (type 4). In this form, there is a qualitative or quantitative defect in aldosterone secretion (Table 30-6).[296]

Treatment. In proximal RTA, huge amounts of alkali at frequent intervals may be needed to sustain adequate correction of the acidosis. The starting dose is between 5 to 10 mmol/kg/day. Administration of potassium is usually necessary. In very severe forms of RTA, alkali therapy alone may be ineffective, and the use of diuretics like hydrochlorothiazide has been successfully used. In distal RTA, the dose of alkali is about 1 to 3 mmol/kg/day, but when there is associated bicarbonate wasting, the requirement of alkali is larger and could be greater than 10 mmol/kg/day for normal growth to be maintained.[297-299] The normal growth pattern is usually achieved by 6 months after sustained correction of the acidosis. Recently, Griger and coworkers suggested that measurement of plasma lysyl oxidase levels may be useful as a marker of adequate alkali therapy.[300] This section will deal with primary forms.

The primary proximal (infantile, transient) form occurs predominantly in males and has its onset in infancy with the cardinal features of recurrent vomiting and failure to thrive. These children will excrete an acid urine when the serum bicarbonate is below the renal threshold (patients with the distal tubular form cannot lower urinary pH to less than 6 with acidosis). The diagnosis in children with proximal RTA involves documentation of a lowered bicaronate threshold and normal capacity of distal acidifying mechanisms. Standardized testing procedures for the latter are available.[299] In general, the acid loading is done with oral ammonium chloride at doses of 75 mmol/m² in infants and 150 mmol/m² in children; five 1-hour urine samples are then collected with blood samples obtained 3 to 4 hours after the ammonium chloride ingestion. In normal infants, urinary pH of 5.0 or less is achieved, with mean values for titratable acid and ammonium of 62 to 57 μmol/min/1.73 m² respectively.

Patients with primary distal RTA (persistent, adult) are generally females with onset of disease usually from 2 years of age to ·adult life. Occasionally, the patient may present in infancy with failure to thrive, vomiting, anorexia, polyuria, constipation, and dehydra-tion. Rickets and osteomalacia may occur; nephrocalcinosis is a common finding and may, by renal tissue damage, lead to decreased GFR. In the face of a metabolic acidosis or under acid-loading conditions, urinary pH usually remains 6.0 or greater, and low levels of titratable acid and ammonium are excreted in the urine. Urinary concentrating ability ultimately is lost, although this may be reversible in early stages prior to nephrocalcinosis and tubular damage.

Incomplete forms of renal tubular acidosis have been described:[301] the patients had nephrocalcinosis without systemic acidosis but with a defect in urinary acidification. This form may present with recurrent nephrolithiasis, idiopathic hypercalciuria, or with symptoms of potassium deficiency.

The renal morphology in patients with proximal RTA reveals no histologic abnormality. In autopsy studies on renal tissue from a patient with distal RTA, calcium deposition was noted in the collecting tubules. Biopsy studies on adults have revealed no pathology.

Primary proximal renal tubular acidosis is not always genetically determined. Primary distal RTA appears to be transmitted by an autosomal dominant mode of inheritance. Most cases, however, are sporadic.

Prognosis. Patients with the proximal variety respond well to therapy; in the majority, recovery occurs, and therapy may be eventually discontinued.[299] In patients with primary distal RTA, early therapy may prevent development of nephrocalcinosis (the degree of nephrocalcinosis, nephrolithiasis, and consequent renal damage results in a variable life span. With adequate and sustained alkali therapy, patients have attained normal stature.[298]

Oculocerebrorenal Syndrome (Lowe's Syndrome)

This entity was first described in 1952,[303] and a comprehensive review appeared in 1968.[304] The typical syndrome consists of cataracts (bilateral, always present at birth), glaucoma, mental retardation, hypotonia with absent or depressed deep tendon reflexes, failure to thrive, and amino aciduria.

GFRs are normal. Tubular defects are variable. Glycosuria may occur; proteinuria usually is an alpha₂ or beta₂ microglobulin. Microscopic hematuria, pyuria, and cylinduria may be present. Biochemically, the patients

Table 30-6. Physiologic Characteristics of Prototypical Disorders of Renal Acidification.

	Renal Tubular Acidosis (RTA)				
	Type 1 RTA ("Distal RTA")	HCO₃ Wasting Classic RTA (Type 3 RTA)	Type 2 RTA ("Proximal RTA")	Type 4 RTA	Uremic Acidosis
Acidemia	Present	Present	Present	Present	Present
Net renal H secretion at normal ($HCO_3)p$	Nearly normal or minimally reduced	Moderately reduced	Greatly reduced	Moderately reduced	Nearly normal to greatly reduced
Bicarbonaturia (% of filtered HCO_3 excreted at normal $(HCO_3)\overline{p}$	3%–5%	5%–10%	>15%	2%–15%	<3% to >30%
$TA + NH_4^+$ excretion at normal $(HCO_3^-)p$	Reduced	Reduced	Reduced	Reduced	Reduced
Therapeutic alkali requirement (mmol HCO_3/kg of body weight per day)	1–3	5–10	2 to >10	1–2	1–3
Urinary acidification during acidosis	Impaired	Impaired	Intact	Intact	Intact
$TA + NH_4^+$ Excretion during acidosis	Subnormal	Subnormal	Not invariably reduced	Not invariably reduced	Subnormal
Bicarbonaturia (% of filtered HCO_3^- excreted during acidosis)	<3%	5%–10%	None	None	None
Serum potassium concentration	Normal or reduced	Usually reduced	Normal or reduced	Greatly or moderately increased	Normal or moderately increased
GFR	Normal or reduced	Normal	Normal or reduced	Normal or reduced	Greatly reduced

(Adapted from Sebastian et al. In The Kidney. Philadelphia, WB Saunders, 1976) have a hyperchloremic acidosis. A sex-linked recessive mode of transmission is suggested. No mechanism currently exists for identification of the heterozygote.

Renal biopsy and autopsy data have been reviewed.[305,306] Early in life, no abnormalities are seen; at 6 months to 5 years nonspecific glomerular atrophy, sclerosis, and hyalinization are observed. The metabolic acidosis is believed to be secondary to renal tubular dysfunction—a proximal renal tubular acidosis.

Prognosis. The patient may die of renal insufficiency, dehydration on intercurrent infection. Survival to adulthood is possible.

Therapy. Adequate fluid management plus alkali therapy for control of acidosis are necessary. Vitamin D therapy is usually needed for prevention or correction of rickets, doses ranging from 500 to 1,500 IU per day to as high as 50,000 to 100,000 IU per day. Dihydrotachysterol or 1,25-di-OH D may be used instead of vitamin D. Ophthalmologic therapy has consisted of cataract removal, iridectomy for glaucoma, and, in some patients, enucleation.

Galactosemia

Galactosemia is a genetically transmitted disease characterized by an inability to metabolize galactose in a normal manner. Infants with the common type of galactosemia present with failure to thrive, jaundice, hepatomegaly, and cataracts. There may be associated mental retardation.

Proteinuria of an alpha$_2$-globulin type exists in almost all patients early in life and may reach values of 1 g per day. It disappears rapidly when galactose is removed from the diet. There is a generalized aminoaciduria which also disappears, although much less rapidly than the proteinuria, with elimination of dietary galactose. Hyperchloremic RTA of the secondary proximal renal tubular type may occur.

Inheritance is by autosomal recessive mode,[306,307] the large majority of patients having a defect in the enzyme galactose-1-uridyl transferase. Heterozygotes are detected by enzyme assay. Another type with a deficiency of galactokinase has also been reported.[308–310]

Clinical findings. Infants with galactose-1-phosphate uridyl transferase deficiency fail to thrive, have gastrointestinal dysfunction, cataracts, hepatomegaly, evidence of liver dysfunction with or without jaundice, and mental retardation. The renal abnormalities appear to be related to the toxic action of galactose-1-phosphate.

Unlike the patients with transferase deficiency, infants with galactokinase deficiency thrive normally but form cataracts later in life if placed on unrestricted diets. There is no hepatic or kidney damage and mental retardation is not a feature.

Diagnosis. Galactosemia suggested by the presence of galactose in blood and urine and demonstration of the specific enzyme deficiency in peripheral blood cells. Intrauterine diagnosis is possible for the homozygote.[311]

Prognosis. The therapy, which includes elimination of dietary galactose, is associated with reversibility of the renal lessions. (See also Chap. 28.)

Cystinosis is a rare, recessively inherited disorder characterized by the widespread deposition of cystine crystals within lysosomes. It exists in infantile (nephropathic), adolescent (intermediate), and benign forms.[312,313]

The benign form is associated with no symptoms and shows neither retinopathy or renal dysfunction. Cystine crystals however are present in the cornea or conjunctiva. In the intermediate form of cystinosis, incomplete tubular dysfunction and slowly progressive glomerular failure develop at a later age.

Clinical findings. The infantile form to be considered here presents with failure to thrive, recurrent vomiting, unexplained fever, metabolic acidosis, polyuria, dehydration, glucosuria, generalized aminoaciduria, and hyperphosphaturia. Hypophosphatemic rickets is seen in the early stages followed by hyperphosphatemic osteodystrophy when chronic glomerular insufficiency occurs. Hepatosplenomegaly may occur. Photophobia is common.

Pathophysiology. The syndrome is primarily a proximal renal tubular dysfunction, presumably secondary to cystine deposition, the basic mechanism for cystine deposition being unknown. There is phosphaturia, proximal renal tubular acidosis, glucosuria, and generalized aminoaciduria. Biochemically, there is metabolic acidosis with hyperchloremia and hypokalemia.

Diagnosis. The diagnosis rests on demonstration of cystine crystals in bone marrow, peripheral leukocytes, liver, spleen, or lymph nodes. In the majority of instances, they may also be seen in the cornea by slit-lamp examination. Elevated levels of cystine occur in peripheral leukocytes and skin fibroblasts but not in plasma. Prenatal diagnosis may be made by determination of cystine in cultured amniotic fluid cells obtained by aminocentesis.[314]

Prognosis is poor, with glomerular failure eventually appearing, leading to uremia and death prior to puberty.

Treatment. Therapy includes specific drugs, low methionine and cystine diet, and renal transplantation.[315] Drugs that have been used include penicillamine, dithiothreitol, and methenamine (Cysteamine). Their efficacy has not been proved. More recently, ascorbic acid has not shown any benefit in the treatment of the disease. Diet therapy is also of no proven value. Recent data suggest that renal transplantation could be successfully performed (see also Chap. 28).[316,317] Alkali therapy (sodium bicarbonate or Shohl's solution) is used for control of acidosis, and vitamin D therapy for rickets. Additionally, diuretic therapy with hydrochlorothiazide plus potassium bicarbonate has resulted in correction of the acidosis and rickets. The dosage of hydrochlorothiazide was 1.5 to 2.0 mg/kg per day with potassium bicarbonate of 20 mmol/day. The apparent mechanism of action of the diuretic in achieving these results is related to the hypovolemia achieved and resulting in increased proximal renal tubular bicarbonate reabsorption and a hypocalciuric effect.[318]

FAILURE TO THRIVE WITH RENAL DISEASE

Growth failure is a documented observation in patients with renal disease. Table 30-7 outlines possible mechanisms. The incidence of growth failure in different studies ranges from 35% to 65%.[319] Growth failure is more frequent and more severe in children with congenital renal disease than in those with acquired disease. Betts and Magrath reported that children with congenital renal disease have severe growth retardation in infancy.[320] However, in acquired renal disease, stature can be maintained above the third percentile until GFR falls below 25 ml/min/1.73 m².

Chronic acidosis is divided into two groups: renal retention or glomerular insufficiency, and renal wasting or tubular dysfunction. Poor growth in children with acidosis and renal disease was recognized some years ago.[321]

Table 30-7. Growth Failure with Renal Disease.[324]

Chronic Acidosis
Inadequate renal excretory function (renal retention)
Polycystic kidneys
Hypoplastic kidneys
Chronic nephritis
Chronic pyelonephritis
Hydronephrosis

Abnormal renal excretion (renal wasting)
Cystinosis
RTA
Oculocerebralrenal syndrome (Lowe)
Chronic pyelonephritis
Hydronephrosis

Chronic Alkalosis
Congenital renal alkalosis
Bartter's syndrome

Negative Nitrogen Balance
Inability to concentrate urine—diminished caloric intake
NDI, chronic renal failure
Protein loss
Nephrosis
Electrolyte disturbances
Potassium depletion
NaCl depletion
Hypophosphatemia
Abnormal renal excretion of phosphate
Vitamin D refractory rickets
Cystinosis
Hypocalcemia, osteodystrophy

Chronic Infection
Pyelonephritis

Hormonal Factors
Decreased somatomedin
Steroid treatment

Experimental animal studies suggested that the pH is not the important variable but rather the excessive loss or decreased intake of such cations as Na, K, Ca, and Mg.[322] Recently, a direct effect of pH on hormone receptor interaction has been advanced.[323] These experimental studies may explain the growth retardation seen in patients with renal alkalosis. Sustained correction of the tubular acidosis with alkali or of the renal alkalosis with sodium chloride, potassium chloride, or both may result in "catch up" growth. However, in those patients having retention acidosis with azotemia, correction of the acidosis has not been associated with resumption of growth. Negative nitrogen balance states, as well as inadequate caloric intake (as in NDI), may obviously be related to poor growth.

Patients with hypophosphatemia with or without rickets are of short stature. Infants with hereditary hypophosphatemia grow normally during the first few months of life when serum phosphate levels are high, secondary to glomerular insufficiency. At about 6 months of age, with the occurrence of hypophosphatemia, the growth rate diminishes. If glomerular insufficiency later supervenes with serum phosphate levels again elevated, growth may increase until acidosis occurs. Osteodystrophy seen in renal insufficiency can cause both deformities and decrease in bone growth. Recent studies suggest that control of calcium and phosphorus balance and administration of 1,25 dihydroxycholecalciferal may result in improvement of stature.

Finally, chronic infection, as with pyelonephritis, may play a role in slow growth rate; however, cation wasting may be associated in such patients.

In summary, the major mechanism of growth failure in renal disease is apparently chronic acidosis, which may be associated with cation losses by the kidney. Other factors, such as inadequate intake of calories or protein, hypophosphatemia, hyperparathyroidism, other hormonal imbalances, and infection, may play a role in selected instances.

REFERENCES

1. **Potter EL:** Normal and Abnormal Development of the Kidney. Chicago, Year Book Publishers, 1972
2. **Winick M, McCrory WW:** Renal Differentiation: A model for the study of development. Birth Defects, Original Article Series, IV:1, 1968
3. **Fetterman GH, Shuplock NA, Philipp FJ, Gregg HS:** The growth and maturation of human glomeruli and proximal convolutions from term to adulthood. Studies by microdissection. Pediatrics, 35:601, 1965
4. **Ljungqvist A:** Fetal and postnatal development of the intrarenal arterial pattern in man. A micro-angiographic and histologic study. Acta Paediatr 52:443, 1963
5. **Tahti E:** Kidney function in early foetal life. Br J Radiol 39:226, 1966
6. **Altschule MD:** The changes in the mesonephric tubules of human embryos ten to twelve weeks old. Anat Rec 46:81, 1930
7. **Ljungqvist A, Wagermark J:** Renal juxtaglomerular granulation in human foetus and infant. Act Pathol Microbiol Scand 67:257, 1966
8. **DeMarino C, Zamboni L:** A morphological study of the mesonephros of the human embryo. J Ultrastruct Res 16:399, 1966
9. **Cameron G, Chambers R:** Direct evidence of function in kidney of an early human fetus. Am J Physiol 123:482, 1938
10. **Kramer I, Sherry SN:** The time of passage of the first stool and urine by the premature infant. J Pediatr 51:373, 1957
11. **Sherry SN, Kramer I:** The time of passage of the first stool and the first urine by the newborn infant. J Pediatr 46:158, 1955
12. **Jones MD, Gresham EL, Battaglia F:** Urinary flow rates in newborn infants. Biol Neonate 21:321, 1972
13. **Arant BS:** Developmental patterns of renal functional maturation compared in the human neonate. J Pediatr 92:705, 1979
14. **Ross B, Cowett R, Oh W:** Renal function and low birth weight infants during the first two months of life. Pediatr Res 11:1162, 1977
15. **Siegel SR, Oh W:** Renal function as a marker of human fetal maturation. Acta Paediatr Scand 65:481, 1976
16. **Oh W, Arcilla RA, Oh MA, Lind J:** Renal and cardiovascular effects of body tilting in the newborn infant. A comparative study of infants born with early and late cord clamping. Biol Neonate 10:76, 1966
17. **Aperia A, Broberger O, Thodenius K, Zetterstrom R:** Developmental study of the renal response to an oral salt load in preterm infants. Acta Paediatr Scand 63:517, 1974
18. **Leake RD, Trygstad CW:** Glomerular filtration rate during the period of adaptation to extrauterine life. Pediatr Res 11:959, 1977
19. **Sertel H, Scopes J:** Rates of creatinine clearance in babies less than one week of age. Arch Dis Child 48:717, 1973
20. **Strauss J, Adamsons K, Jr, James LS:** Renal function of normal full term infants in the first hours of extrauterine life. Am J Obstet Gynecol 91:286, 1965
21. **Papadopoulou ZL, Tina LU, Sandler P, Jose PA, Calcagno PL:** Size and function of the kidneys. In Johnson TR, Moore WM, Jeffries JE (eds): Children Are Different: Developmental Physiology, 2nd ed. Columbus, Ross Laboratories, 1978
22. **Rubin MI, Bruck E, Rapoport MJ:** Maturation of renal function in childhood: clearance studies. J Clin Invest 28:1144, 1949

23. **Horster M, Valtin H:** Postnatal development of renal function. Micropuncture and clearance studies in the dog. J Clin Invest 50:779, 1971

24. **Kleinman LI, Lubbe RJ:** Factors affecting the maturation of glomerular filtration rate and renal plasma flow in the newborn dog. J Physiol 223:395, 1972

25. **Aperia A, Herin P:** Development of glomerular perfusion rate and nephron filtration rate in rats 17–60 days old. Am J Physiol 228: 1319, 1975

26. **Spitzer A, Brandis M:** Functional and morphologic maturation of the superficial nephrons. Relationship to total kidney function. J Clin Invest 53:279, 1974

27. **Solomon S, Capek K:** Regulation of superficial single nephron glomerular filtration rates in infant rats. Proc Soc Exp Biol Med 139:325, 1972

28. **Tavani N, Jr, Zimmet S, Calcagno PL, Einser GM, Flamenbaum W, Jose PA:** Ontogeny of single nephron filtration in the puppy. Pediatr Res 14:799, 1980

29. **Dlouha H, Bibr B, Jezek J, Zicha J:** Single nephron filtration rate ratios of superficial, intercortical and juxtamedullary nephrons in rats during development. Pfluegers Arch 366: 277, 1976

30. **Tucker BJ, Blantz RC:** Factors determining superficial nephron filtration in the mature growing rat. Am J Physiol 232:(2) F97, 1977

31. **Spitzer A, Edelmann CM, Jr:** Maturational changes in pressure gradients for glomerular filtration. Am J Physiol 221:1431, 1971

32. **Calcagno PL, Rubin MI:** Renal extraction of paraaminohippurate in infants and children. J Clin Invest 42:1632, 1963

32a. **Fawer CL, Torrado A, Guignard JP:** Maturation of renal function in full term and premature neonates. Helv Paediatr Acta 34, 11, 1979

33. **Horster M, Lewy JE:** Filtration fraction of PAH during neonatal period in the rat. Am J Physiol 219:1061, 1971

34. **Kleinman LI, Reuter JH:** Maturation of glomerular blood flow distribution in the newborn dog. J Physiol (Lond) 228:91, 1973

35. **Jose PA, Logan GA, Slotkoff LM, Lilienfield LS, Calcagno PL, Eisner GM:** Intrarenal blood flow distribution in canine puppies. Pediatr Res 5:335,1971.

36. **Guignard JP, Torrado A, Da Cunha O, Gautier E:** Glomerular filtration rate in the first three weeks of life. J Pediatr 87:268,1975.

37. **West JR, Smith HW, Chasis H:** Glomerular filtration rate, effective renal blood flow, and maximal tubular excreting capacity in infancy. J Pediatr 32:10, 1948

38. **Renkin EM, Gilmore JP:** Glomerular filtration in Renal Physiology, Handbook of Physiology. In Orloff J, Berliner RW (eds) Wash DC, Am Physiol Soc, 1973.

39. **Calcagno PL, Jose PA:** Maturation of renal blood flow. Proceedings of the 5th Int Congr Nephrol 1:21. Karger, Basel, 1974

40. **Gruskin AB, Edelmann CM, Jr, Yuan S:** Maturation of renal blood flow in piglets. Pediatr Res 4:7, 1970

41. **Davis GS:** Foetal and neonatal physiology. Chicago, Year Book Publishers, 1968

42. **Sulcova B:** Postnatal development of cardiac output distribution measured by radioactive microspheres in rats. Biol Neonate 32:119, 1977

43. **Aperia A, Broberger O, Herin P:** Maturational changes in glomerular perfusion rate and glomerular filtration rate in lambs. Pediatr Res 8:758, 1974

44. **Olbing H, Blaufox MD, Aschinberg LC, Silkolns GI, Bernstein J, Spitzer, A, Edelmann CM, Jr:** Postnatal changes in renal glomerular blood flow distribution in puppies. J Clin Invest 52:2885, 1973

45. **Gruskin AB, Auerbach VH, Black IFS:** Intrarenal blood flow in children with normal kidneys and congenital heart disease; changes attributable to angiography. Pediatr Res 8:561, 1974

46. **Jose PA, Slotkoff LM, Lilienfield LS, Calcagno PL, Eisner GM:** Sensitivity of neonatal renal vasculature to epinephrine. Am J Physiol 226:796, 1974

47. **Jose PA:** Adrenergic control of neonatal hemodynamics. Proceedings of the 4th Int Symposium Pediatr Nephrol. Helsinki, Finland, 1977

48. **Freedman A, Demers L:** Prostaglandin synthetase in the human neonatal kidney (abstr). Pediatr Res 12:394, 1978

49. **Pace–Asciak C:** Prostaglandins and renal function. Proceedings of the 4th Int Symposium Pediatr Nephrol. Helsinki, Finland, 1977

50. **Berlin LJ, Bhattacharyan J:** The effect of prostaglandin synthesis inhibitors on renal blood flow distribution in conscious rabbits. J Physiol 269:395, 1977

51. **Saeed SA, McDonald–Gibson WJ, Cuthbert J, Copas JL, Schneider C, Gardiner PJ, Butt NM, Collier HOJ:** Endogenous inhibitor of prostaglandin synthetase. Nature 270:32, 1977

52. **Matson JR, Robillard JE, Cousamus B, Smith FG:** Role of prostaglandins (PG) in fetal kidney function and blood flow. Proceedings of the 11th Ann Meeting Am Soc Nephrol, p 135 (abstr) 1978

53. Solhaug M, Eisner GM, Calcagno PL, Jose PA: Kinins, modulators of sodium excretion in the canine puppy (abstr). Pediatr Res 13: 521, 1979

54. Jose PA, Slotkoff LM, Montgomery S, Calcagno PL, Eisner G: Autoregulation of renal blood flow in the puppy. Am J Physiol 229:983, 1975

55. Montgomery S, Jose P, Slotkoff L, Calcagno P, Eisner G: Maturation of renal beta adrenergic receptors in the dog (abstr). Proceedings of the 11th Ann Meet Am Soc Nephrol, p 136, 1978.

56. Sassard J, Sann L, Vincent M, Francois R, Cier JF: Plasma renin activity in normal subjects from infancy to puberty. J Clin Endocrinol Metab 40:524, 1975

57. Kotchen TA, Strickland AL, Rice TW, Walters DR: A study of the renin angiotensin system in newborn infants. J Pediatr 80:938, 1972

58. Godard C, Giering JM, Giering K, Valloton MB: Plasma renin activity related to sodium balance, renal function and urinary vasopressin in the newborn infant. Pediatr Res 13:742, 1979

59. Broughton–Pipkin F, Smales OR: A study of factors affecting blood pressure and angiotensin in newborn infants. J Pediatr 91:113, 1977

60. Beitins IZ, Graham GG, Kowarsk A, Migeon CJ: Adrenal function in normal infants and in marasmus and kwashiorkor: plasma aldosterone concentration and aldosterone secretion rate. J Pediatr 84:444, 1974

61. Dillion MJ, Gillin ME, Ryness J, de Sweet M: Plasma renin activity and aldosterone concentration in the human newborn. Arch Dis Child 51:537, 1976

62. Siegel SR, Fisher DA, Oh W: Renal function and serum aldosterone levels in infants with respiratory distress syndrome. J Pediatr 83: 854, 1973

63. Beitins IZ, Bayard F, Levitsky I, Ances IG, Kowarski A, Migeon CJ: Plasma adolsterone concentration at delivery and during the newborn period. J Clin Invest 51:386, 1972

64. Broughton–Pipkin F., Symonds EM: Factors affecting angiotensin II concentrations in human infants at birth. Clin Sci Mol Med 52: 449, 1977

65. Sulyok E, Nemeth M, Tenyi I, Csaba IF, Gyory E, Ertl T, Varga F: Postnatal development of renin-angiotensin-aldosterone system (RAAS) in relation to electrolyte balance in premature infants. Pediatr Res 13:817, 1979

66. Sulyok E, Varga F, Nemeth M, Tenyi I, Csaba TF, Ertl T, Gyory E: Furosemide induced alterations in the electrolyte status, the function of renin angiotensin–aldosterone system and the urinary excretion of prostaglandins in newborn infants. Pediatr Res 14:765, 1980

67. Richer CL, Hornych H, Amieli–Tison C, Relier JP, Giudicelli JF: Plasma renin activity and its postnatal development in preterm infants. Biol Neonate 37:301, 1977

68. Pohlova I, Jelinek J: Components of the renin–angiotensin system in the rat during development. Pfleugers Arch, 351:259, 1974

69. Bailie MD, Derkx FMH, Schalekamp MADH: Release of active and inactive renin by the pig kidney during development. Dev Pharm (in press)

70. Van Acker KJ, Scharpe SL, Deprettere AJR, Neils HM: Renin angiotensin aldosterone system in the healthy infant and child. Kidney Int 16:196, 1979

71. Smith FG, Lupu AN, Barajas L, Bauer R, Bashore RA: The renin angiotensin system in the fetal lamb. Pediatr Res 8:611, 1974

72. Mott JD: The place of the renin angiotensin system before and after birth. Br Med Bull 31:64, 1975

73. Siegel SR, Fisher DA: The renin angiotensin–aldosterone system in the newborn lamb: responses to furosemide. Pediatr Res 11:837, 1977

74. Lumberg ER, Reid GC: Effects of vaginal delivery and cesarian section of plasma renin activity and angiotensin II levels in human cord blood. Biol Neonate 31:127, 1977

75. Osborn JL, Hook JB, Bailie MD: Regulation of plasma renin in developing piglet (abstr). Pediatr Res 13:517, 1979

76. Solomon S, Iaina A, Eliahou H: Possible determinants of plasma renin activity in infant rats. Proc Soc Exp Biol Med 154:309, 1976

77. Siegel SR, Fisher DA: The effects of angiotensin II blockade and nephrectomy on renin angiotensin aldosterone system in the new born lamb. Pediatr Res 13:603, 1979

78. Jose PA, Eisner GM, Medina JV, Calcagno PL: Effects of angiotensin II inhibitor (p-113) on neonatal renal function (abstr). Pediatr Res 7:414, 1973

79. Bender JW, Davitt MK, Jose PA: Angiotensin–1–converting enzyme activity in term and preterm infants. Biol Neonate 34:19, 1978

80. Moore ES, Paton JB, DeLannoy CY, Roan Y, Cevallo E, Ocampo M, Lyons EC: Effect of (Sar^1–Ile^8)–angiotensin II inhibitor on glomerular filtration rate and renal plasma flow in the fetal lamb (abstr). Pediatr Res 8:459, 1974

81. Spitzer A, Schoeneman M: Sodium reabsorption during maturation (abstr). Kidney Int 10:598, 1976

82. Siegel R, Fisher DA: Ontogeny of the renin-

angiotensin-aldosterone system in the fetal and newborn lamb. Pediatr Res (in press)

83. **Prezyna AP:** The renomedullary body—an organ of prostaglandin production—summary of recent observations. Proceedings of Int Conf Prostaglandin, p 181. Florence, Italy, 1975

84. **Day NA, Atallah AA, Lee JB:** Presence of prostaglandin A and F in fetal kidney. Prostaglandins 5:491, 1974

85. **Terragno NA, McGiff JC, Terragno A:** Prostacycline (PGI_2) production by renal blood vessels: Relationship to an endogenous prostaglandin synthesis inhibitor (EPSI) (abstr). Clin Res 26:545, 1978

86. **Tortorolo G, Porcelli G, Cuatalo P:** Urinary kallikreins in premature, small at term and normal newborns and in children. In Pisano JJ, Austen KF(eds): Chemistry and Biology of Kallikrein: Kinin System in Health and Disease, p 433. DHEW (NIH) 76–791 Wash, DC

87. **Sulyok E:** The relationship between electrolyte and acid-base balance in the premature infant during early postnatal life. Biol Neonate 17:227, 1971

88. **Day GM, Radde IC, Balfe JW, Chance GW:** Electrolyte abnormalities in very low birth weight infants. Pediatr Res 10:522, 1976

89. **Roy RN, Chance GW, Radde IC, Hill DE, Willis DM, Sheepers J:** Late hyponatremia in very low birth weight infants (< 1.3 kgs). Pediatr Res 10:526, 1978

90. **Engelke SC, Shah BL, Vasan U, Raye JR:** Sodium balance in very low birth weight infants. J Pediatr 93:837, 1978

91. **Solomon S:** Maximal gradients of sodium and across proximal tubules of kidneys and immature rats. Biol Neonate 25:237, 1974

92. **Broberger U, Aperia A:** Renal function in infants with hyperbilirubinemia. Acta Paediatr Scand 68:75, 1979

93. **Harkavy K, Jose PA, Scanlon J:** The effect of theophylline on renal function in premature infants with apnea. Biol Neonate 35:125, 1979

94. **Janovsky M, Martinek J, Stanicova V:** The distribution of sodium chloride and fluid in the body of young infants with increased intake of NaCl. Biol Neonate 11:261, 1967

95. **Kagan BM, Felix N, Molander CW, Busser RJ, Kalman D:** Body water changes in relation to nutrition in premature infants. An NY Acad Sci 110:830, 1963

96. **McCance RA, Widdowson EM:** Hypertonic expansion of the extracellular fluids. Acta Paediatr Scand 46:337, 1957

97. **Spitzer A:** Renal physiology and functional development. In Edelman CM, Jr (ed): Pediatric Kidney Disease, p 49. Boston, Little, Brown & Co, 1978

98. **Horster M:** Principals of nephron differentiation. Am J Physiol 235:F387, 1978

99. **Dean RFA, McCance RA:** The renal response of infants and adults to the administration of hypertonic solutions of sodium chloride and the urea. J Physiol 109:81, 1949

100. **Kleinman LI:** Renal sodium reabsorption during saline loading and distal blockade in newborn dog. Am J Physiol 228:1403, 1975

101. **Aperia A, Broberger O, Thodenius K, Zetterstrom R:** Development of renal control of salt and fluid homeostasis during the first year of life. Acta Paediatr Scand 64:393, 1975

102. **Tavani N, Jr, Calcagno PL, Eisner GM, Jose PA:** Effect of acute saline loading in single nephron filteration distribution in the dog (unpublished observation).

103. **Solomon S, Hathaway S, Curb D:** Evidence that the renal response to volume expansion involves a blood-borne factor. Biol Neonate 35:113, 1979

104. **Kleinman LI, Banks RO, Gorewitt R:** Role of oxytocin in the natriuretic response to saline expansion in newborn dogs (abstr). Pediatr Res 13:515, 1979

105. **Aperia A, Broberger O, Herin P, Thodenius K, Zetterstrom R:** Renal sodium excretory capacity in infants under different dietary conditions. Acta Paediatr Scand 68:351, 1979

106. **Aperia A, Broberger O, Herin P, Thodenius K, Zetterstrom R:** A comparative study of the response to an oral NaCl and $HaHCO_3$ load in newborn preterm and full term infants. Pediatr Res 11:1109, 1977

107. **Usher R:** Treatment of respiratory distress. In Winters: The body fluids in pediatrics. Boston, Little, Brown & Co, 1973

108. **Simmons MA, Adcock EW, Bard H, Battaglia FC:** Hypernatremia and intracranial hemorrhage in neonates. N Engl J Med 291:6, 1974

109. **Corbett AJ, Adams JM, Kenny JD, Kennedy J, Rudolph AJ:** Controlled trial of bicarbonate therapy in high risk premature newborn infants. J Pediatr 91:771, 1977

110. **Thomas DB:** Hyperosmolality and intraventricular hemorrhage in premature babies. Acta Pediatr Scand 65:429, 1976

111. **Aperia A, Broberger O, Thodenius K, Zetterstrom R:** Developmental study of the renal response to an oral salt load in preterm infants. Acta Pediatr Scand 63:517, 1974

112. **Eisner B, Surwit E, Jose P, Slotkoff L, Lilienfield L:** Response of the canine puppy to acute saline loading (abstr). Proceedings of the 5th Int Congr Nephrol, p 68, 1972

113. **McCance RA, Widdowson EM:** The response

of the newborn piglet to an excess of potassium. J Physiol 141:88, 1958

114. **Schmidt U, Horster M:** Na-K-activated ATPase: activity maturation in rabbit nephron segments dissected in vitro. Am J Physiol 233:F55, 1977

115. **Svenningsen NW, Aronson AS:** Postnatal development of renal concentrating capacity as estimated by DDAVP-test in normal and asphyxiated neonates. Biol Neonate 25:230, 1974

116. **Alexander DP, Nixon DA:** The foetal kidney. Br Med Bull 17:112, 1961

117. **Edelmann CM, Jr, Barnett HL:** Role of the kidney in water metabolism in young infants. J Pediatr 56:154, 1960

118. **Hansen JDK, Smith CA:** Effects of witholding fluid in the immediate postnatal period. Pediatr 12:99, 1953

119. **Trimble ME:** Renal response to solute loading in infant rats: relation to anatomical development. Am J Physiol 219:1089, 1970

120. **Edwards BR, Mendel DB:** Growth of superficial loops of Henle (SLH) and development of urine concentrating ability of rats. Pediatr Res 13:512, 1979

121. **Bursch RL:** Development of renal Na and K activated ATPase in the C 57 BL/6 mouse. Biol Neonate 24:106, 1974

122. **Edelmann CM, Barnett HL, Troupkou V:** Renal concentrating mechanisms in newborn infants. Effect of dietary protein and water content, role of urea, and responsiveness to anti diuretic homeone. J Clin Invest 39:1062, 1960

123. **Calcagno PL, Rubin MI, Weintraub DH:** Studies on the renal concentration and diluting mechanisms in the premature infant. J Clin Invest 33:91, 1954

124. **Wesson LG, Jr:** Physiology of the human kidney. New York, Grune and Stratton, 1961

125. **Janovsky M, Martinek J, Stanincova V:** Antidiuretic activity in the plasma of human infant after a load of sodium chloride. Acta Paediatr Scand 54:543, 1965

126. **Hadeed AJ, Leak RD, Weitzman RE, Fisher DA:** Mechanism of fetal vasopressin hypersecretion during the perinatal period. Clin Res 26:119A, 1978

127. **Hoppenstein JM, Mittenberger FW, Moran WH, Jr:** The increase in blood levels of vasopressin in infants during birth and surgical procedures. Surg Gynecol Obstet 127:966, 1968

128. **Weinberg JA, Weitzman RE, Zakaudin S, Leake RD:** Inappropriate ADH secretion in a premature infant. J Pediatr 90:111, 1977

129. **Kaplan SL, and Fligin RD:** Inappropriate secretion of anti diuretic hormone compli-cating neonatal hypoxic, ischemic encephalopathy. J Pediatr 92:431, 1978

130. **Robillard JE, Weitzman RE, Fisher DA, Smith FG, Jr:** The dynamics of vasopressin release and blood volume regulation during fetal hemorrhage in the lamb fetus. Pediatr Res 13:606, 1979

131. **Fisher DA, Pyle HR, Jr, Porter JC, Beard AG, Panes TC:** Control of water balance in the newborn. Am J Dis Child 106:137, 1963

132. **Robertson GL, Athar S, Shelton RL:** Osmotic control of vasopressin function. In Andreoli TE, Grantham JJ, Rector FC, Jr (eds): Disturbances of Body Fluid Osmolality. Bethesda, Am Physiol Soc, 1977

133. **Hiller H:** The renal function of newborn infants. J Physiol 102:429, 144

134. **Edelmann CM, Jr, Barnett HL, Stark H:** Effect of urea on concentration of urinary non urea solute in premature infants. J Appl Physiol 21:1021, 1966

135. **Schlondorff D, Weber H, Trizna W, Fine AG:** Vasopressin responsiveness of renal adenylate cyclase in newborn rats and rabbits. Am J Physiol 234:F16, 1978

136. **Rajerison M, Butler D, Jard S:** Ontogenic development of antidiuretic hormone receptors in rat kidney: comparison of hormonal binding and adenylate cyclase activation. Mol Cell Encocrinol 4:271, 1976

137. **Lu LT, Bailie MD, Hook JB:** Effect of antidiuretic hormone and theophylline on cyclic AMP in renal medulla of newborn and adult rabbits and dogs. Gen Pharmacol 6:181, 1975

137a. **Jappich R, Kiemann U, Mayer G, Haberle D:** Effect of antidiuretic hormone upon urinary concentrating ability and medullary C–AMP function on neonatal piglets. Pediatr Res 13:884, 1979

138. **McCance RA, Widdowson EM:** The acid-base relationships of the foetal fluids of the pig. J Physiol 151:484, 1960

139. **Edelmann CM, Jr:** Maturation of the neonatal kidney. In Proceedings of the 3rd Int Cong Nephrol, vol. 3, p 1. Wash DC, YS Karger, 1967

140. **Schwartz GJ, Haycock GB, Edelmann CM, Jr, Spitzer A:** Late metabolic acidosis: a reassessment of the definition. J Pediatr 95:102, 1979

141. **Edelmann CM, Jr, Soriano JR, Boichis H, Gruskin AB, Acosta MI:** Renal bicarbonate reabsorption and hydrogen ion excretion in normal infants. J Clin Invest 46:1309, 1967

142. **Tudvad FH, McNamara H, Barnett HL:** Renal response of premature infants to administration of bicarbonate and potassium. Pediatrics 13:4, 1954

143. **Robillard JE, Sessions C, Burmeister L, Smith**

FG: Influence of fetal extracellular volume on renal reabsorption of bicarbonate in fetal lambs. Pediatr Res 11:649, 1977

144. Svenningsen NW, Lindquist B: Postnatal development of renal hydrogen ion excretion capacity in relation to age and protein intake. Acta Paediatr Scand 63:721, 1974

145. Kerpel–Fronius E, Hein T, Sulyok E: The development of renal acidifying processes and their relation to acidosis in low birth weight infants. Biol Neonate 15:156, 1970

146. Svenningsen NW: Renal acid base titration studies in infants with and without metabolic acidosis in the postnatal period. Pediatr Res 8:659, 1974

147. Monnens L, Schrethen E, Van Munster P: The renal excretion of hydrogen ions in infants and children. Nephron 12: 29, 1973

148. Kildeberg P: Disturbances of hydrogen ion balance occuring in premature infants. II. Late metabolic acidosis. Acta Paediatr Scand 53:517, 1964

149. Radde IC, Chance GW, Bailey K: Growth and mineral metabolism in very low birth weigh infants I. Comparison of the effect of 2 modes of NaHCO$_3$ treatment of late metabolic acidosis. Pediatr Res 9:564, 1975

150. Root AW, Harmson HE: Recent advances in calcium metabolism. J Pediatr 88:1, 1976

151. Ghazali, S, Barratt TM: Urinary excretion of calcium and magnesium in children. Arch Dis Child 49:97, 1974

152. Noguchi A, Kleinman LI, Tsang RC: Urinary excretion of calcium (Ca) after acute IV CaCl$_2$ load in newborn and adult dogs (abstr). Pediatr Res 13:517, 1979

153. Schedewie HK, Odell DW, Fisher DA et al: Parathormone and perinatal calcium homeostasis. Pediatr. Res. 13:1, 1979

154. David L, Anast CS: Calcium metabolism in newborn infants. The inter-relationship of parathyroid function and calcium, magnesium and phosphorus metabolism in normal "sick" and hypocalcemic newborns. J Clin Invest 54:287, 1974

155. Dean RFA, McCance RA: Phosphate clearances in infants and adults. J Physiol 107: 182, 1948

156. McCrory WW: Developmental Nephrology. Cambridge, Harvard University Press, 1972

157. Mallet E, Basayu JP, Brumelle P, Demarex AM, Fessard C: Neonatal parathyroid secretion and renal receptor maturation in premature infants. Biol Neonate 33:304, 1978

158. Linarelli LG, Babik J, Babik BS: Newborn urinary cyclic AMP and developmental renal responsiveness to PTA. Pediatrics 50:14, 1972

159. Hillman LS, Rojavasathit S, Slatopolsky E,

Haddad JG: Serial measurements of serum calcium, magnesium, PTH, Calcitonin and hydroxyvitamin D in preterm and term infants during the first week of life. Pediatr Res 11:739, 1977

160. Kodowa S, Sakurai T, Seki A, Mashita Y, Matsuo T: Etiological analysis of neonatal hypocalcemia. Relationship and sensitivity to parathyroid hormone. Kobe J Med Sci 2:69–76, 1975

161. Tudvad F: Sugar reabsorption in premature and full term babies. Scand J Clin Lab Invest 1:281, 1949

162. Brodehl J, Gellissen K: Endogenous renal transport of free amino acids in infancy and childhood. Pediatrics 42:395, 1968

163. Lasley L, Scriver CR: Ontogeny of amino acid reabsorption in human kidney. Pediatr Res 13:65, 1979

164. Blanc WA, Apperson JW, McNally J: Pathology of the newborn placenta in oligohydramnios. Bull Sloane Hosp Women 8:51, 1962

165. Naeye R, Blanc WA: Fetal renal structure and the genesis of amniotic fluid disorders. Am J Pathol 67:95, 1972

166. Moore ES, Galvez MB: Delayed micturition in the newborn period. J Pediatr 80:867, 1972

167. DeLuna MD, Hullet WH: Urinary protein excretion in healthy infants, children and adults. Proceedings of the Am Soc Nephrol, p 16, 1967

168. Rhodes PG, Hammel CL, Berman LB: Urinary constituents of the newborn infant. J Pediatr 60:18, 1962

169. Randolph MF, Greenfield M: Proteinuria. A six-year study of normal infants, preschool and school age populations previously screened for urinary tract disease. Am J Dis Child 114:631, 1967

170. Halverson S, Aas K: Observation on the urine of asphyxiated and dysmature newborn infants. Acta Paediatr Scand 41:417, 1962

171. Tan K, Hull D: The excretion of cells in urine following perinatal asphyxia. Pediatr Res 3: 228, 1969

172. Cruickshank G, Edmond E: "Clean-catch" urines in the newborn—Bacteriology and cell excretion patterns in the first week of life. Br Med J 4:705, 1967

173. Brown DM, Boen J, Bernstein A: Serum ionized calcium in newborn infants. Pediatrics 49:841, 1972

174. Polacek E, Vocel J, Neugebauerova L, Sebrova M, Vechetova E: The osmotic concentrating ability in healthy infants and children. Arch Dis Child 40:291, 1965

175. Edelmann CM, Jr, Barnett HL, Stark H, Boichis H, Soriano JR: A standardized test of

renal concentrating capacity in children. Am J Dis Child 114:619, 1967

176. **Winberg J:** Determination of renal concentration capacity in infants and children without renal disease. Acta Paediatr 48:318, 1959

177. **Emanuel B, White H:** Intravenous pyelography in the differential diagnosis of renal masses in the neonatal period. Clin Pediatr 7:529, 1968

178. **Gilbert EF, Khoury GH, Hogan GR, Jones B:** Hemorrhagic renal necrosis in infancy: relationship to radioopaque compounds. J Pediatr 76:49, 1970

179. **Blaufox MD, Freeman LM:** Radionuclide techniques for the evaluation of diseases of the urinary tract in children. Semin Nucl Med 3:27, 1973

180. **Lyons EA, Murphy AV, Arneil GC:** Sonar and its use in kidney disease in children. Arch Dis Child 47:777, 1972

181. **Ogata ES, Goodiz CA, Phibbs RH:** Angiography and ultrasonographic appearance of cortical and medullary necrosis in the newborn. Pediatr Radiol 3:226, 1975

182. **Adelman DR:** Neonatal renal hypertension. Pediatr Clin North Am 25:99, 1978

183. **Durante D, Jones D, Spitzer R:** Neonatal renal arterial syndrome. J Pediatr 89:978, 1976

184. **Gross RE:** Arterial embolism and thrombosis in infancy. Am J Dis Child 70:61, 1945

185. **Jorgensen L, Neset G, Kjoerheim A, Mageroy K:** Renal vein thrombosis in the newborn. Acta Path Microbiol Scand (Suppl) 148:97, 1961

186. **Avery ME, Oppenheimer EH, Gordon HH:** Renal vein thrombosis in newborn infants of diabetic mothers. N Eng J Med 256:1134, 1957

187. **Oppenheimer EH, Esterly JR;** Thrombosis in the newborn. Comparision between infants of diabetic and non-diabetic mothers. J Pediatr 67:549, 1965

188. **Stuart MJ, Elrad H, Graeber JE, Hakanson DO, Sunderji SG, Barvinchak MD:** Increased synthesis of prostaglandin endoperoxides and platlet hyperfunction in infants of mothers with diabetes mellitus. J Lab Clin Invest 94:12, 1979

189. **Halushka PV, Lurie D, Colville JA:** Increased synthesis of prostaglandin-E-like material by platelets from patients with diabetes mellitus. N Engl J Med 297:1306, 1977

190. **Arneil GC:** Renal venous thrombosis. Contrib Nephrol 15:21, 1979

191. **Wells JD, Margolina EG, Gall EA:** Renal cortical necrosis. Clinical and pathologic features in twenty-one cases. Am J Med 29:257, 1960

192. **Abilgaard CF:** Recognition and treatment of intravascular coagulation. J Pediatr 74:163, 1969

193. **Zueltzer WW, Charles S, Kurnetz R, Newton WA, Fallon R:** Circulatory diseases of the kidneys in infancy and childhood. Am J Dis Child 81:1, 1951

194. **Shah NB, Jenkins ME, Jones GW:** Renal cortical necrosis in a homozygous twin-neonate. J Urol 108:146, 1972

195. **Leonidas JS, Berdon WE, Gribetz D:** Bilateral renal cortical necrosis in the newborn infant: Roentgenographic diagnosis. J Pediatr 79: 623, 1971

196. **Mauer SM, Nogrady MB:** Renal papillary and cortical necrosis in the newborn infant: Report of a survivor with roentgenography demonstration. J Pediatr 74:750, 1969

197. **Chrispin AR, Hulls D, Lillie JG, Ridson RA:** Renal tubular necrosis and papillary necrosis after gastroenteritis in infants. Br Med J 1: 410, 1970

198. **Bernstein J, Meyer R:** Congenital abnormalities of the urinary system. II. Renal cortical and medullary necrosis. J Pediatr 59:657, 1961

199. **Davies DJ, Kennedy A, Roberts C:** Renal medullary necrosis in infancy and childhood. J Pathol 99:125, 1969

200. **Salm R, Voyce MA:** Renal papillary necrosis in the neonate. Br J Urol 42:277, 1970

201. **Levinsky NG, Alexander EA:** Acute renal failure. In Brenner B, Rector F: The Kidney, pp 806–837 Philadelphia, WB Saunders, 1976

202. **Williams GS, Klenk EL, Winters RW:** Acute renal failure in pediatrics. In Winters: The Body Fluids in Pediatrics, pp 523–557. Boston, Little, Brown & Co 1973

203. **Rubin MI, Baliah T:** Urine and urinalysis. In Rubin and Baratt; Pediatric Nephrology, pp 84–104. Baltimore, Williams & Wilkins, 1975

204. **Aranda SK, Northway JD, Crussi FG:** Acute renal failure in newborn infants. J Pediatr 92: 985, 1979

205. **Norman M, Asadi F:** A prospective study of acute renal failure. Pediatrics 63:475, 1979

206. **Guignard JP, Torrado A, Mazouni SM, Gautier E:** Renal function in respiratory distress. J Pediatr 88:845, 1976

207. **Daniel SS, James LS:** Abnormal renal function in the newborn infant. J Pediatr 88:856, 1976

208. **Moore ES, Galvez MD, Paton JB, Fisher DE, Behrman RE:** Effects of positive pressure ventilation on intrarenal blood flow in the primate infant. Pediatr Res 8:792, 1974

209. **McCrory WW:** Renal failure in the newborn. Contrib Nephrol 15:10, 1979

210. **McCrory WW:** Congenital malformations causing renal failure in the neonatal period. Contrib Nephrol 15:55, 1979

211. **Finn WF, Arendshorst WJ, Gottschalk CW:** Pathogenesis of oliguria in acute renal failure. Circ Res 36:675, 1975

212. **Gaudio KM, Kashgarian M, Siegel NJ:** Recovery from postischemic renal injury (abstr). Pediatr Res 13:514, 1979

213. **Bidani AK, Churchill P, Becker–McKenna B, Fleischmann LE:** Age related changes in patterns of mercuric chloride induced acute renal failure (ARF) and their relationship with the determinants of renin angiotensin system (RAS) in developing rat. Proceedings of the 4th Int Symposium Pediatr Nephrol, p 105. Helsinki, Finland, 1977

214. **Anderson RJ, Linas SL, Berns AS, Henrich WL, Miller TR, Gabow PA, Schrier RW:** Nonoliguric acute renal failure. N Engl J Med 296:1134–1138, 1977

215. **Medani CR, Davitt MK, Huntington D, Kramer L, Sivasubramanian KN, Jose PA:** Acute renal failure in the newborn. Contrib Nephrol 15:47, 1979

216. **Greenhill A, Gruskin AB:** In Chan: Laboratory evaluation of renal function. Pediatr Clin North Am 23:661–679, 1976

217. **Calcagno PL, Lowe CU:** Substrate induced renal tubular maturation. J Pediatr 63: 851–853, 1963

218. **Stonestreet BS, Oh W:** Plasma creatinine levels in low birth weight infants during the first three months of life. Pediatrics 61:788, 1978

219. **Miller TR, Anderson RJ, Linas SL et al:** Urinary diagnostic indices in acute renal failure. A prospective study. Ann Intern Med 89:47, 1978

220. **Earley LE, Schrier RW:** Intrarenal control of sodium excretion by hemodynamic and physical factors. In Orloff J, Berliner R: Renal Physiology, pp 721–762. Baltimore, Williams & Wilkins, 1973

220a. **Mathew OP, Jones AS, James E, Blaud H, Grosshong T:** Neonatal renal failure: usefulness of diagnostic indices. Pediatr 65:57,1980

221. **Luke RG, Briggs JD, Allison ME, Kennedy AC:** Factors determining response to mannitol in acute renal failure. Am J Med Sci 259:168–174, 1970

222. **Gordillo–Panigua G, Velasquez–Jones L:** Acute renal failure. In Chan JCM (ed): Pediatric Nephrology. Pediatr Clin North Am 23:817–828, 1976

223. **Gabow PA, Anderson RF, Schrier RW:** Acute renal failure. Cardiovasc Med 2:1161–1175, 1977

224. **Abitbol CL, Holliday MA:** Total parenteral nutrition in anuric children. Clin Nephrol 5: 153, 1976

225. **Tina LU, Calcagno PL:** Edema of the preterm and term infant. Contrib Nephrol 15:67, 1979

226. **Barnes SE, Bryan EM, Harris DA, Baum JD:** Edema in the newborn. Molecular aspects of medicine, vol 1, pp 187–282. Oxford, Pergamon Press, 1977

227. **MacLaurin NC:** Changes in body distribution during the first two weeks of life. Arch Dis Child 41:286, 1966

228. **Cassidy G:** Effect of caesarian section on neonatal body water spaces. N Engl J Med 245:887, 1971

229. **Perrera P, Kurban AK, Ryan TJ:** Development of the cutaneous microvascular system in the newborn. Br J Dermatol 82:Suppl 5, pp 86–91, 1970

230. **Ritchie JH, Matthews B, Fish MB, McMasters V, Grossman M:** Edema and hemolytic anemia in premature infants. A vitamin E deficiency syndrome. N Engl J Med 279:1185, 1968

231. **Baum JD, Eisenberg C, Franklin FA, Meschin G, Battoglin FC:** Studies on colloid osmotic pressure in the fetus and newborn infant. Biol Neonate 18:311, 1971

232. **Kaplan BS, Bureau MA, Drummond KN:** The nephrotic syndrome in the first year of life: is a pathologic classification possible? J Pediatr 85:615, 1974

233. **Benson PF, Parsons V:** Hereditary hypoparathyroidism presenting with edema in the neonatal period. QJ Med 33:197, 1974

234. **Chiswick ML:** Association of edema and hypomagnesimia with hypocalcemic tetany of the newborn. Br J Med III, 15, 1971

235. **Walker RD, Cumming GR:** Response of the infant kidney to diuretic drugs. Can Med Assoc J 91:1149, 1964

236. **Engle MA, Lewy JE, Lewy PR, Metkoff J:** The use of furosemide in the treatment of edema in infants and children. Pediatrics 62: 811–818, 1974

237. **Ross BS, Pollack A, Oh W:** The pharmacologic effect of furosemide therapy in the low birth weight infant. J Pediatr 149–52, 1978

238. **Woo WCR, Dupont C, Collinge J, Aranda JV:** Effects of furosemide in the newborn. Clin Pharmacol Ther 23:266–271, 1978

239. **Aranda JV, Perez J, Sitar D, Collinge J, Portuguez–Malavasi A:** Protein binding and pharmacokinetic disposition of furosemide (F) in newborn infants (abstr). Pediatr Res 12:538, 1978

240. **Wemby PR, Rasmussen LF, Ahlofs CE:** Displacement of bilirubin for human albumin by 3 weeks. J Pediatr 90:647–50, 1977

241. **Harkavy KL, Scanlon JW, Jose P:** The effects of theophylline on renal function in the premature newborn. Biol Neonate 35:126, 1979

242. **Noordewier B, Bailie MD, Hook J:** Pharmacological analysis of the action of diuretics

in the newborn pig. J Pharmacol Exp Ther 207:236–242, 1979

243. **Banks RP, Kleinman LI:** Effect of amiloride on the renal response to saline expansion in the newborn dogs. J Physiol 275:521–534, 1978

244. **Bergstron T, Larson H, Lincoln K et al:** Studies of urinary tract infections in infancy and childhood. XII. Eighty consecutive cases with neonatal infection. J Pediatr 80:858, 1972

245. **Pascual JF:** Neonatal urinary tract infection. Contrib Nephrol 15:41, 1979

246. **Edelmann CM, Jr, Ogwo JE, Fine BP, Martinez AB:** The prevalence of bacteriuria in full term and premature newborn infants. J Pediatr 82:125, 1973

247. **Calcagno PL, D'Albora JB, Tina LU, Papadapoulou ZL, Deasy PF, Hollerman CF:** Alterations in renal cortical blood flow in infants and children with urinary tract infections. Pediatr Res 2:332, 1968

248. **Peckholz I, Semmler L:** Acute interstitial nephritis in infants having died prepartal, perinatal and during infancy. Paediatr Grenzgeb 10:279, 1971

249. **Williams RH, Henry C:** Nephrogenic diabetes insipidus: Transmitted by females and appearing during infancy in males. Ann Intern Med 27:84, 1947

250. **Frasier SD, Kutnik LA, Schmidt RT, Smith FG:** A water deprivation test for the diagnosis of diabetes insipidus in children. Am J Dis Child 144:157, 1967

251. **Cannon JF:** Diabetes insipidus: Clinical and experimental studies with consideration of genetic relationships. Arch Intern Med 96:215, 1955

252. **Miller SS, Winston MC:** Nephrogenic diabetes insipidus. Radiology 87:893, 1966

253. **Macdonald WB:** Congenital pitressin resistant diabetes insipidus of renal origin. Pediatrics 15:298, 1955

254. **Darmady EM, Offer J, Prince J, Stranack F:** The proximal convoluted tubule in the renal handling of water. Lancet, 2;1254, 1964

255. **Fetterman GH:** Microdissection in the study of normal and abnormal renal structure and function. Pathol Ann 5:173, 1970

256. **Robinson MG, Kaplan SA:** Inheritance of vasopressin-resistant ("Nephrogenic") diabetes insipidus. Am J Dis Child 99:164, 1960

257. **Orloff J, Handler JS:** The similarity of effects of vasopressin, adenosine-3', 5'-phosphate (Cyclic AMP) and theophylline on the toad bladder. J Clin Invest 41:702, 1962

258. **Orloff J, Handler JS:** The cellular mode of action of antidiuretic hormone. Am J Med 36:686, 1964

259. **Orloff J, Handler J:** The role of adenosine 3',5'-phosphate in the action of antidiuretic hormone. Am J Med 42:757, 1967

260. **Cooke RE, Ottenheimer EJ:** Clinical and experimental interrelations of sodium and the central nervous system. Acta Paediatr 11:81, 1960

261. **Earley LE, Orloff J:** The mechanism of antidiuresis associated with the administration of hydrochlorothiazide to patients with vasopressin-resistant diabetes insipidus. J Clin Invest 41:1988, 1962

262. **Havard CWH, Wood PHN:** Antidiuretic properties of hydrochlorothiazide in diabetes insipidus. Br Med J 1:1306, 1960

263. **Weiner MW, Weinman EJ, Kashgarian M, Hayslett JP:** Accelerated reabsorption in the proximal tubule produced by volume depletion. J Clin Invest 50:1379, 1971

264. **Schotland MG, Grumbach MM, Strauss J:** The effects of chlorothiazides in nephrogenic diabetes insipidus. Pediatrics 31:741, 1963

265. **Bartter FC, Pronove P, Gill JR, MacCardle RC:** Hyperplasia of the juxtaglomerular complex with hyperaldosteronism and hypokalemic alkalosis. Am J Med 33:811, 1962

266. **Cannon PJ, Leeming JM, Sommers SC, Winters RW, Laragh JH:** Juxtaglomerular hyperplasia and secondary hyperaldosteronism (Bartter's Syndrome): A re-evaluation of the pathophysiology. Medicine 47:107, 1968

267. **Chaimovitz C, Levi J, Better OS, Oslander L, Benderli A:** Studies on the site of the renal salt loss in a patient with Bartter's syndrome. Pediatr Res 7:89, 1973

268. **Fichman MP, Telfer N, Zio P:** Role of prostaglandins in the pathogenesis of Bartter's syndrome. Am J Med 60:785, 1976

269. **Gardner JD, Sinopoulis AP, Lopez A:** Altered membrane sodium transport in Bartter's syndrome. J Clin Invest 51:1565, 1972

270. **Gill JR, Frolich JC, Bowden RE, Taylor AA, Keiser HR, Seyberth VW, Oates JW, Bartter FC:** Bartter's syndrome: a disorder characterized by high urinary prostaglandins and dependence of hyperreninemia on prostaglandin synthesis. Am J Med 61:43, 1976

271. **Gill JR, Bartter FC, Taylor AA, Radfor N:** Impaired tubular chloride reabsorption as a proximal cause of Batter's syndrome (abstr). Clin Res 25:576A, 1977

272. **Halushka PV, Wohltmann H, Privitera PJ, Hurwitz J, Marglolius HS:** Bartter's syndrome urinary prostaglandin E like material and kallikrein; indomethacin effects. Ann Intern Med 87:281, 1977

273. **James T, III:** Editorial: Bartter syndrome. JAMA 235:1966, 1976

274. **Kurtzman NA, Gutierrez LE:** The pathophysiology of Bartter syndrome. J Am Med Assoc 234:758, 1975

275. **McGiff JC:** Perspective. Bartter's syndrome results from an imbalance of vasoactive hormones. Ann Intern Med 87:369, 1977

276. **Norby L, Mork AL, Kaloyanides GH:** On the pathogenesis of Bartter's syndrome: report of studies in a patient with this disorder. Clin Nephrol 6:404, 1976

277. **Robson WL, Arbrus GS, Balfe JW:** Bartter's syndrome. Differentiation into two clinical groups. Am J Dis Child 133:636, 1979

278. **Goodman AD, Vognucci AH, Hartroft PM:** Pathogenesis of Bartter's syndrome. N Engl J Med 281:1435, 1969

279. **Bardgetke JJ, Stein JH:** Pathophysiology of Bartter's syndrome. In Brenner B, Stein J (eds): Acid-base and potassium homeostasis, New York, Churchill Livingston, 1978

280. **Simopoulous AP:** Growth characteristics in patients with Bartter's syndrome. Nephron 23:130, 1979

281. **Simopoulos AP, Bartter FC:** Growth characteristics and factors influencing growth in Bartter's syndrome. J Pediatr 81:56, 1972

282. **Gullner GH, Gill JR, Bartter FC, Chan JCM:** A familial disorder with hypokalemic alkalosis, hyperreninemia, aldosteronism and high prostaglandins that is not Bartter's syndrome (abstr). Clin Res 27:520A, 1979

283. **Calcagno PL, Rubin MI, Esperanca JJ, Mattimore JM:** Congenital renal tubular alkalosis. Am J Dis Child 102:726, 1961

284. **Camacho AM, Blizzard RM:** Congenital hypokalemia of renal origin due to an inherited metabolic defect. Am J Dis Child 100::713, 1960

285. **Camacho AM, Blizzard RM:** Congenital hypokalemia of probable renal origin: A newly described entity due to an inherited metabolic defect. Am J Dis Child 103:44, 1962

286. **Cheek DB, Robinson MJ, Collins FD:** The investigation of a patient with hyperlipemia, hypokalemia and tetany. J Pediatr 59:200, 1961

287. **Fashena GJ, Martin RJ:** Congenital alkalosis of renal origin. Am J Dis Child 79:1127, 1950

288. **Fleisher DS:** Prolonged hypokalemic alkalosis: A specific disorder associated with dwarfism and elevated serum levels of unidentified anions. Am J Dis Child 102:705, 1961

289. **Garella S, Chazant JA, Cohen JJ:** Saline-resistant metabolic alkalosis or "chloride-wasting nephropathy." Report of four patients with severe potassium depletion. Ann Intern Med 73:31, 1970

290. **Houston IB:** Franconi's syndrome with renal salt wasting and alkalosis. Arch Dis Child 44:134, 1969

291. **Rosenbaum P, Hughes M:** Persistent, probably congenital, hypokalemic metabolic alkalosis with hyaline degeneration of renal tubules and normal urinary aldosterone. Am J Dis Child 941:560, 1957

292. **Slater RJ, Azzopardi P, Slater PE, Chute AL:** An unusual case of chronic hypokalemia associated with renal tubular degeneration. Am J Dis Child 96:469, 1958

293. **Calcagno PL:** Congenital renal alkalosis. Pediatr Res 13:1379, 1979

294. **Morris RC, Jr, Sebastian A, McSherry E:** Renal acidosis. Kidney Intern 1:322, 1972

295. **Rodriguez-Soriano J, Vallo A, Garcia–Fuentes M:** Distal renal tubular acidosis in infancy: a bicarbonate wasting state. J Pediatr 86:524, 1975

296. **Sebastian A, McSherry A, Schambelan M, Connor D, Biglieri E, Morris RC, Jr:** Renal tubular acidosis (RTA) in patients with hypoaldosteronism caused by renin deficiency. Clin Res 21:706, 1973

297. **Sebastian A, McSherry E, Morris CM, Jr:** Metabolic acidosis with special reference to the renal acidoses. In Brenner M, Rector F (eds): The Kidney. Philadelphia, WB Saunders, 1976

298. **McSherry E, Morris RC, Jr:** Attainment and maintenance of normal stature with alkali therapy in infants and children with classic renal tubular acidosis. J Clin Invest 61:509, 1978

299. **Rodriguez–Soriano J:** Renal tubular acidosis. In Edelmann C, Jr (ed): Pediatric Kidney Disease, p 995. Boston, Little, Brown and Co, 1978

300. **Griger C, Siegel R, McSherry E:** The effect of acidosis on plasma lysyl oxidase activity in children with renal tubular acidosis. Proc Am Soc Nephrol 11th Ann Meet, p 18A. 1978

301. **Wrong O, Davies HEF:** The excretion of acid in renal disease. Quart J Med 28:259, 1959

302. **Nash MA, Torrado AD, Greifer I, Spitzer A, Edelmann CM, Jr:** Renal tubular acidosis in infants and children: Clinical course, response to treatment and prognosis. J Pediatr 80:738, 1972

303. **Lowe CU, Terrey M, MacLachlan EA:** Organic-aciduria decreased renal ammonia production hydrophthalmos, and mental retardation: A clinical entity. Am J Dis Child 83:164, 1952

304. **Abbassi V, Lowe CU, Calcagno PL:** Oculo-cerebro-renal syndrome: A review. Am J Dis Child 115:145, 1968

305. **Van Acker KJ, Roels H, Beelaerts W, Pasternack A, Valcke R:** The histologic lesions of the kidney in the oculo-cerebro-renal syndrome of Lowe. Nephron 4:193, 1967

306. **Hugh-Jones K, Newcomb AL, Hsia DYY:** The

genetic mechanism of galactosemia. Arch Dis Child 35:521, 1960

307. **Monteleone JA, Beutler E, Monteleone PL, Utz CL, Casey EC:** Cataracts, galactosuria and hypergalactosemia due to galactokinase deficiency in a child. Am J Med 50:403, 1971

308. **Gitzelmann R:** Deficiency of erythrocyte galactokinase in a patient with galactose diabetes. Lancet 2:670, 1965

309. **Gitzelmann R:** Hereditary galactokinase deficiency, a newly recognized cause of juvenile cataracts. Pediatr Res 1:14, 1967

310. **Thalhummer O, Gitzelmann R, Pantlitschko M:** Hyper-galactosemia and galactosuria due to galactokinase definicency in a newborn. Pediatrics 42:441, 1968

311. **Fensom AH, Benson PF, Blunt S:** Prenatal diagnosis of galactosemia. Br Med J 4:386, 1974

312. **Schneider JA, Wong V, Bradley K, Seegmiller JE:** Biochemical comparisons of the adult and childhood forms of cystinosis. N Eng J Med 279:1253, 1968

313. **Goldman H, Scriver CR, Aaoron K, Delvin E, Canlas Z:** Adolescent cystinosis: Comparisons with infantile and adult forms. Pediatrics 47:979, 1971

314. **Schulman JD, Schneider JA, Bradley KH, Seegmiller JE:** Cystine, cysteine, and glutathione metabolism is normal and cystinotic fibroblasts, in vitro, and in cultured normal amniotic fluid cells. Clin Chim Acta 37:53, 1972

315. **Schneider JA, Schulman JD, Seegmiller JE:** Cystinosis and the Fanconi syndrome. In Stanbury JB, Wyngaarden JB, Fredrickson DS (eds): The Metabolic Basis of Inherited Disease. McGraw-Hill, 1978

316. **Lucas JJ, Kempson RL, Palmer J, Korn D, Cohn RB:** Renal allotransplantation in man. II. Transplantation in cystinosis, a metabolic disease. Am J Surg 118:158, 1969

317. **Briggs WA, Kominami N, Wilson RE, Merrill JP:** Kidney transplantation in Fanconi syndrome. N Engl J Med 286:25, 1972

318. **Callis L, Castello F, Fortuny G, Valla A, Ballabriga A:** Effect of hydrochlorothiazide on rickets and on renal tubular acidosis in two patients with cystinosis. Helv Paediatr Acta 6:602, 1970

319. **Potter DE, Greifer I:** Statural growth of children with renal disease. Kidney Intern 14:334, 1978

320. **Betts PR, Magrath P:** Growth pattern and dietary intake of children with chronic renal insufficiency. Br Med J 2;189, 1974

321. **West CD, Smith WC:** An attempt to elucidate the cause of growth retardation in renal disease. Am J Dis Child 91:460, 1956

322. **Cooke RE, Boyden DG, Haller E:** The relationship of acidosis and growth retardation. J Pediatr 57:326, 1960

323. **Holliday MA:** Growth retardation in children with renal disease. In Edelman CM Jr. (ed): Pediatric Kidney Disease, p 336. Boston, Little, Brown, 1978

324. **Holliday MA:** Metabolism and growth in children with kidney insufficiency. Kidney Intern 14:299, 1978

31

Immunology of the Fetus and Newborn

Joseph A. Bellanti and
Attilio L. Boner

INTRODUCTION

Immunology has come a long way since 1905 when the Russian biologist Eli Metchnikoff prophetically wrote[1]

Within a very short period, immunity has been placed in possession not only of a host of medical ideas of the highest importance, but also of effective means of combating a whole series of maladies of the most formidable nature in man and the domestic animals. Science is far from having said its last word, but the advances already made are amply sufficient to dispel pessimism in so far as this has been suggested by the fear of diseases, and the feeling that we are powerless to struggle against them.

Once the branch of medicine that dealt exclusively with the study of protection of the host against microorganisms, immunology now enjoys a much broader biologic scope and is concerned with those processes with which the host recognizes and eliminates "foreignness." In the modern view, immunologic responses serve three functions: **defense** (resistance to infection by microorganisms), **homeostasis** (removal of worn-out "self" cells), and **surveillance** (perception and destruction of mutant cells).[2] Cells of the immunologic system of the fetus and the neonate, once thought to be inactive, manifest a striking

capacity for response to the environment despite the fact that they are not fully developed. However, the fetus and newborn appear to be particularly vulnerable to injury that is either caused directly by immunologic mechanisms or inflicted by infectious agents that take advantage of the relative state of immaturity and inexperience of the immune system. These two concepts, which overlap at times, are clearly different. **Immaturity** refers to the genetically programmed low response or lack of response of the fetal and newborn immune system. **Inexperience** refers to the fact that the newborn immune system has not yet had its first encounter. A knowledge of these processes is particularly essential for those active in the care of newborns because they form the basis for the prevention, diagnosis, and treatment of many disease entities that afflict the fetus and newborn (Table 31-1).

GENERAL DEVELOPMENT OF THE IMMUNE SYSTEM: ROLE OF THE ENVIRONMENT

The development of the immune response may be visualized as a series of adaptive cellular responses to an everchanging and potentially hostile environment, and it may be considered at several levels: the **species,** the **individual,** or the **cell** (Table 31-2). From an

Table 31-1. Applications of Immunology for the Neonatologist.

Type	Example of Immunologic Procedure	Disease
Prevention	Rhogam	Hemolytic disease of the newborn
Diagnosis	Elevated IgM globulins in cord serum	Intrauterine infections
Therapy	Fresh blood transfusions	Acute sepsis of the newborn

evolutionary standpoint, the effect of a hostile macroenvironment provided the selective pressures leading to the survival of those life forms within the species which were best adapted to that environment (**phylogeny**). Within the developing fetus, the microenvironment in which undifferentiated progenitor cells exist (*e.g.,* thymus or the bursa of Fabricius) provides yet another type of inductive environment, permitting the full expression of immunity within the developing infant. The immunologically mature individual may be considered as the best-selected form resulting from this type of development (**ontogeny**). Finally, the molecular environment in which immunologically reactive cells exist (*e.g.,* **antigen**) provides the best-studied inductive stimulus leading to the proliferative and differentiative events commonly associated with cellular immune responses. The establishment of memory cells may be considered the best-adapted form for this environment. Thus, fetal and neonatal development of the immunologic system is best understood against the developmental backdrop of the developing host to his environment.

As shall be discussed, the cells and functions comprising the immune system appear early in fetal life, but at least some of them are fully activated only after birth, following interaction of the neonate with his environment. However, under certain circumstances (*e.g.,* intrauterine infections) the environment of the developing fetus may be so altered that it begins activation *in utero.*

One caveat must be issued to the neonatologist and those entrusted to the care of the newborn: concern must be directed to the current pollution of man's environment. In particular, those agents that may gain access to the fetus during prenatal development are a threat, including maternal drugs, infecting organisms, and other noxious agents, together with those that change the natural environment of the neonate (*e.g.,* hexachlorophene). The obstetrician and the neonatologist, who have already made significant contributions to our understanding of teratogenic effects of these

Table 31-2. Effect of Environment on the Development of the Immune Response.

Target	Inductive Environment	Process	Selected Form
Species	Macroenvironment	Phylogeny	Existing life forms
Individual	Microenvironment	Ontogeny	Immunologically mature individual
Cell	Molecular environment (antigen)	Induction of immune response	"Memory" cells

agents, must be made aware of their effects on the developing immunologic system.

DEVELOPMENT OF THE DIFFERENT COMPONENTS OF THE IMMUNE SYSTEM

For ease of discussion, the immunologic system may be considered under two major headings:

1. The **non-specific mechanisms,** which include phagocytosis, the inflammatory response, and several amplification systems including complement, coagulation, and kinin systems
2. The **specific immune responses,** which consist of cell-mediated (T cell) and humoral (B cell) systems.

It is important to stress that the nonspecific and specific mechanisms are intimately interrelated and interdependent. For example, the activation of the complement system by immunoglobulins (IgM and IgG), or the production of chemotactic factors and other lymphokines, plays a significant role in the whole inflammatory response. The monocyte or macrophage may function in both phagocytic and inflammatory responses as well as play a significant role in the processing of antigen—steps which are essential for the induction of the specific immune response. Thus, the macrophage actually forms part of both the nonspecific and specific immune systems, and is important to both the afferent and efferent limbs of the immune response. The lymphokines are other products secreted by mononuclear cells that play a role in both nonspecific and specific mechanisms.

Nonspecific Immune Mechanisms

There are a number of abnormalities of nonspecific immunity that may affect the newborn infant: (1) the movement of phagocytic cells toward a foreign configuration (**chemotaxis**) and inflammatory response, (2) the preparation of substances for cell ingestion (**opsonization**); and (3) the intracellular destruction of substances (**digestion**). Most of these neonatal impairments of nonspecific immunity occur as expressions of developmental immaturity and may affect systems intrinsic to the neutrophilic leukocyte (**intracellular**) or systems extrinsic to it (**extracellular**).

Inflammatory Response of the Neonate. Fol-

lowing injury of tissue or invasion by micro-organisms, a spectrum of systemic and local events is triggered.

The febrile response is believed to reflect enhanced metabolic activity and is also believed to be related to the release of endogenous pyrogens from host's leukocytes, with hypothalamic response. This is not, however, particularly well developed in the neonate (*i.e.,* functional immaturity of the inflammatory response) and fever is not a valuable sign of infection in this period. Similarly, leukocytosis and an increased rate of sedimentation, commonly associated with bacterial infections in the older infant and child, is not particularly useful in the neonatal period. However, other parameters in the inflammatory response such as the increase in alpha and beta globulins with the elevation of C-reactive protein (CRP) do occur in the neonatal period and are useful in the diagnosis of infectious diseases in the neonate. Moreover, although it is well recognized that an elevation in total neutrophil count is an inconsistent and unreliable index of neonatal sepsis, recent evidence suggests that an increase in total numbers of nonsegmented (band) forms may be a more significant and valuable diagnostic aid. Another important event accompanying non-specific immune responses in the newborn is the activation of the coagulation system with disseminated intravascular coagulation as seen in bacterial sepsis. The measurement of clotting factors or fibrin split products may provide another important predictive marker of infection.

Cellular Component of Inflammatory Response. The cellular responses are carried out primarily by polymorphonuclear leukocytes, macrophages (monocytes), eosinophils, and lymphocytes.

Polymorphonuclear (PMN) Leukocytes. The PMN leukocyte performs three functions: (1) migration, including chemotaxis and random migration or mobility; (2) phagocytosis, and (3) microbicidal activity.

Chemotaxis. The skin of the newborn is relatively deficient in manifesting the expressions of nonspecific immunity. Following introduction of a foreign substance into the skin, for example, a number of inflammatory cells move in a directed fashion toward the foreign configuration, a process referred to as **chemotaxis.** In the adult, a prominent polymorphonuclear leukocyte infiltration is seen during the first 4 to 12 hours, followed by a predominant mononuclear response consisting of macrophages and lymphocytes. In the newborn, however, the shift from a granulocytic to a mononuclear cell response is slower and less intense than in the adult, reflective of a maturational deficiency. Further, in some studies, a curiously high percent of eosinophils is noted in the second- and fourth-hour exudate of newborns older than 24 hours, but not in those less than 24 hours. It is of interest that the lesions of erythema toxicum, well known to neonatologists, consist primarily of eosinophilic leukocytes.

Neonatal PMN leukocytes exhibit less chemotactic activity than do adult cells because of deficiencies of both intrinsic cellular factors and extrinsic humoral factors. The deficiency in complement components C3 and C5 are the primary lacking humoral factors.[3]

Membrane deformability of the newborn's PMN leukocyte is also markedly decreased when compared with those of adults. This increased membrane rigidity may partially explain the defective chemotaxis of the newborn.[4] Random mobility, on the other hand, which refers to the nondirected migration of the PMN leukocyte, is normal in the newborn.

Phagocytosis. Once mobilized, the cells mount an attack on their target by a process of **phagocytosis** (cell-eating). In the mature person, many foreign substances, such as nonvirulent organisms, may be ingested by phagocytic cells through unenhanced processes; others (*i.e.,* virulent organisms) require preparation by specific antibody or complement. The newborn may be compromised in both the cellular and humoral factors involved in phagocytosis. It is only the IgG globulins that are transmitted across the placenta, and complement activity is deficient in the neonate.

There have been a number of conflicting investigations of phagocytosis in the neonate. In some studies, it has been shown that phagocytosis by neonatal leukocytes is abnormal when suspended in neonatal serum. Normal activity is restored when the same cells are resuspended in adult serum, thus suggesting that the primary defect may reside in extracellular factors. However, under certain conditions, both *in vitro* and *in vivo,* neonatal PMN leukocytes are deficient in phagocytic capacity when compared with that of the adult PMN leukocyte.[5] For example, when the con-

centration of serum is varied or when phagocytes are taken from sick full-term infants, phagocytic activity is deficient relative to that seen in normal term neonates.[6]

Bactericidal Activity and Metabolic Activity. Following particle uptake by phagocytes, there is an increase in oxygen consumption and glucose utilization by the hexose monophosphate pathway (HMP).[2] The formation of hydrogen peroxide, the result of increased HMP activity, is believed to be of paramount importance in the killing of many bacteria. The nitroblue tetrazolium dye (NBT) test is a screening procedure for the measurement of HMP activity and is based upon the formation of a blue formazan pigment during phagocytosis of the test dye. Defective HMP with decreased NBT reduction is exemplified by chronic granulomatous disease and is associated with recurrent infections caused by gramnegative organisms and staphylococci. It is of interest that the newborn, who also shows defective shunt activity, is plagued by the same spectrum of infections as in chronic granulomatous disease; thus, the newborn may show similar defects. The data with regard to metabolic activity of the newborn leukocyte, however, are inconsistent. Some have found a decreased metabloic activity of HMP, others a normal activity. Most agree that the reduction of NBT is normal or increased in the newborn, however, and is therefore of little diagnostic value in the newborn period. There is a decrease in NBT dye reduction with maturation during the first 6 months of life followed by a continuous increase of activity with age.[7]

It was also shown that leukocyte glucose-6-phosphate dehydrogenase (G-6-PD) increases with age, and that the activity of this enzyme displays increased thermal lability in infants. Thermal stability increases with age.[7] Similar thermal lability of G-6-PD has been demonstrated in three patients with chronic granulomatous disease.[8] The lability appears to be related to a lack of availability of NADP owing to a diminished or absent NADPH oxidase activity. These two observations could partially account for the increased resistance to infection that occurs with age and may explain the susceptibility of the newborn to infection with certain microbial agents.

The results obtained in studies of bactericidal activity of neonatal PMN leukocytes are similar to those found in phagocytosis, (*i.e.,* results obtained under seemingly normal conditions differ from those obtained under stress). A deficient bactericidal activity was shown in PMN leukocytes from neonates with a variety of clinical abnormalities including sepsis, meconium aspiration, respiratory distress syndrome, hyperbilirubinemia, or premature rupture of the membrane.[9] The situation, therefore, seems much the same as with phagocytosis. When subjected to the demands of adjustment to extrauterine life, relative deficiencies of bactericidal activities may play a significant role in explaining the compromised host defense mechanism of the neonate.

The macrophage, which is a central cell type involved in several immunologic processes, displays a deficient function in the neonate.[10] Recent research has focused on the functional capabilities of monocytes in neonates. Monocyte functions measured in neonates include chemotaxis, phagocytosis, microbial killing, and antibody-dependent cellular cytotoxicity. Of these, only chemotaxis has been shown to be primarily deficient.[11,12] This observation could also explain the newborn's inability to respond to pneumococcal or *Hemophilus influenzae* polysaccharide antigens.

Humoral Component of the Inflammatory Response: Complement System. One of the causes of innate or natural resistance to infection in vertebrates is the complement system. Deficiencies of components of complement can be responsible for severe disorders.

Despite its significant biological role, little is known regarding the complement system in the neonate. The third component of complement, C3, can be synthesized in different tissues in the human conceptus beginning as early as 29 days of gestation.[13] The sites of synthesis for C3 appear to be the fibroblast, the lymphoid cell, and the macrophage. In adults, there is some evidence that the liver is the major producer of C3. Serum concentration of C3 in the fetus rises almost exponentially from 1.9 mg/dl at 5.5 weeks' gestation[13] to a range of 52 to 167 mg/dl between 28 to 41 weeks. The mean level in cord blood is ±90 mg/dl, approximately one-half the maternal levels. Studies of C3 phenotypes indicate that C3 is synthesized *in utero*. The concentration of complement in the newborn falls slightly after birth and recovers before the infant is 3 weeks of age. By the age of 6 months, C3 reaches adult levels. Phagocytosis of bacterial

products enhances production of complement components. Thus, it can be deduced that, after birth, antigen stimulation may play a role in the induction of complement synthesis.

Components C3, C4, and C5 in premature and full-term infants have been found to be deficient when compared with maternal and adult standards. Propp and workers found, in cord blood from full-term neonates, that C1q, C3, C4, and C5 were about 50% of the respective maternal levels.[14] Low levels of properdin, factor B (C3PA), as well as C1, C2, C3, and C4 have also been reported in cord blood.

In summary, C1q, C2, C3, C4, C5, factor B (C3PA), properdin level, and total hemolytic complement levels are all lower in the neonatal period. Most of the biologic effects of complement, including opsonization, immune adherence, complement-dependent viral neutralization, generation of anaphylactic and chemotactic factors, and production of cell membrane lesions, require only the first five complement components. Because the fetus can synthesize each of these components in biologically active form within the first trimester of development (but in smaller quantities than the adult), all these immunologic functions could be affected to one degree or another by complement levels.

• Antibodies: In addition to their direct effect in reacting with antigens, antibodies appear to play a significant role in events mediating inflammatory responses such as phagocytosis, chemotaxis, and the release of mediators. The extent to which the antibodies affect these different functions in the fetus and newborn depends on two main factors: permeability of the placenta to a given antibody (discussed under fetal-maternal relationship) and maturation of the antibody-producing system.

Silverstein and coworkers have studied the maturation of immunologic capability and lymphoid tissues in the normal fetal lamb in utero (Fig. 31-1).[15] They have established the sequence of the antibody response to different antigens. Bacteriophage ϕx174 given on day 37 elicited the earliest antibody response, at 41 days of gestation. This is a remarkable observation because the fetal sheep has little organized lymphoid tissue at this time. At approximately 66 days of gestation, the fetus becomes able to respond to the protein ferritin,

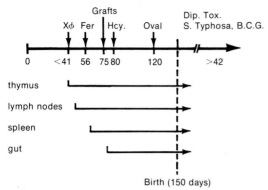

Fig. 31-1. Comparison of immunologic and lymphoid development in the fetal lamb. Numbers on the upper horizontal axis show the earliest times at which antibody responses and graft rejection could be detected. The time at which lymphocytes appear in different tissues is as follows: Xφ = bacteriophage, Fer = horse ferritin, Hcy. = snail hemocyanin, Oval = hen albumin, Dip. Tox. = diphtheria toxoid. (Adapted from Silverstein, Prendergast; In Lindahl–Kiessling K et al: Morphological and Functional Aspects of Immunity. New York, Plenum Press, 1971)

and not until 125 days of gestation can it respond to egg albumin. Antibodies against *Salmonella typhosa* or BCG appear only after birth. These authors also found that they were unable to induce tolerance until the lamb reached the age at which it was able to recognize the antigen and produce antibody. One can draw an analogy between this phenomenon and the known poor response of human newborn infants to the polysaccharide antigens. We must understand these phenomena in the human if we are to develop adequate immunization techniques and prevent allergic diseases.

• Opsonic Capacity: The opsonic capacity of blood refers to the enhancement of phagocytosis and includes the activities of antibodies, complement, and other not well-defined proteins. In general, IgM appears to have higher opsonic activity. Full term human newborns and, to a major degree, prematures appear to be relatively deficient in opsonic activity toward a variety of agents. The degree of deficiency varies with different agents. In part, it probably involves antibodies, particularly of the IgM type; this deficiency of antibodies has been claimed and accounts for the predilection for gram-negative infections of the newborn because IgM antibodies do not

traverse the placenta. However, Miller observed that addition of purified IgM to neonatal sera does not enhance opsonization of yeast particles.[5] It has been shown that complement and other heat-labile factors amplify the opsonic activity of IgM to a much greater extent than they amplify IgG opsonic activity. The deficit in opsonic activity derives from deficiencies of complement, as described above, particularly in components C3, C5, and C3PA. In the premature, it has been suggested that lowered levels of IgG may also play a role in the opsonic deficiency.[6] Rigorously controlled studies of opsonic capacity of the fetus and newborn are needed in order to decide the usefulness of a potentially harmful treatment such as fresh plasma transfusion in the septicemic neonate.

One of the important clinical sequelae of deficient specific antimicrobial antibody is seen in group B streptococcal infection of the newborn. The increased susceptibility of newborns to group B streptococcal infection has been correlated with deficiency of maternal antibody directed against the type-specific polysaccharides of the organism.

Specific Immune Mechanisms

The maturation of specific immune responses in the human begins *in utero* during the eighth to the twelfth weeks of gestation. The differentiation of cells destined to perform these functions appears to arise from a population of progenitor cells, referred to as stem cells, that are located within the yolk sac, fetal liver and bone marrow of the developing embryo (Fig. 31-2). Depending upon the type of microchemical environment surrounding these cells, differentiation will occur along at least two avenues: (1) the **hematopoietic** and (2) the **lymphopoietic.**

Hematopoietic Differentiation. One type of microchemical environment leads to the proliferation and differentiation of stem cells into myeloid, erythroid, and megakaryocyte precursors. The products of these cell lines are the monocytes, granulocytes, erythrocytes, and platelets of the circulation. In the human, granulocytic cells are first noted in the liver of the fetus at about the second month of gestation. Leukocyte production by the fetal liver then declines at about the fifth month of gestation when the bone marrow begins assuming increased activity.

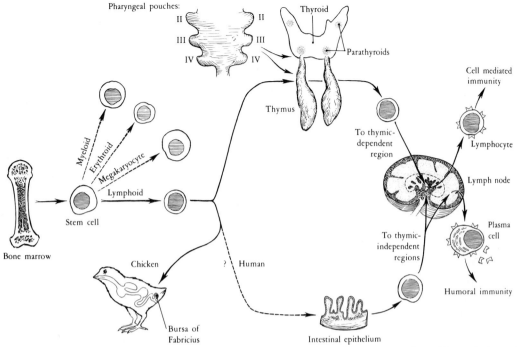

Fig. 31-2. Schematic representation of ontogeny of immune response, showing differentiation of progenitor cells into hematopoietic and immunocomponent cells. (Bellanti JA: Immunology II. Philadelphia, WB Saunders,1978)[2]

Lymphopoietic Differentiation. Classically, the lymphoid system develops along two independent pathways leading to morphologically and functionally distinct populations of immune lymphocytes: (1) the thymus-derived or T system of cell-mediated immunity whose principal effector cells are the T lymphocytes; and (2) the bursal-dependent or B system of humoral or antibody-mediated immunity which is displayed by the B lymphocytes.

The T lymphocyte is commonly identified by its capacity to form rosettes with sheep red blood cells (SRBC). The B lymphocyte is recognized primarily by its surface immunoglobulin.

T-cell System. The basic cell type can differentiate into lymphoid cells when the progenitor cells come under additional types of microchemical environments. The first of these is the thymus, which leads to the differentiation of T cells.[16,17] The thymus gland is derived from the epithelium of the third and fourth pharyngeal pouches at about the sixth week of fetal life. It is noteworthy that the parathyroids also begin their development at about this time from the same pouches (Fig. 31-3).

With further differentiation, a caudal migration of epithelium occurs, and, beginning in the eighth week, blood-borne stem cells enter the gland and are induced into lymphoid differentiation. With further development, the thymus is infiltrated with lymphocytes and is differentiated into a dense cortex containing many small lymphocytes and a less dense, loose central medulla with relatively more epithelial elements. Recent evidence suggests that a hormone (thymosin) is produced by these epithelial cells and may also be operative in the expansion of the peripheral lymphocyte population.[18] Although the characterization of this hormone is quite preliminary, the use of thymosin has intriguing applications to clinical medicine as a means of replacement of immunocompetence.

The clinical importance to the neonatologist of this simultaneous embryogenesis of the parathyroid and thymus is seen in one of the immunologic deficiency disorders of infancy, the Di George syndrome. In this disorder, infants are born not only lacking in thymic function but also without parathyroid glands. Thus, the infant presents not only with re-

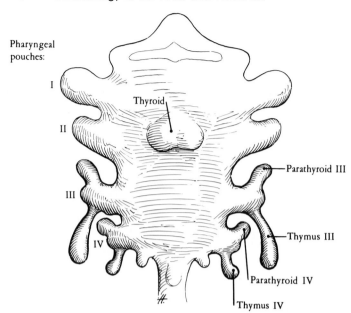

Pharyngeal pouches:

Fig. 31-3. Embryology of the thymus gland from the III to IV pharyngeal pouches. Note close proximity of site of differentiation of thyroid gland (II–III) and parathyroid glands (III–IV). (Bellanti JA: Immunology II. Philadelphia, WB Saunders, 1978)[2]

peated infections caused by monilia or virus but also with hypocalcemic tetany. Moreover, the successful immunologic reconstitution of these infants has been achieved through the use of thymic gland or thymic hormone. A major involvement of the II to III branchial pouches has also been described in congenital absence of the thyroid gland and thymus. Thus, in any infant presenting in the newborn period with either tetany or hypothyroidism, a diligent search for defects in thymic function should also be instituted.

Within the thymus gland, an intense rate of mitotic activity occurs, greater than in any other lymphatic organ. Curiously, over 75% of the cells die within the substance of the gland. The precise explanation for this is unknown, but it has been suggested that its increased mitotic activity may be a reflection of the censorship function of the thymus, eliminating potentially harmful clones. Following emergence from the thymus, the thymic cells acquire new surface antigen markers such as the θ antigen found in the mouse. Although the subject of intense current investigation, the nature and function of these receptors remains unclear, but they are thought to be associated with antigen recognition units on the surface of T cells.

Following emigration of the T cells from the gland, they circulate through the lymphatic and vascular systems as the long-lived lymphocytes (the recirculating pool), which then populate certain restricted regions of lymph nodes, the thymic-dependent subcortical areas, and the periarteriolar regions of the spleen. Removal of the thymus in the neonatal animal (*e.g.,* mouse) renders him deficient in the number of circulating T cells and also leads to a depletion of the thymic-dependent areas in lymphoid tissue. The long-lived nature of these lymphocytes and the degree of competence in the human may explain in part why, following thymectomy, immediate deficits are not usually seen in the newborn period, although they may become apparent much later in life.

After birth, the thymus plays a continually changing role in proportion to body size. It is relatively largest during fetal life and at birth weighs from 10 to 15 g.[2] The gland continues to increase in size, reaching a maximum of 30 to 40 g at puberty, following which an involution is seen. The increased incidence of autoimmunity and malignancy with aging have been thought by some to be related to senescence in thymic function.

Newborns, particularly the premature, have a significantly lower rate and degree of skin sensitization to dinitrochlorobenzene, and rejection of skin allografts is slower in newborns than in normal adults. Delayed hypersensitivity can be induced in newborns, however, during the first month of life. The newborn's inconsistency in this capacity appears to be caused more by a decreased inflammatory response and macrophage function than to depressed T-cell activity. A depressed T-cell function, however, may occur as a consequence of neonatal viral infection, hyperbilirubinemia, corticosteroid therapy, or maternal medications taken late during pregnancy. Specific T-cell immunity can result from antigenic exposure *in utero* to certain antigens such as penicillin, mumps virus, *Escherichia coli,* diphtheria and tetanus toxoids, and dental plaque in the mother. In addition, there are some suggestions that specific cell-mediated immunity can be acquired from the ingestion of T-cells contained in colostrum or breast milk or by way of the placenta. In summary, the proliferative capabilities of immature lymphocytes are well developed early in gestation and, at the time of birth, are equal to or may exceed those of adult lymphocytes; the inflammatory response and macrophage functions, on the contrary, appear to be impaired in the newborn period.

B-cell System. If the progenitor cells come under a second type of microchemical environment, differentiation will occur to produce a population of lymphocytes and plasma cells concerned with humoral immunity or antibody synthesis (Fig. 31-2). This population, referred to as B cells, comes under the influence of a second anatomic site, the bursa of Fabricius, the existence of which is known with certainty only in birds.[19] The bone marrow and the gut-associated lymphoid tissue (GALT) were originally suggested as the equivalent organ. There is now evidence that GALT is not the bursal equivalent. There are also strong suggestions that bone marrow constitutes one of the equivalents of the bursa. However, all the evidence indicates that the human fetal liver is the analogue of the bursa of Fabricius in man.

Fetal liver occupies the central role in B-cell development, as it probably does in T-cell development. Recently Cooper and coworkers using newer data particularly related to IgD development, have postulated a more complete model for mammalian B-cell differentiation, which is illustrated in Figure 31-4. These B cells comprise a much smaller part of the recirculating pool of lymphocytes and populate certain other regions of lymphoidal tissue, the thymic-independent regions, including the germinal centers of lymph nodes. Removal of the bursa or its mammalian equivalent leads to a profound deficiency of gamma globulin with little or no effect on cell-mediated immunity.[20] Antibody provides a major defense against encapsulated high-grade pyogenic pathogens including pneumococcus, *H. influenzae,* and meningococcus. The development of immunity in the fetus and the newborn must not be considered separate from maternal influences but rather should be considered as a maternal-fetal-neonatal unit.

MATERNAL-FETAL-NEONATAL RELATIONSHIPS

In the human, the predominant transfer of antibody occurs by way of the passage of the IgG immunoglobulins from the maternal circulation to that of the fetus. This is accomplished by means of an active transport of this immunoglobulin by virtue of a receptor located on one portion of the molecule. In this manner, the fetus receives a library of preformed antibody from his mother, reflecting most of her experiences with infectious agents. The secretory IgA immunoglobulins found in breast milk also provide local protection on the mucous membranes of the GI tract. Although these antibodies are not absorbed, their unique structure renders them more effective in these sites and may explain the lower incidence of enteric infections seen in breast-fed infants.

Significant numbers of granulocytes and macrophages, as well as B and T lymphocytes, appear in breast milk.[21] The B lymphocytes in human milk have been noted to produce IgA antibodies.[21] Secretory antibodies in milk are directed against antigens occuring in the GI tract: *E. coli* O and K antigens, shigella O antigen, *Vibrio cholerae* O and *E. coli* and *V. cholerae* entertoxins, poliovirus, and rotovirus. There appears to be a direct relationship between the extent of intestinal antigenic exposure and the level of specific secretory antibodies in milk. It is possible that following antigenic stimulation, the lymphoid cells from the Peyer's patches of the GI tract "home," by way of the mesenteric lymph nodes and the blood, to the mammary gland tissue and appear in the milk. As a result of this "homing" mechanism, human milk contains secretory IgA antibodies against many microorganisms

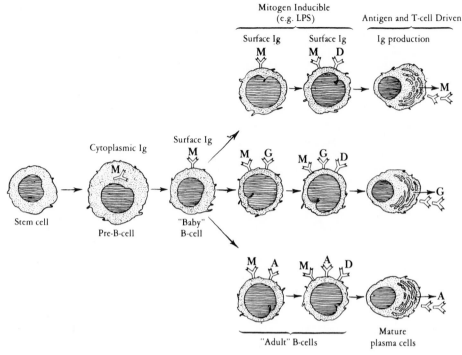

Fig. 31-4. Mammalian B-cell differentiation model. B cells differentiate from a stem cell to a rapidly dividing pre-B cell lacking functional antibody receptors. These cells initially synthesize cytoplasmic IgM that later become surface IgM ("baby" B cells). These "baby" B cells can be easily made tolerant and are pivotal for further differentiation of immunoglobulin-producing cells. While they continue to express surface IgM, they begin to express one of the surface IgG subclasses or IgA, followed later by the appearance of surface IgD. When these "double" or "triple" cells are triggered by antigen, helper T-cells, or B-cell mitogens, they become mature plasma cells or memory cells (not illustrated in this figure). The antigen-dependent T-cell driven stage requires the presence of surface IgD that is lost after antigenic stimulation. (Adapted from Cooper MD et al. In Bellanti JA: Immunology II. Philadelphia, WB Saunders, 1978)

harbored in the maternal intestine at the time of lactation (*i.e.*, microorganisms that the baby is most likely to be exposed to after birth). Because of the same "homing" mechanism, human milk also contains IgA antibodies to many food protein antigens (*e.g.*, cow's-milk proteins). It is possible, particularly in infants with atopic predisposition, that the frequency and magnitude of food allergy may be decreased by a prolonged period of breast feeding.[22] Thus, in the early period of life, when the infant's own secretory IgA system is maturationally deficient, breast-feeding may provide the infant with antibodies that support the local immune defense system. In addition to the protective function provided by secretory IgA antibody in breast milk, other protective factors are present in human milk, such as lactoferrin, lactoperoxidase, *Lactobacillus bifidus* factor, complement components, and leukocytes.

Necrotizing enterocolitis, a disease seen primarily in premature infants who have suffered severe perinatal stress, affects predominantly formula-fed infants. Neonatal rats subjected daily to a short period of hypoxia developed a reproducible model of the disease. All experimental animals died as a result of necrotizing entrocolitis if they had been formula-fed but not if breast-fed. The presence of viable macrophages in their feedings appears to have afforded them protection, and to have prevented the mortality seen in control animals.

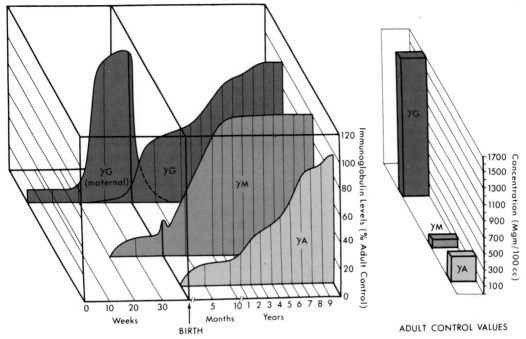

Fig. 31-5. Development of serum immunoglobulins in the human during maturation. (Bellanti JA: Immunology II. Philadelphia, WB Saunders, 1978)[2]

Occasionally, fetal cells or other proteins may gain access to the maternal circulation and thus actively immunize the mother to the paternal allotypes (antigen) found on these substances. This process, referred to as **isoimmunization,** may lead to serious disease in the infant, such as hemolytic disease of the newborn, thrombocytopenia, and leukopenia.

The development of serum immunoglobulins during intrauterine life and postnatally is shown in Figure 31-5. If one analyzes the amount and type of gamma globulin found in the blood of the newborn at birth, one finds that the levels of immunoglobulin are higher than those of the mother and are made up almost exclusively of the IgG immunoglobulins. There are few or no IgA and IgM globulins present in cord sera because the fetus is usually protected *in utero* from antigenic stimuli. If the fetus is challenged *in utero* as a consequence of (*e.g.,* immunization of the mother with salmonella vaccine) or infection (*e.g.,* congenital rubella, cytomegalic inclusion disease, toxoplasmosis), the fetus will respond with antibody production, largely of the IgM variety. The exclusion of other classes of antibody is beneficial to the fetus in many

cases. For example, the exclusion of the IgM isohemagglutinins, leukoagglutinins, or the IgE antibodies of allergy prevents disease which may be produced by these antibodies. However, it also prevents the passage of other maternal antibodies which would be beneficial to the newborn, such as the IgM antibodies important in bacterial defense against gram-negative bacteria (opsonins, agglutinins, and bactericidal antibodies). This may explain, in part, the increased susceptibility of the newborn to infection with gram-negative organisms such as *E. coli.*

There is great variability, however, in the types of antibodies that are obtained in this manner (Table 31-3). This is, in part, reflective of the quantity of antibodies in the maternal circulation, as well as of the molecular size that is present. For example, low molecular weight IgG antibodies (*e.g.,* rubeola antibody), present in high concentrations of maternal serum, are readily transferred. IgG antibodies present in lower concentrations (e.g., Bordetella pertussis) are poorly transferred, while macroglobulin antibody (*e.g.,* Wasserman antibody) are completely excluded.

Because the IgG immunoglobulins are pas-

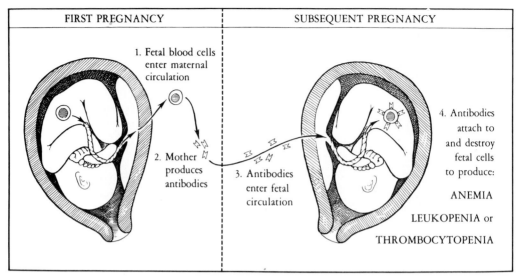

Fig. 31-6. Schematic representation of isoimmunization due to fetomaternal incompatibility. (Bellanti, JA: Immunology II. Philadelphia, WB Saunders, 1978)[2]

sively transferred, they have a finite half-life, between 20 and 30 days, and therefore their concentration in serum falls rapidly within the first few months of life, reaching its lowest level between the second and fourth months. This period is referred to as **physiologic hypogammaglobulinemia.** During the course of the first few years, the levels of gamma globulin increase because of exposure of the maturing infant to antigens in his environment. There appears to be a sequential development in the gamma globulins at different rates. The IgM globulins attain adult levels by 1 year of age,

and the IgA globulins by 10 years of age. This pattern of appearance of immunoglobulins recapitulates that which is seen in phylogeny and also appears to parallel that seen following antigenic exposure during the primary immune response.

Effect of Passive Acquired Antibody. In addition to providing a protective role to the newborn, these passively acquired IgG antibodies may interfere with active antibody synthesis following immunization procedures. Several studies have now confirmed that passively acquired antibody to diphtheria and to

Table 31-3. Relationship of Antibody Type with Transplacental Transfer.

Good Passive Transfer	Poor Passive Transfer	No Passive Transfer
Diphtheria antitoxin	*Hemophilus influenzae*	Enteric somatic (O) anti-
Tetanus antitoxin	*Bacillus pertussis*	bodies (salmonella, shi-
Antierythrogenic toxin	Dysentery	gella, *E. coli*)
Antistaphylococcal antibody	Streptococcus MG	Skin-sensitizing antibody
Salmonella flagella (H) anti-		Heterophile antibody
body		Wasserman antibody
Antistreptolysin		
All the antiviral antibodies		
present in maternal circu-		
lation (rubeola, rubella,		
mumps, poliovirus)		
VDRL antibodies		

Table 31-4. Maternal Antibodies Which Can Lead to Harmful Effects in the Infant.

Maternal Disease	Antibodies	Effect on Newborn
Hyperthyroidism	LATS	Transient hyperthyroidism (exophthalmos)
Idiopathic thrombocytopenia	Platelet antibodies	Transient thrombocytopenia
Isoimmunization (platelets, neutrophils, red blood cells)	Platelet, neutrophil, isohem-agglutinins or $Rh_0(D)$ antibodies	Transient thrombocytopenia, neutropenia, anemia
Lupus erythematosus	Autoantibodies to blood elements (LE cell factor, Coombs test, platelet)	Transient LE cell phenomenon, neutropenia, thrombocytopenia, ?congenital heart disease
Myasthenia gravis	Not defined yet	Transient neonatal myasthenia gravis

(Modified from Bellanti JA (ed): Immunology II. Philadelphia, WB Saunders Co., 1978)

pertussis may actually inhibit active antibody formation following active immunization. This occurred in the case of killed vaccines, appears to be dose related, and can be overcome by increasing the inoculum size. In the case of immunization with live virus vaccines, however, the effect of passively acquired antibody is actually to neutralize the vaccine's virus, thereby inhibiting successful immunization with parenteral live vaccines. From a practical standpoint, immunization at 2 to 3 months of age with killed vaccines (*e.g.*, diphtheria, pertussis, and tetanus), does not appear to be appreciably inhibited by this passive antibody. In contrast, live virus immunization procedures are usually delayed until the end of the first year of life because of the inhibitory effect of the passive antibody.

Another situation in which passive acquired antibody may interfere with active antibody synthesis is in the case of "natural immunity" acquired by the newborn infant from breast milk. IgA in breast milk may interfere with successful immunization with live poliovirus vaccines through neutralization of virus by antibody in the gastrointestinal tract. From a practical standpoint, poliovirus immunizations are not usually delayed, even in breast-fed infants, because, in any case, active immunization would follow subsequent poliovirus administration, according to recommended schedules for immunizations of infants and children. Maternal antibodies can also have harmful effects as shown in Table 31-4.

IMMUNOLOGIC CONSEQUENCES OF INTRAUTERINE INFECTIONS

An intrauterine infection should be suspected whenever an infant manifests the clinical features of petechiae, hepatosplenomegaly, congenital malformation, inguinal hernia, thrombocytopenia, and unusual skin rash. These infections, together with maturational defects postulated to be involved in their genesis, are shown in Table 31-5.

The possibility of intrauterine infection should be suspected in a newborn infant if there is a known exposure of the mother to an infectious disease during pregnancy or if the infant is small for gestational age or fails to thrive. An IgM concentration greater than 20 mg/dl in the cord blood or in the infant serum is considered abnormal. It should be pointed out, however, that occasionally an elevated IgM level may be the result of leakage of maternal blood into the fetus; under these circumstances, the infant's IgA level usually exceeds the IgM level, reflecting the IgA:IgM ratio in maternal blood. In addition, IgM concentrations repeated after 3 to 4 days will disclose a significant fall in the case of maternal transfusion, while IgM actively synthesized by the newborn will increase.

Congenital infections frequently become chronic and persist for weeks and even years with signs and symptoms that are not seen in children or adults with the same infection (Table 31-5). The agents which produce per-

Table 31-5. Infectious Agents Causing Infections in the Fetus and Newborn.

Nature of Infection	Maturational Defect
Acute	
Gram-negative organisms (*E. coli*)	IgM antibody, complement
Gram-positive organisms (Staphylococcus)	
Monilia	Cell-mediated immunity
Chronic	
Herpes simplex	Cell-mediated immunity(?)
Rubella	
Cytomegalovirus	
Toxoplasmosis	
Syphilis	

sistent infection of the human fetus exhibit a predilection for the reticuloendothelial system; an impairment of the functions of its cells may be associated with the development of an immunodeficiency.

The best studied of the congenital infections is the congenital rubella syndrome; congenital infection results from transmission of the virus from the pregnant mother to the fetus in the first 5 months of gestation. The infection of the child continues after birth from 6 months to as long as 3 years despite passive antibody acquired from the mother and active antibody synthesis by the infant. After birth, the child may continue to shed virus while making antibody. A variety of abnormal antibody responses have been reported in children with congenital rubella including increased levels of IgM with low IgG and absent IgA, low levels of IgM with low levels of IgG and absent IgA.[23,24] Moreover, in patients with congenital rubella reports[25,26] have appeared of poor antibody responses as determined by delayed appearance of isohemagglutinins; suboptimal vaccine responses; immune paresis with no response to tetanus or *Salmonella typhi* vaccines; and impaired cell-mediated immunity as demonstrated by impaired lymphoproliferative responses to phytohemagglutinin and decreased lymphocytotoxicity.[27] These abnormal responses have been associated with an increased frequency of infections. Many of the alterations reverted to normal later, when the child was no longer excreting virus.[28] This could represent a form of immunologic blockade while the child is shedding virus.

It should be noted that children who stop shedding virus are also older and may have more mature immunologic systems. Cytomegalovirus and herpes viruses produce infections that persist for years or throughout life when infection is acquired *in utero*. Studies of children with congenital cytomegalovirus infections and several with *in utero* herpes virus infections have shown no immunologic abnormalities.[29] Cell-mediated immunity (CMI) appears to be particularly important in these infections. In a recent study, eight infants with congenital cytomegalovirus infection and six of their mothers showed decreased specific CMI.[30] The decreased CMI in the mothers may have contributed to the transmission of the infection to the infant. It should be stressed that the earlier the infection, the more devastating the effect in the ontogeny of the immune system. If an insult occurs to the thymus in the first trimester, the normal development of T cell function would be affected; however, if the insult occurs in the third trimester, no resulting damage should be expected.

Viral infection of the fetus may be limited by the degree of cellular immune competence, as exemplified by those infants with proven congenital infection and intact cellular responses, who at birth are no longer shedding virus. The cellular competence of the fetus may also modulate the manifestations of intrauterine infection. Intrauterine syphillis, for example occurs only in late pregnancy at which time the body mounts a brisk cellular immune response to the spirochete. In infection early

Table 31-6. Immune Deficiency Disorders Which Can Be Diagnosed in the Newborn Period.

Disorder	Example	Genetics	Time of Onset	Type of Infection
Phagocytic function Quantitative	Neutropenia	Variable	At birth	Virulent bacteria (*e.g.*, staphylococcus)
Qualitative	Chronic granulomatous disease	X-linked, autosomal recessive	At birth	Less virulent bacteria, staphylococcus, monilia
Antibody	Agammaglobulinemia Dysgammaglobulinemia	Variable	>6 months, earlier if premature or small for dates	Virulent bacteria
Cell-mediated (delayed hypersensitivity) function	Congenital aplasia of thymus (Di Georges syndrome)	Variable	At birth	Fungal, viral
Combined antibody and cell-mediated function	"Swiss" agammaglobulinemia	Autosomal recessive, X-linked	At birth	Bacterial, viral, fungal, Pneumocystus carinii
Graft vs. host	Spontaneous abortion			
reactions	Fetal transfusion for hemolytic diseases	Nongenetic	At birth; could be later, but no data available	
Combined	Congenital asplenia	Variable	At birth or later	Gram negative
C_5 complement deficiency or Leiner disease		Variable	At birth	Gram negative
Variable	Ataxia telangiectasia	Autosomal recessive	>6 months	Fungal, viral
	Wiskott–Aldrich syndrome	X-linked recessive	>6 months	

(Adapted from Bellanti JA (ed): Immunology II. Philadelphia, WB Saunders Co., 1978)

in gestation, it may go unnoticed because the spirochete has neither a toxic nor a teratogenic effect on the fetus. It is only teratogenic when the immune response to the organism is activated. Similarly, rubella in very early gestation has primarily teratogenic effects (*e.g.*, congenital defects). In contrast, in later pregnancy (2–4 months), a primarily inflammatory effect is seen (*e.g.*, hepatitis, iridocyclitis, meningitis). These differences may result from an intact cellular immune response characteristic of the older fetus. Nonetheless, in some cases, the immune response of the child may fail to limit or clear these infections.

IMMUNOLOGIC EVALUATION OF THE NEWBORN

The functional significance of the two-compartment system is important to clinical medicine. It provides a useful basis upon which our understanding of the primary immune deficiency disorders rests, as well as a framework for a more logical approach to the management of maturational deficiencies in the newborn period. Selective deficiencies of the thymic-independent B system, so-called agammaglobulinemias, present with recurrent bacterial infections. Selective deficiencies of the

Table 31-7. Reminders for the Clinical Evaluation of Immune System in the Newborn.

History

Previous newborn deaths in the family; history of immune diseases

Previous isoimmunization in mother (due to pregnancy or transfusions [Rh, ABO], gamma globulin administration)

Previous diseases in the mother (autoimmune diseases, *e.g.,* SLE, thyroiditis, myasthenia gravis, idiopathic thrombocytopenic purpura)

History of medications in mother (quinine, guinidine, Sedormid, Clorpromazine)

History of infections during pregnancy (rubella, cytomegalic inclusion disease, toxoplasmosis, syphilis, herpes simplex, UTI, vaginal infections, TB)

Physical Examination

General appearance (assess degree of activity: hyperactivity, consider hyperthyroidism, passive transfer of LATS; hypoactivity or muscle weakness, consider myasthenia gravis with transfer of antibodies to muscle; purpura, consider thrombocytopenia due to the passive transfer of antibodies to platelets.)

Skin (jaundice in first 24 hr; petechiae are characteristic of isoimmunization, *e.g.,* erythroblastosis fetalis)

Eyes (exophthalmos due to LATS)

Chest (pneumonitis seen in many intrauterine infections)

Cardiovascular (evaluate murmurs for congenital heart disease, *e.g.,* infants of LES mothers)

Abdomen (hepatosplenomegaly: seen in severe erythroblastosis fetalis, also in congenital intrauterine infections and GVH reactions, spleen absence)

Extremities (note deformities and other birth defects)

Neurological (convulsions, weakness)

(Bellanti JA (ed): Immunology II. Philadelphia, WB Saunders Co., 1978)

thymic-dependent tissues (the T system) are associated with fungal and viral infections. Patients with combined B and T cell defects are the most serious of all the immune deficiency syndromes, with profound deficiencies in both cell-mediated and antibody-mediated functions; they present with a diversity of infections.

At this point it seems fair to say that evaluation of the immune system during the prenatal period is by no means an easy task. The evaluator must take into consideration the dynamic, rapidly growing, adaptive, and changing parameters of the immune function in response to a changing internal and external environment. In Table 31-6 are shown some of the major classes of immune deficiencies that can be diagnosed in the newborn period together with their time of onset and the type of infections that are typically associated with them. However, a detailed history with emphasis on family background, and a careful physical examination, should offer a solid foundation for interpretation of clinical and research laboratory data. Table 31-7 presents

some suggestions for the clinical evaluation of the newborn. Table 31-8 lists some of the pertinent clinical and historical information that could be useful in the diagnosis of immune deficiency disorders in the newborn period. Although most immunologic defects that we see are not usually clinically apparent until postnatal life, it is not unlikely that in certain instances the result of immunologic deficiency may be intrauterine infection with a resultant damaged baby at birth or an aborted conceptus. Zuelzer and coworkers and others have shown maternal blood-formed elements in fetal circulation.[31] Theorteically, therefore, early passage of immunologically active mononuclear cells from the mother to the fetus could be responsible for graft-versus-host (GVH) reaction. Although direct proof of GVH reactions in the fetus is lacking, several clinical situations suggest that such processes may occur in the newborn and fetus. Among these can be cited the report of a XX/XY chimerism in a 12-week-old abortus of a mother who had a number of repeated "spontaneous" abortions.[32] A case was reported by Naiman, in

Table 31-8. Diagnostic Clues in Suspecting Immune Deficiency Disorders in the Newborn Period.

Finding	Comments
Hypocalcemic tetany Absence of thymic shadow Moniliasis	DiGeorge syndrome—diagnosed by DNCB skin testing, *in vitro* lymphocyte stimulation with phytohemagglutinin, and MLR
History of immune deficiency in other family members	Most immunologic defects genetically determined, and sex-linked most common
Agammaglobulinemia	Quantitative immunoglobulins not useful because of passive transfer of IgG, determination after 2 to 4 months helpful in establishing diagnosis; allotypes helpful
Chronic granulomatous disease	NBT helpful as screening test only because may be nonspecifically elevated; tests of bactericidal function fail to reach normal values in presence of adult sera
Poor growth, splenomegaly, hepatomegaly, diffuse dermatitis, diarrhea	GVH—laboratory findings include anemia, decrease in serum complement, histiocytic infiltration of bone marrow and erythrophagocytosis
Howell Jolly bodies in peripheral smear, absence of spleen, shadow in x-ray film	Congenital absence of spleen and other associated malformations
Seborrheic dermatitis	C5 deficiency (Leiner disease)
Chronic diarrhea	Defect in phagocytosis of Baker's yeast particles, secondary to failure of sera to opsonize yeast

which, following three exchange transfusions, the infant developed jaundice, aplastic anemia, and marked histiocytosis.[33] This infant also had chimerism, with one line representing donor cells.

Evaluation of the Humoral Immune System

Table 31-9 summarizes the evaluation of the humoral immune system. In general, pure humoral immune deficiency syndromes are not clinically manifested in the prenatal period because of the protective effect of maternal IgG. However, very premature infants, particularly those born at less than 32 weeks' gestation, may have IgG serum levels below 400 mg/dl. Small-for-date infants also have decreased IgG, some impairment of specific antibody responses (*e.g.*, to attenuated polio virus), reduction in specific IgG secretory antibody responses, and an increased incidence of antibodies to food.[34] Another factor

to be considered is hypogammaglobulinemia in the mother, which, although rare, would lead to inadequate levels of IgG in the newborn. Other ways to evaluate the humoral immunologic system are described below.

Evaluation of the Cell-Mediated Immune System

Table 31-10 summarizes the evaluation of the CMI system of the newborn. Evaluation of the CMI system begins with a total and differential white cell count. Lymphopenia is seen in most of the CMI deficiencies, but at times the lymphocyte count may be normal. Erythrocyte rosette-forming cells (E^+RFC) should be quantitated and the total number of T lymphocytes calculated from the WBC value and the percentage of lymphocytes. It should be stressed that E^+RFC determinations do not constitute a functional test. Technical details and adequate age-adjusted controls are necessary, because normal numbers for different

Table 31-9. Diagnostic Tests for Evaluation of the Humoral
Immune Function in Neonates.

Test	Comment
Quantitative measurement of immunoglobulins	May reveal elevated IgM or IgA, does not distinguish maternal from fetally produced IgG
B cell mitogen stimulation (*e.g.,* pokeweed)	As with PHA (routine test) Ig's synthesis determined in supernatant (research tool) or cell stained with intracytoplasmic immunofluorescence techniques
Genetic typing (Gm and Inv.)	Of help in determining origin of circulating immunoglobulins in newborn (not routine test)
IgG subclass determination	IgG_3 increases in prenatal period and reaches adult levels after 3 months; $IgG_{1,2,4}$ close to adult levels many months (years) later
Determinations of total number of B cells by EAC or direct immunofluorescence	Does not necessarily correlate with decreased Ig synthesis; helpful to elucidate level of B cell defect
Specific antibody responses de novo sensitization (*e.g.,* salmonella)	O antigen induce IgM; H antigen induce IgG
Regional lymph node biopsy after immunization	Helpful for humoral as well as CMI
Coculture of purified B cells from patient with normal T cells	No production of Igs indicates defective Ig production or release
Regional lymph node biopsy after immunization	Helpful for humoral as well as CMI

ages have not yet been established. B-cell determination should be done, using EAC (erythrocyte-antibody-complement complex) rosettes and by direct immunofluorescence. EAC techniques take advantage of the receptors of B cells for C3b and C3d complement components. The antibody anti-red cell used should be of IgM rather than IgG type to overcome the problem of EA (erythrocyte-antibody complex) rosettes, formed by lymphocytes with receptors for the Fc part of IgG. Fc receptors for IgG are present not only in B cells but also in T and "null" cells. Therefore, apparently normal or augmented numbers of B cells can be detected. The direct immunofluorescence uses antiserum against the B-cell surface immunoglobulins. We prefer to use the Fab'_2 fraction of rabbit antihuman immunoglobulins. The use of whole rabbit IgG antihuman immunoglobulins, as well as EA complex, can yield misleading results, particularly in cases of severe combined immune deficiency (SCID); this approach can show apparently normal numbers of B cells, which in reality represent Fc receptor-positive cells that have recognized the Fc part of the IgG molecule. If E+RFC are low, a thymosin induction of E^+RFC will give a good indication, although not definite proof, of the patient's probable response to thymic hormones. If CMI deficiency is suspected before birth, cord blood lymphocytes can be used in thymosin induction of E^+RFC. Normally, cord blood contains lymphocytes that can be induced to E^+RFC when incubated with thymosin. Absence of this response indicates a probable lack of E^+RFC precursors. A very low initial level of E^+RFC with a brisk thymosin response is more evidence to suggest a probable CMI deficiency syndrome that could respond to thymic hormone. Recently Shore and coworkers reported a patient with partial CMI deficiency whose bone marrow lymphocytes responded to thymosin only after an "inductive" incubation period in a monolayer culture of epithelial thymic cells.[38] This patient also had a larger

Table 31-10. Diagnostic Tests for Evaluation of Cell-Mediated Immunity in Newborns.

WBC and differential	Normal lymphocyte count does not rule out CMI deficiency; low count compatible but not diagnostic
Skin testing with DNCB	Positive result practically rules out CMI deficiency
	Negative or weak result does not confirm diagnosis of CMI deficiency
Immunization with antigens (*e.g.*, diphtheria or tetanus toxoid)	Positive in vitro lymphoblastic response to same antigen used for immunization; or MIF release by same Ag compatible with at least partially CMI is present (not routine test)
Determination of absolute number of E+RFC	No functional test but correlates well with CMI status
Coculture of normal lymphocytes, or T lymphocyte, with lymphocytes from suspected patient	Can indicate defective Ig's production due to increase suppressor T-cell activity or decrease in helper T-cell activity
Mitogen stimulation of lymphocytes (*e.g.*, PHA)	Optimum, suboptimum as well as over optimum concentrations of PHA should be used
MLR	Could be positive in absence of responses to PHA
Determination of human lymphocyte-transforming antigen (HLTA)	Could be helpful in elucidating level of T cell impairment (not routine lab test, may be research tool)
Stimulation of HLTA and E+RFC in PBL or BM	Good response suggests probable response to thymosin treatment (as above)
Thymic hormones determination in blood	Decrease in amount definitely makes diagnosis of thymic insufficiency; if present in normal amount would not necessarily rule out CMI deficiency (as above)
Lymph node biopsy after stimulation with *de novo* organism	To see if dependent areas are normal
Biopsy of thymus	To be performed in patients with obvious CMI; helps to elucidate different types of CMI deficiencies that could orient new therapeutic measures

than normal thymus, which at biopsy showed a lack of Hassall corpuscles.

Tests of lymphoproliferative responses should be performed, using different concentrations of T-cell mitogens, such as concanavalin A and phytohemagglutinin. Newborn lymphocytes seem to respond better than those of adults at low dosages of mitogens; at higher concentrations, they are less responsive than adult lymphocytes.[35] Mixed lymphocyte culture (MLC) reactions may also be helpful in diagnosing CMI deficiencies. A dissociation of low phytohemagglutinin, with normal MLC, can be seen in some patients with CMI deficiency. On the basis of phylogeny and ontogeny, we may speculate that such a defect originates at a higher level of T-cell differentiation. Lack of MLC responses theoretically suggests a defect occurring earlier in ontogenic development. Determinations of enzymes such as adenine deaminase (ADA) and nucleoside phosphorylase may help to clarify some of the cases of SCID and orient the clinician toward enzyme replacement therapy.

Radiologic examinations can show bony abnormalities in immune deficiencies with ADA deficiency, or absence of thymus, which is useful to the diagnostician only when observed

Table 31-11. Diagnostic Tests for PMN Function in Newborns.

Peripheral blood count and differential	Often of help, count important, Ex/Neutropenia; morphology of cells important, Ex/Chediak–Higashi
Skin window—Rebuck	May give general clue to defect of inflammatory function, particularly ability to marshal leukocytes to site of infection
Phagocytosis	Results vary with assay used; particle being phagocytized critical; assay used must distinguish humoral and cellular components of process
Chemotaxis	Decreased in cellular and humoral activity during neonatal period
Quantitative NBT	Screening test; if normal or high, does not rule out CGD
Bactericidal activity	Measured by direct killing assay; CGD can be diagnosed during neonatal period
Measurement of specific WBC enzymes	Not done routinely

in newborns younger than 4 days who have not been previously stressed. A barium swallow may reveal diffuse esophagitis, usually caused by monilia.

Skin testing with fungal, bacterial, and viral antigens for delayed hypersensitivity has not proved useful in the study of the newborn. Skin testing with PHA is claimed to be somewhat more sensitive.[36] Contact sensitization to dinitrochlorobenzene (DNCB) offers advantages over intradermal testing. DNCB is positive in 90% of normal individuals. If any doubt exists regarding humoral immunity, the least resort is antigenic stimulation with a variety of vaccines: salmonella or other antigens, followed by a regional lymph node biopsy looking for B- and T-dependent areas. Paired serum specimens taken prior to and after immunization should be studied for specific antibodies. Virus infections sometimes depress CMI, and some of the patients who are referred to us may show anergy because of persistent viral infections. In these cases, sound medical judgment, patience, and repeated studies are necessary. Fetal growth retardation and malnutrition also depress CMI and humoral responses for several months after birth.[34] Evaluation of the nonspecific immune responses in the newborn is almost limited to testing polymorphonuclear leukocyte function with the Rebuck skin-window technique (Table 31-11),

which has not yet been standardized for the newborn. The NBT test may be used as a screening test for chronic granulomatous disease (CGD); the results should be confirmed by bactericidal assay. Lowered numbers of complement components have been described in the prenatal and cord blood, as mentioned above. The extent to which these reflect actual functional abnormalities of complements is uncertain. Phagocytic tests should include evaluation of influences of C3 and C5. Separate evaluation of the complement effects on phagocytosis, chemotaxis, and bactericidal activities must be made. A functional deficiency of C5 activity has been described in Leiner disease. Finally, monocyte function, although important, is not usually clinically evaluated because of a lack of adequate methods. Recently Poplack and coworkers have shown that in humans antibody-dependent cellular cytotoxicity (ADCC) activity against red blood cells is dependent only on the monocyte.[37] We hope that this test will prove to be of significance in the evaluation of the monocyte.

CONCLUSION

The neonate is not "immunologically null"; he is immunologically nonexperienced and has only a relatively immature immune system. Most of the known immunologic mechanisms develop early in fetal life. At birth, some are not fully developed, but maturation proceeds quickly, probably in response to environmental influences. Although the nonspecific defense mechanisms are of vital importance, observations of children with defects of the cell-mediated immune or humoral systems provide definitive proof that the development of specific acquired immune mechanisms is indispensible for survival in normal individuals. Today, as in the early age of immunology, studies of infections can contribute to our understanding of the basic mechanisms of immunity. The question that remains to be answered is what is the difference immunologically between the newborn that develops septicemia and the newborn that does not. Detailed study of pathogenesis and immunity in intrauterine or perinatal infections such as CMV infections, herpes simplex infection, *E. coli* neonatal septicemia, and streptococcus in the newborn will yield a fuller explanation of inexperience and relative immaturity of immune mechanisms in the fetus and newborn infant. Of equal importance is the study of "experiments of nature." Better methods for evaluation of immunologic compromise in the newborn are urgently needed. The human neonatal macrophage (monocyte) is the prime candidate for study. Impaired activity of this cell system would explain a number of unusual immune responses observed in the newborn and might provide the basis not only for new therapeutic approaches but for prevention of infectious diseases as well as allergic disorders.

REFERENCES

1. **Metchnikoff E:** Immunity in Infective Diseases. London, Cambridge University Press, 1905
2. **Bellanti JA:** Immunology II. Philadelphia, WB Saunders, 1978
3. **Miller ME:** Chemotactic function in the human neonate: Humoral and cellular function. Pediatr Res 5:487, 1971
4. **Miller ME:** Development maturation of human neutrophil motility and its relationship to membrane deformability. In Bellanti JA, Dayton DH (eds): The Phagocytic Cell in Host Resistance, p 285. New York, Raven Press, 1975
5. **Miller ME:** Phagocytosis in the newborn infant: Humoral and cellular factors. J Pediatr 74:255, 1969
6. **Froman ML, Stiehm ER:** Impaired opsonic activity but normal phagocytosis in low birth-weight infants. N Engl J Med 281:926, 1969
7. **Bellanti JA, Cantz BE, Yang MC et al:** Biochemical changes in human polymorphonuclear leukocytes during maturation. In Bellanti JA, Dayton DH (eds): The Phagocytic Cell in Host Resistance. New York, Raven Press, 1975
8. **Bellanti JA, Cantz BE, Schlegel RJ:** Accelerated decay of G-6-PD activity in CGD. Pediatr Res 4:405, 1970
9. **Wright WC, Jr, Ank BJ, Herbert J et al:** Decreased bactericidal activity of leukocytes of stressed newborn infants. Pediatrics 56:578, 1975
10. **Blaese RM;** Macrophages and the development of immunocompetence. In Bellanti JA, Dayton DH (eds): The Phagocytic Cell in Host Resistance, p 309. New York, Raven Press, 1975
11. **Klein RB, Fisher TJ, Gard SE et al:** Decreased mononuclear and polymorphonuclear chemotaxis in human newborns, infants, and young children. Pediatrics 60:467, 1977
12. **Weston WL, Carson BS, Barkin RM et al:** Monocyte–Macrophage function in the newborn. Am J Dis Child 131:1291, 1977
13. **Gitlin D, Biasucci A:** Development of gamma G, gamma M, beta 1_c, beta 1_a, C'l esterase inhibitor, ceruloplasmin, transferrin, hemopexin, haptoglobin, fibrinogen, plasminogen, alpha–1 antitrypsin, orosomucoid, beta–lipoprotein, α 2 macroglobulin and pre–albumin in the human conceptus. J Clin Invest 48:1433, 1969
14. **Propp RP, Alper CA:** C'3 synthesis in the human fetus and lack of transplacental passage. Science 162:672, 1968
15. **Silverstein A, Uhr J, Kramer K et al:** Fetal response to antigenic stimulus: II. Antibody production by the fetal lamb. J Exp Med 117:799, 1963
16. **August CS, Berkel AJ, Driscoll et al:** Onset of lymphocyte function in the human fetus. Pediatr Res 5:539, 1971
17. **Stites DP, Carr MC, Fudenberg HH:** Development of cellular immunity in the human fetus: Dichotomy of proliferative and cytotoxic responses of lymphoid cells to phytohemagglutinin. Proc Natl Acad Sci USA 69:1440, 1972
18. **Goldstein AL, Guha A, Zatz MM, Hondy MA, White A:** Purification and biological activity of thymosin, a hormone of thymus gland. Proc Natl Acad Sci USA 69:1800, 1972
19. **Cooper MD, Lawton AR:** The mammalian "Bursa Equivalent": does lymphoil differential along plasma cell lines begin in the gut-associated lymphoepithelial tissues (GALT) of mammals? In Hanne MG (ed): Contemporary

Topics in Immunobiology, p 49. New York, Plenum Press, 1972

20. **Cooper MD, Lawton AR, Kincade PW:** A two stage model for development of antibody producing cells. Clin Exp Immunol II: 143, 1972

21. **Smith EV, Goldman AS:** The cell of human colostrum: I. In vitro studies of morphology and functions. Pediatr Res 2:103, 1968

22. **Hanson LA, Ahlstedt S, Carlsson B, Fallstrom SP:** Secretory IgA antibodies against cow's milk proteins in human milk and their possible effect in mixed feeding. Int Arch Allergy Appl Immunol 54:457, 1977

23. **Bellanti JA, Artenstein MS, Olson LC, Buescher EL, Kuhrs CE, Milstead KL:** Congenital rubella: Clinicopathologic, virologic, and immunologic studies. Am J Dis Child 110:464, 1965

24. **Alford CA, Jr:** Studies on antibody in congenital rubella infections. Am J Dis Child 110:455, 1965

25. **South MA, Montgomery JR, Rowls WE:** Immune deficiency in congenital rubella and other viral infections. Birth Defects 9:234, 1975

26. **Michaels RH:** Suspension of antibody response in congenital rubella. J Pediatr 80:583, 1972

27. **Fuccillo DA, Steele RW, Henson SA, Vincent MM, Hardy JB, Bellanti JA:** Impaired cellular immunity to rubella virus in congenital rubella. Infec Immun 9:81, 1974

28. **Stern LM, Forbes IJ:** Dysgammaglobulinemia and temporary immune paresis in case of congenital rubella. Aust Paediatr J 77:38, 1975

29. **Montgomery JR, Flauders RW, Yow MD:** Congenital anomalies and herpes-virus infection. Am J Dis Child 126:364, 1973

30. **Rola–Pleszczynski M, Frenkel LD, Fuccillo DA,** Hensen SA, Vincent MM, Reynolds DW, Stagno S, Bellanti JA: Specific impairment of cell-mediated immunity in mothers and infants with congenital infection due to cytomegalovirus. J Infect Dis 135:386, 1977

31. **Cohen F, Zuelzer WW:** Mechanism of isoimmunization. II. Transplacental passage and postnatal survival of fetal erythrocytes in heterospecific pregnancy. Blood 30:796, 1967

32. **Taylor AI, Polani PE:** XX/XY mosaicism in man. Lancet 1:1226, 1965

33. **Naiman TL, Punnet HH, Lischner HW et al:** Possible graft-versus-host-reaction after intrauterine transfusion for Rh erythroblastosis fetalis. N Engl J Med 281:697, 1969

34. **Chandra RH:** Fetal malnutrition and postnatal immunocompetence. Am J Dis Child 129:450, 1975

35. **Stites DP, Wybran J, Carr MC et al:** Development of cellular immunocompetence in man. In Porter R, Knight J (eds): Ontogeny of Acquired Immunity: Ciba Foundation Symposium, p 113. North Holland Elsevier, Excerpts Medic, 1972

36. **Bonforte RJ, Topilsky M, Siltzbach LE et al:** Phytohemagglutinin skin test: A possible in vivo measure of cell-mediated immunity. J Pediatr 81:775, 1972

37. **Poplack DG, Bonnard GD, Holiman BJ et al:** Monocyte-mediated antibody-dependent cellular cytotoxicity: A clinical test of monocyte function. Blood 48:809, 1976

38. **Shore A, Dosch H, Huber J et al:** *In vitro* and *in vivo* definition of a new variant of severe combined immunodeficiency disease (SCID). Pediat Res 11:494, 1977

32

Bacterial and Viral Infections of the Newborn

George H. McCracken, Jr.

Infections of the newborn and young infant are a significant cause of mortality and long-term morbidity. The etiologic agents of neonatal infections have changed during the past four decades in part because of increased usage of antimicrobial agents, the availability of new techniques to diagnose viral and protozoan infections, and the advent of complex resuscitation and respiratory equipment which act as fomites of nosocomial infection. The prognosis of these diseases can be improved if recognized early and if appropriate therapy is promptly instituted. However, successful therapy must also depend upon the physician's familiarity with the historic experience of the nursery and his knowledge of the pharmacokinetic properties of antimicrobial agents in newborn infants.

The purpose of this chapter is to present pertinent epidemiologic and pathogenetic concepts of specific infections, clinical manifestations, and diagnostic workups of patients with these diseases, and a rational approach to therapy and control of neonatal infections.

PHARMACOLOGIC BASIS OF ANTIMICROBIAL THERAPY

Selection of antimicrobial therapy for neonatal infections must be based upon; (1) pharmacokinetic properties of antibiotics in new-born infants, (2) antimicrobial susceptibilities of commonly encountered pathogens, and (3) the natural history of the infectious disease being treated. In the past, antibiotics were selected on the basis of anecdotal experience and data extrapolated from studies of normal adults. Failure to apply data from neonatal pharmacologic studies to clinical therapy has resulted in "therapeutic orphans" and disasters such as the gray syndrome of chloramphenicol, kernicterus from sulfonamides, and osseous and dental complications of the tetracyclines.

The newborn infant is unique from a physiologic and pharmacologic standpoint.[1] An expanded extracellular fluid volume, immaturity of enzyme systems, changing renal function, and alterations of body fluid composition may profoundly affect absorption, conjugation, inactivation, and excretion of antibiotics in newborn infants. Failure to recognize the unique pharmacologic status of the newborn may affect efficacy and safety of antimicrobial therapy. Dosage and frequency of administration of antibiotics must be determined for infants of different gestational and postnatal ages. When antibiotics are properly selected on the basis of neonatal pharmacologic data, morbidity and mortality resulting from infectious diseases and from potential drug toxicity are greatly reduced.

Table 32-1. Source of Common Neonatal Infections.

Maternal*	Environment	Both
Groups B and D streptococcus (early-onset form)	Group B streptococcus (late onset form)	Gram-negative pathogens
E. coli	E. coli	Coxsackie virus
L. monocytogenes (early-onset form)	L. monocytogenes (late onset form)	Echovirus
Gonococcus†	Enteropathogenic E. coli	Adenovirus
Haemophilus influenzae	S. aureus	
Pneumococcus	Group A streptococcus	
Meningococcus	Respiratory syncytial virus	
Syphilis		
Campylobacter (Vibrio) fetus		
Toxoplasmosis		
Rubella		
Cytomegalovirus		
Herpes simplex		
Hepatitis B		

* Acquired either tranplacentally or at the time of delivery.
† There has been one documented gonococcal nursery epidemic in which transmission was by means of infected fomites.

As a rule, a single antibiotic should be used to treat specific infections such as penicillin G for group B beta-hemolytic streptococcal disease, ampicillin for *Listeria* and enterococcal infection, and methicillin for penicillinase-producing staphylococci. On the other hand, combining two drugs is good medical practice when initiating therapy for systemic bacterial disease prior to laboratory confirmation. Thus, ampicillin and an aminoglycoside are combined to treat suspected septicemia or meningitis before identification of the pathogen. Once the susceptibilities have been determined, a single appropriate antibiotic is usually satisfactory for treating most infections.

Although antibiotics are commonly used in an attempt to prevent infection, they are effective prophylactically only when directed against a single pathogen. For example, penicillin G is effective in preventing group A beta-hemolytic streptococcal infection in patients with previous rheumatic fever; sulfonamides are useful in prophylaxis against infection caused by susceptible meningococci; and topical tetracycline prevents ophthalmia neonatorum. Additionally, a single dose of penicillin G given intramuscularly at birth reduces the incidence of early-onset group B streptococcal disease. This has been confirmed by a prospective, controlled study conducted in our institution during the past two and a half years.

On the other hand, when antibiotics are used as "broad-spectrum coverage" against many potential pathogens, they are rarely effective. This umbrella method of chemoprophylaxis encourages the emergence of resistant strains among previously susceptible bacteria, causes alteration of the normal flora of the gastrointestinal and respiratory tracts with overgrowth of potentially virulent organisms, and may lead to the development of drug hypersensitivity. Furthermore, broad-coverage prophylaxis may partially suppress a bacterium, thereby masking the development of clinical disease. This in turn may lead to neglect of important surgical measures or to serious delay in administering more effective therapy.

NOSOCOMIAL BACTERIAL INFECTIONS

The two principal sources of newborn infection are the mother and the nursery environment. Infection is acquired from the mother transplacentally, at the time of delivery, or in the postnatal period. The infant may acquire infection postnatally from environmental sources such as nursery personnel, respiratory equipment, sinks, and incubators. The sources of commonly encountered neonatal bacterial and viral infections are presented in Table 32-1. (Congenital infections are discussed in Chapter 33.)

When an infectious disease caused by the same organism appears in several infants from the same nursery over a short period of time, nosocomial infection should be suspected. The sick infants should be isolated and cultured in order to identify the pathogen. If a single, specific pathogen is responsible for the outbreak, epidemiologic investigations to determine the source of infection must be initiated. Specific typing of organisms such as phage typing of staphylococci or pyocin typing of *Pseudomonas* can usually be performed by county or state laboratories. The physician must determine the extent and possible sources of infection in the nursery unit and what measures should be taken to prevent further colonization and disease.

Staphylococcal Infection. Phage group I *Staphylococcus aureus* (phage types 29, 52, 52A, 79, 80, and 81) caused significant hospital disease in the late 1950s and early 1960s. Disease ranging from pustules and cellulitis to pneumonia, septicemia, and meningitis occurred in neonates during this period. Although the majority of infants are colonized with the epidemic strain during staphylococcal outbreaks, disease occurs in only a small percentage of these infants. Over the past several years, disease caused by phage group I staphylococci has diminished. This decrease may be partially explained by a change in the virulent characteristics of the organism and in techniques used in nurseries to prevent infection.

Disease caused by phage group II *Staphylococcus aureus* (phage types 3A, 3B, 3C, 55, and 71) in newborn and young infants has been encountered recently. Clinical manifestations caused by this organism have been broadly classified into the expanded scalded skin syndrome.[2] Nursery epidemics of bullous impetigo or toxic epidermal necrolysis or both caused by group II staphylococci have been reported.[3] The source of one outbreak was traced to a carrier of the organism among the nursery staff, while an infant reservoir of infection and a change in bathing technique may have contributed to other outbreaks.

During 1979, several nurseries in North America experienced outbreaks of disease caused by multiply resistant *S. aureus* strains. These organisms were resistant to the antistaphylococcal penicillins, cephalosporins, lincomycins, and aminoglycosides and are sus-

ceptible only to vancomycin and rifampin. In such circumstances, vancomycin is the preferred therapy (see below).

When staphylococcal disease occurs in a nursery, the extent of infection must first be determined. All infants and personnel associated with the index patient and a random smapling of the other infants are cultured. The nasopharynx and umbilicus of the infant and the anterior nares, and possibly the hands of all personnel should be cultured. All staphylococcal isolates are tested for coagulase production and phage type. A change in the percent of infants colonized with *S. aureus* and an increase in the carriage of the specific virulent strain are observed during nursery staphylococcal epidemics. As a general rule, fomites play a relatively minor role in nosocomial staphylococcal outbreaks. Carriage of organisms on hands of personnel has been implicated in several nursery epidemics.

It is often necessary for the physician to take certain precautionary measures before the complete cultures and phage typing are available. Selection of the one or several measures necessary to control a nursery epidemic must be individualized. The measures commonly employed are

1. Isolation of all symptomatic and asymptomatic infants colonized with the virulent staphylococcus. Formation of a cohort system in the nursery for exposed, but not as yet colonized, infants and for all new admissions to the nursery. These separate cohorts are maintained until discharge from the nursery; infected infants are removed from the cohort and placed in isolation.
2. Use of antimicrobial agents. Topical antimicrobial therapy may be used for asymptomatic infection; parenteral antistaphylococcal therapy should be used for serious systemic disease.
3. Initiation of routine bathing with antistaphylococcal cleansing agents such as 3% hexachlorophene or application of triple dye to the umbilicus of all new admissions to the nursery, as well as for colonized infants.
4. Artificial colonization of infants with a less virulent staphylococcus such as the 502A strain of *S. aureus* (bacterial interference).
5. Closing of the nursery.

Enteropathogenic **E. coli.** Because diarrhea caused by enteropathogenic strains of *E. coli* occurs rarely during the first week of life, nosocomial disease is usually confined to premature nurseries. The mother is frequently the source of infection for the index case; subsequent cases are usually transmitted from infant to infant by nursery personnel. The epidemiology, symptoms, treatment, and control measures for enteropathogenic *E. coli* diarrhea are considered below.

Group A Streptococcal Infection. The group A beta-hemolytic streptococcus was a common cause of puerperal and neonatal sepsis in the 1930s and early 1940s. With the advent of penicillin and its frequent use in maternity and nursery units, neonatal infections caused by this organism have become relatively uncommon.[4] The primary source of the group A streptococcus in nursery outbreaks is either an attendant (nurse or physician) working in the unit or the mother. Once group A streptococci are introduced into a nursery, many infants become colonized but few develop clinical disease. The most common clinical manifestation is a low-grade granulating omphalitis which fails to heal despite local measures. However, more significant disease may occur including extensive cellulitis, pneumonia, septicemia, and meningitis.

One neonate with group A streptococcal colonization is enough to warrant investigation of the nursery as a potential source of disease. All infants in close contact with the index case, a random sampling of other infants, and nursery personnel should be cultured. Nasopharyngeal and umbilical cultures from infants, and nasopharyngeal, skin, and rectal cultures from personnel should be obtained. Because nursery and maternity personnel are frequently interchangeable, the epidemiologic workup should be coordinated with the obstetric service of the hospital.

Infants with streptococcal disease should be treated with aqueous penicillin G. During nosocomial outbreaks, all asymptomatic infants colonized with group A streptococci should also receive penicillin. The prophylactic use of penicillin for new admissions to the nursery may also be indicated. Benzathine penicillin G has been used effectively as prophylaxis against group A streptococcal infection in one nursery outbreak.

Gram-negative Infections. Routine nasopharyngeal and rectal cultures from normal newborn infants usually reveal one or several coliform organisms. These bacteria and others represent the normal flora of the neonate's gastrointestinal tract. It is likely that the gastrointestinal tract is a source of systemic neonatal infections caused by coliform and other gram-negative bacteria.

Over the past decade, a number of nursery outbreaks caused by specific gram-negative bacteria have been described. Among the organisms incriminated were *Klebsiella pneumoniae, Flavobacterium meningosepticum, Pseudomonas aeruginose, Proteus mirabilis,* and *E. coli.* A common feature of these outbreaks was that the majority of colonized infants were asymptomatic; those who developed disease usually had pneumonia, septicemia, or meningitis. During the past decade, *Pseudomonas aeruginosa* and *Klebsiella–Enterobacter* strains have been the most common gram-negative pathogen causing nosocomial infections.

Infected fomites represent the single most common source of nursery outbreaks caused by gram-negative bacteria. Contaminated faucet aerators, sink traps, and drains, suction equipment, bottles containing distilled water, cleansing solutions, humidification apparatus, and incubators have been incriminated. In addition, colonized infants may act as a source of infection, and the organism is transmitted from infant to infant by way of hands or gowns of personnel. During epidemics, asymptomatic colonization of infants with the specific pathogen is quite variable and ranges from 0 to 90%.

The general approach to nursery outbreaks caused by gram-negative organisms is similar to that caused by *S. aureus.* Identification of an infant in a nursery or intensive care unit with a potentially virulent pathogen such as *P. aeruginosa* should serve as a warning. This infant should be segregated, preferably outside of the nursery, from the other infants and managed appropriately. All infants in the same unit should be cultured. If additional infants are discovered to be asymptomatic carriers of the organism, they should be segregated from other infants in the nursery and an epidemiologic investigation initiated. Resuscitation and inhalation equipment, cleansing solutions, washing facilities, and other objects in the patient's environment are cultured in order to identify the source of nosocomial infection. It may become necessary to close the nursery to new admissions until the source of infection is identified and appropriate measures have been taken to prevent new cases.

NOSOCOMIAL VIRAL INFECTIONS

A number of viral agents have been incriminated in nursery outbreaks of infection.[5,6] The original source of infection in these outbreaks is frequently the mother who transmits the viral agent either transplacentally or by direct contact postnatally. A second common source of nosocomial viral disease is nursery personnel, particularly nurses and aides who have intimate contact with infants, and resident physicians who are assigned to nurseries for extended periods of time. Although the mechanisms accounting for spread of virus from infant to infant are not well defined, it appears likely that respiratory viruses are spread by the airborne route. In contrast, viruses causing diarrhea may be transferred from infant to infant by way of the hand-oral route with the intermediary being nursery personnel. Viruses excreted in the urine in high concentrations may be aerosolized when diapers or sheets are changed. As a general rule, infected infants placed in closed incubators can transmit virus to other infants in open bassinets within the same unit, because filtered air is brought into the closed isolettes under slight positive pressure, thus causing leakage of potentially contaminated air back into the environment. Resuscitation and respiratory equipment, cleansing solutions and other objects in the infant's environment have not been shown to play a significant role in transmission of viral agents during nosocomial outbreaks.

During a nursery outbreak of viral infection, most infected infants are asymptomatic and serve as reservoirs for perpetuation of infection. Even more important, infants with minimal symptoms and signs of disease such as sneezing, stuffy nose, or several loose stools may contribute significantly to transmission of virus by way of the airborne or fecal-oral routes.

Coxsackie Viruses. There have been a number of well-documented nursery outbreaks of the encephalomyocarditis syndrome associated with Coxsackie B viruses.[7] Five of the six Coxsackie viruses of the B group (B1 through B5) have been etiologically associated with this illness, and virus has been isolated from multiple organs including the myocardium, brain, blood, kidney, and liver. The severe involvement found in many infants explains the relatively high mortality rate of this condition. The clinical picture is one of abrupt onset of fever, listlessness, and feeding difficulty. Respiratory distress and cyanosis are noted frequently and cardiac signs such as tachycardia, cardiomegaly, murmurs and gallop rhythm are present in the majority of patients. Hepatosplenomegaly is common and signs and symptoms referrable to central nervous system involvement are present in one-third of the patients. The newborn can apparently acquire his Coxsackie infection either *in utero* or after birth. The postnatally-acquired disease has been traced to direct contact with either the mother or an attendant suffering from an illness which was clinically compatible with or proven to be caused by the Coxsackie agent.

Echoviruses. Occasionally, a number of echo types have been found to cause illness in premature and newborn infants. However, considering the frequency with which infection occurs in the older infant and child, the newborn would generally appear to be extraordinarily resistant.

The clinical manifestations of echovirus infection are varied and range from mild diarrhea to overwhelming hepatic necrosis. Separate nursery outbreaks caused by the same echovirus type may produce different clinical diseases. For example, echovirus type 19 produced respiratory illness in a premature nursery outbreak associated with x-ray findings of cystic emphysema.[8] In a separate outbreak of echovirus type 19, the initial clinical picture was strikingly similar to that of sepsis neonatorum and was characterized by overwhelming infection and hepatic necrosis.[9] This disparity in the clinical diseases that characterize separate nosocomial outbreaks has been observed also for echovirus type 11.

Adenovirus Infection. Infections with this group of agents appear to occur relatively rarely, except during sharply defined epidemics. Nursery outbreaks have been caused by adenovirus types 1, 2 and 3.[10] Illness caused by these viruses varied from "stuffy nose syndrome," caused by the Type 1 virus, to mild diarrhea, caused by adenovirus type 3.

In one nursery outbreak, maternal antibodies acquired transplacentally did not completely protect against clinical disease.

Respiratory Syncytial Virus Infection. This virus has caused nursery outbreaks of bronchiolitis and pneumonia.[11] The patients initially demonstrated coryza and cough lasting several days, followed by the acute onset of dyspnea associated with roentgenographic evidence of pneumonia in the majority of infants. Bronchiolitis was diagnosed clinically in those not demonstrating x-ray findings. In a community outbreak in Rochester, N.Y., 35% of infants in a nursery acquired respiratory syncytial virus infection.[12] Illness was often atypical, especially in infants under 3 weeks of age in whom lower respiratory tract involvement was less common. Four infants died; two unexpectedly after acute illness had subsided. Infection was also acquired in 34% of the nursery staff who appeared to be important in the spread of virus within the nursery. Several epidemics of respiratory illness due to **influenza viruses** have been described in newborn infants. It appears that the influenza virus may be acquired either congenitally or during the postnatal period.

When viruses are suspected as the cause of a nursery outbreak of illness, the affected infants should be isolated. Infants in close association with the index cases should be carefully observed and kept as a cohort separate from other infants in the nursery. All new admissions to the nursery should be isolated from infected infants and their cohorts. If virus isolation cannot be obtained within the institution, specimens should be sent to the county or state laboratory for identification. It may become necessary to close the nursery to admissions if new cases of disease continue to occur despite isolation and cohort measures.

SEPSIS NEONATORUM

Sepsis neonatorum is a disease of infants who are less than 1 month of age, are clinically ill, and who have positive blood cultures. The presence of clinical manifestations distinguish this condition from the transient bacteremia observed in some healthy neonates.

The incidence of sepsis neonatorum is approximately 1 case per 1000 live full-term births and 1 per 250 live premature births.[13] These incidence rates vary from nursery to nursery and depend upon conditions predisposing to infection.

Pathogenesis. Maternal, environmental, and host factors determine which infant exposed to a potentially pathogenic organism will develop sepsis, meningitis, or both. There are many prepartum and intrapartum obstetric complications that have been associated with increased risk of infection in the newborn. The most significant of these are premature onset of labor, prolonged rupture of fetal membranes, chorioamnionitis, and maternal fever. Although maternal bacteremia prior to delivery has been documented for many microorganisms, infants born to these individuals usually remain well. This is most likely explained by a balance between the presence of maternal antibody and the virulence of the microorganism.

With improved supportive care of the sick neonate has come increased opportunity for microorganisms of relatively low virulence to cause systemic disease. The use of arterial and venous umbilical and peripheral catheters, hyperalimentation catheters, and endotracheal tubes provides an access to the debilitated infant for organisms present in the respiratory or gastrointestinal tract, on the skin, or in respiratory support equipment.[13]

Animal models have been utilized in an effort to define the host-bacteria interactions that determine pathogenesis of disease. Blood stream infection in infant rats or mice caused by *E. coli* K1 or any of the Group B streptococcus serotypes can be prevented by pretreatment with type-specific capsular polysaccharide antibody. The orogastric route for *E. coli* K1 in the infant rat and the inhalation of amniotic fluid infected with Group B streptococci in the rhesus monkey produce illnesses that closely parallel the human syndromes.

Investigations of the host-parasite relationship in humans with the Group B streptococcus have focused on measurement of specific antibody in the serum of infected and colonized individuals. Protective levels of BIII antibody were found in 68% of women whose newborn infants were well, but in only 13% of women whose neonates developed sepsis or meningitis caused by this organism. Opsonic activity against the infecting Group B strains has also been shown to be absent from the sera of a small number of patients with systemic disease. On the other hand, opsonic activity was present in 50% of 27 asymptomatically colonized mothers and infants. Further evidence that colonization is associated with antibody formation is the demonstration of protective antibody in the serum of men colonized with the BIII organism and the lack of antibody in those not colonized.

Clinical Manifestations. Most infants with septicemia present with nonspecific signs and symptoms that are usually first noted by the nurse or mother rather than by the physician. The most common of these vague signs are temperature instability, lethargy, and poor feeding. The presence of temperature elevation above 100°F is significant in the neonate; it is unusual to note fever above 102°F. The signs and symptoms in some infants may suggest respiratory or gastrointestinal disease (*e.g.*, tachypnea and cyanosis, or vomiting, diarrhea, and abdominal distention). Septicemia must always be included in the differential diagnosis when evaluating an infant with these findings.[13]

Although it is tempting to recommend a workup for septicemia in all infants with nonspecific clinical manifestations, this is both impractical and unnecessary in many cases. A complete history and physical examination coupled with clinical experience are the best guides in determining the extent of workup. If doubt exists, a blood culture should be obtained. The presence of hepatosplenomegaly, jaundice, and petechiae are classic signs of neonatal infection, but represent late manifestations.

Etiology. Over the past decades, the major organisms responsible for sepsis neonatorum have changed. Group A beta-hemolytic streptococci were most common in the 1930s and early 1940s and were replaced by coliform organisms in the late 1940s and 1950s. In the late 1950s and early 1960s coagulase-positive *S. aureus* caused significant neonatal disease. Group B beta-hemolytic streptococci and coliforms, particularly *E. coli,* have been the most common causative organisms during the past decade. More recently, group D streptococci, *H. influenzae* and *Klebsiella–Enterobacter* species have been incriminated.[13] Familiarity with the historic experience of a nursery or intensive care unit is invaluable in guiding selection of antimicrobial therapy for suspected bacterial disease.

Streptococcal Disease. The group B beta-hemolytic streptococcus is presently the most common gram-positive bacterium isolated from blood of infants with septicemia. The epidemiology, pathogenesis and clinical features of group B streptococcal disease have been recently defined.[14] The organism is a common inhabitant of the female genital tract and can be isolated from cervical cultures of 5% to 30% of asymptomatic pregnant women. The identical serotype can be isolated frequently from uretheral cultures of the sexual partners of these culture-positive women. Although the great majority of infected pregnant females have normal, healthy infants, 1% to 2% result in either stillbirths or infants with neonatal disease. Vertical transmission of group B organisms occurs in approximately 50%–70% of mother-infant pairs, resulting in neonatal colonization rate of from 8% to 25%.

The early onset Group B streptococcal syndrome occurs within the first 72 hours of life and 65% of reported cases are premature infants. Onset is sudden and follows a fulminant course with the primary focus of inflammation in the lungs, although meningitis may rarely be present. Apnea, hypotension, and disseminated intravascular coagulation cause rapid deterioration and often lead to the patient's demise within 24 hours. It is difficult to identify the infant with respiratory distress caused by Group B streptococcal infection because, in 60% of infected patients, the chest roentgenogram shows a reticulogranular pattern with air bronchograms indistinguishable from that seen with uncomplicated hyaline membrane disease, (see Chapter 20). The mortality rate is said to be from 40% to 80%, but is considerably lower (15%–30%) in institutions with advanced intensive care facilities. A similar syndrome has been reported to be associated with the Group D streptococci.

A late onset syndrome caused by Group B streptococci or *Listeria monocytogenes* occurs most frequently at 2 to 4 weeks of age, but may be seen as late as 16 weeks. The onset is insidious; poor feeding and fever are the most frequent presenting symptoms. Rarely, infants with late onset meningitis caused by Group B streptococcus present with hydrocephalus. These infants may appear to have uncomplicated hydrocephalus with a normal lumbar CSF. Examination of ventricular fluid reveals pleocytosis and the organism is recovered on culture. Spinal fluid cultures of infants with meningitis caused by gram-positive organisms are usually sterile within 24 to 36 hours of therapy and the mortality rate is 10% to 15%.

Miscellaneous Syndromes. Approximately 20% of neonatal infections caused by Group B streptococci do not fit into the early or late onset syndromes and extend over a broad clinical spectrum involving many different organ systems. The following manifestations have been observed: cellulitis, scalp abscess, impetigo, breast abscess, conjunctivitis, orbital cellulitis, ethmoiditis, otitis media, pneumonia complicated by empyema, endocarditis, hepatitis, septic arthritis, osteomyelitis, and asymptomatic transient bacteremia.[15] The latter is remarkable because these infants appear clinically well and are cultured because of a history of maternal obstetric complications. A repeat blood culture done prior to the institution of antibiotics is frequently sterile.

Staphylococcal Disease. The phage group I *S. aureus,* which was common in the late 1950s is still present in some nurseries and occasionally causes serious systemic neonatal disease. The pathogenicity of this organism is based on its ability to invade the skin and musculoskeletal system producing furuncules, breast abscesses, and osteomyelitis. Septicemia is usually secondary to local invasion. When *S. aureus* is recovered from blood cultures of neonates, a careful search should be made for a primary focus.

In the early 1970s, phage group II coagulase-positive staphylococci emerged as a common cause of neonatal infection. Although this organism may be invasive, pathogenicity depends principally upon production of an exotoxin. Common areas of primary infection include the umbilical stump, conjuctiva, and throat. Clinical disease may take one of several forms including bullous impetigo, toxic epidermal necrolysis, Ritter's disease, and non-streptococcal scarlatina. Collectively, these diseases have been referred to as the expanded scalded skin syndrome.[1]

The initial finding in Ritter's disease is generalized erythema associated with edema and tenderness on palpation. After several days, a distinctive desquamation of large sheets of epidermis occurs, which is different from the fine desquamation observed in the second and third weeks of streptococcal scarlet fever. Large flaccid bullae are commonly observed in Ritter's disease which, upon rupture, leave a tender, weeping erythematous base. Some

infants may appear quite toxic with the generalized form of disease.

Listeria Monocytogenes. The pathogenesis and clinical diseases caused by *L. monocytogenes* are similar to those caused by group B streptococci. A fulminant, disseminated disease may occur during the first several days of life (granulomatosis infantiseptica). The pathogen is acquired transplancentally or by aspiration at the time of vaginal delivery, and multiple organ systems are involved. The infant frequently presents with hypothermia, lethargy, and poor feeding. A characteristic rash consisting of small, salmon-colored papules scattered primarily on the trunk may be observed in some infants. The chest roentgenogram shows parenchymal infiltrates suggestive of aspiration pneumonitis in most infants. A miliary-type of bronchopneumonia can also be seen in some cases. There are no reports of acute onset listeriosis mimicking the roentgenographic picture of hyaline membrane disease. Listeria serotypes Ia, Ib, and IVb produce the early onset disease, while serotype IVb is the predominant type in late onset meningitic disease.

A delayed form of neonatal listriosis occurs during the second through fifth weeks of life and primarily involves the meninges. The infected infant usually is the full-term product of an uncomplicated labor and delivery. Onset of symptoms and signs is relatively insidious and indistinguishable from those observed with meningitis caused by other pathogens. The bacteriology laboratory should be forewarned of the clinical suspicion of listerial meningitis because these microorganisms are frequently discarded as contaminants because of their tinctorial and morphologic similarities with diphtheroids. Overnight refrigeration of spinal fluid specimens will frequently enhance growth of this organism.

The peripheral white blood cells count usually shows a brisk leukocytosis with a predominance of polymorphonuclear leukocytes in the differential count.[16] A significant elevation in the number of monocytes to 7% to 21% of the total white cell count has been documented on admission laboratory evaluation of infected infants. Likewise, a monocytosis of this magnitude can be demonstrated in most remaining infants upon repetitive testing of the peripheral white blood cell count. By contrast, monocytes are not typically found in the spinal fluid of infants infected with *L. monocytogenes*. Polymorphonuclear leukocytes predominant in about 75% of cases with a relative lymphocytosis noted in the remaining 25%. As with other pyogenic meningitides, hypoglycorrhacia, and elevated protein concentrations are frequent findings. Examination of the stained smear of spinal fluid has not been rewarding in over 50% of cases. This is a reflection of the relatively low concentrations of organisms in the fluid.

Enterococcal Infection. Enterococci are commonly isolated from blood cultures of newborn infants. Some of these cultures represent contamination from the perineum resulting from poor aseptic technique of drawing blood from the femoral area. The importance of identifying the enterococcus as the etiologic agent in septicemia primarily relates to selection of proper antimicrobial therapy. The frequently used combination of a penicillin and an aminoglycoside antibiotic may not sterilize the blood promptly in this desease. Recent reports have stressed the importance of the group D streptococci in early-onset septicemia. The group D organisms incriminated have been *Streptococcus bovis* and the enterococci (*Streptococcus fecalis*). The nonenterococcal forms are susceptible to penicillin G; while enterococci are normally resistant to penicillin G and the aminoglycosides, but susceptible to ampicillin.

Gram-negative Organisms. *E. coli* are the most common gram-negative bacteria causing septicemia during the neonatal period. *Klebsiella–Enterobacter* strains are second. Annual incidence rates for the past 9 years in Dallas have remained reasonably constant at 0.5 to 1.0 cases per 1000 live births. In contradistinction to illness caused by group B streptococci and *L. monocytogenes*, *E. coli* infections do not fit into distinct clinical syndromes of early- and late-onset disease. Approximately 40% of *E. coli* strains causing septicemia possess Kl capsular antigen and strains identical to those isolated from blood cultures can usually be identified in the patient's nasopharynx or rectal cultures. The clinical features of *E. coli* sepsis are generally similar to those observed in infants with disease caused by other pathogens. Localized *E. coli* infections have included breast abscess, cellulitis, pneumonia, lung abscess, empyema, osteomyelitis, septic arthritis, urinary tract infection, ascending colangitis, and otitis media.

Pseudomonas septicemia may present with a characteristic violaceous papular lesion or lesions which, after several days, develop central necrosis. Although this is most commonly seen in pseudomonas infection, it may also be associated with other organisms. The neonate who receives broad spectrum antibiotics while in an environment potentially contaminated by "water bugs" (respirators, moist oxygen, and so on) is particularly prone to pseudomonas infection.

Laboratory Tests and Findings. During the past decade, a number of screening tests have been described which are purported to aid the physician in making the diagnosis of neonatal infection. Although a few of these tests are helpful in identifying the infant at high risk of developing infection, the diagnosis of septicemia can be made only by recovery of the organism from blood cultures. Therefore, it is imperative that these cultures be obtained by strict aseptic technique. Blood should be obtained from a peripheral vein rather than from the umbilical vessels, the outer several millimeters of which are frequently contaminated with bacteria. Femoral vein aspiration may result in cultures contaminated with coliform organisms from the perineum. The skin above the vein to be punctuated should be cleansed with an antiseptic solution, such as that containing iodine, and allowed to dry for maximal antiseptic effect. The amount of blood drawn is critical and should represent 5% to 10% of the total blood culture volume. Pediatric blood culture sets containing 10 ml of trypticase broth are available commercially; 0.5 to 1 ml of blood is required for optimal results.

It is frequently helpful to obtain cultures of other sites prior to initiating antimicrobial therapy. For example, percutaneous bladder aspiration of urine for culture may be helpful in identifying the urinary tract as the focus of infection. This is particularly true for illness occurring in the second through fourth weeks of life. Nasopharyngeal, skin, and rectal cultures are frequently positive in the early septicemic form of listeriosis and group B streptococcal disease. However, these colonization sites are not predictive of the etiology of bloodstream infection and should not be used to guide antimicrobial therapy. All infants with suspected septicemia should have a cerebrospinal fluid examination and culture prior to therapy.

The peripheral white blood cell count is the most useful of the indirect indicators of bacterial infection. After correction for the nucleated red blood cell count, the total absolute neutrophil count and the ratio of immature to total neutrophilic forms are compared to normal standard values for age. In the absence of maternal hypertension, severe asphyxia, periventricular hemorrhage, maternal fever and hemolytic disease, absolute total neutropenia, and an elevated ratio of immature to total neutrophilic forms, are strongly suggestive of bacterial infection. Gastric aspirate stains and culture, erythrocyte sedimentation rate, C-reactive protein, and the nitroblue tetrazolium test have not proven to be useful singly as indicators of bacterial infection, although, in combination, these tests may offer some guidance. Detection of the soluble antigens of *E. coli* Kl, Group B streptococci, *H. influenzae* type b, *Neisseria meningitidis,* and *Streptococcus pneumoniae* by counterimmunoelectrophoresis (CIE) is useful on identifying the infant infected with these pathogens. However, the absence of antigen does not rule out infection.

Therapy. Once septicemia is suspected, suitable cultures should be obtained and therapy started immediately, using ampicillin and either kanamycin or gentamicin. Ampicillin is administered intravenously or intramuscularly in a dosage of 50 mg/kg/day divided in two doses for infants under 1 week, and 100 to 150 mg/kg/day divided in three doses for infants 1 to 4 weeks age. The selection of the aminoglycoside antibiotic should be based on antimicrobial susceptibilities of enteric organisms isolated from infants in each nursery. Kanamycin is the drug of choice for treatment of infections caused by susceptible gram-negative organisms and is administered intramuscularly in a dosage of 15 to 30 mg/kg/day divided in two or three doses depending on birthweight and chronologic age. However, kanamycin-resistant *E. coli* have been encountered in some nurseries in North America. In these nurseries, or when an isolate from an infant is shown to be resistant to kanamycin, gentamicin sulfate should be used in the place of kanamycin. The dosage of gentamicin is 5.0 mg/kg/day divided into two doses for infants under 1 week and 7.5 mg/kg/day divided into three doses for infants 1 to 4 weeks of age. Recent studies from our nurseries have demonstrated no significant ototoxicity in infants and children who were treated in the neonatal period with kanamycin or gentamicin. However, in premature infants and in those receiving these drugs for prolonged periods, auditory studies (invoked brainstem potential technique) should be performed whenever possible. Furthermore, serum concentrations of the aminoglycosides should be monitored in the low-birth-weight premature infants because of erratic absorption and elimination of these drugs in such infants.

When the type of skin lesions or historic experience suggests the possibility of pseudomonas infection, carbenicillin or ticarcillin with or without gentamicin is the drug of choice (see Table 32-2 for dosage recommendation). If gentamicin is to be administered with carbenicillin, the drugs should not be mixed in the same solution and administered intravenously. Polymyxin B sulfate or colistimethate have been recommended for neonatal pseudomonas infections. Although there are no corroborative data, it is our impression that these two agents are not as effective as carbenicillin therapy with or without the addition of gentamicin.

When staphylococcal sepsis is suspected but not proven, parenteral methicillin or naficillin should be substituted for penicillin or ampicillin because approximately 50% of staphylococci encountered in neonates are penicillin-resistant. Although kanamycin and gentamicin possess activity against most staphylococci, these agents cannot be recommended because there are no studies of their efficacy in neonatal staphylococcal disease. During 1978 and 1979, several nurseries in North America experienced outbreaks of disease caused by multiply resistant *S. aureus* strains. In these infants, vancomycin is preferred therapy (see Table 32-2 for dosage recommendations).

Once the pathogen is identified and its antimicrobial susceptibilites are known, the most appropriate drug or drugs should be selected. As a general rule, kanamycin alone or in combination with ampicillin should be used for susceptible *E. coli* and Klebsiella-Enterobacter species, gentamicin alone or in combination with ampicillin for kanamycin-resistant coliform bacteria, carbenicillin or ticarcillin with or without gentamicin for pseudomonas, ampicillin for *P. mirabilis,* enterococcus, and *L. monocytogenes,* and penicillin for other

Table 32-2. Dosage Schedule for Commonly Prescribed Antibiotics in Newborn Infants.

Antibiotic	Usual Individual Dose	Daily Dosage and Intervals (Number of Divided Doses/24 hr)	
		0–7 Days of Age	*>7 Days of age*
Amikacin	7.5 mg/kg	15 mg/kg (2)	15 (?22.5) mg/kg (2 or ?3)†
Ampicillin			
Septicemia	25 mg/kg	50 mg/kg (2)	75–100 mg/kg/day (3 or 4)
Meningitis	100 mg/kg	200 mg/kg/day (2)	300 mg/kg/day (3)
Carbenicillin	100 mg/kg	200 mg/kg (2)	300–400 mg/kg (3 or 4)
Chloramphenicol	25 mg/kg	25 mg/kg (1)	50 mg/kg (2)
Gentamicin	2.5 mg/kg	5 mg/kg (2)	7.5 mg/kg (3)
Kanamycin	7.5–10 mg/kg	15–20 mg/kg (2)*	20–30 mg/kg (2 or 3)*
Methicillin			
Septicemia	25 mg/kg	50–75 mg/kg (2 or 3)	75–100 mg/kg (3 or 4)
Meningitis	50 mg/kg	100–150 mg/kg (2 or 3)	150–200 mg/kg (3 or 4)
Penicillin G			
Septicemia	25,000 U/kg	50,000 U/kg (2)	75,000 U/kg (3)
Meningitis	50,000 U/kg	100,000–150,000 U/kg (2 or 3)	150,000–250,000 U/kg (3 or 4)
Ticarcillin	75 mg/kg	150–225 mg/kg (2 or 3)*	225–300 mg/kg/day (3 or 4)*
Tobramycin	2 mg/kg	4 mg/kg (2)	4 (?6) mg/kg (2 or ?3)†
Vancomycin	15 mg/kg	30 mg/kg (2)	45 mg/kg (3)

* Smaller dose for infants <2000 g, larger dose for infants >2000 g.
† Additional studies required before larger dose can be recommended

gram-positive organisms, except penicillin-resistant staphylococci, for which methicillin or nafcillin is the drug of choice.

Guidelines for determining duration of therapy in the neonatal period are often lacking because objective evidence of illness may be minimal. Culture of the blood should be repeated 24 to 48 hours after initiation of therapy; if positive, alteration of therapy may be necessary. In the absence of deep tissue involvement or abscess formation, treatment is usually continued 5 to 7 days after clinical improvement. When multiple organs are involved or clinical response is slow, treatment may need to be continued for 2 to 3 weeks.

MENINGITIS

Neonatal Meningitis

Neonatal meningitis is relatively uncommon; the incidence is generally reported to be 0.4 cases per 1000 live births but rates as high as 1 per 1000 live births have been reported in a few nurseries.[13] The disease is seen more commonly in premature infants, males, and infants born to mothers with complicated pregnancies and/or deliveries.

Etiology. The bacteria causing neonatal meningitis are similar to those of sepsis neonatorum. Group B beta-hemolytic streptococci and *E. coli* presently account for approximately 65% of all cases. The next most common etiologic agent is *L. monocytogenes*.

Pathology. The pathologic findings are similar regardless of bacterial etiology. The most consistent finding at necropsy of meningitis cases is a purulent exudate coating the meninges and ependymal surfaces of the ventricles.[18] The inflammatory response of neonates is similar to that observed in adults with meningitis, with the exception that babies have a sparsity of plasma cells and lymphocytes during the subacute stage of meningeal reactions. Perivascular inflammation is also noted. Hydrocephalus and a noninfectious encephalopathy can be demonstrated in approximately 50% of infants dying with meningitis. Subdural effusions occur rarely in neonates. By contrast, effusions are observed in approximately 10% to 20% of infants with meningitis who are 3 to 12 months of age. Varying degrees of phlebitis and arteritis of intracranial vessels can be found in all infants. Thrombophlebitis with occlusions of veins may occur in the subependymal zone. Ventriculitis can be demonstrated in virtually all infants dying of meningitis and in approximately 75% of infants at the time of diagnosis.

Clinical Manifestations. The signs and symptoms of central nervous system infection are frequently indistinguishable from those associated with neonatal septicemia. Lethargy, feeding problems, and altered temperature are the most frequent presenting complaints, and respiratory distress, vomiting, diarrhea, and abdominal distention are common findings. Seizures are observed frequently and may be caused by direct central nervous system inflammation or may be associated with hypoglycemia or hypocalcemia. Signs suggesting meningeal involvement are uncommon; bulging fontanelle is noted in 17%, opisthotonus in 33%, stiff neck in 23% and convulsions in 12%.

Pathogenesis. The propensity of certain bacterial strains to cause meningitis in neonates is poorly understood. Although there are more than 100 K types of *E. coli*, only one, *E. coli* K1, accounts for greater than 70% of meningitis cases.[19] Likewise, among the different serotypes of group B streptococci, the B_{III} organisms account for greater than 80% of cases of neonatal group B streptococcal meningitis.[14] Although it is likely that protection from invasive disease by these two pathogens is mediated by type-specific antibody acquired transplacentally from the mother, absence of this antibody alone can not explain the unique proclivity of these organisms to cause meningitis. Both organisms possess capsular polysaccharides comprised of sialic acid: the K1 envelope is a homopolymer of sialic acid while the B_{III} capsule contains approximately 30% sialic acid. Whether this constituent is important for specific meningeal binding, or whether these capsules provide a unique virulence for the neonate remains to be clarified.

The Neonatal Meningitis Cooperative Study group has recently reported that there is no beneficial effect of lumbar intrathecal or of intraventricular instillation of gentamicin in the therapy of meningitis caused by gram negative organisms.[22] Indeed, the mortality rate in infants given intraventricular gentamicin was threefold greater than that in infants treated with systemic therapy only. The explanation for this finding is unknown, but may relate to the procedure for instilling the drug into the ventricles or to toxic concentrations in the CSF space, or to both possibilities.

Chloramphenicol has been advocated for therapy of neonates with meningitis caused by coliform bacilli. Its superior diffusibility is attractive for this purpose. However, this agent is bacteriostatic against gram-negative enteric bacilli compared to the aminoglycosides which are bactericidal. Emergence of resistance may occur during chloramphenicol therapy, and there is evidence from animal studies that chloramphenicol and gentamicin, when administered concomitantly, are antagonistic in eradicating coliforms from cerebrospinal fluid. Every infant treated with chloramphenicol, particularly those in whom phenobarbital is also given, must have serum concentrations monitored constantly in order to be certain that the dosage is safe and therapeutic. For all these reasons, chloramphenicol should not be considered a first-line drug for management of neonatal infections.

Guidelines for determining the duration of therapy during the neonatal period are often lacking because objective evidence of illness may be minimal. In the absence of deep tissue involvement or abscess formation, therapy for sepsis neonatorum is usually continued for 5 to 7 days after clinical improvement. Therapy for meningitis is continued for a minimum of 2 weeks after sterilization of cerebrospinal fluid cultures. From a practical standpoint, this equates to 14 days of therapy for meningitis caused by gram-positive organisms and a minimum of 21 days of therapy for meningitis caused by gram-negative pathogens.

Attention to general supportive therapy is of upmost importance in caring for infants with meningitis and is the single most important factor that accounts for the improved outcome during recent years. Disturbances of fluid and electrolyte balance are common, particularly in the first several days of illness when inappropriate antidiuretic hormone secretion may lead to fluid retention and hyponatremia. In addition, hypoglycemia, hypocalcemia and hyperbilirubinemia are frequent complications. Ventilatory assistance is frequently necessary and blood pressure should be carefully monitored. During the course of illness, hemoglobin and hematocrit values should be checked frequently because infection may exaggerate and prolong the anemias of infancy, particularly in premature infants. Because of the occurrence of bleeding diathesis, platelet counts as well as prothrombin time (PT) and partial prothrombin time (PTT) should be followed. Exchange transfusion with fresh whole blood has been recommended as a means of providing factors to bolster host resistance such as complement and opsonins. This may be especially beneficial if the blood used has a high titer of antibody directed against the infecting organism.

Laboratory Findings. Interpretation of cerebrospinal fluid values in newborn infants may be difficult. Any one or a combination of the following cerebrospinal fluid values should alert the pediatrician to the possibility of meningeal infection: (1) greater than 32 WBC/mm^3 of which more than 60% are polymorphonuclear cells, (2) CSF glucose less than 50% to 75% of a simultaneous serum glucose, (3) protein greater than 150 mg/dl, or (4) presence of microorganisms on gram-stained smears of CSF.[20]

It is important to carefully examine a stained smear of the cerebrospinal fluid of every infant with suspected meningitis. In babies with meningitis caused by group B streptococci or coliform bacteria, each oil-immersion field usually contains several to many bacteria. This is because there are from 10^4 to 10^8 bacteria per milliliter of spinal fluid (average 10^7/ml) present at the time of diagnosis. By contrast, listeria are often difficult to identify on stained smears because the bacterial counts are frequently on the orders of 10^3/ml.

Blood and urine cultures should be obtained from every infant suspected of meningitis.

Treatment. Considerable data have been gathered recently on the pharmacokinetic properties of antibiotics in neonates with meningitis.[1,21,22] After an intramuscular dose of 2.5 mg/kg of gentamicin, peak levels in lumbar cerebrospinal fluid and ventricular fluid are approximately 1 to 2 μg/ml. If lumbar intrathecal gentamicin is added to this regimen, values of 20 to 40 μg/ml or greater, several hours after instillation, may be observed in the lumbar area. Intraventricular administration of 2.5 mg results in ventricular fluid levels of 20 to 80 μg/ml, and in lumbar spinal fluid values of 10 to 50 μg/ml 1 to 4 hours later. With kanamycin, peak CSF values of 6 to 10 μg/ml are observed 4 to 6 hours after an intramuscular dose of 7.5 mg/kg. On the other hand, peak values of 10 to 30 μg/ml are demonstrated in cerebrospinal fluid approximately 2 to 4 hours after a 50 to 70 mg/kg/dose of ampicillin. It is apparent that the minimal inhibitory concentration (MIC) values for the common pathogens are frequently greater than the antibiotic levels achieved in cerebrospinal fluid. For example, an *E. coli* with a gentamicin MIC value of 2.5 or 5 μg/ml is considered susceptible when treating bloodstream infection, but may be resistant when treating meningitis. This is because peak cerebrospinal and ventricular fluid gentamicin levels following parenteral therapy may be considerably lower than this MIC value. Therefore, alternative therapeutic regimens must be considered, such as adding a second antibiotic, selecting a different antibiotic class, changing the route of administration.

At the present time, ampicillin and gentamicin are recommended for initial therapy of neonatal meningitis. The dosage of ampicillin is 100 mg/kg per day in two divided doses during the first week of life and 200 mg/kg per day in three divided doses thereafter. The dosage for gentamicin is the same as for septicemia. All infants should have a repeat spinal fluid examination and culture at 48 to 72 hours after initiation of therapy. If organisms are seen on methylene blue or gram stain of the fluid, the patient should be completely reevaluated with regard to alterations in antimicrobial therapy and to obtaining computerized tomography or a technetium brain scan. The radiologic procedures may demonstrate the presence of a subdural empyema, brain abscess, or ventriculitis that requires neurosurgical intervention.

A new beta lactam antibiotic has shown excellent results in therapy of experimental coliform meningitis in rabbits and, in our preliminary experience, in newborn infants. This drug, moxalactam, combined with ampicillin, will be compared to ampicillin and amikacin in the Third Neonatal Meningitis Cooperative Study.

Prognosis. The mortality in neonatal meningitis is considerable. The overall mortality rate is approximately 20% to 40%, but this varies with etiologic agent, infant population, and the nursery or intensive care unit. In our institution, 15% to 20% of infants with coliform and group B streptococcal meningitis die. Increased attention to supportive care and a more rational approach to antimicrobial therapy have accounted for an improved prognosis in neonatal meningitis.

Short- and long-term sequelae of neonatal meningitis are frequent. The acute complications include communicating or noncommunicating hydrocephalus, subdural effusions, ventriculitis, and blindness. Gross retardation may be obvious immediately. However, many infants will appear relatively normal at time of discharge. It is only after prolonged and careful follow-up that perceptual difficulties, reading problems, or minimal brain damage are apparent. It is estimated that 30% to 50% of survivors will have some evidence of neurologic damage.

Aseptic Meningitis

Aseptic meningitis is an acute nonbacterial inflammatory disease of the meninges which is caused principally by viral agents. The illness occurs frequently in older infants and children and is uncommon in newborn infants. Disease in young infants is either sporadic or occurs in sharply defined epidemics. It is important to differentiate aseptic from bacterial meningitis of infancy because therapy and prognosis are different in the two conditions.

It is frequently difficult to clinically separate aseptic meningitis from encephalitis in young infants. The etiology of viral central nervous system disease depends in part on seasonal variation, age, and immune status of the host. In older infants and children, the enteroviruses (Coxsackie B and echoviruses) account for the majority of cases of aseptic meningitis during the summer months, while mumps, lymphocytic choriomeningitis and other viruses are more common during the other seasons. During epidemics of encephalitis such as those caused by St. Louis encephalitis virus, a mild aseptic meningitis may be seen in young infants and occasionally in neonates. The mild nature of the disease in early life may be caused in part by passively transferred antibodies from immune mothers and the relatively isolated status of young infants with regard to community outbreaks. On the other hand, certain viruses appear to cause significant disease primarily in the very young, such as encephalomyocarditis caused by Coxsackie B viruses. In this disease, multiple organs including brain, myocardium, blood, kidney, and liver are involved. In one nursery outbreak, Cosackie B5 caused aseptic meningitis only.[23] Echovirus type II has been etiologically associated with a nursery epidemic of aseptic meningitis[24] and sporadic cases have been caused by echoviruses 9 and 14.

Encephalitis with or without involvement of the meninges may occur in young infants and is caused by the above-mentioned viral agents as well as by other arboviruses, principally Eastern equine encephalomyelitis and Western equine encephalomyelitis. St. Louis encephalomyelitis is rare in newborn infants. Congenital cytomegalovirus, *herpes simplex*, type 2 rubella, and varicella infections produce encephalitis in a varying percentage of infants.

Symptoms. Poor temperature control, lethargy, diminished appetite, and "failure to thrive" are the most common symptoms. In some infants, a shock-like syndrome occurs associated with seizures. It may be difficult to differentiate this clinical illness from that of bacterial meningitis. In a small percent of patients, an erythematous maculopapular eruption with or without petechiae may suggest a viral etiology.

Diagnosis. Aseptic meningitis should be suspected if several infants in a nursery develop illness over a short period of time or if illness is detected in an infant during a community outbreak of aseptic meningitis. Although the outbreak is caused by a single etiologic agent, the clinical manifestations may differ among infected infants. While one infant manifests respiratory symptoms primarily, others may have gastrointestinal illness, and all may have findings indicating involvement of the meninges. Aseptic meningitis is diagnosed in these infants by failure to demonstrate bacteria on stained smears and cultures of cerebrospinal fluid. Although the cerebrospinal fluid white blood cell count is usually lower than observed in bacterial meningitis, high counts with predominance of polymorphonuclear cells may be observed early in illness. The cerebrospinal fluid protein and sugar content are usually within normal limits. A definitive diagnosis is made by isolation of a viral agent from cultures of cerebrospinal fluid or from the throat or rectum, accompanied by a significant rise in serum antibody titer to the specific agent.

At the present time, there is no specific antiviral therapy for postnatally acquired viral aseptic meningitis (see Chap. 33). Intensive supportive care is frequently necessary with particular attention to maintenance of pH and electrolyte balance, respiratory assistance, and adequate nutrition. When one or more infants develop illness in a newborn nursery, every effort should be made to define the etiology and source of infection. The affected infants should be isolated and treated as cohorts until discharge.

OSTEOMYELITIS AND SEPTIC ARTHRITIS

Because of the unique nature of the vascular supply of the neonatal skeletal system, osteomyelitis and septic arthritis frequently occur concomitantly and therefore will be considered together in this section. During the first 12 months of life, capillaries perforate the epiphyseal plate of long bones and provide a communication between the metaphysis and joint space.[25] Therefore, infections originating in one anatomic location easily spread to the other. This is not true after approximately 1 year of age when the perforating capillaries disappear.

The capsules of the hip and shoulder attach below the metaphysis of the femur and humerus respectively. Infection of the epiphyseal cartilage may rupture through the periosteum and enter the joint space, producing purulent arthritis. Because the capsular articulation of the hip and shoulder are permanent, osteomyelitis and septic arthritis may coexist, making the origin of infection difficult to determine.

Infections of the musculoskeletal system are uncommon in the neonate; incidence figures are not available.

Etiology and Pathogenesis. The infecting organisms in osteomyelitis and septic arthritis are varied, but the predominant ones are *S. aureus* and gram-negative enteric organisms such as klebsiella, proteus, and *E. coli*. Group B streptococci also cause suppurative disease of bone and joints. Whereas gonococcal arthritis and tenosynovitis were commonly encountered in previous decades, they are seen only occasionally today. Other etiologic agents associated with newborn infection are salmonella, pseudomonas, and *Candida albicans.*

Osteomyelitis and arthritis have been reported consequent to several invasive procedures in newborns. These include heel puncture, femoral venipuncture, exchange transfusions, fetal monitoring electrodes, and umbilical artery catheterization.[26-29] Osteomyelitis of cranial bones has complicated infected cephalhematomas. In most cases the origin is unknown and presumed to be hematogenous.

Clinical Presentation. Nonspecific symptoms of infection such as lethargy, irritability, and poor feeding may be the initial manifestations of neonatal musculoskeletal infection. Diminished movement of the affected limb unrelated temporally to birth trauma is probably the most common clinical sign. Heat, erythema and swelling are late manifestations. Occasionally, the diagnosis is made unsuspectingly when purulent material is obtained on attempted aspiration of the femoral vein. In this instance, the needle enters the swollen hip capsule.

Although blood cultures are frequently positive, the infants are usually not clinically toxic. The exception is group A beta-hemolytic streptococcal infection in which the infant may appear gravely ill.

Laboratory Tests and Findings. Blood cultures should be obtained from all infants with suspected infection of the musculoskeletal system. A diagnostic aspiration of the joint or subperiosteal space should be attempted in all patients, and the material obtained should be gram-stained and cultured. The identification of the organism is particularly important because it may be necessary initially to treat with more than one potentially nephrotoxic drug until the causative bacterium has been isolated.

The peripheral white blood cell count is frequently elevated and juvenile forms may be present. There is little information regarding the erythrocyte sedimentation rate during the neonatal period. In older infants and children, the sedimentation rate is accelerated in osteomyelitis; its return toward normal is a rough indicator of therapeutic success.

Roentgenograms of the affected bone or joint taken early in illness may be normal or show widening of the the articular space. Later in the course of disease, subluxation and destruction of the joint is common. If osteomyelitis is present, the normal fat markings on x-ray of the deep tissues may be obliterated, indicating inflammation. Lifting of the periosteum from the bone may also be observed, but cortical destruction is unusual before the second week of illness. Resolution of bone changes is considerably slower than clinical improvement. Although radioisotope scans (technetium or gallium) of bone are useful in early diagnosis of osteomyelitis in infants and children, their value in the newborn has not been established.

Therapy. Selection of initial antimicrobial therapy should be based upon results of gram and methylene blue stains of aspirated purulent material and associated clinical findings, such as furuncles or cellulitis. If gram-positive cocci are observed on stained smears, methicillin or nafcillin should be started. Either kanamycin or gentamicin are indicated if gram-negative organisms are observed. If no organisms are identified on stained smears, a combination of an antistaphylococcal drug and an aminoglucoside are used. Once the organism has been identified and susceptibility studies are available, the most appropriate antibiotic or combination of antibiotics should be used. Direct instillation of an antimicrobial agent into the joint space is unnecessary because most antibiotics will penetrate the inflamed synovium and adequate concentrations are achieved in purulent material.[30] This also applies to treatment of osteomyelitis; direct instillation of antibiotics into infected bone is unwarranted.

As a general rule, infection of the joint space and bone should be drained either by repeated aspiration or by surgery. Suppurative arthritis of the hip and shoulder is best treated with incision and drainage in order to prevent vascular compromise or extension of infection into the metaphysis. Orthopedic consultation must be obtained for all patients.

Antimicrobial therapy of neonatal musculoskeletal infections caused by the staphylococcus or coliform organisms should be continued for approximately 3 weeks and, in some patients, for a longer period of time. The duration of therapy must be individualized. In general, systemic symptoms usually disappear within several days of initiating therapy and drainage, while local signs such as heat, erythema, and swelling may persist for 4 to 7 days. Full range of motion of the involved limb may not return for several months. Because of this, physical therapy should be instituted early in order to prevent contractures. Complete resolution of roentgenographic changes may take several months.

Prognosis. Mortality from these diseases is unusual. However, morbidity may be considerable, particularly when weight-bearing joints such as the hip are involved. Contractions and muscle damage may be permanent.

CUTANEOUS INFECTIONS

Most infections of the skin and subcutaneous tissues in neonates are caused by *S. aureus.* There are three major presentations of superficial staphylococcal disease. The *first* and most common are **pustules** and **furuncles,** which may be either solitary or appear in clusters during the neonatal period. Pustules are frequently in the periumbilical and diaper areas and may coalesce gradually and spread to other areas of the body. Blood-stream or organ invasion is unusual unless the cutaneous infection involves extensive areas. Omphalitis is usually caused by staphylococci or streptococci and infected circumcisions are usually caused by *S. aureus.* These relatively limited cutaneous infections may be caused by any of the many different phage-types of staphylococci although phage group I strains predominated in past years.

The occurrence of staphylococcal skin infections in several infants from the same nursery should alert the physician to the possibility of nosocomial infection caused by a single, virulent strain of *S. aureus.* Cultures of lesions for identification, susceptibility studies, and phage typing are mandatory. If these infections are caused by the same strain of staphylococcus, prompt measures should be instituted to determine the source of infection and to prevent further colonization and disease.

Therapy of cutaneous staphylococcal disease depends upon the extent of the lesions and the general clinical condition of the infant. Small, isolated pustules can be managed by local care using a mild cleansing agent or an antiseptic agent, such as hexachlorophene or povidone-iodine. Infants with more extensive cutaneous involvement, systemic signs and symptoms of infection, or both, should be treated with parenteral antimicrobial agents. The selection of the proper penicillin is based upon historic experience and antimicrobial susceptibility studies of staphylococci isolated from the nursery unit. It should be pointed out that multiply resistant strains of *S. aureus* have been responsible for five or six nursery outbreaks during 1978 and 1979. This number may conceivably increase during the next 5 years.

The second form of neonatal staphylococcal disease has been described as the **expanded scalded skin syndrome.**[2] This group of illnesses includes bullous impetigo, toxic epidermal necrolysis, Ritter's disease, and nonstreptococcal scarlatina, usually caused by phage group II staphylococci. The pathogenesis of these entities appears to be related to release of an exotoxin which acts primarily on the stratum granulosa of the epidermis causing a generalized erythema, edema, and tenderness, frequently progressing to desquamation and formation of flaccid bullae. The usual sites of staphylococcal infection are conjunctivae, throat, or umbilicus. Cultures of blood, nasopharynx, eyes, and other areas should be obtained prior to therapy. Because phage group II staphylococci are frequently resistant to penicillin, methicillin is the initial drug of choice. Vancomycin should be used for multiply resistant strains.

The third form of staphylococcal disease is **necrotizing fasciitis,** which may be associated with streptococci in the older infant and child.[31] Necrotizing fasciitis, an unusual disease of newborns, when observed, is frequently associated with surgical procedures, birth trauma, or cutaneous infection. Staphylococci either alone or associated with streptococci are frequently causative. In this condition, subcutaneous tissue including muscle layers are invaded and the organism spreads along the fascial planes. Overlying skin may appear violaceous and the borders of the lesion are usually indistinct. Extensive surgery involving resection of the destroyed tissue is imperative in treating necrotizing fasciitis. Blood and tissue cultures should be obtained and the patient started on methicillin. The necrotic fatty tissue may combine with calcium, resulting in tetany and convulsions.

URINARY TRACT INFECTION

Improved methods for obtaining sterile specimens have made it possible to define more accurately the incidence of neonatal urinary tract infection. Bacteriuria may be demonstrated in 0.5% to 1.0% of full-term infants and up to 3% of premature infants utilizing bladder aspiration technique.[32] Urinary tract infections are more common in babies born to bacteriuric mothers and in neonatal males, in contrast to the predominance of females beyond this period of life.

Etiology. E. coli is the most common etiologic agent of urinary tract infection. Approximately 70% of E. coli strains belong to one of eight common 0 antigen groups similar to those found in older patients. Several polysaccharide capsular antigens (K1, K2, K12, and K13) are found more often in infants with upper tract disease. This particularly pertains to the K1 antigen.[33] *Klebsiella* and *Pseudomonas* species are encountered less frequently.

Gram-positive bacteria, with the exeption of enterococci, are rare causes of urinary tract infections.

Clinical Manifestations. Many infants with significant bacteriuria are asymptomatic. When symptoms are present they are usually nonspecific and consist of poor weight gain, altered temperature, cyanosis or gray skin color, abdominal distention, and poor feeding. In a small number of patients, jaundice and hepatomegaly may be the presenting features of urinary tract infection. Thrombocytopenic purpura is found in some of these infants. Localizing signs suggesting urinary tract involvement are unusual; when present, they usually consist of a weak urinary stream and/or an abdominal tumor from bladder distention or hydronephrosis.

Diagnosis. The diagnosis of urinary tract infection is confirmed by examination and culture of urine. The result of these tests depends largely on the method of urine collection. Most pediatricians obtain urine with a sterile, plastic receptacle applied to the cleansed perineum. However, urine obtained by this method may have an elevated cell count because of recent circumcision, vaginal reflux of urine or contamination from the perineum. Neonatal asphyxia may also increase the urinary cell count. Further, white blood cells must be differentiated from round epithelial cells which appear in the urine in appreciable numbers during the early days of life. Although pyuria commonly accompanies significant bacteriuria, there are both false-positive and false-negative results. Direct microscopic examination of uncentrifuged, fresh urine is useful. If bacteria are readily seen in each oil-immersion field, there are generally greater than 10^5 bacteria per milliliter. Glitter cells are felt by many to be diagnostic of urinary tract infections.

Quantitative urine cultures from infants with documented disease contain greater than 50,000 colonies per milliliter (usually 100,000 colonies per milliliter or greater), but occasionally one finds a small number of organisms. Any number of bacteria in a urine specimen obtained by needle puncture of the bladder should be considered significant. This latter procedure is the single best source of urine for culture and is safe in most newborn infants.

Treatment. There are a number of approaches to the treatment of neonatal urinary tract infections. Antimicrobial agents should initially be administered parenterally because septicemia is found in approximately 20% of infants and absorption after oral administration may be erratic in neonates. In addition, the physician must assume that there is infection of renal parenchyma resulting from hematogenous spread.

Antibiotic selection should be based upon results of antimicrobial susceptibility studies. In general, kanamycin or gentamicin are effective against the commonly encountered coliform bacteria. Because urinary concentrations of these drugs are considerably higher than those seen in serum, the usual dosages may be halved: for kanamycin, 5 to 7 mg/kg/day; and for gentamicin, 2 to 3 mg/kg/day are satisfactory. Ampicillin and kanamycin or gentamicin should be administered to symptomatic infants with pyuria prior to results of culture and susceptibility tests.

A repeat urine culture should be sterile 36 to 48 hours after initiation of appropriate therapy. Infants with persistent bacteriuria must be evaluated for possible abscess formation with or without urinary obstruction. In the uncomplicated patient, therapy is usually continued for a period of approximately 10 days. Blood urea nitrogen and serum creatinine levels should be determined at the initiation and completion of therapy. If there is evidence of renal failure, dosage and frequency of administration of the drugs, particularly the aminoglycosides, may need to be reduced. Approximately 1 week after discontinuing therapy, a repeat urine culture is obtained. If the culture is positive, therapy is reinstituted and a thorough investigation of the urinary tract made in order to rule out obstruction or abscess formation.

All infants with documented urinary tract infections should have radiologic evaluation of the urinary tract. An intravenous pyelogram is obtained at the outset of therapy to rule out the possibility of gross congenital abnormalities of the urinary system. If obstruction is demonstrated, urologic procedures to ensure proper drainage are mandatory if therapy is to be successful. A voiding cystourethrogram is usually obtained several weeks after therapy has been completed. (See Chap. 35.)

Prognosis. It is the physician's responsibility to be certain that neonates with documented urinary tract infections do not have congenital abnormalities of the urinary system. In such patients, recurrent urinary tract infections are common and physical growth may be retarded until definitive surgery has been performed. Every patient must have careful long-term follow-up studies in order to detect recurrent infections, many of which will be asymptomatic.

NEONATAL SYPHILIS
(see Chap. 33)

NEONATAL OPHTHALMIA

Infections of the eye of the newborn may be caused by a variety of microorganisms including *Neisseria gonorrheae, Chlamydia trachomatis, S. aureus,* and *Pseudomonas aeruginosa.* From a review of over 300 cases of eye infections in newborns at Grady Memorial Hospital in Atlanta, it was determined that 29% were caused by chlamydia, 14% by gonococci, 10% by staphylococci, 2% by chemical reactions, and 1% by mixed gonococcal and chlamydial infections.[34] The remaining 44% were of uncertain causation. This frequency distribution of etiologic agents is typical of the experience at large urban general hospitals.

The incidence of ophthalmia neonatorum has not paralleled the almost astronomic increase in gonococcal disease rates among adolescents and young adults. This is almost certainly a result of universal neonatal gonococcal prophylaxis using 1% silver nitrate solution, antibiotic ointment, or systemic penicillin G. We rarely see today the invasive, destructive ophthalmitis described so vividly in the old literature. A number of agents have been shown to be effective prophylactically against gonococci: 1% silver nitrate and erythromycin or tetracycline ophthalmic ointments. Penicillin applied topically or administered intramuscularly is also effective although the ointment is no longer available commercially.

Clinical Manifestations. Gonococcal ophthalmia usually becomes apparent within the first 5 days of life and is characterized initially by a clear watery discharge. Conjunctival hyperemia and chemosis are associated with a copious discharge of thick, white, purulent material. Both eyes are usually involved, but not necessarily to the same degree. Untreated gonococcal ophthalmia may extend to involve the cornea (**keratitis**) and the anterior chamber of the eye. Corneal perforation and blindness may eventuate. Before the introduction of adequate prophylactic measures, ophthalmia neonatorum was the most frequent cause of acquired blindness in the United States.

Differential Diagnosis. Any infants presenting with a conjunctival discharge should be evaluated carefully to determine the etiology. Three tests should be performed: (1) gram and methylene blue stain of the exudate, (2) culture of the exudate, and (3) Giemsa stain of scrapings made from the lower palpebral conjunctiva after exudate has been wiped away. Appropriate therapy should be instituted on the basis of the results of the stained smears.

Conjunctivitis occurring in the first days of life can be either chemical or bacterial in nature. Chemical irritants such as silver nitrate cause transient conjunctival hyperemia and a watery discharge which rarely turns purulent.

If gram-negative rods are seen in the stained exudate, the greatest concern is *P. aeruginosa* because of the virulent, necrotizing endophthalmitis that can result. In this condition, a relatively mild conjunctivitis can progress to infection of the entire globe within 12 to 24 hours. Prompt diagnosis and immediate institution of appropriate antimicrobial therapy is mandatory.

Conjunctivitis during the second or third week of life may be caused by viral, bacterial or chlamydial agents. Viral conjunctivitis is frequently associated with other symptoms of respiratory tract disease, such as rhinorrhea, cough and rash, and several persons in the family or nursery may have simultaneous disease. In general, the discharge in viral conjunctivitis is watery or mucopurulent, but rarely purulent. Preauricular adenopathy is common. Staphylococci, streptococci, and occasionally, gonococci cause conjunctivitis in this age group. A smear of purulent material is helpful in differentiating these bacterial agents. However, the presence of bacteria on a gram-stained smear of exudate is not necessarily related etiologically to the conjunctivitis. Normal inhabitants of the skin and mucous membranes such as staphylococci, diphtheroids, and neisseria may be observed.

Chlamydial eye infection may begin in the first days of life, but usually does not come to the attention of the physician until the second or third week.[35] Clinical manifestations of chlamydial infection vary from mild conjunctivitis to intense inflammation and swelling of the lids associated with copious purulent discharge. Pseudomembrane formation and a diffuse "matte" injection of the tarsal conjunctiva are common. The cornea is rarely affected and preauricular adenopathy is unusual. In the early stages of disease, one eye may appear more swollen and infected than the other, but both eyes are almost invariably involved. Diagnosis is made by scraping the tarsal conjunctiva and looking for typical cytoplasmic inclusions within epithelial cells.

Therapy. Initial therapy is based on the results of stained smears of exudate and epithelial cells. If gonococci are seen, parenteral penicillin is employed. If staphylococci are seen, methicillin or another penicillinase-resistant penicillin analog is used. Topical antibiotics are unnecessary because ample antibiotic to inhibit bacteria is present in eye secretions.

During the past year, gonococci resistant to penicillin have started to appear in the United States. These strains are susceptible to spectinomycin, erythromycin, and most cephalosporin derivatives. There is no experience in treating gonococcal ophthalmia with these drugs nor are there pharmacologic data for spectinomycin in the newborn. Consequently, it is recommended that a cephalosporin administered parenterally be used for disease caused by these pencillinase-producing gonococci.

Pseudomonas eye infection should always be treated with parenteral therapy consisting of carbenicillin and gentamicin. Additionally, gentamicin ophthalmic drops are used for simple pseudomonas conjunctivitis, and subconjunctival or subtenon injections of gentamicin are given daily when endophthalmitis is present.

Optimal treatment of chlamydial infection has not been determined. Preliminary data suggest that erythromycin or sulfisoxazole given orally eradicates the organism more rapidly and more completely than does topical antibiotic therapy.

Patients with gonococcal ophthalmia should be segregated and strict handwashing techniques should be employed because of the highly contagious nature of the exudate. The eyes should be irrigated with saline to remove the purulent material.

DIARRHEAL DISEASE

Although diarrheal disease during the neonatal period is usually brief and self-limited, it may cause significant morbidity in some infants and represents a potential danger to other infants in the nursery unit.

Etiology and Pathogenesis. The most common cause of diarrhea in young infants is alteration of diet and feeding practices, rather than specific bacterial or viral pathogens. Of the infectious causes of diarrhea, reo-like viruses (rotavirus) have been shown recently to be the most important etiologic agents in infantile diarrheal disease.[36,37] Their significance in the neonatal period has not been determined except in several isolated outbreaks. Enteropathogenic *E. coli* serotypes are probably the most common bacterial agents responsible for diarrhea in young infants. Failure to demonstrate enteropathogenic serotypes of *E. coli* in rectal cultures does not rule out coliform disease. Enterotoxigenic strains of *E. coli* with non-enteropathogenic serotypes have been identified in nursery outbreaks of diarrheal disease.[38] These organisms inhabit the small bowel where they attach to, but do not invade, the intestinal mucosa. The enterotoxin produced by these organisms stimulates cyclic AMP, which in turn inhibits Na and Cl transport across the intestinal wall. As a result, these salts are lost into the lumen of the upper bowel followed passively by water, causing a net loss of stools high in electrolyte content. *Vibrio cholera,* some *E. coli* serotypes (almost exclusively nonenteropathogenic strains), and *Vibrio parahemolyticus* are examples of bacteria that cause diarrhea by this mechanism.

A second mechanism for bacterial diarrhea involves invasion of the intestinal mucosa. Shigella dysentery is the classic example of this disease. Colonic invasion with subsequent destruction of the mucosa causes an outpouring of polymorphonuclear cells and mucous. The resultant diarrhea is usually bloody and contains mucous and pus. Salmonella species also invade the intestinal mucosa, but extensive destruction does not occur. The epithelial lining is left intact and the organisms reach the lamina propia, where an inflammatory response is elicited.

Epidemiologic Control. Although serotyping of *E. coli* to identify the traditional enteropathogenic strains has been questioned recently, we currently take the position that the epidemiologic evidence is strong enough to support a pathogenic role for these strains even though the mechanism of pathogenicity is unknown. When an index case of enteropathogenic *E. coli* diarrhea is recognized in a nursery, secondary cases are likely to ensue. Any nursery infants with diarrhea should be suspected of having a potentially communicable disease. All infants in proximity of the index case should have rectal swabs tested by culture, and preferably by fluorescent antibody technique, which is more sensitive for identifying asymptomatic carriers of enteropathogenic *E. coli.* Ill and healthy colonized infants should be segregated and treated with orally administered neomycin (100 mg/kg/day in four divided doses) or with colistin sulfate (15 mg/kg/day in three divided doses) for 5 days. Neomycin causes rapid disappearance of the organism and abbreviates the period of diarrhea, but approximately 20% of infants revert to the asymptomatic carrier state after treatment. Repeated surveillance of infants is necessary until it has been shown that the pathogenic strain has been eliminated from the nursery.

Clinical Manifestations. Although the etiology of diarrhea in infants and children may be differentiated on clinical grounds, this is usually not possible in newborn infants. As a general rule, diarrhea caused by enteropathogenic strains of *E. coli* is insidious in onset, is associated with seven to ten green, watery stools daily and is usually without blood or mucous. The infants do not appear acutely ill. Complications are rare and are related primarily to dehydration and electrolyte disturbances. Shigella infection is uncommon and usually episodic in neonates, and does not spread within nurseries. Shigellosis in the newborn may present as a diarrheic or dysenteric syndrome or may be evidenced only by a septic or toxic infant. Suppurative complications are rare, but dehydration and electrolyte disturbances are common and need immediate and constant attention.

Reo-like virus infection has been described in newborn infants as a sporadic disease or as part of a nursery outbreak. Infection may be asymptomatic or associated with vomiting and diarrhea. The infants are usually afebrile but temperature elevation up to 39°C may be seen. Vomiting is present in most patients and the diarrhea is characterized by watery stools containing mucous and no blood. Moderate to severe dehydration may occur, which, in some infants, results in significant electrolyte disturbance. Fatal disease has been described in a small number of infants.

Therapy. The most important aspect of therapy for diarrheal disease of newborn infants is maintenance of hydration and electrolyte balance. As a rule, parenteral solutions containing appropriate electrolytes should be administered during the time of active diarrhea and the infant should be examined and weighed frequently to ensure proper rehydration and prevention of complications. Estimation of fluid loss from diarrhea and vomiting should be carefully recorded and used as a basis for replacement therapy.

Selection of appropriate antimicrobial therapy depends in part on the mechanism of diarrhea. In general, an absorbable antibiotic such as ampicillin is indicated for disease caused by invasive bacteria (shigellosis), while orally administered, nonabsorbable drugs, such as neomycin or colistin sulfate, are used for noninvasive organisms which produce enterotoxin (some *E. coli*).[39]

Antimicrobial therapy for salmonella gastroenteritis is controversial. Antibiotics do not alter the course of illness and will usually prolong intestinal carriage of the organism. Additionally, clinical relapse is more common in antibiotic-treated infants. Therefore, we do not currently recommend antibiotic therapy for uncomplicated salmonella gastroenteritis. Therapy is probably indicated for those with prolonged illness and for infants with systemic symptoms suggesting bloodstream invasion. Ampicillin or amoxicillin is usually satisfactory.

Ampicillin was formerly the antibiotic of choice for shigellosis, but in recent years significant resistance to this agent has been observed in many areas of the country. Most strains are susceptible *in vitro* to trimethoprim-sulfamethoxazole, and infants respond clinically and bacteriologically to a regimen of 10 mg trimethoprim-50 mg sulfamethoxazole/kg/day in two divided doses given for 5 days. However, we have very limited experience with this agent in newborn infants, and the drug should not be used in jaundiced infants.

Any infant with diarrhea must be isolated from other babies in the nursery. Surveillance of all infants in contact with the index case and adoption of strict infection control measures are mandatory.

LOWER RESPIRATORY TRACT INFECTION

Lower respiratory tract infection is an important cause of morbidity in the neonate and is demonstrable on postmortem examination of approximately 10% of neonatal deaths.

Pneumonias can be divided into 3 categories on the basis of route of acquisition and age at presentation. The first category is **transplacental pneumonitis** which is acquired *in utero* and presents clinically in the early hours of life. Pneumonia may be part of a generalized congenital infection caused by cytomegalovirus, herpesvirus, rubellavirus, toxoplasma, and *L. monocytogenes*. *Treponema pallidum* produces a severe, usually fatal pneumonitis (pneumonia alba) and mycoplasma has caused a rare form of fatal congenital pneumonia. These infants usually have many organ systems involved which may clinically obscure the pneumonitis. Clinical findings may include hepatosplenomegaly, cutaneous manifestations such as rash or petechiae, neurologic abnormalities, and teratogenic effects.

The second category, **aspiration pneumonia,** is acquired in the immediate perinatal period, and onset of illness occurs within the first several days of life. Pathogenesis is by way of aspiration of amniotic fluid or material from the maternal cervix during the period immediately before or during delivery. The vast majority of infants with roentgenographic evidence of aspiration have not swallowed infected material and therefore do not require antimicrobial therapy. This is also true of meconium aspiration where the pneumonitis is on a chemical basis. The bacterial pathogens most commonly encountered are the group B beta-hemolytic streptococci, group D streptococci, pneumococci, and coliform organisms. Infants with these infections may present in the first 12 hours of life with acute respiratory distress with or without shock. The mortality is considerable in this condition even when appropriate antimicrobial therapy has been instituted early.

The third category of pneumonias are **acquired** during delivery or in the postpartum period and usually beyond the first week of life. This pneumonitis may be caused by viral, chlamydial, or bacterial agents and is most frequently bronchopneumonic or interstitial in type. The respiratory syncytial virus is the most important pathogen of lower respiratory tract disease in young infants. The para-influenza viruses and adenoviruses also cause bronchiolitis and pneumonia during early infancy. Bronchiolitis, pneumonia, or both usually occur in epidemics among premature and full-term nursery infants or in the community.

Documented nursery outbreaks of lower respiratory tract disease have been associated with respiratory syncytial virus, adenovirus, echovirus type 22, influenza A and B viruses, and parainfluenza virus infections. During these outbreaks many infants are colonized with the epidemic virus strains but only a few manifest clinical disease.

S. aureus and coliform organisms are the cost common bacterial pathogens of postnatally-acquired pneumonia. Disease caused by *S. aureus* and *K. pneumoniae* may occur sporadically or in epidemic fashion during the neonatal period. Pyogenic complications such as septicemia, osteomyelitis, and meningitis are frequently associated with the epidemic form of these infections.

Acquisition of *Chlamydia trachomatis* in the intrapartum period may result in conjunctivitia (inclusion blennorrhea) or in pneumonia usually presenting between the fourth and twelfth weeks of life. The pneumonia is associated with a staccato cough often terminating in vomiting or cyanosis and with tachypnea, and the infants are usually afebrile.[40] Rales are present and there may be a history of the infant having conjuctivitis in the newborn period. Eosinophilia is present in approximately half of the patients.

Clincial Manifestations. The early signs of lower respiratory tract disease in the neonate and young infant are frequently nonspecific and include change in feeding status, listlessness or irritability, and poor color. More specific findings which may not be present at the onset of illness are tachypnea, dyspnea, cyanosis, hypothermia, cough, and grunting. Accentuation of the normal irregularity of breathing is a common finding in neonates.

The physical findings of pneumonia are variable. Flaring of the alae nasi, rapid respirations, and sternal and subcostal retractions are frequently observed. When cough is present, it is indicative of lower respiratory tract involvement; a brassy cough is frequently found in viral disease. Percussion dullness is difficult to demonstrate, but when present, it is indicative of consolidation, effusion, or both. Auscultation may reveal diminished breath sounds over the affected area. Rales and/or wheezes can usually be heard on deep inspiration (or when the baby is crying) but may be absent early in the illness. The clinician is frequently surprised by the meager clinical signs in the face of clearly demonstrable and sometimes extensive roentgenographic findings of pneumonia.

Diagnosis. The white blood cell count may be helpful in differentiating viral from bacterial pneumonia. Infants with early-onset bacterial pneumonia with sepsis may have leukopenia with an increased number of band forms. Chorioamnionitis has been demonstrated in some infants with congenital pneumonia.

Cultures of blood and material from the trachea are frequently helpful in defining the etiologic agent of neonatal pneumonia. Results of cultures from the ear canal, throat, and other external sites are most helpful and may be misleading in defining the cause of pneumonia in newborn and young infants. Lung puncture should be considered in infants with consolidated pneumonia when the etiology is unknown or when the infant fails to respond to conventional antimicrobial therapy. Material obtained at puncture should be gram stained for direct visualization of bacteria and cultured.

A chest film is indicated in all infants with nonspecific signs of infection. Roentgenographic evidence of pneumonia may be present in the absence of physical findings. Although it is not usually possible to determine the etiology of neonatal pneumonia from chest films, certain roentgenographic patterns may be associated with specific diseases. A consolidating bronchopneumonia with pneumatoceles with or without empyema suggests staphylococcal disease. This is particularly true when the x-ray findings advance markedly in a few hours. When a lobar infiltrate is associated with bulging fissures on the film, *K. pneumoniae* infection should be considered. In contrast, a miliary-type of bronchopneumonia in a septic neonate is characteristic of listeriosis.

It should be emphasized that a bronchopneumonic infiltrate is most commonly encountered in the first month of life. This can be caused by aspiration of sterile or infected fluid, by viral, chlamydial, or bacterial pathogens, or can represent patchy atelectasis.

Staphylococcal pneumonia. Staphylococcal pneumonia is found most commonly in young infants: 30% of cases occur under 3 months of age and 70% before 1 year. Epidemics of staphylococcal disease caused by phage group I organisms are encountered infrequently today. In the epidemic setting, many infants are colonized with a virulent strain, but few manifest disease. Outbreaks of staphylococcal disease in several nurseries during 1978 and 1979 may be evidence of a resurgence of staphylococcal activity in closed populations of hospitalized patients. Many of these organisms have been resistant to the antistaphylococcal penicillins, cephalosporins, and aminoglucosides.

Staphylococci cause a confluent bronchopneumonia characterized by extensive areas of hemorrhagic necrosis and irregular areas of cavitation. The pleural surface is usually covered by a thick layer of fibrinopurulent exudate. Multiple small abscesses are scattered throughout the lungs. Rupture of a small subpleural abscess may result in a pyopneumothorax, which in turn may erode into a bronchus, producing a bronchopleural fistula.

The onset of illness in staphylococcal pneumonia is abrupt with fever, cough, and respiratory distress as the major manifestations. Tachypnea, grunting respirations, retractions, cyanosis, and anxiety are usually present. Severe dyspnea and a shock-like state may occur. Rapid progression of symptoms is characteristic of staphylococcal pneumonia. Physical examination may be misleading, particularly in the young infant, in whom meager physical findings are disproportionate to the degree of tachypnea. Moist scattered rales, diminished breath sounds and rhonchi may be heard early in the illness. With the development of pleural effusion, dullness on percussion associated with diminished breath sounds is found.

Most patients with staphylococcal pneumonia will have roentgenographic evidence of bronchopneumonia early in the illness. The infiltrate may be patchy and limited in extent or be dense and homogenous involving an entire lobe or hemithorax. Pleural effusion or empyema will be noted in most infants. Pneu-

matoceles of varying size are common. Although no radiographic change can be considered diagnostic, progression over a few hours from bronchopneumonia to effusion or pyopenumothorax with or without pneumatoceles is highly suggestive of staphylococcal pneumonia.

Treatment. All diagnostic procedures and cultures should be obtained before initiating therapy. Methicillin is the initial drug of choice for staphylococcal pneumonia and should be administered parenterally in a dosage of 100 mg/kg/day divided in two or three doses for infants under 2 weeks of age, and 200 to 250 mg/kg/day divided in four to six doses for older infants. When infection extends to the pleural surfaces, surgical intervention usually becomes necessary. With small amounts of effusion, repeated pleural taps may be successful in removing fluid, but empyema is best treated with closed drainage, using a chest tube of the largest possible caliber. For pneumonia caused by *K. pneumoniae* or other coliforms, kanamycin or gentamicin should be used in a total dosage of 15 mg/kg/day or 5 to 7.5 mg/kg/day respectively. Treatment for listeria pneumonia is parenteral ampicillin in a dosage of 50 to 100 mg/kg/day divided in two doses for infants under 1 week of age, and 100 to 150 mg/kg/day divided in three doses for older neonates. Infants with group B streptococcal septicemia and pneumonia should be given penicillin in a dosage of 50,000 units/kg/day divided in two doses for infants under 1 week of age, and 75,000 to 100,000 units/kg/day divided in three or four doses for older infants. Chlamydial pneumonia is probably best treated with orally administered erythromycin. This agent has been shown to shorten the course of illness and abruptly eradicate shedding of the organisms from the nasopharynx.

Pneumonia may be one manifestation of generalized congenital viral infections. It is important to differentiate these infections from congenital syphilis and bacterial pneumonias resulting from aspiration. There is no convincing evidence that antiviral chemotherapy is effective in infants with congenital cytomegalovirus or herpesvirus infections.

The majority of infants with aspiration pneumonia do not require antimicrobial therapy. It is frequently difficult to differentiate infants with aspiration of sterile fluid from those aspirating infected materials. If doubt exists, therapy with penicillin and kanamycin or gentamicin should be initiated and continued until results of cultures are available.

REFERENCES

1. **McCracken GH, Nelson JD:** Antimicrobial Therapy for Newborns. Practical Application of Pharmacology to Clinical Usage. New York, Grune and Stratton, 1977
2. **Melish M, Glasgow L, Turner M:** The staphylococcal scalded skin syndrome: Isolation and partial characterization of the exfoliatin toxin. J Infect Dis 123:129, 1972
3. **Albert S, Baldwin R, Czekajewski S, van Soestkergen A, Nachman R, Robertson A:** Bullous impetigo due to group II Staphylococcus aureus. Am J Dis Child 120:10, 1970
4. **Dillon HC:** Group A type 12 streptococcal infection in a newborn nursery: Successfully treated neonatal meningitis. Am J Dis Child 112:177, 1966
5. **Overall J, Glasgow L:** Virus infections of the fetus and newborn infant. J Pediatr 77:315, 1970
6. **Eichenwald HF, McCracken GH, Kindberg S:** Virus infections of the newborn. Progr Med Virol 9:35, 1967
7. **Javett SN, Heymann S, Mundel B et al:** Myocarditis in the newborn infant. J Pediatr 48:1, 1956
8. **Butterfield J, Moscovici C, Berry C, Kempe CH:** Cystic emphysema in premature infants. N Eng J Med 268:18, 1963
9. **Philip A, Larson E:** Overwhelming neonatal infection with echo 19 virus. J Pediatr 82:391, 1973
10. **Eichenwald HF, Kotsevalov O:** Immunologic responses of premature and full-term infants to infection with certain viruses. Pediatrics 25:829, 1960
11. **Berkovich G, Taranko L:** Acute respiratory illness in the premature nursery associated with respiratory syncytial virus infections. Pediatrics 34:753, 1964
12. **Hall CB, Kopelman AR, Douglas RG, Gelman JM, Meagher MP:** Neonatal respiratory syntytial virus infection. N Eng J Med 300:393, 1979
13. **Wientzen RL, McCracken GH:** Pathogenesis and management of neonatal sepsis and meningitis. Current Problems in Pediatrics VIII, December 1977
14. **Baker CJ:** Group B streptococcal infections in neonates. Pediatrics in Review 1:5, 1979
15. **Howard JB, McCracken GH:** The spectrum of group B streptococcal infections in infancy. Am J Dis Child 128:815, 1974
16. **Manroe BL, Rosenfeld CR, Weinberg AG, Browne R:** The differential leukocyte count in the assessment and outcome of early-onset neonatal group B streptococcal disease. J Pediatr 91:632, 1977
17. **McCracken GH, Shinefield H:** Changes in the pattern of neonatal septicemia and meningitis. Am J Dis Child 112:33, 1966
18. **Berman PH, Banker BQ:** Neonatal meningitis: A clinical and pathological study of 29 cases. Pediatr 38:6, 1966
19. **Robbins JB, McCracken GH, Gotshlick EC, Ørskov F, Ørskov I, Hanson LA:** *Escherichia coli* K1 capsular polysaccharide associated with neonatal meningitis. N Eng J Med 290:1216, 1974
20. **Sarff LD, Platt LH, McCracken GH:** Cerebrospinal fluid evaluation in neonates: Comparison of high-risk infants with and without meningitis. J Pediatr 88:473, 1976
21. **McCracken GH, Mize SG:** A controlled study of intrathecal antibiotic therapy in gram-negative enteric meningitis of infancy. Report of the Neonatal Meningitis Cooperative Study. J Pediatr 89:66, 1976
22. **McCracken GH, Mize SG:** Intraventricular therapy of neonatal meningitis caused by gram negative enteric bacilli (abstr). Pediatr Res 13:831, 1979
23. **Brightman V, Scott T, Westphal M, Boggs T:** An outbreak of Coxsackie B-5 virus infection in a newborn nursery. J Pediatr 69:179, 1966
24. **Miller D, Gabrielson M, Bart K, Opton E, Horstmann D:** An epidemic of aseptic meningitis primarily among infants caused by echovirus II-prime. Pediatrics 41:77, 1968
25. **Ogden JA, Lister G:** The pathology of neonatal osteomyelitis. Pediatrics 55:474, 1975
26. **Asnes RS, Arendar GM:** Septic arthritis of the hip: A complication of femoral venipuncture. Pediatrics 38:837–841, 1966
27. **Nelson DL, Hable KA, Matsen JM:** *Proteus mirabilis* osteomyelitis in two neonates following needle puncture. Am J Dis Child 125:109–110, 1973
28. **Qureshi ME, Puri SP:** Osteomyelitis after exchange transfusion. Br Med J 2:28–29, 1971
29. **Overturf GD, Balfour G:** Osteomyelitis and sepsis: Severe complications of fetal monitoring. Pediatrics 55:244–247, 1975
30. **Nelson JD:** Antibiotic concentrations in septic joint effusions. N Engl J Med 284:349, 1971
31. **Wilson HD, Haltalin K:** Acute necrotizing fasciitis in childhood. Am J Dis Child 125:591, 1973
32. **Nelson JD, Peters PC:** Suprapubic aspiration of urine in premature and term infants. Pediatrics 36:132, 1965
33. **Weintzen RL, McCracken GH, Petruska ML,**

Swinson SG, Kaijser B, Hanson LA: Localization and therapy of urinary tract infection of childhood. Pediatrics 63:467, 1979

34. **Platou R:** Treatment of congenital syphilis with pencillin. Adv Pediatr 4:39, 1949

35. **Rowe DS, Aicardi EZ, Dawson CR, Schacter J:** Purulent ochlar discharge in neonates: Significance of *Chlamydia trachomatis*. Pediatr 63:628, 1979

36. **Ryder RW, McGowan JE, Hatch MH, Palmer EL:** Reovirus-like agent as a cause of nosocomial diarrhea in infants. J Pediatr 90:698, 1977

37. **Middleton PJ, Szymanski MT, Petrie M:** Viruses associated with acute gastroenteritis in young children. Am J Dis Child 131:733, 1977

38. **Boyer KM, Peterson NJ, Farzaneh I, Patternson CP, Hart MC, Maynard JE:** An outbreak of gastroenteritis due to *E. coli* O142 in a neonatal nursery. J Pediatr 86:919, 1975

39. **Nelson JD, Kusmiesz HT:** A double-blind study of neomycin, ampicillin and placebo for enteropathogenic *Escherichia coli* diarrheal disease. Pediatrics (in press)

33

Chronic Congenital and Perinatal Infections

David W. Reynolds,
Sergio Stagno, and
Charles A. Alford, Jr.

INTRODUCTION

Infections of pregnancy involving mother and offspring have long attracted the attention of physicians. In the past, acute bacterial and communicable viral diseases dominated this interest because of clinical recognition, often fulminate courses, and, in the case of the bacteria, available therapy. These agents contribute to the problems of pregnancy wastage through direct invasion of the fetus and neonate or through early termination of pregnancy secondary to profoundly disturbed maternal physiology by mechanisms poorly understood. However, the impact of low-grade, chronic, recurrent, and latent infections of pregnancy is less well defined, mainly because manifest disease is either absent or too subtle to be recognized in the great majority of mothers and their offspring. Yet, these "silent" infections occur more commonly during pregnancy and, therefore, represent diseases of potentially greater medicosocial importance than do the acute forms.

The acute infections are self-limiting with outcomes ranging from death to complete recovery occuring during the acute phase. During convalescence, the pathogen is eliminated by the host, terminating the infectious process and related morbidity. Therefore, damage secondary to these infections has been assessed mainly in the immediate postinfection period and possible sequelae inadvertently overlooked. In contrast, the infections to be discussed here are characterized by chronicity, recurrence, or both, in either mother or baby or both, and posses the potential to inflict continued injury. Adequate assessment of their impact on both mother and offspring requires long-term longitudinal evaluation. This discussion will focus primarily on the results of such investigations, relating pathogenetic phenomenon to the observed developmental disabilities in infected offspring. The agents involved include rubella virus, *Toxoplasma gondii,* cytomegalovirus (CMV), herpes simplex virus (HSV), and *Treponema pallidum.* Likewise, congenital tuberculosis, trypanosomiasis, and malaria share the feature of chronicity but are

Supported in part by a program project grant (HD10699) from the National Institute of Child Health and Human Development, by research grants (CA13148 and CA16424) from the National Cancer Institute, by the National Foundation-March of Dimes (6-180), and by the Robert E. Meyer Foundation.

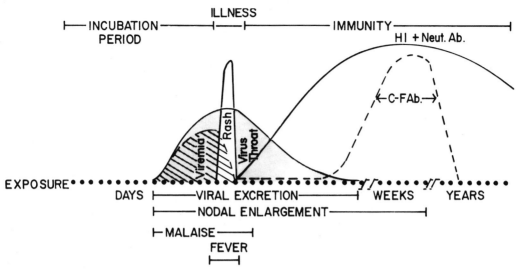

Fig. 33-1. Relation of viral excretion, clinical findings, and antibody response in postnatally acquired rubella.

deleted because of the rarity of the former and the limited geographic distribution of the latter two.

RUBELLA

Epidemiology

Rubella is worldwide in distribution and has a seasonal pattern of epidemicity (*i.e.*, springtime), although endemic disease in the general population may persist throughout the year at low levels.[1,2] Congenitally infected infants who may shed virus for months after delivery also probably contribute to the spread of infection during endemic periods. This seasonal pattern of incidence is totally unexplained, as is the occurrence of pandemics at 6- to 9-year intervals which peak and abate over a 2- to 3-year period. Though the spontaneous appearance of strains of increased virulence has been offered as a reason for the pandemic situation, convincing evidence of this is yet to be presented.[3,4]

Seroepidemiologic studies have confirmed clinical observations that rubella is primarily a disease of school-age children with peak incidence in 5- to 14-year olds.[1,2,5] In developed countries, only 5% to 20% of women entering the child-bearing age group remain susceptible to this infection.[1,2] However, in certain tropical island communities, susceptibility rates in this all-important group may approach 25% to 75%.[6] Conversely, in some South American countries, practically the entire population has experienced this infection by early adulthood.[6] The low infection rates in preschool children belie the relative importance of this age group in relation to congenital infection because they constitute an important source of virus for young pregnant women. Epidemics are common, even among adults, when large numbers of susceptibles congregate in close quarters such as military recruit camps and college campuses.

Humans are the only known host for rubella virus and postnatal transmission occurs by way of respiratory secretions, by droplet spread, by direct contact, or perhaps by fomites freshly soiled with secretions. Airborne transmission is also possible.

Nature and Diagnosis of Maternal Infection

It is necessary to understand the virologic and immunologic findings of both the postnatally and congenitally acquired infections if their pathogenetic, clinical, and diagnostic features are to be appreciated. The most pertinent of these parameters for postnatal infection are depicted in Figure 33-1. Although clinical disease does not manifest until 14 to 21 days (mean, 18 days) following exposure, excretion of virus from nasopharynx, urine, cervix, and feces as a consequence of viremic seeding has been occurring for approximately one week.[7,8] It is most prolonged and at highest levels in pharyngeal secretions, wherein shedding is consistent for 2 weeks and may rarely be detected for upward of 5 weeks. Knowledge of this excretion is crucial when determining the degree of risk following exposure in relation to the stage of illness of the index case, and in assessing the duration of contagiousness. Also of major importance with regard to exposure histories is an appreciation of the fact that inapparent primary infection is common, perhaps one to two asymptomatic involvements for every one clinically apparent case as assessed serologically.

Rubella is a systemic infection; hence, viremia is a consistent feature usually demonstrable when excretion begins from the pharynx; it is terminated as serum antibodies appear some 14 to 18 days after acquisition of infection.[9] Circulation of virus in the serum, prior to the onset of illness, is responsible for placental involvement with primary infections in pregnant women.[10] This is usually the initial event leading to fetal infection. Presumably there is multiple organ system involvement with minimal functional disturbance, except for the relatively common arthralgia and arthritis accompanying synovial infections or the rare encephalitic or thrombocytopenic syndromes.[9,11] Virus is present in the exanthematous lesions; whether because of replication in the skin, blood vessels, or both is unclear.[12] These findings translate clinically into a characteristic, though unfortunately not pathognomonic, picture of fever, a 3-day rubelliform rash, and postoccipital and preauricular adenopathy. When synovial inflammation, especially of the smaller peripheral joints is also present, some degree of clinical specificity is achieved. Given a known exposure history, the correct incubation period, and the presence of epidemic rubella in the community, a presumptive diagnosis can be entertained. However, a definitive assessment should include an appropriate serologic work-up, a mandatory procedure if a therapeutic abortion is being considered.

Because viral replication is widespread throughout the body at least a week before illness begins, specific antibodies can be detected in the serum during the disease or occasionally even before; in the case of asymptomatic infection, they are first demonstrable 14 to 18 days following exposure.[1,7,8,13,14] Antibody levels peak within a week to a month after the onset of illness depending on the type measured. Hemagglutination inhibition (HI) antibodies peak soon after illness, usually within a week or two, followed shortly by fluorescent (FA) and neutralizing (NA) antibodies.[13,14] Complement-fixing antibodies (CF) rise more slowly, peaking approximately a month or two or rarely, 5 to 6 months, following disease.[14] HI and NA antibodies usually persist for years, if not permanently, except in a small percentage (1% to 3%) of patients in whom they wane slowly.[1,15,16] In the latter group, reinfection may occur resulting in a short term, low level of virus replication in the pharynx without demonstrable viremia; a booster antibody response rapidly terminates the new infection and is thought to limit systemic spread of virus.[1] Whether or not this is true is currently an important question with regard to the possibility of infecting the conceptus during the course of maternal reinfection or vaccination.[1,17] Reinfection is, presumably, far less dangerous to the fetus than primary infection because of decreased likelihood of placental exposure to virus.[18]

Recognition of the differential antibody response can prove diagnostically valuable in pregnant women who first present a few weeks following a nondescript rash disease or too long after exposure for one to demonstrate a diagnostic increase in HI antibody in infections without rash. The slower response of the CF antibody can be used to prove infection under these circumstances. The fact that the CF antibody, in contrast to HI and NA, usually disappears a few years after primary infection and is less responsive to reinfection, can also be used to advantage diagnostically.[13] This is especially so in identifying the booster antibody response of reinfection or determining whether seropositivity is of long-term origin. In some cases, a CF antibody response is elicited with vaccination or reinfection.

In those fortunately rare instances in which the foregoing serologic analyses have not proven definitive, the determination of IgM-specific rubella antibody in acute and convalescent sera is indicated. IgM antibody appears in the serum quite early in the course of primary infection, peaks at about 2 weeks, and then disappears a month or two thereafter.[19] It does not appear, or does so only briefly,

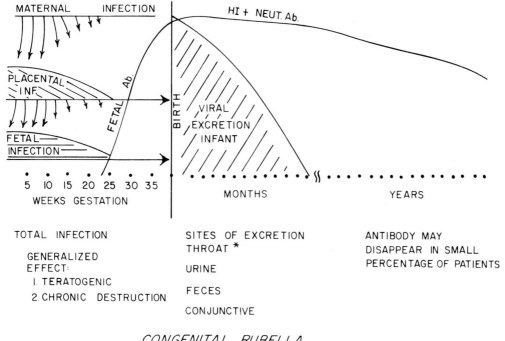

CONGENITAL RUBELLA

(CHRONIC INTRAUTERINE INFECTION)

Fig. 33-2. Summary of virologic and serologic parameters of congenitally acquired rubella. (Alford CA: Diagnosis of chronic perinatal infection. Am J Dis Child 131:456, 1975)

during the antibody response of reinfection. Of the various methods for identifying this antibody, an indirect fluorescent technique appears the most sensitive;[20] but, as with the other methods, is only performed in research laboratories. All of the foregoing should point to the obvious fact that the optimal benefit of serologic analysis is to be had only by evaluation of the patient as soon as possible after exposure or illness with rash.

Nature and Diagnosis of Congenital Infection

Knowledge concerning the dynamic interaction between rubella virus and the fetal host, though incomplete, is far more extensive than that accumulated for the other infections in this chapter. It will, therefore, be presented in detail to serve as a prototype for the discussions to follow.

Virologic Events. Some of the more important sequential virologic and immunologic changes that accompany congenital acquisition are summarized in Figure 33-2. The feature of chronicity clearly distinguishes the congenital infection from the postnatal.[10,21] During the period of maternal viremia, the placenta may become infected and then act as a seed source of virus for the fetus. Virus persists in the placenta for months but is most often cleared or markedly reduced in quantity or distribution in late gestation so that recovery from the placenta at birth is infrequent.[22] In contrast, once the fetus is infected, the virus persists throughout gestation and for months postnatally.[9,10,21] It can infect many fetal organs or only a few.[10] In infected infants, virus can be excreted from multiple sites (pharynx, urine, conjunctiva, feces) and is detectable in the cerebrospinal fluid (CSF) and in bone marrow or circulating white blood cells.[9,10,21] As in the postnatally acquired infections, pharyngeal shedding of virus is more common, prolonged, and intense and, thus, pharyngeal swabs represent the best material for attempted viral diagnosis. Conjunctival swabs and CSF also give high yields, but only if disease is evident in the eye or protein and cell elevations are present in the CSF. Viral shedding diminishes with time; consequently, for maximal diagnosis, isolation attempts should be made as soon as possible (within the first 3 months) after delivery. Persistence in the eye and CSF may be more prolonged.[23,24]

Chronic conceptal infection, the most important pathogenetic feature, is not inevitable even with primary maternal infections.[10,25] In fact, outcome of maternal infection may be as follows:

1. No infection of the conceptus
2. Resorption of the embryo (seen with infections occurring only in the earliest stages of pregnancy)
3. Spontaneous abortion
4. Stillbirth
5. Infection of the placenta without fetal involvement
6. Infection of both placenta and fetus

The infected liveborn can have obvious multiorgan system involvement or, more commonly, no evident disease.[25,26]

Gestational age of the conceptus at the time of maternal infection is the single factor most often cited as influencing the outcome of pregnancy.[10,27] Chronic placental and fetal infections are more common with maternal infection acquired in the first 8 weeks of gestation. In this period, placental infection has been documented in as many as 85% of exposures, with concomitant demonstrable fetal infections in 50%. Transmission to the fetus decreases sharply after the eighth week; placental infection also decreases but less rapidly.[10] Thus, after the eighth to tenth week, isolated placental infection (30%) is more common than fetal infection (5%–10%). The exact significance of isolated placental infection is presently unknown, but postnatal patterns of infection and disease parallel intrauterine events. Abortion and stillbirth result more often with fetal infections acquired in the first 8 weeks. The infection rate, as serologically documented in infants, declines from a high of 54% in the first 8 weeks, to 34% between 9 and 12 weeks, and reaches a low of 10% between 13 and 24 weeks. Afterward, chronic infection of the fetus is rare.

Not only infection rates but pathologic potential is also modulated by gestational influences. Among infected infants born after maternal rubella in the first 8 weeks, as many as 85% have detectable defects by 1 to 4 years of age; these figures are 52% for 9 to 12 weeks,

approximately 16% for 13 to 20, and none after 20 weeks.[26] Because of the further detection of hearing defects with time, these percentages would increase in all gestational categories. Obviously, the disease is more severe with a greater tendency to multiorgan involvement (expanded rubella syndrome) when acquired early. However, normal-appearing infected infants are born following exposures at any gestational age and, commonly so, after the eighth week.[25,28,29,30]

The exact nature of the gestational influences are unknown; speculations are as follows:

1. Immature cells are more easily infected and support the growth of virus better than older cells.
2. Because of rapid maturation during the first trimester, the placenta becomes increasingly more resistant to infection and more capable of limiting viral spread when infected.
3. Maturing fetal host defense mechanisms become capable of confining and clearing the infection. The latter is probably partially true after 18 or 20 weeks of gestation but seems unlikely in the latter half of the first trimester when attenuation of the conceptal rubella seemingly first begins. Likely, a combination of these factors and others will be found responsible for decreasing virulence of fetal infection with advancing gestational age.[10]

Immunologic Events. Because two humoral immune mechanisms, placental and fetal, develop *in utero,* they both must be considered in judging the host response to any intrauterine infection.[31] In congenital rubella, this consideration is complicated by the fact that both the placenta and the fetus almost always become chronically infected in their earliest formative stages.[10] There is a potential danger, then, for interfering with the normal sequence of events that leads to final maturation of either the placental transfer mechanism(s) for shunting maternal antibody or the ability of the fetus to manufacture antibody.

Placental transfer mechanisms mature normally in spite of chronic rubella infection.[32] However, even under normal circumstances, they are severely dampened in the first half of gestation and only minimal amounts of maternal antibody are available to combat the spread of virus.[33] From a practical standpoint, only IgG maternal antibodies are normally transferred by the placenta, but not in substantial amounts until around 16 to 20 weeks of gestation. Levels of antibody in the fetal blood prior to that are only 5% to 10% of those in maternal serum with or without rubella infection.[34] This critical situation remains for many weeks following viral invasion of the conceptus. The placental transfer mechanisms mature rapidly around midgestation.[35] By delivery, levels of IgG rubella antibodies in cord sera are equal to or greater than those in the maternal sera, whether the infant is prematurely born or not. In fact, the dominant antibody present at delivery of rubella-infected infants is maternal IgG rubella antibody.[32] This, of course, complicates serologic diagnosis of congenital rubella because most normal babies (85%) are also born with comparable levels of maternally derived antibody.

The early development of the fetal humoral immune system, like that of the placenta, is also normally too slow to combat spread of virus. Cells with membrane-bound immunoglobulins of all three major classes—IgM, IgG, IgA—appear in the fetus as early as 9 to 11 weeks of gestation.[36] This antibody represents the early acquisition of receptor or recognition sites for antigen. Even cytoplasmic antibody production, although relatively delayed, begins around 15 to 19 weeks of gestation.[36] During the early preparatory period, however, the number of cells capable of making a specific immune response is deficient or else their overall metabolism must differ from that seen in later life. Thus, circulating fetal antibody levels remain low in the face of high levels of rubella virus, while in the mother a prompt serum antibody response is elicited.[32]

Perhaps the poor fetal and placental immune responses account, in part, for the virus' greater ability to invade in early gestation, and contribute to its much increased virulence in utero. Moreover, chronicity would be favored in intrauterine rubella by allowing the virus to gain a stronger foothold at the outset.

The fetal humoral immune mechanisms mature sufficiently so that a serum antibody response is usually elicited beginning around midgestation. Specific fetal IgM antibody is detectable about this time and increases until it may constitute a major or at least a significant portion of the pools of antibody in cord sera.[32]

If the antigenic stimulus is sufficient, usually with very severe infections, fetal IgA antibody may also be present at birth, but far less commonly than fetal IgM and always in lesser amounts.[31,32] Very likely, fetal IgG production is also stimulated, but the fetus' contribution of this antibody type is buried in the large pool of maternal IgG and is therefore difficult to demonstrate.

The antigenic stimulus provided by rubella infection of the conceptus, similar to that provided by other chronic intrauterine infections, not only results in specific IgM antibody production in utero but may cause the total pool of IgM in fetal serum to become increased, so that at or shortly after delivery, elevated levels of this immunoglobulin can be detected in the infected neonate.[31,32,34] Total IgA levels are also occasionally elevated, but seldom is the IgG (mainly maternal in origin) increased over that found in normal babies. The patterns of the immunoglobulin elevations, then, tend to reflect patterns of specific fetal antibody production with IgM being the most markedly stimulated.[31] The demonstration of fetal IgM antibody in cord sera signifies fetal infection and can be employed as an important confirmatory diagnostic tool. Detection of elevated total IgM, which is more widely available and economical, is also helpful diagnostically but is nonspecific and can, therefore, be used only as a high-risk monitor. Both of these testing methods can be employed as screening tools for searching out infants whose infections are asymptomatic at birth. However, levels of total IgM and IgG specific antibody are quite variable between infected infants, with higher levels being detected in the more severely involved infants. This must be taken into consideration when immunologic monitors are used diagnostically in the newborn.

As noted in Figure 33-3, in the first 3 to 5 months following delivery of a rubella-infected neonate, levels of IgM antibody usually increase, while IgG antibody quantities diminish because of the catabolism of the maternal fraction.[32] IgM can even become the dominant variety during this period. Later, as viral excretion wanes and disappears, so does the IgM antibody, and IgG again becomes the dominant and persistent type. The level of total antibody as measured by such serologic tests as HI, NA, CF, and FA remains virtually unchanged throughout the first year, in spite of the con-

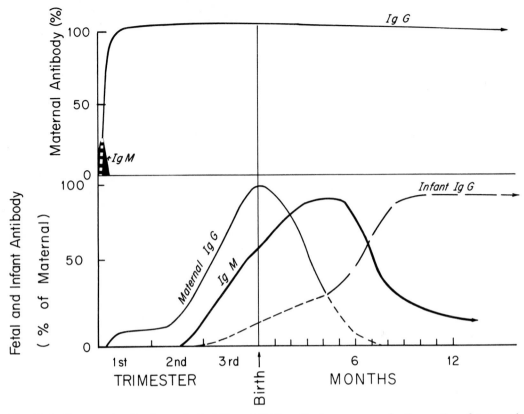

Fig. 33-3. Comparative Ig class rubella NA and HAI antibody responses in the mother, fetus, and infant following early gestational acquisition of infection.

stant changes in its molecular makeup. High levels of IgG antibody are usually maintained for a number of years after cessation of detectable virus excretion, suggesting continued antigenic stimulus provided by the chronic infection often produces a state of relative hypergammaglobulinemia during the early years of life, particularly with respect to IgM and IgG.[37] Serum levels of both of these immunoglobulin classes may, therefore, mature much more rapidly than in the normal child.

In approximately 10% to 20% of infants congenitally infected by rubella, specific rubella HI antibody may wane slowly and disappear between 1 and 4 years of age. This group of patients possesses a peculiar inability to respond to live rubella vaccination with a booster antibody response; in contrast, those with postnatal infections, in whom antibody wanes, respond promptly to reinfection or vaccination. This has led some to think that

a form of immune tolerance develops in a small percentage of patients with congenital rubella. Whether this is true or not remains to be seen, but the phenomenon can be used to advantage diagnostically in older children with signs of congenital rubella who are seronegative at the first visit.

Pathology. Angiopathy is the most characteristic lesion found in fetal tissue as well as in placental.[38,39] Small blood vessels and capillaries frequently show pathologic change with extensive damage to the endothelium, especially in the chorion. It has been postulated that infected clumps of chorionic endothelial cells may act as a seed source of virus to the fetus as well as eliciting fetal tissue injury through vascular obstruction.[38] Intrinsic functional vascular damage in the fetal vessels is evidenced by petechiae and the presence of hemosiderin-laden phagocytes in the surrounding tissues.

In addition to this mechanism, direct cytolysis probably also plays some role in tissue injury. Characteristic findings include cytoplasmic eosinophilia, nuclear pyknosis, or karyorrhexis and cellular necrosis. Such cellular lesions can be found in most organs, including the epithelial cells of the lens, inner ear, and teeth. Relative to the degree of virus-induced tissue damage, inflammation is quite minimal, consisting mainly of small lymphocytes. Clearly, then, vascular insufficiency rather than viral cytolysis or inflammation is more important in the genesis of the rubella syndrome.[38-40] This suggestion is further supported by the observation that rubella virus has a low pathologic potential for cells growing *in vitro,* including those of human origin. In fact, chronically infected human fetal cell lines may be maintained for months to years without loss of viability or evidence of cytopathology.[41] However, these cells may manifest chromosomal breaks, reduced multiplication time, and elaborate a protein inhibitor which arrests mitosis in selected cell types.[41,42] If operative *in vivo,* these effects could account at least in part for the virus' embryopathic potential and the common occurrence of intrauterine growth retardation.[43]

The total pathologic process is progressive, in keeping with the chronic nature of congenital rubella, so that in older conceptal specimens both healing and fresh lesions are seen. The pathologic changes are highly variable in quantity and in organ distribution between embryos, and the location and nature of fetal organ lesions depend, somewhat, on the gestational age at the time of initial infection. In this sense, pathologic changes parallel the enormous variability of clinical disease seen in infected newborns and are apparently worsened by earlier acquisition of infection.

Clinical Findings and Outcome. The extensive studies following the pandemic of the mid-1960s have identified congenital rubella as a chronic infection with a huge range of pathologic potential.[44] The infection may cause intrauterine death or severe multiple organ system disease at birth or, conversely, produce no obvious neonatal illness. In fact, silent infections in the young infant are more common than symptomatic ones. In a unique prospective study of 4005 neonates born during the 1964 epidemic, congenital infection was documented in 2%, of whom two-thirds were clinically asymptomatic.[28] However, 71% of those silently infected developed evidence of disease in the first 5 years of life. Clearly, morbid conditions can be overlooked in early infancy and, in fact, may progress with time in association with prolonged viral replication.[45,46]

Even among the symptomatic newborns, the range of disease is enormous as exemplified by the possible findings summarized in Table 33-1. The only prominent defects usually ascribed to the teratogenic action of rubella are cardiac malformations and cataracts. Although gross anatomic defects may occur in many other organ systems, they are relatively rare and are often missed in young infants.

Other defects, probably more commonly encountered than the gross anatomic abnormalities, include intra- and extrauterine growth retardation, hepatosplenomegaly, thrombocytopenia with purpura, adenopathy, active encephalitis, retinopathy, deafness, interstitial pneumonia, and bony radiolucencies. The rubella syndrome, as expressed in the newborns, should now be expanded to include combinations of these more recently emphasized findings rather than just congenital heart lesions, cataracts, and deafness. By doing so, the index of suspicion will be markedly increased as will true incidence.

The "salt and pepper" retinopathy, the discrete bluish-red lesions of dermal erythropoiesis, the disportionately elevated protein-to-cell ratio of the active encephalitis, findings of cataracts, glaucoma, cloudy cornea, bony radiolucencies, and typical heart lesions (pulmonary arterial and ductal), or the occurrence of a myocardial infarction pattern on ECG (resulting from necrotic lesions of the heart), all lend a degree of specificity to clinical diagnosis.[44] Therefore, careful ophthalmologic and spinal fluid examinations, radiologic bone surveys, and detailed cardiac evaluations should be performed on all suspect newborns, whether symptomatic or not.

Certain lesions carry a poor prognosis for survival. Included among these are severe prematurity, gross cardiac lesions with early heart failure, rapidly progressive hepatitis, extensive meningoencephalitis, fulminant interstitial pneumonitis, and other major life-threatening anatomic defects as recorded in Table 33-1. Obviously, these lesions must be carefully excluded because they may be compensated for during the neonatal period only

Table 33-1. Summary of Clinical Findings and Their Estimated Frequency of Occurrence in Young Symptomatic Infants with Congenitally Acquired Rubella.

Clinical Findings	Frequency	Clinical Findings	Frequency
Prematurity	+	*Hematologic*	
Intrauterine growth retardation	+ + +	Anemia	+
Extrauterine growth retardation	+ +	Thrombocytopenia c/s purpura	+ +
Hepatosplenomegaly	+ + +	Dermal erythropoiesis (Blueberry	+
Jaundice (regurgitative)	+	muffin syndrome)	
Hepatitis	±	Leukopenia	+
Immunologic dyscrasias	±	Adenopathies	+ +
Chromosomal abnormalities	Unknown		
Interstitial pneumonitis	+ +	*Genitourinary*	
(acute, subacute, chronic)		Undescended testicle	+
Bony radiolucencies	+ +	Polycystic kidney*	±
Malformations	+ + +	Bilobed kidney with reduplication	±
		ureter*	
Central Nervous		Unilateral renal agensis*	±
Encephalitis (active)	+ +	Renal artery stenosis with hyper-	±
Microcephaly	±	tension*	
Brain calcification	±	Hydroureter and hydronephrosis*	±
Bulging fontanel	+		
Neurologic deficit	+	*Bone*	
Retinopathy	+ +	Micrognathia	+
Cataracts	+ +	Extremities	±
Cloudy cornea	±		
Glaucoma	±	*Others**	
Microphthalmia	+	Esophageal atresia	
Hearing defects (severe)	+ +	Tracheoesophageal fistula	
Peripheral		Anencephaly	
Central		Encephalocele	
		Meningomyelocele	
Cardiovascular		Cleft palate	
Pulmonary arterial hypoplasia	+ + +	Inguinal hernia	
Patent ductus arteriosus	+ +	Asplenia	
Myocardial necrosis	+	Nephritis (vascular)	
Coarctation of aortic isthmus	+	Clubfoot	
Interventricular septal	±	Others	
Others	±		

* Rarely associated with rubella syndrome (whether caused by infection unknown); incidence seemingly increased in infants with congenital rubella

Frequency Classification

±	Rare
+	0% to 20%
+ +	20% to 50%
+ + +	50% to 75%
+ + + +	75% to 100%

to decompensate later. Some, such as the intersititial pneumonitis, can even be slowly progressive and, on this basis, apparently cause their major functional difficulties months after birth. Serial assessment for immunologic dyscrasias are necessary during this period because the humoral defects may be masked by the presence of maternal immunoglobulin. Even cataracts may not become apparent until some months after delivery. Prognosis, obviously, must be guarded in the early months of life.

Others of the abnormalities are self-limiting and relatively harmless. Hepatosplenomegaly, anemia, retinopathy, thrombocytopenia, leukopenia, dermal erythropoiesis, adenopathy, and bony radiolucencies fall in this category.[44] All of these lesions are more important from a diagnostic than from a prognostic standpoint.

Many lesions of congenital rubella are missed in the first year of life because of their silence or lack of methods for their detection.[26,45,46] Table 33-2 summarizes the most common defects in this category. Because of their frequency, the most important problems are the hearing defects and psychomotor difficulties.

Hearing defects can occur as both peripheral and central defects and are often associated with impaired language development that may lead to a false impression of mental retardation.[47,48] Appropriate hearing aids, speech therapy, and special education programs are frequently required for such children, especially if psychomotor or hearing problems coexist.[9,47] Obviously, serial psychological and perceptual testing should be performed beginning as soon as feasible after birth, and continuing throughout childhood.

Clearly, in keeping with its chronicity, congenital rubella should be managed as a dynamic rather than a static disease state and a continuing effort made on the part of the physician in charge to define the true extent of the problem initially and to remain alert to the possibility of progressive disease or the unmasking of problems later in life.

Prevention and Therapy

With the advent of live attenuated rubella virus vaccine, the control, if not the eradication, of congenital infection now seems possible. Routine childhood immunization is based on the concept of achieving herd immunity in the population and thereby limiting the spread of infection to pregnant women by severely curtailing the circulation of virus in the community.

The immunogenicity of vaccines in current use as measured by serologic response or clinical protection appears adequate.[18] Further, reactions to the vaccines have been within acceptable limits from the consumer standpoint. Clinical side effects do occur in a small percentage of recipients, the most distressing of which is joint inflammation. This

Table 33-2. Congenital Rubella Abnormalities Commonly Associated with Expression of Disease after First Year.

Hearing defects
  Peripheral
  Central
Psychomotor defects
  Motor
  Intellectual
Dental defects
Language disorders
Retinopathy
Genitourinary tract abnormalities
Bony abnormalities
Diabetes mellitus

(Adapted from Alford CA: Congenital rubella. In Remington JS, Klein JO (eds): Congenital and Perinatal Infection, Philadelphia, WB Saunders, 1974.

problem is seen in children of all ages but increases in severity and perhaps duration with advancing age, especially in adult women.[18] For the most part, articular involvements are short lived but occasionally may persist for weeks and, in a few vaccinees, may recur over prolonged periods. Potential recipients should be apprised of this possibility but also reassured of its rarity.

The more direct approach of immunizing women in the child-bearing age group has been advocated and, in fact, practiced in some countries.[1] However, because vaccine virus may infect the fetus and apparently induce tissue injury,[49,50] every precaution must be taken to insure that pregnancy does not supervene for at least 2 months postvaccination. Administration of vaccine in the immediate postpartum period is one such approach. Proof of candidates' susceptibility, as determined by the absence of serum HI antibody, is an absolute prerequisite.

Some concern has arisen regarding efficacy of the childhood rubella immunization program as a result of the recognition of the reduced immunogenicity of the attenuated virus.[1] Clinically inapparent reinfection occurs much more commonly following vaccine-induced, as opposed to natural, immunity both in closed[15] and in open populations.[51] Obviously, the crucial question over such reinfection is whether viremia of a sufficient degree to infect the fetus occurs to any significant extent. This important concern remains undefined. Further concern has been generated out of findings of an apparent failure of herd immunity to limit the spread of virus to susceptibles.[15,51] These observations have established the need for continued close surveillance of the present program but in no way negate its current validity. Present recommendations should be rigorously followed.

The efficacy of passive immunization in the prevention of congenital infection is and will likely remain controversial.[18] Its use should probably be confined to women in the first trimester of pregnancy who have been exposed to rubella and find therapeutic abortion an unacceptable alternative should infection supervene. Because its major effect is to prevent viremia, it should be administered as soon after exposure as possible with the recognition that clinical disease in the mother may be aborted without eliminating viral replication. Therefore, an appropriate serologic workup for infection should follow.

No effective chemotherapeutic agent for the treatment of either postnatal or congenital rubella is currently available.

A discussion of the moral and medical issues involved in the pros and cons of therapeutic abortion for maternal rubella is far beyond the scope of this writing. Needless to say, decisions for such practice must be carefully weighed by the physician and his patients, the father as well as the mother. In order to handle the question of therapeutic abortion in an objective way, the physician will need a thorough understanding of what is known about the pathogenesis of congenital rubella and, most important, deep compassion for the persons involved in these decisions.

TOXOPLASMOSIS

Epidemiology

In order to appreciate the epidemiologic features of this infection, an understanding of the life cycle of this unique protozoan must be acquired.[52,53] Toxoplasmosis is a worldwide zoonosis involving many vertebrate species. However, only members of the cat family serve as the complete or final host. In the domestic cat, ingestion of the organism results in intestinal replication with the development of mature sexual forms of oocysts. These cysts, shed in the feces for several days fol-

lowing recent infection, are quite resistant to adverse influences in the external environment and may retain infectivity in the soil for long periods.[52] If these oocysts are ingested by other animals or birds (incomplete or intermediate host), actively proliferating forms (trophozoites) are released into the gut and subsequently disseminate throughout the body. Following a rapid multiplication in many tissues, the trophozoites form inactive cysts and chronic, clinically inapparent infection ensues. These species do not support sexual stages in gut epithelium and therefore constitute "dead-end" hosts unless their carcasses are fed upon by a carnivore. In this circumstance, the tissue cysts become fully infectious in the gut lumen and the process is repeated. In addition to transmission by means of carnivorism or ingestion of infected soil or fomites, a potential role for coprophilic invertebrates, serving as uninfected carriers, has been suggested based on experimental work.[54] From this brief overview, several potential routes of transmission to humans emerge (1) consumption of raw or undercooked meat, (2) oral contact with cat feces or contaminated soil and, (3) ingestion of food or other material made infectious by contact with invertebrate carriers. Evidence for the first mode is quite conclusive[55,56] and is rapidly accumulating for the second.[57,58,59] A definitive role for invertebrate transport hosts remains to be established. Human-to-human transmission does not occur except in the case of mother to fetus.

The incidence of toxoplasmosis varies widely within human communities depending on meat cooking preferences, cat exposure, climatic, and soil conditions (oocysts survive better in warm, moist conditions), and other variables yet to be determined. In Paris, where the consumption of fresh raw or undercooked meat is common, 50% to 90% of women have been infected by the time of early adulthood.[55] Parenthetically, it should be noted that freezing, as well as heating, adversely affects the viability of tissue cysts. In other areas in which custom dictates that meat be well cooked, similar high rates of acquisition have been noted, probably because of frequent cat exposure and favorable soil conditions.[53]

In this country, previous experience with this infection among women in the child-bearing years is less common, ranging from 15% to 40%.[60,61]

Nature and Diagnosis of Maternal Infection

Upon initial exposure to the protozoan, a parasitemia ensues with resultant seeding of most organs, including the placenta. Interesting to note is that, despite an acute phase of active tissue parasitism, overt clinical disease appears to be a rare occurrence.[62,63] Even among those with illness, a correct diagnosis is infrequently made, probably because of inadequate index of suspicion. Primary infection can elicit protean manifestations, including one or more of the following: fever, myalgia, pneumonitis, encephalitis, myo- and pericarditis, hepatitis, maculopapular rash, and lymphadenopathy.[62] The most common presentation, however, is localized or generalized lymphadenopathy(-itis).[62] Localized infection of the lymph nodes may occur at any site but is most common in the posterior cervical chain. Generalized involvement when accompanied by fever, malaise, lymphocytosis, and atypical lymphocytes mimics infectious mononucleosis. A negative result in the heterophil agglutination test should reasonably suggest toxoplasmosis as the etiologic agent, although other viruses including CMV can also produce this clinical picture.[62] Symptoms usually appear 8 to 13 days following a natural exposure.[56] This lack of clinical specificity and the total absence of related illness in most gravidas[63] place an absolute premium on laboratory diagnosis.

With the appearance of serum antibodies at 2 to 3 weeks following acquisition, the acute illness and presumably parasitemia abate rapidly in most patients, although residual constitutional, muscular, lymphadenitic symptoms may progressively wane over a period of weeks. Likewise, organisms may continue to circulate in the blood of some patients for prolonged periods, possibly protected from antibody by an intracellular residence in leukocytes.[64] With the encystment of organisms in the various tissues, a stage of permanent latent infection supervenes which, however, may occasionally reactivate, particularly in individuals with compromised immune systems who may suffer a disseminated and potentially lethal recrudescence.[62] In the normal host, recurrences are localized (*e.g.,* retina and myocardium) and hematogenous spread is thought not to occur.

From the foregoing, it is obvious that maternal infection can be diagnosed in the vast majority of instances only by an appropriate serologic investigation. In patients with lymphadenopathy, trophozoites, pathognomonic histologic changes in lymph node biopsies, or both have been reported, but recognition of these findings requires considerable expertise.[65] Isolation of the organism by inoculation of mice with infected tissue (*e.g.,* lymph node biopsy) is entirely unfeasible technically and lacks specificity for primary infection because infectious tissue cysts may persist in extraneural tissue for months or even years.[66]

A humoral response, as measured by the Sabin–Feldman dye test or indirect immunofluorescent (IF) technique, is initiated at 2 to 3 weeks, peaks 2 to 3 months later, and thereafter gradually wanes, but rarely if ever to undetectable levels. Therefore, the demonstration of the *de novo* appearance (**seroconversion**) of antibody by either of these tests constitutes definitive evidence of primary infection. Rising antibody levels are strongly suggestive of recently acquired infection but lack complete specificity because reactivation of infection may also elicit this response. High stable titers ($\geq 1/1000$) in single or paired sera should arouse suspicion of primary infection in the recent past; however, some individuals may maintain high antibody levels for long periods. From the practical standpoint, women with high stable titers during pregnancy carry little risk for transmitting infection to the fetus when compared to those with antibody rises.[63] In nebulous situations, an assay for the presence of IgM antibody by the IF test may prove useful.[66] Macroglobulin antibody production, in response to primary infection, mirrors that observed for the total or IgG moieties described above except in regard to persistence. It may disappear completely a few weeks to many months after onset or be intermittently manufactured, a finding in keeping with the chronic nature of toxoplasmosis. Thus, while the presence of this antibody cannot be taken as definitive evidence of recent primary infection, its absence speaks against this occurrence. Defining the interval between onset of infection and the assessment of the patient's humoral immune response is crucial for accurate diagnosis, but unfortunately it is only rarely possible because of the asymptomatic nature and endemic pattern of the infection. An optimal diagnostic approach, then, would entail large-scale serologic screening of pregnant women for toxoplasma antibody as early in gestation as possible. Those without previous infection should be serially studied during pregnancy, or only at delivery, to assess for seroconversion and antibody increases, thereby identifying neonates at risk.

Routes of Transmission

Congenital infection is believed to occur only as a consequence of primary maternal infection acquired during pregnancy by a mechanism similar to that described for rubella (*i.e.,* parasitemia → placentitis → hemotogenous spread to the fetus).[63] The prevalence of fetal infection then varies from locale to locale depending on the frequency of initial exposure to the protozoan among pregnant women. Thus, in Paris where toxoplasmosis is highly endemic, maternal infection remains quite common (5/100 pregnancies per year).[63] In this country, in contrast, more gravidas are susceptible but less frequently infected because of reduced exposure (0.15 to 0.6 per 100 pregnancies per year).[67]

Primary maternal infection does not, however, invariably spread to the fetus. Recent data from France suggest, in fact, that overall rate of transmission approximates 40%, and is inversely related to the time in gestation at which maternal infection occurred.[63] Fetal infection occurred in 66% of third trimester infections, while maternal acquisition in the first and second trimesters culminated in transmission to the offspring in 20% and 30% respectively. The mechanism of reduced transmission rates earlier in gestation is totally unexplained but may relate to a placental barrier effect, as has been postulated for syphilis.

Infection of subsequent offspring is theoretically possible because parasitemia of more than 14 months' duration has been documented; but, in fact, only one instance of infection in successive pregnancies, in which the second conception occurred within a few months of the termination of the first, has been reported.[68] An alternative explanation for this case, purely hypothetical, is the reactivation of infection in the uterus with contiguous spread to the fetus. Whatever the mechanism, such occurrences must be viewed as extraordinarily uncommon.

The causative role for maternal toxoplas-mosis in abortion with or without direct fetal involvement remains controversial. No convincing evidence has been presented linking acute maternal infection to fetal wastage or either primary or chronic involvement to habitual abortion.[63,69] However, a statistical association between chronic infection and sporadic abortion suggests a possible cause-and-effect relationship that is deserving of additional study.[69]

Nature and Diagnosis of Congenital Infection

Pathogenesis and Pathology. Following replication in the placenta, a fetal parasitemia ensues with dissemination to all organ systems. This blood-borne phase is presumably terminated by the appearance of serum antibodies, principally maternal in origin, but by analogy with postnatal toxoplasmosis it may persist for long periods. Early cellular events (only nucleated cells are parasitized) consist of rapid multiplication of trophozoites with resultant cell death and progressive infection of adjacent cells. As with parasitemia, contiguous spread is progressively terminated in the presence of antibody. Trophozoite infestation may, however, persist in fetal tissue for long periods as evidenced by their presence in necropsy material obtained from infants with lethal disease. A phase of slow growth then ensues during which an argyrophilic membrane is laid down forming an inactive tissue cyst.[70] Viable forms may persist in such cysts for years if not for life, retaining the capacity to reactivate.

Although definitive proof does not exist, damage may also be mediated by the host's own response to the parasite. Immune cytotoxicity (delayed hypersensitivity) likely plays a major role in the retinal and CNS pathology attending reactivation of infection in these sites in adults. The *de novo* appearance of chorioretinitis some months after birth in congenitally infected infants provides suggestive evidence for a similar occurrence in congenital infection. Whether this pathophysiologic mechanism is operative during acute fetal infection is unknown. The inflammatory response is variable in degree but consists of cells important in cell-mediated immunity (*i.e.,* lymphocytes, macrophages, and plasma cells).

Extension of parenchymal lesions to surrounding blood vessels may lead to vasculitis with thrombosis and infarction, particularly in the CNS. The genesis of the commonly observed hydrocephalus reveals the remarkable diversity of pathologic pathways available to this agent.[71] Toxoplasma enters the ventricular system from parenchymal lesions and disseminates there. The resulting inflammation of the ependymal cells in the aqueduct of Sylvius may lead to obstruction with the cephalad portion of the ventricular system becoming a functional abscess. With leakage of antigen-rich CSF back into the subependymal tissue, an antigen-antibody reaction occurs in the blood vessels leading ultimately to thrombosis and a periventricular zone of necrosis. Protein levels in ventricular fluid can consequently rise to quite high levels when compared to protein content of CSF obtained by lumbar puncture. Even at this site, though, protein levels are often impressively elevated, attesting to the destruction of brain substance even in the absence of gross changes in cranial volume.

Placentitis consists of small, often microscopic, foci of cellular necrosis with minimal inflammatory response. Vascular damage has not been a major finding.[72] The importance of these lesions, with respect to the tenative finding of increased rates of true gestational prematurity among congenitally infected infants, awaits definition.

The humoral immune response of the infected offspring closely parallels that of the rubella-infected infant with one important exception. Postnatal production of IgM-specific antibody continues for months to years. This probably reflects the continued low-grade nature of this infection.[73] As mentioned previously, whether specific cell-mediated immunity develops *in utero* is, for obvious reasons, unknown. That it is present shortly after birth, however, has been documented by positive reactions to the intradermal skin test.

Factors influencing the outcome of fetal infection are largely unknown. Desmonts has established that infection acquired earlier in gestation (2–6 months) is more likely to result in overt disease even though it is less likely to be transmitted during this time.[63] Severe or mild disease was observed in 80% and 50% of infants delivered of mothers who acquired infection in the first and second trimesters, respectively; whereas mild disease occurred in only 10% of their late-infected cohorts. The remaining patients in each gestational group

were inapparently infected. Virulence differences between strains, although documented experimentally in mice, have not been demonstrated to be a factor in human disease.[52]

Clinical Findings, Outcome, and Diagnosis. As with the other chronic intrauterine infections, clinically expressed disease in the neonatal period is the exception rather than the rule. Perhaps only 10% of infected infants manifest illness recognizable by routine observation. More recent prospective studies suggest, however, that this figure may increase to 30% if careful fundoscopic examinations are performed.[63,73] Those patients symptomatic at birth or shortly thereafter can be generally divided into two categories based on the observations of Eichenwald on 152 infants prospectively and longitudinally studied.[74] Approximately two-thirds manifested principally CNS disease, while in the remainder systemic illness with visceral involvement predominated. It remains to be determined whether these 2 forms are derived from different pathogenetic sequences, or merely reflect a pathologic continuum in which the CNS presentation denotes fetal infection of long standing, in which the visceral lesions have resolved.

The effect of this infection on intrauterine growth has received little systematic evaluation. In one small series of 10 infants with mainly inapparent infection, true gestational prematurity was a significant finding.[73] The true incidence of this complication and, indeed, any association with intrauterine growth retardation await larger studies. Congenital toxoplasmosis appears not to possess significant teratogenic potential.[63,74,75] The observation that maternal infection occurring before the eighth week of gestation is infrequently transmitted to the fetus may offer a partial explanation for this finding.[63]

Major clinical findings are detailed in Table 33-3. Among those with mainly nervous system dysfunction, chorioretinitis, abnormal CSF, convulsions, anemia, and intracranial calcifications are prominent lesions. Generalized involvement elicits manifestations referable mainly to the hemapoietic, reticuloendothelial and pulmonary systems as well as constitutional signs (*i.e.*, fever and vomiting). In this group, however, the occurrence of subclinical meningoencephalitis is quite common, as evidenced by the abnormal CSF findings. Indeed, qualitatively similar inflammatory changes in

Table 33-3. Clinical Findings in infants with Symptomatic Congenital
Toxoplasmosis.

Neurologic Disease 108 Patients		Generalized Disease 44 Patients
Percent	*Clinical Manifestation*	*Percent*
94	Chorioretinitis	66
55	Abnormal CSF	84
51	Anemia	77
50	Convulsions	18
50	Intracranial calcifications	5
29	Jaundice	80
28	Hydrocephalus	0
25	Fever	77
21	Splenomegaly	90
17	Hepatomegaly	77
17	Lymphadenopathies	68
16	Vomiting	48
13	Microcephalus	0
7	Diarrhea	25
5	Cataracts	0
0	Pneumonitis	41
1	Rash	25
2	Hypothermia	21
3	Abnormal bleeding	18
2	Glaucoma, optic atrophy and microphthalmus	0
	Sequelae	
76–100	Psychomotor retardation	76–100
51–75	Severe visual impairment	20–50
<20	Deafness	<20

(Adapted from Eichenwald HF: A study of congenital toxoplasmosis with particular emphasis on clinical manifestations, sequelae, and therapy. In Siim JC (ed): Human Toxoplasmosis. Copenhagen, Munksgaard, 1959)

the spinal fluid occur frequently, even with clinically silent infection. These CSF abnormalities are characterized by a disproportionate increase in protein levels relative to pleocytosis.[73] Likewise, retinal disease is a common pathologic finding regardless of the initial clinical presentation;[63,73] but unlike the inflammation attending CNS invasion, retinal disease may take weeks to months to develop. Therefore, initial lumbar punctures and serial ophthalmologic examinations are mandatory assessments both from the diagnostic and prognostic standpoint in all suspect cases. The spectrum of clinical presentations is tremendously variable, overlapping to a large extent with those of other infectious and noninfectious illnesses, and the individual lesions are not characteristic enough to have major diag-

nostic specificity. Perhaps only the combined findings of the so-called classic triad (*i.e.*, hydrocephalus, chorioretinitis, and periventricular calcifications) constitute sufficient evidence for a clinical diagnosis.

Lethal infection is relatively uncommon (12% in Eichenwald's series) and occurs with equal frequency in the neurologic and generalized forms. Although not well delineated, death results in most cases from severe CNS and occasionally pulmonary dysfunction. Visceral lesions tend to resolve spontaneously with no permanent sequelae in surviving infants.

The prognosis for patients manifesting CNS or eye pathology must be extremely guarded. Severe psychomotor retardation develops in the vast majority of such infants, being more marked in those with gross changes in cranial volume and cortical calcifications. This debilitation is made worse by a superimposed marked diminuition of visual acuity in perhaps 50%. A similar degree of visual handicapping later manifests in those with only eye involvement. Visual loss may range from small scotomata to total blindness, depending on the degree of macular or optic nerve involvement. Deafness poses an additional burden, fortunately in only a small minority of patients.

Even inapparent neonatal infection may not remain clinically silent. Prospective studies have established a late onset of chorioretinitis in some patients; and at least minor degrees of mental incapacitation seem probable given the CSF abnormalities noted during the neonatal period.[63,73] The validity of this assumption was recently suggested by the finding of significantly higher intelligence quotients in treated, as opposed to untreated, neonates when tested at 3 years of age.[73] In this same group of subjects, total ablation and grossly delayed development of IgA was observed in one and two patients, respectively. Whether similar and probably more severe aberrations of immunoglobulin development occur in symptomatic cases, deserves further study.

The chronic nature of this infection elicits concern regarding a continued low-grade pathologic process. The persistence of IgM-specific antibody and the precocious development of immunoglobulins M and G suggest an active, not dormant, infectious process in early life. Therefore, long-term management should provide for serial assessments of mental, motor, and perceptual functions as well as immunologic. If insidious pathology can be shown to be a feature of this infection, then early recognition and institution of effective therapy become all the more important.

The diagnosis of suspect cases is most readily confirmed by serologic testing. In symptomatic cases, attempts to isolate the organism from placental tissue or to demonstrate its presence in this organ by histologic examination can prove rewarding.[63] However, these latter techniques require considerable expertise, are cumbersome and expensive, and most important, offer a relatively low yield. Serial assessment during the first year of life for the persistence of total (Sabin–Feldman dye test) or IgG (IF) toxoplasma antibody will confirm or exclude the diagnosis in all instances. Potential pitfalls in the use of this evaluation include the occasional significant decrease in titer if initial levels were quite high, and the absence of IF IgG antibody in cord serum when maternal infection is acquired late in gestation.[73] In the former situation, titers stabilize after several months, while in uninfected infants, a progressive decline, equivalent to a one- to two-fold dilution per month, will continue until seronegativity is achieved. Late fetal acquisition will result in the appearance and progressive increase in antibody levels during the first few months. The obvious deficiency of this longitudinal approach is delay in diagnosis and consequently therapy; therefore, testing for a fetal humoral immune response (i.e., IgM antibody) offers considerable promise as a rapid means of identifying infected infants.

Macroglobulin antibody can be detected in cord sera of most symptomatic as well as subclinically infected neonates by the IF technique[73,76] and persists for variable periods usually measured in years. In contrast, uninfected neonates with sera reactive in this test will become negative within 1 to 2 weeks after birth.[73] Recent data, however, has demonstrated the fallibility of this assay. Both false positivity (common) and false negativity (rare) can occur even when highly purified batches of anti-human IgM conjugate are employed.[76] Even given these deficiencies, this test remains the best available means for rapid diagnosis and the only definitive method for large scale screening of neonatal populations for this infection. As an alternative screening procedure, quantiation of cord serum total IgM levels may be employed.[73] Most infected neonates, whether symptomatic or not, will manufacture excessive amounts of this immunoglobulin *in utero*. Because this response may reflect normality as well as other intrauterine infections, efforts should be made to diagnose these conditions as well.

Prevention and Therapy

At present, prevention can be achieved only by decreasing the risk of exposure among susceptible gravidas. Women may be screened for toxoplasma antibody as early in gestation as possible, and those found to be at risk should be advised to avoid situations in which acquisition is likely. Specifically, consumption of raw or undercooked meat products of any kind should be strictly terminated during pregnancy and even handling of raw meat might be done with gloved hands or at least followed by careful hand washing to insure against inadvertent ingestion or inoculation through conjunctivae or minor breaks in the skin. Household cats should be kept from hunting and fed only dry, canned, or cooked meat. For added safety, litter pan care should be delegated to someone else with instructions to clean daily before the oocysts have sporulated to an infectious state. Finally, soil potentially contaminated with cat feces should be avoided or handled with gloved hands followed by hand washing.

Prevention of fetal involvement by treating the maternal infection has been advocated and practiced by European workers with moderate success. Using spiramycin, Parisian investigators recently demonstrated a significant reduction in fetal transmission rates in treated, as opposed to untreated, mothers with primary infection; however, the number of symptomatic congenital cases in each group was the same.[63] The apparent inability of this drug to cross the placenta may explain these findings, with the implication that effecting a cure of fetal infection, once established, is not possible. With respect to therapeutic practice in this country, these observations are largely academic at present because spiramycin has not been licensed for this use. The administration of the alternative regimen, sulfadiazine and pyrimethamine, to infected pregnant women is to be assiduously avoided because of the possible teratogenic and other side effects of the latter agent.

In contrast, postnatal therapy with these two agents is recommended in all cases of congenital toxoplasmosis whether symptomatic or not. Although large scale studies demonstrating efficacy are yet to be done, preliminary results are encouraging,[73] and the risks of permanent sequelae far outweigh the acute potential toxicity. Because these synergistic antimicrobials work only on trophozoite forms, early initiation of therapy is essential for maximal benefit, a principle made all the more imperative if this disease proves to be progressive in nature. The dosage regimen consists of sulfadiazine at 100 to 150 mg/kg of body weight per day given in equally divided amounts every 6 hours, and pyrimethamine at 2 mg/kg of body weight per day administered in equal amounts every 12 hours for the first 72 hours, then decreased to 1 mg/kg for the remainder of the course. Both drugs are given orally for approximately 30 days. An intravenous preparation of pyrimethamine is available on request from Burroughs Wellcome & Co.* for the treatment of markedly debilitated infants. In order to avert or at least ameliorate the harmful effects of pyrimethamine (an antifolate) on rapidly growing cells (*e.g.,* bone marrow), folinic acid at a dose of 1 mg/kg of body weight should be administered intramuscularly once every day. Mandatory toxicity monitoring comprises platelet, white blood cell, and reticulocyte counts every 3 days for the duration of therapy.

CYTOMEGALOVIRUS

Epidemiology

Most women (50%–70%) have experienced cytomegalovirus (CMV) infection, as measured by FA antibody, upon entry into the childbearing years.[77,78] Higher rates are found in females of lower socioeconomic class,[79,80] although infection continues at low frequency throughout the child-bearing interval regardless of race or community status. Maternal infection, as monitored by congenital involvement, does not appear to have a seasonal occurrence.[81,82] Because CMV is species specific, man is the only reservoir of the virus, and transmission occurs by direct or indirect person-to-person contact. Sources and routes of transmission, proven and probable, other than intrauterine, include blood transfusion,[83] ingestion of breast milk, direct contact with infected cervical secretions at birth,[84] oropharyngeal secretions and urine postnatally, and venereal contact.[85] Respiratory spread is presumed to be dominant in childhood and possibly during adult life as well, although in adults acquisition by way of a venereal route undoubtedly assumes importance. An accurate measurement of the incubation period has been hampered by the absence of illness; however, estimates of 1 to 2 months have been derived from studies of natal and post-transfusion acquisition.[83,84] The duration of communicability is likely quite prolonged, regardless of time of infection. Viral excretion has

* 3030 Cornwallis Road
Research Triangle Park, N.C. 27709

persisted following congenital infection for as long as 8 years and commonly continues for 2 or more years with the natal and postnatal variety.[84,86] Further, it now appears possible that a given individual may intermittently become infectious for others, especially by way of a venereal route, throughout the reproductive life span.

Nature and Diagnosis of Maternal Infection

The incidence of maternal CMV infection, assessed virologically, is exceedingly high;[77,78] yet, clinically recognizable disease is a rare phenomenon.[79,80] An explanation for this apparent paradox rests with the observation that the great majority of gravidas are probably experiencing reactivation of infection.[77] CMV, like its kindred virus herpes simplex, probably persists in host tissues indefinitely. Chronic infection with intermittent excretion or latent involvement with periodic reactivation, reasonably accounts for the impressively elevated rates seen during pregnancy.[77] Common sites of viral replication in this form of infection (listed in decreasing order of frequency) are cervix, urine, and breast milk.[77,84] Such infection is apparently not accompanied by clinical or serologic evidence of active disease. However, clinical manifestations as yet unrecognized may exist as suggested by analogy with the reactivation syndromes of the herpes simplex and varicella—zoster agents. Even primary infection is usually asymptomatic[79] or nonspecific, although a heterophil agglutination-negative mononucleosis syndrome has been observed following blood transfusion and natural acquisition which, in one instance at least, resulted in transmission to the fetus.[86,87] This illness differs from classic infectious mononucleosis by the minimal-to-absent occurrence of tonsillopharyngeal involvement and lymphadenopathy, but it shares the typical hematologic and liver function test abnormalities. Nonspecific syndromes may present as febrile illness with myocarditis, hepatitis, or pneumonia. Reinfection may also occur, although this has not been adequately documented. Recognition of active maternal infection then entails serial examination for virus and determinations of antibody status during gestation.

In routine practice, at present, only those women manifesting the mononucleosis syndrome can be recognized clinically and definitively diagnosed by serologic testing. For the remainder, who constitute the vast majority, diagnosis is not available short of mass serologic screening done serially during gestation, which of course is impractical using current methodology. Attempts to identify at-risk pregnancies based on isolation of virus from urine, cervix, or both are unfeasible because such excretion is too infrequently associated with intrauterine transmission.[78,84] Recent investigations revealed a frequency of fetal infection consequent to maternal viruria of 38%,[79] 10%,[78] and 0%,[84] while cervical excretion is an even less adequate monitor (1.6%).[84] CMV is rarely present in the oropharynx during pregnancy,[84] and therefore any relationship between this finding and fetal infection awaits definition. Serology, therefore, is the most accurate diagnostic tool for identification of primary infection, which is currently held to pose the greatest risk to the fetus. Even here, limitations exist with regard to the most readily available antibody assay, complement fixation (CF).[88]

Diagnosis of initial infection requires the *de novo* appearance of CF antibody usually present within 2 to 3 weeks after onset of symptoms (mononucleosis) and peaking about 3 weeks thereafter.[86] Fourfold or greater increases in antibody titer reflect active infection which may occur with primary encounter, reactivation,[84] or reinfection, thereby lessening the importance of this finding relative to fetal risk.[77] The specificity of CF antibody appearance or increase has recently been called into doubt by the observation that this antibody moiety is quite labile in healthy adults, falling to undetectable levels with subsequent "diagnostic" increases.[88] Further, the possibility of antigenic differences between strains makes interpretation difficult because usually one strain, AD-169, is employed in the test system.[89] However, until newer antibody measurements achieve respectability, the CF test will remain a valuable, though somewhat tainted, serologic procedure.

Other tests of humoral immunity include neutralization, indirect hemagglutination, and fluorescent antibody (FA). The first is too laborious to be employed routinely and the latter two, although promising, have yet to stand the test of time and are therefore not routinely available. This last antibody assay is reported to be especially advantageous in regard to the diagnosis of primary infection because it can detect specific IgM as opposed to total antibody production. Classically, IgM antibody is made only in response to an initial encounter with a virus and disappears shortly thereafter. However, the unknown duration of IgM antibody response, its possible recurrence with activation and/or reinfection, and the cross-reactivity with other herpes viruses may render this method less diagnostic of a first exposure to this agent than might be expected.[90] It may well prove to be an accurate monitor of the activity of CMV infection regardless of the type of infection involved.

Routes of Transmission

Primary maternal infection often, though not invariably, culminates in transmission to the fetus.[78,79,87] The likely sequence of events is maternal viremia resulting in placentitis with subsequent spread to the conceptus. The relative frequency of fetal involvement given such disseminated maternal infection remains to be established as does the natural history of events (*i.e.*, duration of contagious maternal viremia and placental incubation period and barrier effect). Clearly, transmission may terminate at the placenta in a certain number of cases.[91] The paucity of information concerning the above happenings is mirrored and magnified when maternal reinfection and reactivation of infection are considered.

It is now an established fact, however, that previous CMV infection in the mother may not afford full protection during future pregnancies. In three separate instances, successive infants acquired infection *in utero*.[92,93,94] In one case, the mother became pregnant within 3 months after delivery of the first infected newborn.[92] Because infectious viremia may be quite prolonged, the possibility exists that the inordinately short interval between conceptions allowed for a unique transmission occurrence. Further, the feasibility of reinfection with a different strain of virus was not investigated. In the second case, however, the strains of virus isolated from the two neonates were shown to be quite similar, if not identical, antigenically and the interval between pregnancies approximated 3 years.[93] Therefore, it seems probable that activation of previous infection during gestation may result in fetal involvement. This hypothesis is made more credible by the occurrence of intrauterine infection in two pregnancies in which the mothers were known to be actively infected for a considerable time prior to conception.[92,93] Transmission to the fetus under these circumstances may occur by the following hypothetical routes: (1) transplacentally, by way of maternal viremia or local activation; and (2) transmembranously, by way of endometrial or cervical activation. The relative frequency of fetal infection secondary to primary versus recurrent maternal involvement is completely undefined and in need of urgent resolution because it bears directly on the problem of the feasibility of prevention by vaccination.

Perinatal transmission may occur as a result of exposure to infected cervical secretions at the time of delivery or by ingestion of virus-containing breast milk.[84] The former method of spread may be exceedingly common as evidenced by the 5% to 10% rate of acquisition in a low socioeconomic population in this country.[84] The risk of transmission by this route approximated 50% if virus was present in the cervix at delivery. A period of 4 to 8 weeks elapsed before viruria could be detected in most infants, though shorter and possibly longer intervals were also observed. Nosocomial infection acquired by way of transfused blood or contact with actively infected infants or nursery personnel remains an unproven possibility.

The high incidence of fetal (1 per 100 live births) and perinatal infection has been documented primarily in infants of low-income mothers. Whether gravidas of higher socioeconomic standing possess a similar infectious potential is largely unexplored.

Nature and Diagnosis of Fetal and Perinatal Infection

Pathogenesis and Pathology. Having gained access to the fetus, CMV can invade and replicate in virtually every organ, demonstrating a particular affinity for epithelial cells.[89] Occasionally, typical intranuclear inclusions are recognized in vascular endothelium, and, according to one account, may be especially susceptible if undergoing rapid proliferation.[89] The typical pathologic sequence is cytolysis with focal necrosis and resultant inflammatory response (mainly mononuclear). Healing may occur with fibrosis and occasionally calcification (brain and liver), or with restoration of normal structure in the continued presence of infected cells. The retardation of intrauterine growth has recently been related, in neonates with lethal disease, to a reduction in absolute number of cells in various organs as opposed to a diminution in cell size.[95] A comparable phenomenon occurs to a more striking degree in congenital rubella, possibly secondary to mitotic arrest. It remains to be determined whether CMV possesses a similar capability or whether such pathology is consequent to early cell destruction without replacement or possibly to vascular insufficiency secondary to endothelial injury. Resolution of this problem may further elucidate the embryopathic potential of the virus. Vascular demage (direct or obstructive) in the placental villi is an additional potential mechanism,[96] although here it is reasonable to expect the more classic findings of fetal malnutrition (*i.e.,* reduction in cell size). Such an event could be operative in the infected neonate whose only sign of outward illness is intrauterine growth retardation (IUGR). However, this question is likely to remain unresolved because such infants rarely die.

An immune response by the fetus is evidenced by the presence of elevated IgM levels[82] and specific CMV-IgM antibody[97] in cord serum. Immunoglobulin G antibody, predominantly maternally derived, is typically present in substantial amounts at birth, having been progressively acquired by the fetus since midgestation. Whether specific cellular immunity develops is unknown. Whatever defenses are marshaled, however, appear inadequate, because viral replication and excretion persist throughout intrauterine and long into extrauterine life. Clearly, such chronicity is not the result of the development of antigenic tolerance *in utero* because the production of specific antibody occurs for years, if not for life. Further acquisition of infection in adulthood also results in prolonged viruria.[86] The mechanism involved in this extraordinary example of parasitism is yet to be explained, but it is shared by other members of the herpes virus family. CMV, however, may be unique in its ability to persist in a productive fashion (*i.e.,* continued long-term excretion), giving rise to the concept that this infection may manifest as a chronic process with intermittent excretion in addition to latency with periodic activation. Given this circumstance, the po-

tential for low-grade continued tissue injury is increased.[82] Tissue tropism, local immune defenses, or both may have significance here with regard to sequelae. Excessive production of IgG, even after cessation of viral excretion, suggests the long-term residence of available antigen and hence the possibility of systemic (circulating antigen) or local (fixed-tissue antigen) immune complex disease.[82]

One pathogenetic feature of the natal acquisition of CMV is worthy of comment because of its implications relative to virus-versus-host interaction. This type of infection usually supervenes in the presence of appreciable amounts of maternally derived IgG antibody.[84] This phenomenon also occurs with natal herpes simplex virus type 2 infection. Passive humoral immunity may not be expected to prevent initial invasion and replication at the portal of entry but should, in fact, protect against subsequent viremia. An adequate explanation of this occurrence then presumes either a quantitative disproportion between the virus and antibody or sequestration of virus inside circulating blood elements with resultant protection against antibody. The infected blood element then may become infectious by way of direct cell-to-cell transfer of virus.

It is reasonable to assume, based on the tremendous spectrum of clinical disease, that a number of determinants of outcome, possessing a range of expressivity, must be operative in this infection. Many of these variables, mostly theoretical or inadequately proven, have been discussed in the previous sections. One additional factor, the type of maternal infection, needs to be considered here. Plausibly, infection in a nonimmune host (primary type) is more dangerous than reinfection or reactivation. Whether the severity of maternal illness correlates in any way with outcome, however, is a moot point at present. Regarding nonprimary infection, preexisting immunity seemingly would limit a viremic episode and thereby protect the placenta from the intensive exposure occurring with primary infection. Certainly, circulating antibody would abort extracellular viremia, but leukoviremia (presence of virus in lymphocytes or macrophages) may, indeed, persist in the presence of high levels of antibody.[98] Leukoviremia has been recently demonstrated in adults with apparent latent infection.[99] It remains to be

Table 33-4. Clinical Findings in Infants with Symptomatic Congenital Cytomegalovirus Infection.

Clinical Findings	Frequency
Intrauterine death	±
Prematurity	Unknown
Intrauterine growth retardation	+ +
Reticuloendothelial system	
Hepatitis	+ + +
Direct hyperbilirubinemia	+ + +
Hemolytic and other anemias	+ +
Petechiae-ecchymosis	+ + + +
Disseminated intravascular coagulopathy	±
Hepatosplenomegaly	+ + + +
Adenopathies	Unknown
CNS	
Encephalitis	+ + +
Microcephaly	+ +
Hydrocephaly	±
Intracranial calcifications	+ +
Eye	
Chorioretinitis	+
Congenital malformations	
Inguinal hernias	+ +
First brachial arch derivatives	+
Others	±
Myocarditis	±
Pneumonitis	+
Bone	
Vertical radiolucency	±
Sequelae	
Psychomotor retardation	+ + +
Hearing loss	+ +
Visual impairment	+

Frequency Classification

±	Rare
+	0% to 20%
+ +	21% to 50%
+ + +	51% to 75%
+ + + +	76% to 100%

determined whether such viremia may lead to placentitis or whether infected maternal leukocytes may be rendered infectious after having gained direct access to the fetal circulation. Irrespective of the route (*i.e.*, viremia or local uterine activation) a recurrence of maternal infection can result in fetal acquisition. Transmission secondary to reinfection (*e.g.*, cervical) may also occur, although this has not yet been proven.

Clinical Findings, Outcome, and Diagnosis. The spectrum of disease secondary to fetal infection is quite broad but with a marked skew toward asymptomatic infection at birth. Exact figures are unavailable but a reasonable estimate of subclinical infection would approximate 95% of the total.[79,81,82,100] For those with manifest neonatal illness, stigmata may range from isolated organ system compromise to multi-organ system dysfunction with life-threatening potential. Classically, the sick neonate presents with hepatosplenomegaly, hyperbilirubinemia (usually direct), thrombocytopenia with petechiae, and, occasionally, purpura, IUGR, and encephalitis with or without microcephaly. For the most part, the extraneural pathology is self-limited, with the occasional exception of protracted hepatitis; however, pneumonitis and myocarditis (rarely), severe thrombocytopenic purpura (occasionally), and disseminated intravascular coagulopathy (commonly) possess life-threatening potential. This last process should be excluded in any infant with evidence of a bleeding dyscrasia (including petechiae) because early therapy may significantly improve outcome. Fulminating encephalitis may also be incompatible with survival.

In lieu of microcephaly, neonatal CNS involvement may manifest as seizures, apnea, or focal neurologic signs. The frequency of accompanying cerebrospinal fluid signs of inflammation is undetermined, but clearly they may be absent. It is likely, however, that most symptomatically infected infants have some degree of encephalitis as evidenced by the frequent development of microcephaly and/or other neurologic dysfunction in the early months of life. Occasionally, the disease may have run its course *in utero*, resulting in microcephaly with or without intracranial calcifications in the absence of reticuloendothelial involvement.

Listed in Table 33-4 is a summary of associated clinical findings with expected frequency of occurrence. It is obvious that considerable overlap exists between CMV and the other chronic intrauterine infections, thereby necessitating laboratory confirmation in all cases.

The teratogenic potential of CMV has recently received an excellent review.[101] Defects in virtually every organ system have been associated with intrauterine acquisition of this virus; however, with most anomalies only one or two case reports exist, making a statistically valid cause-and-effect relationship virtually impossible to determine. Exceptions to this observation include inguinal hernia in males and possibly first arch abnormalities, which are more frequent.

To date, perinatal infection acquired through contact with cervical secretions or by other routes has not been associated with acute morbidity.[84,102]

Overt neonatal disease is likely a harbinger of later CNS and perceptual dysfunction.[103-105] Apparently, extraneural organs are spared chronic morbidity, with the possible exception of the liver, despite the fact that viral replication continues in the kidney, at least, for years. Microcephaly, present at birth or developing within the first year of life, is usually, although not invariably, associated with significant mental disability. Brain and perceptual organ pathology may manifest as mental retardation, spastic diplegia, seizures, optic atrophy, blindness, and sensorineural deafness alone or in combination. Such defects may also develop in children without any evidence of CNS involvement at birth. Lesser degrees of handicapping, such as specific defects in perceptual skills, learning disability, minor motor incoordination, and emotional lability, have also been recognized and may indeed become more apparent as more children are followed into the competitive arena of the classroom. Clearly, however, the major social impact of this infection rests with the long-term outlook for the 95% of children with inapparent involvement during the neonatal period.

Data are now accumulating which demonstrate that this type of infection indeed may not remain inapparent. Sensorineural hearing loss occurred in 50% of 18 children longitudinally studied, and in 4 the deficit was either a proven or probable handicap.[82] Further, in this group, there was a tendency toward lower intelligence quotients, with two displaying severe and moderate mental incapacitation, respectively. Retardadion of psychomotor development was found in 10% of another group of 20 young patients recently evaluated in this country.[100] Auditory function was not routinely monitored; however, one child was recognized as having a moderate sensorineural hearing loss. These findings were not corroborated by a third longitudinal investigation recently reported;[106] however, again hearing was not objectively tested. Obviously, additional follow-up is needed to define the scope of the problem, but now there can be little doubt that intrauterine CMV infection contributes significantly to the pool of mental and perceptual retardation heretofore labeled idiopathic.

The morbid potential of this agent *in utero* will be greatly expanded if current suspicions regarding the insidious pathologic course of the infection are confirmed.[82] This supposition is founded on longitudinal virologic and immunologic events. Viruria persists for years in most children despite continued production of specific antibody. In fact, excessive production of IgG may be a characteristic feature of this parasitism.[82] Two possible mechanisms for low-grade, long-term pathology then exist: direct cytolysis secondary to cellular viral replication, and immune complex injury. A precedent for such sequelae has been established with fetal rubella infection following the recent demonstration of late onset and possibly continued hearing loss in these children.[107]

Whether a similar morbid potential exists for natal or early postnatal CMV infection awaits delineation. Based on the similar patterns of viral excretion, it is reasonable to envision resultant morbidity.

The diagnosis of congenital infection is best confirmed by isolation of the virus, preferably during the first few days of life. Acquisition of virus at birth may result in shedding as early as 3 weeks[84] and, frequently, by 8 weeks, thereby rendering this assay less specific for intrauterine infection with advancing age of the patient. The preferred site for isolation attempts is urine, although virus is recoverable from throat, conjunctival, and rectal swabs as well as from white blood cells. The transport of specimens is best accomplished by packing in wet ice. Inoculated cultures should be observed for 4 weeks even though most will demonstrate cytopathologic effect (CPE) within 7 days. Lack of immediate access and expense of this test pose significant obstacles to its general use.

Cytologic examination of the urine sediment has the advantages of relative simplicity and availability, but its value is considerably decreased by the high rate of false-negatives even among neonates with classic disease.[89] The presence of large, intranuclear inclusion-bearing cells is presumptive evidence of infection, especially in the neonatal period; thereafter, similar cells may be shed secondary to adenovirus infection, resulting in a loss of specificity as well. This test may be employed for early diagnosis only when definitive virologic and serologic methods are unavailable and must be confirmed by serial assessment of the antibody status.

Serologic confirmation of overt neonatal infection can usually be obtained by demonstrating the presence of FA-IgM antibody in cord or baby sera.[97] However, the possibility that such antibody is of maternal origin, acquired either by maternofetal transfusion or by "placental leak" should be excluded by repeat determinations at 7 and 14 days. A significant drop in titer will occur in the former situation and macroglobulin activity will, of course, totally disappear if the latter phenomenon pertains. This caveat is issued because of recent data suggesting that maternal IgM antibody may persist for months following primary infection.[90] Although an IgM antibody response might reasonably be expected in all cases, with the exception of acquisition just prior to delivery, in fact, many neonates with inapparent infection show no macroglobulin antibody.[100] Whether this is a real phenomenon based on reduced viral mass or whether it represents technical difficulties is yet to be answered. Persistence of IgM is variable but likely measured in months. Its presence after the second month of life should not, however, be taken as evidence of intrauterine infection because infants acquiring infection at birth or shortly thereafter probably also respond with IgM antibody production. At present, technical difficulties severely limit the general availability of this laboratory aid.

The time-honored and technically easiest diagnostic method entails serial examination of the patient's serum for persistence of IgG antibody. In the absence of fetal or perinatal infection, maternally derived CF antibody will disappear from the infant's serum at the rate of approximately 1 dilution per month (IgG half-life is roughly 30 days). Because maternal antibody titers, in the absence of primary infection, rarely exceed 1:128, disappearance of passively transferred antibody would be expected by 6 months in the great majority of uninfected infants. Representative patterns of CF antibody response and viral excretion with various types of infection are displayed in

Figure 33-4. Antibody levels during the first 6 months of life are determined by the relative rates of catabolism of maternally derived antibody versus production of the patient's own antibody; therefore, the intensity of the infant's humoral response may dictate trends of increase, stability, or decrease in CMV specific immunoglobulin. Severe disease with presumably an increased replicating viral mass may be associated with vigorous early antibody production which can be sustained for prolonged periods (Fig. 33-4). Inapparent neonatal infection recognized in the basis of an elevated cord IgM level produces a similar response, although at lower production rates. Asymptomatic infants without an increase in total macroglobulin at birth (? reduced antigenic load) may respond in this fashion or manufacture antibody at rates commensurate with a substantial decrease in antibody titer. This latter pattern is typical for natally acquired infection as well, necessitating virologic proof in the neonatal period if congenital involvement is to be definitively confirmed. It should be noted, however, that most, if not all, patients maintain antibody activity throughout the first year. Thereafter, CF antibody gradually wanes. Unresolved, however, is the question of reappearance of this antibody in later years. In contrast to the varied antibody responses, viral excretion appears to be uniformly prolonged regardless of the initial presentation or subsequent antibody development.

Prevention and Therapy

Active prevention of fetal CMV infection is currently not possible. Although initial steps toward development of a live virus vaccine have been taken,[108] considerably more information concerning epidemiologic, pathogenetic, oncogenic, and virologic features of this infection must be acquired before deployment can ever be instituted. The administration of gamma globulin or hyperimmune sera holds little promise as a preventive, primarily because of our inability to recognize maternal infection. The only preventive measure currently available is the termination of pregnancy when *primary* maternal infection is diagnosed early in gestation.[87] This radical procedure, however, cannot be generally recommended until definitive information relative to transmissibility and outcome of infection are forthcoming.

Three antiviral chemotherapeutic agents,

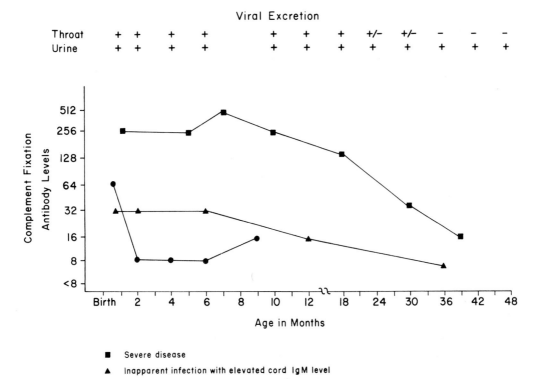

Viral Excretion

Throat	+	+	+	+		+	+	+	+/−	+/−	−	−	−
Urine	+	+	+	+		+	+	+	+	+	+	+	+

Fig. 33-4. Postnatal virologic and serologic events in congenital cytomegalovirus infection.

cytosine arabinoside (ara-C), 5-iodo-2′-deoxyuridine (IDU), and adenine arabinoside (ara-A), are currently being evaluated for use in this infection. Only the first of these agents is a licensed product. All appear to exert a virostatic effect with marginal improvement in clinical status. Significant toxicity occurs rapidly with ara-C and IDU while ara-A appears to have a much greater margin of safety, and thereby offers the most promise.[109] Chemotherapy may be employed only with a tremendous respect for the drugs' toxicity and then only in infants with marked morbidity. However, until current trials are completed, and safety and efficacy established, no recommendations can be made with respect to drug preference or dosage.

HERPES SIMPLEX VIRUS

Epidemiology

There are two distinct strains of herpes simplex virus (HSV) designated types 1 and 2, based on differing biologic, antigenic, and epidemiologic characteristics.[110] Type 1 virus

is spread by close personal contact, infects primarily the oropharynx, and is usually acquired during early childhood with increased rates among those in the lower socioeconomic strata.[111,112] In such a population, more than 75% of persons have been infected by adulthood, in contrast to 50% or less of those more well-to-do.[110,113] Type 2, in contrast, is transmitted venereally, infecting the genitalia, and is first seen at the time of initiation of sexual activity. The frequency of HSV-2 antibody among adults from low socioeconomic groups is between 20% to 60% in contrast to only about a 10% incidence in those achieving a higher position in the community.[110,113] Thus, many individuals' first contact with the genital strain (HSV-2) occurs subsequent to HSV-1 infection. The importance of this observation relative to fetal and neonatal transmission is considered in a later section.

Routes of transmission, other than direct personal contact, have not been demonstrated; in particular, it appears unlikely that breast feeding or blood transfusion are involved. The incubation period varies from 2 to 20 days with a mean of 6 days. The period of contagion is not so easy to define, although an approximation coincides roughly with the presence of lesions. The difficulty arises from the fact that most contagious subjects are unaware of their infectious potential (subclinical recurrence) and may serve as intermittent carriers and, therefore, silent disseminators for life.

Genital infection during pregnancy is quite common. Prospective cytologic and virologic screening of low-income gravidas established an overall rate of 1% while involvement at or near term fell to between 1/250 and 1/1000.[114] Similar data for private obstetric patients are unavailable but estimates of infection occurring at any time during gestation approximate 1 of every 1000 pregnancies.[114]

Nature and Diagnosis of Maternal Infection

Because the great majority of neonates acquired this infection at or immediately preceding birth from exposure to infected genital secretions,[115] this discussion will be essentially limited to maternal infection at this site. Although both herpes simplex virus (HSV) types 1 and 2 can infect the genitalia, the latter strain is the resident pathogen by virtue of being transmitted venereally.[113] As with CMV, HSV is a latent agent with a well-defined reactivation cycle; therefore, genital involvement during pregnancy may represent primary or recurrent infection (reactivation or possibly reinfection). Although subclinical disease is more likely with the latter process, unrecognized infection is also common upon first exposure to the genital strain.[114] One explanation for this occurrence in some patients is an ameliorating effect of previous Type 1 infection.[111,113] The ratio of inapparent (cytologically proven) to clinically recognizable disease approximates 2 to 1.[115] Distinction between primary versus nonprimary involvement is more than of academic interest because the former actively persists for a longer period of time and poses a greater risk for the perinate.[115]

Symptomatic primary infection is characterized by fever, malaise, local pain and tenderness, inguinal adenopathy (often painful) and vesiculoulcerative lesions.[116] Vesicles on erythematous bases may occur at any genital site and tend to ulcerate rapidly in moist locations (*i.e.,* vagina and cervix), thereby considerably lessening their specificity. Severe involvement may lead to coalescence with bullous formation, much erythema and edema, and, occasionally, a fungating cervical mass. The rash may persist for 3 to 6 weeks (average time of virus excretion, 30 days), accompanied by constitutional signs and symptoms for usually less than 1 week.[113,115,116] Nonspecific findings include dysuria, leukorrhea, and pelvic pain. A recurrence rarely elicits constitutional complaints, and lesions are often inconspicuous and difficult to identify. Typical involvement consists of localized patches of small vesicles with an erythematous halo accompanied by local pain and burning. Healing occurs within 7 to 10 days (mean excretion time, 16 days).[115] Rarely, a reactivation may be as incapacitating as that seen with the primary type. It bears repeating that clinical recognition of either type of infection is likely the exception rather than the rule because of their subclinical nature and the frequent localization to the cervix and vagina, which are relatively "silent" areas. Virologic and/or cytologic screening methods, therefore, are necessary to identify most cases of maternal HSV genital infection.

Although a variety of other localized (normal host) and disseminated (compromised host) infections occur in adults,[117] such maternal involvement has not been conclusively linked with transmission to the fetus or perinate and will not be considered here.

The gravida with symptomatic lesions (usually external) can often be diagnosed on clinical grounds alone. Accompanying constitutional signs strongly suggest primary infection, while with recurrent disease a history of a similar bout of illness is confirmatory. Definitive diagnosis can be made by isolation of the virus in tissue culture or by cytologic examination of cells obtained from the peripheral base of a lesion. The former test is relatively rapid (24–96 hours) and completely specific, but generally unavailable. However, the recent development of satisfactory transport media at ambient temperature should obviate this logistical problem.[118,119] Vesicular fluid obtained by needle aspiration or on a swab is the best source of virus. Cytologic diagnosis by conventional staining techniques is predicated on finding multinucleated giant cells and intranuclear inclusions.[120] Recently, a rapid and apparently type-specific test for HSV in cell scrapings has been devised using direct immunofluorescent staining.[121] For those women with silent cervical, vaginal, or both kinds of infection, identification necessitates screening with the virologic (cervicovaginal swab) or cytologic (Papanicolaou smear) laboratory aids.

Confirmation of maternal infection by serologic means is not a practical, or in fact a necessary, approach. Its main value rests with the differentiation of primary versus recurrent infection, but even in this circumstance, serial virologic assessments provide much more definitive information relative to clinical management. All the presently available assays, with the exception of CF, are technically intricate and generally unavailable.

Routes of Transmission

In contrast to the other agents discussed in this chapter, neonatal HSV infection is acquired primarily during the birth process by contact with infected genital secretions at delivery or by way of ascending infection following rupture of membranes.[115,122] Evidence for this observation rests mainly with the fact that 75% of neonates studied virologically with respect to the type of HSV were infected with type 2.[122] Factors favoring transmission include the presence of clinically overt genital lesions, primary infection as opposed to recurrence, and prolonged rupture of membranes. An increase in inoculum size probably accounts for the greater risk in the first two circumstances. Further, with primary infection, the absent or low levels of passively transferred maternal antibody may allow for the establishment of infection once exposed. The hazard posed by the loss of integrity of the protective membranes is obvious but deserves special emphasis because ascending spread may be quite rapid. In fact, transmission following rupture of membranes for 6 hours or longer is common, whereas abdominal delivery within 4 hours of membrane breakage prevents intrauterine spread in most instances (see prevention).[122] The onset of illness ranges from birth to 21 days, with a mean of 6 days.

The risk of transmission to the offspring when genital **lesions** are present at delivery has been estimated at 40% in one large prospective study.[114] However, long-term surveillance data gathered by these same investigators suggest that this figure may be too high. Indeed, the incidence of clinically apparent genital infection was 1 per 1000 deliveries, while recognizable neonatal disease occurred in only 1 in 7500 live births over a 9-year interval.[122] The possibility that inapparent or atypical neonatal cases go undetected could offer a partial explanation for this discrepancy. Transmission rates attending asymptomatic or unrecognized genital infection at term, which may occur as frequently as 1 in 250 to 450 pregnancies,[114]* have not been ascertained but are likely low compared to overt maternal involvement.

Fetal infection antedating the immediate perinatal period is exceedingly uncommon. Only a handful of cases have been described in which the presenting signs at birth (*i.e.,* microcephaly, intracranial calcifications, and chorioetinitis) suggested intrauterine infection of long standing.[123] In one of these cases, serologic and clinical evidence of primary maternal HSV-2 genital infection in early pregnancy was obtained, suggesting a blood-borne transplacental route of spread to the fetus.[124] This route is given further credence by the recent demonstration of HSV-2 in the buffy coat of two nonpregnant women with primary infection.[125] Unanswered is whether congenital transmission is associated only with primary maternal infection or whether local genital recurrences may spread directly to the conceptus with the protective uterine barriers intact. In either case, powerful inherent protective mechanisms must be operative considering the extraordinary rarity of this infection. Such factors may include a low incidence of primary HSV infection with either type during pregnancy, accompanied by a viremia of low magnitude and brief duration, the probable absence of viremia attending recurrences, fetal membrane and placental barrier effect, and the high rate of previous type 1 infection.

Transmission in the nursery from other infected infants or nursery personnel clearly may occur, although there is minimal evidence to support it. Recently, type 2 infection was documented in a 42-day old infant indirectly exposed in the nursery by means of shared nursing personnel to two other neonates with type 2 infection.[126] Further, the higher incidence of type 1 in neonatal infection (25% of total cases definitively studied) compared to genital infection (9%) may suggest acquisition in the nursery or at home.[122] However, in view

*Stagno S, Reynolds DW: unpublished observations, 1974

of the common occurrence of recurrent oral herpes in nursery personnel (estimated at 1% per week) and the general population,[126] it is somewhat surprising that more cases of type 1 neonatal infection are not documented. Protection occurring from passively acquired maternal type 1 antibody and awareness of the infectious nature of their lesions among nursery personnel may offer a partial explanation for this apparent paradox.

Nature and Diagnosis of Perinatal Infection

Pathogenesis and Pathology. The virologic and immunologic events of neonatal HSV infection generally resemble those of the other intrauterine viral infections and only the findings unique to this agent or of major pathogenetic or diagnostic import will be presented.

Following direct exposure, the neonatal host may limit the infection to the portal of entry (*i.e.,* skin, mouth, or eye) by mechanisms unknown, or suffer a disseminated process if initial defenses are inadequate. In the latter event, hematogenous spread occurs. Whether blood-borne virus has an intra- or extracellular residence is unknown but of considerable interest in view of the inability of passively transferred maternal antibody to uniformly block this occurrence.[115] In addition to viremia, adjacent sites can be involved by contiguous spread or possibly by a neurogenic route (brain or retina). With respect to the latter possibility, it is noteworthy that virus is rarely isolated from the CSF in cases of localized CNS infection, while recovery from this site is common with the disseminated form.[122]

Tissue injury occurs through direct and, in the case of many visceral organs, extensive cytolysis. Cell pathology is characterized by clumping of the nuclear chromatin and intranuclear eosinophilic inclusion bodies. Multinucleated giant cells may also be found. The inflammatory response of lymphocytes, plasma cells, and histocytes is usually present, though not invariably, in visceral lesions and surrounding smaller blood vessels. Areas of hemorrhagic infarction are common, suggesting that vasculitis may be an additional mechanism of tissue injury.

The recrudescence of corneal and skin disease is best explained by reactivation of virus which is latent in the sensory ganglion.[110] However, the appearance of new skin lesions suggests an alternative phenomenon such as chronically infected lymphocytes which periodically seed the integument.

With regard to virulence factors, the type of maternal infection is the most important determinant. As a generalization, primary maternal genital infection is likely to be associated with a higher rate of transmission and worse disease because of a greater inoculum (more extensive lesions) and the paucity of maternally transferred antibody in the neonate's serum. That passive acquisition of maternal antibodies is not completely protective, however, has been demonstrated in a small number of infants.[115] In order to clarify this issue, an attempt should be made to classify the type of maternal infection by serologic means in every case by analysis of paired maternal and cord sera. Ascending infection following rupture of membranes may also give rise to more severe infection by virtue of increasing the size of the infectious dose, gaining access through multiple sites, and theoretically by spreading to the fetus transplacentally.

Possible differences in the innate virulence of type 1 versus type 2 strains must be considered, but to date the severity and ultimate outcome of 74 HSV-2 and 31 HSV-1 infections have been virtually indistinguishable.[122] The one exception has been the occurrence of chorioretinitis only with type 2 infections; however, this may reflect simply the relatively small number of neonates virologically studied. Intrastrain variability with respect to virulence remains an undefined possibility.

With regard to host factors, it is interesting to note that localized infections have similar courses in neonates and older patients, while disseminated disease is a rarity in the immunologically competent adult and child. This finding evoked the concept of a functional deficit in cell-mediated immunity, specifically macrophages, in neonates. Animal data demonstrating protection of newborn mice following receipt of adult macrophages, the greater ability of virus to grow in neonatal as opposed to adult mice macrophages, and protection afforded suckling mice by BGG vaccination offer supportive evidence for this contention.[122]

Clinical Findings, Outcome, and Diagnosis. Neonatal HSV infection is almost invariably symptomatic and usually lethal; in fact, only two cases of inapparent infection have been

Table 33-5. Clinical Findings in Neonates with Herpes Simplex Virus
Infection.

Disseminated (½ to ⅔ of cases)		Localized (⅓ to ½ of cases)
Frequency	*Clinical Findings*	*Frequency*
	Constitutional	
+ +	fever	±
	Reticuloendothelial system	
+ +	Jaundice	Absent
+ +	Hepatomegaly	Absent
+	Splenomegaly	Absent
	Hematologic system	
+	Hemolytic or other anemias	Absent
+ +	Bleeding	Absent
	Central nervous system	
+ + +	Encephalitis	+ + +
+	Microcephaly	+
+	Intracranial calcifications	+
±	Meningitis	±
	Eye	
+	Conjunctivitis	+
+	Keratoconjunctivitis	+
+	Chorioretinitis	+
±	Cataracts	±
	Skin	
±	Maculopapular exanthem	Absent
+ +	Vesicular exanthem	+ + +
+	Vesicular enanthem	+
	Lung	
+	Pneumonitis	Absent
	Heart	
±	Pericarditis	Absent
±	Arrhythmia	Absent
+ + + +	Lethal outcome	+
	Sequelae	
+ + +	Psychomotor retardation	+ +
+	Visual impairment	+

Frequency Classification

±	Rare
+	0% to 20%
+ +	21% to 50%
+ + +	51% to 75%
+ + + +	76% to 100%

documented despite large-scale prospective attempts to identify such patients.[122] For prognostic, therapeutic, and pathogenetic considerations, sick infants may be divided into two groups based on the extent of involvement (see Table 33-5).[122] In the disseminated form, the illness usually commences at about 1 week of age with the onset of constitutional signs and symptoms, irritability or seizures, respiratory distress, jaundice, petechiae, or ecchymoses, a shock-like syndrome (rare), or vesicular exanthem alone or in combination. The vesicular rash, of major importance because of its diagnostic specificity, unfortunately occurs as the presenting sign in only a small number of infants; however, vesicles subsequently appear in almost 50%. In the absence of this dermatologic manifestation, a clinical diagnosis becomes exceedingly difficult because of the similarity of clinical findings relative to other infectious and noninfectious entities.

CNS involvement occurs in 50% of disseminated cases and commonly manifests as seizures, irritability, or both occasionally associated with bulging fontanel, opisthotonus, and pyramidal tract signs. Cerebrospinal fluid abnormalities typically consist of a moderate pleocytosis (50–200 WBCs/mm³) and a disproportionate elevation in protein levels (500–1000 mg/dl). A neurologic death supervenes in two-thirds of such patients.

In those without CNS lesions (as well as many with it), pathology of the hemapoietic, reticuloendothelial, and pulmonary systems are the prominent features of this illness. Of particular concern here, because of morbid potential, are pulmonary infection and a bleeding diathesis. Progressive pulmonary disease accounts for one-half of all deaths in this group with a shock-like syndrome often associated with evidence of disseminated intravascular coagulopathy comprising the lethal insult in the remainder.[127] The mortality rate with either form of disseminated infection (untreated) approximates 75% to 80%.

Between 30% and 50% of neonates will manifest disease in the CNS, eye, skin, or oral cavity without evidence of visceral involvement. Of infants diagnosed clinically to date (as opposed to those examined at necropsy) one-half of the total fell into this category, which may represent a more accurate ratio of localized to disseminated infection.[122]

The CNS disease resembles closely that seen in infants with visceral infection except for a later onset (11 days), the appearance of herpetic skin vesicles in virtually all cases, and the rarity of isolation of virus from the CSF (recovery common in the disseminated form). A fatal outcome can be expected in approximately one of every two patients.

Ocular involvement (uncommon as the primary site of infection) may present as conjunctivitis, keratoconjunctivitis, or more rarely chorioretinitis. The presence of corneal dendritic ulcers offers some diagnostic specificity. Chorioretinitis may appear without preceding external ocular infection.

Infection clinically limited to the integument

has been observed in approximately 10% of cases. Typical manifestations are discrete vesicles on erythematous bases varying in size from 1 mm to 1 cm in diameter; clusters of lesions are common. Presenting parts at delivery (*i.e.,* scalp and buttocks as well as the extremeties) are most frequently involved although eruptions may occur anywhere. Vesicles in neonates rapidly ulcerate, thereby lessening their diagnostic specificity. Such lesions occasionally induce scar formation. A unique feature of skin, oral, and perhaps corneal infection is a tendency for recurrences. Reappearance of lesions at the same and less frequently new sites have been observed for as long as 5 years after onset of the illness.[122] A vesicular enanthem is quite uncommon as an isolated finding but occurs in association with disseminated or other localized disease in as many as 30% of cases.

The prognosis for survivors with encephalitis, either the disseminated or localized form, is bleak. Psychomotor retardation, often severe, develops in 50% to 75% of such cases occasionally in association with microcephaly, hydrocephaly, or porencephalic cysts. These tragic sequelae may also supervene in those without clinically manifest CNS disease, although to a much lesser extent. Ocular infection may result in visual handicaps as a result of corneal scarring, chorioretinitis, cataracts, and in one instance, optic atrophy. Apparently isolated skin involvement is usually benign, although psychomotor retardation and serious ocular sequelae have been observed in some of these cases, suggesting that subclinical infection at other sites may induce significant pathology.[122] Whether damage can be progressive, as has been advocated for CMV, is uncertain at present; however, the recurrent nature of this infection, at least in the skin and eye, reasonably suggests the possibility of such an occurrence.

The diagnosis of this infection is difficult unless skin, oral, or corneal lesions are present. Even with the occurrence of these lesions, the diagnosis is often not entertained because the stigmata are overlooked or the index of suspicion is inadequate. A history of genital lesions in the mother or her sexual consort(s) may be helpful if present.

The appropriate deployment of laboratory aids is necessary to establish the etiology in most cases. Cytologic examination of material obtained from skin, mouth, conjunctival, or corneal lesions provides the most readily available and rapid means of confirming the diagnosis when such lesions are present (50% of cases). The peripheral base of the lesion is the preferred sampling site. Smears should be fixed in alcohol immediately, stained by the Papanicolaou method, and examined by a trained cytologist.[120]

The most definitive assessment of HSV infection entails recovery of the virus. Obviously, visible lesions are the preferred sites for isolation attempts. However, additional sites (i.e., throat, stool, conjunctivae, urine, and CSF) should be sampled to assess the extent of infection. For transport, clinical specimens should be frozen at −70°C and shipped in dry ice. Transport at ambient temperature is also possible with the use of selected media.[118,119] Herpes grows readily in virtually all tissue culture systems and, therefore, most virology laboratories can provide this diagnostic service. Determination of the type (i.e., 1 or 2) of the infecting strain requires more specialized assays but should be attempted in all cases for epidemiologic and pathogenetic considerations.[110] Direct identification of the virus in clinical or necropsy specimens including perhaps CSF leukocytes can also be accomplished by immunofluorescent techniques.[110,122] In order to determine the source of infection, a cervicovaginal sample from the mother should be assessed for the presence of virus by virologic, cytologic, or both methods.

As with the other congenital infections, assessment of this infection by classic serologic means is made impossible in many cases by the presence of maternally transferred IgG antibody which early on may mask the infant's own IgG response. Only in those instances in which the mother acquires primary genital infection late in gestation, before significant transfer of antibody to the fetus occurs, can an early diagnostic rise in antibody be demonstrated. Even in this instance, the delay in the infant's response will make this laboratory aid less rapid than those previously discussed. Serial assessment of the patient's sera during the first year for antibody levels to types 1 and 2 will eventually confirm the diagnosis even if type 1 infection supervened in the interim. Persistence of type 2 antibody into the latter half of the first year is absolutely confirmatory because the risk of infection with this agent during that time period is essentially nil. In fact, the demonstration of type 2 humoral immunity at any time before the onset of sexual activity constitutes presumptive evidence of perinatal acquisition. This finding cannot be interpreted as definitive evidence of neonatal infection because type 2 infection has been documented in children as a result of contact with infected adults.[128] Multiple serologic tests are available (i.e., CF passive hemagglutination, neutralization, inhibition passive hemagglutination, and immunofluorescence [IF]). The last three can be employed to detect type-specific antibodies but are available mostly in research laboratories.[122]

Analysis of infants's IgM specific-antibody response is the most rapid serologic means of establishing the infection.[129] As assessed in the IF test, this antibody moiety appears 1 to 2 weeks following onset of infection and persists for 6 to 12 months. The rarity of type 1 and certainly type 2 infection in infants less than 6 months of age makes the finding of IgM antibody in this age group suggestive of neonatal infection.

Therapy and Prevention

The previous general comments regarding the therapy of congenital CMV infection also pertain to neonatal herpes with a few important exceptions. Even given the unknown efficacy of these agents, the severe nature of the localized CNS and disseminated forms of this infection make therapy advisable in such cases.[122] Whether infants presenting with infection localized to the skin, mouth, or eye also should be treated is a moot point at present. Many of these patients do show a progression of infection with frank dissemination or spread to the CNS or internal portion of the eye. Hopefully, current studies will tell us when to treat, with which drug, and by what regimen.[130] For maximal therapeutic benefit, drug therapy must be initiated as soon as the diagnosis is established. Other therapies, including gamma globulin, hyperthermia, interferon stimulants, and BCG vaccine, have been advocated but as with the antiviral drugs, have yet to be adequately tested in infected neonates.

Active prevention of this infection by immunization of susceptible females is a desirable but currently unrealistic goal. Another approach would entail the eradication of virus from the genital tract by chemotherapeutic or other means; however, at present, no such measure is available. Clearly, therapeutic abortion as a preventive measure in cases of primary or recurrent genital or nongenital herpes in early pregnancy is absolutely contraindicated. Therefore, the only preventive approach of major promise is delivery by cesarean section when genital herpes is diagnosed close to the time of delivery. The effectiveness of this procedure is suggested by recent data demonstrating that only 1 of 16 infants delivered abdominally within 4 hours of membrane rupture developed infection, while transmission occurred in one-half of 20 infants delivered vaginally and in 6 of 17 delivered by cesarean section 6 or more hours following membrane breakage.[122] The great majority of these mothers, however, had clinically recognizable infection. The decision whether to intervene surgically when asymptomatic genital infection is fortuitously diagnosed by virologic or cytologic methods near term is an unresolved question. That silent genital infection can be transmitted to the offspring is suggested by the occurrence of type 2 infection in many neonates whose mothers denied genital lesions,[122] but the frequency of such occurrences is completely unknown. These findings suggest that cesarean section is warranted if genital lesions, especially internal, are present at the onset of labor but create a problem with respect to intervention in silent maternal infection. The latter instances must be individualized, considering the risk of the operative procedure against the outcome of infection in the infant. Attempts should be made, using a serologic assay, to determine whether the maternal infection is primary or recurrent because in the latter instance the risk to the infant is lessened. A similar assessment should be made with respect to maternal infection diagnosed earlier in the third trimester, thus allowing for an estimate of the duration of excretion, (*i.e.* 2–12 weeks with primary infection and 1–4 weeks with recurrent). More definitive information as to persistence should be sought, if possible, by serially assessing the presence of virus by tissue culture inoculation. Once the decision is made to intervene, cesarean section should be accomplished as soon after rupture of membranes as possible in order to abort ascending infection.

SYPHILIS

Syphilis, especially the congenital form, and its causative organism, *Treponema pallidum,* despite having been clinically recognized and actively investigated for generations, remains a medical enigma from many standpoints, not the least of which is pathogenesis. Huge gaps in knowledge, inadvertently maintained by the advent of effective antimicrobial therapy, persist with respect to an adequate delineation of the natural history of this disease entity. This is undoubtedly accounted for in large measure by the inadequate tools available to the investigators of the 1920s and 1930s and the lack of clinical material and resultant disinterest on the part of modern researchers. Therefore, this presentation of necessity will undertake a very pragmatic approach to the problem with major emphasis on the diagnosis of maternofetal infection.

Epidemiology

Syphilis, a classic example of a sexually transmitted or venereal disease, is currently increasing in frequency on a global scale.[131] The reasons for this burgeoning incidence are multiple and beyond the scope of this writing; suffice it to say that perinatologists must appreciate this fact and refamiliarize themselves with pertinent epidemiologic and clinical parameters of this infection. *T. pallidum* is transmitted (excluding fetal infection) only by direct contact with persons having lesions containing the organism.[132] Such contact almost invariably takes place during sexual intercourse or play. Acquisition by way of blood transfusion has all but been eliminated because of the universal serologic screening of blood donors. Indirect contact with contaminated fomites is of no practical significance. Postnatal infection, therefore, is essentially limited to sexually active persons with the highest rates of primary acquisition in this country: 15- to 25-year-old urban dwellers.[131] Although syphilis is now prevalent in all socioeconomic groups, low income persons, especially males, are at greater risk because of more promiscuous sexual habits.[131]

The mean incubation period to onset of clinical disease (*i.e.,* primary stage) is 21 days with a range of 10–90 days. Thereafter, for epidemiologic purposes, an infected individual experiences two or three additional stages of the disease process. The discussion here as well as in the clinical section to follow will be concerned only with early infectious syphilis (*i.e.,* primary, secondary, and early latency) because of its causal relationship with fetal infection. The secondary stage, also highly communicable if active lesions are present, usually commences 6 weeks (range, 2–24 weeks) following primary involvement. Though clinical relapses and subclinical spirochetemia may recur following this stage of clinical dissemination, the treponema commonly enter into a phase of stable symbiosis with the host which usually lasts for life. Clinical or asymptomatic recurrences (spirochetemia), when present, gradually diminish to virtual nonexistence within the first 2 to 4 years after initial infection;[133] this stage has been termed **early latency** and is of importance to the epidemiologist and perinatologist because such an individual remains a source of infection for the community at large as well as for her fetus in the case of pregnancy. In contrast, individuals with infection in later stages rarely transmit the disease vertically or horizontally.

Nature, Diagnosis, and Therapy of Maternal Infection

An adequate discussion of the clinical events of early infectious syphilis is impossible because of space limitations; therefore, only a few salient points referable to primary and secondary disease will be presented. The first concerns the location of the chancre, the typically painless, indurated ulcer occurring at the portal of entry. This lesion is often overlooked by the female patient and her physician because of its frequent location in the vagina or cervix, and also may be misdiagnosed by the physician if it is in an unusual location. The variety of sexual habits in vogue today may allow for its occurrence on the lip, tongue, tonsil, nipple, fingers, and anus in addition to the genital tract. To provide for the greatest index of suspicion, any ulcer appearing *de novo* during pregnancy at any site likely to have been involved in sexual activity should be considered syphilitic until proven otherwise by darkfield microcscopy.[132] Likewise, one

should view a generalized cutaneous eruption irrespective of its morphology as being caused by *T. pallidum* until the contrary is established. The ratio of asymptomatic to clinically apparent primary and secondary infection has not been well delineated. Thus, the physician must place great reliance on a diagnosis by serologic means. In order to use this laboratory tool most effectively, a basic understanding of the humoral immune reponse to *T. pallidum* is required.[132,134–136]

The antibody response is commonly measured against nontreponemal or reagin antigen, the widely used and studied assay being the VDRL (Venereal Disease Research Laboratory), although the RPR (rapid plasma reagin) is gaining increasing popularity. Although both employ a laboratory prepared cardiolipin, lecithin, and cholesterol mixture, the addition of choline chloride and finely divided carbon increases the sensitivity of the latter test by two- to eightfold in most laboratories. The disadvantages of these assays are the occurrence of occasional false-positive reactions following acute infections, immunizations, autoimmune disease, drug exposure and old age, and the tendency of the host with longstanding infection to discontinue production of these antibodies. These detriments are more than compensated for by universal availability, ease of performance, and most important, by the fact that reagin antibody responses most accurately reflect the host's response to antimicrobial therapy.

Specific or treponemal antibody assays circumvent the problem of false-positive reactions. Of these various tests, the fluorescent treponemal antibody-absorbed (FTA-ABS) assay offers the most sensitivity and a high degree of specificity, as well as measuring an antibody of apparent permanent duration. It is currently the method of choice for establishing the existence of humoral immunity to *T. pallidum.* In contrast to the VDRL antibody which is quantitated and expressed in terms of the highest dilution of serum which remains reactive, the FTA-ABS antibody is reported only qualitatively.

The dynamic aspects of the VDRL antibody response in relation to the progression of early infectious syphilis and therapeutic intervention is depicted in Figure 33-5. Usually within 1 week following the clinical manifestations of

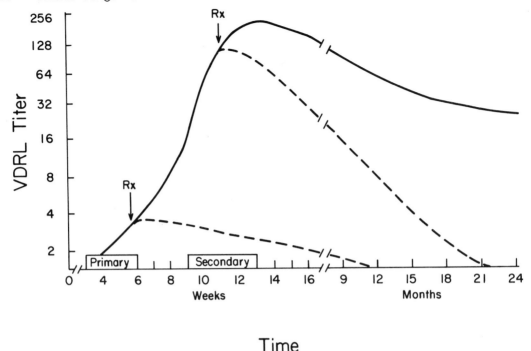

Fig. 33-5. VDRL antibody response in early syphilis according to therapy.

the primary stage, this antibody moiety appears in the serum, and with resolution of this phase approximately 75% to 90% of patients will become seropositive at low dilutions (*i.e.,* 2–8 dils). With onset of the secondary stage, the production of VDRL antibody to usually high levels (*i.e.,* 64 to 256 dils) is universal. Thereafter, this reagin antibody response gradually wanes to such a point that 30% to 50% of patients with late infection will become seronegative. Effective antimicrobial therapy during the primary and secondary stages will result in prompt resolution of clinical illness and a gradual reversion of the VDRL to negative in approximately 1 and 2 years in most cases.[132] Failure to serorevert during this interval is grounds for retreatment in the minds of a minority of syphilologists.[137] Adequate treatment of early latent (occasionally) and late latent or tertiary (frequently) fails to effect a seroreversal and the individual is said to be serofast. The events of FTA-ABS antibody development mirror those of the VDRL except for the important exceptions of permanent persistence and lack of responsiveness to therapy.[134]

Stability of the VDRL and certainly increases in titer following therapy of early infectious syphilis must be viewed as either relapse or reinfection. Though often difficult, distinction between the two should be attempted because the former necessarily implies treatment failure with the attendent specter of antimicrobial resistance (unproven to date) while the latter carries significance with regard to continued spread in the community. Reinfection is more likely to occur the earlier in the course of disease therapy was instituted; in general, exogenous reacquisition following the resolution of the secondary stage is uncommon. Estimates of the incidence of recurrent infection in this country within 2 years following therapy of primary or secondary stages approximate 10% of which about 67% represents reinfection.[138]

Benzathine penicillin in a single intramuscular dose of 2.4 million units remains the treatment of choice of early infectious adult syphilis. Some recommend repeating this regimen at 1 week following the first course; while still others contend that 10 daily doses of 600,000 units of procaine penicillin are necessary to effect a 100% cure rate.[137] Treatment with the first regimen has been shown to be quite efficacious regarding maternal and fetal infection.[139,140] though rare instances of fetal treatment failure have been documented when maternal disease is treated quite late in the third trimester. For the gravida with substantive evidence of penicillin allergy, erythromycin, given 4 times daily for 10 to 15 days for a total dosage of 30 g, is the alternative drug of choice at present.* Limited data suggest that inadequate fetal therapy with this drug may be not uncommon, probably because of relatively poor placental passage of the agent. Irrespective of the type of antimicrobial employed, careful initial and longitudinal evaluation of the offspring for evidence of infection becomes *mandatory*. The adequacy of maternal therapy should likewise be longitudinally assessed by serologic means, particularly during pregnancy. This becomes especially important in view of the high recurrence rate.

Diagnosis and management of the gravida with clinical, epidemiologic, microbiologic or serologic evidence of early infectious syphilis then poses no significant problem. Diagnostic dilemmas most often arise concerning the clinically asymptomatic gravida or parturient with low levels of VDRL antibody and no history of or treatment for syphilis. A check with the VD clinic of the local health department will frequently uncover dispositional information. In our experience, such a patient is usually found to have serofast syphilis following one or more courses of appropriate therapy. With this condition, the woman presents virtually no risk to her fetus, unless of course relapse or reinfection have supervened. This can be adequately assessed by comparing her present reagin antibody level to the most recent previous result. It should be noted that VDRL results *cannot* be compared to RPR levels in this situation, because of the relative difference in sensitivity. Rises in titer should be viewed as active infection and the neonate assessed accordingly. Should the VD clinic inquiry prove unfruitful, a determination of FTA-ABS antibody will provide a definitive answer regarding whether or not syphilis is present. A positive result would warrant therapy and referral of the mother to the VD clinic. Because

staging of this type of maternal infection is often impossible, the risk to the fetus cannot be ascertained and agressive follow-up is warranted.

Route of Transmission

From the practical standpoint, fetal acquisition of this infection occurs only by way of transplacental passage consequent to maternal spirochetemia. In assessing fetal risk, therefore, accurate staging of the maternal infection and, of course, previous therapy assume ultimate importance. Primary and secondary syphilis pose a high risk to the conceptus with transmission rates decreasing in a more or less linear fashion to quite low levels at the end of the early latent stage. In no case in untreated infection, however, can the risk factor be assumed to be zero; isolated instances of congenital transmission occurring as long as 20 years after primary maternal infection have been documented. Under such circumstances, the mother may lack reagin antibody. Another situation in which fetal infection may occur notwithstanding a negative VDRL result in the mother is when maternal infection supervenes quite late in gestation. Because the treponema is capable of widespread dissemination within hours or at least days after gaining access to host tissues, it is entirely possible for the pathogen to invade the fetus some weeks before clinical or serologic evidence of infection manifest in the mother.

Another factor often quoted as influencing fetal infection is gestational age. Maternal treponemia occuring before the 16th to the 20th weeks of pregnancy is thought not to result in transmission to the fetus.[141] Whether this is because of the protective barrier afforded by the layer of Langerhans or merely because of an inhospitable fetal tissue milieu, and whether or not this concept invariably pertains is, and will likely remain, a moot point. Others have suggested that this protective effect may be more apparant than real because recognition of lethal infection in young fetuses may be hampered by the absence of the characteristic inflammatory response.[142] The finding of normal abortion rates among syphilitic women, however, lends credence to this axiom.

Natal acquisition by means of contact with active maternal genital lesions represents another potential mode of transmission for offspring who escaped intrauterine infection.

Nature and Diagnosis of Congenital Infection

Pathogenesis and Pathology. Initial fetal invasion apparently begins with placental villitis manifested by intense proliferation of endo- and perivascular tissues as well as the supporting stroma.[143] Both processes may lead to vascular obliteration. Grossly, these changes result in nonedematous enlargement of the placenta, a finding which should suggest the possibility of fetal syphilis. Pathologic sequelae attending such placental abnormalities have not been adequately delineated but could well be manifest in the high rates of gestational prematurity. The role of placental injury in the genesis of fetal death remains unclear. It is interesting to note that inadequate nutrient transfer leading to IUGR seems not to occur.[144]

Subsequently, the organisms disseminate widely in fetal tissues. The duration of the spirochetemia and host factors influencing its termination are subjects of pure speculation but likely include the development of immobilizing antibody and perhaps cell-mediated immunity. Morphologic evidence for both events is suggested by the characteristically intense infiltration of plasma cells and lymphocytes into infected areas. The mechanisms whereby the treponema induces tissue damage are completely undefined. Although the production of a mild exotoxin has been implied, there is no direct evidence to support it. Unfortunately, the inability to grow *T. pallidum in vitro* severely limits study of all organism-related virulence factors. The host's contribution to his own morbidity, (*i.e.*, immunologic injury) has been adequately documented with respect to renal glomerular disease.[145] Whether a similar mechanism is operative with respect to other organ systems demands intensive investigation. Therefore, while the salubrious effects of the immature host's immune response to this infection remain in doubt, their existence, at least with regard to the humoral limb, is incontrovertible. Elevated total macroglobulin, often, and pathogen-specific IgM antibody, invariably, develop postnatally—depending on the duration of the disease *in utero*.[146] Further, the active production of IgG moieties against reagin, as well as treponema-specific antigens, uniformly occurs. The contribution of cell-mediated immunity toward outcome, either favorable or detrimental, remains completely unexplored. One indisputable fact, however, is that host defenses unaided by chemotherapy are incapable of terminating the infection in a sizable number of cases, as evidenced by the development of late stigmata (*e.g.*, interstitial keratitis).

Histopathologically, the interaction of the microbe and host produces characteristic findings consisting of obliterative endarteritis and intense infiltration of the interstitial stroma.[132] These reactions occur in virtually every organ system but are most intense in the liver, spleen, bone, pancreas, and kidney. The end result of this potent inflammatory response is necrosis resulting from vascular occlusion and compression atrophy.

Parameters influencing outcome of established infection, other than appropriate therapy, cannot even be speculated on at present, with the possible exception of the stage of maternal disease. A less intense fetal exposure may be reasonably expected with the transient spirochetemias of advanced disease.

Nature and Diagnosis of Congenital Infection. In contrast to the other chronic intrauterine infections, syphilis as a rule manifests itself clinically within the first few months of life; however, only a small percentage of infected infants will display signs or symptoms of diagnostic significance during their nursery stay.[133,147] The exception to this generalization is most often the premature infant, either by virtue of a more severe disease process or long nursery sojourn. Therefore, initial suspicions of the perinatal physician are usually grounded on positive maternal serologic results.

The common and most important clinical features of early congenital syphilis are displayed in Table 33-6.[132,133,147,148] As with the other infections previously discussed, the spectrum and nature of abnormalities overlap considerably with other disease entities. However, syphilis is unique among this group in that it induces several lesions of considerable diagnostic significance. The most clinically recognizable of these is dermal eruption. Though rashes may be quite pleomorphic in nature, discrete, symmetrical, papulosquamous lesions are the most common, and predilection for oral, anogenital, and intertriginous areas as well as palms and soles offer specificity. Raised, flat, moist plaque-like lesions, grayish in color, are virtually pathognomonic. Though not often a clinical finding, except in instances of pseudoparalysis (*i.e.,* inactivity resulting from pain on motion of affected extremities), long bone involvement produces pathognomonic radiographic changes consisting of irregular calcification of the distal metaphysis (osteochondritis) and periosteal elevations in the same region (periostitis). The occurrence of generalized adenopathy, an uncommon response in early infancy, should suggest a syphilitic cause. Other classic stigmata, only occasionally present should strongly implicate *T. pallidum* infection; these include purulent snuffles, hemorrhagic rhinitis and rhagades (radiating scars around the anus and corners of the mouth). Cerebrospinal fluid pleocytosis, protein elevations, and/or positive reagin titers are frequently encountered but infrequently forebode manifest acute CNS pathology.[147] When CNS disease does supervene, prominent features are spasticity, bulging fontanel, behavioral changes, and, occasionally, seizures. The relative rarity of an associated glomerulopathy leading to nephrotic syndrome belies the extraordinary importance of the recent finding of an immune complex etiology for this entity.[145] The implications of this discovery with respect to long-term sequelae in untreated and perhaps even treated patients should undoubtedly draw considerable research interest in the coming years.

The mortality in untreated early infection is high, ranging from 10% to 30%.[147,148] In spite of this, causes and mechanisms of death have been inadequately studied or at least reported; therefore, an assessment of prognosis based on the pathology at the time of presentation is unclear to the authors. Clearly, though, profound CNS and pulmonary embarrassment portend an unfavorable outcome, as does marasmus and general obtundation. The long-term morbidity attending untreated late congenital syphilis can be quite incapacitating when the brain and perceptual organs are involved. These pathologic phenomena (*i.e.,* neurosyphilis, eighth nerve deafness, and interstitial keratitis) commonly manifest around the time of puberty, and this quite prolonged latent period has given rise to speculation concerning an immunopathologic etiology.

Diagnosis in the immediate neonatal period then must rely heavily on appropriate serologic investigation of all instances of positive reagin tests in maternal or cord blood samples. In

Table 33-6. Clinical Findings in Infants with Symptomatic Early Congenital Syphilis.

Clinical Findings	Frequency
Intrauterine Death	+ +
Prematurity	+ +
Intrauterine growth retardation	?
Reticuloendothelial system	
Hepatitis	+ + +
Direct hyperbilirubinemia	+ +
Hemolytic and other anemias	+ + +
Petechiae	+
Disseminated intravascular coagulopathy	?
Hepatosplenomegaly	+ + +
Adenopathy	+ + +
CNS	
Abnormal cerebrospinal fluid	+ +
Meningoencephalitis	+
Hydrocephalus	±
Skin	
Polymorphic rashes	+ + +
Mucocutaneous lesions	+ +
Bone	
Osteochondritis	+ + + +
Periostitis	+ + +
Eye	
Iritis	±
Chorioretinitis	±
Pneumonitis	+
Myocarditis	±
Renal	
Glomerulopathy	±
Sequelae	
Psychomotor retardation	+
Sensorineural hearing loss	+
Corneal inflammation	+
Teeth deformities	+
Bone deformities	+
Joint disease	+

Frequency Classification

±	Rare
+	0% to 20%
+ +	21% to 50%
+ + +	51% to 75%
+ + + +	76% to 100%

each case of suspect congenital syphilis, one's initial efforts should be directed toward establishing the existence, stage, and therapy of maternal infection as a necessary first step toward evaluating the occurrence of fetal involvement. A logical scheme for the investigation of maternal infection has been previously described.

Because reagin antibody (*e.g.,* VDRL) is comprised primarily of IgG, positive results in cord or baby serum may merely reflect maternal infection; therefore, confirmation of fetal infection necessitates the demonstration of persisting reagin antibody (beyond the time passive antibody would catabolize) and/or the presence of specific IgM antibody by the immunofluorescent technique.[146] Initial findings in the infant's reagin test *suggestive* of fetal involvement are titers of $\geq$ 32 dils and/or levels fourfold or greater than that simultaneously observed in maternal serum. Conversely, it must be remembered that on rare occasions, a neonate may be infected *in utero* and not possess reagin antibody in his serum. The presence of *T. pallidum*-specific IgM antibody, as determined by the FTA-ABS IgM assay, is confirmatory. A recent prospective study from South Africa, where congenital syphilis remains endemic, unequivocally demonstrated the diagnostic value of this test, allowing for a clear differentiation between infected infants and those pseudoinfected by virtue of having been delivered of a mother with reagin antibody.[149] This test, however, is technically difficult and quite variable in sensitivity and reproducibility, depending on the quality of the fluorescein conjugated antihuman IgM antibody. Both false-positive and false-negative results may occur. Until the vagaries of antigen, conjugate, and reference human serum can be standardized, it is suggested that suspect sera be analyzed by a reference laboratory such as the Venereal Disease Research Laboratory of the Center for Disease Control in Atlanta. Macroglobulin antibody production usually commences shortly though variably after dissemination of the pathogen, and therefore its presence in the circulation may be delayed in some instances for a few days to weeks following birth.[146]

In addition to the initial serologic approach, the following should be obtained on all suspect cases: darkfield microscopy of all suspicious lesions (best specimen is expressed lesion fluid followed by deep scrapings of the periphery), lumbar puncture, histopathologic examination of the placenta, and, most important, x-ray films of the long bones. It must be emphasized that the pathognomonic radiographic changes will not be manifest until after the second to the fourth week in most cases. Diagnostic follow-up for nebulous cases, which comprise the majority of VDRL positive infants, is best accomplished by weekly or at least fortnightly assessments of reagin and IgM antibody levels, clinical status, and radiography of the long bones. The frequency of follow-up may be modified according to the risk imposed by the nature of the maternal infection.

Prevention and Therapy

The cornerstone, obviously, of prevention and therapy of fetal syphilis is prompt recognition and treatment of maternal infection. This is best accomplished by assaying maternal serum for reagin antibody at the **first prenatal visit** and again **at delivery.** Even this surveillance system will not allow for detection of a large percentage of syphilitic infants (*i.e.,* those infected mothers not availing themselves of prenatal care) which in 1973 accounted for 50% of the total cases.[131] Bringing these gravidas into the fold of medical care remains one of the most challenging problems for the whole of preventive perinatology.

An adequate understanding of the therapeutic disposition of the infection requires the recognition of two important, interrelated facts. First, the replicative time of *T. pallidum* by binary fission is approximately 30 to 33 hours. Second, the organism is extraordinarily sensitive to low levels of penicillin (*i.e.,* 0.001 to 0.01 μg/ml of serum).[140] The import of these findings is that effective penicillinemia may only require small amounts of drug, but such levels must be maintained for prolonged periods empirically estimated at 10 days or more based on animal experimentation.[139]

Treatment, therefore, of the syphilitic woman with 2.4 million units of benzathine penicillin either before or during the first 16 weeks of pregnancy may be presumed to effect prevention of fetal infection, assuming of course that neither treatment failure nor reinfection occurred in the interim before delivery. These events can and should be checked for by appropriate serologic and clinical follow-up of the gravida during pregnancy. After the sixteenth week, fetal cure is achieved in most instances with this regimen, in which maternal levels of 0.03 μm/ml of serum will be maintained for at least 2 weeks. Of the alternative antimicrobials—tetracycline, cephaloridine, and erythromycin—the last currently appears the most suitable because of enamel hypoplasia with the first and potential fetal nephrotoxicity with the second agent. Any of the 3 available forms of erythromycin appear suitable for preventive fetal therapy; however, the estolate agent is recommended when one is attempting cure of fetal infection.* Any and all forms of maternal therapy should be viewed as inadequate for the fetus until the contrary is established upon longitudinal follow-up. This is especially important in instances of late third trimester acquisition.

The chemotherapeutic management of postnatal congenital syphilis in relation to severity of disease has been discussed above. One additional comment should be made here. Late stigmata of congenital infection,[150,151] and indeed in one case report persistence of active infection,[152] have been documented, penicillin notwithstanding. These provocative findings demand long-term and longitudinal follow-up of all treated infants with the aim of better understanding the peculiar relationship between this interesting microbe and its host.

REFERENCES

Rubella

1. **Horstmann DM:** Rubella. The challenge of its control. J Infect Dis 123:640, 1971
2. **Witte JJ, Karchmer AW, Herrmann KL et al:** The epidemiology of rubella. National Communicable Disease Center, Health Services and Mental Health Administration, Atlanta, Ga, 1969
3. **Potter JE, Banatvala JE, Best JM:** Interferon studies with Japanese and U.S. rubella virus. Br Med J 1:197, 1973
4. **Best JM, Banatvala JE:** Studies on rubella virus strain variation by kinetic hemagglutination-inhibition tests. J Gen Virol 9:215, 1970
5. **Rawls WE, Melnick JL, Bradstreet CMP et al:** WHO collaborative study on the seroepidemiology of rubella. Bull WHO, 37:79, 1967
6. **Dowdle WR, Ferreira W, Gomes LFD et al:** WHO collaborative study on the sero-epidemiology of rubella in Caribbean and Middle and South American populations in 1968. Bull WHO 42:419, 1970
7. **Heggie AD, Robbins FC:** Rubella in naval recruits. A virologic study. N Engl J Med 271:231, 1964
8. **Green RH, Balsamo MR, Giles JP et al:** Studies of the natural history and prevention of rubella. Am J Dis Child 110:348, 1965
9. **Cooper LZ:** Rubella. A preventable cause of birth defects. Birth Defects, Original Article Series, National Foundation—March of Dimes 4:23, 1968
10. **Alford CA, Neva FA, Weller TH:** Virologic and serologic studies on human products of conception after maternal rubella. N Engl J Med 271:1275, 1964
11. **Hildebrandt HM, Maassab HF:** Rubella synovitis in a one-year-old patient. N Engl J Med 274:1428, 1966
12. **Heggie AD:** Pathogenesis of the rubella exanthem. Isolation of rubella virus from the skin. N Engl J Med 285:664, 1971
13. **Plotkin SA:** Rubella virus. In Lennette CH, Schmidt NS (eds): Diagnostic Procedures for Viral and Rickettsial Infections 4th ed, pp 364–413. Am Pub Health Assoc, 1969
14. **Lennette EH, Schmidt NJ:** Neutralization, fluorescent antibody and complement fixation tests for rubella. In Friedman H, Prier JE (eds): Rubella, pp 18–32. Springfield, Ill, Charles C Thomas, 1973
15. **Horstmann DM, Liebhaber H, LeBouvier GL et al:** Rubella. Reinfection of vaccinated and naturally immune persons exposed in an epidemic. N Engl J Med 283:771, 1970
16. **Horstmann DM, Pajot TG, Liebhaber H:** Epidemiology of rubella. Subclinical infection and occurrence of reinfection. Am J Dis Child 118:133, 1969
17. **Strannegard O, Holm SE, Hermodsson S et al:** Case of apparent reinfection with rubella. Lancet 1:240, 1970
18. **Krugman S (guest ed):** Proceedings of the International Conference on Rubella Immunization, Am J Dis Child 118:133, 1969
19. **Ogra PL, Kerr-Grant D, Umana G et al:** Antibody response in serum and nasopharynx after naturally acquired and vaccine-induced infection with rubella virus. N Engl J Med 285:1333, 1971
20. **Forghani B, Schmidt NJ, Lennette EH:** Demonstration of rubella IgM antibody by direct fluorescent antibody staining, sucrose density gradient centrifugation and mercaptoethanol reduction. Intervirology 1:48–59, 1973
21. **Rudolph AJ, Yow MD, Phillips A et al:** Transplacental rubella infection in newly born infants. JAMA 191:843, 1965
22. **Catalano LW Jr, Fuccillo DA, Traub RG, Sever JL:** Isolation of rubella virus from

---

* Rein MF: Personal communication. Venereal Disease Control Division, Center for Disease Control, 1974

placentas and throat cultures of infants: A prospective study after the 1964–65 epidemic. Obstet Gynecol 38:6, 1971

23. Menser MA, Harley JD, Hertzberg R et al: Persistence of virus in lens for three years after prenatal rubella. Lancet, 2:387, 1967

24. Monif GRG, Sever JL: Chronic infection of the central nervous system with rubella virus. Neurology 16:111, 1966

25. Horstmann DM, Banatvala JE, Riordan JT et al: Maternal rubella and the rubella syndrome in infants. Am J Dis Child 110:408, 1965

26. Peckham GS: Clinical and laboratory study of children exposed in utero to maternal rubella. Arch Dis Child 47:571, 1972

27. Alford CA Jr: Congenital rubella: A review of the virologic and serologic phenomena occurring after maternal rubella in the first trimester. South Med J 59:745, 1966

28. Schiff GM, Sutherland J, Light L: Congenital rubella. In Thalhammer O (ed): Prenatal Infections, pp. 31–36. International Symposion of Vienna, Sept 2–3, 1970. Stuttgart, Georg Thieme Verlag, 1971

29. Phillips GA, Melnick JL, Yow MD et al: Persistence of virus in infants with congenital rubella and in normal infants with a history of maternal rubella. JAMA 193:1027, 1965

30. Butler NR, Dudgeon JA, Hayes K et al: Persistence of rubella antibody with and without embryopathy: A follow-up study of children exposed to maternal rubella. Br Med J 2:1027, 1965

31. Alford CA Jr: Immunoglobulin determinations in the diagnosis of fetal infection. Pediatr Clin North Am 18:99, 1971

32. Alford CA Jr: Studies on antibody in congenital rubella infections, I. Physicochemical and immunologic investigations of rubella neutralizing antibody. Am J Dis Child 110:455, 1965

33. Gitlin D: The differentiation and maturation of specific immune mechanisms. Acta Paediatr Scand 172 (suppl):60, 1967

34. Alford CA, Blankenship, WJ, Straumfjord, JV, Cassady G: The diagnostic significance of IgM-globulin elevations in newborn infants with chronic intrauterine infections. Birth Defects 4:5, 1968

35. Gitlin D, Biasucci A: Development of γG, γA, γM, β1C/β_1A, C'l esterase inhibitor, ceruloplasmin, transferrin, hemopexin, haptoglobin, fibrinogen, plasminogen, α_1-antitrypsin, orosomucoid, β-lipoprotein, α_2-macroglobulin, and prealbumin in the human conceptus. J Clin Invest 48:1433, 1969

36. Lawton AR, Self KS, Royal SA, Cooper MD: Ontogeny of B-lymphocytes in the human

fetus. Clin Immunol Immunopathl 1:104, 1972

37. Alford CA Jr: Fetal antibody in the diagnosis of chronic intrauterine infections. In Thalhammer O (ed): Prenatal Infections, pp. 53–69. International Symposium of Vienna, Sept. 2–3, 1970. Stuttgart, Georg Thieme Verlag, 1971

38. Töndury G, Smith DW: Fetal rubella pathology. J Pediatr 68:867, 1966

39. Driscoll SG: Histopathology of gestational rubella. Am J Dis Child 118:49, 1969

40. Dudgeon JA: Teratogenic effect of rubella virus. Proceedings of the Royal Society of Medicine 63:1254, 1970

41. Boué A, Boué JG: Effects of rubella virus infection on the division of human cells. Am J Dis Child 118:45, 1969

42. Chang TH, Moorhead PS, Boué JG et al: Chromosome studies of human cells infected in utero and in vitro with rubella virus. Proc Soc Exp Biol Med 122:236, 1966

43. Naeye RL, Blanc W: Pathogenesis of congenital rubella. JAMA 194:1277, 1965

44. Krugman S (ed): Rubella symposium. Am J Dis Child 110, 1965

45. Forrest JM, Menser MA: Congenital rubella in schoolchildren and adolescents. Arch Dis Child 45:63, 1970

46. Sheridan MD: Final report of a prospective study of children whose mothers had rubella in early pregnancy. Br Med J 2:536, 1964

47. Ames D, Plotkin SA, Winchester RA, Atkins TE: Central auditory imperception: A significant factor in congenital rubella deafness. JAMA 213:419, 1970

48. Weinberger MM, Masland MW, Asbed R, Sever JL: Congenital rubella presenting as retarded language development. Am J Dis Child 120:125, 1970

49. Wyll SA, Herrmann KL: Inadvertent rubella vaccination of pregnant women: Fetal risk in 215 cases. JAMA 225:12, 1973

50. Fleet WF, Benz EW Jr, Karzon DT et al: Fetal consequences of maternal rubella immunization. JAMA 227:621, 1974

51. Abrutyn E, Herrmann KL, Karchmer AW et al: Rubella vaccine comparative study: Nine-month follow up and serologic response to natural challenge. Am J Dis Child 120:129, 1970

Toxoplasmosis

52. Jacobs L: Toxoplasma gondii: Parasitology and transmission. Bull NY Acad Med 50:128, 1974

53. Frenkel JK: Toxoplasma in and around us. BioScience 23:343–351, 1973

54. **Wallace GD:** Experimental transmission of *Toxoplasma gondii* by cockroaches. J Infect Dis 126:545, 1972

55. **Desmonts G, Convreur J, Alison F et al:** Etude Epidemiologique sur la toxoplasmose: De l'influence de la cuisson des viandes de boucherie sur la frequence de l'infection humaine. Rev Franc Etud Clin Biol 10:952, 1965

56. **Kean BH, Kimball AC, Christenson WN:** An epidemic of acute Toxoplasmosis. JAMA 208:1002, 1969

57. **Peterson DR, Tronca, E, Bonin P:** Human toxoplasmosis: Prevalence and exposure to cats. Am J Epidemiol 96:215, 1972

58. **Reynolds D, Stagno S, Stubbs K et al:** Prevalence of toxoplasmosis in pregnant women: The cat as a vector. Program and Abstracts, 14th Interscience Conference on Antimicrobial Agents and Chemotherapy, 1974

59. **Wallace GD, Marshall L, Marshall M:** Cats, rats, and toxoplasmosis on a small Pacific island. Am J Epidemiol 95:475, 1972

60. **Feldman HA:** Toxoplasmosis: An overview. Bull NY Acad Med 50:110, 1974

61. **Feldman HA:** Toxoplasmosis. N Engl J Med 279:1370, 1431, 1968

62. **Remington JS:** Toxoplasmosis in the adult. Bull NY Acad Med 95:211, 1974

63. **Desmonts G, Couvreur J:** Congenital toxoplasmosis: A prospective study of 378 pregnancies. N Engl J Med 290:1110, 1974

64. **Miller MJ, Arouson WJ, Remington JS:** Late parasitemia in asymptomatic acquired toxoplasmosis. Ann Intern Med 71:139, 1969

65. **Dorfman RF, Remington JS:** Value of lymphnode biopsy in the diagnosis of acute acquired toxoplasmosis. New Engl J Med 289:878, 1973

66. **Remington JS, Miller MJ, Brownlee I:** IgM antibodies in acute toxoplasmosis: II. Prevalence and significance in acquired cases. J Lab Clin Med 71:855, 1968

67. **Kimball AC, Kean BH, Frech F:** Congenital toxoplasmosis: A prospective study of 4,048 obstetric patients. Am J Obstet Gynecol 3:211, 1971

68. **Garcia AGP:** Congenital toxoplasmosis in two successive sibs. Arch Dis Child 43:705, 1968

69. **Kimball AC, Kean BH, Fuchs F:** The role of toxoplasmosis in abortion. Am J Obstet Gynecol 111:219, 1971

70. **Jacobs L:** Propagation, morphology, and biology of toxoplasmosis. Bull NY Acad Sci 64:154, 1956

71. **Frenkel JK:** Pathology and pathogenesis of congenital toxoplasmosis. Bull NY Acad Med 50:182, 1974

72. **Driscoll SG:** Fetal infections in man. In Benirschke K (ed): Comparative Aspects of Reproductive Failure. New York, Springer-Verlag, 1967

73. **Alford CA, Stagno S, Reynolds DW:** Congenital toxoplasmosis: Clinical, laboratory and therapeutic considerations, with special reference to subclinical disease. Bull NY Acad Med 50:160, 1974

74. **Eichenwald HF:** A study of congenital toxoplasmosis with particular emphasis on clinical manifestations, sequelae, and therapy. In Siim JC (ed): Human Toxoplasmosis. Copenhagen, Munksgaard, 1959

75. **Talhammer O:** Die Angeborene toxoplasmose. In Kirchhoff H, Kraubig H (eds): Toxoplasmose. Stuttgart, Georg Thieme Verlag, 1966

76. **Remington JS, Desmonts G:** Congenital toxoplasmosis: Variability in the IgM fluorescent antibody response and some pitfalls in diagnosis. J Pediatr 83:27, 1973

CMV

77. **Stagno S, Reynolds DW, Smith R, Alford CA:** Cervical cytomegalovirus excretion in pregnant and nonpregnant women: Suppression in early gestation. Program and Abstracts, 13th Interscience Conference on Antimicrobial Agents and Chemotherapy, 1973

78. **Nankervis GA, Cox FE, Kumar ML, Gold E:** A prospective study of maternal cytomegalovirus and its effect on the fetus. Pediatr Res 6:125, 1972

79. **Stern H, Tucker SM:** Prospective study of cytomegalovirus infection in pregnancy. Br Med J 2:268, 1973

80. **Montgomery R, Youngblood L, Medearis DN:** Recovery of cytomegalovirus from the cervix in pregnancy. Pediatrics 49:524, 1972

81. **Starr JG, Bart RD, Gold E:** Inapparent congenital cytomegalovirus infection: Clinical and epidemiologic characteristics in early infancy. N Engl J Med 282:1075, 1970

82. **Reynolds DW, Stagno S, Stubbs KG et al:** Inapparent congenital cytomegalovirus infection with elevated cord IgM levels: Causal relation with auditory and mental deficiency, N Engl J Med 290:291, 1974

83. **Lang DJ, Hanshaw JB:** Cytomegalovirus infection and the postperfusion syndrome: Recognition of primary infections in four patients. N Engl J Med 280:1145, 1969

84. **Reynolds DW, Stagno S, Hosty TS, et al:** Maternal cytomegalovirus excretion and perinatal infection. N Engl J Med 289:1, 1973

85. **Jordan MD, Rousseau WE, Noble GR et al:** Association of cervical cytomegaloviruses

with venereal disease. N Engl J Med 288: 932, 1973

86. **Klemola E, Essen VR, Wager O et al:** Cytomegalovirus mononucleosis in previously healthy individuals. Ann Intern Med 71:11, 1969

87. **Davis LE, Tweed GV, Stewart JA:** Cytomegalovirus mononucleosis in a first trimester pregnant female with transmission to the fetus. Pediatrics 48:200, 1971

88. **Waner JL, Weller TH, Kevy SV:** Patterns of cytomegaloviral complement-fixing antibody activity: A longitudinal study of blood donors. J Infect Dis 127:538, 1973

89. **Weller TH:** The cytomegaloviruses: Ubiquitous agents with protean clinical manifestations. N Engl J Med 285:203, 267, 1971

90. **Langenhuysen M:** IgM levels, specific IgM antibodies and liver involvement in cytomegalovirus infection: Report of 17 patients. Scand J Infect Dis 4:113, 1972

91. **Hayes K, Gibas H:** Placental cytomegalovirus infection without fetal involvement following primary infection in pregnancy. J Pediatr 79: 401, 1971

92. **Embil JA, Ozere RL, Haldane EV:** Congenital cytomegalovirus infection in two siblings from consecutive pregnancies. J Pediatr 77: 417, 1970

93. **Stagno S, Reynolds DW, Lakeman A et al:** Congenital cytomegalovirus infection: Consecutive occurrence due to viruses with similar antigenic compositions. Pediatrics 52: 788, 1973

94. **Krech U, Konjajev Z, Jung M:** Congenital cytomegalovirus infection in siblings from consecutive pregnancies. Helv Paediatr Acta 26:355, 1971

95. **Naeye RL:** Cytomegalic inclusion disease: The fetal disorder. Am J Clin Pathol 47:738, 1967

96. **Monif GR, Dische RM:** Viral placentitis in congenital cytomegalovirus infection. Am J Clin Pathol 58:445, 1972

97. **Hanshaw JB:** Congenital cytomegalovirus infection: Laboratory methods of detection. J Pediatr 75:1179, 1969

98. **Lang DJ:** Cytomegaloviremia following congenital infection. J Pediatr 73:812, 1968

99. **Diosi P, Moldovan E, Tomescu N:** Latent cytomegalovirus infection in blood donors. Br Med J 4:660, 1969

100. **Melish ME, Hanshaw JB:** Congenital cytomegalovirus infection: Developmental progress of infants detected by routine screening. Am J Dis Child 126:190, 1973

101. **Hanshaw JB:** Developmental abnormalities associated with congenital cytomegalovirus infection. Adv Teratol 4:64, 1970

102. **Levinsohn EM, Foy HM, Kenny GE:** Isolation of cytomegalovirus from a cohort of 100 infants throughout the first year of life. Proc Soc Exp Biol Med 132:957, 1969

103. **McCracken GH, Shinefield HR, Cobb K:** Congenital cytomegalic inclusion disease: A longitudinal study of 20 patients. Am J Dis Child 117:522, 1969

104. **Weller TH, Hanshaw JB:** Virologic and clinical observations on cytomegalic inclusion disease. N Engl J Med 266:1233, 1962

105. **Medearis DN:** Observations concerning human cytomegalovirus infection and disease. Bull Johns Hopkins Hosp 114:181, 1964

106. **Kumar ML, Nankervis GA, Gold E:** Inapparent congenital cytomegalovirus infection. N Engl J Med 288:1370, 1973

107. **Peckham CS:** Clinical and laboratory study of children exposed in utero to maternal rubella. Arch Dis Child 47:571, 1972

108. **Elek SD, Stern H:** Development of a vaccine against mental retardation caused by cytomegalovirus infection in utero. Lancet, 1:1, 1974

109. **Ch'ien LT, Cannon NJ, Whitley RJ, Diethelm AG et al:** Effect of adenine arabinoside on cytomegalovirus infections. J Infect Dis 130: 32, 1974

Herpes Simplex

110. **Nahmias A, Roizman B:** Herpes simplex viruses. N Engl J Med 289:667, 719, 781, 1973

111. **Nahmias A, Josey W, Naib Z et al:** Antibodies to Herpesvirus hominis types 1 and 2 in humans: I. Patients with genital herpetic infections. Am J Epidemiol 91:539, 1970

112. **Smith IW, Peutherer JF, MacCallum FO:** The incidence of Herpesvirus hominis antibody in the population. J Hyg 65:395, 1967

113. **Rawls WE, Gardner HL, Flanders RW et al:** Genital herpes in two social groups. Am J Obstet Gynecol 110:682, 1971

114. **Nahmias AJ, Josey WE, Naib ZM:** Significance of herpes simplex virus infection during pregnancy. Clin Obstet Gynecol 15: 929–938, 1972

115. **Nahmias AJ, Josey WE, Naib ZM et al:** Perinatal risk associated with maternal genital herpes simplex virus infection. Am J Obstet Gynecol 110:825, 1971

116. **Kaufman RH, Gardner HL, Rawls WE et al:** Clinical features of herpes genitalis. Cancer Res 13:1446, 1973

117. **Nahmias AJ:** Infections caused by Herpesvirus hominis. In Hoeprich PD (ed): Infectious Disease, pp 841–852. Hagerstown, Harper & Row, 1972

118. **Nahmias A, Wickliffe C, Pipkin J et al:** Transport media for herpes simplex virus types 1 and 2. Appl Microbiol 22:451, 1971

119. **Rodin P, Hare MJ, Barwell CF, Withers MJ:**

Transport of herpes simplex virus in Stuart's medium. Br J Vener Dis 47:198, 1971

120. **Naib ZM, Nahmias AJ, Josey WE, Zaki SA:** Relation of cytohistopathology of genital herpesvirus infection to cervical anaplasia. Cancer Res 13:1452, 1973

121. **Rubin SJ, Wende RD, Rawls WE:** Direct immunofluorescence test for the diagnosis of genital herpesvirus infection. Appl Microbiol 26:373, 1973

122. **Nahmias AJ, Visintine AM:** Herpes simplex. In Remington JS, Klein JO (eds): Infectious Diseases of the Fetus and Newborn Infant, pp 156–190. Philadelphia, WB Saunders, 1976

123. **Florman AL, Gershon AA, Blackett PR, Nahmias AJ:** Intrauterine infection with herpes simplex virus. JAMA 225:129, 1973

124. **South MA, Tompkins WAF, Morris CR, Rawls WE:** Congenital malformations of the central nervous system associated with genital type (type 2) herpesvirus. J Pediatr 75:13, 1969

125. **Craig CP, Nahmias AJ:** Different patterns of neurological involvement with herpes simplex virus types 1 and 2: Isolation of herpes simplex virus type 2 from the buffy coat of two adults with meningitis. J Infect Dis 127:365, 1973

126. **Francis DP, Herrmann KL, MacMohon JR, Chavigny KH:** Maternal and hospital acquired neonatal herpesvirus hominis infections: A report of four fatal cases. 1974

127. **Miller DR, Hanshaw JB, O'Leary DA, Hnilicka JV:** Fatal disseminated herpes simplex virus infection and hemorrhage in the neonate. J Pediatr 76:409, 1970

128. **Nahmias AJ, Dowdle WR, Naib ZM et al:** Genital infection with herpesvirus hominis types 1 and 2 in children. Pediatrics, 42:659, 1968

129. **Nahmias A, Dowdle W, Josey W et al:** Newborn infection with herpesvirus hominis types 1 and 2. J Pediatr 75:1194, 1969

130. **Ch'ien LT, Whitley RJ, Nahmias AJ et al:** Antiviral chemotherapy and neonatal herpes simplex virus infection, a pilot study: Experience with adenine arabinoside (Ara-A). Pediatrics 55:678,1975

Syphilis

131. **Today's VD Control Problem. New York, American Social Health Association,** 1974

132. **Syphilis:** A synopsis. Washington, D.C., Public Health Service Publication No. 1660, U.S. Department of Health, Education and Welfare, 1968

133. **Whipple DV, Dunham EC:** Congenital syphilis, part I: Incidence, transmission and diagnosis. J Pediatr 12:386, 1938

134. **Sparling PF:** Diagnosis and treatment of syphilis. N Engl J Med 284:642, 1971

135. **Wilkinson AE:** Recent progress in venereal disease: Serology of syphilis. Br Med J 2:573, 1972

136. **Wallace AL, Norins LC:** Syphilis serology today. In Stefanini M (ed): Progress in Clinical Pathology, Vol. 2, pp 198–215. New York, Grune & Stratton, 1969

137. **Fiumara NJ:** Venereal diseases. In Charles D, Finland M (eds): Obstetric and Perinatal Infections, pp 456–478. Philadelphia, Lea & Febiger, 1973

138. **Schroeter AL, Lucas JB, Price EV, Falcone VH:** Treatment for early syphilis and reactivity of serologic tests. JAMA 221:471, 1972

139. **Jackson FR, Vanderstoep EM, Knox JM, Desmond MW, Moore MB:** Use of aqueous benzathine penicillin G in the treatment of syphilis in pregnant women. Am J Obstet Gynecol 83:1389, 1962

140. **Idsoe O, Guthe T, Willcox RR:** Penicillin in the treatment of syphilis. Bull WHO 47:1972

141. **Dippel AL:** The relationship of congenital syphilis to abortion and miscarriage and the mechanism of intrauterine protection. Am J Obstet Gynecol 47:369, 1944

142. **Silverstein AM:** Ontogeny of the immune response. Science, 144:1423, 1964

143. **Russell P, Altshuler G:** Placental abnormalities of congenital syphilis. Am J Dis Child 128:160, 1974

144. **Naeye RL:** Fetal growth and congenital syphilis: A quantitative study. Am J Clin Pathol 55:228, 1971

145. **Wiggelinkhuizen J, Kaschula ROC, Uys CJ, Kuijten RH, Dale J:** Congenital syphilis and glomerulonephritis with evidence for immune pathogenesis. Arch Dis Child 48:375, 1973

146. **Alford CA Jr, Polt SS, Cassady GE, Straumfjord JV, Remington JS:** γM-Fluorescent treponemal antibody in the diagnosis of congenital syphilis. N Engl J Med 280:1086, 1969

147. **Platou RV:** Treatment of congenital syphilis with penicillin. Adv Pediatr 4:39, 1949

148. **Nabarro D:** Congenital Syphilis. London, Edward Arnold, 1954

149. **Rosen EU:** A reappraisal of the value of the IgM fluorescent treponemal antibody absorption test in the diagnosis of congenital syphilis. J Pediatr 1975

150. **Oksala A:** Interstial keratitis after adequate penicillin therapy. Br J Vener Dis 33:113, 1957

151. **Bernfeld WK:** Hutchinson's teeth and early treatment of congenital syphilis. Br J Vener Dis 47:54, 1971

152. **Rayn SJ, Hardy PH, Hardy JM, Oppenheimer EJ:** Persistence of virulent treponema pallidum despite penicillin therapy in congenital syphilis. Am J Ophthalom 73:258, 1972

34

Surgery of the Neonate

Judson G. Randolph,
R. Peter Altman,
and Kathryn D. Anderson

To bring any major neonatal surgical procedure to a successful conclusion, cooperation between the neonatologist and pediatric surgeon is of great importance. The regulation of parenteral fluid and electrolytes, antibiotics, and other supportive drugs is best directed, as in the case of adult surgery, by the surgeon. Intrathoracic procedures and the chest tube, bowel anastomoses, and the intraperitoneal status are examples of occasions when mechanical considerations in the healing surgical patient must be considered in the postoperative decisions. When respiratory support is needed and for the special metabolic considerations in the premature optimal care is provided when the neonatologist and surgeon work in close cooperation. Together they can assure comprehensive care throughout the postoperative phase.

General Considerations

Because gastric emptying occurs rapidly in the infant, prolonged preoperative starvation is not warranted. Extended periods without food and water may result in dehydration in small babies. In the normal infant, 6 hours of fasting is adequate to assure that the stomach will be empty.[1]

Fluid administration during major surgery requires an intravenous tubing of adequate size. In all but the smallest premature infants, a cannula adapted to a No. 18 needle can be used. This is introduced by cutdown or, when possible, percutaneous puncture. Central venous pressure monitoring by way of a catheter advanced to the superior vena cava is feasible and provides important information relating to fluid and blood replacement during and after major surgery.[2] In neonates, cannulation of the radial or superficial temporal artery provides access for serial blood gas monitoring.[3]

The most critical intraoperative concern is the thermolability of the infant. The temperature of the operating room itself must be kept uncomfortably warm for the surgical team in order to provide a safe environment for the baby. Many operations on premature infants can be done in the isothermic environment of an infant warmer. In the operating room, cautious, direct surface warming by heat lights will prevent cooling during the induction of anesthesia as well as during emergence from surgery. Precautions must be exercised to prevent burning from heat lamps.

When the need for blood is anticipated, it is prewarmed, as are irrigating solutions prior to use. The temperature is monitored by means of a rectal or cutaneous thermocouple and the surgical team strives for maximal efficiency, especially when the bowel or thoracic viscera are exposed and body heat can be lost. When the environmental temperature falls below the thermoneutral zone for an infant, his metabolic activity increases.[4] The increased metabolic work required to restore normal body temperature results in an accumulation of potentially toxic metabolites detrimental to the infant. The importance of maintaining the infant in a warm thermoenvironment cannot be overemphasized.

Throughout the surgical procedure, blood must be replaced with precision. Sponges are weighed or carefully estimated with the realization that the amount of blood absorbed in one or two sponges can account for profound hypovolemia in a neonate.

Postoperative monitoring implies meticulous attention to fluid balance including those losses induced surgically by creation of enterostomies. Serial measurements of hematocrit and electrolytes as well as serum osmolality serve as a guide for fluid replacement in the postoperative phase. Although the infant's kidney is an efficient organ, his ability to concentrate urine is not as well developed as the adult's. Even in a dehydrated baby, the urine osmolality rarely exceeds 500 mosm/liter. Serial measurement of urine volume, osmolality, and specific gravity permit one to recognize important trends in the dynamics of fluid equilibrium.[5]

Postoperative fluid therapy includes maintenance requirements and replacement of losses. Gastrostomy and ileostomy drainages are measured, their electrolyte content determined and replacement tailored to the individual needs. The infant's losses are replaced regularly at 8-hour intervals because the deficits incurred in 24 hours can be excessive. The successful management of many of these fragile subjects depends upon strict adherence to the principles of management outlined above.

LESIONS OF THE HEAD AND NECK

Congenital abnormalities of the head and neck occur commonly in the newborn. Because of the short, fat neck of the baby some of these lesions are not immediately apparent and the examiner must be alert to their possibility in order to detect them.

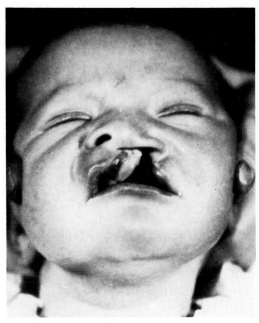

Fig. 34-1. Complete congenital cleft of the lip with associated cleft of the palate extending forward through the alveolar ridge.

Cleft Lip

Congenital clefts of the face are most common in the upper lip.[6] They occur because of improper fusion of the anterior and lateral processes which develop into major components of the face between the fourth and eighth weeks of fetal life. The defect is more common in males and there seems to be an ill-defined hereditary relationship.

Single clefts in the lip range from a simple notching to a complete defect extending from the border of the lip through the floor of the nostril on either side of the midline. A complete cleft of the lip may occur with no additional defect of the palate or may be associated with a partial or complete cleft palate. (Fig. 34-1) Bilateral congenital clefts occur about half as often as do single clefts. Bilateral or double-lip clefts are almost always associated with a bilateral defect in the alveolar ridge and usually with a cleft in the palate. Bilateral cleft lip and clefts of the alveolar ridge cause the entire premaxilla to extend forward, presenting a bizarre appearance and a more complicated problem in reconstruction.

In rare instances, a cleft is observed in the midline of the upper lip. This is almost always associated with microcephaly and poor brain development and careful neurologic evaluation is necessary in children with this unusual finding.

Treatment. Although repair of a cleft lip can be accomplished in the first day of life, the approach favored by many is to wait 2 to 6 weeks before surgery is undertaken. This delay has salutory features. Congenital anomalies not immediately apparent may come to light. A second major benefit is psychological; if the mother sees, recognizes, and takes home her baby for a period of time to love and establish the maternal-infant bond, then improvement by subsequent surgery reinforces this relationship. Conversely, if the baby is operated upon immediately, the mother may view the subsequent scar and necessary imperfection with resentment and negativity.

There are a number of different types of repair for the single complete cleft lip.[7] All have as their major goal the restitution of the cupid's-bow shape of the vermilion border of the lip, and a rejoining of the labial musculature to derive optimal appearance and function. This is usually accomplished with a series of measured flaps of skin, mucous membrane, and muscle so constructed as to minimize scarring.

Bilateral lip clefts are more complicated because of the absence of tissue and the forward thrust of the entire premaxilla. While early closure of the skin is possible, major revisions of the bony arch of the alveolar ridge, the premaxilla, and the palate require a number of additional procedures during the growing years of the child.[6] Reconstructive surgery is much more successful today than it was in past decades, but the family must be prepared for some facial disfigurement, and the possibility of nasal speech which requires years of training to circumvent. With any kind of predictable permanent facial disfigurement, it is important for the pediatrician to prepare the family so that they, in turn, can support the baby and child throughout the developmental years to assure that personal skills and strong personality traits are acquired.

Cleft Palate

A cleft palate may exist in any degree from partial to complete. Embryologic fusion of the palate probably terminates at the uvula because many clefts involve only the uvula and a portion of the soft palate. A complete defect encompasses the soft palate, the bony palate, and extends forward through the gingival ridge on one or both sides of the premaxilla.[7]

Treatment. A complete cleft of the palate may cause difficulty in swallowing because the whole nasopharynx is exposed to the oral cavity. A special nipple with a tube extension reaching into the pharynx usually obviates problems with feedings and prevents choking or aspiration.

Most surgeons feel that the best time for palatal reconstruction is between 12 and 15 months. This allows the child to grow as large as possible before beginning meaningful speech. For simple palatal repairs, lateral incisions allow closure of the vascularized palatal flaps in the midline. When the defect is wider, flaps of pharyngeal mucosa and muscle can be rotated medially, closing the posterior portion of the palatal defect. Another method used to obtain the important posterior palatal tissue is the so-called "push-back" procedure in which the muscular attachments of the hard palate are pushed posteriorly to allow for functional closure between the nasopharynx and oral pharynx. The major function of the palate is to provide a barrier between the nasal pharynx and the oral pharynx so that phonation can be entirely an oral function, yielding normal speech patterns. Palatal reconstructive surgery must be coupled with years of supervised speech training to ensure the best possible palatal function.

Cleft Palate Coupled with Mandibular Hypoplasia (Pierre–Robin Syndrome)

Mandibular hypoplasia forces a posterior positioning of the tongue, which in turn creates a partial barrier to normal respirations. Coupled with cleft palate, underdevelopment of the mandible is hazardous and can be fatal to the neonate if the posteriorly placed tongue becomes lodged above the palatal defect. The diagnosis is suspected whenever a receding chin or short jaw is noted during the neonatal examination. The integrity of the palate is immediately determined. Thereafter, precautionary measures are undertaken and the baby maintained in an intensive care environment.

The face-down position favors a clear airway for babies with the Pierre–Robin syndrome. This can be achieved with appropriate rolls under the chest and axillae and a doughnut-roll support for the forehead. The most dangerous times for the baby are during feedings which are commonly attended by bouts of choking, gasping, and obvious respiratory distress. Proper positioning of the infant and use of gavage feeding may overcome the respiratory hazards imposed by oral intake. Usually, however, the circumstances are more urgent. When there is severe respiratory distress in the early days of life, some have advocated placing a large suture through the middle muscular portion of the tongue, bringing the two ends of the suture out of the mouth attached to a surgical clamp so that the nursing personnel can grasp this whenever the baby is in distress.[8] For those patients in whom respirations are satisfactory except at feeding times, a gastrostomy has been recommended until the mandible grows sufficiently. Dennison has devised a plaster of Paris cap which stretches the baby into the most advantageous position for breathing.[9] In those babies in whom respiratory obstruction is a continual life-endangering threat, a tracheostomy may be necessary. The mandible grows rapidly, and an adequate airway and space for the tongue is predictable by 6 months to a year of age. Thus, all management is geared to achieving this age with safety.[10,11]

Thyroglossal Duct

The embryologic development of the thyroid gland results as an outgrowth from the thyroglossal duct. This structure originates as an outpouching of the foregut, beginning at the base of the tongue at the foramen cecum and passing downward and forward through the hyoid bone to the normal anatomic position of the thyroid gland (Fig. 34-2**A**). Persistence of a portion of the thyroglossal duct allows the formation of a midline cervical mass known as a thyroglossal duct cyst (Fig. 34-2**B**). Ultimately, these cysts become troublesome because of repeated infection. However, such infection is rarely seen in the neonate and, as a matter of fact, the discovery of a thyroglossal duct cyst is extraordinary in this age group. Rather, it is more commonly seen in the 2- to 4-year-old child when the baby fat subsides and irregularities in the neck are more readily apparent. The cyst is almost always found in the midline except when repeated infection and scarring cause some retraction laterally.

The occurrence of a thyroglossal duct cyst in a neonate almost always occurs in one or two presentations: as an anterior cervical abscess with imminent external rupture or as a mass at the base of the tongue in the foramen cecum.

In infants, infected thyroglossal duct cysts are treated with intensive antibiotic therapy and abscess formation promptly drained. Weeks later, when infection has completely subsided, removal of the cyst and the entire thyroglossal duct including the middle portion of the hyoid bone is carried out.[12] It is rare that this operation is necessary in the neonatal period.

When a thyroglossal duct cyst is discovered in the mouth at the base of the tongue, early excision under intratracheal anesthesia is recommended to avoid potential respiratory obstruction. A midline mass in the neck or in the base of the tongue which is thought to be a thyroglossal duct cyst may be ectopic thyroid tissue. If a normal thyroid can not be palpated with certainty, a thyroid scan is performed because it is probable that this mass represents all of the thyroid. Excision can be deferred and the patient treated with thyroid extract which, in most instances, results in decrease in size of the ectopic thyroid mass.

Branchial Cleft Anomalies

Branchial clefts are those embryologic grooves that ultimately form the lower face and neck. Abnormal persistence of any portion of the branchial apparatus leads to specific anomalies about the face and neck.[13]

Preauricular Tabs and Sinuses. Persistent preauricular anomalies are common, representing about a third of all congenital branchial abnormalities. They are seen as dimples, small sinus openings in the skin, or protruding skin tags just in front of the ear at the level of the auditory canal. A small flap of skin with contained cartilage requires simple excision. A preauricular sinus usually has a harmless blind end, but in every instance it must be traced carefully to its termination to prevent recurrent infection in the tract.

Cervical Fistula. A fistula originating low in the anterolateral neck is another manifestation of the branchial cleft anomalies. The location of the tract confirms the second branchial cleft as the embryologic origin because the fistula extends from the skin of the lower neck upward

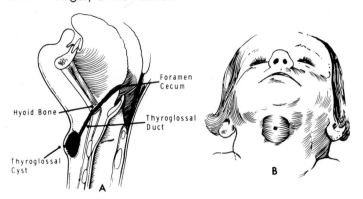

Fig. 34-2. A. The tract of the thyroglossal duct is depicted, showing relationship to tongue, hyoid bone, and anterior neck. **B.** As shown, the thyroglossal duct cyst usually presents in the midline at about the level of the thyroid cartilage. (Nardi GL, Zuidema GD: Surgery 3rd ed. Boston, Little, Brown and Co., 1972)

along the sternocleidomastoid muscle, then inward between the internal and external carotid arteries to attach to the posterolateral pharynx just below the tonsillar fossa (Fig. 34-3). The presenting complaint is usually related to persistent or intermittent drainage onto the neck. Complete surgical extirpation is necessary for cure. A large incision in the neck can be avoided by the use of two or three small, neat transverse "stair-step" incisions.

Branchial Cyst. About 10% of persistent branchial deformities are cystic. These invariably arise low in the anterior triangle of the neck and present as smooth cysts anterior to the sternocleidomastoid muscle. Dissection and excision is curative.

Cervical Cutaneous Tabs. Occasionally a baby presents with a cutaneous tab in the skin of the anterior aspect of the neck. A small, irregular formation of cartilage may be contained in the skin tab. The cartilage is never associated with fistula and so there is no urgency to have this small appendage removed.

Cystic Hygroma

Cystic hygroma arises as a result of congenital deformity of development of lymphatic channels (Fig. 34-4). About 65% of these watery cysts occur in the neck, and most are located posterior to the sternocleidomastoid muscle. Other sites of occurrence are the groin, the axilla, and the mediastinum. The term **hygroma** suggests the watery fluid contained in the endothelial-lined spaces. The cyst may be unilocular but more often there are numerous cysts of various sizes which permeate the surrounding structures and distort the local anatomy. Supporting connective tissue often shows extensive lymphocytic infiltration. Except in the case of single large cysts, no clear-cut cleavage plane is found between the hygroma and normal tissue.

The lesion is almost always evident at birth.

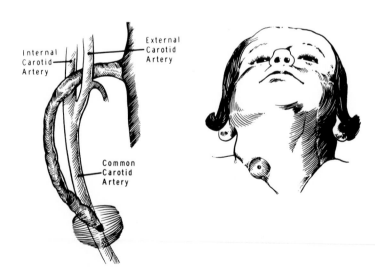

Fig. 34-3. Brachial cleft cyst, which presents low in the neck as a mass and/or an opening in the skin, extends upward and laterally in the neck, passing between the branches of the carotid artery to connect with the pharynx below the tonsillar fascia. (Nardi, GL, Zuidema GD: Surgery 3rd ed. Boston, Little, Brown and Co., 1972)

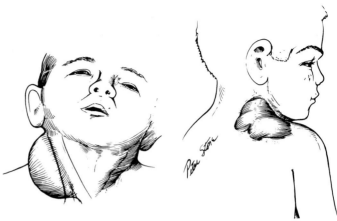

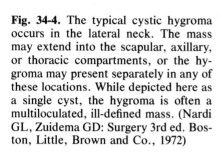

Fig. 34-4. The typical cystic hygroma occurs in the lateral neck. The mass may extend into the scapular, axillary, or thoracic compartments, or the hygroma may present separately in any of these locations. While depicted here as a single cyst, the hygroma is often a multiloculated, ill-defined mass. (Nardi GL, Zuidema GD: Surgery 3rd ed. Boston, Little, Brown and Co., 1972)

Occasionally, the mass occupies the entire submandibular region, distorting the subglottic area and compromising the airway. Not infrequently, a supraclavicular mass is seen which may become prominent with the Valsalva maneuver. This form of cystic hygroma is usually associated with a mediastinal component.

Symptoms are related entirely to the location and size of the mass. Disfigurement is often severe. Sudden enlargement of a hygroma generally indicates hemorrhage into a cyst. Infection in the mass may lead to dangerous regional cellulitis but when the infection subsides, the resultant intracystic fibrosis and scar may significantly reduce the size of the tumor mass.

Repeated aspiration of the cyst and injection of sclerosing agents such as hypertonic glucose solution or sodium morrhuate may be useful in an occasional isolated cyst. As original therapy this approach is not advised.

Surgical excision offers the best chance of cure. Total excision is often impractical because of the extent of the hygroma and proximity to vital structures. Important nerves and vascular structures must not be sacrificed in an attempt to achieve total excision of this benign lesion; rather, multiple repeated excisions of the residual hygroma are preferable.

DISTRESS FROM RESPIRATORY OBSTRUCTION

Neonatal respiratory distress from partial obstruction in the larynx or trachea may arise suddenly and threaten the life of the infant or may be subtle, mild, or intermittent and require special techniques to define its etiology.[14] In-spiratory stridor, though an alarming symptom in the newborn, is often self-limiting and requires no specific therapy. Before this reassurance can be given, however, an orderly diagnostic evaluation is required to exclude mechanical causes which may represent a threat to the infant.

The newborn infant has several inherent disadvantages in respiratory mechanics. The diameter of the trachea and bronchi is small; thus the risk of major obstruction from a mucous plug is increased. The musculature of the chest wall is relatively weak; thus, coughing is less efficient than in older subjects.

The infant is an obligatory nose breather and patency of the nares must be established by catheter whenever airway obstruction is suspected. Obstruction at the larynx is best determined by direct laryngoscopy which reveals structural abnormalities of the larynx and epiglottis, obstructing webs as well as polyps. The latter are rare, and can usually be managed locally, restoring full airway patency. Hemangiomas involving the vocal cords or trachea can also compromise the airway. Surgical excision of hemangiomata situated in such positions is often impossible. When obstructive symptoms are severe, a course of parenteral steroids is tried in an attempt to accelerate involution of these vascular anomalies.

An overpenetrated chest film is useful in defining the location and patency of the trachea and its major divisions. Extrinsic pressure defects or major displacement of the trachea are readily appreciated on this study. All infants with respiratory distress should have a barium swallow in the lateral projection to demonstrate compression by vascular structures within the mediastinum (vascular ring). Most symptoms of vascular entrapment of the trachea and esophagus are referable to swallowing, but the airway can be compromised and ventilation impaired. Because of interference with swallowing, aspiration with pneumonia is commonly seen as a cause of respiratory distress in this group of infants.

Laryngotracheomalacia. In some infants, the combination of a narrow tracheal diameter and the lack of firm cartilagenous support, permits compromise of the lumen with each inspiration. Momentary collapse of the larynx and cervical trachea results in a characteristic stridor. This is accentuated when respiratory efforts are most vigorous, such as when the infant is crying. Although alarming, the stridor associated with laryngotracheomalacia is usually self-limiting, requiring no specific treatment. It generally resolves by 6 to 8 months of age as the cross-sectional diameter of the tracheal lumen increases and the supporting cartilage matures.

Laryngoscopy is performed to observe the motions of the larynx during inspiration. This is best done with the infant awake. The flexible bronchoscope can be introduced through the infant's nose with minimal discomfort. Laryngotracheomalacia is a diagnosis which is made only after obstructing tracheal lesions are ruled out.

Parents of infants with laryngotracheomalacia are advised that respiratory infections, with resultant edema of the mucous lining of the larynx and trachea, may accentuate the symptoms. A humidified environment and antibiotics are key factors in therapy whenever such babies contract respiratory infection.

Though spontaneous resolution of laryngotracheomalacia is the rule, an occasional infant expends an inordinate amount of energy in the work of breathing. This caloric loss necessarily occurs at the expense of growth. Infrequently, the amount of inspiratory obstruction is so severe that cyanosis and even cardiac instability result. In these rare instances, tracheostomy may be required as a life-saving procedure.

Congenital Lobar Emphysema. Congenital lobar emphysema can produce severe, life-threatening respiratory embarrassment as a result of hyperexpansion of a single lobe of the lung.[15] Air is permitted into the involved lobe but denied egress. Consequently, the lobe becomes emphysematous, resulting in compression of adjacent pulmonary parenchyma and mediastinal displacement. Symptoms may appear shortly after birth but are usually delayed for several weeks or months. The etiology is unknown. An inherent, cartilaginous defect in the bronchus has been postulated; however, the bronchial abnormality is not always recognizable in the resected specimen.

A chest x-ray film is characteristic, showing hyperaeration of the involved lobe with a mediastinal shift away from the affected side. The lobar distribution of the hyperaeration can be appreciated and adjacent pulmonary parenchyma is seen to be compressed. The upper lobes are most frequently involved but the condition is seen in the right middle lobe in about 10% of cases.

Treatment is surgical and prompt thoracotomy and lobectomy are undertaken when the diagnosis is made. An infant may remain compensated for some weeks and then deteriorate rapidly from acute hyperinflation of the involved lobe. For this reason, there is no place for expectant management of congenital lobar emphysema.

Tracheostomy. Acute respiratory emergencies in infants can usually be managed by the temporary placement of an endotracheal tube. An endotracheal tube is surprisingly well tolerated by the infant, even for extended periods of time.[16,17,18] Thus, rarely is emergency tracheostomy necessary in the newborn period. Only when the respiratory crisis extends beyond 3 to 4 weeks is the infant considered for tracheostomy. The operation is always undertaken in the operating room. An endotracheal tube or bronchoscope is put in place to assure stabilization of the delicate trachea and provide good control of the infant's airway until the trachea can be identified and opened. Proper placement of the tracheostomy is essential. The tube is at the level of the second or third tracheal ring, thus avoiding the cricoid, yet not so low that the tube is in the mediastinum when the neck is flexed. The incision is made transversely between the second and third tracheal cartilages. Alternatively, a vertical incision may be made through two cartilages, but tracheal substance is never resected. Stay sutures are placed on the incised margins of the trachea to facilitate insertion of the tracheostomy tube and to serve as traction sutures should the tube become dislodged in the early postoperative period. With the development of the newer silastic tracheostomy tubes, problems relating to erosion and postoperative stenosis have been minimized.[19,20]

When embarking upon tracheostomy, it is understood by the care team and by the parents that decannulization may be difficult. When tracheostomy becomes necessary in an infant, the baby may be committed for many months and, in some cases, even years, before the tube can be removed safely. Complications can be minimized if postoperative surgical care is meticulous and silastic tubes are utilized. Therefore, the alternative of extended endotracheal intubation need not be abandoned unless the cause of respiratory obstruction has been shown to be unduly protracted.

Diaphragmatic Hernia. Failure of development of the posterolateral portion of the diaphragm results in persistence of the pleuroperitoneal canal or foramen of Bochdalek.[21] This defect accounts for 70% of congenital diaphragmatic hernias. The lesion occurs once in every 3,000 live births with equal frequency in males and females. Diaphragmatic hernia of Bochdalek is almost always encountered on the left side.[22]

Typically, babies with congenital Bochdalek hernia present dramatically with cyanosis and severe respiratory distress immediately after birth. Because the abdominal viscera are dislocated through the defect into the chest, the abdominal contour is scaphoid. Breath sounds are diminished or absent and, because the mediastinal structures have been displaced, the heart sounds are heard in the right chest. As the bowel fills with gas, respiration and cardiac action are further compromised, hypoxia and respiratory acidosis are increased and death is inevitable unless surgical intervention is undertaken. In some instances, the infants remain relatively asymptomatic in the early hours and days of life and, rarely, a diaphragmatic hernia is an incidental finding in an older child. The respiratory symptoms demand an immediate x-ray film, which is diagnostic. Typically, the air-filled bowel is seen occupying the left hemithorax with resultant displacement of the mediastinum to the right (Fig. 34-5). The abdomen is airless. No further x-rays are necessary and contrast studies for additional confirmation are contraindicated.

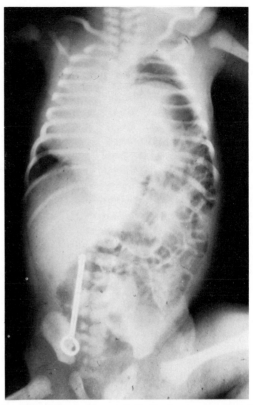

Fig. 34-5. X-ray film of left diaphragmatic hernia with loops of bowel well up into the chest. While most diaphragmatic hernias do not have a sac, the smooth curve of the sac in this instance is visible. Note the displacement of the heart all the way to the border of the right chest.

In the baby with respiratory embarrassment, survival depends on prompt reduction of the hernia allowing the mediastinum to assume a normal position and the contralateral lung to expand.[23,24] Concomitantly, therapy is directed at correction of the combined metabolic and respiratory acidosis.[25] While administration of buffering agents, such as bicarbonate or tromethamine (THAM), may temporarily restore acid-base balance, a favorable outcome depends upon the ability of the opposite lung to support the infant. The surgical findings are usually those of a posterolateral defect in the left diaphragm with most or all of the abdominal viscera in the chest. The hernia is reduced gently by withdrawing the viscera from the chest. If a sac is present, it is delivered and excised. There is usually adequate diaphragmatic tissue to accomplish direct suture repair.

If a significant portion of the diaphragm is lacking, repair is still managed by using the portion of the muscle which is present anteriorly and the endothoracic fascia posteriorly. The use of prosthestic material in this defect is occasionally necessary. Before completion of the repair, a small chest tube is placed in the left hemithorax and brought out through an intercostal space.

The temptation to expand the compressed lung at the time of the initial surgery must be resisted. The lung has been described as "hypoplastic."[26] It is, however, potentially normal, and gradually expands in 7 to 14 days. Aggressive attempts at expansion at the time of surgery can result in pneumothorax on the contralateral side, which, if unrecognized, is a disastrous complication. In many centers, a chest tube is placed prophylactically on the contralateral side.

The abdominal viscera have been located in the thorax throughout the developmental period of the fetus. Therefore, there is insufficient room to accommodate the intestine after the diaphragmatic repair without increasing dangerously the intraabdominal pressure, thereby compressing the vena cava and compromising respirations by elevating the diaphragm. To avoid these potential problems, anatomic closure of the abdominal wall is omitted. Rather, skin flaps are quickly mobilized and the skin is closed. The ventral pouch thus created accommodates the intraabdominal organs; diaphragmatic action and venous return are unimpeded. The ventral defect can be repaired easily in 10 days to 2 weeks, at which time both lungs are fully expanded and respiratory physiology is normal.

Reduction and repair of the hernia can also be accomplished through a thoracotomy incision.[27] However, the ability to decompress the abdomen by creation of a ventral pouch is lost.

Ten percent of infants with Bochdalek hernias present with the defect on the right side. The difference in incidence on the two sides is probably explained by the presence of the liver, which at least partially blocks the pleuroperitoneal canal, thus limiting the amount of bowel which can herniate into the chest. Symptoms in babies with right-sided hernias are almost always less severe, but when a right diphragmatic hernia of Bochdalek presents as an emergency, it is managed as described above.

After the abdominal incision is closed, the infant is moved to the intensive care unit in which therapy is directed toward correcting the acid-base derangement. In those infants distressed in the early hours of life, respiratory and metabolic acidosis, hypoxia, and hypercarbia are anticipated. For correction, intermittent support with a volume respirator is sometimes necessary. Despite aggressive therapeutic efforts, the mortality remains high in this group. Pulmonary hypertension often supervenes and may not respond to antihypertensive drugs such as tolazoline hydrochloride (Priscoline). Right-to-left shunts occur through the foramen ovale and patent ductus arteriosus, leading to further anoxia and an increase in pulmonary pressures. In the future, the membrane oxygenator may find use as a lifesaving temporary pulmonary support during the hours immediately following surgical repair. Babies who present after the first day of life with signs and symptoms leading to a diagnosis of diaphragmatic hernia are almost always hardier subjects with greater pulmonary reserve and they can be expected to make a satisfactory recovery.

The anterior retrosternal hernia of Morgagni is rarely encountered in the newborn. The diagnosis is confirmed by chest film in the lateral projection. A correct treatment is surgical reconstruction beginning with an abdominal approach through a thoracoabdominal incision. The prognosis is almost always favorable and these lesions are not associated with the severe cardiopulmonary complications seen with Bochdalek hernias in the neonatal period.

THE ESOPHAGUS

The esophagus is subject to a variety of congenital malformations. Each produces a characteristic clinical picture. Prompt recognition of an esophageal abnormality and accurate determination of the anatomic features are important determinants in the outcome of surgical correction.

Esophageal Atresia with Lower Segment Tracheoesophageal Fistula[28,29]

Anatomy. Atresia with associated tracheoesophageal fistula accounts for nearly 90% of all anatomic malformations of the esophagus (Fig. 34-6A). The blind-ending upper esophageal segment usually extends only into the upper portion of the thorax. Typically, the proximal end of the lower portion of the esophagus is connected to the trachea, usually at or just above the tracheal bifurcation. This connection is usually 3 to 5 mm in cross-sectional diameter, easily admitting inspired air, or, in a retrograde fashion, the acidic gastric juice.

Associated anomalies occurring at the same time in the embryologic calendar are common. In nearly 20% of the babies born with esophageal atresia, some variant of congenital heart disease occurs, while imperforate anus is found in about 10%.

Clinical Signs. The earliest and most obvious clinical sign of esophageal atresia is regurgitation out of the infant's mouth and nose of saliva or the first offered feeding. Aspiration of feeding is often followed by choking and coughing. Abdominal distension is a prominent feature in these babies, occurring as inspired air is transmitted through the fistula and distal esophagus into the stomach. Regurgitated gastric juice passes through the fistula and into the trachea and pulmonary alveoli, leading to a chemical pneumonia. The pulmonary problems are magnified by atelectasis which occurs from diaphragmatic elevation secondary to gastric distension.

These clinical findings are obvious from the earliest hours after birth. Observers with the best advantage are the nursing personnel, for it is they who are feeding the baby and also observing for longer periods of time behavioral patterns such as the accumulation of mucus or saliva around the lips. The pediatrician making his initial newborn examination probably will not feed the baby and therefore may miss this diagnosis unless he attempts to pass a tube into the stomach of all babies he examines.

Upon the first suspicion of esophageal atresia, the diagnosis can be made by passing a catheter through the nose or mouth. Tiny flexible feeding catheters are not used because they may coil up and give the misleading impression that they have advanced into the stomach. A larger catheter, slowly advanced, meets the obstruction.

X-ray study confirms the diagnosis and, in most instances, offers specific information concerning the deranged anatomy. The most helpful study is a lateral view with 1 ml of contrast

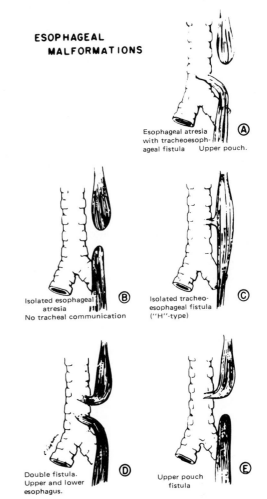

ESOPHAGEAL MALFORMATIONS

Esophageal atresia with tracheoesophageal fistula Upper pouch. (A)

Isolated esophageal atresia No tracheal communication (B)

Isolated tracheo-esophageal fistula ("H"-type) (C)

Double fistula. Upper and lower esophagus. (D)

Upper pouch fistula (E)

Fig. 34-6. Representation of the various forms of esophageal malformations shown in the order of the frequency in which they occur. (Nardi GL, Zuidema GD: Surgery, 3rd ed. Boston, Little, Brown and Co., 1972)

media instilled into the pouch to outline the blind upper esophagus (Fig. 34-7A). The barium is aspirated immediately to prevent any spillover into the lungs. This x-ray study can be expected to show the length of the upper pouch and its exact extension into the chest. These facts are of importance to the surgeon in planning reconstruction of the esophagus. Air which has entered the stomach through the fistula will be seen, and, in some instances, air may outline the lower esophageal segment. The existence of pneumonia and atelectasis is also important information.

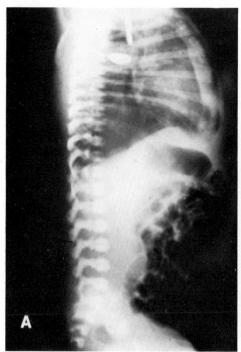

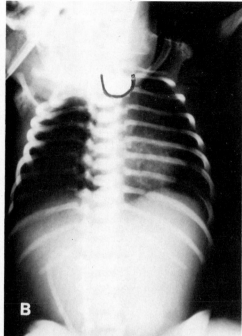

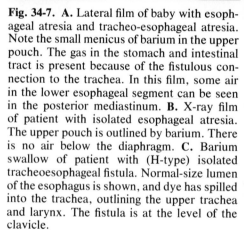

Fig. 34-7. **A.** Lateral film of baby with esophageal atresia and tracheo-esophageal atresia.
Note the small menicus of barium in the upper
pouch. The gas in the stomach and intestinal
tract is present because of the fistulous connection to the trachea. In this film, some air
in the lower esophageal segment can be seen
in the posterior mediastinum. **B.** X-ray film
of patient with isolated esophageal atresia.
The upper pouch is outlined by barium. There
is no air below the diaphragm. **C.** Barium
swallow of patient with (H-type) isolated
tracheoesophageal fistula. Normal-size lumen
of the esophagus is shown, and dye has spilled
into the trachea, outlining the upper trachea
and larynx. The fistula is at the level of the
clavicle.

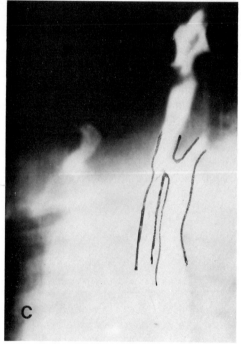

Management

With the diagnosis secure, the following measures are instituted immediately:

1. Isolette care
2. Cut-down for intravenous therapy
3. Antibiotics (even if pneumonia is not yet clinically manifest)
4. 30° Head-up position
5. Sump catheter suction in the upper pouch (Replogle tube)[30]
6. Oxygen as indicated by clinical need and blood gas studies

Gastrostomy is a useful adjunct in the management of most babies before operative repair of the esophagus is undertaken. Many surgeons list gastrostomy with the six primary steps in stabilizing all patients with esophageal atresia and tracheoesophageal fistula.

At this point, all babies are considered surgical candidates and fall into one of three categories of surgical treatment:[31]

1. Prompt surgical correction
2. Short-term delay with subsequent primary repair
3. Long-term delay with staged repair.

The factors determining the surgical plan rest on (1) maturity of the infant, (2) the condition of the lungs, and (3) the presence of other major anomalies.

If other clinical factors dictate that the baby is not an immediate candidate for surgery and that he must be placed in category 2 or 3, then a gastrostomy is done to afford immediate decompression of the air accumulating in the stomach. With the baby in the head-up position and the upper pouch suction established, most of the immediate deleterious effects of the anomaly are annulled.

Category 1: Prompt Surgical Correction. If the infant is of adequate weight and maturity, has no significant pneumonia, and is not shown to have other major congenital anomalies, then primary repair can be undertaken safely. At the option of the surgeon, the right thoracotomy can be performed in either a transpleural or extrapleural manner. The transthoracic route has the virtue of speed. The retropleural approach, though somewhat more tedious, is advantageous should a leak at the anastomosis occur. The lower segment of the esophagus is detached from the trachea and this fistula meticulously closed by sutures which must not

compromise the tracheal lumen. The blind upper pouch is mobilized and its end opened; a union between the two segments is then accomplished. Surgeons vary as to the specific type and placement of sutures used to make the anastomosis. Many prefer the Haight anastomosis, wherein a second layer of muscle is developed in the upper pouch and this muscular sleeve brought down over the inner anastomotic layer. If the transthoracic operative route is used, a tube is left in the pleural space and connected to suction. If the retropleural approach is used, a small tube is left in the posterior mediastinum and remains open for drainage. If the baby has tolerated the procedure well and a gastrostomy has not been done previously, it may be carried out as a complimentary procedure under the same anesthesia.

Category 2: Short-Term Delay. If the patient has pneumonia, cardiac disease or other serious anomaly, then these temporarily take precedence. The infant is placed in category 2 for short-term stabilization and further evaluation. In this group, a gastrostomy is always performed, often under local anesthesia. If the contraindication to immediate surgery is pneumonia or atelectasis, then 2 to 3 days is usually given to conservative care, employing upper pouch suction, the head-up position, antibiotics, intravenous feeding, and gastrostomy drainage (Fig. 34-8). Infants with congenital heart disease may require digitalis and diuretics. The baby may be safely managed in this way for about 1 week, and some surgeons feel that this temporizing may be kept up for a longer period without undue risks. Thoracotomy and repair is carried out after the infant has been stabilized and is judged to be a satisfactory risk for anesthesia.

Category 3: Staged Repair. Although staged repair is used much less frequently than the delayed primary repair, this approach still has merit for a very sick infant, for a premature infant who weighs less than 1500 g, or for an infant with a severe congenital heart problem. There are several methods for staging the repair of esophageal atresia.

Retropleural Division of the Fistula.[32] In this operation, the retropleural approach is used to divide the tracheoesophageal fistula. No effort is made to repair the esophagus at this time. The baby is then sustained with gastrostomy feeding and upper pouch suction.

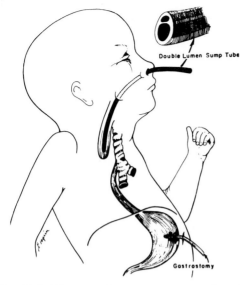

Double Lumen Sump Tube

Gastrostomy

Fig. 34-8. Diagram of temporary care of patient with esophageal atresia and tracheoesophageal fistula. Patient is in the upright position. A gastrostomy is in the stomach and a double lumen sump tube is in the upper pouch to clear secretions and saliva.

Although this situation requires intensive nursing care, it can be safely maintained for months. Later, at the time of election, a transthoracic operation is performed and the esophageal anastomosis is carried out. Undoubtedly, this method of management has resulted in the salvage of a number of babies.

Intravenous Hyperalimentation. This technique of sustaining babies has increased neonatal salvage in a wide variety of conditions; it has been advocated as a way of handling babies whose esophageal repair is to be delayed. This form of nutritional support is coupled with gastrostomy for drainage and continued suction of the upper pouch. A serious negative feature of this method, however, is the continued exposure of the lungs to gastric acid reflux, which may occur in spite of gastrostomy drainage as long as the fistula remains open.

Gastric division and double gastrostomy.[33] Division of the stomach with double gastrostomy is another method of staging the repair. The stomach is transected high on the fundus, sparing the great vessels and the major trunk of the right vagus nerve. The two ends of the stomach are oversewn and gastrostomy tubes are led from both gastric pouches at the greater

curvature. The tube from the upper gastric pouch is placed under water-seal drainage. The baby is fed through the distal gastrostomy tube. This method isolates the tracheoesophageal fistula effectively and has the advantage of sparing the infant a thoracic procedure. At the appropriate time, when the clinical condition requiring staging permits, repair of the esophagus may be carried out safely in a virgin operative field. Later the stomach is reconstructed by a simple end-to-end anastomosis of the two severed units. Gastric division is also useful in isolating the esophagus and encouraging healing when a major leak follows primary repair of an esophageal atresia in the infant.

Complications

The most frequent complication following surgical repair of esophageal atresia and tracheoesophageal fistula is the formation of stenosis at the site of the anastomosis. This may occur weeks or even months later and become apparent with increasing difficulty in swallowing, spitting of ingested liquid, and finally fever secondary to aspiration and pneumonia. Most patients with esophageal stricture can be managed with only occasional dilatations during the first year or two of life. In such instances, general anesthesia is preferred and graduated tapered dilators can be guided down the esophagus with safety. When frequent repetitive dilatations are needed, the gastrostomy is maintained, with a string led through the esophagus and out the nose and gastric vent. These patients may then have a set of linked graduated rubber dilators pulled retrograde through the gastrostomy and up the esophagus to accomplish dilatation, and resection with a new anastomosis is advised.

A less frequent but more serious complication of esophageal anastomosis for atresia is disruption of the suture line with leakage. Gastrostomy drainage and upper esophageal sump suction are reinstituted. The retropleural or intrathoracic suction are utilized to evacuate the material leaking from the esophagus. There can be no feeding by mouth and, in many instances, feeding by gastrostomy is hazardous because of reflux through the leaking esophagus. The magnitude of the leak is best determined by barium swallow, carefully monitored under fluoroscopic control. If the leak is small, the chance of spontaneous closure is good and conservative management is warranted. This may involve the use of intravenous hyperalimentation for nutrition over a period of weeks. Alternatively, gastric division may be selected to allow isolation of the leaking esophagus and safe feeding through the distal gastrostomy tube. If the leak is so large as to overwhelm the baby with massive drainage into the chest and attendant sepsis, then esophageal continuity is abandoned and the proximal esophagus diverted to the neck as an esophagostomy. This commits the child to esophageal replacement with a gastric or colonic conduit at a later date.

The treatment of babies with esophageal atresia and tracheoesophageal fistula is curative in about 85% of the affected neonates. This high salvage results from two main factors: (1) a well-informed pediatric community which recognizes the anomaly promptly and (2) surgeons experienced in managing neonates, with a flexible approach to their treatment guided by the clinical factors and anatomical features.

Isolated Esophageal Atresia

About 8% of babies with esophageal anomalies present with isolated esophageal atresia (Fig. 34-6**B**). No fistula to the respiratory tract is present. An important anatomic feature in these infants is that the short nubbin of lower esophagus barely protrudes above the diaphragm. This feature is of clinical significance because it contraindicates an early, fruitless exploratory thoracotomy in the hope that the ends will reach.[34]

Signs and Symptoms. As in other forms of esophageal atresia, these infants cannot handle their saliva or feedings. Babies with isolated esophageal atresia present a scaphoid abdomen because the gastrointestinal tract is devoid of air. The x-ray finding of a blind upper pouch and the absence of air below the diaphragm is pathognomonic of isolated esophageal atresia without fistula (see Fig. 34-7**B**). There have been exceedingly rare instances when a tracheoesophageal fistula was present but became plugged with mucus, leading to an erroneous diagnosis of pure atresia. This clinical occurrence is so rare that maneuvers to disprove the possibility in all babies with isolated atresia of the esophagus are unwarranted.

Management. Esophageal replacement by a colon segment or gastric tube is necessary in babies with isolated atresia.[35,36] Prompt esophagostomy with the upper esophageal pouch brought to the skin of the left neck allows drainage of saliva and prevents aspiration. A gastrostomy is performed and serves for feeding until esophageal replacement can be safely undertaken, usually at about 1 year of age.

Reconstruction of the esophagus is usually carried out by interposition of the colon, which can be placed in the chest behind the root of the left lung and brought out through the upper thorax behind the clavicle to join the stump of the esophagus; alternatively, the colon may be placed in the substernal position. Positioning the colon in the posterior chest is more anatomic but can compromise expansion of the left lung. On the other hand, the substernal position, while not embarrassing the left lung, requires an anterior angle of the upper colon making subsequent esophagoscopy more difficult. Another method of esophageal replacement more recently adapted to pediatric patients is the construction of a tube from the greater curvature of the stomach. With any of these procedures, normal growth and development can be expected for most infants in whom esophageal replacement has been necessary. Reports of bougienage of the upper and lower pouches suggest that, in selected cases, delayed primary repair may be possible.[37]

Isolated ("H" Type) Tracheoesophageal Fistula

In rare instances (1% or 2% of infants with congenital abnormalities of the esophagus), an isolated congenital fistula may persist, connecting the trachea and the esophagus (Fig. 34-6**C**).[38] The connection between the esophagus and trachea almost always occurs at the level of the clavicle. The opening in the trachea may vary from a few millimeters to nearly a centimeter while the opening in the esophagus is usually larger. In most cases both the trachea and the esophagus are otherwise normal with no narrowing or obstruction.

In contrast to babies with esophageal atresia, these infants usually swallow all offered food and liquid without difficulty. The clinical features are more subtle and infants are usually several weeks or even months old before a correct diagnosis is made. A triad of symptoms is usually found: (1) choking when feeding, (2) excessive gas in the stomach and intestine, and (3) frequent bouts of aspiration pneumonia. A number of diagnostic maneuvers have been suggested to define accurately the H-type tracheoesophageal fistula. Barium swallow in the face-down position is successful in demonstrating the communication in about half the cases (Fig. 34-7C). This examination can be augmented by inserting a Foley catheter to the midesophagus and gently blowing up the balloon so that the column of barium remains above the obstruction, affording a better chance for its passage through the fistula. Simultaneous esophagoscopy and bronchoscopy, utilizing a colored dye instilled into the trachea, are usually successful. However, when these diagnostic measures fail and there remains a high index of suspicion on the basis of the clinical features, surgical exploration of the neck is justified.

Treatment. Because most of the isolated tracheoesophageal fistulae occur at or just below the level of the clavicle, the incision is placed low in the lateral right neck; a thoracotomy is usually unnecessary. The steroncleidomastoid muscle is retracted or transected, exposing the posterior and lateral aspects of the trachea and the anterior portion of the esophagus. Most of the fistulous connections can be seen at this location so that thoracotomy is avoided. Definitive treatment consists in dividing the fistula and closure of the esophagus and trachea, with special care to avoid any encroachment on the lumen of the trachea.

In a few instances, double fistulae have occurred, with the second one occurring lower so that thoracotomy is necessary for its surgical correction. Cases have also been reported in which there is a cleft defect between the esophagus and trachea extending from the larynx to the bifurcation of the trachea. Surgical cure of this extensive lesion has been disappointing in most instances, but the two structures have been separated successfully in several patients. As might be expected, patients with extensive tracheoesophageal clefts have severe respiratory distress and thus are brought to the attention of the pediatrician and surgeon shortly after birth.

Esophageal Atresia with Double Fistulae

Atresia with double fistula is exceedingly rare. Both the upper and lower blind ends of the esophagus enter the trachea. Esophageal

atresia with a short, blind lower segment and only the upper pouch entering the trachea through a fistula has also been described (Fig. 34-6 **D** and **E**). In both of these variants, saliva drains directly into the lungs, increasing the pulmonary hazard for the infant. The surgical considerations are similar to those above but the mortality is high.

Gastroesophageal Reflux (GER), "Chalasia," and Hiatal Hernia

In 1947, Berenberg and Neuhauser defined a condition they termed "chalasia," or abnormal relaxation of the gastroesophageal junction.[39,*] Babies so afflicted manifest relentless regurgitation which may present as spitting, mild vomiting, or very vigorous vomiting after every feeding. The deleterious effect of reflux in infants has been recognized with increasing frequency in the past few years.[40–42] The spectrum of symptoms from GER is distinctly different in the infant than in the adult. In infants, the main symptoms of GER are regurgitation, significant growth retardation, aspiration pneumonia, apneic spells, and esophagitis.[39,*] Clinical observations have confirmed that the radiologic or endoscopic visualization of gastric herniation through the hiatus is not a prerequisite for the diagnosis of pathologic gastroesophageal reflux in infants. The single abnormality is the absence of a normal valvular mechanism at the GE junction which in turn allows unimpeded reflux of gastric content.

A majority of infants with GER can be treated successfully by propping them in a semiupright position.[41] It is noteworthy that reflux, which leads to major symptoms and is demonstrable on barium swallow x-ray studies, may often disappear when the baby assumes the upright position at 10 to 15 months of age.[39,41] Because GER in the infant often has a spontaneous resolution sometime after 1 year of age, the condition has mistakenly been regarded as normal or insignificant. The debilitating nutritional disturbances occurring in a very significant percentage of these infants during their first and most important year of development[43] may have a lifetime of consequences.[44]

Most infants with GER have some form of vomiting from birth. In some babies, the vomiting is projectile in character and initially

---

* Leape LL: unpublished data

suggests the diagnosis of pyloric stenosis. Weight loss or delayed weight gain with retardation of developmental landmarks comprise the second most common presenting symptom, occurring in approximately 80% of our patients. These babies rank below the 10th percentile on their growth chart or show a marked falling off of growth progression. A small group of infants with GER are so severely malnourished as to require hospitalization because of marked debilitation. In such patients, a vigorous positional and feeding therapy should be undertaken by the nursing staff. In this selected group of infants, if control of aspiration, dehydration and nutrition is not achieved in a period of three weeks, operation is advised. Recurrent aspiration with pneumonia occurs in nearly half of all infants with pernicious GER. More patients are now being recognized with apneic episodes who have GER as the underlying cause.

Most infants can be safely treated medically for at least 3 months before being judged as failures of conservative treatment. The medical regimen consists of thickening all formula feedings with rice cereal and propping the infant for one to two hours after each feeding. If this does not control the vomiting, the infant may be propped for 24 hours/day. In such cases, it is necessary to support the baby's head with a doughnut or other padding to ensure that the head does not become flattened. Rarely, operation may be necessary because of severe esophagitis; this condition is manifested in the infant by constant fussiness or apparent "colic." It is also necessary to operate on those patients who have major displacement of the stomach in the chest whenever this anatomic deformity is discovered.

The criteria used for operation are persistent vomiting after sustained rigorous medical regimen, plus one of the following: (1) absent or markedly depressed weight gain; (2) severe malnutrition and no response to 2 weeks of intensive medical treatment in the hospital; (3) recurrent pneumonia; (4) apneic spells; or (5) major anatomic displacement of the stomach in the chest.

In most patients, when surgical treatment is necessary, the Nissen fundoplication has proven remarkably effective (Fig. 34-9).[45] Surgical correction of reflux has usually been followed by gratifying clinical improvement including prompt gain in weight and other

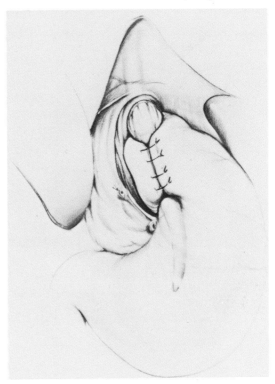

Fig. 34-9. A successful method for the surgical correction of gastroesophageal reflux employs gastric fundoplication described by Nissen.

growth parameters: relief of pneumonia, prevention of apneic spells, and healing of esophagitis (Fig. 34-10).[39,43,46]

Neuromuscular Dysfunction

Interference with the normal propulsive movements of the esophagus can occur as a result of intracranial pathology. Dysphagia, regurgitation, or failure of the baby to feed avidly is typical. Aspiration with subsequent bronchopneumonia and atelectasis is common. The symptom complex is often confused with simple feeding problems or GER. The diagnosis is usually made by careful anteroposterior (AP) and lateral cine fluoroscopic observation of the esophagus during barium swallow. This study discloses discoordinate, ineffective peristalsis with poor transport of the ingested material into the stomach. There is no specific therapy to correct this problem. In some infants gastrostomy may be necessary if starvation and overwhelming aspiration are to be prevented.

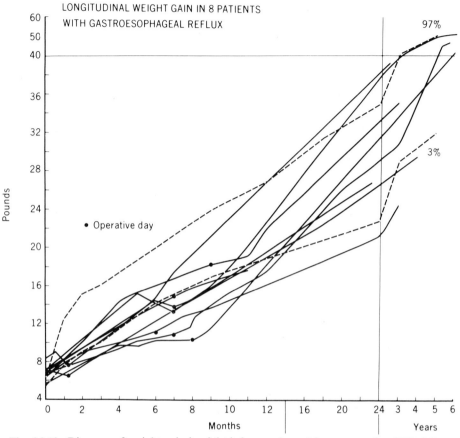

Fig. 34-10. Diagram of weight gain in eight infants selected for surgery for GER followed to 24 months of age. Most show a dramatic postoperative change in weight gain and growth when pernicious GER has been manifest.

Vascular Ring

Vascular rings are considered in more detail in the section on cardiovascular disease but deserve mention here as another important cause of partial obstruction of the esophagus.[47,48] The common types that cause dysphagia are the true ring double aortic arch and right aortic arch with a persistent left ligamentum arteriosum. Because both of these defects entrap the trachea as well as the esophagus, respiratory obstruction may be more clinically obvious than the difficulty with swallowing. The aberrant right subclavian artery originates as a persistent fourth branch of the descending aorta and passes behind the esophagus on its way to the right shoulder; this vessel is usually asymptomatic but occasionally causes partial obstruction of the esophagus and dysphagia. Anomalies of the aortic arch are best defined

by barium esophageal swallow, tracheogram, and contrast studies of the aortic arch (angiography). Esophagoscopy and tracheoscopy are sometimes helpful in determining the magnitude of obstruction and the dynamic features of the transmitted pulsations in the wall of the esophagus and trachea. Appropriate surgery affords complete relief in nearly all babies with an obstructing vascular ring.

Achalasia

Achalasia (without relaxation) describes the condition of the terminal esophagus seen as a tightening or overactivity of the musculature causing partial obstruction of the esophagogastric junction. Even in babies, the esophagus may be dilated for part or all of its length above the constriction. The condition usually affects the young adult but, while rare in the newborn, has been reported and is part of any differential diagnosis concerned with obstruction of the distal esophagus. Pressure dilatation of the constricted area of the esophagus has been effective in many older patients but this treatment must be repeated at intervals. Because patients can be completely and permanently relieved by a direct operation on the esophageal muscle similar to a Ramstedt pyloromyotomy, this has been the treatment selected for most babies with achalasia.

ABDOMINAL SURGERY — GENERAL

The hallmarks of the surgical abdomen are distension and bilious vomiting. To these should be added the scaphoid contour seen when there is high intestinal obstruction or when the abdominal viscera are in an ectopic location such as in those infants with congenital diaphragmatic hernia. Extreme degrees of abdominal distension are associated with intestinal perforation, particularly gastric. Tenderness signifying peritoneal irritation can be elicited by careful examination. A tender, erythematous abdominal wall is a reliable sign of an intraabdominal catastrophe with resultant peritonitis and ischemic intestine. Reliance on bowel sounds can be misleading. Peristalsis can be present despite peritonitis or absent when intestinal distension is secondary to mechanical obstruction.

Pertinent radiologic studies to be obtained in all cases of suspected intraabdominal surgical lesions are the flat and upright views of the abdomen. Intestinal obstruction can be diagnosed and the level of obstruction determined by the configuration of the air-fluid levels. Pneumoperitoneum is readily appreciated. Distended bowel and the absence of air fluid levels in intestinal loops of various sizes suggests obstruction secondary to meconium ileus. Unless precluded by a deteriorating clinical condition, a barium enema requires only a short delay which is usually justified by the information obtained. The enema need not be an elaborate study in these precarious subjects. The instillation of a few ounces of contrast material provides information regarding the rotation of the colon in case of suspected volvulus, or the existence of a microcolon confirming distal intestinal obstruction. When the caliber and position of the colon are normal, proximal obstruction or Hirschsprung's disease must be considered.

Radiographic study by contrast medium of the upper intestine is rarely needed. Air is often effective in delineating the stomach and upper portion of the intestine. The progress of a bolus of air is readily followed with serial films and the infant is not subjected to the risks of vomiting and aspiration of other contrast agents. However, incomplete obstructions of the GI tract such as those caused by congenital stenosis or intralumenal webs are often the most difficult congenital lesions to diagnose and may require formal contrast studies of the upper gastrointestinal tract.

Pneumoperitoneum — Gastric Perforation

Spontaneous perforation of a hollow viscus is most frequently seen in distressed neonates who have undergone resuscitation immediately after birth. Although the stomach is the most common viscus to perforate, the presence of free air in the peritoneal cavity may be secondary to perforation elsewhere in the gastrointestinal tract. For that reason, the surgeon approaching the infant with pneumoperitoneum must be prepared to investigate systematically the entire gastrointestinal tract and anticipate diverse problems such as gastric perforation, necrotizing enterocolitis, Hirschsprung's disease, or other ischemic insults to the intestine resulting in perforation.

Following perforation, egress of air in the free peritoneal cavity usually leads to impressive abdominal distension. Elevation of the diaphragm occurs with considerable embarrassment of the infant's respiratory dynamics. A temporizing but life-saving maneuver is needle aspiration of the peritoneal cavity to diminish air under pressure, thereby allowing the diaphragm to return to a more normal position. Usually, there is dramatic relief of abdominal distension and respiratory distress. It is not hazardous to insert a needle adapted to a 50 ml syringe through the anterior abdominal wall. The bowel is usually compressed against the posterior parietes and is not likely to be injured by this maneuver.

Surgical intervention must be prompt. When massive distension of the abdomen occurs, a gastric perforation can be anticipated. Typically, the rent occurs high on the greater curvature of the stomach. Because the perforation may be located on the posterior gastric wall, thorough exploration of the relatively inaccessible areas of the stomach must be carried out. Although it has been suggested that perforation of the stomach results from congenital deficiency of musculature in the gastric wall, this explanation is questionable. The apparent absence of musculature at the margin of perforation probably represents retraction of the muscles of an overdistended stomach with a ballooning of mucosa between the muscle fibers.

Repair is accomplished by direct suture after débridement of the margins of perforation. A gastrostomy tube inserted through a noninvolved area of the stomach is advisable to ensure postoperative decompression. The subsequent course of the infant is usually smooth if the underlying problem for which resuscitation was required is controlled. Cautious feedings can be started within a few days of surgical repair. The diagnosis and management of perforations occurring elsewhere in the gastrointestinal tract are considered under specific headings.

Temporary Diversion of the Intestinal Tract

Newborn intestinal emergencies often demand a temporary vent or enterostomy. Though not as desirable as an end-to-end union of the bowel, these measures may be lifesaving in fragile infants who are depleted by intestinal obstruction or peritonitis, or who are threatened by serious congenital defects. An abdominal stoma in the infant does not carry the same implications as in the adult; this fact must be stressed to allay the fears and doubts of a worried parent. Usually, the procedures are temporizing and the outlook for restoration of complete intestinal continuity is good.

Gastrostomy. The stomach requires venting for two reasons. First, decompression of the gastrointestinal tract is necessary in the face of any abdominal catastrophe. Placement of the gastrostomy obviates the need for a nasogastric tube. It is not only more efficient, but eliminates the danger of pressure necrosis of the alar cartilage of the infant's nose as well as the respiratory hazards which attend nasogastric tubes. Second, the gastrostomy tube provides access for feeding a depleted neonate.

Gastrostomy can, when necessary, be performed under local anesthesia while the baby remains in the isothermic environment of an infant warmer. Frequently, the procedure complements a primary abdominal operation. A simple Stamm gastrostomy is preferred and it is not difficult to remove or replace the tube as an office procedure.

Ileostomy. Temporary ileostomy is less desirable than primary union of the bowel, but there are clinical circumstances when its creation as a temporary diverting procedure is prudent, including: (1) inflammatory necrosis of the distal small bowel with intraperitoneal soiling and peritonitis (2) an ischemic insult with marginal viability of the bowel and (3) marked disparity in lumen size as seen in intestinal atresia or meconium ileus.

A properly performed ileostomy is usually well tolerated and rarely results in skin breakdown. With appropriate supportive care, weight gain and healing proceed and subsequently, intestinal reconstruction can be carried out electively with greater safety for the infant.

In very sick infants, or in babies with other underlying conditions such as meconium ileus, the double barrel enterostomy of Mikulicz has proven valuable. The common wall which has been created is gradually crushed with a special clamp, partly reestablishing intestinal continuity. Subsequently, complete closure of the bowel can be achieved without the necessity of reentering the peritoneal cavity. Another effective technique of intestinal venting which permits access to the distal gastrointestinal tract is the end-to-side enteroenterostomy described by Bishop and Koop. This technique has particular application for lesions in the proximal gastrointestinal tract such as jejunal or high ileal atresia.

Colostomy. The four usual indications for colostomy in the neonate are (1) impending or actual perforation of the colon, (2) colonic atresia with huge disparity of the bowel lumen, (3) Hirschsprung's disease, and (4) high imperforate anus. The loop colostomy is favored by many and has the advantage of simplicity and speed in critically ill babies. An endcolostomy is mechanically sound, easily managed, and avoids spillover into the distal loop. This latter characteristic is an advantage in Hirschsprung's disease and imperforate anus. A diaper neatly covers the colostomy during the early months of life until definitive surgical correction of the primary problem is accomplished and the colostomy closed.

Hypertrophic Pyloric Stenosis

The incidence of pyloric stenosis has been estimated at between 1/300 and 1/1000 live births. Despite its frequency, the etiology is obscure. Male infants are affected about four times as frequently as females and the disease seems to have a predilection for the firstborn. There is a familial tendency, with a 7% incidence of pyloric stenosis in children of affected parents. It has been speculated that hypertrophy of the circular muscles of the pylorus results from propulsion of milk curds against the spastic pyloric canal, producing edema, further spasm and subsequently, hypertrophy of the musculature leading to complete obstruction. Some have postulated that the muscle hypertrophy is a response to vagal stimulation. This is somewhat substantiated by the observation that infants undergoing surgery for esophageal atresia and tracheoesophageal fistula seem to have a higher incidence of pyloric stenosis, a result perhaps of vagal nerve irritation in the operative field. No infectious agent has ever been isolated despite the apparent seasonal incidence of the disease. The clinical onset of bile-free projectile vomiting in the firstborn male 2 to 8 weeks of age strongly suggests the diagnosis of congenital hypertrophic pyloric stenosis. Often however, the onset is insidious and these babies can present to the pediatrician as perplexing feeding problems. A typical history reveals intermittent vomiting which gradually increases in frequency and intensity over a period of a week, until the baby vomits most ingested feedings with impressive force.

Abdominal examination is carried out with the stomach empty. It may be necessary to accomplish this by means of a nasogastric tube in order to ensure an adequate examination. The baby can be given a sugar nipple or pacifier for relaxation. The examiner stands to the left, elevating the baby's feet with his left hand to relax the abdominal muscles and then proceeds to palpate gently in the right upper quadrant. The pyloric "olive" is palpable to the experienced examiner in 90% of cases and upper gastrointestinal contrast studies are usually not needed.

Infants with pyloric stenosis are conveniently grouped according to their clinical condition at the time they are seen by the surgeon. About half will be well hydrated and in a satisfactory nutritional state. Serum electrolytes are normal and the urine, though concentrated, is of adequate volume. These babies can undergo surgical correction without preoperative preparation. In the remaining infants, preparation prior to surgery is necessary. The typical pattern of electrolyte disturbance is that of mild to moderate metabolic alkalosis. The hypokalemia may not be reflected in the serum electrolytes, but potassium supplements must be provided before the alkalosis can be corrected. On the average, these moderately dehydrated infants can be corrected after 24 hours of intravenous rehydration with a dextrose-electrolyte solution calculated at 2000 to 2500 ml/m². Replacement of potassium ion must be adequate to restore acid-base equilibrium. This requires 2 to 3 mmol/kg of potassium during the 24-hour period of therapy.

A small number of infants present with severe dehydration and malnutrition and are often well below their birth weight. In this group, extensive rehabilitation is mandatory before surgery. The infants are profoundly alkalotic and potassium deficient. Their protein stores are depleted, urine is scanty and they may be anemic. Intensive therapy of 2 to 3 days is required to bring these infants into proper metabolic balance. Fluids, electrolytes, colloid, and even blood may be necessary.

A Ramstedt–Fredet pyloromyotomy is best performed through a transverse skin incision placed in the right-upper quadrant of the abdomen. This short, safe, surgical procedure accomplishes division of the hypertrophic circular muscles of the gastric outlet and reestablishes patency of the pyloric channel (Fig. 34-11). In most cases, glucose water feedings can be reinstituted 6 hours postoperatively. The initial oral feedings are limited to about 30 ml every 2 hours until the infant demonstrates that this can be tolerated. The following day, the feedings are advanced to diluted formula, again restricting the volume to 30 ml every 2 hours. On the second postoperative day, full-strength formula is offered with similar restrictions on volume. By the third or fourth day, the infants are usually advanced to standard feedings in adequate volumes and can be considered ready for discharge. Typi-

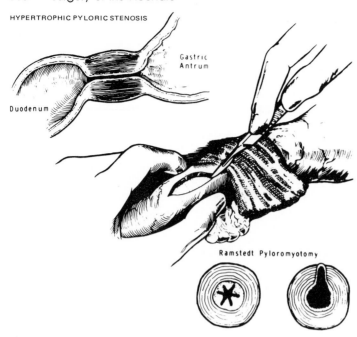

HYPERTROPHIC PYLORIC STENOSIS

Gastric Antrum

Duodenum

Ramstedt Pyloromyotomy

Fig. 34-11. Ramstedt pyloromyotomy, which is made through all layers of the pylorus except the mucosa. The cross-section figure demonstrates how the mucosa of the pylorus open into the defect created, thereby expanding the cross-sectional diameter of the pyloric channel.

cally, the babies enjoy a growth spurt in the immediate postoperative weeks, much to the satisfaction of the parents.

INTESTINAL OBSTRUCTION, ABNORMALITIES OF ROTATION, MALROTATION, AND MIDGUT VOLVULUS

In the developing embryo, as the elongating intestine returns to the coelomic cavity, it must of necessity undergo rotation so that it can be accommodated within the confines of the abdominal cavity. The proximal small intestine assumes the characteristic C-contour and the duodenum is fixed in the upper left abdomen at the ligament of Trietz. The cecum takes a counter-clockwise rotation reaching its final location in the right lower abdomen. Incomplete intestinal rotation with consequent inadequate fixation of the intestinal mesentery may be an asymptomatic occurrence, may give rise to subtle symptoms difficult to diagnose, or may present as a life-threatening intraabdominal catastrophe. An understanding of the mechanism by which the lesion becomes symptomatic is necessary if one is to recognize and prevent the devastating complications which can accompany midgut volvulus.

When rotation is abnormal, bands are formed between the ectopic cecum, located in

the right upper quadrant, and the right lateral abdominal wall. As these bands course from the cecum to the abdominal wall, they traverse the duodenum and can cause intermittent, incomplete duodenal obstruction. Symptoms of partial duodenal obstruction are often baffling. The infant may experience intervals of a normal feeding pattern which are interspersed with exasperating episodes of vomiting. Because the obstruction is high in the gastrointestinal tract, abdominal distension does not occur. The telltale sign of an underlying mechanical problem is the presence of bile in the vomitus. This lesion, more than any other, supports the contention that bile-stained vomitus in the infant necessitates a thorough diagnostic work-up lest a malrotation go undetected and a subsequent midgut volvulus occur.

The most reliable diagnostic study is a barium enema which shows the cecum in the right upper quadrant of the abdomen. An upper gastrointestinal series usually is not necessary for confirmation but, when performed, shows the abnormal course of the duodenum and partial obstruction by the ''bands of Ladd'' which traverse it. Surgical correction of malrotation of the colon prevents a future volvulus of the midgut and relieves the partial duodenal obstruction. The bands binding the cecum to the right abdominal wall are lysed, thereby freeing the large bowel, which is then transposed to the left side of the abdomen. The duodenum is mobilized on its medial aspect where the narrow mesentery is intimately associated with the superior mesenteric artery. As the mesentery of the small bowel is freed medially, it assumes a broad position over the posterior abdominal wall. With the mesentery thus splayed out, potential for torsion is eliminated. It is not necessary to fix the intestine in its new position with sutures. The appendix, however, because it now lies on the left side of the abdomen, is usually removed or inverted.

Malrotation with Midgut Volvulus

When fixation of the mesentery of the small bowel has not occurred normally, the intestine is subject to torsion on the axis of the superior mesenteric artery. This mechanism of obstruction must be considered whenever an infant is seen with bile-stained vomiting, especially when abdominal distension is not present. Abdominal tenderness is an ominous finding.

Roentgenographic abnormalities are often characteristic, with evidence of duodenal obstruction and scanty gas distributed throughout the remainder of the bowel. The air-fluid levels typical of intestinal obstruction elsewhere in the gastrointestinal tract are not usually associated. An airless abdomen is an ominous sign and usually means that infarction of the intestine has already taken place. A barium enema is confirmatory because it shows the cecum abnormally in the right- or central-upper abdomen. If an upper gastrointestinal series is obtained, it shows a corkscrew-like constriction of the third portion of the duodenum. This study is not usually required to establish the diagnosis.

Once the diagnosis of midgut volvulus is made, or if there is sufficient suspicion that it may be the underlying mechanism for the infant's illness, emergency surgical exploration is undertaken. When the findings are favorable and the bowel is viable, the torsion is reduced by counterclockwise rotation and a Ladd procedure, precisely the same as that described for the treatment of malrotation without volvulus, is carried out. The prognosis is favorable as long as the viability of the intestine is not in question. However, when the diagnosis has been delayed or when the

volvulus has been an intrauterine event, intestinal ischemia, infarction, or both may be encountered in the distribution of the superior mesenteric artery. Initial judgments regarding the viability of the intestine are not easy; intestinal resection at the time of initial exploration is contraindicated. The ischemic intestine must be given every opportunity to recover after the torsion has been reduced. Thus, the first operation consists only of untwisting the small bowel and establishing a gastrostomy. This can be accomplished rapidly and under local anesthesia in precarious subjects. Reexploration 24 to 36 hours later is undertaken and areas of obvious infarction are identified. These are resected and appropriate enterostomies are brought out to the abdominal wall; anastomosis is contraindicated. Once again, any intestine of marginal viability is left behind in the hope that it will recover. Reexploration in order to determine recovery or further loss of small bowel is repeated after another interval of 36 to 48 hours. When the full extent of intestinal loss has been established, and the margins of viable bowel exteriorized, one is then faced with the management of a desperately ill infant at risk from sepsis, disseminated intravascular coagulation, and the inevitable nutritional crisis attending a short bowel syndrome.

In 1969, Dudrick, Wilmore and coworkers demonstrated the feasibility of total parenteral nutritional support for such infants.[49,50] A central venous catheter for total parenteral alimentation is established and nourishment is provided by this technique throughout the early postoperative weeks. When the infant has achieved positive nitrogen balance and the reestablishment of intestinal continuity is complete, there is then a difficult period of weaning from parenteral to oral feedings. About 40 cm of residual intestine seems to be required for successful adaptation of the intestine.[51] When the distal ileum and ileocecal valve are intact, slightly less bowel may be tolerated.[52] Infant formulas which are fat free and contain monosaccharides and hydrolysed protein are now available.[53] These require only a minimal absorptive surface and little enzyme activity for assimilation. Gradually, the volume and concentration of these substances may be increased until all calories are taken by mouth. The process of weaning the infant from total intravenous to total oral alimentation may take

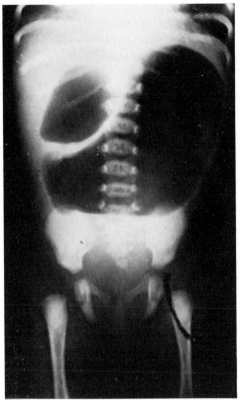

Fig. 34-12. Characteristic "double bubble" of congenital duodenal obstruction.

months. This serves to underscore the devastating complications of a midgut volvulus and indicates the need for vigilance by pediatrician and surgeon in the pursuit of the diagnosis of malrotation.

Intestinal Obstruction

Intestinal obstruction in the newborn occurs from a variety of congenital causes. An early sign is bile-stained vomitus. While there are medical causes of bilious vomiting, such as sepsis, any infant with this complaint is presumed to have a surgical lesion. Only after mechanical causes of intestinal obstruction have been excluded can alternative explanations be accepted. Depending upon the level in the gastrointestinal tract at which the obstruction occurs, the abdomen may or may not be distended. Tenderness can be elicited even in the newborn, and special significance must be accorded this symptom when it accompanies bile vomiting because it usually means that there is an associated peritonitis.

An orderly but expeditious diagnostic approach is undertaken when an infant is suspected of having intestinal obstruction. Flat and upright abdominal x-ray films are always obtained. When circumstances permit, a barium enema or in special cases, a contrast enema (Gastrografin) is a useful adjunct. Information is obtained regarding intestinal rotation, caliber, as well as the presence of inflammation. Radioopaque contrast administered by mouth is ordinarily not necessary and can be hazardous. When upper intestinal contrast studies are needed, the progress of a bolus of 60 ml of air instilled by tube into the stomach provides the necessary information.

Duodenal Obstruction

Duodenal obstruction may be complete or partial and result from intrinsic causes or external compression. An intralumenal diaphragm can cause partial, intermittent obstruction difficult to recognize. Only a carefully performed upper gastrointestinal series outlines an intralumenal web and determines the site of obstruction. Annular pancreas, duodenal stenosis, and congenital bands are other causes of partial obstruction in which the need for early surgical intervention is more apparent.

Duodenal atresia results in complete obstruction. In instances of complete duodenal obstruction, swallowed air is prevented from passing beyond the duodenum, and therefore the mid- and lower abdomen is scaphoid. The characteristic x-ray finding is that of a double bubble of ingested air filling the stomach and blind-ending duodenum (Fig. 34-12). Duodenal atresia is often seen in association with Down syndrome (trisomy 21).

Unless the underlying cause of obstruction is related to malrotation, an initial period of nasogastric drainage and resuscitation with intravenous fluids and electrolytes is appropriate before embarking upon surgical correction of duodenal obstruction. Surgical therapy is tailored to the particular lesion encountered. The intralumenal web can be resected through a transduodenal approach. It may be necessary to perform a gastrotomy or duodenotomy through which a Foley catheter with the balloon minimally inflated is passed, in order to identify the site at which the web is attached. Obstruction secondary to annular pancreas is best treated by creating a duodenojejunos-

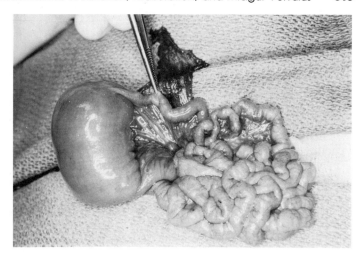

Fig. 34-13. Jejunal atresia, showing dilated proximal segment and narrow distal jejunum.

tomy, bypassing the obstruction. Efforts to resect the pancreatic tissue have usually resulted in dangerous complications. Some stenotic lesions can be managed by local duodenoplasty but obstruction from duodenal atresia requires bypass for relief. Following surgery, a long period of duodenal atony can be anticipated. A gastrostomy is therefore advisable at the time of initial surgery to provide decompression until intestinal function returns.

Jejunoileal Atresia

Atresia of the bowel probably results from an ischemic insult to the intestine during its developmental stages.[54] The atresia may be discrete involving only a short segment of jejunum or ileum (Fig. 34-13) or may involve the intestine over many centimeters.[55] Atretic areas are sometimes multiple and, although the intervening bowel is normal, considerable length may be absent. Abdominal distension and bile-stained vomiting are the usual presenting symptoms. X-ray films show air fluid levels distributed throughout the abdomen (Fig. 34-14). In cases of distal ileal obstruction, the barium enema adds further confirmation, showing the typical microcolon.

A short period of restoration with fluids, electrolytes and colloid may be necessary but this should never exceed a few hours. Surgical correction is best accomplished by resecting a short segment of the bulbous end of the bowel which is just proximal to the atresia. End-to-end reconstruction after appropriate tailoring of the small distal segment is the most desirable goal.[56,57] End-to-side anastomosis,

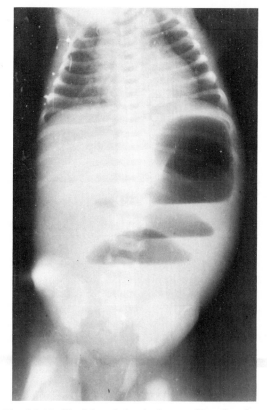

Fig. 34-14. Upright, abdominal x-ray film of patient with jejunal atresia. There is gastric distension and approximately three other loops of bowel with no gas beyond the obstruction.

described by Bishop and Koop, has proven safe and effective and has the added advantage of providing access to the gastrointestinal tract for irrigations postoperatively.[58] This type of repair is particularly helpful when there is a major disparity in the size of the ends of the intestine. A Mikulicz enterostomy or simple end-enterostomy may be lifesaving in critically ill, depleted newborns with distal bowel obstruction.

Incomplete obstruction resulting from stenosis of the bowel can be both puzzling and hazardous because there is a confusing clinical picture.[55] The infants feed poorly, occasionally vomit, or become distended without pattern. These symptoms continue despite changes in the formula. The pediatrician considers food allergies, nonspecific failure to thrive, and even "nervous mother" as the underlying cause. Finally, the obstruction becomes complete or the bowel perforates. Surgical exploration may be needed to confirm a diagnosis of ileal stenosis and this approach is considered even if x-ray examinations of the intestine have been normal but the clinical course of the infant suggests this diagnosis. Cure is achieved by resection of the stenotic segment or by appropriate intestinal tailoring procedures such as a Y-V plasty or longitudinal incision and transverse closure (Heineke–Mikulicz principle).

Duplications

A less common cause of intestinal obstruction in the newborn is that arising secondary to duplications of the bowel. These can exist in any level of the intestine and may cause obstruction when the lumen is compromised by the gradually expanding duplication. Because they occur on the mesenteric aspect of the bowel, duplications are intimately involved with the blood supply to the normal intestine. Small, cystic duplications are easily resected along with a segment of the adjacent bowel. However, extensive fusiform or intramural duplications may tax the surgeon's ingenuity. In these instances, resection of the common wall with creation of a single conduit may enable the surgeon to preserve an extensive segment of normal intestine. Gastric mucosa can exist within a duplication and, although an infrequent complication, may result in gastrointestinal hemorrhage. This cause of gastrointestinal bleeding is considered in the evaluation of a baby with melena.

Meconium Ileus

Intestinal obstruction resulting from viscid meconium impacted in the terminal ileum is seen as the earliest manifestation of cystic fibrosis. This problem arises in about 10% of the cystic fibrosis population. Infants with meconium ileus subsequently develop other complications of their underlying disease; however, the latter respiratory sequelae are not necessarily more severe.[59]

The clinical presentation of meconium ileus is not unlike that seen with other forms of distal intestinal obstruction. Abdominal distension and bile-stained vomitus are characteristic. The upright film of the abdomen is especially helpful in this form of intestinal obstruction in the newborn. The characteristic soap bubble mass in the right-lower abdomen as well as a paucity of air-fluid levels despite the presence of many gas-filled loops of intestine is pathognomonic (Fig 34-15). The air-fluid levels characteristic of obstruction do not develop because air is trapped by the tenacious meconium and a clear interface is not produced. The barium enema shows a microcolon, unused because of the distal ileal obstruction. Concretions of meconium in the terminal ileum immediately proximal to the ileocecal valve are often seen.

In the past, surgical intervention was required for relief of obstruction. More recently, it has been shown that rectal installation of Gastrografin will often eliminate the obstructing bolus of meconium.[60] This radiopaque contrast material contains a wetting agent (Tween 80) in which the thick meconium is soluble. Thus, if the Gastrografin can be successfully advanced through the microcolon and into the obstructed distal ileum, there is reasonable expectation that meconium will be passed spontaneously with relief of obstruction. This kind of enema is not without risk. Because of the hyperosmolarity of the agent, dehydration secondary to fluid shifts into the lumen of the intestine must be prevented.[61] The infant's hydration is maintained throughout the procedure by a continuous intravenous infusion. When the first attempt moves some meconium out but the infant's obstruction is not completely relieved, a second enema is justified several hours later. When these maneuvers fail to relieve the obstruction or meconium peritonitis is present, surgical exploration is the only accepted treatment.

When surgical correction is necessary, technical problems associated with evacuating the tar-like meconium from the distended distal ileum and also establishing intestinal continuity between the dilated proximal intestine and the distal microcolon have been solved in various ways. Irrigation with dilute n-acetylcysteine has proven effective. A rapid and safe anastomosis using the Bishop–Koop technique is well suited for this problem. A Mikulicz enteroenterostomy has the virtue of speed while also providing decompression and establishment of continuity. These techniques allow access to the distal intestine for irrigations in the postoperative period with n-acetylcysteine. With use, the colon has the potential to function normally, and the vent established by the Mikulicz or Bishop–Koop procedure is closed surgically. In the postoperative period, the infant is subject to respiratory difficulty secondary to impacted secretions. These may require tracheal suctioning or bronchoscopy for relief. When oral feedings are instituted, exogenous pancreatic supplements are provided to assure digestion and utilization of calories.

Hirschsprung's Disease

The clinical presentation of Hirschsprung's disease (aganglionic megacolon) may be subtle and, in fact, go unrecognized for months or even years until the classic symptoms of constipation and abdominal distension are unmistakable.[62] It is important to note, however, that the history of constipation goes back to the early days of life in most patients with Hirschsprung's disease. The consequences of aganglionosis can be of such magnitude as to be life-threatening in the newborn period. The absence of ganglion cells modifies neuromuscular conduction and prevents proper evacuation of the bowel. Abdominal distension or debilitating enterocolitis brings the infant to the surgeon's attention.

Failure of an infant to pass meconium in the first 36 hours of life should alert the pediatrician to the possibility of Hirschsprung's disease. Retention of a meconium plug requiring mechanical assistance for its evacuation is another presumptive sign that the colon may be aganglionic. A positive barium enema, even in a newborn, can be a reliable indication of the diagnosis of Hirschsprung's disease. The characteristic terminal narrow segment, with transition to dilated bowel in the area of the rectosigmoid, are classic findings. However,

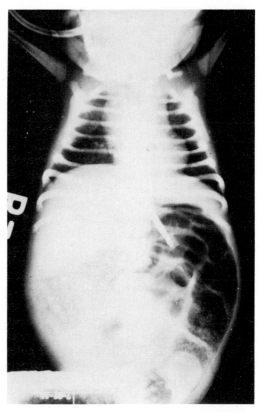

Fig. 34-15. X-ray of newborn infant with meconium ileus. There are many gas-filled loops, but little fluid is seen. Note that the right-lower quadrant is filled with a large loop of intestine distended by meconium. Gas trapped in the meconium gives the typical "ground-glass" appearance.

a normal barium enema in the neonate does not exclude the diagnosis of aganglionosis, and confirmatory evidence must be obtained by rectal biopsy.

Several techniques of biopsy have been described, but one which provides an adequate specimen of the rectal wall can serve to establish the diagnosis.[63] The absence of ganglion cells in the submucosal or muscular plexis confirms the diagnosis. Experienced pathologists can interpret the more superficial biopsies which include only the submucosal tissue. The advantage of partial thickness biopsy is that there is less intramural scarring to complicate the definitive surgical procedure for correction of Hirschsprung's disease. Recently, a suction biopsy technique has become available which is readily adapted for use in infants.[64] This bedside procedure provides adequate submucosal tissue for interpretation by an experienced pediatric pathologist. Additionally, a histochemical technique estimating acetylcholinesterase activity has been helpful in establishing the diagnosis and has the added advantage of using only tiny fragments of bowel tissue.[65]

The clinical presentation of Hirschsprung's disease is varied. Intestinal obstruction is not always typical. Enterocolitis is often the presenting complaint in a newborn and this may be confused with the necrotizing enterocolitis seen primarily in premature infants with respiratory distress. The effects of enterocolitis associated with Hirschsprung's disease can be devastating unless recognized and treated appropriately.[66] Whether the symptoms are those of obstruction or enterocolitis, once the diagnosis has been established, the safest course of action is the performance of a colostomy in an area of ganglionic bowel. The majority of babies have a transition somewhere in the rectosigmoid and a high sigmoid colostomy usually assures normal innervation. The presence of ganglion cells at the site of the colostomy should be verified at the time of surgery. In desperately ill infants, the condition may be so precarious as to preclude a controlled laparotomy with frozen section confirmation of the transition area. In these babies, a right transverse colostomy can be performed under local anesthesia. This proximal colostomy will assure that ganglionic bowel has been exteriorized in 98% of cases. The few remaining infants will have total colonic aganglionosis or aganglionic small bowel and will present special problems in management.[67] In these infants, barium enema is helpful, showing marked foreshortening of the entire colon. The basic surgical principle, however, is to achieve exteriorization of the most distal normally enervated bowel.

Definitive surgical therapy is deferred until the infants are managed through the initial crisis and have achieved a weight of about 7 to 9 kg. At that time, the ganglionic intestine is transposed to the anus by one of several pull-through techniques now available. These include the classical operation described by Swenson or the modification popularized by Duhamel.[68] Many centers now favor the endorectal pull-through of Soave.[69]

In those infants having ''short-segment'' Hirschsprung's disease, in which only the terminal rectum is aganglionic, it may be possible to achieve satisfactory bowel evacuation without colostomy. Reliance on laxatives and enemas is not necessary but colostomy can be avoided before the definitive surgical procedure is carried out. Stripping of the muscular layers of the rectum and utilizing a sacral approach is the definitive treatment of ultra-short-segment Hirschsprung's disease.

One of the most dangerous complications of Hirschsprung's disease is enterocolitis. This often presents with diarrhea and signs of collapse. Sepsis may be fatal if not promptly recognized and treated. The enterocolitis can sometimes be controlled by careful rectal lavage using quarter-normal solutions of saline. This lavage should be done by a physician mindful of the dangers of water intoxication and dilutional hyponatremia or excess sodium absorption. It is vital that the volume of solution instilled be recovered during the lavage. The diseased colon is at risk of perforation and the first signs of peritonitis demand surgical intervention and colostomy.

When the index of suspicion of Hirschsprung's disease is high, the diagnosis will be made early. In general, the outlook for these infants is favorable because currently available operations have now become standardized and there is hope that the babies with congenital megacolon will achieve an excellent functional result.

Enterocolitis

Until recently, this entity has received little attention. Apparently, advances in the techniques of management of severely distressed infants have resulted in a population of newborns at risk from this condition. Necrotizing enterocolitis has been encountered with increasing frequency as more infants with respiratory distress are salvaged. (See also Chap. 42.)

The etiology, pathogenesis, and pathophysiology remain controversial.[70] Necrotizing enterocolitis probably results from an ischemic insult to the intestine. Umbilical artery catheters usually placed for blood gas monitoring may contribute to the development of the syndrome. However, whether the catheter *per se* is the inciting factor or is incidental in distressed, hypoxic infants requiring monitoring is not known. The disease also occurs in infants in whom there has been no indwelling arterial line. Most infants who develop this disease have been fed and especially hypertonic formulas have been implicated in its etiology. The stressed, premature infant is at great risk for necrotizing enterocolitis and constant observation for the early signs of the disease is mandatory.

Progression to the florid syndrome of necrotizing enterocolitis is often gradual and insidious. The earliest signs include poor feeding, gastric distension and the presence of bile in the gastric aspirate. These findings, albeit nonspecific, should alert the medical and surgical staff to an underlying ischemic insult to the intestine with impending necrotizing enterocolitis. There follows abdominal distension, often associated with erythema of the abdominal wall. The abdomen may be tender and loops of distended intestine may be visible through the abdominal wall. Ultimately, the intestine may undergo ischemic necrosis with perforation and peritonitis. Evolution of this pathologic state can be rapid and perforation can occur within a few hours of the first symptom; more often, 24 to 36 hours elapse before peritonitis develops.

X-ray films taken early in the course of the disease show generalized small bowel distension without obstruction. The loops of distended intestine may be separated, indicating edema of the wall. The roentgenographic finding of air in the wall of the intestine is the hallmark of necrotizing enterocolitis. Pneumatosis intestinalis may not be apparent early in the course of the disease and the absence of this finding does not rule out necrotizing enterocolitis. The x-ray finding of air in the portal system used to be regarded as an ominous sign, signifying a far-advanced ischemic insult. This is not invariably true, and infants with this finding may recover.

The management of these infants throughout the pathophysiologic stages of this illness presents a dilemma for both pediatrician and surgeon. Premature surgical exploration confirms the diagnosis of ischemic intestine, but unless there has been perforation, there is little the surgeon can do to improve the course of the baby.[71] Furthermore, the subsequent ability to assess the progression of abdominal tenderness or the presence of free air in the abdomen is lost after surgical exploration. The indications for surgery are intestinal perforation, or intestinal infarction without free perforation. These intraabdominal events are not always easy to recognize, and delay subjects the infant to the risks of peritonitis with secondary sepsis, disseminated intravascular coagulation, and death. Successful management requires meticulous observations of the infant's status with frequent x-ray evaluation for the sudden development of free abdominal air. While this finding indicates the need for immediate surgical exploration, the clinical assessment of the infant is equally important. If abdominal tenderness worsens or the infant's condition is obviously deteriorating, surgery may be elected with the expectation of encountering infarcted intestine. The development of thrombocytopenia may indicate an underlying disseminated intravascular coagulation incited by the ischemic bowel. Careful monitoring of serial platelet counts has proven useful in identifying the infants in whom these intestinal changes were evolving. Persistent acidosis and the need for ventilator support of respiration may well be early indicators of the development of gangrene of the intestine. The recent finding of turbid brown fluid with bacteria on gram stain after peritoneal lavage is regarded by some authors as a reliable indicator of gangrene.[72]

Pathologic findings may be those of diffuse involvement of the gastrointestinal tract including even the stomach and large bowel, or the disease can be segmental in distribution and restricted only to a short segment of small intestine (Fig. 34-16). In some, areas of involvement in the small intestine alternate with relatively normal bowel, while in others the lesion is restricted only to the distal ileum and proximal large bowel. Surgical conservatism is the rule. Areas of intestine of marginal viability are preserved, while obvious necrotic or perforated bowel must be exteriorized. No attempts at primary anastomosis are made at the time of initial exploration because of the hazard of uniting potentially ischemic bowel. Gastrostomy is useful to promote decompression of the intestinal tract postoperatively.

Extended periods of gastrointestinal dysfunction can be anticipated even when there has been no surgical intervention. Parenteral hyperalimentation is usually necessary to maintain the infants in positive nitrogen balance as their bowel recovers from the ischemic insult. After an appropriate period of gastrointestinal rest, usually 3 to 4 weeks, x-ray evaluation of the intestinal tract is advised to

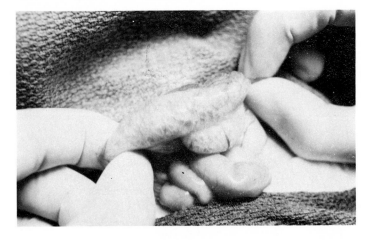

Fig. 34-16. Operative photograph of loop of intestine suffering from necrotizing enterocolitis. Note the gas in the seromuscular layer which distorts the segment of intestine. Normal loops of uninvolved intestine are also present.

determine whether stenosis has developed secondary to necrotizing enterocolitis. As intestinal function returns, the previously created enterostomies are closed, reestablishing gastrointestinal continuity. Cautious feedings are then begun. The more elemental formulas containing simple sugars and hydrolysed protein are advised for the initial feedings. Care must be exercised that the infant is not fed a hyperosmolar formula because this too has been implicated in the development of necrotizing enterocolitis.

Successful management of the syndrome of necrotizing enterocolitis with a combination of antibiotics provided through a nasogastric tube as well as by the intravenous route has been reported.[73] This method of therapy has resulted in the reversal of clinical symptoms and a lessening incidence of perforation. Early resumption of feedings has been possible in infants so treated and this method of therapy is worthy of further trial.

Necrotizing enterocolitis has become a major concern to the neonatologist and the pediatric surgeon. Despite an increasing awareness of the disease in the population at risk, the disease is lethal in 50% of the infants affected.

Imperforate Anus

Imperforate anus affects males and females with equal frequency and occurs in about one in every 20,000 live births.[74-79] The lesion results from a failure of differentiation of the urogenital sinus and cloaca. Associated anomalies include urogenital, cardiac, and esophageal anomalies including esophageal atresia and tracheo-esophageal fistula. The latter has an incidence of 10%.

Imperforate anus is considered high or low depending upon the level to which the rectal pouch has descended. High imperforate anus in either sex implies that the rectal pouch is at or above the level of the puborectalis portion of the levator musculature. Low imperforate anus implies that the rectum has descended past this level and is in the normal anatomic relationship to the puborectalis muscle. Infants with low imperforate anus can be expected to have rectal continence. The puborectalis sling must be located in infants with high imperforate anus and a normal relationship to the rectum established surgically for continence to be achieved.

In the female, 90% of infants have imperforate anus of the low type. Usually, the rectum terminates by means of a fistula, which presents anterior to the normal location of the anus, on the perineum (Fig. 34-17A), the vaginal fourchette (Fig. 34-17B), or low in the vagina. Because the termination of colon is accessible and colostomy is not necessary, early therapy can be directed at decompression of the bowel by catheter irrigation and dilatation of the fistula.

It is feasible to transpose the anus from the posterior vagina or perineum to its normal location in the newborn period. This is not always necessary if the baby is easily decompressed or can stool spontaneously through the fistula. A judicious interval is appropriate so that the baby is able to gain in size before the definitive operation is carried out. Definitive repair usually can be accomplished by

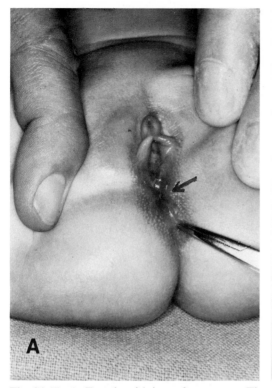
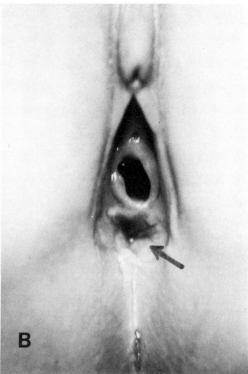

Fig. 34-17. A. Female with imperforate anus. The arrow demonstrates perineal fistula opening. The clamp is at the point where a normal anus would open. **B.** The close-up of female with imperforate anus and an introital fistula just inside the labia minora and immediately beneath the hymenal ring. This is the most common form of fistulous opening in female imperforate anus.

means of a perineal operation because the rectum is properly related to the muscles of continence. However, for low imperforate anus with a vaginal fistula, a sacroperineal approach is preferable since the dissection of the fistula and separation of the distal rectum from the vagina is more readily accomplished from the posterior aspect. In instances in which the fistula cannot be identified, it is usually high in the vagina and not accessible to dilatation or surgical revision in the newborn period. The rectum is located above the puborectalis sling. In this 10% of female infants, a colostomy is necessary. Definitive therapy for high imperforate anus in the female is deferred until the baby weighs 7–9 kg.

In the male, the distribution of high and low imperforate anus is equally divided. About half the babies present with a fistula placed ectopically on the perineum, anterior to the normal location of the anus. The fistula can terminate as far forward as the ventral surface of the penis. At birth, the opening of the fistula is not always apparent and an interval of 12 to 24 hours may be required until the bowel fills with air or meconium reaches the distal-most point in the gastrointestinal tract (Fig. 34-18A). When a spot of meconium or beads of mucus can be identified on the ventral penis or scrotum, there is assurance that the rectal pouch is low, implying that the rectum has traversed the levator sling and continence is expected. In these babies, a perineal anoplasty in the newborn period accomplishes decompression of the bowel and no colostomy is needed.

When no fistula is visible on the perineum, the infant can be presumed to have high imperforate anus. In these, the fistula usually communicates with the posterior urethra. A colostomy is needed for decompression and the definitive pull-through operation is generally deferred until the baby is about a year old.

The use of the upside-down (Wangensteen–Rice) x-ray film in the diagnosis of the

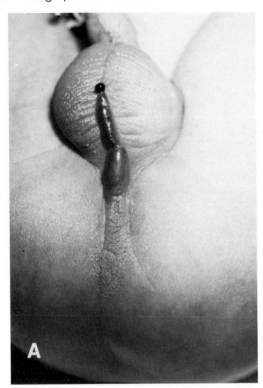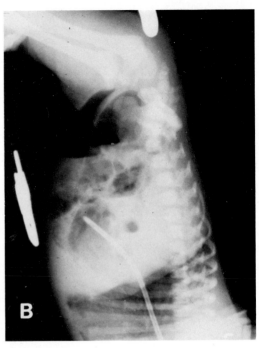

Fig. 34-18. **A.** Male with imperforate anus and perineal fistula, partly covered, which opens on scrotum. When such a fistula is present, the presence of a "low pouch" is certain, and the rectum has traversed the leveator sling musculature properly. **B.** Upside-down film technique of Wangensteen–Rice. The metal market at the anus shows the distance between the rectal pouch and the anal skin. It is clearly above a line drawn between the pubis and lower border of the sacrum. Note that there is a second gas-containing space anterior to the rectum. This indicates the presence of a rectourethral fistula with air trapped in the bladder.

level of imperforate anus is limited (Fig. 34-18B). Although it may help when it shows the rectal pouch at or near the perineum, it can also be misleading if the distal rectum is filled with meconium preventing air from reaching the distal-most aspect of this pouch. Thus, complete reliance on this view for the selection of therapy is ill-advised. Ultrasound may be helpful in locating the rectal pouch.

In the rare instance that the level of the rectal pouch cannot be determined accurately, a colostomy is advised. A colostomy performed on a low imperforate anus is preferable to prejudicing the chances for a successful pull-through by an ill-advised perineal exploration in the newborn period. With realization of the importance of the accurate transposition of the rectal pouch to the perineum, successful restoration of these infants has become the rule.

Obstructive Jaundice
(See also Chap. 24)

The majority of jaundiced infants fall into the category of physiologic jaundice, and spontaneous resolution can be anticipated. A variety of neonatal cholestatic syndromes overlap in presentation with obstructive jaundice from biliary atresia. Many conditions causing direct hyperbilirubinemia have been grouped into the generic heading "neonatal hepatitis." To some extent, this is misleading because hepatitis implies an inflammatory process within the liver. It is preferable to separate the infants into a group with cholestatic syndromes and another group with obstruction from biliary atresia. In the former group, specific disease entities are further identified by serologic testing or metabolic screening. Thus, the infant being evaluated for obstructive jaundice should have screening for intrauterine infections by TORCH titer determination. Among the most common metabolic conditions which can cause neonatal jaundice is alpha$_1$-antitrypsin deficiency. Screening for this inherited disorder is recommended for all infants with conjugated hyperbilirubinemia.[80]

Recent advances in hepatobiliary imaging using 99M technetium PIPIDA have made it possible to discriminate between cholestatic and obstructive jaundice with a high degree of accuracy.[81] A plethora of diagnostic blood tests have been recommended but none is completely reliable and most represent unnecessary procrastination. For any infant in whom the cause of jaundice is thought to be biliary atresia, or if the diagnosis is not known, surgical exploration is recommended.

Laparotomy is undertaken using an anesthetic technique which does not subject the infant to the risk of hepatic toxicity. Nitrous oxide, oxygen, and curare have proved to be a safe combination. An x-ray cassette is placed beneath the baby before commencing surgery. An initial exploration is planned through a limited right subcostal incision. If a normal gallbladder is seen, a transcholecystic cholangiogram is obtained. If the extrahepatic biliary tree appears normal, a liver biopsy is obtained and the incision closed.

When the gallbladder is atretic or the liver is obviously cirrhotic, suggesting an obstructive process, the incision is enlarged to permit formal exploration of the extrahepatic biliary system. Any remnant of the gallbladder or extrahepatic biliary duct through which a cholangiogram can be performed is utilized. In the infant with extrahepatic biliary atresia, only thread-like remnants of the biliary tree are identified. The atretic ducts are transected at their confluence deep in to the porta hepatis, and an anastomosis is created to a segment of the small intestine. When the operation is performed in infants under 3 months of age, there is expectation that bile will be drained into the intestine.[82-84]

In the series reported from the Children's Hospital National Medical Center, bile drainage was achieved in 35 of 54 infants having Kasai's operation for so-called "noncorrectable" biliary atresia.[85] Of these, 16 currently survive, jaundice-free, 1 to 6 years postoperatively.

Other causes of jaundice which can be relieved surgically are choledochal cysts, common duct stones, or inspissated sludge in the bile ducts. True choledochal cysts are rarely encountered in the newborn period. However, cystic dilatation of the biliary tree ending blindly without communication into the gastrointestinal tract has been described in some of the older infants. Resection of the cyst with anastamosis of the intestine is technically feasible and results in cure. Bile peritonitis, consequent to spontaneous rupture of the bile duct, may resemble a choledochal cyst to the unwary surgeon. The flimsy saccular collection of bile in the porta hepatis may appear contained with a true cyst when actually a wall of inflammatory tissue unsuited for intestinal anastomosis exists. This condition is seen in younger infants and must be recognized because attempted intestinal anastomosis has met uniformly with disaster. These babies require only drainage of the area with anticipation that the perforation will heal spontaneously, while the infant is maintained on antibiotics.[86]

Biliary hypoplasia is another condition which has received considerable attention. A gallbladder remnant is usually present. The ducts appear to be patent, in contradistinction to the thread-like structures encountered in complete biliary atresia. A cholangiogram confirms the patency of these structures as well as their narrow caliber. Liver biopsy invariably shows cholestasis and there is often a paucity of intrahepatic bile ducts. Speculation that there is an inflammatory component associated with biliary hypoplasia, and that it represents a phase of a dynamic process leading perhaps toward total biliary obstruction, has prompted the use of corticosteroids for treatment. In some instances, this seems to have been helpful, in that the jaundice has resolved and subsequent biopsies have reverted to normal.

On the other hand, biliary hypoplasia is a descriptive term for the radiologic finding of a diminutive extrahepatic ductal system. This may be a secondary rather than primary condition resulting from intrahepatic cholestasis. Biliary hypoplasia has been associated with intrahepatic disease conditions such as the cholestasis seen in alpha$_1$-antitrypsin deficiency.[87]

In the light of these new developments in the surgical therapy of obstructive jaundice, the prognosis has been changing. It is expected that with continued cooperation between neonatologists and surgeons in both the diagnostic and therapeutic phases of the management of these infants, these advances will be furthered and sustained.

Hernia and Hydrocele

Inguinal hernia and hydrocele occur commonly, especially in male infants. They result from the persistence of a patent processus vaginalis. This is a finger-like projection of the peritoneum accompanying the testicle as it descends into the scrotum. In the female, the peritoneal extension accompanies the round ligament and can remain patent, becoming a potential hernial sac. Hydrocele is often associated with inguinal hernia. The fluid may be in communication with the peritoneal cavity, and the hydrocele may therefore wax and wane in size, or it may be separated and completely isolated in the scrotum, in the inguinal canal, or, in females, the canal of Nuck. A hydrocele may present as an isolated finding without an associated hernia. Often, the hernia is of such size that it is easily appreciated as a swelling in the groin or scrotum. The mass can usually be reduced back into the abdominal cavity. Occasionally, the hydrocele component is irreducible while the main mass in the groin is appreciated as a hernia. The hernia usually becomes apparent as a lump in the groin of a baby described as "fussy" by the mother. Because of the special anatomic relationships in infants, they are at particular risk from incarceration of a hernia. The internal inguinal ring is narrow and intestine finding its way into the hernial sac in the inguinal canal can become trapped and reduce only with great difficulty. In some infants, there is a strong history of a recurrent lump in the groin, but this is not easily appreciated at the time of examination. In these babies, careful palpation by gently rubbing the structures in the inguinal canal in a perpendicular direction to the long axis of the canal allows one to appreciate the peritoneal lining or hernial sac (silk-glove sign). A hydrocele presents a smooth contour, cylindrical in shape, with the superior margin generally distinct. It is not tender and is often asymptomatic. When there is diagnostic confusion between an incarcerated hernia and a hydrocele, a rectal examination with bimanual palpation of the internal inguinal ring delineates the structures passing through the ring into the inguinal canal. The vas deferens is a constant reference point and the presence of intestine adjacent to the vas and between the examining fingers confirms the diagnosis of a hernia. Surgical repair is indicated in all cases of inguinal hernia.

Because the infant is at risk of incarceration, surgery must be scheduled at the earliest convenience of the family. If the baby presents with incarceration, the hernia is reduced and surgery delayed 24 to 48 hours until the local edema secondary to incarceration has resolved. Reduction of an incarcerated hernia is almost always successful if the baby is adequately sedated to achieve relaxation. Moderate, bimanual pressure, applied by compressing the sac from below while a gentle counterforce downward is provided from the examiner's hand above the inguinal ring usually achieves reduction. Occasionally, these hernias reduce spontaneously after sedation is given and the continuous struggling and crying is terminated. Should the hernia fail to reduce, or, in cases of obvious intestinal obstruction and systemic toxicity, emergency operation, surgical reduction, and repair are necessary.

An inguinal hernia in the female is often diagnosed by palpation of a nontender ovoid mass in the groin. The mass represents an ovary herniated into the open sac. Although the gonad can usually be reduced back into the abdomen, it often prolapses in and out until surgical repair is carried out. In about 10% of females, the ovary and fallopian tube constitute one wall of the hernia sac (sliding hernia) and in these cases the ovary can be reduced only at the time of operation.

Bilateral hernia repair is carried out on all infants under 1 year of age unless precluded by a coexisting medical condition. One can expect to encounter a hernia on the asymptomatic or contralateral side in about 25% of cases. This number is reported to be up to 60% in infants less than one year of age.

Undescended Testicle

One or both testicles may be absent from the scrotum on examination of a newborn male. The empty scrotum can mean incomplete descent or atrophy of a testicle.[88] Evaluation is best carried out with the baby comfortable and warm because an active cremasteric reflex may cause the gonad to retract into the inguinal canal. Sometimes, the testicle can be felt as a discrete bulge in the inguinal canal. Efforts are then made to milk it out of the canal and into the scrotum. If this is not possible, the diagnosis of undescended testicle is established.

Though not usually a surgical consideration in the neonate, about 10% of undescended testicles are accompanied by a troublesome hernia. The hernia may demand surgical attention even in the very young. In such instances, the testicle is mobilized and brought into the scrotum. The parents are forewarned that the testicle may subsequently retract and require a second procedure for repositioning within the scrotum.

Because the undescended testicle lacks scrotal fixation, it is at risk from torsion. The physical finding of a tender, undescended testicle usually signifies that this has occurred. This situation demands immediate surgical intervention to prevent ischemic necrosis of the gonad.

When the undescended testicles are bilateral or occur in association with hypospadias, a careful evaluation must be undertaken to be sure that there is no form of intersexual abnormality (see below).

ABNORMALITIES OF THE UMBILICUS AND ABDOMINAL WALL

Umbilical Hernia

Umbilical hernia is a common condition of the newborn, present as a central fascial defect beneath the umbilicus. Incarceration is a rare complication in patients with umbilical hernia but occurs more commonly in patients with smaller defects of the fascia, such as those seen in the neonate. Umbilical hernias are more common in Blacks, in premature infants, and in patients with congenital deficiencies of thyroid hormone.

Most babies with umbilical hernia require no surgical treatment because the hernia disappears spontaneously by 2 or 3 years of age. With persistence of the hernia until 3 years of age, repair is indicated. In a few patients there is progressive enlargement of the skin of the umbilicus until a prominent proboscis is produced. In such patients, surgical repair is indicated early. A simple repair suffices for all of these patients and can be accomplished through a small semilunar incision made in the curve of the umbilicus. Complicated fascial flap repairs such as may be required in adults

are unnecessary and therefore contraindicated in young patients. The umbilicus is never excised.

Adhesive dressings with coins and metallic or plastic objects have no place in the management of umbilical hernia because they are ineffective and merely cover the defect at the expense of irritating the surrounding skin.

Primary Infection of the Umbilicus (Omphalitis)

With the advent of sound perinatal care, the incidence of infection around the umbilicus has been markedly reduced. Potentially serious complications can result from infections in this area. Cellulitis of the abdominal wall, with direct spread into the peritoneal cavity and resultant peritonitis of the newborn, has been recorded. The most serious consequence is ascending infection along the umbilical vein to the portal system and liver. In preantibiotic days the resultant multiple hepatic abscesses were often fatal. A more common sequela is portal vein thrombosis, which is a major cause of portal hypertension in children. In the past, this was a significant cause of esophageal varices in young patients, and while this condition is now reduced in frequency, it must be assiduously avoided by prompt local and systemic antibiotic treatment of suspected infections in and around the umbilicus.

Umbilical Granuloma

The formation of weeping granulation tissue at the umbilicus is not unusual in the newborn. Failure of the umbilical epithelium to grow over the severed stump of the umbilicus results in a persistent crusting mass of granulomatous tissue. Cauterization with silver nitrate is both diagnostic and therapeutic. Applications of silver nitrate twice weekly for 1 month clear up most umbilical granulations. With persistence of fluid at the umbilicus, the presence of a patent omphalomesenteric duct or patent urachus is a consideration.

Patent Omphalomesenteric Duct

During fetal development the omphalomesenteric duct forms a connection from the intestinal tract to the placenta. If this duct fails to involute, a tubular attachment persists connecting the ileum to the abdominal wall (Fig. 34-19). Liquid ileal content refluxes out of this duct.

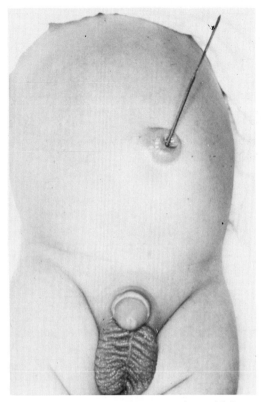

Fig. 34-19. Probe in umbilical opening, which connects with the intestinal tract (patent omphalomesenteric duct).

Diagnosis of a congenital fistula at the umbilicus is made by inspection and probing of the tract. The introduction of radiopaque material into the ostium at the umbilicus demonstrates a connection to the intestinal lumen on lateral x-ray view of the abdomen.

Treatment for patent omphalomesenteric duct is elective abdominal exploration with division and closure of the fistula at its origin in the ileum and total excision of the fistula including its attachment to the undersurface of the umbilicus. This procedure must not be postponed because there is a potential for intestinal volvulus to occur around the post-like attachment between the umbilicus and the ileum.

In rare instances, when the patent omphalomesenteric duct opening is large, the peristaltic activity of the bowel can result in eversion of proximal intestine, as in intussusception, through the opening onto the abdominal wall. Clinically this appears as a mucosal-covered extrusion, and the resulting mass is easily confused with a small ruptured omphalocele. Careful inspection of the neck of the defect at the border of the abdominal skin discloses the true nature of the lesion. The bowel has in effect turned inside out and prolapsed through the patent omphalomesenteric duct. Immediate operation with reduction and repair is indicated.

Patent Urachus

During embryologic development, there is a free communication between the urinary bladder and the abdominal wall. Persistence of this tract establishes a communication between the urinary bladder and the umbilicus through which urine may pass. Although this passage is small, the umbilicus is constantly wet. The first sign of a patent urachus may be urinary infection. In some patients, a portion of the urachus has obliterated with only a partially patent remnant or cyst remaining beneath the umbilicus.

In the diagnostic work-up of a newborn suspected of having a patent urachus, the cystogram in lateral projection demonstrates the abnormal tract. Another diagnostic technique is the introduction of a colored dye into the bladder through the urethral catheter. The appearance of dye on the abdominal wall then confirms the connection between the umbilicus and the bladder.

Treatment. Extraperitoneal surgical exploration of the infraumbilical area allows complete excision of the urachal tract and closure of the bladder. Partial urachal remnants, sinus tracts, or cysts are also easily excised.

Omphalocele

Developmental arrest of those somites, which form the peritoneal, muscular, and ectodermal layers of the abdominal wall, results in a central defect termed an omphalocele.[89] The defect is covered by a translucent membrane overlying the bowel and solid viscera, and may vary in size from a small "hernia of the cord" measuring 1 or 2 cm to a huge mass containing essentially all of the abdominal viscera (Fig. 34-20). Usually the sac remains intact, but occasionally it is ruptured during delivery.

The diagnosis of this lesion is made entirely by inspection for it is readily apparent imme-

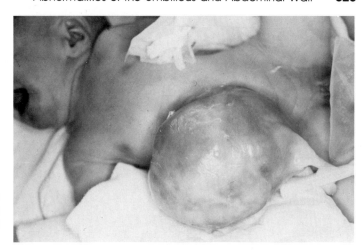

Fig. 34-20. Large omphalocele. Note covering of the sac and its relationship to the umbilicus which protrudes from the lower portion.

diately after delivery of the baby. The abdomen is wrapped carefully with well-padded saline-soaked gauze and an outer dry layer in preparation for transport. No pressure is placed on the omphalocele in an attempt to "reduce" it. This is not only hazardous to the integrity of the sac, but may interfere with venous return and may stifle the child's respiratory efforts.

Surgical Treatment. Small omphaloceles are usually amenable to complete one-stage surgical repair. For larger omphaloceles (greater than 6 cm) a sheet of silastic with interwoven Marlex can be sewed around the edge of the defect to envelop the omphalocele.[90-92] Steady pressure on the prosthesis over a period of days brings about gradual reduction of the omphalocele so that surgical closure can be accomplished. Irrigation with povidone-iodine (Betadine) solution has been effective in reducing surface contamination throughout the time the prosthesis is required.[93]

Conservative (Nonoperative) Management. Coexisting anomalies such as extrophy of the cloaca or congenital heart disease may make surgical closure inappropriate. Painting the omphalocele sac with 4% mercurochrome promotes a firm, strong crust to cover the defect. This protection is designed to serve until the natural process of epithelialization occurs. More recently, success with plastic material has obviated the need for the painting method, but this is still a useful treatment in certain instances.

Congenital malrotation of the colon is almost always present in patients born with omphalocele. While in itself of no great moment, this anomaly can lead to midgut volvulus. Thus, symptoms of intestinal obstruction in a baby who has previously been well recovered from treatment of omphalocele must be considered a dire emergency.

Gastroschisis

Originally confused as a type of omphalocele, gastroschisis is now recognized as a separate entity. It differs embryologically in that the abdominal wall has completed its development but a defect remains at the base of the umbilical stalk, through which a portion of the intestinal tract has escaped. An alternative hypothesis is that gastroschisis always occurs as a defect lateral to the base of the umbilicus and represents an isolated congenital defect in the abdominal wall. A third theory of the embryogenesis of gastroschisis holds that closure of the coelomic cavity has been completed while a portion of the intestinal tract remained trapped outside of the abdomen in the base of the umbilical cord. It is postulated that this hernia of the cord then ruptures, allowing the intestine to float freely in the amnion while the umbilical arteries and vein remain attached to the baby. The escape of the intestine into the free amniotic cavity apparently can occur at different times in fetal development. This conclusion follows the observation that in some infants the intestines are glistening and normal looking, as if they had escaped a coelomic envelope just prior to birth. Many infants with gastroschisis, however, are born with edematous and matted intestinal loops which appear to have been

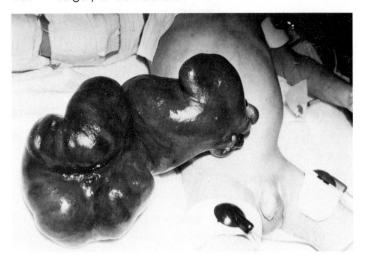

Fig. 34-21. Patient with gastroschisis. Note edematous, matted bowel, the result of the intestines floating freely in the amniotic fluid. Remarkably, these distorted viscera will ultimately fit back into the abdominal cavity and will finally assume a normal appearance and function.

exposed to the amniotic fluid for many weeks (Fig. 34-21).

Treatment. Immediate treatment in the delivery room consists in wrapping the baby and the exteriorized intestine in saline-soaked gauze and dry sterile dressings. Prompt surgical repair is undertaken. In about half the cases, all of the viscera can be returned to the abdomen and secure closure obtained. Gastrostomy is a useful adjunct. In favorable cases, peristalsis returns in a few days and normal bowel function can be expected. When the bowel is matted and edematous, it may take many weeks before intestinal function recovers. Nutrition can now be successfully supported during this interval by intravenous hyperalimentation. Previously, many of these babies died from malnutrition before intestinal function returned.

When the abdominal wall cannot be closed without undue tension, which embarrasses the respiration and interferes with venous return, then an extra-abdominal prosthetic compartment must be fashioned. As in staged omphalocele repair, silastic-covered Marlex is well-suited for this purpose because its surface is inert and does not adhere to the bowel.[90-92] Once the prosthesis is fastened to the fascial margins, the capacity of the plastic compartment can be gradually reduced until complete surgical closure is possible, usually within 7 to 10 days. This staged maneuver, coupled with intravenous alimentation, has resulted in an increased percentage of survivors from a previously hopeless anomaly.[92,93] Intestinal atresia occurs in about 10% of patients with omphalocele. In these babies, the clinical course is one of early complete obstruction, which requires abdominal exploration if the lesion has been inadvertently overlooked at the time of initial repair of the omphalocele.

Congenital Deficiency of the Abdominal Muscle (Prune-belly Syndrome)

A rare but troublesome anomaly is that involving deficient abdominal musculature. This condition is readily apparent in the newborn because of the thin, lax abdominal wall which sags and bulges at the flanks (Fig. 34-22). In severely affected infants, there is marked wrinkling of the skin of the abdomen and no muscular substance beneath. Lower abdominal musculature is most frequently and severely involved. Histologic studies have shown that all of the muscular layers are present. Babies born with this congenital abdominal wall defect usually show major abnormalities of their urinary collecting system. The bladder is characteristically large and the ureters dilated and tortuous. The kidneys may be hypoplastic, but usually there is adequate renal parenchyma in one or both kidneys. In embryologic considerations, it has been proposed that all of these infants have some degree of urethral obstruction with resultant overdistension of the bladder and abnormal pressure on the developing muscular somites. Conversely, others have suggested that pri-

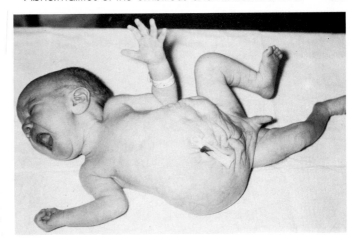

Fig. 34-22. Infant with congenital deficiency of the abdominal musculature, showing typical "wrinkled belly" appearance.

mary deficiency in the abdominal musculature allows overdistension of the bladder with secondary changes in the ureters. It is probable that neither of these explanations is completely valid and some more comprehensive explanation exists for the coexistence of the unusual abdominal deficiency and the distortion of the collecting system.

The outlook for these babies has improved over the past fifteen years because of advances in techniques of urinary reconstruction. Treatment consists of direct attack on the bladder outlet and urethra with simultaneous reconstruction of the ureters and reconstruction of the vesicoureteral mechanisms as needed. Various surgical procedures have been devised to shorten the lax abdominal musculature and reduce the redundancy of the abdominal wall. While not entirely normal, adequate appearance and muscular support can now be achieved and satisfactory growth attained.

Exstrophy of the Cloaca (Vesicointestinal Fissure)

This constellation of anomalies represents one of the severest forms of interruption of normal embryologic development. The group of abnormalities classed as the exstrophic anomalies have been described in the past as resulting from a failure of the fusion in the midline. This concept is probably an oversimplification because all of the abdominal and pelvic musculature and the pelvic bones are well formed. It appears that the cloaca had extruded anteriorly, preventing the normal ventral closure of the pelvis and abdominal wall. Major components of cloacal exstrophy or vesicointestinal fissure are (1) omphalocele; (2) exstrophy of the bladder; (3) external intestinal fistula between the bladder halves, usually emanating from the remaining portion of a Meckel's diverticulum or omphalomesenteric duct; (4) epispadias in the males; (5) imperforate anus; and (6) short colon. Frequently there is a deformity in the distal leg and foot on one side. The summation of these physical defects is such that many of the newborns are not hardy enough to survive. Yet many of these physical defects are correctable or at least can be rehabilitated.

Treatment. Early surgical intervention may become necessary because of intestinal prolapse through the intestinal fistula. In such circumstances, an ileostomy is required. If laparotomy discloses a significant length to the colon, it can be temporarily exteriorized as a mucous fistula. The omphalocele can be excised and closed or treated with a scarifying agent which leads to subsequent spontaneous epithelialization. There is no urgency about repair of the exstrophied bladder and reconstruction of the urinary system need not be completed until the patient is 2 or 3 years of age.

The many discouraging reports in the literature with respect to treatment of this set of anomalies are now being offset by aggressive early surgical treatment and long-term rehabilitation measures. While most patients suffer a number of physical limitations, many have normal intellect and can lead useful lives.

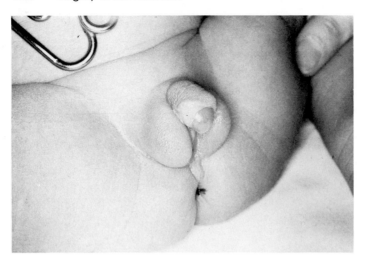

Fig. 34-23. Infant born with ambiguous genitalia. From this photograph it is difficult to tell whether this patient has an atypical penis with penoscrotal hypospadias or whether there is extreme masculinization of the clitoris and scrotal changes of the labia majora.

Ambiguous Genitalia: Intersex
(See also Chap. 44)

The presence of a confusing or ambiguous appearance of the external genitalia requires investigation of the intersex phenomenon (Fig. 34-23). These patients may be grouped into several categories, which are helpful in dealing with the hermaphrodite syndrome.

1. True hermaphrodite (coexisting testicular and ovarian tissue)
2. Male pseudohermaphrodites (testicular gonads only) with hypospadias, one or both testes undescended, and various persistent Mullerian duct remnants
3. Female pseudohermaphrodites (ovarian gonads only).

Every infant born with indeterminate sex demands a thorough evaluation. Diagnostic procedures, even including laparotomy, can be completed by the time the infant is 2 weeks of age. The situation can then be reviewed with the family and a proper sex assignment made. Delay in sex assignment causes unnecessary embarrassment and confusion to the parents. Hurried assignment of sex role without adequate understanding of the patient's anatomy, endocrine physiology, and chromosome constitution can lead to a mistaken diagnosis with tragic consequences in later years.

Diagnosis. Family history and history of the pregnancy, with attention to drug ingestion, is obtained. The genitalia are inspected and all orifices carefully defined. Rectal examination suggests the presence or absence of uterus or cervix. Roentgenographic examination of the urethra and vagina with radiopaque material discloses the presence and size of these structures. Intravenous pyelography and (for older subjects) bone age films are obtained. Chromosomal studies offer important information about genotypic sex, but this information alone should never form the final basis for sex assignment without consideration of the anatomical and endocrine status of the patient.[94] Urinary pregnanetriol and 17-ketosteroid excretion are diagnostic of the presence of congenital adrenal hyperplasia. In some patients, a laparotomy and biopsy of gonadal tissue is necessary for final diagnosis and sex assignment. While some have recommended laparoscopy at this stage, we believe that a careful pelvic exploration is to be favored in these complicated patients. The laparotomy is for diagnosis only, and excisional or corrective surgery is avoided at this stage.

Versatility in a number of surgical procedures must be part of the armamentarium of any surgeon dealing with this group of infants. Many of the males require hypospadias repair and excision of contradictory sexual structures such as remnants of the Mullerian ducts. In true hermaphrodites removal of the inappropriate gonad is necessary. Surgical revision of the enlarged clitoris may be necessary.[95] A revision of the vaginal introitus is often needed in infancy to eliminate urinary infection, and a second revision may be required in the premarital years. In some masculinized females, the distal vagina is congenitally absent, and extensive reconstruction to unite the perineal skin and the upper vaginal passage is needed. Severe penile hypoplasia and cryptorchidism occurs in a small number of males. The testicles are histologically normal and the chromosome studies reveal normal male genotype, but the phallus is a tiny clitoral-like structure. Such patients usually have a vagina. Because the phallus is inadequate for the male role, these patients are more successfully reared as females.

Problems of intersex require effective teamwork between neonatologist, endocrinologist, geneticist, and surgeon to accomplish prompt and correct sex assignment, hormonal management, and plan for appropriate reconstruction of the deformed parts. When the diagnosis is missed in the newborn period, the psychiatrist becomes a necessary part of the team.

REFERENCES

1. **Altman RP, Randolph JG:** Neonatal surgery: Criteria for success. Med Ann DC 38:477, 1969
2. **Lister J, Altman RP, Win MS:** Homeostatic responses to alterations of blood volume in puppies. J Pediatr Surg 2:241, 1967
3. **Tooley WH:** What is the risk of an umbilical artery catheter? Pediatrics 50:6, 1972
4. **Roe CF, Santulli RV, Blair CS:** Heat loss in infants during general anesthesia and operations. J Pediatr Surg 1:266, 1966
5. **Rowe MI:** The role of serial serum osmolality measurements in the management of the neonatal surgical patient. Surg Gynecol Obstet 6: 333, 1971
6. **Stark RB, Ehrmann NA:** Development of the center of the face with particular reference to surgical correction of bilateral cleft lip. Plast Reconstr Surg 21:177, 1958
7. **Matthews DN:** Hare lip and cleft palate. In Mustardé JC (ed): Plastic Surgery in Infancy and Childhood. Philadelphia, WB Saunders, 1971
8. **Douglas B:** Treatment of micrognathia asociated with obstruction by plastic procedures. Plast Reconstr Surg 22:94, 1958
9. **Dennison WM:** The Pierre Robin syndrome. Pediatrics 36:337, 1965
10. **Farnsworth PB, Pacik PT:** Glossoptotic hypoxia and micrognathia—The Pierre Robin Syndrome reviewed. Clin Pediat 10:600, 1971
11. **Davies PA:** Management of the Pierre Robin syndrome. Dev Med Child Neurol 15:359, 1973
12. **Sistrunk WE:** The surgical treatment of cysts of the thyroglossal tract. Ann Surg 71:121, 1920
13. **McPhail N, Mustard RA:** Branchial cleft anomalies: a review of 87 cases treated at the Toronto General Hospital. Can Med Assoc J 94:174, 1966
14. **Gans SL, Berci G:** Advances in endoscopy of infants and children. J Pediatr Surg 6:199, 1971
15. **Hendren WH, McKee DM:** Lobar emphysema of infancy. J Pediatr Surg 1:24, 1966
16. **Mattila MAK, Suutarinen T, Sulamaa M:** Prolonged endotracheal intubation of tracheostomy in infants and children. J Pediatr Surg 4:674, 1972
17. **Tunstall ME, Carter JI, Thomson JS et al** Ventilating the lungs of newborn infants for prolonged periods. Arch Dis Child 43:486, 1968
18. **Aberdeen E:** Mechanical pulmonary ventilation in infants. Proc R Soc Med 58:900, 1965
19. **Talbert JL, Haller JA, Jr:** Improved silastic tracheostomy tubes for infants and young children. J Pediatr Surg 3:408, 1968
20. **Haller JA, Jr, Talbert JL:** Clinical evaluation of a new silastic tracheostomy tube for respiratory support of infants and young children. Ann Surg 171:915, 1970
21. **Bochdalek V:** Einiege betrachtungen ueber die einstellung des angeborenen awerchfellbruches als beitrat zue pathologischen anatomie der hernien. Vrtljhrsb Prakt Heilk 19:89, 1848
22. **Gross RE:** Congenital hernia of the diaphragm. Am J Dis Child 71:579, 1946
23. **Meeker IA, Jr, Snyder WH, Jr:** Management of diaphragmatic defects in infants. Am J Surg 104:196, 1962
24. **McNamara JJ, Eraklis A, Gross RE:** Congenital partero-lateral diaphragmatic hernia in the newborn. J Thorac Cardiovasc Surg 55:55, 1968
25. **Boix—Ochoa J, Peguero A, Seijo G, Natal A, Canals J:** Acid-base balance and blood gases in prognosis and therapy of congenital diaphragmatic hernia, J Pediatr Surg 9:49, 1974
26. **deLorimier AA, Tierney DF, Parker HR:** Hypoplastic lungs in fetal lambs with surgically produced congenital diaphragmatic hernia. Surgery 62:12, 1967
27. **Koop CE, Johnson J:** Transthoracic repair of diaphragmatic hernia in infants. Ann Surg 136: 1007, 1952
28. **Haight C, Towsley HA:** Congenital atresia of the esophagus with tracheoesophageal fistula: extrapleural ligation of fistual and end-to-end anastomosis, esophageal segments. Surg Gynecol Obstet 76:672, 1943
29. **Holder FM, Cloud DT, Lewis JE, Jr et al:** Esophageal atresia and tracheoesophageal fis-

tula: a survey of its members by the surgical section of the Am Acad Pediatr. Pediatrics, 34:542, 1964

30. **Replogle RL:** Esophageal atresia: plastic sump catheter for drainage of the proximal pouch. Surgery 58:725, 1965

31. **Randolph JG, Altman RP, Anderson KD:** Selective surgical management based upon clinical status in infants with esophageal atresia. J Thorac Cardiovasc Surg 74:335, 1977

32. **Holder TM, McDonald VG, Jr, Wooley MM:** The premature or critically ill infant with esophageal atresia: increased success with a staged approach. J Thorac Cardiovasc Surg 44:344, 1962

33. **Randolph JG, Tunell WP, Lilly JR, Altman RP:** Gastric division; another surgical adjunct in selected problems with esophageal anomalies. J Pediatr Surg 6:657, 1971

34. **Koop CE:** Recent advances in the surgery of oesophageal atresia. Progr Pediatr Surg 2:41, 1971

35. **Sherman CD, Jr, Waterston D:** Oesophageal reconstruction in children using intrathoracic colon. Arch Dis Child 32:11, 1957

36. **Burrington JD, Stephens CA:** Esophageal replacement with a gastric tube in infants and children. J Pediatr Surg 3:246, 1968

37. **Woolley MM, Leix F, Johnston PN et al:** Esophageal atresia types A and B; upper pouch elongation and delayed anatomic reconstruction. J Pediatr Surg 4:148, 1969

38. **Moncrief JA, Randolph JG:** Congenital tracheoesophageal fistula without atresia of the esophagus. J Thorac Cardiovasc Surg 51:434, 1966

39. **Randolph JR, Lilly JR, Anderson KD:** Surgical treatment of gastroesophageal reflux in infants. Ann Surg 180:479, 1974

40. **Bettex M, Kuffer F:** Long-term results of fundoplication in hiatus hernia and cardioesophageal chalasia in infants and children. Report of 112 consecutive cases. J Pediatr Surg 4:526, 1969

41. **Carre IJ:** Postural treatment of children with a partial thoracic stomach (hiatus hernia). Arch Dis Child 37:569, 1960

42. **Filler RM, Randolph JG, Gross RE:** Esophageal hiatus hernia in infants and children. J Thorac Cardiovasc Surg 47:551, 1964

43. **McNamara JJ, Paulson DL, Urschel HC, Jr:** Hiatal hernia and gastroesophageal reflux in children. Pediatrics 43:527, 1969

44. **Cravioto J, Delicardie ER, Birch HG:** Nutrition, growth and neurointegrative development: an experimental and ecologic study. Pediatrics 38:319, 1966

45. **Nissen R, Rossetti M:** Zur indickation der fundopliatio and gastropexix bie der hiatushernie. Schweiz med Wehschr 92:533, 1962

46. **Vos A, Boerema I:** Surgical treatment of gastroesophageal reflux in infants and children. J Pediatr Surg 6:101, 1971

47. **Eklof O, Ekstrom G, Eriksson BO et al:** Arterial anomalies causing compression of the trachea and/or the oesophagus; a report of 30 symptomatic cases. Acta Paediatr Scand 60:81, 1971

48. **Lincoln JCR, Deverall PB, Stark J et al:** Vascular anomalies compressing the oesophagus and trachea. Thorax 24:295, 1969

49. **Dudrick SJ, Rhoads JE, Vars HM:** Growth of puppies receiving all nutritional requirements by vein. Fortschr Parenteral Ernahrung 2:16, 1967

50. **Wilmore DW, Dudrick SJ:** Growth and development of an infant receiving all nutrients exclusively by vein. JAMA 203:860, 1968

51. **Clatworthy HW, Jr, Salleby R, Lovingood C:** Extensive small bowel resection in young dogs: its effect on growth and development. Surgery 32:341, 1952

52. **Benson CD, Lloyd JR, Krabbenhoft KL:** The surgical and metabolic aspects of massive small bowel resection in the newborn. J Pediatr Surg 2:227, 1967

53. **Weinberger M, Rowe MI:** Experience with an elemental diet in neonatal surgery. J Pediatr Surg 8:175, 1973

54. **Barnard CN, Louw JH:** The genesis of intestinal atresia. Minn Med 39:745, 1956

55. **Fonkalsrud EW, deLorimier AA, Hays DM:** Congenital atresia and stenosis of the duodenum—a review compiled from the members of the surgical section of the American Academy of Surgery. Pediatrics 43:79, 1969

56. **Louw JH:** Jejunoileal atresia and stenosis. J Pediatr Surg 1:8, 1966

57. **deLorimier AA, Fonkalsrud EW, Hays DM:** Congenital atresia and stenosis of the jejunum and ileum. Surgery 65:819, 1969

58. **Bishop HC, Koop CE:** Management of meconium ileus: resection, Rouxen-Y anastomosis and ileostomy irrigation with pancreatic enzymes. Ann Surg 145:410, 1957

59. **LoPresti JM, Altman RP, Kulczycki L:** Meconium Ileus: Operative therapy and pulmonary complications in the newborn. Clin Proc Child Hosp DC 28:221, 1972

60. **Noblett HR:.** Treatment of uncomplicated meconium ileus by gastrografin enema: a preliminary report. J Pediatr Surg 4:190, 1969

61. **Rowe MI, Seagram G, Weinberger M:** Gastrograin-induced hypertonicity: the pathogenesis of a neonatal hazard. Am J Surg 125:185, 1973

62. **Swenson O:** Pediatric surgery, Vol 1. New York, Appleton–Century–Crofts.

63. **Swenson O, Fisher JH, Gherardi GJ:** Rectal biopsy in the diagnosis of Hirschsprung's disease: experience with one hundred biopsies. Surgery 45:690, 1959

64. **Campbell PE, Noblett HR:** Experience with rectal suction biopsy in the diagnosis of Hirschsprung's disease. J Pediatr Surg 4:410, 1969

65. **Tobon F, Reid NCRW, Talbert JL et al:** Nonsurgical test for the diagnosis of Hirschsprung's disease. N Engl J Med 278:188, 194, 1968

66. **Fraser GC, Berry C:** Mortality in neonatal Hirschsprung's disease: with particular reference to enterocolitis. J Pediatr Surg 2:205, 1967

67. **Martin LW:** Surgical management of total colonic aganglionoisis. Ann Surg 176:343, 1972

68. **Duhamel B:** Retrorectal and transanal pull-through procedure for the treatment of Hirschsprung's disease. Dis Colon Rectum, 7: 455, 1964

69. **Soave F:** Hirschsprung's disease: technique and results of Soave's operation. Br J Surg 53:1023, 1966

70. **Touloukian RJ, Posch JN, Spencer R:** The pathogenesis of isochemic gastroenterocolitis of the nenoate: slective gut mucosalischemia in asphyxiated neonatal piglets. J Pediatr Surg 7:194, 1972

71. **Touloukian RJ, Berdon WE, Amoury RA et al:** Surgical experience with necrotizing enterocolitis in the infant. J Pediatr Surg 2:389, 1967

72. **Kosloske AM, Lilly JR:** Paracentesis and Lavage for Diagnosis of Intestinal Gangrene in Neonatal Necrotizing Enterocolitis. J Pediatr Surg 13:135, 1978

73. **Bell MJ, Kosloske AM, Martin LW et al:** Prevention of perforation in necrotizing enterocolitis of the newborn. J Pediatr Surg (in press).

74. **Stephens FD:** Congenital Malformations of the Rectum, Anus and Genito-urinary Tract. Edinburgh, E & S Livingstone, 1963

75. **Santulli TV, Kiesewetter WB, Bill AH, Jr:** Anorectal anomalies: a suggested international classification. J Pediatr Surg 5:281, 1970

76. **Wangensteen OH, Rice CO:** Imperforate anus: a method of determining the surgical approach. Ann Surg 92:77, 1930

77. **Kiesewelter WB:** Rectum and Anus. In Ravitch MM, Welch KJ, Benson CD, Aberdeen E, Randolph JA (eds): Pediatric Surgery, Vol 2, pp 1059–1081. Chicago, Year Book Medical Publishers, 1979

78. **Rehbein F:** Imperforate anus: experiences with abdomino-perineal and abdomino-sacral-perineal pull-through procedures. J Pediatr Surg 2:99, 1967

79. **Kieswetter WB:** Imperforate anus. II. The rationale and technic of the sacro-abdominoperineal operation. J Pediatr Surg 2:106, 1967

80. **Talamo RC:** Basic and clinical aspects of the alpha-1-antitrypsin. Pediatrics 56:91, 1975

81. **Majd M, Altman RP, Reba RC:** Hepatobiliary scintigraphy with Tc99m PIPIDA in infants and children. J Nucl Med 20:680, 1979

82. **Kasai M, Kimura S, Asakura Y et al:** Surgical treatment of biliary atresia. J Pediatr Surg 3: 665, 1968

83. **Lilly JR, Altman RP:** Hepatic portoenterostomy (The Kasai Operation) for biliary atresia. Surgery 78:76, 1975

84. **Odievre M, Valayer J, Razemon–Pinta M et al:** Hepatic partoenterostomy or cholecystostomy in the treatment of extrahepatic biliary atresia. J Pediatr 88:774, 1976

85. **Altman RP:** The portoenterostomy procedure for biliary atresia—a five year experience. Ann Surg 188:35, 1978

86. **Lilly JR, Weintraub WW, Altman RP:** Spontaneous perforation of the extrahepatic bile ducts and bile peritonitis in infancy. Surgery 75:664, 1974

87. **Altman RP, Chandra R:** Biliary hypoplasia consequent to alpha-1-antitrypsin deficiency. Surg Forum 37:377, 1976

88. **Kieswetter WB, Shull WR, Fetterman GH:** Histologic chances in the testis following anatomically successful orchidopexy. J Pediatr Surg 4:59, 1969

89. **Gross RE:** A new method for surgical treatment of large omphaloceles. Surgery 24:277, 1948

90. **Schuster SR:** A new method for the staged repair of large omphaloceles. Surg Gynecol Obstet 125:837, 1967

91. **Allen RG, Wrenn EL, Jr:** Silon as a sac in the treatment of omphalocele and gastroschisis. J Pediatr Surg 4:3, 1969

92. **Gilbert MG, Mencia LF, Brown WT et al:** Staged surgical repair of large omphaloceles and gastroschisis. J Pediatr Surg 3:702, 1968

93. **Wesselhoeft CW, Jr, Randolph JG:** Treatment of omphalocele based on individual characteristics of the defect. Pediatrics 44:101, 1969

94. **Hung W, Jacobson CB, Wigger HR, Randolph JG:** Chromosome studies in a chromatin-negative, YW true hermaphrodite. J Urol 96:565, 1966

95. **Randolph JG, Hung W:** Reduction clitoroplasty in females with hypertrophied clitoris. J Pediatr Surg 5:224, 1970

35

Abnormalities of the Genitourinary System

A. Barry Belman

EMBRYOLOGY

The most significant developmental step in the formation of the urinary tract is the budding of the ureter from the Wolffian (mesonephric) duct. This occurs early, at the 3 to 5 mm stage (4th–5th gestational week), even before completion of the division of the cloaca by the urorectal septum. The ureteral bud then meets the nephrogenic mass to stimulate renal development. Simultaneously, the Wolffian duct becomes absorbed into the urogenital sinus carrying the ureter with it (Fig. 35-1). The ureteral orifice then finds its way to the bladder base and becomes incorporated in the formation of the superficial detrusor **(trigone).** The distal Wolffian duct forms the internal male genital structures (vas deferens, seminal vesicles, ejaculatory ducts) or becomes resorbed in the female; there the only remnant, its most distal segment, is represented by Gartner's duct.

Failure of the budding of the ureter precludes formation of ipsilateral renal tissue. Absence of the Wolffian duct results in failure of both ipsilateral renal and internal male structural development (absent vas deferens, epididymis, seminal vesicle), although a testis would be present. Failure of formation of the urogenital ridge is responsible for renal, internal male

genital, and testicular absence. With the above knowledge, one can predict the embryologic misadventures responsible for various pathologic states.

The urinary bladder forms relatively late in fetal development, at about 6 weeks of gestation. Budding of the ureters has already begun by this time, and the genital tubercle has fused. The bladder becomes a separate entity when the urorectal septum divides the cloaca.

At about the seventh gestational week, the genital tubercle begins to enlarge under the stimulus of fetal testosterone. The urorectal septum has completely divided the cloaca, and the urogenital membrane ruptures with the urogenital ostium appearing between the urogenital folds on the ventral aspect of the phallus. Towards the end of the first trimester the urethral groove is becoming closed and formation of the urethra itself completed.

RENAL ABNORMALITIES

Bilateral Renal Agenesis

Bilateral renal agenesis is obviously incompatible with survival. Renal agenesis should be considered when urinary output is nil after 24 hours of life and a distended bladder is not palpable. Often times, these children have Potter's facies. This is an uncommon abnormality occurring about once in 3000 births.[1]

Causes of renal agenesis include failure of formation of the urogenital ridge (a most rare occurence also resulting in failure of ipsilateral internal genital formation), failure of budding of the ureter, absence of the nephrogenic blastema, and failure of vascularization. In the latter two circumstances, some degree of ureteral formation may be present.

The diagnosis of renal agenesis is definitively made with umbilical artery angiography. Renal arteries will not be present. Urography and renal scanning are not diagnostic in this circumstance because failure of function of existing kidneys can also produce complete nonvisualization, yet kidney substance is present. Ultrasonography in the newborn is worthwhile for delineating masses, but may not offer sufficiently sensitive resolution to determine the presence or absence of small kidneys.

Survival in these infants can be distressingly prolonged. Unless death occurs from failure of some other organ system, they may live for several days. The high incidence of other associated urinary anomalies and the extremely poor results in this age group obviates consideration for transplantation or dialysis.

Unilateral Renal Agenesis

Unless associated with some other abnormality or condition leading to urologic evaluation, the diagnosis of unilateral renal agenesis is not likely to be made because it is not associated with symptoms. Its incidence is in the general range of 1 in 500.[2] Although a single kidney is adequate for a normal life span, congenital absence of one renal unit suggests a higher incidence of disease in the remaining kidney. Emmanuel and coworkers reviewed a series of 74 children with known unilateral agenesis.[3] Five died within the newborn period and one-third required surgical procedures on the solitary unit. However, in all of these, some reason existed for evaluation in the first place; thus it is a selected population.

Nonurologic abnormalities are frequently associated with unilateral renal agenesis. It is the commonest nonskeletal anomaly seen in children with supralevator imperforate anus,[4] is associated with congenital scoliosis, and vaginal and uterine agenesis.

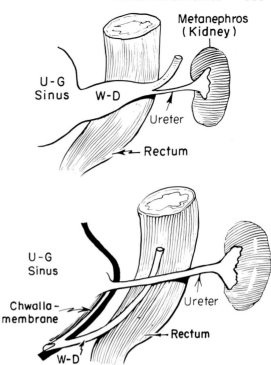

Fig. 35-1. Incorporation of wolffian (mesonephric) duct (**W-D**) into urogenital sinus (**U-G**; Kelalis PP, King LR, Belman AB (eds): Clinical Pediatric Urology, Vol. 1. Philadelphia, WB Saunders, 1977)

If suspected, screening can be carried out most safely with ultrasonography. Confirmation can be obtained by renal scan to rule out ectopia.

Supernumerary Kidneys

Many people confuse duplication of the urinary collecting system, a common abnormality (see below), with the presence of an additional kidney. The presence of a third, separate kidney is a rare anomaly, one which this author has never seen. Its presence would be picked up as an incidental finding, unless it was palpated as a mass and its significance would depend upon any associated pathology.

Malrotation

Renal malrotation results in the kidney maintaining its fetal position with the pelvis pointing anteriorly. It poses no clinical significance other than adding difficulty to the interpretation of the excretory urogram.

Table 35-1. Classification of Renal Parenchymal Cysts

I. Polycystic Disease
  A. Infantile polycystic disease
    1. Polycystic disease of early infancy
    2. Polycystic disease of childhood
    3. Congenital hepatic fibrosis
  B. Adult polycystic disease

II. Renal Cysts in Hereditary Syndromes
  A. Tuberous sclerosis complex and von Hippel-Lindau disease
  B. Meckel syndrome
  C. Zellweger cerebrohepatorenal syndrome and Jeune asphyxiating thoracic dysplasia
  D. Cortical cysts in syndromes of multiple malformations

III. Renal Medullary Cysts
  A. Uremic medullary cystic disease complex
    1. Familial juvenile nephronophthisis
    2. Medullary cystic disease
    3. Renal-retinal dysplasia
  B. Medullary sponge kidney

IV. Renal Cysts of Differing Causes
  A. Simple cysts, solitary and multiple
  B. Segmental and unilateral cystic disease

V. Renal Dysplasia
  A. Multicystic and aplastic dysplasia
    1. Unilateral multicystic kidney
    2. Bilateral multicystic dysplasia
  B. Cystic dysplasia, diffuse and segmental
  C. Cystic dysplasia associated with lower urinary tract obstruction

(Harrison JH et al (eds): Campbell's Urology, 4th ed. Philadelphia, WB Saunders, 1979)

Renal Ectopia

Abnormal renal position often presents itself as an abdominal mass. In older children, minimal trauma may lead to hematuria, although this would not be expected in the newborn. The most common ectopic position is the true pelvis. Vesicoureteral reflux and ureteropelvic junction obstruction are common.

Genital abnormalities are often associated with pelvic ectopia. Hypospadias in the male and vaginal and uterine agenesis in the female are not uncommon.[5] Vaginography should be performed in the female child found to have a pelvic kidney, particularly if she has a solitary pelvic kidney.

Fused Kidneys

Midline renal fusion in the form of horseshoe kidneys, pancake kidneys, and so on may present as an abdominal mass. Ureteropelvic junction obstruction associated with abnormal vessels or compression by the isthmus may result.

Crossed fusion is uncommon. The crossed kidney can generally be found below the normally positioned one. As in all abnormally positioned kidneys, vesicoureteral reflux and obstruction should be ruled out. Additionally, abnormalities of other organ systems, particularly spinal and cardiac, are frequently present.

Renal Cystic Disease

This is an extremely complex subject. Although many forms of cystic renal disease exist, the two types seen in the neonatal period include the multicystic kidney (cystic dysplasia) and infantile polycystic disease (Table 35-1). Adult type polycystic disease, a true Mendelian dominant trait, can also present in the newborn, but very rarely.

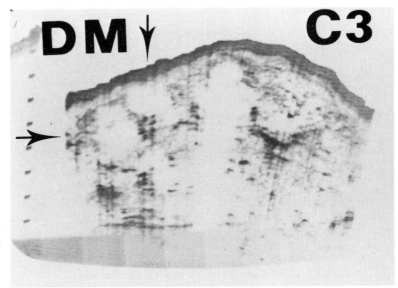

Fig. 35-2. Transverse abdominal ultrasound carried out in prone position 3 cm (**C3**) above the iliac crest in infant (**DM**) with left multicystic (cystic dyplastic) kidney. Note multiple echo free areas (**arrows**).

Multicystic Kidney (Cystic Dysplasia)

The multicystic kidney presents as a flank mass in the newborn which does not function on excretory urography. The underlying etiologic process is related to total urinary obstruction because either ureteropelvic or upper ureteral atresia is virtually always present.[6] The incidence of multicystic kidney disease about equals that of hydronephrosis as a cause for an abdominal mass of renal origin in the newborn.[7]

The diagnosis is presumed when renal nonfunction is associated with the typical picture noted on ultrasonography of a multiseptated fluid filled mass (Fig. 35-2). Confirmation can be achieved only by surgical removal of the typical grape-like cluster representing the dysplastic kidney (Fig. 35-3). Histologically, true dysplastic elements exist with primitive tubules present (Fig. 35-4).

Controversy exists as to the necessity for removal of the cystic dysplastic kidney. There is no known incidence of malignancy and the mass does not enlarge with age.[8] The only advantage to surgery is that of diagnostic confirmation, ruling out other possibilities including mesoblastic nephroma.

Infantile Polycystic Disease

Inherited as an autosomal recessive, this category of bilateral cystic disease apparently encompasses several forms.[6] Hepatic fibrosis is a significant component of this complex and may result in portal hypertension in those newborns who survive the pulmonary complication of having such large intraabdominal masses, because the kidneys may fill the entire abdomen. Urography is usually diagnostic when the typical sun-ray or streak appearance is noted (Fig. 35-4). However, as the child gets older, the radiographic picture changes, with distortion of the collecting system becoming a more prominent feature.

Adult-type Polycystic Disease

This is the more common variety, is an autosomal dominant, and is virtually always associated with a family history of fatal renal disease. Adult-type polycystic disease is extremely uncommon in infancy, although there have been reports of it appearing in neonates.[9] Hypertension is a prominent feature of polycystic disease with complications usually leading to death within 10 years of diagnosis. However, clinical recognition of polycystic disease of the adult type does not usually occur until the fourth to fifth decades. Although hepatic cysts do coexist, interference with liver function is not a feature.

Renal Tumors

Wilm's tumor (nephroblastoma) is not an entity often seen in the newborn; however reports of its occurrence exist.[10] More common, although still a relatively rare lesion, is the congenital mesoblastic nephroma. Tumors

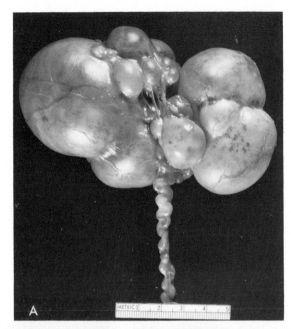

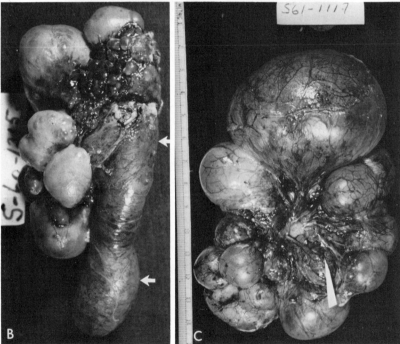

Fig. 35-3. Three examples of the variety of multicystic disease. **A.** Multicystic kidney with a tortuous atretic ureter. The cysts vary in size and appear to be held together by fibrous tissue. **B.** Multicystic kidney from a 1-month-old girl. The **arrows** indicate the dilated pelvis and proximal ureter. **C.** Multicystic kidney from a 4-day-old female. No ureter was found during the nephrectomy. (Kelalis PP, King LR, Belman AB (eds): Clinical Pediatric Urology, vol. 2. Philadelphia, WB Saunders, 1977)

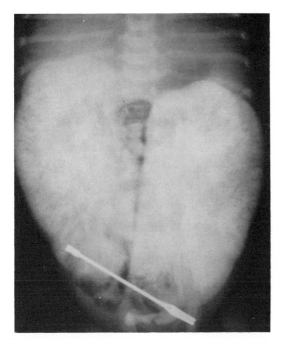

Fig. 35-4. Excretory urogram from a 2-day-old girl with infantile polycystic kidney disease. Notice the sunray appearance of the contrast material and the enormous renal size. (Kelalis PP, King LR, Belman AB (eds): Clinical Pediatric Urology, vol 2. (Philadelphia, WB Saunders, 1977)

present as a flank mass. However, as compared to the cystic dysplastic kidney, radiographic visualization of a portion of the kidney is usually present. Distortion of the collecting system by an intrinsic mass is the rule.

Excision of the mesoblastic nephroma is curative in almost every instance; however, these "benign" tumors apparently rarely have the potential for direct invasion. Because the differential diagnosis of mesoblastic nephroma versus Wilm's tumor cannot be made preoperatively, exploration and excision should be carried out as soon as the newborn is considered a favorable operative risk.

Renal Vein Thrombosis

Hemoconcentration in the newborn as the result of dehydration or in infants of diabetic mothers may result in sludging of cells in the intrarenal venules and thrombosis. When this is relatively extensive, the involved kidney becomes enlarged, hematuria results, and there is hematologic evidence of intravascular

coagulation. Platelet levels fall, fibrin split products are elevated, and fragmented red cells can be seen.[11] If both kidneys are extensively involved, the baby may become uremic; however, in most instances some renal tissue is either uninvolved or spared from permanent damage. Survival is the rule.

Operative intervention is no longer considered necessary in this group because the thrombotic process originates in small vessels and, therefore, caval or main renal vein thrombectomy serves no useful purpose. The main therapeutic maneuver is to correct the abnormal state of hydration which led to the original problem. Anticoagulation probably should not play a role in treatment.

THE URINARY DRAINAGE SYSTEM

Anomalies of Number (Duplication of the Urinary Collecting System)

One of the most common urinary tract developmental abnormalities is duplication of the collecting (drainage) system. Duplication of the ureteral bud as it comes off the mesonephric duct leads to two completely separate ureters and pyelocaliceal systems (Fig. 35-5). Complete duplication occurs in 1 in 500 individuals.[1] If the ureter bifurcates after it has budded, incomplete duplication results. This usually is of no clinical significance. Complete duplication, however, is associated with a higher risk of urinary pathology than the normal and may be associated with urosepsis in the newborn.

Vesicoureteral reflux into the lower renal segment is common, and, although duplication occurs in 1 in 500 of the general population, it is seen in 1 in 4.5 of the total population with vesicoureteral reflux (Fig. 35-6).[12] Our own review supports this, with a ratio of 1 in 6.

On the other hand, when the upper renal segment of a duplication is abnormal, obstruction is the rule. A renal (hydronephrotic) mass may be noted in the newborn because of this obstruction; however, that is uncommon. Most present for evaluation with urinary infection in infancy or early childhood.

Ureteral Ectopia

As the Wolffian duct migrates and is absorbed into the base of the bladder, the ureter normally becomes separated from it. However,

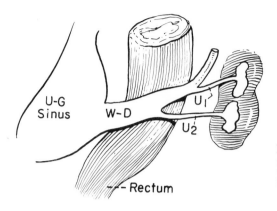

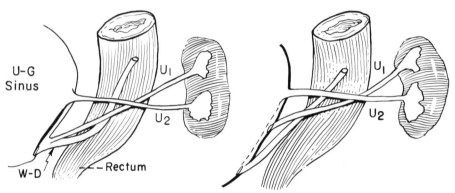

Fig. 35-5. Development of ectopic ureter. **U-G** = urogenital; **W-D** = wolffian duct; **U** = ureter. (Kelalis PP, King LR, Belman AB (eds): Clinical Pediatric Urology, vol 1. Philadelphia, WB Saunders, 1977)

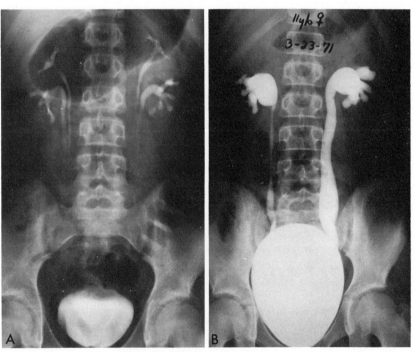

Fig. 35-6. A. Intravenous urogram in girl with complete, bilateral duplication of collecting system. Note blunting of lower calyces. **B**. Cystogram in same child demonstrating reflux into both lowering collecting systems only. (Belman AB: Pediatr Clin North Am 23:710, 1976)

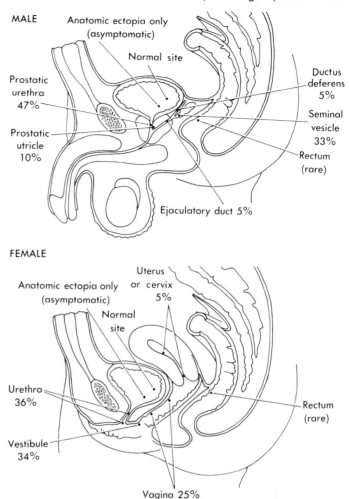

Fig. 35-7. Sites of ectopic ureteral orifices and their relative frequencies of occurrence in men and women. (Gray SW, Skandalakis JE: Embryology for Surgeons. Philadelphia, WB Saunders, 1972)

if this separation fails to occur, it has the potential of carrying the ureter with it, producing an ectopic orifice. The ureter of the upper renal segment of a duplicated system stands the highest risk for this developmental abnormality. Ureteral ectopia in the female may occur into any of the Müllerian structures, including the uterus, vagina, and introitus (Gartner's duct). In the male, Wolffian structures which may harbor an ectopic ureter include the prostate and seminal vesicals (Fig. 35-7). Urethral and bladder-neck ectopia can occur in either sex; however, in boys ectopia does not occur below the urogenital diaphragm.

Ectopic ureters are often obstructed and at risk for urinary infection. Obstruction of the upper renal segment of a duplicated system

may also be the result of an ectopic ureterocele. A ureterocele is an unusual dilatation of the distal ureter, often associated with a stenotic orifice (Fig. 35-8). These children also often present with urinary infection, but seldom in the newborn nursery. Rarely, when the ureterocele is extremely large, it may prolapse from the female urethra and is visible. This may lead to urinary retention. Confusion between urethral prolapse, sarcoma botryoides, and a prolapsing ureterocele may occur. However, urography with delayed studies generally resolves that question. The typical "dropping lily" configuration is seen when the hydronephrotic upper renal segment pushes the functioning lower segment downward. That picture, in addition to the bladder-filling defect produced by the ureterocele, should identify

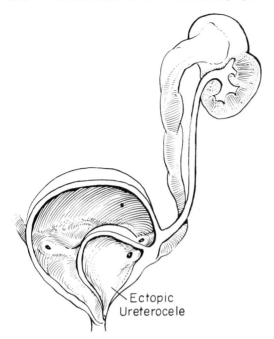

Fig. 35-8. Ectopic ureterocele (Malek RS, Kelalis PP, Burke EC et al: Simple and ectopic ureterocele in infancy and childhood. Surg Gynecol Obstet 134: 611-616, 1972. By permission of Surgery, Gynecology and Obstetrics.)

the child with obstruct d, duplicated system (Fig. 35-9).

Ectopic ureters may also exit outside the bladder sphincter mechanism. In girls, this causes continuous urinary dribbling and should be kept in mind as the underlying problem in the child with a constantly wet diaper. Pus draining from the vagina may be the result of an infected, partially obstructed, ectopic system. Unusual vaginal drainage in girls should always be evaluated with urinary x-ray films.

An ectopic single ureter (*i.e.,* one not associated with duplication of the urinary collecting system) is an extremely rare phenomenon. Urinary obstruction with little chance of a salvagable renal unit results when the ureter pursues a course which brings it through the bladder neck (internal sphincter mechanism). When both ureters of single systems are ectopic, the body of the bladder may develop poorly. Urinary control (bladder neck function) is nonexistent. Renal survival is likely in those with bilateral ectopia but hope for urinary control in the future is poor.

URETERAL OBSTRUCTION

Multicystic Kidney (Cystic Dysplasia)

This entity is discussed under renal cystic diseases. However, the etiology is most likely complete ureteral obstruction (atresia), and, therefore, falls into the spectrum of obstructive renal disease.

Ureteropelvic Junction Obstruction

Obstruction of the urinary tract is the single most common cause of an abdominal mass in the newborn. In a variety of series, hydronephrosis and cystic dysplasia account for about equal numbers.[7] The multicystic kidney (cystic dysplasia) does not function, and, therefore, projects as a negative image on both renal scan and urography. The differentiation of various masses of renal origin is outlined in Table 35-2.

Obstruction at the ureteropelvic junction, usually the result of a congenital narrowing, produces hydronephrosis which can be quite extensive (Fig. 35-10). The mass is smooth, firm, functional on delayed scans or excretory

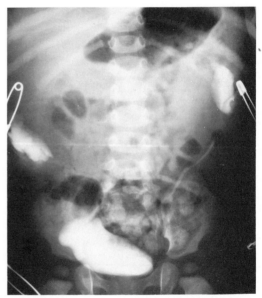

Fig. 35-9. Excretory urogram in infant with duplication. Ectopic ureters from upper segments produced massive displacement of lower segments, leading to misdiagnosis of abdominal mass and neuroblastoma. (Kelalis PP, King LR, Belman AB (eds): Clinical Pediatric Urology, vol 1. Philadelphia, WB Saunders, 1976)

Table 35-2. Abdominal Masses of Renal Origin.

Mass	Texture	Renal Scan or Excretory Urogram	Ultrasound
Hydronephrosis	Smooth	Delayed drainage	Sonar lucent
Multicystic kidney (cystic dysplasia)	Irregular	Nonfunction	Multiple large and small cysts
Polycystic kidney	Smooth (infantile), irregular or smooth (adult)	Delayed function distortion of collecting system	Diffuse small cysts (infantile) Multiple large and small cysts (adult)
Tumor	Smooth	Distortion of collecting system	Solid
Renal Vein Thrombosis	Smooth	Poor to nonfunction	Relatively normal renal architecture; kidney enlarged

urograms, and has a high potential for surgical correction. The diagnosis is made radiographically when delayed visualization on renal scan or urogram is associated with a sonar lucent mass on ultrasonography (Fig. 35-11). Differentiation between the multicystic kidney and hydronephrosis is made on the basis of function.

As soon as the child is stable, definitive therapy should be carried out. Although there occasionally may be situations in which an intubated (nephrostomy) or nonintubated (cutaneous pyelostomy) form of high urinary diversion may be indicated, these are extremely uncommon. The choice is primary correction with pyeloplasty. The general rule is to conserve renal tissue in infants. Regardless of the extent of hydronephrosis it is worthwhile attempting repair; the favorable results in the majority support this approach.

Ureterovesical Obstruction

Hydroureteronephrosis secondary to ureterovesical obstruction is relatively common but rarely presents in the newborn nursery (Fig. 35-12). Although the degree of hydronephrosis can be severe, it does not usually manifest itself as a mass and, unless vesicoureteral reflux is also present, urinary sepsis is uncommon.

As compared to ureteropelvic junction obstruction, ureterovesical obstruction may *occasionally* not require immediate operative intervention. This applies particularly to those with ureterectasis but little or no caliectasis. Obviously, close observation is imperative and surgical intervention may well be necessary if the dilatation is noted to progress. During the observation interval, continuous urinary prophylaxis with low-dose antimicrobials should be instituted, particularly in the child in whom the uropathy was discovered upon evaluation for urinary tract infection.

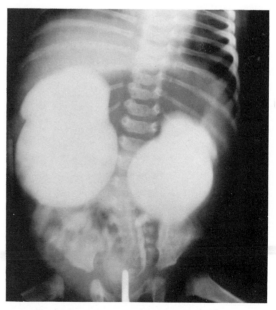

Fig. 35-10. Severe bilateral hydronephrosis secondary to ureteropelvic junction obstructions.

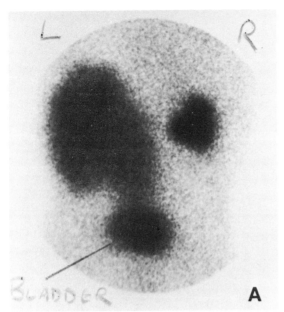 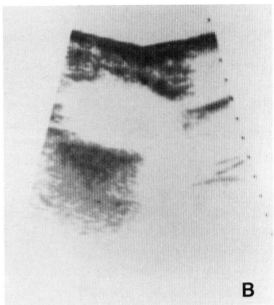

Fig. 35-11. A. Delayed renal scan in newborn with massive left hydronephrosis secondary to ureteropelvic junction obstruction. Renal pelvis extends all the way to child's true pelvis. **B.** Longitudinal abdominal ultrasound demonstrating single large echo-free region consistent with hydronephrosis.

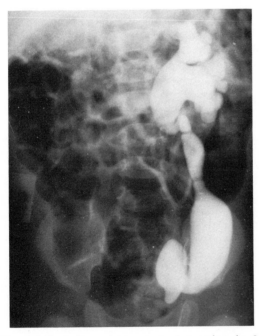

Fig. 35-12. Left ureterovesical obstruction in 3-month-old boy presenting with unresponsive diarrhea. Urine culture was positive and radiographic evaluation demonstrated significant pathology seen above. The diarrhea dissolved with treatment of the urinary infection. The ureterovesical obstruction was treated surgically. (Kelalis PP, King LR, Belman AB (eds): Clinical Pediatric Urology, Vol. 1. Philadelphia, WB Saunders, 1977)

Vesicoureteral Reflux

By far the most common anatomic abnormality seen in the pediatric urinary tract is vesicoureteral reflux. Its actual incidence is unknown, since the diagnosis is made only in those presenting with symptoms for evaluation; however, it has been estimated to occur in 1 in 200 of the general pediatric population.

Because reflux is a primary congenital abnormality in all but those with bladder outlet obstruction, the highest incidence must exist in the newborn. However, efforts to determine its incidence in both full-term and prematures has not been successful.[13,14] Vesicoureteral reflux has been identified in the fetus as an incidental finding during intrauterine exchange transfusions.[15] Roberts and Riopelle have also noted that 80% of infant Rhesus monkeys have reflux that resolved spontaneously by 36 months in all.[16]

Vesicoureteral reflux is a ureteral bud abnormality which appears to be genetically determined.[17] Some have even suggested that the siblings of all children with reflux should be screened radiographically because the likelihood of its presence is about 25%.[18] The normal ureterovesical junction incorporates a flap-valve mechanism dependent upon the ureter pursuing a submucosal course from the muscular bladder hiatus to the ureteral orifice

(Fig. 35-13). Intravesical pressure closes this valve, preventing bladder urine from reentering the ureters.

In the neonate, reflux becomes apparent when a baby is evaluated following urosepsis. The incidence of reflux in this group approaches 50%.[19] In some groups, it is recognized that ureteral bud abnormalities are more common and cystography should be performed as soon as convenient. This particularly includes those with imperforate anus. Children with posterior urethral valves have cystography to confirm the primary diagnosis; however reflux will also be noted in about one-half.

The question of timing of the cystogram (which should be done in the x-ray department with the child awake) often arises. Cystography should not be carried out while the child is actively infected because the high-pressure study may well result in further renal infection and bacteriuria. In the neonate, it is imperative, nevertheless, to establish the presence or absence of vesicoureteral reflux before discontinuation of antibiotics.

If reflux is demonstrated, the baby should be maintained on long-term suppressive medication. Unfortunately, the choices are limited in the newborn period and during the first few months of life. Amoxicillin may be used, although it is not an effective long-term prophylactic agent. At the earliest opportunity, the child should be switched to sulfa until the reflux is noted to resolve or antireflux surgery

is carried out. However, under no circumstances should the infant with reflux who has been found to be susceptible to urinary tract infection be without some means of protecting his or her urinary tract.

It has become increasingly apparent that the infant kidney is most at risk for scarring from bacterial pyelonephritis. We can prevent this damage only in those whom we identify as being at risk and aggressively treat (either medically or surgically). Current evidence does not support the concept that the back pressure of sterile reflux alone injures kidneys.[20] Therefore, prevention of infection is an adequate means of insuring renal growth. Uncontrollable breakthrough infection while on prophylaxis, on the other hand, suggests the need for early corrective surgery.

The Urinary Bladder

Abnormalities of the urinary bladder itself are rare. Agenesis of the urinary bladder is incompatible with survival unless the ureteral orifices have implanted elsewhere and urinary obstruction is absent. Duplication anomalies and bladder septa may be associated with complete or incomplete genital duplication. These are complex problems which require detailed and comprehensive evaluation.

Bladder exstrophy is probably the most common bladder abnormality. Yet even this occurs in only 1 in 10,000 to 1 in 50,000 births. The birth of a child with an exstrophic bladder is a shocking experience for all involved. However, tremendous strides have been made and the chances for a closed, functional bladder are quite good. Surprisingly, the remainder of the urinary tract is usually normal in these children, although virtually all have an associated epispadias (Fig. 35-14).

The cause of bladder exstrophy is unknown. However, it is not a developmental arrest but rather the consequence of a fetal accident. The result is an anterior abdominal wall defect filled by the opened bladder. The ureteral orifices can be seen as can the entire urethra, including the prostatic urethra in the male. The pubic symphysis is widely separate resulting in a stubby penis which has a distinctive upward tilt. Variations of bladder exstrophy include the superior vesical fissure and superior vesical fistula in which the bladder neck and urethra are intact. These forms are much milder and even more rare than the standard variety.

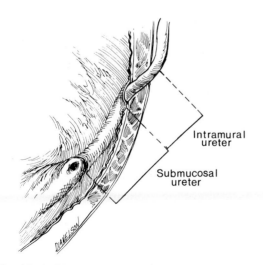

Intramural ureter

Submucosal ureter

Fig. 35-13. Normal ureterovesical junction. (Harrison JH et al (eds): Campbell's Urology, 4th ed. Philadelphia, WB Saunders, 1979)

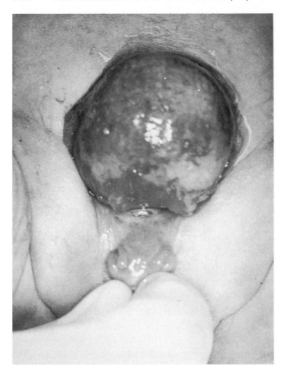

Fig. 35-14. Complete bladder exstrophy in male child. Note that penis is epispadiac, short, and stubby.

The desired treatment of bladder exstrophy is closure with the establishment of urinary continence. Incredible success in this area is being achieved, with over half achieving urinary control.[21] However, some are not candidates for closure, bladder size being the determining factor.

Functional closure is a staged procedure with the actual turning in of the bladder and approximation of the anterior rectus fascia achieved as a first step. No effort is made to produce urinary continence at that time. However, in the male the penis is also released at this time to normalize its appearance and redirect its angle of intent. Occasionally, a male with exstrophy has an extremely short penis with little or no corporal tissue present. Serious consideration should be given to raising this child as a female with castration performed at the time of bladder closure and vaginal construction carried out at puberty.

Many urologists are now carrying out closure in the immediate newborn period: within 48 hours of birth. The advantage to this approach resides in the flexibility of the pelvic girdle in the newborn and the ability to forcibly approximate the symphysis pubic. Beyond 48 hours, bilateral iliac osteotomies are required to achieve this essential maneuver. Bearing this in mind, pediatric urologic consultation should immediately be obtained in children born with this abnormality.

To achieve urinary continence, bladder neck revision with bilateral ureteral reimplantations is performed sometime in the second or third year of life. It is at this time that definitive urethroplasty can be carried out in the male, although this may be deferred as a third and separate step. The alternative to functional closure is urinary diversion. Internal diversion, placing the ureters into the intact colon (ureterosigmoidostomy), is the second choice, allowing a form of urinary control. However, a risk of malignancy occurring 10 or more years later has been recognized. Regular follow-up of individuals with ureterosigmoidostomy is required. The final alternative is cutaneous urinary diversion, which should be saved as the last choice when all else fails.

The unclosed urinary bladder, a choice obviously unacceptable, is at exceedingly high risk for adenocarcinoma occuring in the second to third decade of life. Function closure obviates this risk.

Cloacal Exstrophy (Vesicointestinal Fissure)

Perhaps the most severe anomaly compatible with survival in either the genitourinary or gastrointestinal tract includes both systems. In cloacal exstrophy, the exstrophic bladder flanks a midline strip of exstrophic cecum (Fig. 35-15). Ileum is seen to prolapse inferiorly and the child has an imperforate anus with little or no large bowel present. Oftentimes, the small intestine is severely foreshortened, a fact which may interfere with the baby's survival.

The abdominal and pelvic defect interferes with fusion of the genital tubercle in this group, resulting in widely separated corporal bodies. Although these are approximated when surgical repair is carried out, it is unlikely that a functioning penis will result. It is advised that consideration be given to raising all of these children as girls.

Gaining a functional anus with this problem is virtually impossible. Bowel diversion is the rule. Oftentimes, the absorptive problems related to a permanent ileostomy can be improved upon by using the distal remnant of colon as an end colostomy. Attempts at rectal pull-through are probably not justifiable.

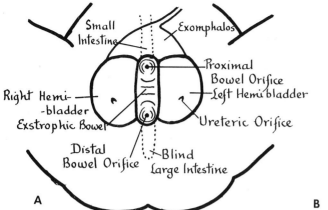 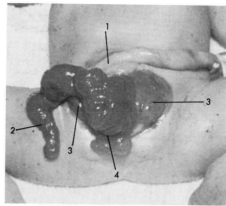

Fig. 35-15. Exstrophy of the cloaca. **A.** Diagram of the external anatomy. **B.** Photograph of a patient showing exomphalos. (**1**) Prolapsed ileum, (**2**) hemibladders lying on either side of exstrophic bowel, (**3**) distal bowel orifice, and (**4**) absence of anus and external genitalia. (Johnston JH, Penn IA: Br J Urol 38: 302-307, 1966)

Bladder closure may be attempted. Again, this is a staged reconstruction with removal of the midline colonic segment and permanent bowel diversion as the first step. At a later date, the bladder is turned in, accompanied by iliac osteotomy to achieve the abdominal closure. Urinary control is unlikely. However, continence by means of intermittent catheterization or the possible insertion of an artificial sphincter device are all possibilities for the future. The majority of the survivors, however, will probably require cutaneous urinary diversion.

The Urachus

A persistent patent urachus is also uncommon. In the presence of complete distal obstruction, as might occur in the prune-belly syndrome when urethral obstruction coexists, the presence of a patent urachus may be the only reason functioning renal tissue develops. Otherwise, total outflow obstruction precludes the formation of significant normal renal tissue. The diagnosis of a patent urachus is made on voiding cystourethrography.

A urachal sinus may present in the neonatal period as an umbilical discharge. This is the result of infection in an incompletely obliterated urachal remnant.

The treatment of both patent urachus and urachal sinus is complete excision of the tract. It is probably advisable to also excise any portion of the urachus present at the bladder dome, including a cuff of bladder at that junction. Bladder adenocarcinoma in the urachal remnant is a possible risk for the future.

THE PENIS

The development of the penis is dependent upon hormonal stimulation. Testosterone, secreted by the fetal testis, is the normal force which produces enlargement and masculinization of the genital tubercle. Other sources of testosterone, including that produced as a by-product of excessive adrenal production or by maternal ingestion, can produce partial to complete masculinization in the female.

Ambiguous Genitalia
(See also Chap. 44)

Sexual differentiation is a spectrum, the extremes of which are easily recognizable. The degree of expectation of normal genital development is so great that it is natural for a new parent first to be asked, "Is it a boy or a girl?" and not, "Is the baby well?" Therefore, it is extremely difficult for the pediatrician or obstetrician to respond, "I don't know," to the parents' expected question regarding the sex of their new offspring.

When a child is born with an incompletely developed phallus, the first maneuver which will help determine the genetic sex is a search for scrotal gonads. The presence of two palpable gonads in the scrotal compartments is reliable assurance that the genetic sex is male. If, on the one hand, only one scrotal gonad is present, the possibility exists for true hermaphroditism or one of the forms of gonadal dysgenesis. On the other hand, if no gonads are palpable, there is strong likelihood that the child is a female pseudohermaphrodite, and one must immediately rule out adrenal hyperplasia.

Rapid screening in all should include urine electrolyte determination, 17-ketosteroid production, buccal smear, and chromosomal analysis to identify the sex chromosomes. The results of these studies must be available within a few days to allow a definitive assignment of sex. Additionally, cystourethrography can often outline internal female structures, confirming the impression of the presence of a uterus at the time of rectal bimanual examination (Fig. 35-16).

Definitive differentiation in the male pseudohermaphrodite may still require abdominal exploration with gonadal biopsy before final gender assignment. Generally, this is carried out during the newborn period with removal of any female structures if phallic development is such that adequate penile reconstruction is possible and the gonads are normal testes.

The group with a negative sex chromatin pattern and 45,XO/46,XY mosaicism are most likely to have mixed gonadal dysgenesis. Most commonly, a testis and contralateral streak gonad are found with a well formed Müllerian system. Because of the high risk of gonadal malignancy and short stature in this group, castration and female gender assignment are recommended.[22]

A number of syndromes exist, the majority of which are familial, in which a defect in steroid synthesis results in defective testosterone production. In addition, another group exists in which androgen action is ineffective, either because of lack of protein binding of dihydrotestosterone, with the result that masculinization is completely absent (testicular feminization syndrome), or because virilization is incomplete. Finally, a group exists in which testosterone cannot be converted to the more potent dihydrotestosterone, also resulting in abnormal development of the external male genitalia. The interested reader is referred to the excellent chapter by Wilson and Walsh for further clarification.[22]

Penile Agenesis

Agenesis of the penis is rare and suggests a very early embryologic accident resulting in failure of development of the genital tubercle (Fig. 35-17**A**). The urethra may exit on the perineum or into the rectum (Fig. 35-17**B**).

Needless to say, these children should be raised as females with castration and external reconstruction performed at an early age.

Penile Duplication

Duplication of the penis may be complete or incomplete. When complete the urethra and bladder may also be involved and reconstruction then involves a choice between the more functional segment. More commonly, when a duplication anomaly exists, the penis is bifid, involving the glans or a portion of the distal phallus (Fig. 35-18).

Penoscrotal Transposition

Occasionally, the penis is found to lie between the scrotal folds (Fig. 35-19). Although usually accompanied by hypospadias, the transposition can, very rarely, be complete (Fig. 35-20). Severe genital abnormalities of this type are frequently accompanied by urinary anomalies and complete urologic evaluation is indicated.

Penile Torsion

Torque of the penis is almost always to the left (Fig. 35-21). The abnormality is primarily one of misalignment of the midline skin. It is often associated with hypospadias but may be an isolated finding. It constitutes no severe functional threat, although the direction of penile erection is abnormal and urination is misdirected.

Repair is achieved by dissecting the penile skin off the shaft and then realigning it. Circumcision can be carried out at the same time.

Microphallus

One of the more difficult problems to deal with is the male born with an abnormally small phallus. Microphallus is frequently associated with bladder and cloacal exstrophy, but is rare as an independent entity. The cause is most likely hypogonadism and may be either primary or secondary. If gonadic function is lost following completion of penile formation, further growth will be interfered with, the result being a completely formed but diminutive phallus.

The normal newborn phallus measures about 3.75 cm *stretched* length from symphysis to tip of glans.[23] However, the microphallus usually measures no more than 1 cm. During infancy, as the pubic fat pad increases, the

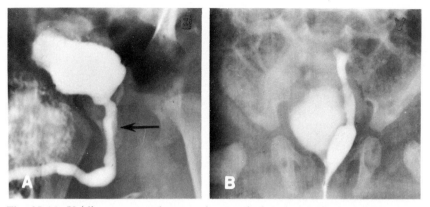

Fig. 35-16. Voiding cystourethrogram in genetic female totally masculinized by adrenal hyperplasia. **A.** Utriculus masculinus **(arrow)** as would normally be expected in a male. **B.** Retrograde vaginohystogram revealing normal vagina and uterus as well as overflow of contrast into urinary bladder **(midline)**.

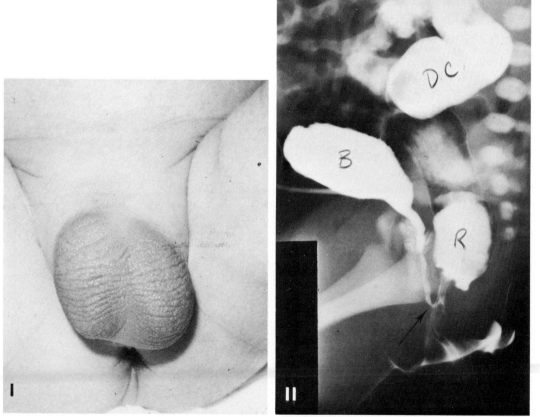

Fig. 35-17. I. Genetic male born with complete penile agenesis. **II.** Antegrade cystourethrogram in genetic male with penile agensis. Filled bladder **(B)**, communication between urethra and rectum **(arrow)**, rectum **(R)**, descending colon **(DC)** filled with voided contrast material.

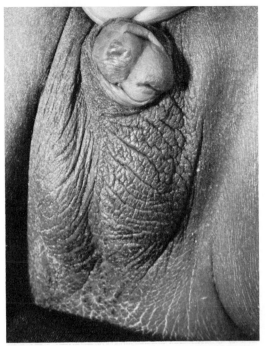

Fig. 35-18. Duplication of the glans in a 2-year-old boy. (Kossow JH, Morales PA: Duplication of bladder and urethra and associated anomalies. Urology 1:71-73, 1973. By permission.)

penis may become withdrawn and appear to be very small. The actual size can be appreciated by compressing the fat on each side of the shaft against the symphysis, extending the penis.

Treatment of microphallus is difficult because it is unlikely that full growth potential will be reached in adulthood. Hormonal stimulation either with 2.5% to 10% local testosterone or gonadotropin will at least determine whether the penis has the potential for a relative increase in size.[24] If no response is noted within 2 to 3 weeks or if, on initial examination, no corporal tissue is felt, it is probably in the best interests of the child to be raised as a female with castration and formation of a vagina in later years. This is a decision which must be made before the child is named and discharged from the hospital.

The Foreskin

The final step in penile formation is completion of formation of the prepuce. Therefore, one commonly sees absence of the ventral foreskin in those with hypospadias and absence of dorsal foreskin in those with epispadias. Normal development of the foreskin

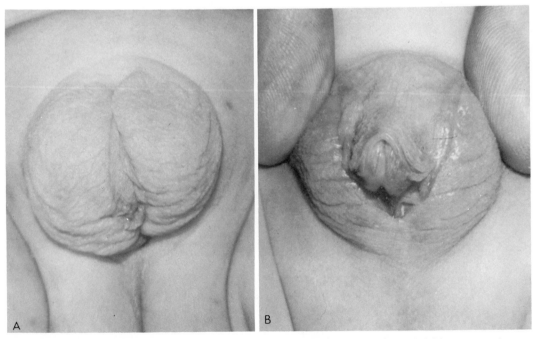

Fig. 35-19. Doughnut scrotum in a 1-year-old boy. **A.** Frontal view. **B.** Scrotal folds separated to expose the hypospadiac penis.

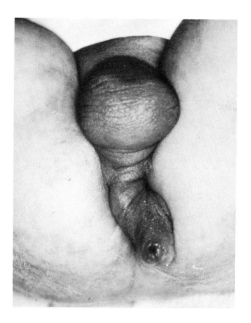

Fig. 35-20. Complete transposition of the penis and scrotum. This child survived only a few weeks, having only minimal renal tissue developed. A saccular urethra was found proximal to a severe distal stenosis. (Belman AB: Urol Clin North Am 5:17, 1978)

appears to require glanular urethral development.

At birth, the inner layer of the foreskin is adherent to the glans to a greater or lesser degree. The meatus of the prepuce is also smaller than the diameter of the glans itself. Retraction of the foreskin in the newborn requires dilation of its orifice as well as disruption of the adhering layers. Some people interpret this constellation as phimosis. True phimosis is an inability to retract the foreskin because of an acquired circumferential scar.

Natural History of the Foreskin

In those Western countries in which circumcision is not carried out as routine, the opportunity exists to evaluate the natural history of the foreskin. Øster reported on 9545 uncircumcised boys, finding that complete retraction of the foreskin did not occur in many until adolescence.[25] Meanwhile, the orifice of the prepuce gradually stretches to accommodate the dimensions of the glans. Frequently, desquamated epithelial cells accumulate between the two layers producing subcutaneous pearls which have the appearance of sebaceous cysts.

These spontaneously "drain" as the overlying skin becomes more and more retracted.

In our society, however, the covered glans is apparently a cause for great anxiety. Those who are not circumcised at birth then fall prey to the primary physician who is convinced the foreskin should be completely retractable in infancy. Forcible retraction becomes the rule. This results in minute tears along the orifice of the foreskin which, when the penis is returned to the diaper, become inflamed and scarred. The result is a self-fulfilling prophecy: the foreskin is retracted forcibly to prevent phimosis, a circumferential scar results, and iatrogenic phimosis occurs.

Circumcision

It is fruitless to discuss the pros and cons of newborn circumcision. Americans have adopted this as a tribal mark, thereby eliminating it as a medical decision. One must nevertheless remain aware that this is an operative procedure with inherent risks. Complications are uncommon, but when they occur

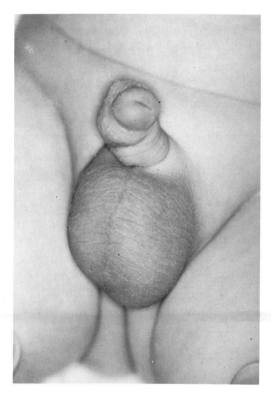

Fig. 35-21. Torsion of the penis. (Belman AB: Urol Clin North Am 5:17, 1978)

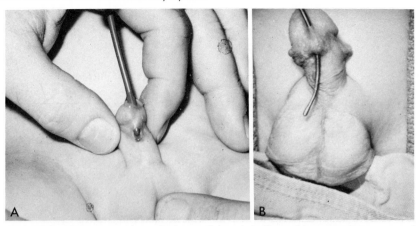

Fig. 35-22. Two examples of circumcision injuries with secondary coronal fistulae. (Belman AB: Urol Clin North Am 5:17, 1978)

can be serious. Urethral fistulae and complete or incomplete amputation are the more severe complications (Fig. 35-22). One commonly seen complication is complete or incomplete adherence of the skin of the shaft to the denuded glans resulting in dense scarring (Fig. 35-23) or fibrous bands (Fig. 35-24). This is the result of the penis either retracting within the pubic fat or inadequate skin removal. This complication can be avoided by having the

parents retract the remaining skin daily until healing is complete, a postoperative instruction rarely given.

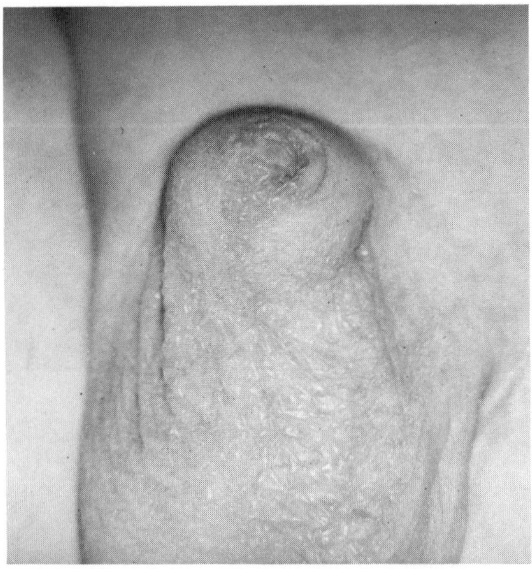

Circumcision in the newborn is a blind procedure done either with one of the various clamp devices or with a plastic ring. The ring is left on, causing necrosis of the surrounding skin. Athough the risk of fistula is slim, inflammation from the foreign body occurs and the overall complication rate is higher in this group.[26]

When circumcision is carried out beyond the newborn period, hospitalization and an anesthetic agent become necessary. This adds an additional risk to life and increases the cost astronomically. It is therefore advisable to carry out circumcision in the newborn period in those in whom it cannot be avoided, and to teach proper care of the penis in the remainder. This includes careful attention to hygiene with the child taught to withdraw his foreskin as far as he comfortably can, wash the exposed glans, and return the skin over the glans. Gradually, full retractability will result without scarring. Adequate hygiene will prevent the majority of the problems associated with being uncircumcised.

THE URETHRA

Hypospadias

Male urethral developmental is under hormonal control. Inadequate testosterone production or poor responsiveness may be the cause for incomplete formation. In most in-

Fig. 35-23. Circumcision injury. Excessive skin of shaft healed over retracted glans, obscuring the glans. The appearance is that of amputation of the glans. (Belman AB: Urol Clin North Am 5:17, 1978)

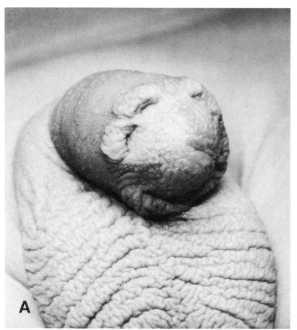 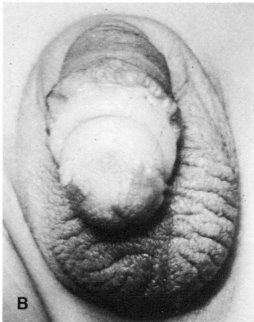

Fig. 35-24. Adhesions between distal foreskin and glans penis before **(A)** and after **(B)** surgical transection.

stances, hypospadias is an isolated abnormality; however, its occurrence can be familial. Bauer and coworkers[27] determined that the chances of having a second child with hypospadias is 11%, while the incidence of hypospadias in the general population is 3.2 per 1000 births.[28] Probands with more severe hypospadias are more likely to have siblings with hypospadias.

The severe forms of hypospadias are immediately recognizable and may lead to confusion of sex assignment. Again, if two gonads are palpable in the scrotum, there is little question of the genetic sex.

In less severe hypospadias, one of the first clues as to the presence of a urethral abnormality is the appearance of the foreskin. Incomplete formation of the ventral prepuce is an almost universal concomitant of hypospadias, even in its mildest, glanular form.

The location of the meatus is oftentimes difficult to find, as it can be quite stenotic. A trick in locating the meatus is to hold the penis firmly upwards with the left hand, while pulling the ventral skin in the opposite direction with the right (Fig. 35-25). The meatus will automatically open because it is abnormally at-

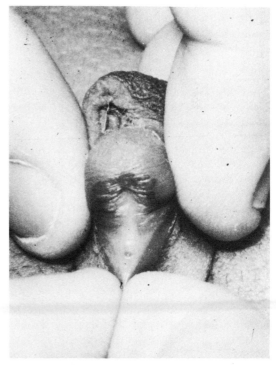

Fig. 35-25. Demonstration of hypospadiac meatal position by pulling ventral shaft of skin away from penis.

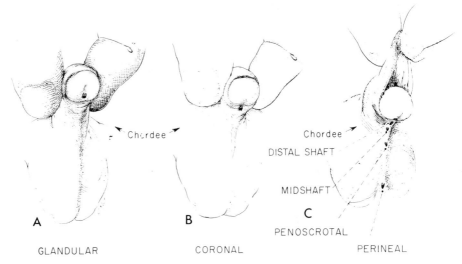

Fig. 35-26. Classification of hypospadias based on anatomic location of urethral meatus. Associated chordee is best described in terms of its severity: mild, moderate, or severe. (Kelalis PP, King LR, Belman AB (eds): Clinical Pediatric Urology, vol 1. Philadelphia, WB Saunders, 1977)

tached to the skin. It is easy to be fooled into believing there is urethral duplication by a groove and/or dimple in the glans, a rare abnormality, or that the meatus is further distal than it really is.

Hypospadias is amenable to surgical correction. The primary physician serves three important functions in dealing with this problem. First, he must protect the child from circumcision, even when the severity of the abnormality appears mild. Second, he reassures the family as to the expectations of a favorable outcome. Finally, he must refer that child to a surgeon experienced in the correction of hypospadias. Unfortunately, a boy too often becomes a hypospadiac cripple in the hands of a surgeon ill-equipped to manage the complexities and delicacy of penile reconstruction.

Hypospadias is a triad named for the abnormal urethral location but accompanied always by the incompletely formed prepuce and, in one-third, by chordee, the ventral bending of the penis accentuated by erection. Hypospadias should ideally be defined by meatal position and severity of chordee (Fig. 35-26). Therefore, one may say that a boy has coronal hypospadias with or without chordee or midshaft hypospadias with moderate or severe chordee. This is much clearer than referring to first-, second-, or third-degree hypospadias.

Repair of hypospadias is being carried out in single-stage procedures by more and more surgeons. The age at which this is recommended varies. However, without question, the plan should be to have the reconstruction completed by the time the boy starts school. Therefore, surgical repair should be begun by age 3 at least.

It is advisable to have the child seen by the surgeon in the first few months of life. Questions in reference to age of repair, types of procedures which may be applicable, and reassurance that the child will be functionally normal should be addressed to assuage parental anxiety.

Associated Anomalies

We have all been taught to look for additional urinary abnormalities after noting the presence of one. Fortunately, this is not the case with hypospadias. The incidence of urinary abnormalities in boys with hypospadias is no higher than the general population.[29] Therefore, urography is *not* indicated in this group as a routine.

Epispadias

Isolated epispadias, without exstrophy, is even more uncommon than the exstrophy-epispadias complex (Fig. 35-27). Urinary control may be affected when the abnormality

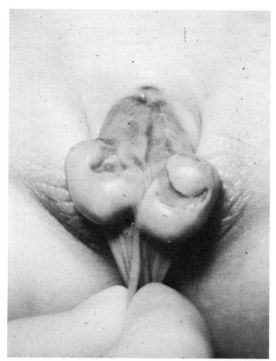

Fig. 35-27. Isolated epispadias without exstrophy. Bladder neck is intact in this child with good but not excellent urinary continence. Note also the incomplete duplication of glans.

extends into the bladder neck. Repair includes penile lengthening by freeing the corpora from the puboischial rami and release of the dorsal fibers contributing to the reverse chordee.[30] The result is a longer penis which points outwards, rather than upwards. At a later date, urethral construction is carried out with bladder neck revision if urinary continence is a problem.

Accessory Urethra

Urethral duplication may be complete or incomplete. The extra meatus is usually located dorsally and may be blind ending. This is particularly true in hypospadias where the functional urethra is on the ventral aspect of the penis.

When duplication is complete, urinary control becomes a problem only if the accessory channel communicates with the bladder outside of the sphincter mechanism. In the majority with this altogether rare abnormality, the urethra is incompletely duplicated, forming a Y-junction with two streams as a result. Treat-ment involves either excision of the more abnormal urethra or disruption of the common septum.

Urethral Agenesis or Atresia

Absence of the urethra, when complete, is incompatible with normal development of the urinary tract unless there is another means of egress of fetal urine. Patency of the urachus or an accessory urethra therefore have to coexist. The accessory urethra may then have a perineal or rectal communication resulting in an "H" or "Y" fistula abnormality. Reconstruction will ultimately achieve closure of the abnormally located urethra as well as construction of a more normally situated penile urethra.[31]

Urethral Valves

Obstruction to the outflow of bladder urine in the newborn is most commonly secondary to obstructive urethral valves. Although valves of the anterior (distal) urethra occur, the most common valve is the type I posterior urethral valve (Fig. 35-28).

The child with obstructing valves voids poorly after birth and typically has a large, thick-walled, distended urinary bladder which is easily recognized on newborn examination if the lower abdomen is palpated. Various degrees of hydroureteronephrosis may coexist, and vesicoureteral reflux is present in about 50%. Paradoxically, the infant recognized in the first year of life as having posterior urethral valves has a *worse* prognosis than those picked up later. The older children, who have a less severe degree of obstruction and pathology, become recognized when they become infected or have difficulty with toilet training.

The diagnosis of obstructing valves is made radiographically by voiding cystourethrography. After catheterizing the *awake* infant with a 5F feeding tube, the bladder is gradually filled with dilute contrast material. The catheter is not removed until voiding is noted to occur around it, at which time spot films are taken and the tube removed. Voiding will usually continue and the classic configuration is noted (Fig. 35-29). Reflux, if present, is documented. The management of the child with posterior urethral valves has progressed markedly in the past decade.[32] Temporary urinary diversion by way of nephrostomy

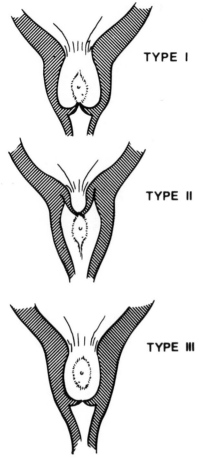

TYPE I

TYPE II

TYPE III

Fig. 35-28. HH Young's classification of valves into three types. (Kelalis PP, King LR, Belman AB (eds): Clinical Pediatric Urology, vol. 1. Philadelphia, WB Saunders, 1977)

drainage or loop-cutaneous ureterostomy (a form of high tubeless drainage in which the ureter is brought directly to the skin like a colostomy) is rarely indicated. The infant with sepsis, fluid and electrolyte imbalance, or both is drained short term with an in-dwelling urethral catheter and treated medically until he can tolerate an anesthetic. Advances in miniature fiberoptic cystoscopes allow visualization and direct transurethral resection of the obstructing valve in virtually all patients. In the exceptional situation, direct tubeless bladder drainage (vesicostomy) may be indicated.

Postoperative diuresis may require special fluid management. Dilatation of the urinary tract remains for months to years, and vesicoureteral reflux will require correction in

about half of those ureterovesical junctions which were originally incompetent.

Observation over several years is imperative. To avoid infection in these large, dilated systems, long-term antibacterial prophylaxis is recommended. Those who present with evidence of renal insufficiency will, in all likelihood, not improve with time. They will, in fact, have renal deterioration as they grow. Many of these children have congenital renal dysplasia, a product of the intrauterine urinary obstruction. Acidosis, poor growth, the potential for renal rickets, and anemia should be monitored and appropriately managed.[33] In addition, some of these children have difficulty with urinary control. Many can anticipate improvement as they become pubertal and have growth of their prostate.

The Scrotum and its Contents

Scrotal abnormalities *per se* are uncommon. Penoscrotal transposition has been previously mentioned. Clefting of the scrotum is usually seen as part of the hypospadias complex in the more severe cases and is corrected at the time of urethroplasty.

Testicular abnormalities other than maldescensus (this is discussed elsewhere) are also uncommon in the newborn. **Neonatal torsion,** however, is relatively common. Torsion in the newborn is generally of the extravaginal type. That is, the entire tunica vaginalis and its contents twist as a result, in all likelihood, of their incomplete attachment to the scrotum or as an accident of descent. Presentation is as a hard, dark nontransilluminating mass. Exploration is probably of no value because it is too late for restoration of circulation and testicular survival. Contralateral exploration and simple orchidopexy is *not* indicated in this type of torsion.

Intravaginal torsion, on the other hand, is the result of a poor congenital attachment of the testis to its tunica vaginalis. This is called the bell-and-clapper abnormality because the testis then lies free within its tunic and can rotate on its spermatic cord, causing ischemia. This type of torsion is rare in the newborn, occurring for the most part in pubertal boys.

Testis Tumors

The incidence of tumors of the testis peaks in infancy and again in early adulthood. In infants, two types of germinal cell tumors

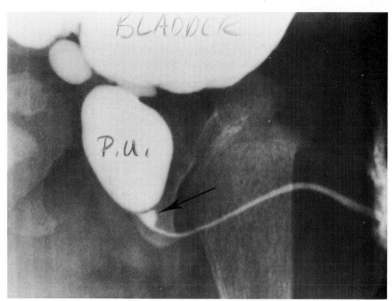

Fig. 35-29. Voiding cystourethrogram in newborn male
with posterior urethral valve
(arrow). Prostatic urethra **(PU)**
dilated and bladder trabecu-
lated with multiple diverticula
(upper left).

occur. The **orchioblastomas** (embryonal carcinoma) are malignant and must be treated
aggressively with radical orchiectomy and retroperitoneal node dissection. The use of postoperative chemotherapy in all is debatable
because some suggest that those with negative
retroperitoneal lymph nodes do not need additional treatment. This author's feeling is that
all should be treated with chemotherapy. **Teratomas,** on the other hand, are benign and
require excisional biopsy only. Both types of
tumors may be present at birth and both should
always be approached through an inguinal
incision to avoid scrotal contamination if a
malignant tumor is found.

URINARY TRACT INFECTION

There is a sex reversal in the incidence of
bacteriuria in the newborn. The overall incidence of neonatal urinary infection has been
recorded as 1.4 to 5.0 per 1000 live births. The
males:female ratio has been cited as 2.8:1 to
5:1.[19,34,35] The explanation for this reversed
sex ratio remains unclear, although it has been
reliably documented and is even more apparent in low-birth-weight and premature
newborns.[36,37]
Newborn males have a higher incidence of
sepsis than newborn females, in approximately
the same ratio as that for bacteriuria.[38] The
source of the bacteriuria in this age group is
thought to be primarily hematogenous and not
ascending from the urethra.[39]
Although the mature kidney prevents the
filtration of bacteria from blood into urine,[39]
it would appear that in newborns, and particularly in prematures, circulating bacteria may
indeed enter the urine by filtration. One group
feels that this is substantiated by the recent
observation that in late-onset neonatal sepsis
(>72 hours of age), bacteriuria without bacteremia is common; whereas, in the early-
onset group (<72 hours of age), bacteremia
without bacteriuria was more frequently
seen.[40] Time had not allowed bacteria to enter
the urinary tract in the early-onset group.
There is strong evidence to support the
necessity for radiographic evaluation in newborns with culture documented, significant
bacteriura (>10⁵). Vesicoureteral reflux has
been noted in about half of those *appropriately*
evaluated.[19,35] Additionally, significant obstructive uropathy must be recognized at an
early date to minimize renal damage and maximize the potential for functional return.
Evaluation includes visualization of renal
excretory ability which, in the newborn, is
best achieved by radioisotope. Excretory urography is often difficult to interpret because of
poor renal concentrating ability and excessive
bowel gas in neonates (Fig. 35-30). One of
these studies should be performed as soon as
infection is controlled.

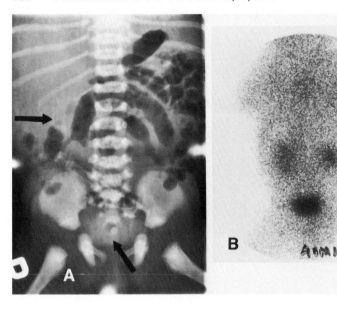

Fig. 35-30. A. Excretory urogram in newborn. Right kidney barely concentrates contrast **(arrow)** with no evidence of left kidney. Contrast apparent in bladder **(arrow). B.** Isotope renal scan the next day demonstrates presence and function of two kidneys. Child was ultimately normal.

No evaluation is complete in boys or girls with a history of bacteriuria until a voiding cystogram is performed. In boys, visualization of the urethra is imperative as a part of this study to rule out posterior urethral valves (see above). Cystography in boys and girls should be done awake with catheterization by use of a small (5F) feeding tube. Anesthesia is not necessary and may even be contraindicated. Identification of those with vesicoureteral reflux at an early age is extremely advantageous. It is then possible to prevent recurrent urinary infection and the potential for pyelonephritis by maintaining these children on long-term suppressive antibacterial prophylaxis (see above).

Urologic Management of the Newborn With Myelodysplasia

The child born with myelodysplasia is almost assured of having urinary bladder involvement. In the newborn period, this may be of no consequence unless the bladder becomes distended and overflow incontinence results. Untreated, this may lead to hydroureteromephrosis, urinary infection, or both. In the majority, suprapubic bladder expression (Credé maneuver) is successful in periodically emptying a bladder temporarily flaccid from spinal shock. Spontaneous emptying will be regained in the majority.

Rarely in a newborn, bladder emptying does not occur even with suprapubic expression. The current means of management to achieve bladder emptying in children and infants with neurogenic disease is clean intermittent catheterization.[41] This can be performed in both infant males and females on a regular basis using 5 to 8F feeding tubes.

All children with myelodysplasia should have a baseline evaluation of renal presence and function. A renal scan (or excretory urogram) before hospital discharge with arrangements for periodic follow-up is mandatory. Urine culture should be carried out every 3 months and repeat radiographic evaluation at 6 to 12 months.

REFERENCES

1. **Campbell MF:** Anomalies of the kidney. Urology, 2nd ed. W.B. Saunders, Philadelphia, 1964
2. **Longo VJ, Thompson GJ:** Congenital solitary kidney. J Urol 68:63, 1952
3. **Emanuel B, Nachman R, Aronson N, et al:** Congenital solitary kidney: A review of 74 cases. Am J Dis Child 127:17, 1974
4. **Belman AB, King LR:** Urinary tract abnormalities associated with imperforate anus. J Urol 108:823, 1972
5. **Malek RS, Kelalis PP, Burke EC:** Ectopic kidney in children and frequency of association of other abnormalities Mayo Clin Proc 46:461, 1971

6. **Bernstein J, Gardner KD:** Cystic disease of the kidney and renal dysplasia. In Harrison JH, Gittes RF, Perlmutter AD, Stamey TA, Walsh PC: Campbell's Urology, 4th ed. WB Saunders, Philadelphia, 1979

7. **Kaplan GW:** Abdominal masses. In Kelalis PP, King LR, Belman AB (eds): Clinical Pediatric Urology. WB Saunders, Philadelphia, 1976

8. **Bloom DA, Brosman S:** The multicystic kidney. J Urol 120:211, 1978

9. **Filmer RB, Taxy JB:** Cysts of the kidney, renal dysplasia and renal hypoplasia. In Kelalis PP, King LR, Belman AB: Clinical Pediatric Urology. Saunders, Philadelphia, 1976

10. **Govan DE, Donaldson SS, Wilbur J:** Pediatric oncology. JH Harrison et al: Campbell's Urology, 4th ed. WB Saunders, Philadelphia, 1979

11. **Belman AB:** Vascular and related disorders. In Kelalis PP, King LR, Belman AB (eds): Clinical Pediatric Urology. Saunders, Philadelphia, 1976

12. **Ambrose SS, Nicholson WP:** Ureteral reflux into duplicated ureters. J Urol 92:439, 1964

13. **Lich R, Howerton LW, Goode LS, Davis LA:** The ureterovesical junction in the newborn. J Urol 92:436, 1964

14. **Peters PC, Johnson DE, Jackson JH:** The incidence of vesicoureteral reflux in the premature child. J Urol 97:259, 1967

15. **Booth EJ, Bell TE, McLain C, Evans AT:** Fetal vesicoureteral reflux. J Urol 113:258, 1975

16. **Roberts JA, Riopelle AJ:** Vesicoureteral reflux and the primate, II. Maturation of the ureterovesical junction. Pediatrics 59:566, 1977

17. **Burger RH, Burger SE:** Genetic determinants of urologic disease. Urol Clin North Am 1: 419, 1974

18. **Dwoskin JY:** Sibling uropathology. J Urol 115: 726, 1976

19. **Drew JH, Acton CM:** Radiologic findings in newborn infants with urinary infection. Arch Dis Child 51:628, 1976

20. **Ransley PB, Risdon RA:** Reflux and renal scarring. Br J Radiol (Suppl.) 14: 1978

21. **Jeffs RD:** Exstrophy and cloacal exstrophy. Urol Clin North Am 5:127, 1978

22. **Wilson JD, Walsh PC:** Disorders of sexual differentiation. In Harrison JH et al (eds): WB Saunders, Philadelphia, 1979

23. **Feldman KW, Smith DW:** Fetal phallic growth and penile standards for newborn male infants. J Pediatr 86:395, 1975

24. **Klugo RC, Cerny JC:** Response of micropenis to topical testosterone and gonadotropin. J Urol 119:667, 1978

25. **Øster J:** Further fate of the foreskin. Arch Dis Child 43:200, 1968

26. **Gee WF, Ansell JS:** Neonatal circumcision: A ten year review. Pediatrics 58:824, 1976

27. **Bauer SB, Bull MJ, Retik AB:** Hypospadias: A familial study. J Urol 121:474, 1979

28. Editorial: Genetics of hypospadias. Br Med J 4:189, 1972

29. **Felton CM:** Should intravenous pyelography be a routine procedure for children with cryptorchidism or hypospadias? J Urol 81:335, 1959

30. **Johnston JH:** Epispadias. In Harrison JH, et al (eds): Campbell's Urology, 4th ed. WB Saunders, Philadelphia, 1979

31. **Belman AB:** The repair of a congenital H-type urethrorectal fistula using a scrotal flap urethroplasty. J Urol 118:659, 1977

32. **Kaplan GW:** Obstructive uropathy: The posterior urethra. In Kelalis PP, King LR, Belman AB (eds): Clinical Pediatric Urology. WB Saunders, Philadelphia, 1976

33. **Lewy PR:** Renal function and renal failure. Ibid. In Kelalis PP, King LR, Belman AB (eds): Clinical Pediatric Urology. WB Saunders, Philadelphia, 1976

34. **Bergstrom T, Larson K, Winberg J:** Studies of urinary tract infections in infancy and childhood. J Pediatr 80:585, 1972

35. **Maherzi M, Guignard J-P, Torrado A:** Urinary tract infection in high-risk newborn infants. Pediatr 62:521, 1979

36. **Thrupp LD, Hodgman JE, Karelitz M, et al:** Transurethral reflux during cleansing procedure for clean voided urine specimens in low birth weight infants. J Pediatr 82:1057, 1973

37. **Edelmann CM, Jr, Ogwo JE, Fine BP, et al:** The prevalence of bacteriuria in full term and premature newborn infants. J Pediatr 8:125, 1973

38. **Beutow KC, Klein SW, Lane RB:** Septicemia in premature infants. Am J Dis Child 110:29, 1965

39. **Stamey TA:** Urinary infections, pp 1, 130. Williams and Wilkins, Baltimore, 1972

40. **Visser VE, Hall RT:** Urine culture in the evaluation of suspected neonatal sepsis. J Pediatr 94:635, 1979

41. Action Committee on Myelodysplasia, Section on Urology, Am Acad Pediatr: Current approaches to evaluation and management of children with myelomenigocele. Pediatr 63: 663, 1979

36

Neoplasia in the Neonate and the Young Infant

Jeffrey G. Rosenstock and
Audrey E. Evans

Tumors or masses are relatively common in the neonatal period but are rarely malignant. It is difficult to determine the exact incidence of cancer in childhood because most statistics are derived from death certificates. The annual death rate is 7 per 100,000 in children up to 15 years of age with the peak at 4 years of age; the incidence is probably 9 per 100,000. Fraumeni and Miller reviewed the death certificates for all children dying from cancer within the first 28 days of life in the United States from 1960 to 1964.[1] There were 130 certificates representing 0.6% of all childhood cancer deaths; 86 of these deaths were caused by solid tumors and 44 by leukemia (Tables 36-1 and 36-2). Because these figures represent only those who died within the first month of life, the true incidence is considerably higher. Not only do certain neoplasms, such as teratomas, present more commonly during the neonatal period, but they often have a natural history different from that in the rest of childhood. Some tumors, neuroblastoma for example, have a much better prognosis if present at birth, while others, such as leukemia, are much more resistant to treatment. The reader

This work was supported in part by Grants Nos. CA08147 and RR 05506-0 from the U.S. Public Health Service.

interested in age as a prognostic factor is referred to the various discussions by Wells,[2] Bollande,[3] and Smithers.[4] Awareness of this age difference is important in the selection of treatment because the very young infant may be more at risk from the deleterious effects of chemicals and radiotherapy, although remarkably able to tolerate major surgical manipulation. In some cases, the prognosis is excellent if proper treatment is instituted; therefore, early diagnosis is essential and a feeling of hopelessness is not warranted.

Differential Diagnosis [5,6]

As stated previously, the likelihood of encountering a malignant disease in the neonatal period is very small. There is no valuable routine screening test for making or excluding the diagnosis of cancer, and probably it is most helpful to remember that the possibility exists when confronted with the acutely ill neonate. The detailed differential diagnosis of cancer is included in the various chapters dealing with the different organ systems. There are one or two syndromes, seen at birth or shortly thereafter, that are the result of malignant disease. Although the child with anemia, hepatosplenomegaly, and bleeding manifestations is much more likely to have a blood group incompatibility or to have been exposed to an intrauterine infection, both true leukemia and pseudoleukemia in infants with trisomy 21 are seen. Massive enlargement of the liver, accompanied by subcutaneous nodlues can result from metastatic neuroblastoma. A large abdominal mass is usually the result of congenital malformation of the gastrointestinal or urogenital systems, but it can on occasion be caused by a retroperitoneal teratoma, neuroblastoma, or Wilms' tumor. Infants with congenital defects have a higher incidence of renal neoplasms.

Diagnostic Workup[7,8]

The diagnostic studies to determine the nature of a hematologic disorder or a mass lesion are no different in the neonatal period from later in childhood. Ultrasound is a good noninvasive technique to separate cystic from noncystic lesions. Also the umbilical vessels serve as easy access for angiographic studies. They are given in more detail under the headings of the individual tumors. The routine x-ray studies, including an IVP for abdominal mass, should also include a chest film and a skeletal survey to look for the presence of metastases. The blood count should include a platelet estimation because occasionally benign and malignant tumors, particularly in the liver, may trap platelets and lead to secondary thrombocytopenia. A bone marrow aspiration can sometimes be helpful in making the diagnosis of leukemia or metastatic neuroblastoma;

Table 36-1. Mortality from Malignant Neoplasms in the United States Under 5 Years as Compared with Under 28 Days of Age, 1960 to 1964.

Neoplasms	No. Deaths Under 5 Years	Deaths Under 28 Days		
		No.	Rate Per 10^6 Live Births	%*
Leukemia	4592	44	2.11	1.0
Neuroblastoma	1049	29	1.30	2.5
Brain tumor	1035	7	0.34	0.7
Wilms' tumor	696	9	0.43	1.3
Liver cancer, primary	196	10	0.48	5.1
Teratoma	111	9	0.43	8.1
Sarcoma, type specified	1940	12	0.58	1.2
Other		12	0.58	
TOTAL	9619	130	6.24	1.4

* Percent of neonatal deaths among type-specific cancers under 5 years of age (*e.g.*, for leukemia = $(44 \times 100)/4592 = 1.0$).

(From Fraumeni, JF, Miller RW.: Amer J Dis Child 117:186, 1969) [1]

other solid tumors are not usually seen in the bone marrow aspirates unless there is x-ray evidence of bone metastases. The catecholemines in the urine will be markely elevated in the majority of infants with neuroblastoma.

Table 36-2. Deaths from Neonatal Cancer According to Specific Diagnosis, Age, and Sex.

Neoplasms	Age			Sex	
	24 hours	1 to 6 days	1 to 4 weeks	Male	Female
Leukemia	10	9	25	21	23
Neuroblastoma	13	2	12	15	12
Sarcoma	7	1	4	7	5
Liver cancer, primary	4	3	3	6	4
Wilms' tumor	1	6	2	6	3
Teratoma	7	1	1	4	5
Brain tumor	3	1	3	4	3
Other	6	5	1	4	8
TOTAL	51	28	51	67	63

(Fraumeni, Miller) [1]

NEOPLASMS

Teratomas [9,10,11,12,13]

Teratomas are developmental masses, often diagnosed at birth, approximately 50% being diagnosed during the first month of life. Willis defines teratomas as being true tumors or neoplasms, composed of multiple tissues of kinds foreign to the part in which they arise.[11] Greater than 50% of all teratomas are sacrococcygeal. Overall, only about 10% are malignant and these are predominantly in the sacrococcygeal region. They can occur anywhere in the body, but most frequently are seen in the midline or arise in germinal tissues such as testis and ovary.

Teratomas are usually large, averaging 8 cm in diameter, can be cystic or solid, and frequently contain both cystic and solid areas. The solid tissues are often a mixture of mature, well-developed tissues that resemble their normal homologous counterparts and immature areas showing various stages of embryonic development. The mature solid areas contain all three germinal layers in which the most commonly identified tissues are skin, skin appendages, fat, smooth muscle, glial tissue, cartilage, and bone. Greater than one-third of these tumors contain calcium identifiable by x-ray film. Tumors that are predominantly cystic are only rarely malignant, while those that are predominantly solid have a greater than 75% chance of being malignant. Such tumors show frankly neoplastic tissue that has an embryonal adenocarcinomatous appearance. This has been called the endodermal sinus pattern or *yolk sac tumor.* Because of the variability from one area to another in such large tumors, it is important that numerous sections be examined.

Much has been noted about the marked female predominance of teratomas, but this is only true for sacrococcygeal teratomas. Congenital anomalies have been noted in association with teratomas such as spina bifida, hemihypertrophy, imperforate anus, meningomyelocele, and cardiac defects. The etiology of these tumors has caused a great deal of speculation. In the past, they were felt to represent incomplete twinning resulting from the frequent formation of mature tissues that are at sites distant from the homologous tissue. Presently, the general consensus is that these tumors represent germinal tissues that migrated incorrectly and grew without normal control of embryologic development.

Sacrococcygeal Teratomas.[14-20] Sacrococcygeal teratomas have an incidence of approximately 1 per 40,000 births and are most frequently noted at birth. Seventy-five percent occur in females. They usually present as large cystic, well-encapsulated, lobulated tumors protruding externally from the coccyx. There is frequently an associated large intrapelvic extension or the tumor may be totally intrapelvic.

The infant with a large cystic external sacrococcygeal mass rarely presents a major problem of differential diagnosis. Pressure on a meningomyelocele usually causes bulging of the anterior fontanelle, and vertebral roentgenograms may show defects associated with meningomyeloceles. An intrapelvic teratoma needs to be differentiated from other pelvic masses such as dermoid cysts, anterior meningomyeloceles, lipomas, angiomas and duplications of the rectum. Because a mass in the buttock can be mistaken for an abscess, a complete workup should be performed before any surgical measures are undertaken because the lesion could be malignant. Solid, intrapelvic teratomas occur more frequently in males than in females, are often diagnosed some time after birth, and have a high incidence of malignancy. Histologic subtypes also relate to prognosis. They frequently cause bowel or bladder dysfunction or show evidence of venous or lymphatic obstruction—all signs that are highly suggestive of malignancy.

The burden of treatment rests upon the surgeon, and removal should be as complete as possible. The coccyx, which is the origin of the tumor, should also be removed because failure to do so leads to a significant recurrence rate, the majority of the recurrences being malignant. Simple but total removal of benign teratomas is adequate therapy. The results with malignant lesions are very poor, with only a few survivors reported. Teratomas are considered to be relatively radioresistant, but in the face of an incomplete resection radiation should be employed with a dose not more than 2000 rads in combination with chemotherapy. Hopefully, such combined treatment will make the primary lesion more sensitive to radiation and growth of any distant metastases which have already occurred may be suppressed. Agents such as actinomycin D, cyclophosphamide, and vincristine have been used in this manner with some benefit. Because all chemotherapy has its unfortunate side effects, and the infant's bone marrow is particularly sensitive, these agents should be given only by pediatric chemotherapists experienced in their use.

Ovarian Teratomas. Mass lesions of the ovaries are very rarely identified during the early neonatal period.[21-25] Marshall, in his thorough review of ovarian teratomas in 1965, found reports of only 23 during the first month of life.[24] At the Children's Hospital of Philadelphia between 1947 and 1961, 25 ovarian masses were diagnosed, and 3 of these were seen during the neonatal period. In contrast to those seen later in childhood, these early lesions are rarely malignant. The lesions are usually identified as a mass in the abdomen during routine palpation and rarely cause any symptoms. Signs of endocrine dysfunction, such as pseudohermaphroditism, which often accompanies a granulosa cell tumor, are extremely rare.

The treatment of these tumors is surgical removal and the opposite ovary should be examined because the lesion is bilateral in 10% of cases.

Testicular Teratomas.[26] Testicular tumors are also rare in the neonatal period. They present in infancy as a painless, scrotal swelling, upward of 25% having an associated hydrocele that will transilluminate. A significant number will be malignant, with the embryonal cell carcinoma being the most frequent malignant variant. Benign teratoma should be treated by simple orchiectomy. Malignant tumors are dealt with in greater detail below.

Teratomas in Other Sites.[27-36] Although teratomas usually occur in the midline or in organs containing germinal tissue, they can sometimes develop in other areas, presumably resulting from a developmental abnormality. Lesions are seen in the nasopharynx, the face, and in the parotid region. Gifford described five cases of teratoma of the face, all presenting at birth, with large lesions extending from the ear to the chin.[27] Of the five lesions, four transilluminated light and two showed calcification on x-ray film. Though all were histologically benign at the initial surgery, two had local recurrence of a malignant tumor and both died. During the neonatal period, teratomas are occasionally seen as masses markedly distorting the orbit with the lids stretched over the mass. They do not have intracranial extensions in contrast to the base of the skull. Total surgical excision is required, for these orbital teratomas can recur locally. Cervical teratomas usually present as nontender cervical masses that displace the trachea laterally, often causing airway obstruction. These lesions may cause severe respiratory distress at birth and may be responsible for stillbirths. Attempts at tracheostomy may be fatal because of the distorted anatomy. More than 50% of these lesions have calcium identifiable by roentenograms, and this is helpful in the differential diagnosis.

Teratomas of the pericardium can occur during infancy, producing cardiac effusion with tamponade. The neonatal lesions are usually benign, in contrast to the myocardial rhabdomyosarcoma that is occasionally seen during childhood. Unfortunately, the diagnosis during the neonatal period is rarely made prior to surgery or postmortem examination. Examination of the pericardial effusion should include cytology that may be suggestive of the presence of a teratoma. Total surgical removal is often feasible and appears to be curative. Lesions of the anterior mediastinum are usually benign but may be so large as to cause respiratory difficulty.

Renal Neoplasms

Renal masses seen during the neonatal period are almost always caused by congenital malformations such as hydronephrosis and cysts.[37-47] True malignant tumors are very rare. The "malignant" renal tumor seen during early infancy is usually the more benign variant of a Wilms' tumor, the mesoblastic nephroma. Such a lesion can be quite large and has been seen even in premature infants at the time of birth. It has been stated that the prognosis for Wilms' tumor in infancy is excellent, but in retrospect it is difficult to determine the exact influence of age as an independent prognostic factor because it is likely that some lesions previously reported as Wilms' tumor may have been mesoblastic nephromas, which are essentially benign (though rare recurrences have been reported). However, Wilms' tumor does occur, even though rarely, during the neonatal period. Though such children have been known to die of metastatic disease, the proportion of infants who have localized disease is high; thus, the overall prognosis is excellent.

The diagnosis of an intrarenal neoplasm is made on the basis of an intravenous urogram. This is best done by an injection in the foot, so that a simultaneous inferior vena cavagram is obtained. Treatment of a mesoblastic nephroma is simple surgical resection and no other measures appear necessary. For a classic Wilms' tumor, treatment depends on the stage and the histology of the disease when first diagnosed. Patients with totally encapsulated lesions which are removed do not need postoperative radiation. Chemotherapy is indicated to eliminate microscopic metastases. Recent results from the National Wilms' Tumor Study show that chemotherapy with two agents, actinomycin D and vincristine, given for only 6 months will produce survival in 90% of all such patients. In those cases in which resection was incomplete, or the paraaortic lymph nodes contained tumor, postoperative irradiation combined with actinomycin D and vincristine should be employed. It is customary for some radiation therapists, experienced in the treatment of malignant disease in children, to give reduced doses of radiation therapy to the very young because such doses appear adequate for eradication of local disease and are less damaging for the bone and soft tissue. In the rare case of the infant who has metastases when first diagnosed, treatment with actinomycin D and vincristine, and x-ray therapy to both the renal fossa and metastatic lesions is likely to be successful in curing the patient. There are several anomalies, both hereditary and sporadic, associated with Wilms' tumor. In one report, over 25% of all children with severe sporadic aniridia developed Wilms' tumors. With such a close association, all infants with severe sporadic aniridia should be followed prospectively and systematically in order to diagnose the tumor at the earliest possible time.

Neuroblastoma

Neuroblastoma is the commonest congenital malignant tumor identified during the neonatal period.[48-53] In the review of congenital malignant neoplasms by Wells in 1940, one-quarter of the 150 patients reported had neuroblastoma.[2] If it presents at birth or soon thereafter, the signs are usually those of an abdominal mass, resulting from the primary tumor or massive hepatomegaly, or multiple skin nodules with an abdominal primary that may not be palpable. Rarely is there evidence of hemorrhage resulting from thrombocytopenia secondary to trapping of platelets in a liver heavily infiltrated with metastatic disease or decreased production caused by bone marrow involvement. A review of 234 patients with neuroblastoma seen at the Children's Hospital of Philadelphia and in the participating institutions in Children's Cancer Study Group A determined that 29% were diagnosed during the first year of life and slightly more than half of this number were metastatic when first seen. The pattern of disease spread which occurred most frequently in the infants diagnosed in the first months of life, was a small primary tumor in the adrenal and metastatic disease to the liver or skin. It appears likely that neuroblastoma is present at birth in the majority of children with the disease, but it must grow to a significant size before symptoms or signs bring it to the attention of the physician. The median age at diagnosis of neuroblastoma is 2 years.

The diagnosis in the neonatal period is relatively easy once the possibility is included in the differential. During early infancy, the primary tumor is usually in the abdomen and can be detected by an IVP. Not infrequently, patients with massive hepatic involvement have no detectable primary tumor. Catecholamines are almost always elevated in the urine, and a VMA spot test is useful in making a rapid diagnosis. Quantitive measurement of the catecholamines should be performed. The diagnosis should be confirmed by biopsy of the primary or metastatic lesions. In the patient with metastases, elevation of the urinary catecholamines, together with tumor cell clusters in the bone marrow, are sufficient to make a definite diagnosis.

With neuroblastoma there is a strong influence of age upon survival. This fact should be kept in mind when determining the amount of treatment necessary. There is no place for heroic surgical or radiotherapeutic measures in the management of the infant with neuroblastoma. If the disease is localized, surgical resection as complete as possible is indicated; a small amount of irradiation may be given if gross tumor is left behind. The prognosis for children with localized neuroblastoma in the neonatal period is excellent, with almost 90% survival including numerous patients who, by most criteria of "good cancer therapy," received very inadequate treatment. In the review of 234 patients, the infants with metastatic disease involving liver, skin, and marrow, but without evidence of bone involvement (Stage IVS), did as well as those children with localized disease (Stage I). In fact, only 2 in 20 infants with this Stage IVS pattern of spread expired during the first year of life, and apparently the death of these 2 infants was related to chemotherapy and infection. It is in this group of patients, particularly in those with disease of the skin, where spontaneous regression of neuroblastoma has been seen. Although for children with metastatic disease in the liver some pediatric oncologists would recommend an attenuated course of radiation therapy to the liver followed by chemotherapy, it should be remembered that infants are very sensitive to both modalities and such treatment should be employed very cautiously. Once regression of discernable disease is initiated, one can be confident that it will continue and most likely lead to long-term survival.

Children with metastases to bone do not have as good a prognosis as those whose metastases are in skin and liver, and such children do require more aggressive chemotherapy. However, their chance of survival is better than the older child with bone metastases from neuroblastoma, so that aggressive treatment is indicated. Unless the disease is very widespread, about one-fourth of these infants can be retrieved. Several chemotherapeutic agents, used alone or in combination, have caused regression of neuroblastoma. Vincristine, imidazole carboxamide (DTIC), and cyclophosphamide have produced remissions of several months to, occasionally, years. Nitrogen mustard, once commonly used, has more recently been supplanted by cyclophosphamide. The antibiotics daunomycin and adriamycin have also been found to be effective. If patients survive free of disease for 2 years, they are, in all probability, cured.

One other interesting aspect of neuroblastoma should be mentioned. Beckwith and Perrin reported an autopsy study of infants who died of disease unrelated to neuroblastoma.[48] They found an increased incidence of neuroblastoma *in situ* that was approximately 40 to 50 times the expected rate. This suggests that neuroblastoma, at least in microscopic amounts, may be quite common but regresses spontaneously.

Hepatoblastoma[54–63]

Primary malignant neoplasms of the liver occur rarely in neonates. Hepatomegaly resulting from malignant disease is more likely to occur from neuroblastoma or leukemia. However, it can be seen from Table 36-1 that primary liver tumors do form 8% of the cancer fatalities in the first month of life (10 in 130).[1] They are seen in association with certain congenital malformations such as hemihypertrophy and extensive hemangiomata. Histologically, hepatic tumors can be divided into the infantile type, hepatoblastoma, rarely seen after 2 years of age, and the adult type, hepatocellular carcinoma, rarely seen before the age of 5 years. Hepatoblastoma is two to three times more common in males and occurs rarely in Blacks.

The most frequently presenting sign is asymptomatic abdominal enlargement. Poor appetite, failure to gain weight, and pallor are common. While jaundice is rarely seen, evidence of bleeding in the skin or abdominal cavity may be present because of platelet trapping and secondary thrombocytopenia. Precocious puberty has been reported in males, the youngest reported being 1 year of age. X-ray films of the abdomen will demonstrate an enlarged liver, sometimes with areas of calcification and displacement of the abdominal contents. A hepatic angiogram and a liver scan are important in determining the type and degree of liver involvement. Such investigations may define a large hemangioma or, in the case of a malignant lesion, determine its resectability. Liver function tests are usually normal, and a serum α-fetoprotein is likely to be high. The child with precocious puberty will have elevated levels of ketosteroids and chorionic gonadotropins.

The diagnosis should be confirmed by open biopsy. A needle biopsy is not indicated because of the danger of hemorrhage from a hemangioma. Extensive preparations should be made before surgery so that partial hepatectomy can be performed if the tumor is localized to one lobe of the liver. Resection is the only method of cure currently practiced. If primary resection is not feasible, irradiation combined with chemotherapy may make a previously inoperable lesion resectable. Such was the experience recently at this institution. The tumor in an 11-month-old infant responded to 2000 rads, combined with actinomycin D, vincristine, and cyclophosphamide. Complete resection was possible 3 months after the initiation of treatment. In patients with tumors too extensive for resection, radiotherapy and chemotherapy may cause temporary response. There is no chemical agent or combination of agents that has produced consistent results in hepatoblastoma. Any of those drugs currently used for sarcomas in childhood can be tried. During a period of whole liver irradiation, a careful watch should be kept on liver enzymes and the platelet count in anticipation of radiation hepatitis.

Retinoblastoma[64-69]

Retinoblastoma, the commonest eye tumor of childhood, is also the most common congenital ocular neoplasm. There are slightly over 100 new cases diagnosed per year in the United States. Because more cured persons now reach their reproductive years, this genetically transmitted malignancy will be seen in increasing numbers. The present frequency is 1 in 17,000 to 34,000 new births. The genetics of retinoblastoma have only recently been fully understood. There seems to be a high rate of spontaneous mutation, since only 4% of new cases seen at the Institute of Ophthalmology, Columbia Prebsyterian Hospital, have a family history of retinoblastoma. In families with a positive history, the penetrance of this dominant gene is variable. Offspring of affected parents with bilateral disease have a very high rate of penetrance approaching 100%; those of a parent with unilateral involvement have a 50% or lower manifestation of the gene in their offspring. Therefore, their children will have less than 25% chance of being affected. The carrier state seems to occur because occasionally more than one child of phenotypically normal parents may be affected. The risk of a child of phenotypically normal parents developing retinoblastoma where a sibling has the disease is estimated to be 4%.

Though this is a congenital tumor, the median age at diagnosis is 18 months. The physician caring for the child of an affected parent or with an affected sibling should carefully and regularly examine the retina, under general anesthesia if possible, to make the diagnosis early. In this manner cases can be detected in the first few months of life. The typical signs are (1) a white or "cat's eye" reflex, (2) strabismus, and (3) unilateral dilated pupil.

The lesion frequently arises in the region of the ora serrata, making visualization through the undilated pupil in the infant extremely difficult. Use of mydriatics and general anesthesia is mandatory in order to confirm the diagnosis. Approximately 30% of cases are bilateral at presentation, increasing the morbidity and mortality. Calcification occurs in approximately 75% of the cases, which can be appreciated roentgenographically. Ellsworth[64] and Reese have developed a system for staging the tumors according to size, position, and presence of vitreous seeding, all of which have prognostic value. The overall mortality rate is less than 20%, even though almost one-third of the patients present with bilateral disease.

In general, the treatment for unilateral disease, after full examination of the uninvolved eye, is enucleation. If a child with a positive family history is diagnosed very early, radiotherapy might be employed to preserve the eye. In the presence of bilateral disease, it is customary to remove the more seriously involved eye and treat the other with irradiation. Intracarotid triethylenemelamine was formerly used for patients with more extensive disease. The data are difficult to interpret. More recently, adjuvant chemotherapy is being tried in prospective trials in children with a high likelihood of developing metastatic disease. If the second eye is so involved that useful vision cannot be expected, enucleation is recommended. Distant metastases occur in approximately 15% of patients. They respond to the same agents used for neuroblastoma.

Early diagnosis through frequent examination of patients with a family history of retinoblastoma, full examination of infants and children with signs of retinal disease, and genetic counseling of adults who are cured of their disease, are the best means for decreasing the incidence, mortality, and morbidity of this congenital tumor.

Rare Miscellaneous Tumors[70-89]

Although **brain tumors** account for 5% of neonatal deaths (see Table 36-1), they are seldom diagnosed antemortem. These tumors cause a rapidly enlarging head, the speed of growth being much greater than that seen with congenital hydrocephalus. Vomiting is not common because of the ability of the head to expand. Approximately 50% of the reported cases have been teratomas. Survival with normal intellect and motor ability can occur.

Soft tissue sarcomas are usually of muscle or fibrous tissue origin and tend to be undifferentiated. Rhabdomyosarcomas can occur at any site and are particularly associated with the pelvic organs and testicles. They are best treated surgically, but since the advent of effective chemotherapy, multilating resection is no longer necessary. The lymph node drainage area should be explored. Incomplete resection should be followed by radiotherapy, but if the primary tumor arises in an organ such as the uterus or bladder and the margins of excision are clear, probably the benefits of irradiation are outweighed by the damage caused in the young infant. It has been shown that multiagent chemotherapy with actinomycin D and vincristine decreases the metastatic rate of rhabdomyosarcoma and should be administered even though the lymph nodes are normal. In the neonate, some of these tumors appear to be of neurogenous origin or to have neurogenous elements.

Fibrosarcomas have rarely been reported in the neonatal period, and without multiple histologic sections they are difficult to distinguish from the fibromatoses. Kauffman and Stout [82] report 3 in 23 patients with juvenile fibrosarcoma occurring at birth.[82] When encountered, they are often large and amputation is the only possible surgical procedure. An interesting variant of fibrosarcoma seen in infancy occurs on the medial aspect of the digits, sometimes on two contiguous surfaces.

Leukemia [90–97]

True congenital leukemia is extremely rare and usually rapidly fatal. The differential diagnosis in the newborn period should include all those diseases that cause anemia, thrombocytopenia, bleeding, and hepatosplenomegaly. Bluish skin infiltrates are also seen, the picture being similar to metastatic neuroblastoma. The white count is invariably elevated, often over 100,000/mm^3, the elevation usually being the result of circulating immature myeloid cells. It is important to differentiate true leukemia from a nonmalignant severe myeloid

proliferative disorder and also from the "pseudoleukemia" seen in infants with Down's syndrome, (trisomy 21). To fulfill the criteria of true neonatal leukemia, it is necessary to demonstrate leukemia infiltration of nonhemapoietic tissues such as skin or muscle. In the infant with anemia, thrombocytopenia, and a high white count, every effort should be made to rule out an infectious etiology causing a leukemoid reaction.

If indeed the patient appears to have acute leukemia, treatment is in order with agents such as prednisone, vincristine, 6-mercaptopurine and cytosine arabinoside. Full cytochemical, enzymatic, and antigenic evaluation of the cells is necessary to type the cells. Morphologic criteria alone are inadequate. Intensive supportive measures may be necessary because it is likely that such a child will succumb before antileukemic treatment can have any effect. Because the response rate to treatment is reported to be very poor in the neonatal period, such an infant is best under the care of an experienced pediatric hematologist. During the first few months of life, acute lymphocytic and monomyelocytic leukemia are rarely seen. Even with lymphocytic disease, the infant does not do as well as the slightly older child. The burden of disease is greater, with a high WBC and marked hepatosplenomegaly, and it is now becoming clear that the prognosis for long-term survival of children with lymphocytic leukemia depends a great deal on the clinical status of the disease when first treated.

The infant with trisomy 21 with pseudoleukemia requires no treatment because this is a self-limiting disease. Treatment of the child with a leukemoid reaction is that of the underlying infection. Supportive care should also be used here and platelets should be given to the thrombocytopenic patient with evidence of bleeding.

A problem that occasionally faces the neonatologist or pediatrician is the risk to the fetus from a mother who has leukemia. Many cases of pregnancy and leukemia have been reported in the literature, of which only one infant has had leukemia at birth. The factors that seem to be most important to the newborn of a mother with leukemia is her general state of health, the specific drugs taken to treat the disease and the desires of the parents. Apparently, women with leukemia rarely conceive, either because of drug-induced sterility, loss of libido from ill health, or family planning. In most cases of leukemia diagnosed early in pregnancy, therapeutic abortion is elected because of the potential teratogenic effects of many of the chemotherapeutic agents. Leukemia diagnosed later in pregnancy can cause problems for the newborn such as prematurity, intrauterine growth retardation, and drug effects (*e.g.*, adrenal suppression from steroids). These problems are self-limiting, if the infant can be properly supported.

Histiocytosis X [98–103]

The term histocytosis X is applied to a spectrum of clinical entities often broken into eosinophilic granuloma of bone and the Letterer–Siwe and Hand–Schuller–Christian syndromes. Whether these three clinical entities are related pathologically and etiologically remains open to speculation.

Eosinophilic granuloma, with its limited bone involvement, is rarely diagnosed during infancy and, overall, has an excellent prognosis no matter how treated. The more extensive forms of these diseases, included under the term histiocytosis X, though rarely diagnosed at birth, are often seen during the first year of life. Over 20% of the cases occur during the first 6 months of life, and another 20% during the second half of the first year. The disease has no sex or racial predilection. Though histiocytosis is extremely rare, leading to a probability of death by 3 years of age, of about 3.6 per 1,000,000, there have been several reports of multiple cases within siblings. A death certificate study of the 270 deaths attributed to Letterer–Siwe disease in the United States from 1960 to 1964, revealed five pairs of siblings, including one set of twins.[99] This suggests that the risk of a sibling's developing the disease is estimated to be 1400 times normal. This is a much higher risk than in any other childhood malignancy, except possibly retinoblastoma.

The clinical picture during infancy is usually a multisystem disease with involvement of skin, liver, spleen, lungs, bone marrow, and lymph nodes. Recurrent fever is common. The natural course of this disease is variable. In some children, there is a rapidly progressive course while others have a much slower progression, or a spontaneous remission. The diagnosis must be confirmed by biopsy of an involved organ, preferably not skin or bone marrow because these areas are sometimes atypical.

Examination of the histologic material may help in differentiating benign from malignant histiocytes. The differentiation is important because those with benign lesions have a better prognosis. Evidence of organ dysfunction is also of value in predicting an unfavorable outcome. The age of the child affects the course of the disease, the younger infants doing less well.

Therapy of generalized histiocytosis should be based upon the number of "systems" involved, evidence of organ dysfunction, and the histologic appearance. Obviously, the same treatment is not indicated for the child with seborrhea and running ears as for the one with hepatosplenomegaly and dyspnea from pulmonary disease. Some physicians leave the child with asymptomatic disease untreated, while others recommend a short course of prednisone with methotrexate or 6-mercaptopurine. The more seriously affected child should probably have more aggressive treatment because the death rate overall is 30% and even higher in those less than 6 months of age. Agents such as vincristine, vinblastine, prednisone, methotrexate, and 6-mercaptopurine have all been helpful in some cases. Because the disease is variable, it is difficult to determine which are the most effective regimens or the ideal duration of treatment.

REFERENCES

1. **Fraumeni JF, Jr, Miller RW:** Cancer deaths in the newborn. Amer J Dis Child, 117:186, 1969
2. **Wells HG:** Occurrence and significance of congenital neoplasms. Arch Pathol 30:535m 1940
3. **Bolande RP:** Benignity of neonatal tumors and concept of cancer repression in early life. Am J Dis Child 122:12, 1971
4. **Smithers DW:** Maturation in human tumors. Lancet 2:949, 1969
5. **Hope JW, Koop CE:** Differential diagnosis of mediastinal masses. Pediatr Clin N Am 6:379, 1959
6. **Griscom NT:** The roentgenology of neonatal abdominal masses. Am J Roentgen 93:447, 1965
7. **Melicow MM, Uson AC:** Palpable abdominal

masses in infants and children: A report based on a review of 653 cases. J Urol 81: 705, 1969

8. **Lara FR, Fernandez AG:** Aortografia transumbilical en el recien nacido con tumoracion abdominal. Bol Med Hosp Infant 35:1077, 1978

9. **Berry CL, Keeling J, Hilton C:** Teratoma in infancy and childhood: A review of 91 cases. J Pathol 98:241,1969

10. **Carney JA, Thompson DP, Johnson CL, Lynn HB:** Teratomas in children, clinical and pathologic aspects. J Pediatr Surg 7:271, 1972

11. **Chappell JS:** Teratomas in infancy and childhood. S Afr J Surg 8:77, 1970

12. **Willis RA:** The Borderland of Embryology and Pathology. Butterworth's, London, 1958

13. **Zimmerman FA, Stemp AF, Meister P:** Teratome in Kindesalter. Z Kinderchir 21:203, 1977

14. **Altman RP, Randolph JG, Lilly JR:** Sacrococcygeal Teratoma. American Academy of Pediatrics Surgical Section Survey—1973. J Ped Surg 9:389, 1974

15. **Dillard BM, Mayer JH, McAlister WH, McGavrin M, Strominger DB:** Sacrococcygeal teratoma in children. J Pediatr Surg 5: 53, 1970

16. **Donnellan WA, Swenson O:** Benign and malignant sacrococcygeal teratomas. Surgery 64:834, 1968

17. **Exelby PR:** Sacrococcygeal teratomas in children. CA 22:202, 1972

18. **Gonzalez-Crussi F, Winkler RF, Mirkin DL:** Sacrococcygeal Teratomas in Infants and Children. Arch Pathol Lab Med 102:420, 1978

19. **Mahour GH, Landing BH, Woolley MD:** Teratomas in Children: Clinicopathologic Studies in 133 Patients. Z Kinderchir 23:365, 1978

20. **Vaez-Zadeh K, Sieber WK, Sherman, FE, Kiesewetter WB:** Sacrococcygeal teratomas in children. J Pediatr Surg 7:152, 1972

21. **Carlson DH, Griscom NT:** Ovarian cysts in the newborn. Am J Roentgenol 116:664, 1972

22. **Hyman RA, VonMicsky LI, Finby N:** Ovarian teratoma in childhood. Am J Roentgenol 116: 673, 1972

23. **Kobayashi RH, Moore TC:** Ovarian teratomas in early childhood. J Pediatr Surg 13: 419, 1978

24. **Marshall JR:** Ovarian enlargements in the first year of life. Ann Surg 161:372, 1965

25. **Reis RL, Koop CE:** Ovarian tumors in infants and children. J Pediatr 60:96, 1962

26. **Colodny AH, Hopkins TB:** Testicular tumors in infants and children. Urol Clin North Am 4:347, 1977

27. **Gifford GH, Jr, MacCollum D:** Facial teratoma in the newborn. Plas Reconstr Surg 49: 616, 1972

28. **Bartholdson L, Johanson B, Mortensen K:** Congenital teratoma of the orbit. Scand J Plast Reconstr Surg 1:90, 1967

29. **Birt BD, Knight-Jones EB:** Respiratory distress due to nasopharyngeal hamartoma. Br Med J 3:281, 1969

30. **Casanovas R:** Congenital teratoma of the orbit. Arch Ophthalmol 77:795, 1967

31. **Goodwin BD, Gay BB, Jr:** The roentgen diagnosis of teratoma of the thyroid region. Am J Roentgenol 95:25, 1965

32. **Hoyt WF, Joe S:** Congenital teratoid cyst of the orbit. Arch Ophthalmol 68:196, 1962

33. **Jensen OA:** Teratoma of the orbit. ATA Ophthalmol 47:317, 1969

34. **Stone HH, Henderson WD, Guidio FA:** Teratomas of the neck. Am J Dis Child 113:222, 1967

35. **Towne BH, Mahour GH, Woolley MM, Isaacs H Jr:** Ovarian cysts and tumors in infancy and childhood. J Pediatr Surg 10:311, 1975

36. **Tuson KWR:** Epignathus: Basicranial teratoma. Br J Surg 58:935, 1971

37. **Beckwith JB:** Mesenchymal renal neoplasms of infancy revisited. J Pediatr Surg 9:803, 1974

38. **Beckwith JB, Palmer AF:** Histopathology and prognosis of Wilms' tumor. Cancer 41:1937, 1978

39. **Bolande RP:** Congenital and infantile neophasia of the kidney. Lancet 2:1497, 1974

40. **D'Angio GJ, Beckwith JB, Breslow N, Sinks L, Sutow W, Wolff J:** Results of the Second National Wilms' Tumor Study, Am Assoc Clin Oncol (abstr) 20:309 (C-74), 1979

41. **D'Angio GJ, Evans A, Breslow N, Beckwith B, Bishop H, Feigl P, Goodwin W, Leape L, Sinks L, Sutow W, Tefft M, Wolff J:** The treatment of Wilms' tumor, results of the National Wilms' Tumor Study. Cancer 38: 633, 1976

42. **Favara BE, Johnson W, Ito J:** Renal tumors in the neonatal period. Cancer 22:845, 1968

43. **Fu Y-S, Kay S:** Congenital mesoblastic nephroma and its recurrence. Arch Pathol 96: 66, 1973

44. **Klapproth HJ:** Wilms' tumor: A report of 45 cases of an analysis of 1351 cases reported in the world literature from 1940 to 1958. J Urol 81:633, 1959

45. **Miller RW, Fraumeni JF, Jr, Manning MD:** Association of Wilms' tumor with aniridia, hemihypertrophy and other congenital malformations. N Eng J Med 270:922, 1964

46. **Pilling GP:** Wilms' tumor in seven children with congenital aniridia. J Pediatr Surg 10: 87, 1976

47. **Waisman J, Cooper PH:** Renal neoplasms of the newborn. J Pediatr Surg 5:407, 1970

48. **Beckwith JB, Perrin EV:** In situ neuroblastomas. Am J Pathol 43:1089, 1963

49. **Catalano PW, Newton WA Jr, Williams TE Jr, Clatworthy WJ, Kilman JW:** Reasonable surgery for thoracic neuroblastoma in infants and children. J Thorac Cardiovasc Surg 76: 459, 1978

50. **D'Angio GJ, Evans AE, Koop CE:** Special pattern of widespread neuroblastoma with a favorable prognosis. Lancet 1:1046, 1971

51. **Evans AE, Chard R, Baum E;** Do children with IV-S neuroblastoma require treatment? Am Assoc Clin Oncol (abstr) 19:367, (C-243), 1978

52. **Jaffe N:** Neuroblastoma: Review of the literature and an examination of factors contributing to its enigmatic character. Cancer Treat Rev 3:61–82, 1976

53. **Schneider KM, Becker JM, Krasna IH:** Neonatal neuroblastoma. Pediatrics 36:359, 1965

54. **Alpert ME, Seeler RA:** Alpha fetoprotein in embryonal hepatoblastoma. J Pediatr 77: 1058, 1970

55. **Behkle FC, Mantz FA, Jr, Olson RY, Trombold JC:** Virilization accompanying hepatoblastoma. Pediatrics 31:265, 1963

56. **Exelby PR, Filler RM, Grosfeld JL:** Liver tumors in children in the particular reference to hepatoblastoma and hepatocellular carcinoma. J Pediatr Surg 10:329, 1975

57. **Fraumeni JF, Jr:** Primary carcinoma of the liver in childhood: An epidemiologic study. J Natl Cancer Inst 40:1087, 1968

58. **Fraumeni JF, Jr, Rosen PJ, Hull EW, Barth RF, Shapiro SR, O'Connor JF:** Hepatoblastoma in infant sisters. Cancer 24:1086, 1969

59. **Herman RE, Lonsdale D:** Chemotherapy, radiation and hepatic lobectomy for hepatoblastoma in an infant. Surgery 68:383, 1970

60. **Ishak KG, Glunz PR:** Hepatoblastoma and hepatocarcinoma in infancy and childhood. Cancer 20:396, 1967

61. **Kasai M, Watanabe I:** Histologic classification of liver-cell carcinoma in infancy and childhood and its clinical evaluation. Cancer 25:551, 1970

62. **MacMahon RA, Lambert TF, Bevan M:** Problems in the diagnosis and management of hepatoblastoma. Austr Paediatr J 7:111, 1971

63. **Van Vaerenberg P, Thijs L, Delbeke MJ, Craen M:** A case of malignant hepatoma with precocious puberty. Acta Paediatr Belg 26: 78, 1972

64. **Ellsworth RM:** Current concepts in the treatment of retinoblastoma. In Peyman GA, Apple DJ, Sanders DR (eds): Intraocular Tumors, p 335. Appleton, Century, Crofts, New York, 1977

65. **Editorial:** The changing pattern of retinoblastoma. Lancet 2:1016, 1971

66. **Leelawongs N, Regan CDJ:** Retinoblastoma. Am J Ophthalmol 66:1050, 1968

67. **Lonsdale D, Berry DH, Holcomb TM, Nora AH, et al:** Chemotherapeutic trials in patients with metastatic retinoblastoma. Cancer Chemother Rep 52:631, 1968

68. **Sagerman RH, Cassady JR, Tretter, P, Ellsworth RM:** Radiation induced neoplasia following external beam therapy for children with retinoblastoma. Am J Roentgenol Radium Ther Nucl Med 105:529, 1969

69. **Thompson RW, Small RC, Stein JJ:** Treatment of retinoblastoma. Am J Roentgenol Radium Ther Nucl Med 114:16, 1972

70. **Abell MR, Holtz F:** Testicular neoplasms in infants and children. Cancer 16:965, 1963

71. **Barsky P:** Congenital astrocytoma: Definitive diagnosis at 30 days of age, with survival. Can Med Assoc J 98:216, 1968

72. **Buck BE, Mahboubi S, Raney RB Jr:** Congenital neurogenous sarcoma with rhabdomyosarcomatous differentiation. J Pediatr Surg 12:581, 1977

73. **Castro J:** Lymphadenectomy and radiation therapy in malignant tumors of the testicle other than pure seminoma. Cancer 24:87, 1969

74. **Cooperman E, Marshall KG, Haust MD:** Congenital astrocytoma. Can Med Assoc J 97:1045, 1967

75. **Craig JM:** Tumors of the lower genitourinary tract. Pediatr Clin North Am 6:491, 1959

76. **Farwell JR, Dohrmann GJ, Flannery JT:** Intracranial neoplasms in infants. Arch Neurol 35:533, 1978

77. **Finck FM, Antin R:** Intracranial teratoma of the newborn. Am J Dis Child 109:439, 1965

78. **Fuste FG, Snyder DE, Price A:** Congenital spongioblastoma of the pons. Am J Clin Pathol 47:790, 1967

79. **Green DM, Jaffe N:** Progress and controversy in the treatment of childhood rhabdomyosarcoma. Cancer Treat Rev 5:7, 1978

80. **Holdsworth CMH, Favara BE, Holton CP, Rainer G:** Malignant Mesenchymoma in infants. Am J Dis Child 128:847, 1974

81. **Houser R, Izant RJ, Jr, Persky L:** Testicular tumors in children. Am J Surg 110:876, 1965

82. **Kauffman SL, Stout AP:** Congenital mesenchymal tumors. Cancer 18:460, 1965

83. **Matsumoto K, Nakauchi K, Fujita K:** Radiation therapy for the embryonal carcinoma of testis in childhood. J Urol 104:778, 1970

84. **Rashkind R, Beigel F:** Brain tumors in early infancy—probably congenital in origin. J Pediatr 65:727, 1964

85. **Reye RD:** Recurring digital fibrous tumors in childhood. Arch Pathol 80:228, 1965

86. **Tefft M, Vawter GF, Mitus A:** Radiotherapeutic management of testicular neoplasms in children. Radiology 88:457, 1967
87. **Walsh PC, Kaufman JJ, Coulson WF, Goodwin EW:** Retroperitoneal lymphadenectomy for testicular tumors. JAMA 217:309, 1971
88. **Woods JE, Murray JE, Vawter GF:** Hand tumors in children. Plast Reconstr Surg 46:130, 1970
89. **Young PG, Mount BM, Foote EW, Jr, Whitemore WF:** Embryonal adenocarcinoma in the prepubertal testis. Cancer 26:1065, 1970
90. **Cangir A, George S, Sullivan M:** Unfavorable prognosis of acute leukemia in infancy. Cancer 36:1973, 1975
91. **Cramblett HC, Friedman JL, Najjar S:** Leukemia in an infant born of a mother with leukemia. N Engl J Med 259:727, 1958
92. **Dalgaard JB, Kass A:** Congenital leukemia with cirrhosis of the liver. Acta Pathol Microbiol Scand 37:465, 1955
93. **Finklestein JZ, Higgins GR, Rissman E, Nixon GW:** Acute leukemia during the first year of life. Clin Pediatr 11:236, 1972
94. **Irvin L, Campbell JW:** Congenital Leukemia. South Med J 71:1445, 1978
95. **Pierce MI:** Leukemia in the newborn infant. J Pediatr 54:691, 1959
96. **Rosner F, Lee S:** Down's syndrome and acute leukemia. Am J Med 53:203, 1972
97. **Wolk JA, Stuart MJ, Davey FR, Nelson DA:** Congenital and neonatal leukemia—lymphocytic or myelocytic? Am J Dis Child 128:864, 1974
98. **Ahnquist G, Holyoke JB:** Congenital Letterer-Siwe disease (reticuloendotheliosis) in a term stillborn infant. J Pediatr 57:897, 1960
99. **Glass AG, Miller RW:** U. S. mortality from Letterer-Siwe disease, 1960–1964. Pediatrics 42:364, 1968
100. **Lahey ME:** Histiocytosis X—analysis of prognostic factors. J Pediatr 87:184, 1975
101. **Lahey ME:** Histiocytosis X—comparison of three treatment regimens. J Pediatr 87:179, 1975
102. **Starling KA, Donaldson MH, Haggard ME, Vietti TJ, Sutow WW:** Therapy of histiocytosis X with vincristine, vinblastine and cyclophosphamide. Am J Dis Child 123:105, 1972
103. **Vogel JM, Vogel P:** Idiopathic histiocytosis: A discussion of eosinophilic granuloma, the Hand-Schuller-Christian syndrome and the Letterer-Siwe syndrome. Semin Hematol 9:349, 1972

37

Congenital Malformations

Murray Feingold

Approximately 4% of children are born with some major birth defect. There are various causes of these malformations including genetic abnormalities, dysmorphogenesis, and infectious and toxic effects on the fetus.

TYPES OF INHERITANCE

Autosomal Dominant Inheritance

In this type of inheritance, there is no carrier state, and, if the gene is present, the patient will be affected. However, manifestations vary depending upon the expressivity and penetrance of the gene. Generally each person has two genes for each specific genetic trait, and each parent gives one of the two genes to the fetus. Therefore, if one of the genes is abnormal (*e.g.*, autosomal dominant gene for achondroplasia) the infant will have a one out of two chances of inheriting this gene from the affected parent (Fig. 37-1). This 50 percent chance occurs with each pregnancy and is not related to the sex of the child. If the infant does not inherit the abnormal gene, it will not be passed on to his children.

If neither of the parents is affected and if their child is born with an autosomal dominant condition, it is most likely secondary to a mutation. Before one can be certain about this, it is mandatory that both parents be examined to be sure that they do not have the disease in a mild, undetected form. Parents who have a child with an autosomal dominant syndrome secondary to a mutation are unlikely to have a second affected child with the same condition, although the chances are perhaps slightly greater than with the general population.

Autosomal Recessive Inheritance

In this type of inheritance, the parents of the affected child do not have the disease but are carriers of the abnormal gene. For example, both parents of a child with cystic fibrosis carry the recessive gene but they are not affected because their "normal" gene has a greater influence over the action of the recessive gene. Their chances of having another child with cystic fibrosis are one out of four with each pregnancy (Fig. 37-2). A child who does not have cystic fibrosis but whose parents are carriers has a two out of three chance of being a carrier of cystic fibrosis. If he is a carrier, it is necessary for his mate also to be a carrier before his children will have cystic fibrosis. In order to predict the possibilities of this occurring, it is necessary to know the gene frequency for cystic fibrosis (*i.e.*, the number of people in the general population who are carrying the gene for cystic fibrosis). If it is a

	A	a
a	Aa	aa
a	Aa	aa

Fig. 37-1. Autosomal dominant inheritance.
Aa—Has the disease.
aa—Does not have disease and is not a carrier
Chance of recurrence: 1 out of 2

	B	b
B	BB	Bb
b	Bb	bb

Fig. 37-2. Autosomal recessive inheritance.
BB—Normal (1 out of 4)
Bb—Normal but carrier (2 out of 4)
bb—Has the disease (1 out of 4)
Chance of recurrence: 1 out of 4

fairly common gene, such as the gene for cystic fibrosis, the chances of one carrier marrying another are greater than when it is a rare gene.

In certain autosomal recessive diseases, such as those listed below, the carrier state can be detected.

α_1-Antitrypsin deficiency
Argininosuccinic aciduria
Brancher deficiency
Cystinosis
Galactosemia
Gaucher disease
Glycogenosis types I, III, IV
GM_1-gangliosidosis
GM_2-gangliosidosis
Goitrous certinism
Histidinemia
Homocystinuria
Hypervalinemia
Maple syrup disease
Metachromatic leukodystophies
Methylmalonic acidemia
Mucolipidosis II (I-cell disease)
Mucopolysaccharidoses I-H, I-S, III
Pyruvate kinase deficiency

X-linked Inheritance

X-linked recessive conditions occur more frequently than do X-linked dominant ones. Some of the more common X-linked recessive syndromes are

Albright's hereditary osteodystrophy
Ectodermal dysplasia, hypohidrotic
Fabry's disease
Focal dermal hypoplasia (Goltz's syndrome)
Hemophilia A and B

Lesch–Nyhan syndrome
Menkes syndrome (kinky hair disease)
Mucopolysaccharidosis II (Hunter syndrome)
Muscular dystrophy, Duchenne type

In this type of inheritance, the abnormal gene is present on one of the female's two X chromosomes. Because the affected gene is recessive, the normal gene on the other X-chromosome prevents the expression of the abnormal gene. Very little genetic material is presently known to be carried on the Y-chromosome; therefore, if a male inherits his mother's X-chromosome containing the abnormal gene, he will be affected. For example, parents of a child with hemophilia or Duchenne type muscular dystrophy will have a one out of four chance of having an affected child with each pregnancy (Fig. 37-3). In providing genetic counseling for the sister of a male with

	X	X˙
X	XX	XX˙
Y	XY	X˙Y

Fig. 37-3. X-linked inheritance.
XX—Normal female (1 out of 4)
X˙X—Normal female but a carrier (1 out of 4)
XY—Normal male (1 out of 4)
X˙Y—Has the disease (1 out of 4)
Chance of recurrence: 1 out of 4.

Table 37-1. Frequency of Down Syndrome.

Age	Age
20—1/1923	35—1/365
21—1/1695	36—1/287
22—1/1538	37—1/225
23—1/1408	38—1/177
24—1/1299	39—1/139
25—1/1205	40—1/109
26—1/1124	41—1/85
27—1/1053	42—1/67
28—1/990	43—1/53
29—1/935	44—1/41
30—1/885	45—1/32
31—1/826	46—1/25
32—1/725	47—1/20
33—1/592	48—1/16
34—1/465	

(Hook EB, Chambers GM: Birth Defects: Original Article Series XII (3A), Alan R. Liss, New York, 1977)

hemophilia or any other X-linked recessive condition, it is important to determine whether she is a carrier. This cannot always be done with certainty. The normal male sibling of a child with hemophilia does not inherit the X-chromosome containing the gene for hemophilia and will not only be normal but also will not be a carrier. In X-linked dominant diseases, both males and females can be affected, as demonstrated in vitamin D-resistant rickets. The chances of an affected person having affected children are 50%.

Polygenic or Multifactorial Inheritance

This type of inheritance is responsible for many genetic conditions including cleft lip, cleft palate, meningomyelocele, and various congenital heart defects. In autosomal dominant and X-linked recessive inheritance, only one gene is necessary to have an affected child; in autosomal recessive inheritance, two genes are necessary. However, in polygenic inheritance, many genes from both parents are necessary before the child will be affected. Therefore, the chance of recurrence in the latter case is much less than in the other forms of inheritance. Parents who have a child with an isolated cleft lip (with or without a cleft palate), have a 3% to 5% statistical chance of recurrence. If a second child is affected, the possibility of a third occurrence is 14%.

CHROMOSOMAL ABNORMALITIES

Chromosomal aberrations occur in approximately 1 out of every 200 deliveries, although many of these patients are phenotypically normal. Approximately 40% of all spontaneous abortions have some type of chromosomal abnormality.

Nondisjunction is probably the most common cause of chromosomal syndromes. The result of nondisjunction is usually the presence of an extra chromosome, as illustrated in **Down syndrome** (trisomy 21). Chromosomes undergo reduction during meiosis, at which time their number decreases from 46 to 23. They then divide, producing daughter cells which also have 23 chromosomes. At this stage, both the egg and sperm contain 23 chromosomes and are ready for fertilization which results in the fetus having a total of 46 chromosomes, half coming from the mother and half from the father. In Down syndrome of the nondisjunction type, chromosomes 21 do not separate during meiosis. At fertilization, these two chromosomes join with the single chromosome 21 of the mate resulting in three chromosomes 21 or trisomy 21. The reason why both chromosomes 21 do not separate during meiosis is not known, but maternal age is certainly a factor (Table 37-1). There is evidence that in couples younger than age 30 who have a Down syndrome child, the extra 21 chromosome comes from the father approximately 20% to 30% of the time. The most common types of nondisjunction abnormalities associated with the autosomes are trisomies 21, 18, and 13.

Translocation. Chromosomal material may also break off from one chromosome and translocate onto another. It is important to determine whether a translocated chromosome is present because that chromosome can be passed on from parent to child. Translocation of a chromosome 21 onto either a D group (13–15) or G group (21–22) chromosome is responsible for approximately 3% of children with Down's syndrome. If the mother is a carrier of the translocated chromosome, there is about a 10% chance of recurrence in her next pregnancy. However, if the father is a carrier the chances are only approximately 2%. Many translocation syndromes do not present classic clinical findings and therefore may be difficult to diagnose. Manifestations are usually present when the translocation is unbalanced, resulting in the presence of extra chromosomal material. In the carrier state **(balanced translocation),** manifestations are usually not present.

Deletion occurs when chromosomal material is missing (deleted) from either the upper (p) or lower (q) arms of a chromosome. An example of a deletion is the *cri du chat* syndrome, in which material is missing from the upper arm of chromosome 5 (5p−). A partial trisomy occurs when there is an extra p or q (*e.g.,* 11q+: partial trisomy syndrome).

An abnormal number of X and Y chromosomes occurs with some frequency, as seen in Turner and Klinefelter syndromes. In Turner syndrome, because of the absence of one X chromosome, there are only 45 chromosomes. In contrast to patients who are missing an autosome **(monosomy),** survival can take place if an X chromosome is missing. However, a high percentage of chromosomal abnormalities resulting in spontaneous abortion have an XO or Turner karyotype. Mosaicism occurs when there is more than one cell line (*e.g.,* some cells containing an XO line and other cells containing an XX line). This frequently occurs in Turner syndrome, resulting in such mosaics as XO/XX and XO/XX/XY. Although the classic XO Turner syndrome patient generally cannot reproduce, this is not always true in patients with mosaic Turner's.

Klinefelter syndrome is the most common chromosomal aberration in males and usually consists of 47 chromosomes (XXY). Although it may be difficult to diagnose during the newborn period, two helpful clues are radioulnar synostosis and abnormal genitalia. There are numerous other abnormalities involving the X and Y chromosomes including the XYY karyotype, which occurs in approximately 1 out of 700 deliveries. This syndrome has been reported to be associated with an increased tendency for criminal behavior, but the true significance of this finding is not known.

EVALUATING THE MALFORMED INFANT

Before examining the infant, it is important to obtain all pertinent historic data. Pregnancy history provides valuable information, especially if there is a history of frequent spontaneous abortions or exposure to infections, medications, alcohol, or x-ray examinations.

Details concerning labor, delivery, birth weight, Apgar score, placenta, and number of umbilical vessels are also helpful. Family history, especially regarding mental retardation, chromosomal abnormalities, skeletal dysplasias, and so on are useful in making a diagnosis. A family pedigree should be obtained routinely.

Initially, on physical examination, the child should be examined for major defects.

Facies. It is important to get an overall impression of the facies. Is the face normal in configuration? Is it triangular, as seen in patients with marked loss of subcutaneous fat (The triangular facies of patients with progeria and diencephalic syndrome are not apparent in the newborn period.) A rounded facies may be present in patients with the Prader–Willi, Laurence–Moon–Biedl, and *cri du chat* (deletion of chromosomal material from the upper arm of the chromosome 5) syndromes. In myotonic dystrophy the face is expressionless, and, in the newborn period, drooling frequently occurs. Other terms used to describe the face include bird-like (Seckel dwarf and Hallermann–Streiff syndromes), elfin facies (Williams syndrome and leprechaunism), flattened facies (Potter syndrome and congenital syphillis), coarse facies (congenital hypothyroidism, GM_1-gangliosidosis and mucolipidosis II), and facial dysostosis (Apert, Crouzon, and Chotzen syndromes). Patients with the various types of mucopolysaccharidoses are not included because they generally do not have coarse facial features in the newborn period.

The Head. The size and shape of the head should be noted. If the head size is significantly small (microcephaly), DeLange syndrome rubella, toxoplasmosis, cytomegalic inclusion disease, cebocephaly, and various chromosomal abnormalities should be considered. The most common cause of an enlarged head is hydrocephalus which may or may not be associated with a meningomyelocele. Hydrocephalus may also be found in achondroplasia, cerebral gigantism, hydrancephaly, and congenital toxoplasmosis. Another cause of an enlarged head is macrocephaly which is present in achondroplasia, cerebral gigantism, osteopetrosis, Conradi–Hünermann syndrome, and pycnodysostosis. An enlarged anterior fontanel is present in a variety of syndromes including osteogenesis imperfecta, Conradi syndrome, pycnodysostosis, congenital hypothyroidism and congenital syphilis. Other abnormalities of the head including a prominent frontal bone, flattened occiput, prominent occiput, and premature closure of sutures should be noted. The latter is found in Apert, Saethre–Chotzen, and Crouzon syndromes but may also be an isolated finding.

The size and shape of the infant's skull are helpful in determining the correct diagnosis in a patient suspected of having a skeletal dysplasia. For example, in achondroplasia, thanatophoric dwarfism, cleidocranial dysplasia, and achondrogenesis, a large head is present. However, in spondyloepiphyseal dysplasia, a fairly common type of dwarfism, the head size is normal, as it is in the Ellis–van Creveld syndrome.

The Eyes. The eye examination can be divided into an external and internal examination. It is difficult and frequently not practical for the physician to do a complete ophthalmologic examination on all newborn infants. However, it should be thorough enough to alert the physician to the possibility of any ocular abnormalities so that a more extensive evaluation can be done by an ophthalmologist.

On external examination, the presence of colobomas of the iris and lid should be noted. A coloboma of the upper lid raises the question of the Goldenhar syndrome, while in the Treacher Collins syndrome the lower lid is involved. Cataracts may be the result of an intrauterine infection or an inherited biochemical defect. They may not be present in the newborn period but occur later (*e.g.,* galactosemia). Long eyelashes are unusual in the newborn, but are present in patients with the Cornelia DeLange syndrome, which also includes synophrys (eyebrows meeting in the midline). Structural iris abnormalities may be found at birth (Rieger syndrome), but heterochromia or iris bicolor associated with the Waardenburg syndrome do not occur until at least 3 months of age. The size of the eyes should be noted; if they are small consider trisomy 13, Hallermann–Streiff syndrome, and congenital toxoplasmosis. Some external abnormalities that may occur include nystagmus, ptosis of the lids, megalocornea, Brushfield spots, and dermoids. The presence of epicanthal folds may be difficult to interpret because the newborn usually has a broad bridge of the nose, giving the appearance of an epicanthal fold. Epicanthal folds are frequently associated with Down, *cri du chat,* Noonan, and the Smith–Lemli–Opitz syndromes.

An important factor to consider in the eye examination is whether the eyes are too far apart (ocular hypertelorism) or too close together (ocular hypotelorism). These findings have important clinical significance not only because of the numerous syndromes associated with both but also because there is a much higher incidence of mental retardation in hypotelorism. Some of the syndromes associated with hyper- and hypotelorism are listed in Table 37-2. The manner in which the interpupillary distance can be determined is found in Figure 37-23.

Observe the slant of the palpebral fissures to determine whether a mongoloid (upward and outward) or antimongoloid (downward and outward) slant is present. Because it is difficult to quantitate the slant of the eyes, it is mainly a clinical impression. Some of the conditions associated with an antimongoloid

Table 37-2. Syndromes Associated

With Ocular Hypertelorism		With Ocular Hypotelorism
Aarskog	Fetal hydantoin	Cebocephaly
Apert	Fetal warfarin	Ethmocephaly
Cerebrohepatorenal	Idiopathic infantile hypercalcemia	Oculodentodigital
Chromosome 4p–	Larsen	Trisomy 13
Cleidocranial dysplasia	Leprechaunism	Holoprosencephaly
Coffin–Lowry	Multiple lentigenes (Leopard)	
Craniometaphyseal dysplasia	Median cleft face	
Cri du chat (Cat-cry, 5p–)	Otopalatodigital	
Crouzon	Robinow	
	Turner	

slant include the Rubinstein–Taybi, Treacher Collins, Noonan, otopalatodigital, and ring chromosome 18 syndromes.

Abnormalities on internal (funduscopic) examination of the eye may also lead the examiner to suspect a possible diagnosis. For example, the finding of chorioretinitis suggests the possibility of an intrauterine infection, and, if microcephaly is also present, the possibility becomes even stronger. Look for such other findings as presence of a cherry-red spot, corneal opacities, iritis, macular degeneration, optic atrophy, and retinitis pigmentosa.

The Ears. A variety of ear abnormalities are associated with syndromes, and it is important to note whether they are unilateral or bilateral. For example, patients with Goldenhar syndrome and hemifacial microsomia usually have unilateral ear involvement, while patients with Treacher Collins syndrome have bilateral abnormalities. There is also a higher incidence of renal anomalies present in patients with unilateral ear and facial bone abnormalities. Other abnormalities including the length of the ear (increased in cerebral gigantism and decreased in Down syndrome), prominent helix (deletion of chromosome 18), absence of ear lobes (Seckel dwarf syndrome), and square ears (Down syndrome). Low-set ears are found in numerous genetic syndromes including Apert, Crouzon, Turner, Noonan, and Rubinstein–Taybi, and trisomies 13 and 18. There are various methods used to determine whether the ears are low set. Our method consists of extending a line from both medial canthi to the ear and determining the percentage of the ear above this line. A graph can then be used to determine if the ear is low set (see Fig. 37-25).

The Nose. There are numerous terms used to describe the shape of the nose including **beaked** (Apert, Crouzon, Hallermann–Streiff, and Treacher Collins syndromes), **upturned** (achondroplasia, DeLange, Smith–Lemli–Opitz), **bulbous** (trisomy 13), and **pinched** (oculodentodigital). The nasolabial distance (philtrum) varies greatly and the same distance may be present in both the neonate and adult. Prominence of the philtrum is characteristic of various conditions including the DeLange and Smith–Lemli–Opitz syndromes. A broad bridge of the nose is a common finding and occurs in Down syndrome, Williams, achondroplasia and Conradi syndrome.

The Oral Region. The most obvious abnormalities involving the oral region are cleft lip and cleft palate, which are usually inherited in a polygeneic manner. It is important to examine such patients for the presence of lip pits, which are indentations or depressions located on the lower lip. When present, and associated with a cleft lip, the chance for recurrence changes from approximately 4% to 50% because it is then inherited in an autosomal dominant fashion. Other oral abnormalities include natal teeth (pycnodysostosis), serrated gingivae (Ellis–van Creveld) and high-arched palate (Treacher Collins, Apert, Crouzon, Smith–Lemli–Opitz, Marfan, Turner, and Noonan syndromes, and familial microcephaly). The tongue also provides clues to syndrome diagnoses. An absent tongue may be noted in the aglossia-adactylia syndrome. A large tongue is found in Beckwith syndrome, gangliosidosis, congenital hypothyroidism, isolated macroglossia, and angiomas and hamartomas of the tongue. In dysautonomia, there is absence of the fungiform papillae. Clefts of the tongue are seen in the orofaciodigital, Meckel, and glossopalatine ankylosis syndromes.

Various terms are used to describe the shape of the mouth including **broad** (Williams), **fishlike** (Treacher Collins, Prader–Willi, Silver syndromes), **open** (Down syndrome, Apert syndrome, myotonic dystrophy), and **small** (Schwartz–Jampel syndrome, Hallerman–Streiff, craniocarpotarsal dystrophy). Micrognathia occurs in many conditions including the Pierre Robin, Treacher Collins, and Hallermann–Streiff syndromes, and trisomies 13 and 18. Prognathism (prominence of the mandible) is frequently seen in Crouzon, Apert, and Rieger syndromes and in cerebral gigantism.

The Neck. On examination of the neck, note should be made as to whether it is short (Turner syndrome, Noonan syndrome, spondyloepiphyseal dysplasia, Klippel–Feil syndrome, trisomy 13), **webbed** (Turner, Noonan, and Down syndromes and trisomy 18), or both. Deafness should be suspected in patients with branchial cleft sinuses located along the anterior border of the sternocleidomastoid muscle associated with cup-shaped ears.

Skeleton. Cardiopulmonary and abdominal abnormalities are described in Chapters 23 and 34. There are a large number of skeletal abnormalities secondary to birth defects or genetic syndromes. They may be isolated (polydactyly) or part of a syndrome (polydactyly

Table 37-3. Some Hand Abnormalities Present in the Newborn.

Hand Abnormalities	Syndrome	
Arachnodactyly	Marfan	
	Contractual arachnodactyly	
	Homocystinuria	
Brachydactyly	Down	Achondroplasia
	Coffin–Lowry	Congenital hypothyroidism
	Multiple epiphyseal	Diastrophic dwarfism
	dysplasia	Ellis–van Creveld
	Laurence–Moon–Biedl	Hypochondroplasia
	Pseudoachondroplasia	Orofaciodigital
	Robinow	Turner
	Silver–Russell	DeLange
Polydactyly	Achondrogenesis	Focal-dermal hypoplasia
	Asphyxiating thoracic dyspla-	Fetal Alcohol
	sia	Laurence–Moon–Biedl
	Cerebrohepatorenal	Meckel
	Ellis–van Creveld	Short-rib polydactyly
	Trisomy 18	
	Trisomy 13	
	DeLange	
Abnormal thumbs		
Broad	Rubinstein–Taybi	
	Larsen	
	Otopalatodigital	
Proximally placed	DeLange	
	Trisomy 13	
	Diastrophic dwarf	
Finger-like and triphalangeal	Hypoplastic congenital anemia	
	Fetal hydantoin	
	Heart-hand	
	VATER association	
	Holt–Oram	
Stub thumb	Isolated autosomal dominant	
Thumb sign	Marfan	
	Ehlers–Danlos	
	Mucosal neuroma syndrome	
Dorsal swelling	Turner	
	Noonan	
	Congenital hypothyroidism	
	Thrombocytopenia, absent radius	
Shortened metacarpals	Albright hereditary osteodystrophy	
	Cri du chat	
	Turner	
	Basal cell nevus syndrome	
	Sjogren–Larsson	

type of polydactyly is postaxial (*i.e.*, the extra digit or digits are on the ulnar side of the middle finger or toe). Syndactyly, which also occurs in many syndromes, most frequently is an isolated finding involving the second and third toes. The hand is very accessible for examinations and frequently provides clues to syndrome diagnoses (Table 37-3). Other hand abnormalities that should be looked for include clinodactyly, broad hands, camptodactyly (bent fingers), tapered fingers, and abnormal dermatoglyphics. The nails should also be observed (*e.g.*, dysplasia associated with Ellis–van Creveld syndrome, ectodermal dysplasia, hereditary osteoonycho dysplasia, and focal dermal hypoplasia).

The majority of the skeletal dysplasias can be suspected in the newborn period. It is very difficult to keep abreast of the changing classifications of the skeletal dysplasias, but the pediatrician should have a general approach to these problems in order to raise the possibility of such a diagnosis.

The most common and also the most over-diagnosed skeletal dysplasia is achondroplasia.

associated with trisomy 13). The most common An infant who dies in the newborn period and resembles an achondroplastic dwarf, most likely had thanatophoric dwarfism or achondrogenesis and not achondroplasia. X-ray findings and microscopic examination of the cartilage differ in each syndrome. A general way of differentiating achondroplasia from other types of skeletal dysplasia, as described earlier, is by head size. Some of the bone dysplasias that have manifestations at birth associated with dwarfism are listed in Table 37-4. Patients with thanatophroic dwarfism and achondrogenesis do not survive the newborn period. In asphyxiating thoracic dysplasia and the camptomelic syndrome, respiratory distress is present. It is important to note whether the long bones are shorter proximally (achondroplasia) or distally (Ellis–van Creveld) and whether the chest is narrow. X-ray examination will confirm the diagnosis.

For a compilation of inherited disorders in humans, see McKusick.[1] Malformations of particular organs are described in Chapters 23, 34, 35, and 40.

Table 37-4. Skeletal Dysplasias Present in the Newborn Period.

	Large Head	Narrow Chest	Inheritance
1. Achondrogenesis	+	+	AR, −
2. Achondroplasia	+	+	AD
3. Asphyxiating thoracic dystrophy	−	++	AR
4. Camptomelic syndrome	−	++	AR
5. Cleidocranial dysplasia	+	−	AD
6. Chondrodysplasia punctata, rhizomelic type	+/−	−	AR
7. Chondrodysplasia punctata, Conradi–Hünermann type	+/−	−	AD
8. Diastrophic dwarfism	−	−	AR
9. Ellis–van Creveld	−	++	AR
10. Metatropic	−	+	AD/AR
11. Osteogenesis imperfecta congenita	+	−	AR
12. Pycnodysostosis	+	−	AR
13. Robinow	+	−	AD/AR
14. Spondylocostal dysplasia	−	+/−	AD
15. Spondyloepiphyseal dysplasia congenita	−	−	AD
16. Spondylothoracic dysplasia	−	++	AR
17. Thanatophoric dwarfism	+	++	?

+ present
− absent
AD autosomal dominant
AR autosomal recessive

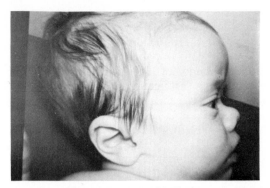

Fig. 37-4. Achondroplasia.

COMMON MALFORMATION SYNDROMES[2-6]

Achondroplasia (Fig. 37-4)

Major manifestations include short stature with the proximal segments of the limbs being more involved than the distal segments. The hands are short and stubby. The head is enlarged which may be secondary to macrocephaly, hydrocephalus, or both. There is a depressed nasal bridge with an upturned nose. The chest cavity appears small. As the child grows older, there is lordosis and the abdomen protrudes. Motor development, such as sitting and standing, may be delayed, but intelligence is usually normal. X-ray examination substantiates the diagnosis. The ilia are square, the sacrosciatic notch is small, the pubic and ischial bones are short, and there is a lack of the normal increase in the interpediculate distance from L1 to L5.

Achondroplasia is inherited as an autosomal dominant, although approximately 80% of the cases are secondary to a new mutation.

Apert Syndrome (Acrocephalosyndactyly; Fig. 37-5)

Major manifestations include craniosynostosis mainly of the coronal sutures, depressed broad bridge of the nose, hypoplasia of the maxilla, apparent hypertelorism, antimongoloid slant of the eyes, and a high-arched narrow palate. Skeletal abnormalities consist mainly of syndactyly of the hands and feet, usually including the second to fifth digits.

Mental retardation is not frequently found although some of the children have dull to normal intelligence. Although most of the cases are sporadic, autosomal dominant inheritance has been reported.

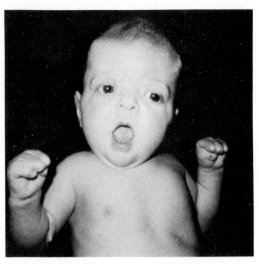

Fig. 37-5. Apert syndrome.

Beckwith Syndrome (Fig. 37-6)

Major manifestations include a birth weight over 3200 g, large tongue and viscera, neonatal hypoglycemia usually after the first day of life, leucine sensitivity, strabismus, and an omphalocele or large umbilical hernia. After an initial weight loss, there is an increase in both height and weight. The hypoglycemia may be severe enough to cause death or slow development. Other findings include microcephaly, indentation or notching of the ear lobes, diaphragmatic eventration, cliteromegaly, and asymmetry.

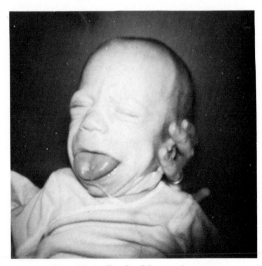

Fig. 37-6. Beckwith syndrome.

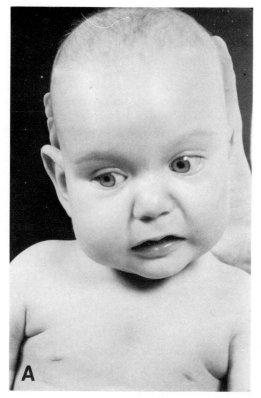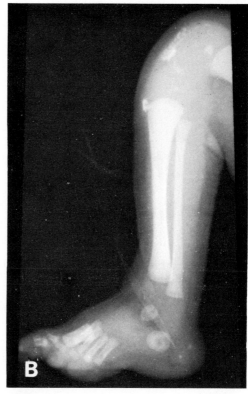

Fig. 37-7, A, B. Chondrodysplasia punctata.

The type of inheritance is uncertain but polygeneic, autosomal recessive, and autosomal dominant inheritance have been reported.

Chondrodysplasia Punctata: Rhizomelic Type (Fig. 37-7)

Present in the newborn period are dwarfism, microcephaly, flat bridge of the nose, puffy cheeks, cataracts, contractures, club feet, dyskeratotic skin lesions, respiratory distress, and congenital heart disease. The limbs may be quite short causing some confusion with achondroplasia or osteogenesis imperfecta. Death may occur within the first year of life. X-ray examination reveals a characteristic deformity of vertebral bodies. The spine has vertical radiolucent bars of cartilage which separate the anterior and posterior ossification centers; shortened femora, humeri, or both; metaphyseal irregularities; and symmetrical strippling.

Chondrodysplasia punctata-Conradi–Hünermann type is much more benign and is inherited in an autosomal dominant manner.

Cri-Du-Chat Syndrome (Fig. 37-8)

Major manifestations are a high-pitched, cat-like cry present during infancy, microcephaly, ocular hypertelorism, rounded face, mental retardation, and deletion of the short arm of

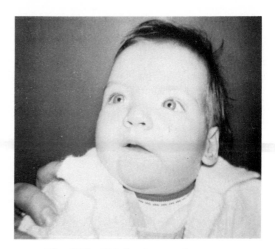

Fig. 37-8. *Cri du chat* syndrome.

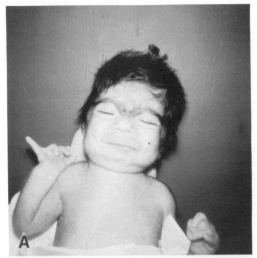

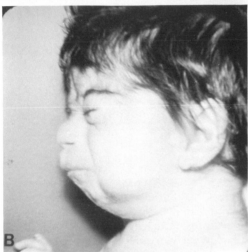

Fig. 37-9, A B. DeLange syndrome.

The cause is unknown and recurrence is unlikely. There have been rare reports of familial translocation abnormalities.

Down Syndrome (Trisomy 21; Fig. 37-10)

Clinical findings include brachycephaly, broad bridge of the nose, speckled iris, epicanthal folds, flattened facies, high-arched narrow palate, protruding tongue, small square ears, short broad hands, short or missing fifth middle phalanx, congenital heart disease, webbing of the neck, and mental retardation.

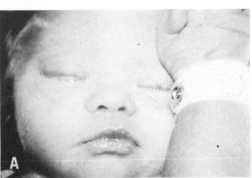

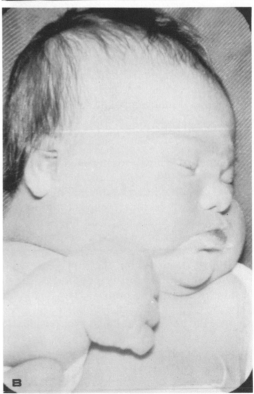

Fig. 37-10, A, B. Down syndrome.

chromosome 5. Other findings include a small-for-dates infant, low-set ears, short metacarpals or metatarsals, and epicanthal folds.

The partial deletion of the short arm of chromosome 5 is usually a sporadic occurrence, although occasionally one of the parents may be a balanced translocation carrier.

DeLange Syndrome (Fig. 37-9)

Manifestations include short stature, hirsutism, synophrys, long eyelashes, prominent nostrils and philtrum, thin lips, congenital heart disease and a variety of skeletal abnormalities. Mental retardation is almost always present, as is microcephaly.

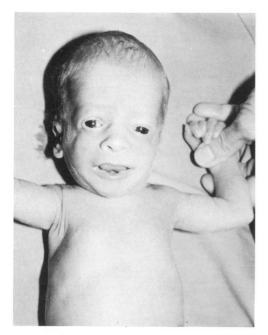

Fig. 37-11. Treacher Collins syndrome. (mandibulofacial dysostosis).

Trisomy 21 is present in approximately 95% of the patients and a translocation abnormality in 2% to 3%. See Table 37-1 for frequency in various age groups.

This syndrome is so familiar that a lengthy description is not included here. Usually moderate mental retardation is a constant feature.

Mandibulofacial Dysostosis (Treacher Collins Syndrome; Fig. 37-11)

Major manifestations include an abnormal facial appearance manifested by an antimongoloid slant of the eyes, coloboma of the lower lid, hypoplasia of supraorbital ridges, facial bone dysostosis, micrognathia, dysplastic ears, conductive hearing loss, defects of auditory ossicles, preauricular tags, flame-shaped projections of hair extending from the ear onto the cheek, and micrognathia. Mental retardation is usually not present.

The syndrome is inherited as an autosomal dominant trait with a varying degree of expressivity.

Osteogenesis Imperfecta Congenita (Fig. 37-12)

Multiple fractures and skeletal deformities present at birth. The skull is soft, and there is a "ping-pong" sensation on palpation of the skull. In very severe cases, the face may be "bird-like." The limbs are usually very small with multiple deformities and hyperextensibility of the joints. Blue sclerae may be present. Hydrocephalus and intracranial hemorrhage are frequent findings. X-ray films of the skull show multiple wormian bones and fractures.

The mode of inheritance in the severe neonatal type is usually autosomal recessive. Osteogenesis imperfecta tarda is inherited in an autosomal dominant manner, and manifestations are generally not present in the neonatal period.

Potter Syndrome (Fig. 37-13)

Major manifestations include a typical facial appearance, absent kidneys, pulmonary hypoplasia and neonatal death. The facies appear flattened with micrognathia, low-set and abnormally shaped ears, flattened, beaked nose, apparent ocular hypertelorism, and a skin fold below the eye. Other malformations include arthrogryposis, abnormal genitalia, lower limb abnormalities, and gastrointestinal malformations. Oligohydramnios and amnion nodosum are associated with this syndrome.

The etiology is unknown and there does not appear to be an inherited pattern.

Smith–Lemli–Opitz Syndrome (Fig. 37-14)

Major manifestations include marked failure to thrive, mental and motor retardation, a classic facial appearance, vomiting and pyloric stenosis, microcephaly, a shrill cry, cryptor-

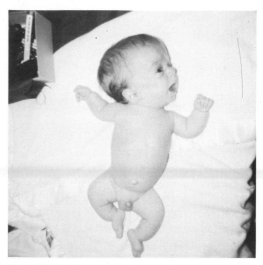

Fig. 37-12. Osteogenesis imperfecta congenita.

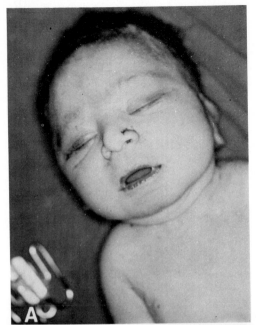

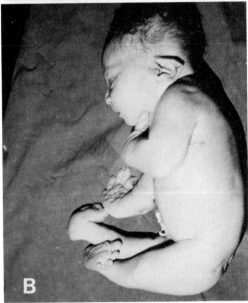

3
4   **Fig. 37-13, A, B.** Potter syndrome.

chidism, hypospadias, small penis, simian line, syndactyly of the second and third toes and abnormal dermatoglyphics. The facial appearance includes ptosis of the eyelids, strabismus, anteverted nostrils, prominent philtrum, and broad maxillary alveolar ridge. There are other less frequently found congenital birth defects including a clenched hand with the index finger

over the middle finger. Many of these children die within the first year of life and few survive beyond childhood. The syndrome is inherited in an autosomal recessive manner and the carrier state is not detectable.

Sturge–Weber Syndrome (Fig. 37-15)

Major manifestation is a port-wine hemangioma involving the distribution of the fifth cranial nerve. The hemangioma may also affect

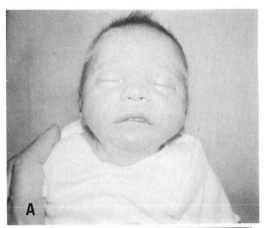

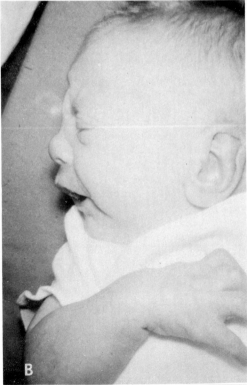

Fig. 37-14, A, B. Smith–Lemli–Opitz syndrome.

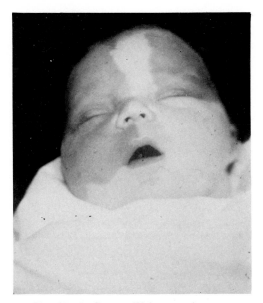

Fig. 37-15. Sturge–Weber syndrome.

the brain, resulting in seizures and intracerebral calcifications. Glaucoma may also be present on the side of the hemangioma. Hemianopia and hemiplegia are frequently present.

The etiology is unknown and there does not appear to be an inherited pattern.

Trisomy 13 (Fig. 37-16)

Major manifestations include marked mental/motor retardation, microphthalmia, low-set malformed ears, microcephaly, cleft lip and/or palate, micrognathia, webbing of the neck, undescended testicles, congenital heart disease, hand abnormalities, capillary hemangioma, and scalp defects. Postmortem examination reveals various renal and gastrointestinal abnormalities, holoprosencephaly, and a bicornuate uterus. There are 47 chromosomes with chromosome 13 being the extra chromosome.

Trisomy 18 (Fig. 37-17)

Common manifestations include prominent occiput, malformed ears, ptosis of the eyes, small palpebral fissures, "Grecian" or upturned nose, narrow palate or clefting of the palate, congenital heart disease, and renal abnormalities. Skeletal anomalies include overlapping of the second over the third fingers, retroflex or distally placed thumb, rocker-

bottom feet, syndactyly, short sternum, and small pelvis. Other findings include failure to thrive, poor suck, and abnormal cry, pyloric stenosis, Meckel's diverticulum, webbing of the neck, and meningomyelocele. Mental retardation and early death are constant findings. The chromosomal abnormality consists of an extra chromosome 18.

Turner Syndrome (Fig. 37-18)

Major manifestations include short stature, webbing of the neck, low posterior hairline, lymphedema on the dorsa of the hands and feet, congenital heart disease usually coarctation of the aorta, abnormal dermatoglyphics, increased number of pigmented moles, dysplastic or hyperconvex fingernails, broad bridge of the nose, ptosis of the eyelids, epicanthal folds, gonadal dysplasia or streaked gonads, lack of secondary sexual characteristics, horseshoe kidneys, and unilateral renal agenesis. Intelligence is normal.

Classically, an X chromosome is missing,

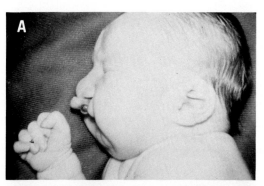

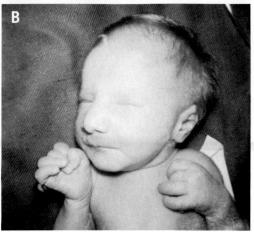

Fig. 37-16, A, B. Trisomy 13.

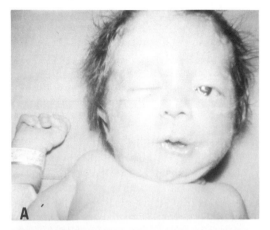

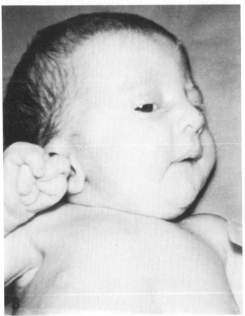

Fig. 37-17, A, B. Trisomy 18.

but isochromosome X and a variety of mosaic forms may be present. Recurrence in the same family is unusual.

Fetal Alcohol Syndrome

Major manifestations includes slow pre- and postnatal growth, mental retardation, microcephaly and a facial appearance characteristic of a child born to an alcoholic mother. Other findings include small palpebral fissures, prominent philtrum, congenital heart defects, congenital dislocated hip and other joint abnormalities, poor motor coordination and tremulousness during the newborn period.

Manifestations can also occur in offspring born to mothers who were moderate drinkers but the symptoms usually are not as marked (Fig. 37-19).

Fetal Hydantoin Syndrome

Major manifestations include slow pre- and postnatal growth, microcephaly, mental retardation, and a facial appearance characteristic of an infant born to a mother who has taken hydantoins during her pregnancy. Other findings include ptosis of the palpebral fissures, upturned short nose with a prominent philtrum, epicanthal folds, apparent ocular hypertelorism, strabismus, wide mouth, cleft lip and palate, and short neck. Various types of congenital heart disease are present. Limb abnor-

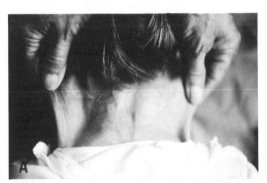

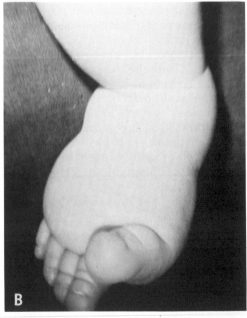

Fig. 37-18, A, B. Turner syndrome.

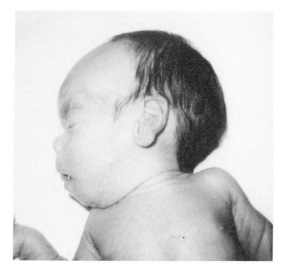

Fig. 37-19. Fetal alcohol syndrome.

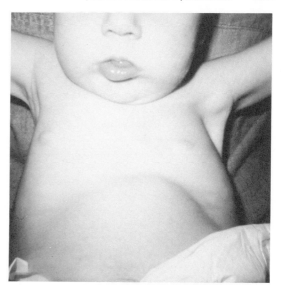

Fig. 37-21. Poland malformation complex.

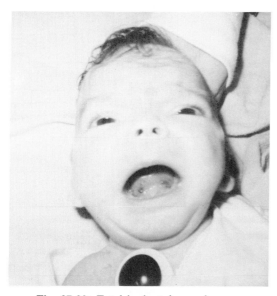

Fig. 37-20. Fetal hydantoin syndrome.

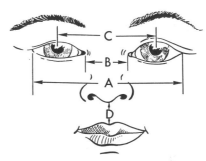

Fig. 37-22. A. Outer canthal distance. **B.** Inner canthal distance. **C.** Interpupillary distance. **D.** Nasolabial distance.

malities include finger-like thumbs, hypoplasia of the distal phalanges, and nail dysplasia. Frequently, only a few of these findings are present (Fig. 37-20).

Poland Malformation Complex

Major manifestations include synbrachydactyly (syndactyly and short digits) and a defect of the pectoralis muscle. All variations of syndactyly and brachydactyly can occur, but the thumb is usually not as severely affected.

The sternal head of the pectoralis muscle on the same side as the hand anomaly is abnormal, while the clavicular head is always present. Other findings include asymmetrical breast development, absent breast on same side, ipsilateral webbing of the axilla, rib abnormalities, shortening of the arm and forearm, and Sprengel deformity (Fig. 37-21).

PHYSICAL NORMS FOR SYNDROMES

One of the difficulties in syndrome identification is the lack of specific descriptive measurements (Fig. 37-22). For example, the definition of low-set ears varies from observer to observer. The same is true in defining other

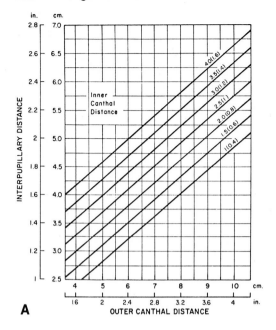

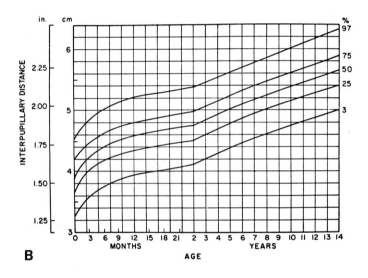

Fig. 37-23. A. Nomogram for computing interpupillary distance from inner and outer canthal distance. **B.** Age-specific norms for interpupillary distance, with key percentiles designated.

facial features. We have studied various physical parameters in a normal population, and the methodology and results are reported elsewhere.[7] A summary of these findings are described below.

Eye Measurements

Although the presence of ocular hypertelorism or hypotelorism is extremely important in syndrome diagnosis, direct interpupillary measurements are difficult to obtain and therefore are unreliable in infants and children.

A graph was prepared to determine the interpupillary distance (Fig. 37-23A). By plotting the inner and outer canthal distances, the interpupillary distance was obtained and plotted against the patient's age (Fig. 37-23B), and the percentile determined.

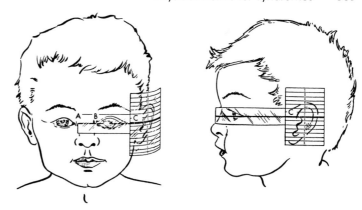

Fig. 37-24. X-ray film device for measuring ear length and computing percent of the ear above and below the inner canthal eyeline.

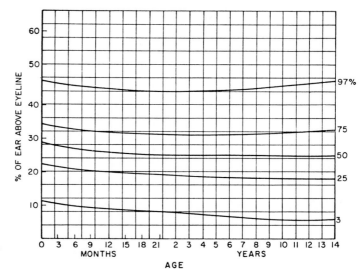

Fig. 37-25. Age-specific norms for percent of ear above the eyeline.

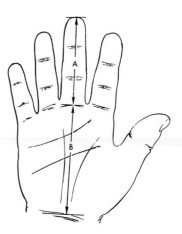

Fig. 37-26. Landmarks used in measuring palm and finger length.

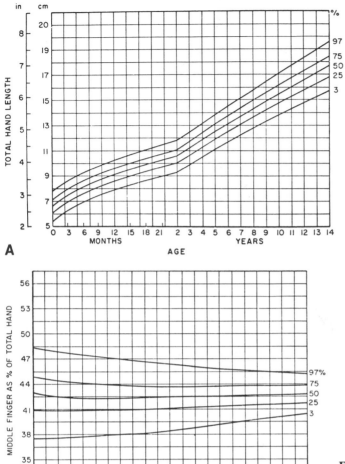

Fig. 37-27. A. Age-specific norms for total hand length. **B.** Age-specific norms for middle finger length as a percent of total hand length.

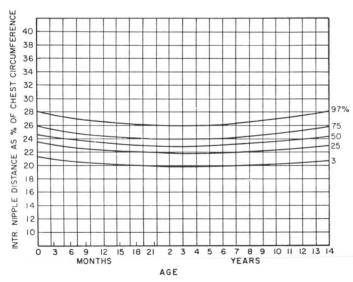

Fig. 37-28. The internipple distance as a percent of chest circumference.

Ear Measurements

Figure 37-24 depicts the instrument (made from x-ray film) utilized in our study and its application. Both sides of the instrument are divided into millimeters allowing the right and left ears to be measured by the same instrument. A central horizontal line is drawn on the instrument and the length of the ear above or below this line is determined. The medial canthi (A and B Fig. 37-24) were used as landmarks instead of the lateral canthi because a mongoloid or antimongoloid slant of the palpebral fissures can provide incorrect landmarks. The central horizontal line is placed over both inner canthi and point C is found by extending this center line to the side of the face. The measuring part of the instrument covers the ear and the length of the ear above or below the center line is determined. The percentage of the ear above the line is determined and this percentage is then related to age by using Figure 37-25 to ascertain the percentile. Because this measurement is more difficult to obtain than the others, at least two measurements should be done to improve reliability.

Hand Measurements

The hands were measured using the landmarks depicted in Figure 37-26. The length of the middle finger as a percentage of the total hand size (Fig. 37-27A) remained fairly constant from the newborn period to 14 years of age (42%–43%). This measurement is useful in determining if the fingers are longer than normal. The total length of the hand was plotted against age (Fig. 37-27B).

Internipple Distance

An increase in internipple distance has been claimed in various syndromes (e.g., Turner syndrome). The internipple distance as a percentage of the chest circumference is plotted in Figure 37-28. This percentage was highest during the newborn period and then remained fairly constant.

REFERENCES

1 **McKusick VA:** Mendelian Inheritance in Man, 5th ed. Johns Hopkins Press, Baltimore, 1978
2 **Warkany J:** Congenital Malformations. Year Book Medical Publishers, Chicago, 1971
3 **Smith DW:** Recognizable Patterns of Human Malformation, 2nd ed. WB Saunders, Philadelphia, 1976
4 **Gorlin RJ, Pindborg JJ, Cohen MM:** Syndrome of the Head and Neck, 2nd ed. McGraw-Hill, New York, 1976.
5 **Temtamy S, McKusick V:** The Genetics of Hand Malformations. The National Foundation—March of Dimes, Birth Defects Original Article Series XIV (3), Alan R. Liss, New York, 1978.
6 **Bergsma D:** Birth Defects Compendium, 2nd ed. The National Foundation—March of Dimes, Alan R. Liss, New York, 1979.
7 **Feingold M, Bossert WH:** Normal Values for Selected Physical Parameters. Birth Defects Original Article Series X (13). The National Foundation/March of Dimes, 1974.

38

Orthopedics in the Newborn

Paul P. Griffin

The orthopedic or musculoskeletal examination of the newborn is a significant part of the evaluation of the neonate. Normal variations in contour, size, relationships, and range of motion of joints are influenced by genetic factors and by *in utero* position. These must be distinguished from congenital anomalies and traumatic lesions. The basic principle, that the earlier appropriate treatment is started the better the correction, makes it incumbent upon those caring for the neonate to make the diagnosis early and to obtain appropriate consultation promptly.

PHYSICAL EXAMINATION

The musculoskeletal system is examined first by inspection, looking for anomalies in contour and position, and observing the spontaneous and reflex movements of the infant; and second, by palpation and manipulation to determine whether there are abnormalities of passive motion. This is followed by stimulation, where indicated, to observe active motion.

A routine for examining a newborn should be developed so that the examination will be complete. This routine may vary with each physician, but each part of the musculoskeletal system should be examined systematically.

Head and Neck

The neck is examined passively for rotation, lateral flexion, anterior flexion, and extension. Rotation of 80° and lateral flexion of 40° should be present. Both of these motions are normally symmetrical to the right and left. Extension and flexion are difficult to measure, but in flexion the chin should touch or nearly touch the chest wall, and on extension the occiput should touch or almost touch the back of the neck. When there is asymmetrical rotation or lateral flexion, or when motion is limited, radiographs of the neck should be made.

Upper Extremities

The clavicle and shoulder girdle including the scapula and proximal humerus, elbow, forearm, and hand are inspected and palpated, looking for anomalies in contour and postural attitudes. Range of motion of the shoulder girdle is evaluated. Flexion and abduction of the shoulder is 175° to 180°. Extension, internal rotation, and external rotation of the shoulder should be at least 25°, 80° and 45° respectively.

The elbow is next inspected and its motion is evaluated. Normally the newborn's elbow lacks 10° to 15° from going to full extension and flexes 145°. The forearm should pronate and supinate at least 80°. Limitation of these two motions can be easily missed. Supination and pronation are tested by holding the humerus at the side of the trunk with the elbow held flexed 90° with one hand, while supination and pronation are checked with the other. The wrist flexes 75° or 80° and extends 65° to 75°. The normally clenched fist of the newborn should have full passive extension of the thumb and all fingers. Active finger extension may be elicited if necessary by a pinprick to the palm. Extension should be to 0° at the metacarpal phalangeal joint, but active extension of the interphalangeal joint usually lacks 5° to 15° from going to 0°.

Spine

In the newborn, congenital anomalies of the spine are not readily detectable on physical examination. However, gross anomalies can be recognized by inspection of the spine, and by passive flexion, extension and lateral bending of the spine. Flexion and extension should be smooth and regular, but lateral flexion may be slightly asymmetrical secondary to *in utero* position. A hairy patch, cutaneous vascular pattern, or lipomatous masses are frequent telltale signs of underlying axial anomalies.

Lower Extremities

The lower extremities are observed for symmetry, variations in contour, position, and size. The hips of a newborn will flex 145° and generally have a flexion contracture as shown by the Thomas test. This test is performed by flexing both hips fully, then extending the hip to be tested while the opposite hip is held in flexion to lock the pelvis. The number of degrees that the extended thigh lacks from going to 0° extension is the degree of flexion contracture present. It is normal for the newborn to have a 25° to 30° flexion contracture. The hip flexion contracture gradually diminishes during the first 12 weeks or so of life but on occasion will be present longer than 3 months. The stability of the hip must always be evaluated by doing an Ortolani test (see Fig. 38-14). Internal and external rotation of the hip in general will range between 40° and 80°, and abduction between 45° and 75°, while normal adduction is between 10° and 20°.

Babies who have not been in the breech position will generally have a knee flexion contracture of 10° to 25° with additional ability to flex to 120° to 145°. In those born breech,

the knees will usually hyperextend 10° to 15° and have limitation of flexion.

Examination of the ankles and feet should include observation of the resting position, stimulation for active motion by stroking the sole, dorsum, medial, and lateral sides of the foot to observe the range of active motion. Passive motion of the ankle in both dorsiflexion and plantar flexion varies depending on the *in utero* position, but dorsiflexion to above neutral should always be present and plantar flexion of less than 10° below neutral would generally be abnormal. Abduction and adduction of the forefoot is at least 10° to 15°, and the hindfoot has 5° to 10° or more of motion in both varus and valgus.

MUSCULOSKELETAL ANOMALIES

It is not within the scope of this text to discuss all of the congenital and acquired abnormalities of the musculoskeletal system seen in the neonate. Most of the common abnormalities are covered in this chapter.

Anomalies of Duplication and Reduction

Supernumerary parts, absence or reduction anomalies of the extremities, and segmentation defects of the limb should offer no problem in diagnosis. These anomalies seldom need immediate attention, but should be seen early by the orthopedist to plan appropriate therapy and discuss prognosis with the family. This is true in both the upper and lower extremities.

Syndactylism is a common anomaly and easily recognized. A synchondrosis or synostosis may be associated with syndactyly. It is important to determine whether or not there is union between two or more digits because this affects the timing of surgical treatment. Correction of the syndactylism is usually done after 3 years of age, but where a synostosis interferes with growth or is creating a deformity of one finger, repair needs to be done earlier.

Polydactyly is correctable by surgery. Timing of surgical treatment depends upon the extent of the duplication. When the duplication does not contain bone or cartilage it should be removed in infancy. Where there is a question of function, surgical correction should wait until one can be certain of the degree of

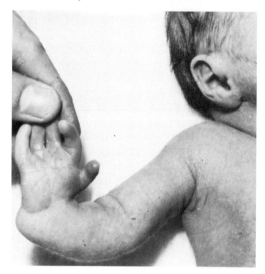

Fig. 38-1. Congenital absence of the radius.

function present in each of the duplicated digits.

Absence of the radius, commonly called **radial club-hand,** is easily recognized (Fig. 38-1). The wrist and hand are deviated 90° or more. Early treatment by corrective splints may be sufficient to correct the radial deviation and prepare the extremity for surgery at a later date. Absence of the radius may be bilateral or unilateral and is frequently associated with aplastic anemia. The thumb may be present, absent, or hypoplastic.

Congenital absence of the thumb occurs as an isolated anomaly or may be associated with a radial club-hand. When unilateral, little, or no treatment is needed, but when the absence is bilateral, pollicization of the dominant hand will improve function.

Anomalies of the Neck

Klippel–Feil is a defect in segmentation of the cervical vertebrae. There is both a decrease in the number of vertebrae and fusion of two or more of the vertebrae. The neck appears shorter than normal and motion is limited in all directions. The limitation of motion depends upon the number of fused segments, and is frequently asymmetrical in both rotation and lateral flexion. The asymmetrical motion may simulate muscular torticollis but x-ray examination of the neck can confirm the presence of the Klippel–Feil deformity. Treatment

started early and consisting in passive stretching of the neck to improve rotation, lateral bending, and flexion-extension, if done several times a day, may improve the range of motion of the neck.

Torticollis of the noenate may be one of several types. The typical muscular torticollis (Fig. 38-2A) has a mass that appears in the sternocleidomastoid at 2 weeks of age. The mass gradually disappears during the next 8 to 10 weeks. This mass may go unnoticed and the torticollis not be recognized until there is facial asymmetry and limited motion of the neck. The physical findings of muscular torticollis are limited rotation of the neck toward the side of the lesion (Fig. 38-2B and C) and limited lateral flexion away from the lesion. In well-established, persistent torticollis, there is flattening of the maxillary and frontal bones on the side of the lesion and of the occiput on the opposite side. The asymmetry is not present in the newborn but may become apparent as early as 2 or 3 weeks and is progressive until the tightness is corrected.

Initial treatment of torticollis is by passive exercises and appropriate positioning of the infant in bed. The neck should be gently but firmly stretched, four or five times each day, toward the direction of limited rotation and lateral flexion. Sandbags or some similar objects may be used to position the baby's head to prevent it from assuming the position that the tight muscle encourages.

There is a type of congenital torticollis that is associated with neither a mass in the sternocleidomastoideus nor cervical spine abnormalities. In these infants, there is a myostatic contracture of the sternocleidomastoideus probably secondary to *in utero* position. This type of torticollis is often associated with scoliosis, an abductor contracture of one hip and adductor tightness of the opposite hip, and there may be acetabular dysplasia opposite to the hip with abductor tightness (Fig. 38-3). The torticollis will usually correct with little or no treatment. However, the tight abductor and adductor should be treated by passive stretching, particularly the abductor, plus the use of multiple diapers or some other abduction device. It is rare for the dysplasia to progress to dislocation but it may happen as in this case. When there is scoliosis with asymmetrical lateral flexion, exercises to improve flexibility of the spine should also be done.

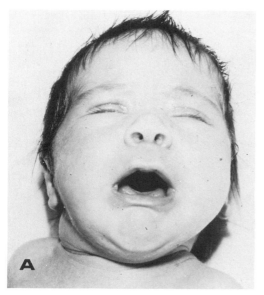

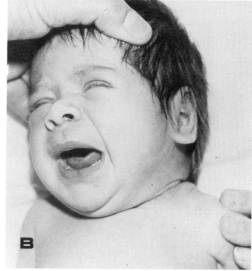

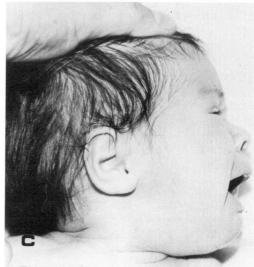

Fig. 38-2. **A.** Congenital muscular torticollis. There is a fibrous mass in the right sternocleidomastoideus muscle. **B.** Rotation toward the right is limited by the tightness in the right sternocleidomastoideus muscle. **C.** Rotation toward the left is normal.

Spine

Most congenital anomalies of the spine are not recognized in the newborn by physical examination, but are diagnosed by radiographs that are made for other reasons. Exceptions to this are anomalies such as rigid scoliosis, kyphosis, and a myelomeningocele (dysraphism), or where there is an abnormality of the skin over a defect in the spine. These can all be appreciated by palpation and inspection. The lower extremities may be affected when there is a severe congenital axial skeletal anomaly.

Treatment of **congenital scoliosis** should be-

gin in the first few weeks of life, by having the baby sleep in an apparatus that keeps the trunk laterally flexed toward the convexity and by passively bending the trunk toward the convexity several times a day. When the curve is progressive, spinal fusion will be needed and should be done before the curve becomes severe enough to be cosmetically or functionally significant. Fusion of a short segment may be done as early as 2 or 3 years of age if necessary. Congenital scoliosis has a high incidence of associated genitourinary anomalies, and an excretory pyelogram should be done on all patients with this abnormality.

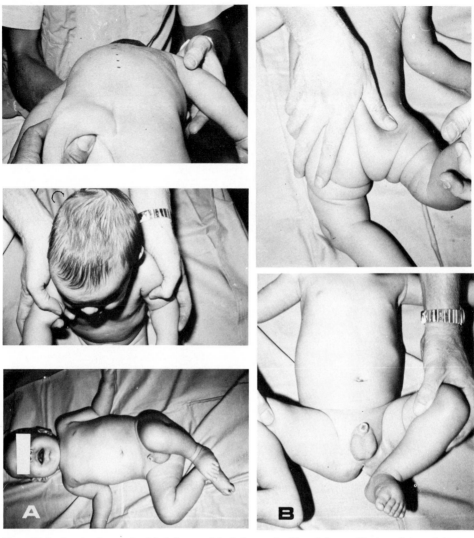

Fig. 38-3. A. A 6-month-old infant with left torticollis, left scoliosis, right abductor contracture, and left adductor tightness. **B.** The right abductor is tight. The left adductor is tight.

Meningomyelocele. Diagnosis of a meningomyelocele generally poses little problem when there is a skin defect (Fig. 38-4). However, the skin is not always defective, and any soft mass in the middle of the spine or off the midline must be examined closely to determine whether or not it is a meningomyelocele. Lipomas, however, always have good skin coverage and may be off the midline.

The care of the infant born with a meningomyelocele is complex and requires input from several specialties. (See also Chap. 40.) It is important to determine immediately after birth the level of involvement of the meningomyelocele. This can be done by inspection of the back, review of radiographs, and a careful examination of the muscle function of the lower extremities. If the meningomyelocele is to be surgically closed, it should be done a few hours after birth, but after the radiographs and muscle evaluation have been done.

The most common lower extremity deformities associated with meningomyelocele are in the feet. Initial treatment of the deformed foot is with plaster cast correction. When correction is not possible by this method, surgical

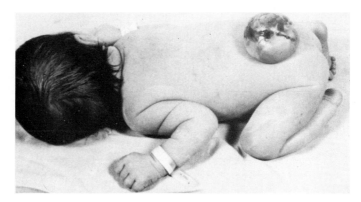

Fig. 38-4. Meningomyelocele.

releases are usually effective. Transfer of muscle insertions are frequently needed to maintain the postsurgical correction and these may be done at almost any age.

Flexion or extension deformities of the knee can be treated by splinting and gentle passive exercises. New splints need to be made every 2 or 3 days as the deformity improves.

Dislocated hips in the patient with a lesion of L3–L4 or below should be treated first in the same way as the ordinary congenital hip. Early traction followed by cast immobilization after reduction is satisfactory. In lesions above L2, reduction, if easily obtained, may be maintained by immobilization of the hips in abduction and extension. The flexed, abducted, externally rotated position should not be used in treating dislocated hips in the infant with lesion above L2 because this position frequently leads to the development of fixed contractures that prevent the hips from extending and adducting.

There is now a philosophy developing related to the wisdom of aggressive treatment of the child with a meningomyelocele. The infants with high lumbar—low thoracic meningomyeloceles have a very high early mortality, and this is significantly lowered by early surgical closure of the meningomyelocele. The evidence gathered on the degree of disability and mental retardation can be correlated very well with the level of the defect, the presence and degree of the hydrocephalus, and the presence of a bony kyphosis. Lesions above L1, in an infant with increased head circumference who has a kyphosis, will almost without exception be accompanied by severe mental and motor disability. Some physicians are proponents of discussing the prognosis with the family, and,

with their concurrence, of withholding surgical closure, and treating the infant with general life-supporting measures only.

Upper Extremities

Sprengel's deformity (congenital elevated scapula) is one of the more common congenital anomalies of the shoulder girdle. It may be bilateral or unilateral and is usually associated with other anomalities such as Klippel–Fell, congenital anomalies of the upper thoracic vertebrae, or anomalies of the ribs. The asymmetry of the shoulder with unilateral involvement makes recognition easier. On palpation, the scapula is high and rotated outward and downward so that its vertebral border lies superiorly and more horizontal than normal. Shoulder abduction and flexion is usually but not always limited. The early conservative treatment is passive range of motion exercises. Surgical correction at 3 or 4 years of age and up to 16 years of age generally improves appearance and function. The overall improvement from surgery is better in the younger child.

The clavicle has two congenital malformations. These are congenital pseudarthrosis and congenital absence of part or all of the clavicle. The physical signs of congenital pseudarthrosis are angulation of the clavicle, and a painless bulbar mass in the midclavicle area (Fig. 38-5). Palpation will confirm both of the above. The shoulder girdle is hypermobile and there is motion in the clavicle at the site of the pseudarthrosis. Early treatment is not needed. Surgical correction by grafting of the defect at 3 or 4 years of age is usually successful, but the need for such treatment is controversial and each patient needs to be individualized.

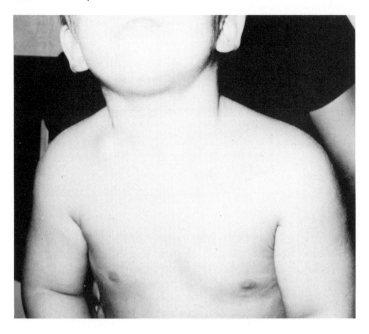

Fig. 38-5. A 2-year-old child was seen with pseudarthrosis of the clavicle.

Partial or complete absence of the clavicle may be recognized by palpation and by the presence of scapulothoracic excessive motion (Fig. 38-6). The completely absent clavicle is usually associated with cranial dysostosis or with a widened pubic symphysis. There are no symptoms and no treatment is needed. With partial absence of the clavicle, the end of the bone may irritate the brachial plexus. In such case, the fragment will need to be excised. Whereas congenital pseudarthrosis is usually an isolated anomaly, partial absence of the clavicle is almost always associated with an axial or appendageal skeletal anomaly.

Defects of Limb Segmentation

Synostosis of the elbow and synostosis of the radius and ulna are two of the more common skeletal anomalies in this group. The elbow synostosis is easily recognized by the lack of motion, and, in addition, the extremity is almost always significantly smaller than its

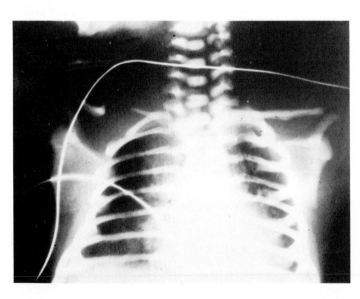

Fig. 38-6. Partial absence of the right clavicle.

opposite member. Synostosis of the radius and ulna is seldom diagnosed in the nursery and it is not uncommon for the child to be several years old before anyone recognizes the abnormality. This is particularly true if the defect is bilateral because the child will not appreciate a difference in the two arms. Supinating and pronating the forearm in the initial examination of the newborn should demonstrate this anomaly.

Lower Extremities

Variations in contours and postural attitudes of the lower extremities in general and the foot in particular are frequent causes of concern. The feet *in utero* seldom rest at a neutral position, being either dorsiflexed, plantarflexed, inverted, or everted, or having a combination of these positions. At times, it may be difficult to determine whether or not there is a structural deformity present.

Feet. Metatarsus adductus may be either a positional deformity (Fig. 38-7) with no bony abnormality or a structural deformity. It is not always easy to determine whether a metatarsus adductus is positional or structural. The decision becomes easier with time because the positional metatarsus adductus corrects fairly rapidly by passive exercises or even without treatment. The structural deformity does not spontaneously correct, and usually becomes more rigid with time.

The differentiation between a postural and structural metatarsus adductus is made mostly by physical examination. In the structural metatarsus adductus (Fig. 38-7A), the base of the fifth metatarsal and the cuboid are prominent. There is an impressive, well-defined skin crease on the medial side of the foot at the first metatarsal-cuneiform joint. The lateral and medial borders of the foot in a positional metatarsus adductus are curved more gently than in the structural deformity. However, the most significant physical finding is the presence or absence of rigidity of the forefoot as determined by its resistance to abduction. In the structural deformity, the forefoot usually cannot be abducted beyond the midline (Fig. 38-7B), whereas in the positional deformity the forefoot is more flexible and can be abducted (Fig. 38-7C). The heel of the structural metatarsus adductus foot is usually, but not always, in valgus and in the positional deformity it is likely to be in varus or at neutral. The valgus

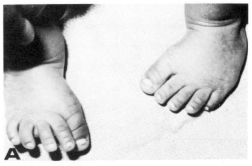

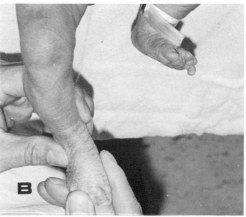

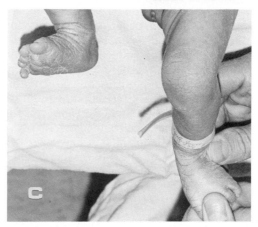

Fig. 38-7. A. Structural metartarsus adductus. **B.** Structural metatarsus adductus. The forefoot does not abduct beyond neutral. **C.** Positional metatarsus. The forefoot abducts beyond the midline.

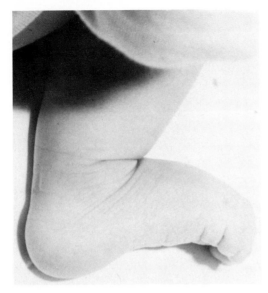

Fig. 38-8. Talipes calcaneovalgus.

position of the hindfoot can be seen on clinical evaluation and, if necessary, confirmed by x-ray studies.

Treatment of the positional flexible deformity is either observation or passive stretching. Stretching the forefoot into abduction is done with the foot held as in Figure 38-7**B.** The structural metatarsus adductus generally needs to be treated with repeated cast changes.

Talipes calcaneovalgus is not a structural deformity but rather a reflection of the foot's *in utero* position (Fig. 38-8). The sole lies against the uterine wall, and the foot is dorsiflexed so that its dorsal skin lies against the anterior surface of the tibia. The fibula is prominent and appears to be dislocated posteriorly, being pushed backward by the excessive dorsiflexion. There is a depression over

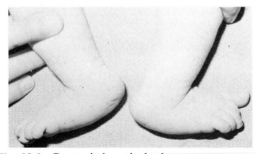

Fig. 38-9. Congenital vertical talus.

the sinus tarsus. The calcaneovalgus foot is flexible and passively plantarflexes at least to neutral and, in most, to 5° to 10° beyond neutral.

Treatment of the calcaneovalgus foot is either by passive exercises or corrective plaster cast according to the severity of the deformity. Mild cases are treated with exercises which stretch the foot into equinus and varus. The motion is repeated 15 to 20 times at four to five sessions daily.

The more severe resistant deformities, those that flex only to neutral plantarflexion, are treated by repeated application of plaster cast for 8 weeks. Casts are changed as needed with growth, and, at each cast change, the foot is placed in equinus and varus with a mold placed in the arch to relax the plantar ligaments and posterior tibialis muscle. The problem to be avoided by cast treatment is that, with the foot held dorsiflexed and everted *in utero*, the plantar ligament and posterior tibialis tendons are stretched out so that their function of supporting the medial-plantar arch is compromised. Early plaster treatment appears to give these children a better chance at having strong feet.

It is important that the positional calcaneovalgus foot not be confused with **congenital vertical talus,** a rare but serious anomaly. In congenital vertical talus the forefoot is dorsiflexed and the hindfoot is in equinus (Fig. 38-9). The talus is rigidly fixed in plantar flexion and if the examiner places one thumb on the talus and with the other hand dorsiflexes and plantarflexes the foot, the talus will remain almost stationary as the forefoot moves around it. The forefoot cannot be plantarflexed as much as in the calcaneovalgus foot, and seldom can it be plantarflexed more than 5° beyond neutral. An x-ray examination of the foot will demonstrate the hindfoot equinus and forefoot dorsiflexion plus the other radiographic characteristics of this anomaly. Although treatment will not create a normal foot, the results are far better with early treatment.

The classical **clubfoot** is a developmental anomaly of the entire foot (Fig. 38-10). There is varus of the hindfoot, varus and adduction of the forefoot, and equinus that is not apparent until the varus and adduction are corrected to neutral. This is a structural deformity, and resists correction; it is easily recognized by its rigidity. There is a positional equinovarus foot

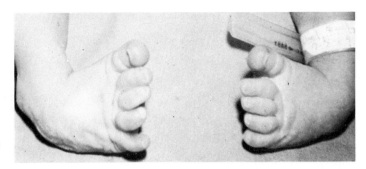

Fig. 38-10. Talipes equinocavovarus foot (club-foot).

that may resemble the true clubfoot but it is flexible and can be corrected beyond neutral with little difficulty. Treatment of the structural clubfoot is by repeated manipulation and strapping, or by manipulation and application of a cast. Treatment should start on the day of birth. When conservative measures are unsuccessful in correcting the foot, surgical correction is necessary.

Tibia and Fibula. Significant deformities of the tibia and fibula do not occur frequently and are not difficult to recognize when present. Congenital absence of the tibia or fibula, congenital amputation, and congenital bowing are all easily recognized. When the tibia is absent, the foot is in varus, and when the fibula is absent the foot has an equinovalgus deformity. These deformities should be seen by the orthopedist early because conservative and supervised treatment of the foot deformities is indicated in some of these children, and in others early amputation is the treatment of choice.[1,2,3]

Anterior bowing of the tibia is a serious deformity (Fig. 38-11). The bone of the tibia is of poor quality, and in most cases it is either sclerotic with partial or complete obliteration of the intermedullary space or has cystic areas that contain material which is similar to fibrous dysplasia. There may be a pseudarthrosis present at birth or a fracture is likely to occur within the first 2 years of life. A pseudarthrosis always follows the fracture. Protection of the tibia by casts and braces is important and may be sufficient to prevent a fracture. Although the case shown in Figure 38-11 is mild, there is a narrowed intramedullary canal, and the bone needs protection, for should it fracture, it is not likely to heal. There is no tendency for these cases to spontaneously improve.

Conversely, the tibia that is bowed poste-riorly corrects spontaneously, seldom fractures, and, if a fracture does occur, it usually heals. The posteriorly bowed tibia needs only to be observed (Fig. 38-12).

The majority of babies have an inward or medial torsion of the leg distal to the knee and outward rotation above the knee. The medial torsion below the knee may occur in the knee, tibia, ankle, or a combination of these, and, except in extreme cases, no treatment is necessary because alignment will progressively improve.

Knee. Significant deformities of the knee are very rare. Recurvatum, a frequent positional

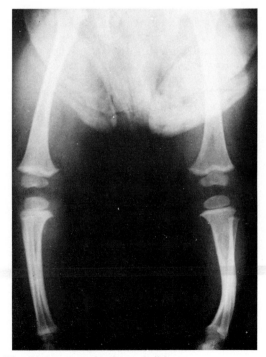

Fig. 38-11. Anterior bowed tibia.

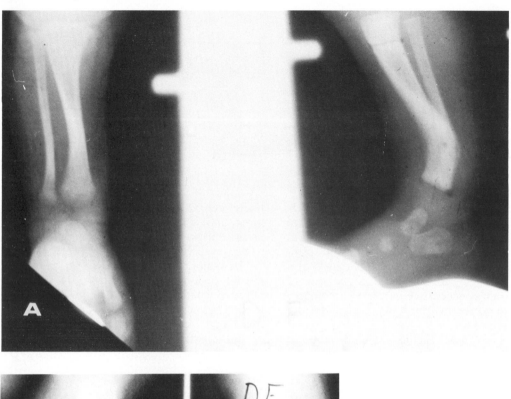

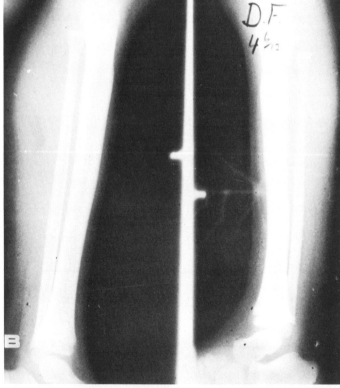

Fig. 38-12. A. Posterior bowed tibia in a 1-month-old infant. B. The same patient at 4 years of age.

deformity associated with a breech delivery, is not serious and will respond to gentle exercising. However, a congenital dislocation of the knee is a serious deformity which superficially may resemble a recurvatum deformity. It is important that the two be differentiated because the dislocation needs to be relocated and the tibia realigned with the femur. In the congenital dislocation, the tibia is usually anteriorly dislocated on the femur and can be hyperextended but cannot flex beyond neutral. One can demonstrate by palpation that the tibia is anteriorly displaced and an x-ray film of the knee will confirm the dislocation.

Congenital fibrosis of part of the quadriceps is an anomaly that if present will prevent knee flexion. Children having congenital fibrosis generally lie with the knee in extension. Active and passive flexion is limited and is seldom more than 40°. When there is limitation of knee flexion, this condition should be suspected as a possible cause. Treatment is by surgical excision of the fibrous mass.

Hip. **Congenital dislocation of the hip** should be diagnosed and treatment started before the baby is discharged from the nursery. Treatment is easier on the family and child and the results are far better than when treatment is started several months or years later. There are two basic types of congenital dislocated hips. The more common of the two is the perinatal or postnatal type, and the other is a teratogenic dislocation that occurs early in fetal life.

Congenital dislocation of the hips occurs more frequently in females. It is usually unilateral with the left hip more frequently affected, but may be bilateral. The dislocation is almost always reduced in flexion and abduction, and is usually but not always stable if held flexed 90° or above and then abducted. In the newborn, radiographs of the hip are not necessarily diagnostic, although, in some, the hip appears laterally displaced in the AP projection as in Figure 38-13.

In the newborn, the typical dislocated hip does not have the classic signs of dislocation, such as asymmetrical skin folds, limited abduction, and shorter-appearing femur (Galeazzo sign). These signs are secondary and develop usually by the end of 6 weeks of life as the hip migrates laterally and superiorly. Diagnosis in the newborn is made by demonstrating that the femoral head can be lifted into the acetabulum as the thigh is abducted in flexion (Fig. 38-14**A**), and that it dislocates as the hip is adducted (Fig. 38-14**B**). This is the Ortolani's test and is positive in the dislocated hip until 6 to 8 weeks of age and sometimes even longer. In addition to feeling the dislocation as the thigh is adducted, the examiner should reduce the hip by abduction in flexion and, while maintaining the same degree of abduction, extend the thigh and the hip will dislocate. In each instance, whether dislocation is obtained by adducting or by extending the thigh, the examiner not only can feel the hip dislocate but see the sudden jerk that occurs as the femoral head rides out of the acetabulum.

Not all hips that dislocate on adduction in the newborn are destined to remain dislocated. If, on the first day, the hip has a positive Ortolani, it should be reexamined at 3 and at 5 days. If the hip is stable at 3 to 5 days (*i.e.,* the hip is neither dislocated nor dislocatable on adduction), no treatment is needed. If at 5 days the Ortolani is still positive, the hip needs to be treated in a splint that will hold it flexed to 90° or above and abducted. Hip x-rays in both the AP and horizontal planes should be taken with the child in the splint to determine that the hip is held reduced. Rarely, the hip dislocates posteriorly in the splint but appears to be reduced in the AP view; only the horizontal view will show the dislocation in this instance.

All infants should have follow-up hip examinations at 6 and 12 weeks. The Ortolani's test may still be positive, but more common late physical signs of congenital dislocation of the hip are asymmetrical folds, an apparent leg length discrepancy (caused by pelvic obliquity and a high riding femoral head), limited abduction, and a palpable defect anteriorly in the groin where the femoral head should be if normal. These signs, plus a high trochanter and piston or telescoping motion, are sufficient to make the diagnosis. Roentgenograms should be made to confirm the diagnosis, and whenever there is doubt.

The teratogenic dislocation presents an entirely different problem. The hip dislocates early in fetal life and ordinarily will not reduce by flexion and abduction because the femoral head is displaced proximally. Therefore, the Ortolani's sign is usually not present in the teratogenic dislocation. If the dislocation is unilateral, there is asymmetry of abduction of

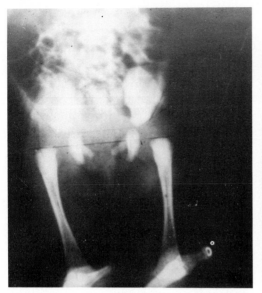
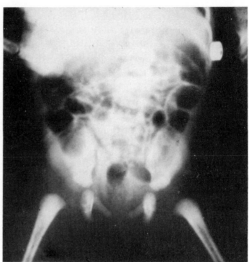

Fig. 38-13. Bilateral congenital dislocation of the hip.

the hips. The dislocated hip will have more extension than the opposite hip and rotation may also be limited. When the dislocation is bilateral, the diagnosis is more difficult because there is no asymmetry. Abduction of both hips is limited, the thighs appear short in relation to the lower legs and the perineum appears wider than normal. The diagnosis is usually made by x-ray examination which in the teratogenic dislocation is always abnormal.

Proximal femoral focal deficiency, commonly called PFFD, is an anomaly of serious magnitude. It may be either unilateral or bilateral. The degree of deficiency is variable and ranges

from absence of the diaphysis and upper metaphysis and femoral head to a very short femur with coxa vara of the neck and head. It is not uncommon for the fibula to be absent and the foot deformed in the more severely affected infant. The shortness of the femur is obvious on inspection. Motion of the hip may be limited. Early referral to the orthopedist who will give the definitive treatment is important. Initial treatment may include stretching exercises, traction, or both to correct contractures about the hip. Definitive surgical management depends upon the potential for function in the extremity, and ranges from

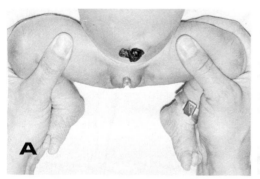
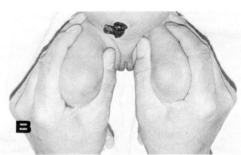

Fig. 38-14. A. Ortolani's sign. The fingers are on the trochanter and thumb grips the femur as shown. The femur is lifted forward as the thighs are abducted. If the head was dislocated it can be felt to reduce. **B.** The thighs are adducted and if the head dislocates it will be both felt and seen as it suddenly jerks over the acetabulum.

measures to correct leg length discrepancy to fusion of the knee and amputation of the foot to create a stump for an above knee prosthesis.

GENERALIZED MUSCULOSKELETAL ANOMALIES

The many syndromes that primarily involve either the epiphysis, epiphyseal plate, metaphysis, or diaphysis are, with few exceptions, easily recognized by their phenotypes. There is similarity of all of the chondrodystrophies, but there are important differences in prognosis. Because the classification of the various types is generally made by the x-ray appearance of the skeleton, roentgenograms of the spine, skull, and extremities should be examined before making a diagnosis and discussing prognosis with the parent.[4] There is little that needs to be done for most of these syndromes, but where there is a deformity, treatment should be undertaken early.

Achondroplasia, chondroectodermal dysplasia (Ellis–van Creveld disease), and **epiphyseal dysostosis (diastrophic dwarfism)** are three of the more common congenital generalized skeletal affectations recognizable at birth that are associated with dwarfism. Children with large heads, short extremities, excessive or restricted motion of joints, unusual appearing faces, and short, stubby phalanges raise suspicion that a skeletal dysplasia is present which can usually be identified by radiographs of the skull, spine, and extremities.[5] However, infants affected by certain skeletal ''dysplasias'' and by metabolic skeletal affectations appear normal at birth, with the skeletal anomalies appearing later in infancy and childhood.

Osteogenesis imperfecta is a generalized disturbance of the skeleton manifested by soft, fragile bone (Fig. 38-15). It is very obvious at birth if severe, but may be mild enough not to be diagnosed until the child is several years old. It involves the skeleton but also affects the skin, ligaments, tendons, sclera, nose, ear, platelet function and probably other systems.[6,7]

The diagnosis of osteogenesis imperfecta is not difficult when there are multiple fractures, a very soft skull, paradoxic respirations, and bluish gray sclera. For those who survive the delivery, gentle handling to prevent further injuries and skin traction to align the extremities are important considerations. It is possible to align all four extremities simultaneously with traction. The fractures heal rapidly and by 9 or 10 days, the traction can usually be discontinued.[8]

Arthrogryposis multiplex congenita (Fig. 38-16) is an uncommon but easily recognizable affectation of the musculoskeletal system. All four extremities and the trunk may be affected or the abnormalities may be limited to the arms or legs. The hallmark of this entity is the lack of active and passive motion in the affected extremities.

The microscopic picture of the muscle in arthrogryposis shows changes of denervation and fibrofatty replacement. Secondary to the muscle weakness and dysfunction, there is distortion of the joints, as well as limitation of motion. Frequently, these infants have dislocation of the hips, knees, or radial heads or combinations of the three. In addition many have either clubfeet or vertical talus, both of which are more resistant to treatment than those not associated with arthrogryposis. Treatment should begin in the nursery, and is directed at increasing the motion of all affected joints by passive exercises done 6 to 8 times each day. Joint dislocation and the hand and foot deformities should be treated early by appropriate plaster splints, casts, or by traction.

BIRTH INJURIES

Long, difficult labor, particularly with the breech position, a large infant, or fetal distress requiring rapid extraction make birth injuries frequent. Birth fractures almost always involve the clavicle, humerus, or femur. It is rare for birth fractures in a normal infant to occur below the elbow or below the knee. The fracture is more likely to be through either the diaphysis or the epiphyseal plate, so that the epiphysis and epiphyseal plate are separated from the metaphysis. At times the fractures are painless and diagnosis is made incidental to a radiograph taken for unrelated indications. In others, the fracture is painful and is a cause of pseudoparalysis, with the limb lying limp and not moving on stimulation.

Diaphyseal Fractures

Fractures of the diaphysis of the humerus are generally diagnosed by the obstetrician, who hears and feels the snap when the humerus fractures as the baby is being extracted. The

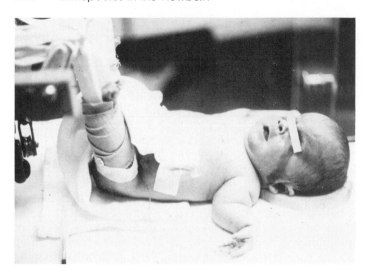

Fig. 38-15. Osteogenesis imperfecta.

same can be said about fractures of the femoral shaft. A radiograph confirms the fracture.

A fracture of the shaft of the humerus is treated by immobilization of the arm by the side. Soft padding is placed between the arm

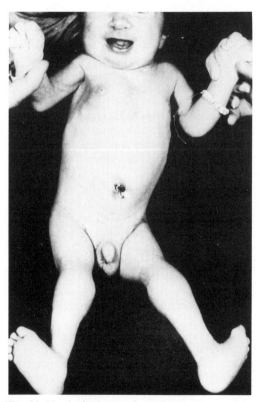

Fig. 38-16. Arthrogryposis multiplex congenita.

and the chest and the elbow is held at 90° flexion.

Fractures of the femoral shaft can be held with a posterior splint that extends from below the knee to over the buttock and is held in place with an elastic bandage for 10 to 14 days.

Fractures of the clavicle may be asymptomatic if undisplaced and need no treatment except care in handling the infant. If the fracture is displaced, it is usually painful. The fracture can be treated either by strapping the arm to the chest with padding placed in the axilla and the elbow flexed 90°, or by a figure-of-eight bandage made of stockinette used to immobilize the fracture. In 8 to 10 days, the callus is sufficient for the immobilization to be discontinued.

Epiphyseal Injuries

The epiphyseal separation or fracture occurs through the hypertrophied layer of cartilage cells in the epiphysis. A fracture through the proximal epiphyseal plate of the humerus is one of the more common skeletal injuries associated with a difficult delivery (Fig. 38-17A). The diagnosis has to be made primarily on the clinical findings of swelling about the shoulder, and crepitus and pain when the shoulder is moved. Motion is painful and the arm lies limp by the side. The proximal humeral epiphysis is not ossified at birth and is therefore not visible on x-ray. This makes diagnosis by x-ray very difficult. If there is complete or almost complete separation of the epiphysis,

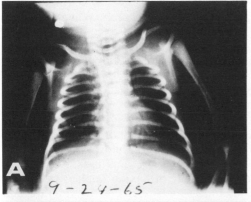

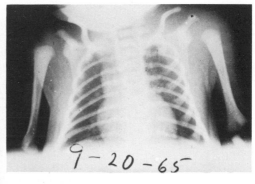

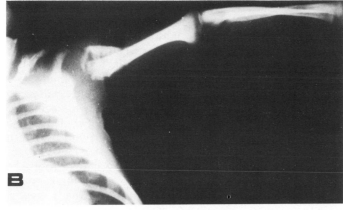

Fig. 38-17. A. This injury to the left shoulder, the **top** shows only swelling. The **bottom** film 4 days later shows the clavicle obviously fractured. **B.** Ten days after birth a callus formation is visible.

the metaphysis appears displaced in relation to the glenoid of the scapula, but usually the separation is minimal and there are no x-ray changes except soft tissue swelling. After 8 to 10 days, callus appears and is visible on x-ray (Fig. 38-17**B**).

The treatment for a fracture of the proximal epiphysis of the humerus is immobilization of the arm by the side with soft padding in the axilla for 8 to 10 days. Healing is rapid and remodeling is such that a striking angulation will progressively improve to where the contour appears normal. If a complete separation is present, manipulation and reduction by gentle traction should probably be attempted.

A fracture separation of the distal humeral epiphysis is very rare. It is difficult to diagnose by x-ray because this epiphysis, like the proximal epiphysis, is completely cartilaginous. When an injury is present there will be swelling about the elbow with pain and crepitus on passive motion. If the epiphysis is displaced, the AP radiogram will show that the olecranon is displaced medially or laterally in its rela-

tionship with the long axis of the humerus. A fracture of the distal epiphysis is more likely to have a significant residual deformity than is a fracture of the proximal humeral epiphysis. Traction on the forearm for 9 to 10 days is my preference for treatment of this injury.

Fracture of the proximal femoral epiphysis is an uncommon problem but one that can cause confusion if it is not recognized. It is often confused with a congenital dislocation or with acute pyarthrosis. The epiphyseal plate of the proximal femur is a crescent-shaped line extending from the greater to the lesser trochanter and includes the cartilaginous epiphysis of the trochanter, neck, and femoral head. Swelling about the hip is difficult to appreciate and suspicion of the presence of this injury should be aroused when the baby does not move the extremity on stimulation. This is confirmed by the presence of pain and crepitus when the hip is moved passively. The radiograph of the hip will show the upper end of the femoral metaphysis to be displaced laterally, and, if the separation is complete,

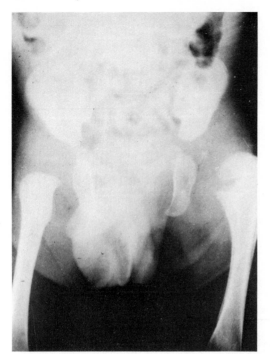

Fig. 38-18. A 3-week-old infant had a birth fracture of the proximal epiphysis of the femur.

the metaphysis is likely to be displaced above the center of the acetabulum as well as displaced laterally. After several days of incomplete separation, the hip will no longer be painful, and, in my experience, most of these have been recognized only after callus formation is seen on an incidental radiograph or after a large massive callus presents as a firm tumorous mass in the groin or upper thigh (Fig. 38-18). If the diagnosis is recognized before healing is underway, the hip should be manipulated gently and immobilized in flexion and abduction for 10 to 14 days. When the diagnosis is uncertain, aspiration of the joint will help differentiate the fracture from the congenital dislocation and acute pyarthrosis. If a fracture is present, blood should be found in the joint.

The diagnosis of a fracture separation of the distal femoral epiphysis can be made by x-ray studies. Ossification of the distal femoral epiphysis is present at birth and even slight displacement and angulation can be recognized. If there is swelling around the knee and pain on passive motion, a radiograph will confirm the diagnosis. Treatment is by im-

mobilization in plaster for 10 to 14 days, if displacement is not severe. When displacement or angulation is excessive, traction should be applied to the leg for reduction and immobilization of the fracture.

Brachial Plexus Injuries
(See also Chap. 41)

Traumatic neuropathy of the brachial plexus is one of the more common birth injuries. It is the result of traction and lateral flexion of the neck. In vertex presentations, it occurs by traction and lateral flexion applied to deliver the shoulder, and in breech by traction and lateral flexion to deliver the head.

The clinical picture is easily recognized by the absence of motion of the involved extremity in the moro reflex. There may be supraclavicular swelling and the clavicle may be fractured in addition to the plexus injury.

There are three types of obstetric palsy and the clinical findings are different in each. The upper plexus type is called Erb–Duchenne (Fig. 38-19), and in this the C5 and C6 nerve roots are affected. In the lower plexus type, known as Klumpke's, the C8 and T1 roots are involved. The third type is a total involvement of all roots that make up the plexus. If the C5 and C6 roots are affected, the shoulder is held internally rotated with the forearm supinated and the elbow extended and the wrist and fingers flexed. When the lower roots, C8 and T1, are involved, the hand is flaccid with little or no control. When the entire plexus is affected, the total extremity is flaccid.

The early treatment of the obstetric palsy is conservative. Myelography and surgical exploration have little to offer in the management of this problem. Recovery of function depends of course on the degree of injury. When the injury is a neuropraxia, complete recovery over several weeks usually takes place. When there is a neurotomesis no recovery takes place. Because it is not possible to say which degree of injury is present, all should be treated by prevention of further injury to the plexus by gentle handling. The arm needs protection for the first 4 or 5 days until swelling has subsided. After this period, the joints of the arm may be carried through a passive range of motion several times each day to maintain flexibility. The paralyzed muscles should be supported in a position of relaxation for most of each day, care being taken that a contraction

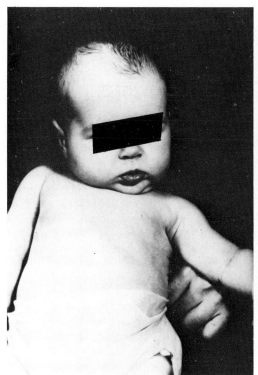 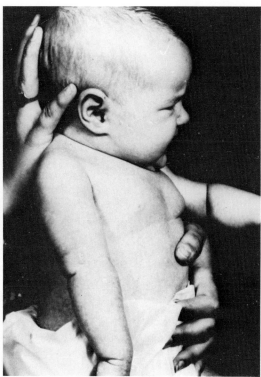

Fig. 38-19. An Erb–Duchenne type of brachial plexus injury.

of the protected muscles does not occur. Denervated muscles undergo fibrosis which can become contractured, producing a fixed deformity.

Passive exercises, protection, and progressive active exercises should be continued for months and years, as long as there is some progressive improvement. At 3 to 5 years, certain residual deformities can be improved surgically.

BONE AND JOINT INFECTIONS

Osteomyelitis and acute septic arthritis occur in the neonate although not as frequently as in older infants. The priorities of treatment are different in osteomyelitis and septic arthritis and the differences are of paramount importance.

Osteomyelitis occurs almost always by hematogenous spread from either a cutaneous, oral, or other lesion. Staphylococcus and streptococcus are the most frequent causative organisms. The infection begins in the metaphysis of long bones. Bacteria reach the metaphysis through the nutrient artery, which terminates in the sinusoids adjacent to the epiphyseal plate.[9,10] The rate of flow in the sinusoid is slower, creating an ideal situation for bacteria to settle and begin to multiply. Edema, vascular engorgement, and cellulitis is followed by thrombosis and abscess formation, with destruction and absorption of trabeculae. The purulent exudate in the metaphysis spreads by way of Volkmann canals to the periosteal space and elevates the loosely attached periosteum, which responds by laying down new bone over the original cortex. The new bone is the envolucrum. In infants, unlike older children, the exudate perforates the cortex of the metaphysis early and does not spread down the diaphysis, sparing the endosteal and haversian vessels, and therefore does not cause massive sequestrum as readily as in older children.

In children beyond infancy, the epiphyseal plate acts as a barrier that prevents spread to the epiphysis. In the infant, Trueta has shown that vessels cross the epiphyseal plate, so that infection of the metaphysis may spread to the epiphysis and cause irreparable damage to the secondary center of the ossification, and the epiphyseal plate.[9]

The neonate with hematogenous osteomyelitis presents with varied complaints and findings. Movement of the affected part may provoke crying. There may be loss of active motion of the affected extremity (pseudoparalysis), or the baby may have unexplained fever. Swelling of the extremity is apparent very early after the onset of bone infection; it is visible in a soft-tissue x-ray film and is palpable. In the newborn, the swelling may be massive, including the entire extremity before visual changes in the bone are apparent on x-ray evaluation. In a newborn with extensive swelling of an extremity, osteomyelitis must be strongly considered as the diagnosis until proven otherwise. Alternatively, the child may be so overwhelmed that he responds very little to stimulation and may even be afebrile. In any child who is seriously ill or who is failing to thrive, careful examination of the extremities should be done, looking for evidence of tenderness, pain, and swelling that may indicate the presence of osteomyelitis.

Treatment early with appropriate antibiotics and immobilization will usually control the infection. If treatment is started too late, abscess formation will occur and requires surgical drainage. Before surgery, the general status of the infant should be good. Dehydration should be corrected and temperature decreased before anesthesia is given.

Acute septic arthritis has even greater urgency in treatment than osteomyelitis in the neonate, although delay in either may cause irreparable damage to the secondary center of ossification. Joint infection is usually by hematogenous spread, although the hip is occasionally infected by needle during attempted femoral vein puncture.

The neonate with septic arthritis is generally very ill but may be so overwhelmed that there is no fever. Failure to thrive, as in osteomyelitis, may be the reason for admission. Pseudoparalysis, pain on passive motion, and swelling and increased warmth are the usual physical findings. Diagnosis is difficult when the hip is affected, for visible swelling and palpable warmth are minimal. X-ray examination will show the joint effusion and distension with widening of the joint space. The hip will frequently be subluxated and, if diagnosis is delayed several days, the intraarticular pressure will cause dislocation of the hip. When dislocation occurs secondary to pyarthrosis, the joint is usually severely and permanently damaged.

Treatment of an infected joint in an infant should generally be by surgical decompression and parenteral antibiotics as soon as the diagnosis is confirmed. If the hip is infected, there is no acceptable alternative to early decompression and débridement. A delay in surgical decompression may cause the hip to dislocate by the increasing accumulation of joint fluid. The blood supply to the femoral head is vulnerable both to the increased pressure and to the products of the infection, and delay in adequate débridement may cause occlusion of the vessels, which will result in further deterioration of the femoral head. Both of these complications can be prevented by early diagnosis and surgical decompression. In other joints, repeated needle aspiration and irrigation may sufficiently debride, but one never knows whether there is pannus covering the joint surface which must be removed to prevent further destruction of the articular cartilage. Because of this open surgical decompression and débridement is a more reliable method than needle aspiration. Infected extremities should be in traction for immobilization and protection. If the hip is affected, traction should pull the thigh into abduction and moderate flexion with the traction force just sufficient to overcome muscle spasm. Great care should be taken not to over-pull the hip so as to cause further distraction. If the hip joint is tending to dislocate, immobilization in abduction and flexion in a spica cast may be needed to maintain reduction of the hip.

REFERENCES

1. **Brown, FW:** Construction of a knee joint in congenital total absence of the tibia. J Bone Joint Surg, 47-A:695, 1965
2. **Farmer AW, Laurin CA:** Congenital absence of the fibula. J Bone Joint Surg 42-A:1, 1960
3. **Wood WL, Zlolsky N, Westin GW:** Congenital absence of the fibula: treatment by Syme amputation-indications and technique. J Bone Joint Surg 47-A:1159, 1965
4. **Ruben P:** Dynamic Classification of Bone Dysplasia, Chicago, Year Book Publishers, Inc., 1964

5. **Fairbank HAT:** An Atlas of General Affectation of the Skeleton. Edinburgh, E & S Livingstone, Ltd. 1951

6. **McKusick VA:** Heritable Disorders of the Connective Tissue, 3rd ed. St. Louis, CV Mosby, 1966

7. **Weber M:** Osteogenesis imperfecta congenita: A study of its histopathogenesis. Arch Pathol, 9:984, 1930

8. **Sofield HA, Miller EA:** Fragmentation, realignment and intramedullary rod fixation of deformities of long bones of children. J Bone Joint Surg 41-A:1371, 1959

9. **Trueta J:** The three types of acute hematogenous osteomyelitis: A clinical and vascular study. J Bone Joint Surg 41-B:671, 1959

10. **Trueta J:** The normal vascular anatomy of the human femoral head during growth. J Bone Joint Surg 39-B:358, 1972

11. **Griffin PP:** Bone and joint infections in children. Pediatr Clin North Am 3:533, 1967

39

Neurologic Disorders

Joseph J. Volpe and
Richard Koenigsberger

This chapter is devoted to the neurologic aspects of neonatal medicine. The first sections concern the neurologic evaluation of the neonate. Separate consideration is given to the findings associated with normal neurologic development and to the abnormal neurologic findings resulting when such development is deranged by disease or by an inborn error in the developmental program. The next two sections treat separately two common and often perplexing neurologic manifestations: apnea and periodic breathing, and seizures. The remainder of the chapter deals with the most important pathologic categories of neurologic disease, hypoxic-ischemic perinatal brain injury, intracranial hemorrhage, and developmental disorders. The important infectious and metabolic derangements are covered in other chapters.

NEUROLOGIC EVALUATION OF THE NEONATE

NORMAL NEUROLOGIC FINDINGS

The neurologic examination of the newborn infant has been the object of intensive study in many centers in the world, but perhaps the greatest contributions overall have come from the clinics and laboratories of Thomas and Saint-Anne Dargassies, Peiper and Prechtl.[1-4] From their work has evolved an approach to the neurologic examination of the newborn that differs in many respects from the approach used with older infants and children. We have attempted to incorporate into our neurologic evaluation of the newborn some of the important contributions of these workers. At the same time, we have adapted the basic framework of the neurologic examination of older infants and children to the newborn because much of our basic understanding of the mechanisms of neurologic abnormalities in the older patient has been gained by that basic approach.

Level of Alertness

Prior to 28-weeks' gestation, the baby is in a state of persistent stupor. However, at approximately 28 weeks, there is a distinct change in the level of alertness.[5] At that time, the baby can be roused from sleep with a gentle, persistent shake and will remain alert for several minutes. Spontaneous alerting also occurs occasionally at this age. By 32 weeks, stimulation is no longer necessary, and frequently the eyes remain open and spontaneous roving eye movements appear. In addition to increased alertness, vigorous crying appears during wakefulness at about 37 weeks. At 40 weeks the baby has distinct periods of attention to visual and auditory stimuli, and by this age it has been possible to study sleep-waking patterns in detail.[6]

Cranial Nerves

Vision. At 28 weeks, the baby consistently blinks to light.[5] By 32 weeks, eye closure to bright light persists for as long as the light is present (dazzle reflex of Peiper).[3] At 37 weeks, visual following cannot be elicited consistently, but the infant will turn his eyes toward a soft light.[5] By term, however, definite visual following of a bright target (*e.g.,* a flashlight held at approximately 2 feet or a shiny silver bell) or of a dangling object (*e.g.,* a red rubber ball) is readily elicited.[7] Opticokinetic nystagmus, elicited by a rotating drum, is present at term and probably appears somewhat earlier.[3]

Fundi. This portion of the examination is too often omitted. With patience and the aid of a nurse, the fundi can be visualized easily in the neonate. The optic disc is paler than in older infants. Retinal hemorrhages occur in as many as 20% to 40% of all newborns and are usually not associated with concomitant CNS injury or sequelae.[3]

Pupils. The size of the pupils in the newborn period is approximately 2 to 3 mm, and they are equal. Reaction to light may appear as early as 29 weeks but is not consistently present until approximately 32 weeks.[8] The reaction of the pupil to light is approximately 1 mm and is readily visible.

Extraocular Movements. In prematures, the eyes are often dysconjugate, one or the other being 1 to 2 mm out. However, even in the full-term baby, minor degrees of dysconjugate eye movements are present and will persist for several months. Spontaneous roving eye movements appear at approximately 32 weeks.[5] The tracking movements of the full-term and older infant are at first rather jerky and do not become smooth and gliding until approximately the third month of life.[3] At approximately 32-weeks' gestation, full movement with doll's head maneuver becomes obvious, and, similarly, caloric stimulation with cold water will lead to deviation of eyes to the side of the stimulated ear, as in adults. Another convenient means of eliciting oculovestibular responses is to spin the baby held in a vertical position; the eyes will deviate in a direction opposite to the spin.

Facial Motility and Sensation. The basic features of facial sensation and movement are assessed as in older infants. **Spontaneous** facial motility is of greatest importance in the assessment of cerebral lesions, and examination of the face should not be limited to observation of crying, the latter being of particular value in the assessment of peripheral lesions. Especial attention should be paid to the **onset** of movement, as well as to its final amplitude.

Hearing. The premature infant of 28 weeks will startle to loud noise.[5] As the baby matures, more subtle responses become apparent: cessation of motor activity, change in respiratory pattern, opening of mouth, wide opening of eyes, and so on.[3] The relation of such responses to the development of hearing has been the subject of considerable controversy, but it is likely that these responses at least represent the presence of some auditory function. Inability to elicit these responses is usually related to the failure to test in a quiet surrounding and while the baby is alert and not agitated or very hungry. Most frequently a baby that does not respond initially will respond upon retesting under more favorable conditions. More detailed evaluation of auditory function is indicated if responses are consistently absent.

Sucking and Swallowing. The act of feeding requires a concerted action of breathing, sucking and swallowing. Sucking requires the function of cranial nerves 5, 7, and 12, and swallowing, cranial nerves 9 and 10.[3] The concerted action of these functions is adequate for oral feeding as early as 28 weeks and the development of vigorous rooting at this age is an important ancillary feature.[5] However, the 28-week-old infant tires so rapidly that oral feeding is difficult and, in fact, dangerous at this early age. By 32 to 34 weeks, however, the normal infant is able to maintain a concerted action for productive oral feeding.

Taste and Smell. We rarely evaluate these parameters in the examination of the neonate, but their development is worthy of mention here in passing. The 28-week-old infant will demonstrate appropriate facial expression of attraction or repulsion to concentrated solutions of sweetness or to sourness-bitterness-saltiness.[3,5] Normal infants of more than 32 weeks of gestation will respond to peppermint extract with sucking, arousal-withdrawal, or both.[9]

Motor Examination

The major features of the motor examination to be evaluated in the neonatal period are muscle tone and its reflection in the posture of limbs, motility and muscle power, deep tendon reflexes and plantar responses, and several of the primary neonatal reflexes. These will be discussed separately below.

Tone and Posture. Muscle tone is best assessed by passive manipulation of limbs. In addition, tone of various muscles will determine, in large part, the posture of limbs in repose, and thus careful observation of the baby's posture is critical for the proper evaluation of tone in the neonatal period. Some investigators have devised various maneuvers of passive manipulation of limbs (*e.g.,* approximation of heel-to-ear, hand-to-opposite ear, or measurement of angles of certain joints such as the popliteal angle) in an attempt to quantitate these parameters.[10] These maneuvers have not been particularly useful for this examiner and are not discussed in detail below.

At 28 weeks, the baby lies with limbs in full extension, and passive manipulation will corroborate the visual impression of minimal tone in flexors and extensors of limbs. However, by 32 weeks' gestation, flexor tone becomes apparent in the lower extremities, and, in repose, the baby lies with extension of upper limbs but with beginning flexion of lower limbs (popliteal angle 150°).[10] By 36 weeks, flexor tone is prominent in the lower extremities, reflected in a popliteal angle of 90°, and can be noted by manipulation of upper extremities. The baby still tends to keep upper extremities in extension, although periods of flexor posture become apparent. By term, all limbs are maintained in flexor posture and passive manipulation affords appreciation of strong flexor tone in all extremities.

Motility and Power. The quality, quantity, and symmetry of motility and muscle power are the parameters of interest. The normal infant at 28-weeks' gestation demonstrates spontaneous movements during the brief periods of wakefulness.[5] The movements are usually either slow twisting of the limbs or the trunk (perhaps inappropriately, but frequently, termed **athetoid**) or rapid, wide-amplitude, whole-limb movements that occasionally have the qualities of myoclonus or chorea as seen in older patients. These interesting movements are replaced by 32-weeks' gestation by flexor movements, especially at hips and knees, often occurring in unison. Head-turning appears for the first time, but neck flexor or extensor power is negligible as judged by complete head lag on pull to sit or when the infant is held in the sitting position. By 36 weeks, the active flexor movements of lower extremities become more vigorous and often occur in an **alternating** rather than symmetric fashion. Flexor movements of upper extremities appear. For the first time, definite neck extensor power can be observed; when the baby is held sitting, the head is lifted off the chest and maintained in upright posture for several seconds. By term, the awake infant is very active, especially when stimulated slightly with a gentle shake. Limbs move in an alternating manner and neck extensor power is still better. Neck flexor power becomes apparent; when the infant is pulled to a sitting position, the neck flexion results in movement of the head nearly to the same plane as that of the thorax.

Deep Tendon Reflexes and Plantar Response. Deep tendon reflexes readily elicited in the newborn are the biceps, knee, and ankle jerks. The knee jerk is often accompanied by crossed adductor responses and this should be considered a normal finding in the first months of life (less than 10% of normal infants demonstrate crossed adductor responses after 8 months of age).[11] Ankle clonus of approximately 10 beats also should be considered a normal finding in the neonatal period, if no other abnormal neurologic signs are present. Clonus normally disappears rapidly, and more than 3 beats at 1 to 2 months is abnormal. The plantar response has long been considered to be extensor in neonates. That this peculiar notion is, in fact, not the case has been shown by Hogan and her coworkers.[12] Of a group of 100 neonates (both full term and premature), the first movement of the great toe (the critical response) was flexor. Optimally, infants should be awake with the head in the midline and the lateral border of the sole should be stimulated. Care must be taken to avoid eliciting the plantar grasp or positive supporting response, both of which result in plantar flexion of toes, or the nociceptive withdrawal response or avoidance reaction, both of which result in dorsiflexion of toes. If such care is taken, plantar flexion is uniformly seen in the full-term neonate and probably also in the premature.

Primary Neonatal Reflexes. The variety of primary neonatal reflexes recorded in the classic literature on the newborn is astounding and will not be discussed here. We have found useful the Moro reflex, the palmar grasps, and the tonic neck response. The Moro reflex is elicited best by the sudden dropping of the baby's head backward in relation to the trunk (the dropping head should be caught by the examiner) and consists in lateral extension of upper extremities (with opening of hands) followed by anterior flexion and audible cry. The first component appears at 28-weeks' gestation and the latter two at 32 weeks.[5] The reflex disappears by 6 months of age in normal infants.[11] Palmar grasp is clearly present at 28-weeks' gestation, is strong at 32 weeks, and of sufficient power at 36 weeks to allow the infant to be lifted from the bed. The palmar grasps become inconsistent after about 2 months of age, when voluntary grasping begins to develop. The tonic neck response, elicited by rotation of head, consists in extension of the upper extremity on the side to which the face is rotated and flexion of the upper extremity on the side of the occiput. Participation of lower extremities is less definite. The response is usually unimpressive in the neonatal period, but becomes prominent 1 month past term. It disappears by approximately 7 months of age.[11]

Sensory Exam. Apart from observation of "withdrawal" of limbs stimulated by a pinprick, careful evaluation of sensory function has rarely been a part of the usual neonatal neurologic exam. It is noteworthy that the premature of only 28-weeks' gestation differentiates touch and pain, the former resulting in alerting and slight motor activity, and the latter in withdrawal and cry.[5] The rooting reflex elicited by tactile stimulation of the perioral region is well-established by 32-weeks' gestation. By 35 to 36 weeks, there is rapid turning of the head away from a pinprick over the side of the face. We routinely assess response of the infant to multiple pinpricks (5–10) over the medial aspect of the extremities. A lower level response is extremely rapid and consists of a stereotyped response, for example, triple flexion at ankle, knee, and hip. There is no clear response decrement with repeated trials. A higher level response has a latency of approximately 1 to 2 seconds and consists in lateral withdrawal from the stimulus and is accompanied by a grimace, a cry, or both. The response tends to "dampen" with repeated trials, and this characteristic of "habituation" is an important feature of the normal neonatal response.[13] Although more data are needed, it appears that the higher level responses may require intact cerebral hemispheres or at least diencephalic structures.

ABNORMAL NEUROLOGIC FINDINGS

The clinical and anatomic implications of abnormal neurologic findings occurring in the neonatal period will now be considered, but a detailed discussion of all possible diagnoses associated with such findings would detract from the objective of this section and will not be attempted. The clinical and/or anatomic basis of many abnormal findings in the neonatal period have not been delineated, but it will become clear that herein lies a basic and promising field for future research.

Level of Alertness

Accurate assessment of the level of alertness of an infant requires that he be at his optimal level, and thus ideally, the exam should not be carried out immediately after a feeding. The child should be aroused by persistent, gentle shaking until a consistent level of alertness is obtained. In characterizing the level of alertness, we have used only the three terms: alert, stupor, or coma. Babies who are alert behave in the fashion described above in the section on normal neurologic findings for gestational age. Babies are considered to be in coma when there is either no response to a shake, pinch, and certain other stimuli (*e.g.,* a bell or bright light), or when there is a response that is only low-level in type (see above). Babies in states of arousal intermediate between alertness and coma are considered to be either slightly, moderately, or severely stuporous. The causes of diminished level of alertness are many and are alluded to in appropriate sections to follow. Coma and related states occur in older patients when there is marked bilateral cerebral disturbance, or disturbance of the activating system of reticular gray matter present in diencephalon, midbrain, and upper pons.[14] Similar correlates probably pertain to the newborn, but as yet the detailed clinical and anatomic correlates of stupor and coma in neonates are not available.

Cranial Nerves

Vision. Consistent and persistent failure to demonstrate visual following (and opticokinetic nystagmus with rotating drum) in a full-term newborn must be considered a disturbing sign because such visual following is the only definite indication of cerebral function in the newborn period. Most commonly, this deficit is part of a constellation of neurologic abnormalities that suggest major disturbance of the central nervous system including, particularly, the cerebral hemispheres. Blindness is by no means the usual finding on follow-up, and more frequently than not, visual following appears later in the first months of life. However, if pendular, searching nystagmus, digital manipulation of the globe, and hand movements before the eyes appear in the first weeks or months of infancy, congenital blindness is likely and the locus of the disturbance of optic pathways must be sought in the usual way.

Funduscopic examination may reveal a variety of abnormalities in the neonatal period. Particularly noteworthy are large **preretinal hemorrhages** indicative of subarachnoid blood, usually under increased pressure, and **chorioretinitis.** The latter is seen most commonly with congenital toxoplasmosis, cytomegalovirus, herpes simplex, or rubella infection. Chorioretinitis with syphilis usually appears later in infancy or childhood. The retinopathy associated with rubella is readily distinguished from the others in that it consists of small areas of depigmentation and pigmentation in the macular area, "salt-and-pepper appearance," rather than the more typical, large, yellow scarred lesions. The earliest changes of retrolental fibroplasia, vasoconstriction of retinal vessels, may be impossible to detect with certainty, but the early intravitreous proliferative changes of this disease are definitely detectable, especially by indirect ophthalmoscopy. Progression of these changes may be an indication for some of the newer forms of therapy of the disease.[15]

Pupils. Abnormal pupillary findings are of great value in clinical neurology in the localization of pathologic events occurring in older infants and young children. However, their significance in the newborn period remains largely an unexplored field. Marked irregularity in pupil size is not a common feature of neonatal neurologic disorders. One situation in which inequality is distinct is the presence of a Horner's syndrome. We have seen this most commonly with severe lower brachial plexus palsies. Unilateral pupillary dilatation is rare and perhaps reflects the rarity of the uncal form of transtentorial herniation. The infrequency of the latter relates both to the pliability of the neonatal skull and sutures and the rarity of large **unilateral** mass lesions. Pupils which do not react to light should raise the possibility of a drug intoxication or infantile botulism. In advanced hypoxic-ischemic injury or with intraventricular hemorrhage, pupils may be fixed to light in the mid- or dilated position.

Extraocular movements. Minor degrees of dysconjugate eye movements are normal in newborns and young infants. Isolated nerve palsies are not frequent, although the third or sixth nerves may be affected occasionally. These are distinguished from tropias by the doll's-head maneuver, which fails to result in full movement of the eye in nerve palsy. (Retraction of the globe and narrowing of the palpebral fissure on adduction of the affected eye, in addition to limitation of eye abduction, are the features of Duane's syndrome.)[16] Gaze palsies, manifested often by conjugate deviation of eyes to one side, can reflect, in an older patient, primary affection of frontal contraversive eye fields or of gaze centers in the pons for ipsilateral eye movement. These palsies are distinguished by the doll's-head maneuver and by caloric stimulation, which will result in movement of eyes in disturbances of cerebral eye fields but not in disturbances of brain stem gaze centers. More usually in the newborn period, tonic deviation of eyes to one side is a manifestation of seizure (see below). Other frequently noted abnormalities of extraocular movement are skew deviation of eyes, characterized by disparity of eye position in the vertical plane. This abnormality is associated in older patients with lesions in the brain stem involving brachium pontis, the medial longitudinal fasciculus, or both.[14] Whether this is the case in the newborn period is unknown; that this seems likely is supported by our frequent observation of skew deviation in severe brain stem disturbances associated with major intraventricular hemorrhage and severe hypoxic or hypoglycemic encephalopathy. **Ocular bobbing** is an abnormality of eye movement described originally by Fisher and is characterized by intermittent bobbing down and up movements of eyes, usually synchronous, and associated primarily with pontine disturbance.[17] We have noted this finding especially in neonates with severe hypoxic or hypoglycemic encephalopathy. Opsoclonus is a remarkable abnormality of eye movement characterized by frequent, irregular, rapid, multidirectional conjugate jerking of eyes and is associated in older patients with disturbance primarily of cerebellum and its immediate connections.[18] Recently, we have observed this remarkable disturbance in two neonates, one with probable intraventricular hemorrhage and the other with maple syrup urine disease.

Facial Movement. Facial symmetry and movement should be assessed when the child is at rest, during spontaneous facial movement, and during crying or grimacing. Facial weakness secondary to disturbance of the central nervous system is usually more obvious with the baby at rest or during the first movements of spontaneous expression, and may be completely inapparent during the full movements of crying. However, nuclear, peripheral nerve or muscle lesions are usually more obvious during elicited facial movement such as grimace or cry. A simple classification of the types of facial weakness which can occur in the neonatal period is given below, according to the level of the lesion.

1. **Central.** The upper face is spared. Other signs of cerebral deficit are usually present, for example, hemiparesis, especially of the arm, and seizures.
2. **Nuclear.** This is primarily a manifestation of Mobius syndrome and, thus, is bilateral, often associated with sixth nerve palsies and with a variety of other neurologic and congenital abnormalities.[19]
3. **Nerve.** Nerve injury is usually related either to intrauterine position during labor (usually left occiput anterior, and thus most of these cases are left facial palsies)[20] or, less commonly, to forceps injury during difficult mid- or high-forceps extractions. The upper face is usually affected as well as lower and eye closure is notably poor.
4. **Neuromuscular junction.** This locus for facial weakness occurs particularly in myas-

thenia gravis. Bilateral facial weakness, often with ptosis, dysphagia, and generalized hypotonia may accompany either the neonatal transient or congenital persistent varieties of myasthenia gravis.[21] Diagnosis is readily made in both cases by observation of response to edrophonium or neostigmine. In neonatal transient myasthenia gravis, the more common variety, the mother also has the disease.

5. **Muscle.** The most common of the muscle diseases associated with facial weakness in the newborn period are (1) hypoplasia of the depressor angularis oris muscle (DAOM), (2) facioscapulohumeral dystrophy, and (3) myotonic dystrophy. Hypoplasia of the DAOM, studied in detail by Eng and coworkers, results in an inability of the corner of the mouth to retract and to be depressed, and this disturbance is especially noticeable during crying.[22] An association with cardiac and other anomalies now seems established.[23] Facioscapulohumeral dystrophy has been shown to present in the newborn period with bilateral facial palsy.[24] Similarly, myotonic dystrophy may have as its first manifestation bilateral facial weakness.[25]

Hearing. Delineation of hearing deficit in the newborn period is extremely difficult. The parameters of hearing function described above indicate that some auditory function is present, but probably cannot differentiate deficits short of deafness from the normal state. The use of evoked EEG potentials has not been clearly shown to be a solution to this problem. Brain stem auditory-evoked responses may prove to be of greater value.[26] Most often, the clinician must rely on close follow-up with careful, repeated examinations in order to find those cases of significant hearing loss that may be missed early. Such case-finding is important because language development will be benefited by early rehabilitative efforts. Deafness accompanies a variety of genetic syndromes, many having accompanying physical stigmata (*e.g.*, Treacher Collins syndrome, Waardenburg's syndrome, trisomy 13, Goldenhar's syndrome), or congenital infections with other characteristic concomitants (*e.g.*, rubella).

Sucking and Swallowing. Most often, disturbances of sucking accompany the more generalized depression of central nervous system function associated with most of the disorders to be discussed below. More specific abnormalities of sucking and of swallowing in the newborn period are much more commonly associated with nonneurologic disturbances, for example, tracheoesophageal fistula. Nevertheless, diseases of peripheral mechanisms, such as myotonic dystrophy and myasthenia gravis, can result in neonatal swallowing difficulties. Werdnig–Hoffman disease, in which affection of lower motor neurons occurs, is a rare cause of disturbance of sucking and swallowing in the newborn period.[27] Visible fasciculation and, perhaps, atrophy of the tongue may also be present in the neonate with Werdnig–Hoffmann disease. Affection of the autonomic nervous system can lead to disturbances of swallowing and may be a manifestation of the Riley–Day syndrome in the newborn.

Motor Examination

Determination of abnormality of **muscle tone** must be made in the frame of reference of the normal development of tone in the newborn (see discussion above). Thus, persistent, generalized decrease in flexor and extensor tone is normal at 28-weeks' gestation but is distinctly abnormal at term. Decrease in upper extremity tone is normal at 32 weeks, but a persistent diminution in lower extremity tone at this age is abnormal.

Hypotonia in the newborn period is most commonly generalized and is most often related to major disturbances of the central nervous system. These disturbances may affect the **central nervous system** primarily, for example, hypoxic-ischemic encephalopathy, serious intracranial hemorrhage, intracranial infection or hypoglycemic encephalopathy. Other disturbances of the central nervous system may be concomitants of systemic disorders such as sepsis or congestive heart failure. Under all of these circumstances, deep tendon reflexes are usually depressed, but present, and ankle clonus may or may not be present. Occasionally, hypotonia is more marked on one side, and this almost always reflects primary central nervous system disease of a focal nature. Much less commonly diminished tone occurs secondary to **anterior horn cell disease,** especially Werdnig–Hoffmann disease.[27] Under these circumstances, deep tendon reflexes are usually totally absent and fasciculations

may be seen in the tongue or in the fingers (if the latter are observed with the wrists slightly hyperextended). Disturbance of **peripheral nerve** as a cause of hypotonia in the newborn has not yet been described, although it is well known in slightly older infants.[28,29] Disease of **myoneural junction,** for example, neonatal transient or congenital persistent myasthenia gravis, can present as generalized hypotonia in the neonatal period; other features are often present (see above). Disorders of **muscle** rarely present in the newborn period as hypotonia; the most common of these is myotonic dystrophy which also often has additional features (see above). To define precisely the presence of disease of anterior horn cell, peripheral nerve, neuromuscular junction, or muscle, EMG and nerve conduction velocity studies are usually necessary.

Hypertonia is less commonly seen in neonates than is hypotonia. When present, hypertonia rarely has the clasp-knife feature of spasticity, but rather there is a plastic increase in tone, which increases with passive manipulation of the limbs and is reminiscent of "gegenhalten" of older patients.[14] We have observed the most striking hypertonia in prematures who have suffered hypoxic-ischemic injury and who have had a week or so of generalized hypotonia after the initial insult. Whether the hypertonia relates to white matter affection, such as periventricular leukomalacia, is not yet known. **Marked** hypertonia may result in retrocollis with arching of the back (*i.e.*, opisthotonus); this posture has been seen most commonly with severe forms of the hypoxic-ischemic injury just noted, bacterial meningitis and massive intracranial hemorrhage. In the latter two cases, a meningeal irritative phenomenon, especially in the posterior fossa, has seemed the most likely basis of the opisthotonus.

Constellations of motor abnormalities in the newborn period may precede the development of motor deficits later in infancy. For example, the combination of accentuated deep tendon reflexes, sustained ankle clonus, markedly accentuated positive supporting reaction, and hyperextension with scissoring of the lower extremities when the infant is held vertically, even in the presence of marked hypotonia, usually evolves over months into spastic quadriparesis.[11] Marked hypotonia secondary to central nervous system disease without the findings just enumerated may also evolve into spasticity, or remain as atonic quadriparesis of cerebral origin.[30] Occasionally, such hypotonia will develop into athetosis, which usually appears after approximately 1 year of age.

Transient Increase in Tone of Limbs. In prematures who often have not sustained major detectable injury to the central nervous system in the newborn period, we have observed frequently in the ensuing months an interesting syndrome characterized primarily by a transient increase in tone of limbs, occasionally with jitteriness, in an otherwise normally developing infant. These infants may conform to the syndrome of "transient dystonia" recently described by Drillien.[31] The syndrome occurs most frequently in the youngest prematures (approximately 50% of infants less than 1500 g at birth), and, in the majority of cases, it resolves completely. Drillien has noted that, in 20% of her cases, abnormal signs may disappear at 1 year of age, only to reappear months or years later in infancy or childhood.[31] The etiology of this phenomenon is unclear.

Abnormalities of motility and power are particularly important to delineate. Particular attention must be paid to the quantity, quality, and symmetry of movement. Weakness in a hip-shoulder distribution in a full-term infant suggests an ischemic injury to brain, whereas ischemic injury in a premature more commonly leads to weakness in the lower limbs (see discussion below). These deficits may not be obvious, but careful observation of spontaneous and elicited motility usually allows definition of the characteristic pattern. Hemiparesis on a cerebral basis is manifested by a paucity of movement of affected limbs that may be accompanied by accentuated fisting of the affected hand. Precise determination of the level of peripheral lesions (*e.g.,* the varieties of brachial plexus palsies), can be established, in large part, by observation of spontaneous and elicited motility of the affected parts.

Abnormalities of the Moro reflex are of limited but definite value in the neurologic evaluation. The precise anatomic substrate subserving the Moro reflex has never been clearly established. Therefore, a Moro reflex that is not as completely developed as expected for the gestational age of an infant does not provide the clinician with localizing information. Nevertheless, it is a useful response to elicit because the Moro reflex is readily assessed and is highly sensitive to a wide variety of insults to the central nervous system. Asymmetry of the Moro response is very useful in assessing root or peripheral nerve injury such as occurs in the varieties of brachial plexus palsies. The striking movements of lateral extension and anterior flexion of upper extremities that characterize much of the Moro response are uniformly absent in brachial plexus injury involving segments C5 and C6. Infants with severe bilateral lesions of cerebrum, originating *in utero* and either destructive (hydranencephaly) or developmental (anencephaly, severe microcephaly) often have Moro responses that are elicited by a *minimal* stimulation (slight drop of the head), are stereotyped and "automatic" in appearance, and do not show habituation, a highly important feature of the normal neonatal response to various stimuli (see above). These easily elicited, stereotyped Moro responses are often misinterpreted as normal and are used as evidence for the claim that the cerebrum does not influence the responses of the neonate. In fact, the modulating influence of the cerebral hemispheres on the other areas of the central nervous system is clearly emphasized by such abnormal Moro responses.

Abnormal palmar grasps also have limited but definite value in the neurologic examination. Their value in assessment of hemiparesis on a cerebral basis has already been alluded to above. In addition, the grasp reflex is totally absent in most cases of brachial plexus palsy in which the affection extends to segments C8 and T1.

The tonic neck response, like the Moro reflex, normally prominent in the 1-month-old infant, may be stereotyped and exaggerated in neonates with severe bilateral cerebral disturbances. The tonic neck response that is more striking with the head to one side may accompany hemiparesis and/or be followed by the emergence of a motor deficit more severe on the side of the greater tonic neck reaction.[11] Persistence of a distinct tonic neck response beyond 7 months of age usually presages either a pyramidal, an extrapyramidal or both types of motor disorders.

Sensory Examination

Abnormalities of sensation are most easily elicited and interpreted in the newborn period in examples of peripheral lesions. The most illustrative of these is the sensory deficit in patients with brachial plexus palsies. We have been able to elicit distinct deficits in response to pinprick in a segmental distribution that usually is less extensive than the deficit of motor function. This is consistent with the usual pathologic finding in these cases of less severe involvement of posterior than anterior roots. Disturbances of sensory function that relate to lesions of the central nervous system have been more difficult to document in the neonate. This relates, at least in part, to the lack of clear clinical documentation of the gamut of normal responses to pinprick or touch in the newborn period. Parameters of interest will include the quality of motor response, the appearance of grimace and/or cry, and the degree to which the response dampens with repeated trials. Correlation of aberrations of these responses with the anatomic level of derangement of the central nervous system are needed.

TRANSILLUMINATION

An important aspect of the neurologic evaluation of every infant is transillumination of the head. Although this is an old procedure, and one whose usefulness has been documented many times,[32-36] it is frequently omitted in the neurologic evaluation of the neonate. The procedure is simple. It requires an ordinary flashlight holding two fresh type D batteries. A rubber attachment around the light rim is used to provide close, flexible contact with the scalp. Higher intensity lamps are not as portable but provide excellent information.

Factors Modifying Transillumination

Extracranial Factors. Certain extracranial factors modify the transillumination.[34] Thus, factors increasing transillumination include sparse, blond hair, fair skin (especially when associated with subcutaneous fat or edema), thin skull, and any clear fluid between the skull and the light (*e.g.,* infiltrated intravenous solution). Factors decreasing transillumination are the opposite: thick, black hair, pigmented skin, thick skull and/or excessive marrow, and blood or other turbid fluid between skull and light (subgaleal hematoma). In the normal newborn, transillumination beyond the rim of the flashlight will rarely exceed 2.5 cm in the frontal area or 1.0 cm in the occipital region.[34] In premature infants these values should be increased by 0.5 to 1.0 cm. Recently, higher intensity lamps have become more popular than the simple flashlight, and glowing beyond the rim of these higher intensity lights is slightly greater than with the flashlight.

Intracranial Factors. Intracranial factors that will alter transillumination in the neonatal period include primarily abnormal fluid collections within the subdural or subarachnoid space or markedly thinned or otherwise decreased cerebral mantle. Abnormal fluid collections within the subdural space include subdural effusion, secondary for the most part to extension of meningeal inflammation, usually bacterial meningitis. Subdural hemorrhage will result in abnormally *decreased* transillumination on the affected side until dissolution of the hemorrhage occurs in 2 to 3 weeks, with resultant formation of subdural effusion. (Abnormally decreased transillumination in an infant with a traumatic delivery, and thus a possible setting for subdural hemorrhage, is much more likely to be secondary to a palpable subgaleal hematoma than to subdural hematoma.) Increased fluid in the subarachnoid space may be related to an arachnoidal cyst. A disproportion between the volume of the cranium and the size of the cerebrum (*i.e.,* a relative increase in subarachnoid space) is probably the major cause of the increased glowing observed in normal prematures.[37] The most common cause of marked glowing secondary to increase in the subarachnoid fluid space occurs when there is marked diminution of cerebral substance, consequent to either severe destructive lesion or to developmental aberration. Destructive lesions may have occurred *in utero:* hydranencephaly, a bilateral lesion which may be related to a major vascular event or inflammatory disease,[38,39,40] or porencephaly, a unilateral lesion which can be caused by a vascular event,[34] usually within the distribution of the middle cerebral artery.[34] Lesions may have also occurred postnatally (*e.g.,* days or weeks after severe hypoxic-ischemic insult). Developmental aberrations of cerebral hemispheres with an increase in the subarachnoid fluid space include marked microcephaly,[34] holoprosencephaly, and schizencephaly. If the destruction or maldevelopment of the cerebrum is severe enough, transillumination is greatly increased and may extend across the whole skull. Under these conditions it is clear that the intraventricular

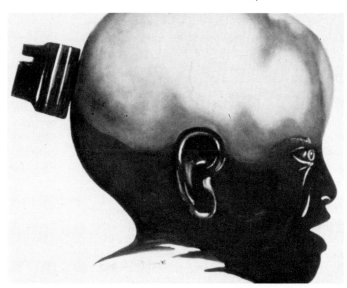

Fig. 39-1. Transillumination in hydranencephaly. The whole cranium transilluminates with a flashlight positioned in the midline posteriorly. (Courtesy of Dr. P. R. Dodge)

fluid is also responsible for the glowing. Complete transillumination of this sort is most commonly seen in the newborn period with hydranencephaly (Fig. 39-1), schizencephaly, or marked hydrocephalus. Transillumination in hydrocephalus relates largely to the degree of thinning of cerebral mantle, and complete transillumination is said to occur when the cerebral mantle is less than 1 cm in thickness.[32,34] Transillumination highly localized to the infratentorial region is highly suggestive of hydrocephalus secondary to the Dandy–Walker malformation. Such infratentorial glowing can also be seen in the newborn period with posterior fossa arachnoidal cysts.

LABORATORY STUDIES

As in older infants and children, pertinent laboratory studies for the neurologic evaluation of a newborn may include skull and other appropriate radiographs, EEG, computerized tomographic (CT) brain scan, radionuclide brain scan, analysis of various metabolic parameters in blood and urine, EMG, and nerve-conduction studies, as well as more complicated air or dye contrast studies such as ventriculography or myelography. Where appropriate, these will be considered below in a discussion of the various pathologic states and will not be discussed in detail here. The broad interpretation of these data is similar to that at later ages and can be gleaned from standard sources. The normal findings for many of the studies differ for the newborn and such differences must be borne in mind in their interpretation.

Examination of the cerebrospinal fluid (CSF) of the neonate does present some particularly difficult problems and these should be discussed briefly. Much of the difficulty in interpretation of the CSF findings in neonates relates to the remarkably wide range of values considered "normal."[41-45] For example, on the basis of such data, some observers consider as normal a few hundred red blood cells per cubic millimeter, less than 30 to 40 white blood cells per cubic millimeter, and a protein concentration between 50 to 130 mg/dl in the full-term infant and "higher" in the premature. These values have been derived from studies which usually have not used rigorous diagnostic techniques, and we consider such values overestimates. Thus, recently we examined prospectively and retrospectively the results of the 394 infants who had received lumbar puncture after being admitted to the neonatal intensive care unit of St. Louis Children's Hospital during the last 3 years.[46] Although all of the patients had one or more illnesses, comparison of their CSF findings, taken as a whole, with those published in the literature for normal infants did not reveal any striking differences. This indicated that previous studies must have had some considerable degree of patient heterogeneity. In fact, we noted that many of our patients had CSF findings that fell within the range considered normal for older children and adults. Thus, approximately one-third of both premature and full-term infants had 0 to 1 white cell per cubic millimeter in their CSF during the first 3 weeks of life, and, by the fourth week, one-half of the prematures and two-thirds of the full-terms had such values. In general, increasing age was associated with decreasing number of cells and lower protein values. The most notable findings were that values of CSF protein and red and white blood cells correlated clearly with the patient's primary disease. Thus, patients with intracranial hemorrhage or bacterial meningitis had the characteristic CSF formulas seen in these well-known states. In another study of infants in a neonatal intensive care unit, mean values for term and preterm infants were 8 and 9 white blood cells per cubic millimeter, a protein concentration of 90 and 115 mg/dl, a glucose concentration of 52 and 50 mg/dl, and a CSF: blood glucose of 0.81 and 0.74.[47]

The essential point is that, in the evaluation of the CSF in the newborn, an *isolated* borderline finding should not be a major determinant for establishing a diagnosis. Constellations of CSF findings, however, can be given considerable weight, especially when they are evaluated in the context of a rigorous clinical and neurologic evaluation.

APNEIC SPELLS AND PERIODIC BREATHING

Apneic spells in the neonatal period have long been considered possible forerunners of brain injury, but the quantitative nature of the relationship has never been established. It is a frequent clinical problem and one that demands the immediate attention of the neonatal physician. Apneic spells in small babies are related to the irregular respiratory pattern known as **periodic breathing.** A discussion of the latter will help our understanding of the former.

Periodic Breathing

In its typical form, periodic breathing occurs in 25% to 50% of prematures, and irregularities of respiration akin to this disturbance occur at one time or another in nearly all small babies.[48-50] Classically, the pattern consists of a period of apnea of 5 to 10 seconds, followed by ventilation of 10 to 15 seconds at a rate of 50 to 60 per minute. The overall respiratory rate is 30 to 40 per minute.[48] During the period of apnea, no changes in heart rate, color, or body temperature occur (in contrast to "apneic spells"). Only minor alterations in blood gases have been noted in association with periodic breathing,[48,51-53] and these are not consistent. The most striking characteristic of the phenomenon is the marked change in frequency with the level of maturation; periodic breathing is more frequent the more immature the baby and becomes dramatically less frequent after 36-weeks' gestational age. The latter has been particularly well-documented by Parmelee and coworkers.[50]

Apneic Spells

Periods of apnea of more than 20 seconds and/or those accompanied by bradycardia and cyanosis are termed **apneic spells.** With prolonged monitoring, at least 25% of the babies in a premature intensive care unit demonstrated such spells.[49] The spells occurred only in conjunction with periodic breathing.[49] Bradycardia and cyanosis are followed by hypotonia and unresponsiveness, the former occurring in most prematures after 20 seconds and the latter after 45. For smaller infants, the time periods may be much shorter. Although the possibility exists that apneic spells can result in brain injury secondary to accompanying hypoxemia and ischemia, very little information is available regarding the neurologic status of infants *during* severe spells. Deuel observed marked suppression of the EEG during apneic spells,[54] suggesting cerebral hemispheral and, perhaps, diencephalic dysfunction. Whether oculovestibular reflexes or other indicators of brain stem function are also disturbed is unknown and is thus an obvious topic for future research.

Provocative Factors. The important clinical settings that provoke the occurrence of apneic spells in our population of newborns in a neonatal intensive care unit are discussed next in decreasing order of frequency.

1. **Extreme immaturity** *per se* is the most common association of severe apneic spells. Such infants are particularly likely to experience apena with changes in skin temperature (especially increases), after feeding, or with rectal or nasopharyngeal stimulation.

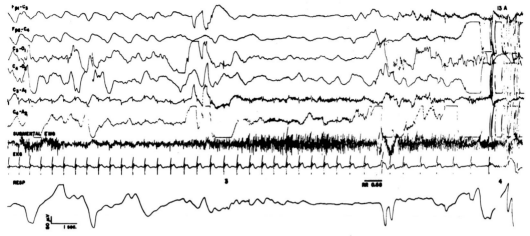

Fig. 39-2. Apnea secondary to hypoxemia and pulmonary insufficiency. Polygraphic recording of EEG (six upper channels), submental EMG, ECG, and respiratory activity in a neonate. See text for details. (Deuel RK: Arch Neurol 28:71, 1973; Copyright 1973, American Medical Association)[54]

Fig. 39-3. Apnea secondary to seizure. Polygraphic recording of EEG (two upper channels), respiratory activity and EKG in a neonate. See text for details. (Deuel, RK: Arch Neurol 28:71, 1973; Copyright 1973, American Medical Association)[54]

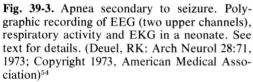

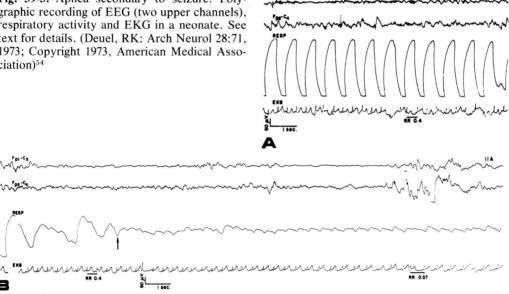

2. **Hypoxemia secondary to airway obstruction or pulmonary disease** is a frequent setting for the occurrence of apneic spells. Excellent studies of patients in this group are available.[49,55,56] Polygraphic recording of EEG, ECG, and respiratory activity of a newborn with an apneic spell secondary to hypoxemia is shown in Figure 39-2. The episode was precipitated by accu-

mulation of respiratory secretions, which resulted in cyanosis, a few irregular respirations and then apnea. The EEG flattened (No. 3, Fig. 39-2), the baby developed opisthotonus and, then, bradycardia (No. 4, Fig. 39-2). Resuscitative efforts were required and apneic episodes became distinctly less common by continuous attention to pulmonary toilet.[54]

3. **Primary disease of the central nervous system,** though often the first diagnosis in the baby with apnea, is not the most frequent clinical setting. Nevertheless, apneic spells can be provoked by a concomitant affection of central nervous system or represent a manifestation of seizure in the neonate. When the latter is the case, other subtle manifestations of seizure (see below) are usually present. A polygraphic recording of EEG, ECG and respiratory activity of a newborn with apnea secondary to seizure is shown in Figure 39-3. The apnea sequence started with spike and slow wave activity in the EEG (Fig. 39-3A), was followed in seconds by 3 irregular respirations (Fig. 39-3B), then respiratory cessation (**arrow**), marked EEG suppression and, finally, bradycardia. Cerebral activity returned to normal after about 2 minutes. Because the abnormal discharge was the primary event, the baby was treated with anticonvulsants and had no further severe apneic spells.[54]

4. **Metabolic aberrations** can lead to apneic spells, and the common denominator of such aberrations appears to be the ability to disturb CNS metabolism. Thus, hypoglycemia, hypocalcemia, acidosis and marked hyperbilirubinemia are the most common of the aberrations, and each of these is usually accompanied by a variety of other manifestations of CNS dysfunction.

Management and Prognosis. The management and prognosis of the baby with apneic spells depends more on the provocative factors recorded above than on the occurrence of apnea per se. The study by Daily and coworkers is relevant to the appropriate management for all neonates with apnea.[49] These workers continuously monitored a group of prematures with apnea, most of whom had no obvious provocative disease. Of all spells recorded (540), 37% aborted spontaneously by 30 seconds after onset, 55% required cutaneous stimulation to so abort, and 8% required bag and mask. Thus, it is clear that continuous monitoring of respiration with a system equipped with an appropriate alarm to alert personnel to the occurrence of apnea is the most critical therapeutic maneuver. As illustrated above, appropriate therapy of pulmonary disease, seizure, or other neurologic disturbance, or metabolic aberration should be instituted when such entities are present. Usage of continuous positive airway pressure, theophylline, or both is discussed elsewhere in Chapter 22.

Pathogenesis. An understanding of the pathogenesis of periodic breathing and apneic spells can be derived from the following considerations. It is now clear that there is a uniform relation of apneic spells with periodic breathing, and these entities can be considered to be at the ends of a spectrum of disturbance of regulation of respiration characteristic of the premature. The discrete temporal characteristics of periodic breathing relating to gestational age indicate that this unusual respiratory pattern occurs during the maturation of a regulatory system within the central nervous system. The anatomic correlates of this regulatory system are unknown. However, present evidence allows formulation of a reasonable hypothesis which is outlined below.

First, it is quite clear that periodic breathing does not closely resemble any of the major respiratory disturbances associated with disease of brain stem, at least as manifested in older patients. The work of Plum and coworkers has established that lesions of the reticular formation of midbrain and pons, ventral to the aqueduct and fourth ventricle, are associated with sustained, regular, rapid, and deep hyperpnea, so-called central neurogenic hyperventilation.[14,57] Lesions of dorsolateral tegmentum of mid- or lower pons are accompanied by apneustic or cluster breathing. Lesions of dorsomedial medulla result most often in ataxic breathing, characterized by an irregular pattern of respiratory rate, rhythm and amplitude. Occasionally seen with low pontine or upper medullary lesions is a form of periodic breathing akin to Cheyne–Stokes breathing (see below). However, this brain stem form of periodic breathing is seen almost invariably in deeply stuporous or comatose patients.[57] Thus, none of these respiratory aberrations associated with brain stem disease seem related to the disturbance of regulation of respiration of the premature infant. Perhaps more important evidence ruling against a brain stem locus of the regulatory disturbance is the presence of numerous manifestations of normal neurologic function of stem (see section on neurologic development above). Moreover, neuroanatomic development, in terms of demarcation and neuronal population of all major nuclear structures, and definition of all major fiber tracts, is very well established in the brain stem of the smallest prematures.

There is, however, good evidence to suggest that periodic breathing is associated with the development of a modulating system in the cerebral hemispheres. Thus, periodic breathing of the neonate bears a very close resemblance to Cheyne–Stokes breathing, a pattern associated in older children with deep, bilateral disturbance of cerebral hemispheres, diencephalon or both.[14] During the gestational time period in question, these areas are undergoing rapid maturational changes in neuroanatomic development and function (see section on neuroanatomic development below).

Thus, we propose that periodic breathing is a result of the influence of a system that modulates respiration and that is not completely developed in the premature. The system has its origins in cerebral hemispheres, perhaps in diencephalon, or both. Periodic breathing results in apneic spells when this vulnerable system is insulted by any of the variety of provocative factors discussed above. Thus, these respiratory phenomena should be envisioned in the same way as other, better-characterized developing systems of the neonate (*e.g.,* hepatic glucuronyl transferase) that may also decompensate when insulted by a variety of provocative factors.

SEIZURES

Seizures are a frequent and often dramatic occurrence in the neonatal period. Unlike the situation with older infants, neonatal seizures do not usually represent a medical emergency because the convulsive activity in the neonate only uncommonly interferes with respiratory activity. However, seizures in the newborn may be sustained for considerable periods and seriously interfere with important supportive measures, such as alimentation and assisted respiration for associated disorders. Recent experimental data suggest that neonatal seizures *per se* may have a deleterious effect on developing brain.[58] In addition, and perhaps most important, the spells often are related to significant illness, and, thus, it is critical to determine their etiology as rapidly as possible and to treat them.

Clinical Features

Pathophysiologic Aspects. Seizure types in newborns differ considerably from those observed in older infants, and the types in prematures differ from those in full-terms. Unlike older infants, newborns rarely have well-organized, generalized, tonic-clonic seizures. Prematures have even less well-organized spells than do full-term infants. The precise reasons for these differences must relate to the developmental state of the nervous system in the perinatal period. As discussed below in the section on development, the most critical neuroanatomic processes occurring during this period are the organizational events. These events are characterized by the attainment of proper orientation, alignment, and layering of cortical neurons; the elaboration of axonal and dendritic ramifications; and the establishment of synaptic connections. These processes must be highly significant in providing the cortical organization to propagate and sustain a generalized seizure. Such a degree of cortical organization is apparently not present in the human neonate. In contrast, in the newborn monkey, the spread of seizure discharges is relatively rapid and well-organized; synchronous, generalized seizures are readily apparent clinically and electroencephalographically.[59] Such propagation and spread may be related to the more advanced cortical organization and to the myelination of interhemispheric commissures present in the neonatal monkey but absent in the human.[60,61] The relatively advanced cortical development apparent in human limbic structures and the connections of these structures to diencephalon and brain stem may underlie the frequency and dominance, as clinical manifestations of seizure, of oral-buccal movements, such as sucking, chewing, or drooling, oculomotor abnormalities and apnea (see below).[62,63] The importance of developmental changes in physiologic parameters has been emphasized by Purpura and coworkers, who have shown, primarily in newborn kittens, that inhibitory synaptic activities are predominant and that excitatory activities develop later.[64–67] Thus, it is clear that the characteristic seizure patterns of the neonate have their basis in the particular state of neuroanatomic and neurophysiologic development cited above and discussed in more detail below in the section on development.

Seizure Types and Jitteriness. In a population of sick newborns that includes both full-terms and prematures, such as those we have seen at St. Louis Children's Hospital, at least five varieties of spells can be observed. In decreasing order of frequency, these types of seizure are

1. **Subtle.** We have chosen to characterize the most frequent type as *subtle,* because the clinical manifestations thereof are readily overlooked. Such manufestations may consist of only tonic horizontal deviation and/or jerking of the eyes; repetitive blinking or fluttering of eyelids; drooling, sucking, or other oral-buccal movements; tonic posturing of a limb; or apnea. Apnea as a manifestation of seizure is almost always accompanied by one of the other subtle manifestations. Occasionally accompanying one of these subtle manifestations are a variety of unusual movements of limbs. As noted by others these movements are more common in upper limbs, are pendular and rhythmic, and often resemble "rowing" or "swimming" movements.[68] When lower limb movements are involved, they often resemble "pedaling." All of these phenomena are readily stamped as seizure because of accompanying EEG correlates and cessation with anticonvulsant medication. The EEG accompaniments are either high voltage slow waves (1–4 cycles/second), sometimes accompanied by positive or negative spikes, a burst-suppression pattern, or a rhythmic alpha-like rhythm.[68] (The latter is often overlooked as an EEG manifestation of seizure in the neonate.) Subtle seizures, in general, are most common in the most premature infants.

2. **Multifocal clonic** seizures are manifested by clonic movements of one or another limb, which migrates to another body part in a nonordered fashion (*i.e.,* left arm jerking may be accompanied or followed by right leg jerking). The multifocal character of these spells is expressed in the EEG by multiple foci of sharp activity or slower rhythmic activity migrating from one area of cortex to the other. This seizure type is common in the full-term infant with hypoxic-ischemic encephalopathy. Approximately three-fourths of neonates with clonic seizures will have definite spikes accompanied by 1 to 4/sec slow waves and/or alpha-like activity.[68]

3. **Focal clonic** seizures are typically well-localized and are not usually accompanied by unconsciousness. The predominant EEG pattern is focal sharp activity, usually including spikes, which may spread to the whole hemisphere. It should be emphasized that in the neonate, focal seizures are more commonly a manifestation of bilateral cerebral disturbance (*e.g.,* a metabolic encephalopathy) than of focal disease.

4. **Tonic.** When generalized, tonic seizures may seem like decerebrate posturing of older patients, but accompany stertorous breathing, eye signs or occasional clonic movements stamp these as convulsions. This is the most common seizure observed in premature infants with intraventricular hemorrhage. In the neonatal period, the major EEG correlates only uncommonly include spikes;[68] the predominant patterns are high-voltage slow waves, sometimes in a burst-suppression pattern, marked voltage suppression, and/or alpha-like activity.

5. **Myoclonic.** Usually synchronous, myoclonic seizures take the form of single or multiple jerks of flexion of upper and/or lower limbs. Often, the EEG accompaniment is the burst-suppression pattern. Neonates with bilateral flexion myoclonus may also develop the syndrome of hypsarrhythmic EEG and infantile, massive myoclonic spasms weeks or months later.

Jitteriness should be distinguished from neonatal seizures. This remarkable state is characteristically a disorder of the neonatal period and is rarely, if ever, seen in similar form at a later age. It may be defined as a movement disorder with qualities primarily of tremulousness but occasionally also of clonus. The distinction of jitteriness from seizure is usually readily made if the following points are remembered:

1. Jitteriness is not accompanied by abnormalities of gaze or extraocular movement; seizures usually are.

2. Jitteriness is exquisitely stimulus-sensitive—seizures are not.

3. The dominant movement in jitteriness is tremor (*i.e.,* the alternating movements are rhythmic, of equal rate, and amplitude); the dominant movement in seizure

Table 39-1. Seizures Occurring in the First 10 Days of Life.

Etiology	Time of Onset*	
	0–3	*4–10*
Perinatal complications	+	
Hypoglycemia	+	
Hypocalcemia†	+	+
Infection		+
Developmental anomalies	+	+

*Postnatal age (days) when seizures most likely to occur
†Two major varieties of hypocalcemia are included (see text)

is clonic jerking (*i.e.,* the movements have a fast and slow component).

4. The rhythmic movements of limbs in jitteriness usually can be stopped by flexion of the affected limb.[69] Convulsive movements will not stop with this maneuver.

Etiology

The causes of neonatal seizures are diverse and long lists can be composed. However, most of the spells are secondary to relatively few etiologies and these will be emphasized here. Determination of etiology is highly critical because it affords the opportunity to treat specifically and also to make a meaningful prognostic statement (see below). The most important etiologies, their usual time of onset and their relative frequency as the major cause of seizures in the newborn are shown in Table 39-1.

Perinatal Complications. These include hypoxic, ischemic, or both forms of encephalopathy; cerebral contusion associated with obstetric trauma; and intracranial hemorrhage. These account for more cases than any other etiologic category, particularly among prematures.[70–72] Because each of these states will be discussed in detail in relevant sections below, only brief descriptions will be given here. Hypoxic and/or ischemic encephalopathy most often occurs secondary to perinatal asphyxia. **Intrauterine** insults are most common. Of the various perinatal complications, hypoxic and/or ischemic injury account for the large majority of cases. These patients usually are initially stuporous or in coma, and often develop seizures on the first postnatal day. Jitteriness may be particularly striking. Cerebral contusion, usually secondary to trauma asso-

ciated with breech deliveries, forceps extractions, or other obstetric difficulties, occurs particularly in large full-term infants. The most common neurologic syndrome consists of focal seizures with focal cerebral signs, subarachnoid hemorrhage, and, occasionally, skull fracture. However, in most obstetric units, this is now an uncommon occurrence. Intracranial hemorrhage, as a cause of seizures distinct from hypoxia or trauma, is difficult to establish unequivocally because of the usual concurrence of these factors. When seizures accompany primary subarachnoid hemorrhage, the infant usually appears remarkably well in the interictal period.[74,77] Periventricular intracerebral hemorrhage, emanating from subependymal veins in the germinal matrix, is a lesion of the premature, often occurring 1 to 3 days after severe hypoxia. Seizures in this context may be part of a rapid deterioration that evolves in a few hours to coma and respiratory arrest. Subdural hemorrhage, secondary either to tear of the tentorium, falx, or superficial cortical veins, a traumatic lesion of large babies, is the least frequent of the clinically important varieties of intracranial hemorrhage. Seizures accompany subdural hemorrhage in about 50% of such cases.[77]

Metabolic Disturbances. These disturbances are the next most frequent cause of neonatal seizures.

Hypoglycemia (*i.e.,* glucose below 20 mg/dl in the premature or 30 mg/dl in the full-term infant) is particularly frequent in small babies, most of whom are small for gestational age, or in infants of mothers who are diabetic or prediabetic. The most critical determinant for the occurrence of neurologic symptoms with neonatal hypoglycemia is the duration of the hypoglycemia and, as a corollary, the time before treatment is begun.[78] Neurologic symptoms consist most commonly of jitteriness, stupor, hypotonia, and apnea, as well as seizures. More than one-half of the small hypoglycemic babies develop neurologic symptoms and 10% to 30% of those symptomatic experience seizures. In such infants, it is often particularly difficult to establish that hypoglycemia is the cause of the neurologic syndrome because perinatal complications (see above), hypocalcemia (see below), or infection (see below) are frequently associated. In contrast to the situation with low-birth-weight babies, neurologic symptoms, including seizures, are much less frequent in hypoglycemic infants of diabetic mothers (10%–20%), possibly because the duration of hypoglycemia in these infants is relatively brief.[79]

Hypocalcemia (*i.e.*, calcium below 7 mg/dl) has two major peaks of incidence in the neonate. The first, in the first 2 to 3 days of life, occurs most often in low-birth-weight infants (both of average and below average weight for gestational age) and often accompanies the hypoxic-ischemic encephalopathy of perinatal asphyxia. Seizures occurring in this context are usually not accompanied solely by hypocalcemia. A therapeutic response to intravenous calcium is of help in determining whether the low serum calcium is etiologically related to the seizures (see Chap. 27). The delineation of hypocalcemia as a major etiologic factor in neonatal seizures is easier when it occurs later in the first week than earlier. These babies are usually large full-term infants, voraciously consuming a milk preparation with a suboptimal P/Ca ratio (*e.g.*, cow's milk). This hypocalcemia of "later onset" has been studied in considerable detail recently by Cockburn and coworkers.[69]

The importance of *hypomagnesemia* in this context has also been emphasized. Thus, of 75 infants with seizures primarily occurring late in the first week and related to abnormal mineral metabolism, 93% had hypocalcemia and of these fully one-half had accompanying hypomagnesemia. *Hyperphosphatemia* was present in about two-thirds of these hypocalcemic babies, and 7% had hypomagnesemia without hypocalcemia. These data have important implications for treatment (see below). These infants with hypocalcemia of later onset demonstrated a neurologic syndrome consisting primarily of hyperactive deep tendon reflexes, ankle, jaw, and knee clonus and jitteriness in addition to seizures.[69] A prolonged QT interval is often apparent on EKG. None demonstrated generalized hypotonia or obtundation.[69] In contrast, infants with hypocalcemia of early onset, and often associated with hypoxic-ischemic encephalopathy, frequently are slightly to moderately stuporous and have generalized hypotonia.

There have been striking differences in the incidence of hypocalcemia, hypomagnesemia, or both as a cause of seizures in various studies. Thus, several older studies have recorded a relatively high incidence (*i.e.*, 20%–55%).[69,73,74,80] In contrast, in our infants with seizures, we have seen an incidence of less than 5% in our prematures and 10% in our full-term infants. It is likely that such differences relate to sampling and feeding differences. The highest incidences of hypocalcemia as the etiology of neonatal seizures occur in large obstetrical divisions or units receiving many referrals from such divisions. A neonatal intensive care unit like our own receives most of its referrals from divisions that tend to care for later onset hypocalcemia and refer more complicated problems. More important, cow's milk feeding has been replaced in large part by feeding of commercial formulas with compositions similar to human milk.

Other Metabolic Disturbances. Metabolic disturbances other than those relative to glucose, calcium, magnesium, and phosphorus are very uncommon causes of seizures in the newborn. Worthy of brief mention though are hyponatremia and hypernatremia, pyridoxine dependency, hyperbilirubinemia, and amino and organic acid abnormalities (drug withdrawal is discussed below). Hyponatremia may result in seizures and occurs most commonly in our experience with inappropriate antidiuretic hormone secretion associated with meningitis. Hypernatremia occurs primarily in severely dehydrated infants or in infants treated with hypertonic sodium bicarbonate. Seizures may occur during rehydration if markedly hypotonic solutions are used, presumably secondary to the development of intracellular edema.[81] Pyridoxine deficiency and dependency, the latter a metabolic defect, may produce severe seizures, recalcitrant to all therapy.[82,83] The best means of diagnosis is a therapeutic trial of pyridoxine, administered IV in a dose of 50 mg, accompanied by simultaneous monitoring by EEG; this is accompanied by cessation of seizure and normalization of the EEG. Hyperbilirubinemia *per se* is a rare cause of seizures; however, in one study, approximately 50% of babies with kernicterus were said to exhibit seizures.[77] Of the amino acid disturbances, maple syrup urine disease and the hyperammonemia syndromes are the most common cause of neonatal seizures. The inadvertent injection of mepivacaine or related local anesthetics into the fetal scalp at the time of placement of paracervical block is another uncommon metabolic cause of seizures in the first hour after birth.[84]

Infection. This is the next most frequent etiologic category. Of the infectious causes, bacterial meningitis is the underlying disease in the majority, with the remainder consisting largely of various encephalitides, including toxoplasmosis, herpes simplex, Coxsackie B, rubella, and cytomegalovirus infection.

Developmental Disorders. The developmental disorders are quite varied, but polymicrogyria and other cerebral cortical dysgeneses (discussed in detail below) constitute the majority.

Passive Addiction to Narcotics or Barbiturates. A problem of increasing frequency, though still relatively uncommon in most centers, is the occurrence of neonatal seizures associated with withdrawal from narcotics[85] or other depressants (*e.g.,* barbiturates).[86] These seizures have their onset most commonly in the first 2 to 3 days of life. Several excellent reports of this problem have come from the groups in New York City[85,87–91] Perhaps most important for the present discussion, seizures are a very infrequent manifestation of narcotic withdrawal in passively addicted infants. Thus, in a large series of 384 infants, approximately 70% exhibited some signs of withdrawal, but only 3% of those symptomatic developed seizures.[85] The most striking signs have included jitteriness and irritability, occurring in approximately 70% or more of the symptomatic babies. Other notable findings have included persistent and high-pitched cry, hypertonicity, hyperactivity, sneezing, vomiting, respiratory distress, low birth weight for gestational age, and diarrhea. The occurrence of symptoms is directly related to the size of the maternal intake of narcotics, the duration of maternal addiction, and the proximity of the last maternal ingestion of drug to the time of birth. The withdrawal signs occur early (*i.e.,* in the first 48 hours, in approximately 85% of those symptomatic). More recently, methadone-addicted infants have comprised an increasingly large proportion of the passively addicted group. Seizures may appear later in the first week in these infants.[92]

Treatment of affected infants has been a subject of some controversy; the major therapeutic agents utilized have included paregoric, chlorpromazine, phenobarbital, and diazepam. Published data do not indicate any striking differences in efficacy among these agents, although the duration of therapy needed may have been somewhat shorter when diazepam was used.[89] We are reluctant to recommend diazepam in the neonate for several reasons (see discussion below of treatment of seizures). One of the problems cited below (*i.e.,* the uncoupling of the bilirubin-albumin complex by the vehicle—sodium benzoate—for parenteral diazepam) has been considered remote in neonates with narcotic withdrawal, because significant jaundice is uncommon in these infants.[85] This fact is probably related to stimulation by the narcotic of the microsomal enzyme, glucuronyl transferase.[90] Nonetheless, because phenobarbital has been proven to be a safe and effective drug in the therapy of neonatal narcotic withdrawal,[87] and in view of the continued uncertainty regarding the safety or necessity of diazepam in the newborn period, we recommend use of the barbiturate in the treatment of this syndrome. (The doses needed are described below.)

Diagnosis

Diagnostic evaluation must begin with a careful history and physical examination. It must be emphasized that the maternal history is very critical and, if possible, should be obtained directly from the mother. This is of particular importance when considering the possibilities of drug withdrawal, intrauterine or postnatal infection, or certain metabolic disorders. Not infrequently, the etiologic diagnosis will become obvious from such pursuits. The most immediate laboratory tests should be directed toward the most dangerous but readily treatable diseases; thus, lumbar puncture and blood sugar (Dextrostix) determination are first on the list. Blood should also be drawn to test for sodium, potassium, blood

Table 39-2. Changing Prognosis in Neonatal Seizures.

Time of Report	Number of Patients	Follow-up Data %		
		Normal	*Dead*	*Sequelae**
Before 1969[70-72,74,77,93,94]	608	41	40	19
After 1969[73,74,95]	347	53	17	30

* Neurologic sequelae include mental retardation, significant motor deficits and/or seizure disorders.

urea nitrogen, calcium, phosphorus, and magnesium. Neurodiagnostic studies, including EEG, are best obtained in the interictal period. Although the interictal EEG is of some value in establishing prognosis in full-term infants (see below), rarely is it of help in determining the etiologic diagnosis. Focal EEG abnormalities are very common in generalized disease and vice versa, and a normal EEG may accompany brain disease severe enough to result in neurologic sequelae.

Prognosis

The overall prognosis of seizures in the neonatal period is shown in Table 39-2, based on approximately 1000 reported cases recorded in reports published before and after 1969. Although the reports are not comparable regarding the number of prematures, nature of the obstetrical population, and so on, it seems reasonable to conclude that a decrease in mortality and, perhaps, an increase in normal survivors are now more common. In large part, this probably reflects improved obstetric practice and neonatal intensive care.

The interictal EEG is helpful in determining the prognosis in some full-term infants.[74,94] For example, in one large series a normal EEG was associated with an 86% chance for normal development at 4 years of age, whereas an EEG with multifocal abnormalities was associated with only a 12% chance.[74] A smaller group of babies, approximately 10% in the series of Rose and Lombroso, demonstrated a striking, periodic, burst-suppression pattern.[74] The pattern consists of alternating periods of marked voltage suppression, interrupted by bursts of high voltage, asynchronous sharp activity, including spikes, and slow waves. It bears a superficial resemblance to the *tracé alternant* of the normal newborn. However, the abnormal pattern just described,

termed *tracé paroxystique* by Monod and Dreyfus-Brisac, is virtually an invariable indication of severe cerebral disease and a poor prognosis.[96] Nevertheless, some caution must be used in attributing a grave prognosis to abnormal paroxysmal patterns with long silent periods in young prematures, especially around 33 weeks of conceptual age.[68] Most important, at least 25% to 35% of neonates with seizures will have EEGs that are either "borderline" or which demonstrate other less marked abnormalities associated with an uncertain prognosis.[74,94] In addition, no studies to date have clearly demonstrated that the EEG is particularly valuable in establishing a prognosis for prematures with seizures.

A far more rational and reliable indicator of ultimate outcome in both prematures and full terms is the nature of the neurologic disease producing the seizures. The relationship of prognosis and the underlying neurologic disease, based on our own experience and that of others in all neonates with seizures, is summarized in Table 39-3.[69,72-74,76,96] Thus, it is clear that perinatal hypoxia and/or ischemia is associated with an approximately 50% chance for normal development, primary subarachnoid hemorrhage with as high as a 90% chance, marked intraventricular hemorrhage with 10% or less chance, hypocalcemia of late onset with an 80% to 100% chance and of early onset with approximately 50% chance, hypoglycemia with approximately a 50% chance, infection with 20% to 50% (depending on the gestational age of the infant and on the organism), and developmental anomalies with no chance.[69,72-74,76,96] It is clear, then, that the task of the neonatal physician is to determine as precisely as possible the nature of the neurologic disease in the convulsing neonate, not only to institute appropriate therapy but also to make as meaningful a prognostic statement as possible.

Table 39-3. Relation of Neurologic Disease to Prognosis in Neonatal Seizures.

Disease	Normal Development*
Hypoxic-ischemic encephalopathy	50%
Primary subarachnoid hemorrhage	90%
Intraventricular hemorrhage	<10%
Hypocalcemia	
early onset	50%
later onset	80–100%
Hypoglycemia	50%
Bacterial meningitis	20–50%
Developmental anomaly	0

* In general, the lower incidence of normal development occurs in prematures, especially with gram-negative infections, and the higher incidence in full-terms, especially with gram-positive infections.

Treatment

Continuous or very frequent seizures in neonates should be treated with urgency. An intravenous line should be established, blood drawn for the metabolites mentioned above and a Dextrostix done immediately (on blood from a separate vessel if dextrose has been given recently through the same line). If hypoglycemia is present, 25% dextrose is given IV in a dose of 2 to 4 ml/kg (0.5 to 1.0 g/kg) and the baby maintained on IV dextrose at a rate as high as 0.5 g/kg/hour if necessary. If hypoglycemia is not present, phenobarbital should be administered IV in a dose of 10 mg/kg over several minutes. This dose may be repeated within 20 minutes if necessary. Occasionally, diphenylhydantoin in similar doses may be necessary as well. If phenobarbital alone is successful, maintenance with 3 to 4 mg/kg/day is indicated. Similar doses of diphenylhydantoin may be necessary for maintenance if this drug was also needed to abort the acute episode. Monitoring of blood levels of these drugs is helpful to achieve adequate maintenance doses.[98] We have found the use of phenobarbital and diphenylhydantoin eminently satisfactory for the acute treatment of prolonged seizure activity and for maintenance in the newborn period. Very occasionally, in less than 5% of cases, rectal or intravenous paraldehyde has been necessary to control prolonged seizure activity. We do not recommend diazepam (Valium) as a first-line drug because

1. The drug has not been shown to be more effective than phenobarbital in the treatment of neonatal seizures.

2. It is a poor drug for maintenance and barbiturate usually must be used.

3. When used with barbiturate, it carries an increased risk of severe circulatory collapse with respiratory failure.[99]

4. The vehicle (sodium benzoate) for intravenous diazepam uncouples the bilirubin-albumin complex and may increase the risk of kernicterus.[100]

5. The therapeutic dose is extremely variable and is not necessarily less than the toxic dose (0.30 and 0.36 mg/kg have led to respiratory arrest in two infants).[101,102]

If hypocalcemia is present, calcium gluconate is administered IV over several minutes in a 5% solution in a dose of 4 ml/kg (200 mg/kg). EKG, or at least cardiac rhythm by auscultation, should be monitored during administration. It is important to recognize that phenobarbital will suppress the seizures of hypocalcemia. If hypomagnesemia is present, 2% to 3% magnesium sulfate is given IV in a dose of 2 to 6 ml, or 50% magnesium sulfate IM in a dose of 0.2 ml/kg per day. Recall that approximately one-half of neonates with seizures secondary to hypocalcemia also have hypomagnesemia. The importance of treating with magnesium is emphasized by the following. The administration of calcium to such infants may increase renal excretion of magnesium,[103] aggravate the hypomagnesemia, and maintain the convulsive state. The administration of magnesium has been shown to correct both the hypocalcemia and hypomagnesemia in some of these babies,[69] perhaps by increasing movement of calcium from bone to plasma.[104] However, magnesium can produce a curare-like neuromuscular blockade, and transient weakness and hypotonia (without plasma magnesium more than 2 SDs above the mean) were noted in nine treated infants in the series of Cockburn and coworkers.[69] Seizures recalcitrant to the above therapies may be related to pyridoxine deficiency or dependency and as noted above, these states should be identified and treated by intravenous pyridoxine (50 mg) with simultaneous EEG monitoring. Control of seizures and return to normal of the EEG pattern occurs within minutes.

Although the treatment of seizures in the neonate should be vigorous, overtreatment can be a serious threat to the baby and must be avoided. Even more important than treatment of the spells is the determination of the specific etiologic diagnosis because the most serious error to be made in the management of the convulsing neonate is to delay or to completely miss the diagnosis and treatment of a correctable disturbance such as hypoglycemia, hypocalcemia, or bacterial meningitis.

HYPOXIC-ISCHEMIC PERINATAL BRAIN INJURY

Scope of the Problem

This is an immense clinical problem, for hypoxic and/or ischemic injuries account for the greatest number of the severe nonprogressive neurologic deficits occurring secondary to perinatal events. These neurologic deficits usually occur in combination and include mental retardation, seizure disorders, spasticity, choreoathetosis, and ataxia. In the following paragraphs, we will discuss the pathogenetic factors of general importance, the prognosis as it can be best determined at the present time, the neurologic syndromes seen in the neonatal period, and the neuropathologic lesions with their accompanying neurologic sequelae.

General Pathogenetic Factors

The neuropathologic lesions that develop consequent to hypoxic-ischemic insults are concomitants of a wide variety of neonatal diseases. Hypoxia (or, more accurately, hypoxemia) occurs most commonly in association with (1) perinatal asphyxia, (2) recurrent apneic spells, or (3) severe respiratory disease. Ischemia (*i.e.*, diminished perfusion of brain, associated usually with systemic hypotension),

occurs most commonly with (1) cardiac arrest or severe bradycardia associated with perinatal asphyxia or recurrent apneic spells, (2) severe cardiac failure, as with congenital heart disease, or (3) vascular collapse associated with sepsis. An additional lesion not to be discussed in this context, porencephaly, is primarily an ischemic lesion associated most commonly with a failure of perfusion *in utero* of a specific cerebral artery or branch thereof.

The precise relationships between the clinical events just noted and the development of hypoxic-ischemic brain injury are still largely unknown. However, considerable insight has been gained from recent studies of birth-related events in the human and, particularly, the subhuman primate. Caldeyro–Barcia and coworkers have studied the relationship of uterine contractions and the fall in fetal heart rate that is largely synchronous with the peak of the contraction (type 1 dips).[105-107] These decelerations of fetal heart rate appear to be related to compression of the fetal head, occurring particularly after rupture of membranes and cervical dilatation when the head becomes engaged. [105,106] Type 1 dips occur during 25% to 40% of uterine contractions under these conditions.[105] In monitoring of fetal EEG and heart rate as well as amniotic fluid pressure, these workers observed the association of slow waves in the EEG with the type 1 dips in fetal heart rate. Similar EEG changes have been noted in fetal animals (*e.g.*, lambs) made anoxic by administration of nitrogen.[108] It has been suggested that the uterine contractions cause deformations in the cranial cavity disturbing blood flow and producing cerebral ischemia and the EEG change. This relationship remains unestablished. Whether these events play a role in the pathogenesis of some cases of hypoxic-ischemic injury to brain occurring at the time of birth is unknown, but the experimental data are of considerable interest in this regard.

Fetal bradycardia, which begins during uterine contraction but reaches a maximum 30 to 60 seconds after the contraction is completed (type II dips)[109] is of definite clinical importance because the fetus exhibiting such late bradycardia is usually severely asphyxiated and depressed at birth.[110,111] Caldeyro–Barcia and coworkers have correlated this bradycardia with fetal hypoxemia by the use of fetal capillary blood samples and tissue oxygen electrodes.[112] Studies in subhuman primates have shown that type II dips are associated not only with fetal hypoxemia but also with acidosis and hypotension.[113] The bradycardia accentuated the hypotension. When fetal oxygenation was improved by administering 100% O_2 to the mother, the bradycardia ceased, and it was concluded that fetal hypoxemia is the essential component producing the late deceleration of heart rate.[113] Hypoxic depression of the myocardium may be the mechanism whereby fetal hypoxemia causes this type of bradycardia.

The potential for the development of CNS injury secondary to the intrauterine hypoxic and ischemic insults just described is obviously great. The evolution of such injury and the mechanisms operative have been studied in the monkey by Myers and his coworkers.[114-118] The basic experimental model involves the production of "partial asphyxia" of the fetus by such means as infusion of excessive oxytocin to the mother to produce frequent, strong uterine contractions or by mechanically constricting the maternal abdominal aorta. Such measures lead to reduction in placental blood flow and, in the fetus, to marked decreases in partial pressure of oxygen and oxygen content, and increases in partial pressure of carbon dioxide and organic acids, resulting in a hypoxic and acidotic state. Fetal late bradycardia (type II dips) develops following uterine contractions, and each one is associated with a lowering of fetal arterial blood pressure. As the asphyxia worsens, so does the fetal bradycardia and hypotension, and the possibility of ischemic injury to the brain becomes great. In addition, ischemic myocardial injury can occur, thus worsening the cardiac and vascular changes, and a vicious cycle becomes operative. The hypoxic-ischemic insults that occur are accompanied in the monkey by brain swelling, and, associated with this phenomenon, impairment in cerebral blood flow, as measured by the use of ^{14}C-labeled antipyrine with autoradiography.[114] The fixed neuropathological lesions described in such monkeys are similar in many ways to those to be described below for full-term human infants considered to have sustained perinatal hypoxic-ischemic insults.

Recent studies of cerebral blood flow in the human infant indicate an exquisite susceptibility to ischemic injury because of impaired vascular autoregulation.[119] In infants only slightly asphyxiated at birth, cerebral blood flow was shown to be pressure-passive, (i.e., when blood pressure fell so did cerebral blood flow). This indicated impaired autoregulation and means that the newborn is incapable of maintaining adequate cerebral blood flow by arteriolar vasodilation when perfusion pressure falls. Thus, the infant is expected to be prone to cerebral ischemia with only modest falls in blood pressure.[120]

Neurologic Syndrome in the Neonatal Period

Clinical Features. The prototype of hypoxic-ischemic insult is intrauterine asphyxia.[121] In the typical case, hypoxemia and ischemia occur simultaneously or in sequence. Frequently, however, it is possible to define either hypoxemia or ischemia as the dominant insult, and such definition is highly important because it allows us to determine the neurologic features associated with each of these two major insults. When intrauterine asphyxia with severe hypoxemia and/or ischemia has occurred, the infant is initially either deeply stuporous or in coma. Irregularity of respiration becomes apparent, and periodic breathing is the most common abnormality. We have considered this analogous to Cheyne–Stokes respiration and indicative of bilateral hemispheral disturbance (see below, *Apnea*). The induction of periodic breathing by administration of lowered oxygen tensions may be analogous to these observations.[53] Pupillary response to light is intact in the baby at more than approximately 32 weeks of gestation (although careful observation is sometimes necessary to detect the response), and spontaneous roving eye movements are present. Occasionally, eye movements are present only to doll's-head maneuver. Only in babies with very severe insults do signs of severe brain-stem disturbance appear (*i.e.,* fixed, dilated pupils, eye movements absent and not elicitable by doll's-head maneuver). Additional, though less common, signs of brain-stem disturbance in very severe hypoxemic-ischemic injury have included ocular bobbing, skew deviation of eyes, ataxic respirations, and opsoclonus. Nevertheless, most often the initial state of stupor or coma is compatible with primarily bilateral hemispheral disturbance. Seizures appear frequently within the first 12 hours after birth.

At approximately 12 to 24 hours of age, the

infant often becomes less depressed, and, associated with this change in level of consciousness, seizures usually become more severe. In the full-term infant, they are most commonly of the subtle and multifocal clonic types (see below, *Seizures*). Jitteriness may be particularly marked. Those infants who have sustained **primarily ischemic** injury have demonstrated the most impressive patterns of motor weakness—full-term infants have exhibited weakness of proximal limbs, with more impressive involvement of upper than lower extremities (see discussion of parasagittal cerebral injury below), and prematures, bilateral lower limb weakness* (see discussion of periventricular leukomalacia below).

At approximately 24 to 72 hours of age, the level of alertness may again become impaired as the baby lapses into deep stupor or coma. Respiratory arrest may ensue. This turn of events may be accompanied by a full anterior fontanel, and, in our experience, most of the babies with severe hypoxic-ischemic injury who die in the neonatal period do so during this deterioration. At postmortem examination, the dominant findings, in the full-term are cerebral necrosis with edema, and in the premature, intraventricular hemorrhage. Those infants who survive show improvement in the level of consciousness by the end of the first postnatal week. The subsequent course is difficult to define clearly but is usually one of gradual improvement over weeks. The rate of improvement is highly variable; however, those infants improving more rapidly tend to make the greatest ultimate gains. The neurologic sequelae to be described below often do not become apparent for many months after the neonatal insult.

Treatment. The most important form of treatment of this malignant form of brain injury is prevention. Careful monitoring of the fetus during labor and considered but prompt intervention at the early signs of fetal compromise are important in preventing intrauterine hypoxia. The immediate care of the asphyxiated newborn has been reviewed, and the importance of establishing adequate ventilation, maintaining body temperature, treating circu-

*These patterns are quite definite but not striking; we suspect that they have been overlooked in the past, by ourselves as well as others, and are in fact common. The lower limb weakness in premature infants is especially difficult to detect.

latory failure, and administering glucose appropriately emphasized.[122]

Seizures should be managed as described in the section above. In hypoxic-ischemic encephalopathy, particularly prefer phenobarbital, not only for its anticonvulsant action but also for its potential benefit in diminishing cerebral metabolic rate.

Treatment of the cerebral edema of neonatal hypoxic-ischemic encephalopathy has not been necessary as frequently as in older children. Presumably, this reflects a diminished risk in the newborn of transtentorial herniation or other sequelae of expansion of cerebral hemispheres. The cranium of the newborn is considerably less rigid than that of the older infant with tighter sutures. Moreover, edema is usually secondary to cerebral necrosis and thus difficult to modify. Administration of fluids at minimal maintenance levels is appropriate, but a role for glucocorticoids or hypertonic solutions remains unproven.

Prognosis. The outlook for the neonate exposed to hypoxic-ischemic insults has been a subject of considerable controversy for many years. The many studies, mainly retrospective, often cited to support or refute a relation between such insults and brain injury will not be reviewed in detail here. We will discuss in detail in the next section the neuropathologic lesions clearly related to such insults, and such data provide unequivocal evidence that hypoxic-ischemic insults do produce significant brain injury. The most important aspects still to be defined are the quantitative relationships between the severity of the insult and the degree of brain injury. It is still unclear how severe an insult in the neonatal period must be to produce an irreversible neurologic deficit. The central problem in the past has been the difficulty of reliably determining the severity of the insult. Continuous monitoring of the level of hypoxemia is obviously very difficult, despite advances in blood gas technology, and even intermittent assessment of the level of ischemia has not been accomplished because of the lack of practical methodology applicable to the neonate. The recent advent of transcutaneous techniques for monitoring tissue oxygen content, of continuous measurements of blood pressure, and of noninvasive measurements of cerebral blood flow may provide critical data on these issues.

A useful source of information concerning

the relation of the neonatal insult to brain injury is the careful analysis of neonates with seizures secondary to hypoxic/ischemic encephalopathy. Obviously, an important bias is introduced because the occurrence of seizures *per se* indicates an insult that has clearly affected the brain in the newborn period. The most recent data suggest that such infants have approximately a 50% chance for normal development.[97] The issue of outlook is reviewed further in Chapter 19.

Neuropathologic and Neurologic Sequelae

The often devastating neurologic sequelae of hypoxic-ischemic injury have as their structural bases a variety of neuropathologic lesions. This presentation is not the appropriate forum for a discussion of these neurologic sequelae because they appear in complete form many months to years after birth. Nevertheless, it should be emphasized that the sequelae include a wide variety of neurologic deficits, such as mental retardation and more discrete intellectual deficits, various motor disturbances (especially spasticity, choreoathetosis and/or ataxia), and seizure disorders. In Malamud's series of 198 severely affected cases evaluated by postmortem examination, 82% of the patients were severely mentally retarded, 81% had epilepsy, 50% spastic quadriplegia, and 7% athetosis.[123] In the large series of Crothers and Paine, those cases of cerebral palsy clearly related to perinatal anoxia were composed of approximately 50% with spastic hemiplegia, "tetraplegia," or "triplegia," and approximately 25% each of "pure extrapyramidal cerebral palsy" and "mixed types."[124] In McDonald's series of more than 1500 babies with birth weights of less than 1800 g, spastic diplegia (comparable to spastic tetraplegia, see discussion below) accounted for approximately 80% of the motor deficits on follow-up and was highly correlated with cardiorespiratory disturbances in the neonatal period.[125] An IQ of less than 90 occurred in 40% to 60% of these infants. Seizure disorders occurred in approximately 20% to 50% of those patients with spastic motor deficits secondary to perinatal injury, whereas only 2% to 3% of those patients with extrapyramidal disorders developed seizures.[124,125] Thus, it is clear from this brief review of the sequelae of hypoxic-ischemic insults in the neonatal period that

significant brain injury and a variety of neurologic manifestations certainly do occur. With this background, we next discuss the neuropathologic substrates for these neurologic deficits.

The neuropathologic sequelae of hypoxemic-ischemic injury in the neonatal period have been described particularly in the writings of Courville,[126] Malamud,[123,127] Banker,[128,129] Towbin,[130,131] and Norman.[132] Many lesions have been described, but at least four basic and clinically important lesions can be recognized. These are selective neuronal necrosis, status marmoratus of basal ganglia and thalamus, parasagittal cerebral injury, and periventricular leukomalacia. The lesions often occur in combination and their pathogenesis may also overlap, but, to a considerable extent, these can be considered pathologic and clinical entities.

Selective Neuronal Necrosis. *Pathological Features.* This is the hallmark of hypoxic injury. There is necrosis of neurons of cerebral and cerebellar cortices. In cerebral cortex, the deeper cortical layers are affected in a laminar pattern, especially in the depths of sulci. In the cerebellar cortex, Purkinje cells are first affected. In mild cases, only hippocampal cerebral cortex (neurons of Sommer's sector) and Purkinje cells are affected, whereas in more severe cases the cerebral cortex is affected diffusely and granule cells of cerebellum may become involved. In more advanced lesions of cerebral cortex, the gyrus may become shrunken, the gray matter replaced with a dense network of glial fibrils, and the immediately subjacent white matter involved with gliosis and paucity of myelin.[132] The margins of the lesions may contain dense collections of myelinated fibers, actually myelinated glial fibers, similar to those to be described below for status marmoratus. This constellation of findings, characteristic of ulegyria or sclerotic microgyria, is often most apparent in arterial border zones (*e.g.,* posterior parietooccipital regions) or in end fields of cerebral arteries (*e.g.,* visual cortex). Much clinicopathologic evidence has been presented to indicate that these are hypoxic lesions. (See Courville for review.[126]) Courville suggests that the cortical lesion is the primary lesion caused by hypoxemia and the white matter disturbance is a secondary vascular phenomenon.[126]

An additional accompaniment in neonatal

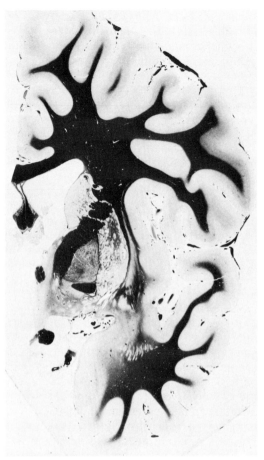

Fig. 39-4. Status marmoratus of basal ganglia. Coronal section of cerebral hemisphere, stained for myelin, from a patient who died years after the insult. Marbled appearance is especially striking in putamen. (Courtesy of Dr. E.P. Richardson, Jr.)

hypoxic-ischemic encephalopathy is injury to neurons of the brain stem.[133-135] Particularly involved are various motor nuclei of cranial nerves.

Clinical Features. The neurologic concomitants are readily predicted from the topography of the lesions. Thus, mental retardation, seizure disorders, and spasticity are related to the cerebral lesions. It is still unclear, though probable, that the ataxic component demonstrable with careful examination of many patients with spastic motor deficits is related to the cerebellar disturbance.[124] Correlates of the brain stem neuronal injury may include disturbances of sucking, swallowing, and facial movement.

Status Marmoratus. Pathologic Features. This lesion represents a very distinctive change of basal ganglia, especially putamen and caudate, and thalamus, characterized by a peculiar marbled appearance of these nuclear structures (Fig. 39-4). In complete form, status marmoratus is a lesion related to perinatal events and is without a similar counterpart at any later stage of life. The major pathologic features are (1) neuronal loss, (2) astrocytic gliosis, and (3) hypermyelination (*i.e.,* an increase of myelinated fibers within structures not normally heavily interspersed with such fibers). The neuronal loss and gliosis are similar to such events occurring in other destructive lesions. The hypermyelination is the unique characteristic of this lesion. Light microscopic observations had suggested previously that the many myelinated fibers were axons, and the idea that such overgrowth was a result of regenerative activity was proposed and accepted for many years.[136] However, Borit and Herndon have used electron microscopic techniques to demonstrate that the myelinated fibers are, in fact, astrocytic processes.[137] Thus, in their material the fibers contained large numbers of approximately 70- to 100-A thick filaments characteristic of astrocytic processes. The absence of the numerous organelles (mitochondria, microtubules, dense core granules, vesicles) found in axons further indicated that the processes were not axonal but astrocytic in type. Thus, it is apparent that the very young brain near the time of normal myelination may respond to injury in this distinctive fashion.

The etiology of status marmoratus is related, at least in part, to hypoxemia. Several lines of evidence support this contention. The lesions are bilateral and symmetrical, as one would expect from hypoxemic injury. They are associated very frequently with other typically hypoxemic lesions (*e.g.,* sclerotic microgyria and hippocampal and cerebellar neuronal loss).[127,132,138] Finally, as described above, a lesion similar to status marmoratus has been produced in fetal monkeys subjected to "prolonged partial asphyxia," which results in fetal hypoxemia. The possible roles of ischemia, acidosis and/or venous stasis are unknown.[139]

Clinical features. The neurologic sequelae will include the features described above for hypoxemic cortical injury if the latter lesion accompanies status marmoratus. However, the striking additional features and those ascribable to the injury of basal ganglia are extrapyramidal disturbances, especially choreoathetosis and rigidity. It is interesting that the extrapyramidal abnormalities usually do not become clearly apparent until about 1 year of age or later.

Parasagittal Cerebral Injury. Pathologic Features. Parasagittal cerebral injury ("watershed infarcts") is most probably the neuropathologic consequence of a generalized reduction in cerebral blood flow in the full-term infant. The areas of necrosis of cerebral cortex and subcortical white matter have a characteristic distribution and include primarily the superomedial aspects of the cerebral convexities. Involvement of posterior cerebrum is greater than that of anterior cerebrum. The lesions extend from the second frontal gyri to the paramedian central regions and to posterior parietooccipital areas. Other areas affected are in temporal lobes and cerebellum, as well as basal ganglia and thalami. These infarcts are principally in the border zones lying between the end fields of the major cerebral arteries. Thus, the lesions of the cerebral convexity are between the supplies of the middle and anterior cerebral arteries, the middle and posterior cerebral arteries and all three major cerebral arteries (posterior parietooccipital region). The lesions in the temporal lobe are between the supplies of the middle and posterior cerebral arteries, in the cerebellum between the superior cerebellar and posterior inferior cerebellar arteries, and so forth.

These border zones are the brain regions most susceptible to a fall in systemic blood pressure. The characteristic topography of the important cerebral lesions was described clearly by Meyer[140] who related the injury to systemic hypotension.[140] The watershed concept, based on the analogy with an irrigation system supplying a series of fields with water, was enunciated by Zulch, who pointed out the vulnerability of the "last fields" when the head of pressure falls.[141] This concept received experimental support in the studies of Brierly and Excell.[142] Profound systemic hypotension was produced in the rhesus monkey by the injection of trimethaphan camsylate (Arfonad) combined with head-up tilt of the table. Normal arterial oxygen saturation was maintained by mechanical ventilation. Typical watershed lesions were produced in the cortex (and cere-

bellum) of these animals and were ascribed to the sharply reduced cerebral blood flow. A particular susceptibility of the human newborn infant to ischemic injury is suggested by the impairment of vascular autoregulation described above.

Although watershed infarction has received wide attention in the neurologic literature of adults, it should be emphasized that Meyer's original study included a case of a child who experienced severe birth asphyxia secondary to tightly wrapped nuchal cord.[140] Other well-documented examples in neonates have been recorded by Norman, and coworkers[143] and are apparent in the material presented by Courville.[126] We have defined this lesion in the newborn period by the use of the technetium brain scan.[144] Affected infants have not been premature, and it is unlikely, in fact, that cerebral infarction in the parasagittal distribution occurs commonly in the premature, for reasons to be outlined below. Thus, it is clear that ischemia in the perinatal period can result in a characteristic pattern of cerebral infarction, and this watershed injury is found in the full-term infant.

Clinical Features. The neurologic sequelae of parasagittal cerebral injury occuring in the perinatal period are unknown. The few cases with some clinical documentation have had concomitant hypoxemic injury, and, thus, the sequelae of the ischemic injury have been difficult to define. However, as noted above, we have defined in the neonatal period the characteristic hip-shoulder pattern of weakness (with greater involvement of upper than lower extremities), predictable on the basis of the topography of the involvement in the region of the motor cortex. The more posteriorly located lesions (*i.e.,* in posterior parietooccipital areas) lie in regions of critical importance for many associative functions, especially those relating to verbal and visual input and output and to various visuomotor phenomena. It is interesting to speculate that some of the examples of the various dyslectic syndromes and other less well-defined perceptual disturbances, presenting at school age, have their origin in perinatal ischemic injury. Certainly, delineation of the neurology of ischemic injury in the full-term neonate is an important area for future clinical research.

Periventricular Leukomalacia. Pathologic Features. Periventricular leukomalacia is the

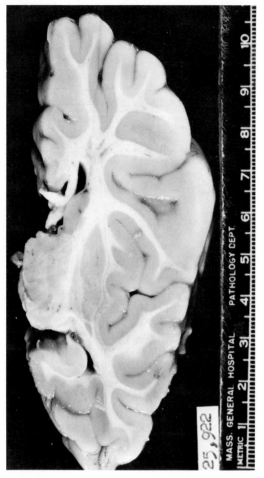

Fig. 39-5. Periventricular leukomalacia. Coronal section of cerebral hemisphere from a 20-month-old child who was the product of a 35-week pregnancy and experienced cardiorespiratory difficulties in the neonatal period. Small cavitated lesions can be seen approximately 5 mm from the external angle of the lateral ventricle of the parietal lobe. (DeReuck J et al: Arch Neurol 27:229, 1972; Copyright 1972, American Medical Association)[145]

neuropathologic consequence of a generalized reduction in cerebral blood flow in the premature infant. It is a common lesion, occurring in 19% of all infants dying before 1 month of age. As many as 75% of the cases are prematures.[128] The areas of necrosis of periventricular white matter have a characteristic distribution and include principally the regions just adjacent to the external angles of the lateral ventricles (Fig. 39-5).[145] The lesions are found most commonly along the frontal horn,

the body, the collateral trigone, and the occipital and temporal horns of the lateral ventricles. In the smallest lesions, the white matter immediately adjacent to the ventricular system is spared, but, in larger lesions, the necrosis may extend from ependyma to (but not including) subcortical arcuate fibers. The evolution of the lesions has been described well by Banker and Larroche and includes initially a coagulation necrosis, followed by astrocytic, endothelial, and macrophage proliferation.[128] These relatively early changes are followed by cavitation and thinning of periventricular white matter with widening of the lateral ventricles. In severe lesions, periventricular cavitation is marked and bears a distinct resemblance to similar cases recorded earlier by Courville,[146] Malamud,[147] and Schwartz.[139]

The pathogenesis of periventricular leukomalacia is now well established. After Virchow's initial description of the entity in 1867,[148] Parrot suggested that the periventricular region is affected because it is farthest from the blood supply.[149] Not until the careful study of Banker and Larroche was the relation of the lesion to vascular border zones emphasized.[128] They considered the periventricular infarcts to be in the border zone between the deep territories of the middle, anterior, and posterior cerebral arteries. The precise nature of these periventricular border zones has been delineated recently.[145,150] By a postmortem colloidal injection-radiographic technique, DeReuck defined three periventricular arterial end zones (Fig. 39-6).[150] The type 2 zone is essentially a border zone between penetrating branches of the middle cerebral artery and the posterior choriodal branches of the posterior cerebral artery. However, the type 1 zone is an arterial end field of penetrating branches of the middle cerebral artery, and the type 3 zone is derived, as depicted, by branches of the middle cerebral artery, which reach the ventricular wall and loop back (ventriculofugal) or end before reaching the ventricular wall (ventriculopetal). These three zones have a characteristic distribution in the periventricular region, and it is precisely within these zones that the lesions of periventricular leukomalacia occur. In addition to these pathoanatomic considerations, it is pertinent to recall the impaired vascular autoregulation and, hence, particular susceptibility of the neonatal brain to ischemic injury.

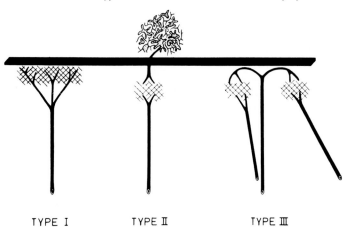

TYPE I   TYPE II   TYPE III

Fig. 39-6. Three types of periventricular arterial endzones (cross-hatching). See text for details (DeReuck J et al: Arch Neurol 27:279, 1972; Copyright 1972, American Medical Association)[145]

Although the pathologic, anatomic, and physiologic data, as well as the clinical correlates, in the neonatal period indicate that periventricular leukomalacia is an ischemic lesion, it remains for us to explain why ischemia in the premature infant does not result in the cerebral cortical watershed infarcts described above for older infants. The relative sparing of cerebral cortex is apparently the result of the presence of many meningeal anastomoses between the anterior, middle, and posterior cerebral arteries, anastomoses characteristic of fetal but not postnatal brain.[151] This explanation is supported by the observation that in the mature cat, which has interarterial anastomoses comparable to those in human fetal brain, periventricular leukomalacia can be produced by experimental occlusion of the basilar artery and subsequent narrowing of one or both carotic arteries.[152]

Clinical Features. The neurologic sequelae of periventricular leukomalacia probably include the most important motor deficit observed in prematurely born infants (*i.e.,* the so-called spastic diplegia syndrome). This constellation of motor disturbances has as its central feature a spastic paresis of extremities which is characterized by greater involvement of lower limbs than upper. The neuropathologic studies of periventricular leukomalacia include only a few cases that survived for several months or more.[128,145] Thus, precise clinicopathologic correlation has not yet been performed. Nevertheless, several lines of evidence indicate that periventricular leukomalacia results in spastic diplegia and its variants. First, the topography of the lesion includes the region of cerebral white matter traversed by descending fibers from motor cortex. Moreover, those fibers subserving lower extremity function are more likely to be affected by the periventricular locus of the necrosis. More severe lesions with lateral extension would be expected to affect upper extremities, also. Indeed, cases of spastic diplegia with significant involvement of upper extremities exhibit other manifestations of more severe clinical disturbance (*e.g.,* more severe intellectual deficits).[125]

A second major line of evidence pertains to the well-established clinical finding that spastic diplegia is the most common motor deficit observed in prematurely born infants on follow-up.[125] Thus, in McDonald's series of more than 1000 infants weighing less than 1800 g at birth, 6.5% exhibited "cerebral palsy" and 81% of these, spastic diplegia.[125] Approximately one-half of these had affection of lower limbs only. The highest incidence of spastic diplegia occurred in the babies with the lowest gestational ages. Moreover, a significant history of cardiorespiratory disturbances in the neonatal period was especially common among these patients. Such disturbances occurred in virtually all of the cases of periventricular leukomalacia documented at postmortem examination by Banker and Larroche[128] and De Reuck and coworkers.[145] Thus, a growing body of clinical data indicates that this ischemic lesion of the premature infant underlies the most common neurologic sequela of premature birth, spastic diplegia.

INTRACRANIAL HEMORRHAGE

Scope of the Problem

This is an important clinical problem simply in terms of its frequency. Indeed, as discussed below, nearly one-half of all premature infants in neonatal intensive care facilities can be shown to have experienced periventricular-intraventricular hemorrhage. At least in the now growing population of small *preterm* infants that survive the early neonatal period, intracranial hemorrhage and the complications thereof appear to be the major determinants of neurologic morbidity.

The prognosis for infants with intracranial hemorrhage varies according to the nature of the hemorrhage and the pathogenetic factors leading to the hemorrhage. Determination of the precise site and extent of the hemorrhage is critical for decisions of therapy and estimation of prognosis. Such determinations are possible with careful clinical assessment and use of the CT scan. Unfortunately, precise quantitative estimation of the injury produced by the pathogenetic factors (*e.g.*, asphyxia, trauma, or both) and separable from the injury produced by the hemorrhage is much more difficult to make in certain cases. These considerations are discussed below in relation to the individual types of hemorrhage.

General Pathogenetic Factors

There are four major clinically important categories of intracranial hemorrhage which occur in the newborn period. These are

1. Subdural hemorrhage
2. Primary subarachnoid hemorrhage
3. Periventricular-intraventricular hemorrhage
4. Intracerebellar hemorrhage

The distinctive pathogenesis of each of these is discussed in the appropriate section below. It should be recognized at the outset, however, that two major pathogenetic themes are operative (*i.e.,* trauma and asphyxia). Subdural hemorrhage is principally related to trauma; intraventricular hemorrhage is principally related to asphyxia. Subarachnoid hemorrhage is related both to trauma and asphyxia; the former may be more important in the full-term and the latter in the premature infant. The pathogenesis of intracerebellar hemorrhage is unclear, although a relation to asphyxia appears to be the best possibility. Although the various types of hemorrhage, as well as the major pathogenetic factors, may occur concurrently, almost invariably a single form of hemorrhage and series of pathogenetic events dominate the clinical syndrome. The major varieties of intracranial hemorrhage are discussed next.

Subdural Hemorrhage

Neuropathological Features. Before summarizing the major varieties of subdural hemorrhage occurring in the newborn period, we shall review briefly the major anatomic features of the veins involved in the production of such hemorrhage. The deep venous drainage of the cerebrum empties into the great vein of Galen at the junction of the tentorium and falx. The confluence of the vein of Galen and the inferior sagittal sinus, the latter running in the inferior margin of the falx, forms the straight sinus. This sinus proceeds directly posteriorly and with the superior sagittal sinus, running in the superior margin of the falx, and the lateral sinus, running in the lateral margin of the tentorium, forms the torcula. Blood from the torcula proceeds by way of the lateral sinus eventually to the jugular vein. The superficial portion of the cerebrum is drained by the superficial cerebral veins which empty into the superior sagittal sinus. Tears of these veins, venous sinuses, or both, occurring secondary to forces to be described below and often accompanying laceration of dura, result in subdural hemorrhage.

The three major varieties of subdural hemorrhage are

1. Tentorial lacerations, with rupture of
   a. straight sinus
   b. vein of Galen
   c. lateral sinus
2. Falx laceration, with rupture of
   a. inferior sagittal sinus
3. Rupture of superficial cerebral veins

With tears of the tentorium, hemorrhage is most often infratentorial.[153,154] This is the case particularly with ruptures of the vein of Galen or straight sinus, or with severe involvement of the lateral sinus. The clot extends into the posterior fossa and very rapidly results in lethal compression of the brain stem.[131,139,153-156] Massive infratentorial hemorrhage from a rupture of the vein of Galen may also occur without visible tear of the tentorium. Tentorial laceration is the most common accompaniment of *severe* subdural hemorrhage in the newborn period.

Laceration of the falx as the sole accompaniment of subdural hemorrhage is very uncommon. The tear occurs usually at a point near the junction of the falx with the tentorium. The source of bleeding that results is usually the inferior sagittal sinus and the clot is located in the longitudinal cerebral fissure over the corpus callosum.

Rupture of superficial cerebral veins, usually near their entrance into the superior sagittal sinus, with hemorrhage over the cerebral convexity, is probably quite common because it is a frequent incidental finding at autopsy in the term newborn.[131] However, clinically significant hemorrhage of this type is considerably less frequent than usually suggested. When such bleeding does occur in considerable amount, it is usually bilateral and accompanied by subarachnoid blood. The trauma that leads to the hemorrhage frequently results also in cerebral contusion, and the latter, in fact, often dominates the clinical picture.

Clinical Features. In contrast to the considerable literature relative to the neuropathologic aspects of subdural hemorrhage, astonishingly little clinical neurologic data are available. However, some important conclusions can be drawn from our own observations and from those recorded by Craig, Fleming, and Haller.[153,154,156]

Tentorial laceration with massive infratentorial hemorrhage is associated with neurologic disturbance from the time of birth. Initially the baby, almost always a full-term, demonstates signs of midbrain-upper pons compression (*i.e.*, stupor or coma), skew deviation of eyes with lateral deviation that is not altered by doll's-head maneuver, unequal pupils with some disturbance of response to light, and rapid respiration. In infratentorial hemorrhage, marked nuchal rigidity with retrocollis or opisthotonus may also be a helpful early sign.[157] Over minutes to hours, as the clot becomes larger, stupor progresses to coma, pupil(s) may become fixed and dilated, and signs of lower brain stem compression appear. Ocular bobbing and ataxic respirations may occur, and

finally respiratory arrest will ensue. Infants who survive the deterioration of the early hours may live long enough to develop severe hydrocephalus secondary to obstruction of flow of CSF through the tentorial notch to the convexities for reabsorption. A less acute syndrome has been described recently and identification by CT scan demonstrated.

No careful description of the clinical course of falx tears with subdural hemorrhage is available. However, it is likely that initially bilateral cerebral signs appear but that striking neurologic findings do not occur until the clot has extended infratentorially. The resulting syndrome is then similar to that just described.

Subdural hemorrhage over the cerebral convexities is associated with at least three clinical states. First, and probably most common, minor degrees of hemorrhage occur and no clinical signs are apparent. Second, signs of cerebral disturbance may occur, especially seizures. The seizures may be focal and are often accompanied by focal cerebral signs (*e.g.*, hemiparesis, deviation of eyes to the side of the hemiparesis—although the eyes will move by doll's-head maneuver because this is a cerebral lesion). Subarachnoid blood is very common, as it is in all forms of neonatal subdural hemorrhage, and a fracture may be apparent. An identical neurologic syndrome can occur without subdural hemorrhage and has been considered secondary to "cerebral contusion."[74] The large majority of these babies are normal on follow-up.[74,159] Convexity subdural hematoma is demonstrated most readily by CT scan. A third clinical presentation, though still not established unequivocally, may be the occurrence of subdural hemorrhage in the neonatal period with few clinical signs and the development over the next several months of a chronic subdural effusion. It is certainly well known that many infants presenting in the first 6 months of life with an enlarging head, increased transillumination and chronic subdural effusion have no known etiology for the lesion and that subdural hemorrhage can evolve into subdural effusion.[160,161] This potential relationship deserves further study, although the difficulties in structure of such a study are obvious.

Pathogenesis. Neonatal subdural hemorrhage is almost exclusively a traumatic lesion of the full-term baby.[153-155] The major factors involved in the production of the traumatic event relate to

1. The relationship of the size of the fetal head to the size of the birth canal
2. Rigidity of the birth canal
3. The duration of labor
4. The manner of delivery

Thus, subdural hemorrhage is most likely to occur when the baby is relatively large and the birth canal relatively small; when the pelvic structures are unusually rigid as in a primiparous or elderly multiparous mother; when the duration of labor is either unusually brief, not allowing enough time for dilatation of the pelvic structures, or unusually long, subjecting the head to prolonged compression and molding; when the head must pass through a birth canal not gradually adapted to it, as in foot or breech presentations; or when delivery requires difficult forceps extraction. Under such circumstances there is excessive vertical molding of the head with frontooccipital elongation. This results in stretching of both the falx and tentorium and a tendency for tearing of the tentorium near its junction with the falx. Even if laceration does not occur, the sinuses into which the vein of Galen drains are placed stretch, and the result is often tear of the vein of Galen or its immediate tributaries. Thus results the first group of subdural hemorrhage described above. Tear of the falx occurs particularly with extreme fronto-occipital elongation, especially that associated with face or brow presentation. Extreme vertical molding underlies most tears of superficial cerebral veins and the formation of convexity subdurals. In addition to the phenomena just described, injudicious use of forceps, particularly mid or high forceps, can result in skull fracture and cerebral contusion by direct compressive effects.

Fortunately, operation of many of these pathogenetic factors has been eliminated by vastly improved obstetric practice in most centers. Thus, on many obstetrical services subdural hemorrhage of any sort is a very uncommon entity.

Primary Subarachnoid Hemorrhage

Neuropathological Features. Primary subarachnoid hemorrhage refers to hemorrhage within the subarachnoid space that is not secondary to extension from subdural or intraventricular hemorrhage. This is a common variety of neonatal intracranial hemorrhage but is usually not of major clinical importance. The source of the bleeding is venous, and, thus, subarachnoid hemorrhage in the neonate is unlike the dramatic arterial hemorrhage of older patients. Small amounts of subarachnoid blood are not infrequently found in postmortem exams of newborns not suspected clinically of having intracranial hemorrhage.[131] Even in major degrees of subarachnoid hemorrhage, signs of significantly increased intracranial pressure with brain stem compression is extremely uncommon (perhaps because the hemorrhage emanates from small veins and not large vessels or arteries) and the only significant sequela clearly related to the hemorrhage is hydrocephalus. The latter is secondary either to adhesions around the tentorial notch, which result in obstruction to CSF flow, or to adhesions over the cerebral convexities, which result in impaired CSF flow and/or absorption.

Clinical Features. It is very difficult to delineate the clinical neurologic features of primary subarachnoid hemorrhage because the lesion is often associated with other factors deleterious to brain function. However, we have defined three major syndromes. First, and most commonly, minor degrees of hemorrhage occur and no signs develop. This is particularly the case with premature infants. The outlook in these babies is probably uniformly good. Second, primary subarachnoid hemorrhage can certainly result in seizures[74,155] The seizures most often have their onset on approximately the second day of life (see *Seizures* above). This is a consistent and very helpful clinical finding. In the interictal period these babies usually appear remarkably well, and the euphemism, "well baby with seizures," often seems appropriate. The outlook in these cases is excellent; approximately 90% are normal on follow-up. A third syndrome, quite rare, is massive subarachnoid hemorrhage with a rapidly fatal course. These infants have often sustained a severe asphyctic insult, sometimes with an element of trauma at the time of birth.[154,155] A few will prove to have a structural vascular lesion, such as an aneurysm or vascular malformation.

Pathogenesis. Neonatal subarachnoid hemorrhage is primarily related to an asphyctic insult. The relationship of the asphyxia to the

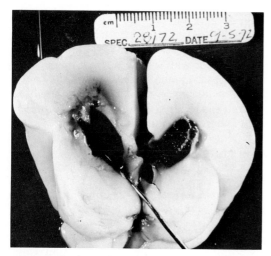

Fig. 39-7. Periventricular hemorrhage with intraventricular rupture at the level of the foramen of Monro; blood fills both lateral ventricles. Site of rupture of hemorrhage from right subependymal region can be seen. (Courtesy of Dr. John Axley)

development of the hemorrhage is probably similar in many ways to that described in detail below for intraventricular hemorrhage.

Periventricular-Intraventricular Hemorrhage

Neuropathologic Features. Although this variety of intracranial hemorrhage is usually termed **intraventricular hemorrhage,** the most descriptive appellation is **periventricular-intraventricular hemorrhage.**[162] Exceptional neuropathologic studies include those of Larroche, Schwartz, Yakovlev, Towbin, and Wigglesworth.[131,139,163,164,165] In its most striking form, this lesion is characterized by hemorrhage into the subependymal germinal matrix, usually at the level of the head of the caudate nucleus and less commonly the body of the caudate or the thalamus, which bursts through the ependyma and fills the ventricular system. However, approximately 20% to 40% of the lesions may be confined to the subependymal region and never enter the ventricular system.[164] The hemorrhage most commonly originates at the level of the foramen of Monro (Fig. 39-7).[163,164] For example, 90% of periventricular–intraventricular hemorrhages originating from a single site were located at the level of the foramen of Monro in Yakovlev's 65 specimens.[164] Hemorrhage at the level

of the frontal horn was next most common and, at the level of occipital and temporal horns, least common. The lesion has been shown to emanate from capillaries in the periventricular vascular network.[165] The initially small hematoma may enlarge because of a large amount of periventricular fibrinolytic activity (see below) and then burst through the ependyma. The hemorrhage may spread throughout the ventricular system, pass through the foramina of Magendie and Luschka and collect in the posterior fossa (Fig. 39-8). Occasionally, hemorrhage extends forward to the optic chiasm.

In those cases that survive the initial hemorrhage, neurologic sequelae often occur. The most common of these is progressive hydrocephalus.[163,166] The most frequent etiologies for the hydrocephalus are obstruction of CSF flow through the aqueduct by organized hemorrhage and necrotic ependyma, or obstruction of flow out of the fourth ventricle or through the posterior fossa by organized hemorrhage in the posterior fossa.

Clinical Features. The dominant clinical feature is the almost invariable association of intraventricular hemorrhage with prematurity, and, in fact, the risk of the lesion increases with decreasing gestational age.[162] The remarkably high frequency of periventricular-

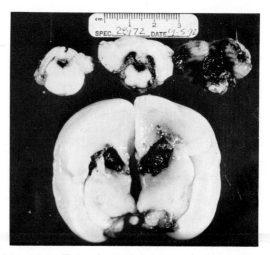

Fig. 39-8. Extension of intraventricular hemorrhage. Same case as shown in Fig. 38-7. Hemorrhage can be seen in lateral ventricles, aqueduct of Sylvius, fourth ventricle, and in subarachnoid space around cerebellum and base of brain. (Courtesy of Dr. John Axley)

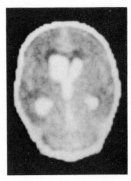

Fig. 39-9. CT scan, marked intraventricular hemorrhage. Note blood in frontal horns, third ventricle, and occipital horns.

intraventricular hemorrhage is demonstrated by the finding of a 40% to 50% incidence in premature infants (less than 1500 g body weight or 32 weeks of gestation), evaluated recently by CT scan in two neonatal intensive care facilities.[167,168]

Two major clinical syndromes associated with intraventricular hemorrhage can be defined: a rapid, catastrophic deterioration, and a more saltatory deterioration. The first syndrome has been well-described in the major writings on intraventricular hemorrhage and is usually associated with major degrees of intraventricular hemorrhage. (The converse is not necessarily true, however; severe hemorrhage need not be accompanied by the catastrophic syndrome.) Onset often appears to depend on the timing of a major asphyctic insult, which precedes the hemorrhage. Thus, if the insult occurs at birth, the deterioration occurs after 24 or 48 hours of life; and if the insult occurs in association with severe respiratory distress syndrome, the deterioration follows in 24 to 48 hours and, thus, after several days of life (and perhaps during the period of recovery from the pulmonary disease).[169]

Evolution of the catastrophic deterioration occurs in minutes to hours and consists usually of deep stupor progressing to coma; hypoventilation going on to respiratory arrest; pupils fixed to light, (pertinent if the child is more than 32-weeks gestation); eyes skewed and/or deviated, often downward, and not readily movable by the doll's-head manuever; and flaccid quadriparasis. Generalized tonic seizures and decerebrate posturing may also occur. Falling hematocrit, a bulging anterior fontanel, and aberrations of blood pressure, temperature, water, and glucose homeostasis are not infrequent. We have attributed much of this syndrome to the movement of blood through the ventricular system. CT scan usually reveals a major hemorrhage (Fig. 39-9), and death or marked hydrocephalus is the usual outcome.

A second important syndrome observed with intraventricular hemorrhage is more subtle in its presentation. Because of its usual stuttering evolution, we have used the term **saltatory deterioration.** Progression occurs over many hours and consists of fragments of the catastrophic syndrome, including subtle aberrations of the level of consciousness, quantity and quality of spontaneous and elicited motility, hypotonia, and skewed deviation or vertical drift of the eyes, usually downward. This syndrome may be so subtle that the hemorrhage, for all intents and purposes, is clinically silent. CT scan may reveal a major intraventricular hemorrhage, but more often demonstrates a less severe lesion (Fig. 39-10). Most of these infants survive the lesion, and only the minority develop hydrocephalus.

Pathogenesis. Concepts of pathogenesis must explain the predilection of intraventricular hemorrhage for prematurity, the distinctive periventricular locus of the lesion, and the strong association with perinatal asphyxia. The association with prematurity relates to the

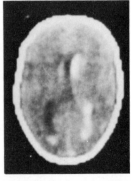

Fig. 39-10. CT scan of moderate intraventricular hemorrhage. Note blood in frontal horns, probably emanating from hemorrhage in germinal matrix over heads of the caudate nuclei, and blood in occipital horns, right more than left.

fact that the subependymal germinal matrix in the human cerebrum does not dissipate until term.[164] This matrix provides very poor support for the small vessels that course through it. In addition, as noted above, vascular autoregulation is impaired in the human premature infant.[119] Thus, when arterial perfusion rises, secondary, for example, to resuscitative efforts, infusion of colloid, hyperosmolar solutions, and the like, the periventricular capillaries will be directly exposed to the burst in pressure and encouraged to rupture.[170] Moreover, the vessels in the periventricular vascular network of the premature infant are relatively thin-walled and fragile.[171] The characteristic **periventricular locus** of the lesion relates to the fact that this is the site of the germinal matrix. Moreover, in this region a peculiar hemodynamic situation exists; there is a peculiar U-turn in the direction of blood flow, as the terminal, thalamostriate, and choroidal veins converge to form the internal cerebral vein. The resulting sharp change in direction of blood flow would be expected to encourage venous stasis, congestion, increased intravascular pressure, and rupture. In addition, an unusual amount of fibrinolytic activity is present in the periventricular white matter in the human newborn, and this may encourage spread of the hematoma.[172] Asphyxia and associated metabolic consequences may act in three ways: (1) the precipitation of circulatory failure and, as a result, venous congestion in brain;[173,174] (2) direct injury to the endothelium of small blood vessels;[174] and perhaps most important; (3) worsening of the impairment of vascular autoregulation.[175] It is likely that the relative roles of these various factors differ for individual infants, but several basic pathogenetic principles seem apparent. Further work will be of particular interest and importance.

Intracerebellar Hemorrhage

Neuropathology. Recent reports suggest that a relatively frequent type of hemorrhage in small premature infants is intracerebellar.[176-179] Thus, in two large series, 15% to 25% of infants of less than approximately 32 weeks of gestation and 1500 g body weight exhibited major degrees of intracerebellar hemorrhage.[176,177] The locus of the hemorrhage within the cerebellum has not been consistent. Both subpial and subependymal distributions have been noted. In most of the major lesions,

the peripheral one-half of the cerebellar hemisphere was particularly involved and the cerebellar cortex and white matter destroyed. Whether these lesions originate from poorly supported small vessels in the germinal cell layers in the subependymal region around the fourth ventricle or in the subpial external granule cell layer remains to be determined. Of particular note is a strong association with marked intraventricular hemorrhage and the recent observations suggesting that the intracerebellar blood may represent *extension from* intraventricular hemorrhage.[179] The clinical frequency and significance of these lesions are unclear, because none has been described in large series of premature infants routinely subjected to CT scan.[167,168]

Clinical Features. Because the diagnosis in all the recently described cases has been made at postmortem examination, clinical details are based on retrospective analysis. There is an almost invariable association with perinatal asphyxia, respiratory distress syndrome, or both. Most of the cases exhibit a catastrophic deterioration, in which apnea, bradycardia, falling hematocrit, and bloody CSF are the most distinctive signs. Onset of the syndrome has varied from the first to the twenty-first postnatal day. Death results in 12 to 36 hours. A similarity to the catastrophic deterioration seen with marked intraventricular hemorrhage is apparent. The apnea and bradycardia that have been defined probably relate to involvement of medulla by the cerebellar mass.

None of the infants recently described have survived. Hydrocephalus has been reported after intracerebellar hemorrhage in full-term infants.[180,181] Careful assessment of cerebellar function will be of particular interest in the follow-up of small premature infants who have sustained intracranial hemorrhage that is not further defined in the neonatal period. It is possible that some of these babies have survived intracerebellar hemorrhage.

Pathogenesis. The pathogenesis of intracerebellar hemorrhage of the small premature infant is unknown. The initial series of patients had all received intermittent positive pressure ventilation by a face mask attached by a band across the occiput.[178] The band caused occipital molding and compression, and Pape and coworkers suggested that the hemorrhage was related to mechanical factors.[178] Subsequent instances did not occur in such a clinical setting.[176,177] The close association between cerebellar hemorrhage and marked intraventricular hemorrhage suggests either that the pathogenesis of these two varieties of hemorrhage is very similar or that the latter, in fact, leads to the former. More data are needed on this issue.

DEVELOPMENTAL DISORDERS

Many of the most startling disorders of the neonate are those reflecting disturbance of development of the nervous system. The diagnosis may be obvious at a glance (*e.g.,* holoprosencephaly with cyclopia). Nevertheless, a basic understanding of such a disorder requires knowledge of the specific developmental process affected, and if the time that such a process was disturbed can be deduced, the physician is alerted to certain other developmental disturbances that might not be so obvious. In addition, we have all been faced with the neonate who "looks funny" (*i.e.,* as if he has a developmental anomaly that may not be immediately apparent). Insight into the qualitative and temporal characteristics of brain development will aid considerably in ruling out or in certain broad categories of developmental disturbances. Thus, in this section an attempt is made to review the basic features of brain development, their time of occurrence, and the disorders that result when these developmental features are disturbed.

Dorsal Inductive Processes

The time period involved is the third and fourth weeks of gestation. The nervous system begins as a plate of tissue differentiating in the middle of the ectoderm. The lateral margins of this neural plate invaginate and close dorsally to form the neural tube. This tube closes first in the region of the medulla and then "zippers" rostrally and caudally. These processes are induced by the underlying notochord and chorda mesoderm, thus the term, "dorsal induction." The neural tissue, in turn, induces the formation of the axial skeleton, vertebrae and skull, from surrounding mesenchyme.

Disorders. If these critical inductive steps are disturbed, there result various errors of neural tube closure, accompanied by alterations of axial skeleton as well as overlying meningovascular and dermal coverings. The resulting disorders in *decreasing* order to severity, are the following:

1. **Craniorachischisis totalis.** This is a very rare disorder. Development has been arrested at the neural plate stage. The neural tube is either abortive or completely unformed, the skull and vertebrae do not cover the lesion, dermal covering is absent and only a meningovascular surface separates the neural tissue from the external environment. These patients are either stillborn or die in the neonatal period.

2. **Anencephaly.** Unfortunately, this is a relatively common disorder. Development has been arrested early in anterior neural tube closure. Cerebral hemispheres may be affected alone, or with diencephalon and midbrain, or with the cerebellum, brain stem, and even spinal cord (similar to craniorachischisis totalis).[132] Secondary degenerative changes occur, and usually the neural tissue is reduced to a mass of highly vascular tissue containing neuronal and glial elements and choroid plexus. The frontal bones above the supraciliary ridge, the parietal bones and the squamous part of the occipital bone are usually absent. This anomaly of skull imparts a remarkable frog-like appearance to the patients when they are viewed face-on. In slightly more than one-half of the cases, disturbance of spinal cord and overlying vertebrae accompany the lesion. These infants usually die in the first days of life.

Anencephaly can be an inheritable condition. Its inheritance is linked to that of myelomeningocele and congenital hydrocephalus. Thus, in a family with one child affected with one of these disorders, the chances for a second sibling's being affected are approximately 6%, based on data obtained in Great Britain.[182] In Lorber's series, 64% of the cases were myelomeningocele, 26% anencephaly, and 10% congenital hydrocephalus.[182]

3. **Myeloschisis.** This also is a relatively common disorder. The arrested developmental process is posterior closure of the neural tube. The spinal cord is represented by a flat neural plate-like structure, overlain by a highly vascularized mass of connective tissue. The vertebral column is defective and the meningovascular covering presents as a raw, velvety surface. The neural tissue may contain some relatively well-organized internal structure in

its ventral half. However, the spinal root ganglia are located in aberrant position in the subarachnoid space and ectopic nerve cells and fibers occupy the dorsal half of the neural plate.[132] These patients have profound neurologic deficits and usually die in the first days of life with infection.

4. **Myelomeningocele** with or without *encephalocele.* These are the most common of the severe dysraphic states and will be considered in detail in Chapter 40. The developmental process disturbed is neural tube closure, and the fact that the majority (80% in Matson's series of 1,380 cases) of myelomeningoceles are located in the lumbar and lumbosacral regions probably reflects the fact that this is the last region of the tube to be "zippered" closed.[161] Encephalocele occurs most commonly in the occipital region, this locus accounting for about 75% of the cases.[161,183] The protruding brain is usually derived from the occipital lobe and is often accompanied by dysraphic disturbances in the posterior fossa involving cerebellum and superior mesencephalon.

An important accompaniment of myelomeningocele, the Arnold–Chiari malformation, presumably also is caused by a disturbance in development during the period of neural tube closure. The major features of this malformation are (1) displacement of the medulla and fourth ventricle into the cervical canal, (2) elongation of the medulla and thinning of upper medulla and lower pons, (3) reduced AP diameter of cerebellum and displacement of its lower portions into the cervical canal, (4) persistence of the "embryonic" flexure of pons and medulla, and (5) a variety of bony defects of occiput, foramen magnum, and cervical vertebrae. Hydrocephalus* of varying severity occurs in 95% of cases, secondary either to aqueductal stenosis (present in 40% of cases) or to obstruction of CSF flow out of the fourth ventricle or region of the foramen magnum. Disturbances of cerebral function will occur not only secondary to hydroceph-

---

* The two other important causes of congenital hydrocephalus are aqueductal stenosis and the Dandy–Walker malformation (secondary to the absence of the foramina of Magendie and Luschka of fourth ventricle). These anomalies are much less common than the Chiari malformation and are less clearly related to the developmental period of dorsal induction.

alus but also to cerebral cortical microgyria which occurs in 55% to 95% of cases.[184] The precise nature of the morphogenetic disturbance giving rise to the Chiari malformation is unclear. List and Russell concluded that the developmental process affected is neural tube closure.[185,186] The associated dysraphic bony phenomena and myelomeningocele support this contention. However, the genesis of this malformation remains a controversial point. Nevertheless, it is apparent that this important malformation has its morphogenetic origin during the time period when neural tube closure is the dominant developmental process and that disturbance of this process is probably directly involved in its evolution.

5. **Spina bifida occulta.** This term refers to a vertebral defect unaccompanied by any visible exposure of meninges or neural tissue. It is extremely common, occurring to some degree in 5% to 25% of the population. Approximately 80% of all examples are located in the lumbar, lumbosacral and sacral regions.[161] These disorders are related to disturbances of caudal neural tube formation, which occurs by the processes of canalization and retrogressive differentiation in the cell mass caudal to the remainder of the neural tube. These processes are active after closure of the latter is complete and continue throughout gestation.[187]

Overlying cutaneous or subcutaneous abnormalities call the lesion to attention. These abnormalities are (1) abnormal growth of hair, often rather coarse or very silky, (2) midline dimple with or without a descending sinus tract, (3) cutaneous angioma, usually of the "port wine" variety, or (4) subcutaneous mass, usually representing a lipoma or, less commonly, a dermoid cyst. When neurologic signs occur, they consist of abnormalities of gait; positional deformities of feet, secondary to various patterns of muscle weakness; or sphincter disturbances. The deficits appear either in late infancy or in later childhood, particularly during the periods of most rapid growth. The pathologic findings in such cases include, in addition to lipoma and dermoid cysts, intraspinal meningioma, dermal sinus, diastematomyelia or prolonged conus and/or filum terminale. These portions of the cord are usually "tethered" and relatively immobile. The neonatologist should be alert to these possibilities, but should also recognize that they are quite uncommon in relation to all cases of spina bifida occulta. If spinal x-ray films reveal vertebral defects, or that a mass is palpable, or that neurologic signs are apparent in lower extremities or in relation to sphincter function, myelography is indicated.

Ventral Inductive Processes

The time period involved is the second month of gestation, particularly the fifth and sixth weeks. The important developmental process is the induction of forebrain by the prechorda mesoderm. This inductive interaction influences formation of face as well as forebrain, and the disorders resulting from disturbances of this process will be manifested by anomalies of nervous system and of facial structure. These anomalies are situated ventrally in the embryo, thus the term ventral inductive processes, as opposed to the dorsally situated dysraphic disorders described above. The major feature of the ventral inductive processes is cleavage of the prosencephalon into (1) paired optic vesicles, olfactory bulbs and tracts; (2) telencephalon; and (3) diencephalon. Telencephalon will include cerebral hemispheres and basal ganglia; diencephalon will include thalamus and hypothalamus.

Disorders. These disorders comprise the faciotelencephalic malformatons, in which face and brain are anomalous. Many of these anomalies are still not well-defined. However, the prototype, holotelencephaly, has been aptly defined, particularly by Yakovlev.[188] The most consistent abnormalities in this disorder are related to varying degrees of failure in evagination and expansion of the cerebral ventricles. In the severe case (Fig. 39-9), there is a spherical forebrain with basal ganglia that are continuous in the midline. Olfactory bulbs and tracts have failed to evaginate but, most critically, the cerebral hemispheres have not been demarcated and the huge expanse of supralimbic neocortex, characteristic of the human brain, does not form.[188] A variety of facial anomalies accompany the neural lesion, the most consistent being cleft lip with or without cleft palate and ocular abnormalities, the latter varying from microphthalmus with ocular hypotelorism to cyclopia.[189] The neurologic syndrome in the neonate usually includes severe apneic spells, myoclonic seizures, hypotonia, and absent auditory responses.[190] The total disturbance is most often

a manifestation of trisomy 13 but has also been seen with deletion of chromosome 18[191] and with normal chromosomes.[192] These unfortunate babies usually die in the first year.

It is not unreasonable to speculate that the spectrum of faciotelencephalic malformations is a broad one. The neonatal physician frequently is confronted by a baby with neurologic and facial abnormalities and the possibility is good that a disturbance of development of face and brain has occurred. Many of these infants have developmental anomalies of other organs and conform to the growing list of eponymic syndromes of multiple congenital anomalies, some of which have accompanying chromosomal aberrations. Certainly one reasonable possibility is that at least one of the developmental processes disturbed in such patients is ventral induction early in the second month of gestation. A precise answer to this question awaits more definitive neuropathologic evaluation of these cases.

Proliferative Events

The time period involved is the second to the fourth months of gestation.[193] Unfortunately, very little is known about the quantitative and kinetic aspects of cell proliferation in the developing brain. All of the neurons and glia ultimately are derived from the periventricular germinal matrix (*i.e.,* the ventricular and subventricular zones) present at every level of the developing nervous system. Clearly this is a highly critical process, one that relates to the ultimate integrity of every system within the nervous apparatus. Currently, we can only infer the disorders of cell proliferation, and even at that, qualitative and not quantitative statements can be made.

Disorders. Clearly, those cases of **true microcephaly**, unassociated with destructive disease of brain or major alteration in form referable to aberration of other major developmental processes, fall into this category of disordered cell proliferation (*i.e.,* marked *decrease* thereof). Quantitative definitions are lacking. Some of these cases are familial; inheritance is usually autosomal recessive but may also be X-linked. The infants in the neonatal period often show few distinguishing features other than the marked microcephaly. This is in contrast to the seizures, marked hypotonia, and other striking neurologic deficits usually seen in cases of severe microcephaly secondary to destructive disease or to other types of developmental aberration.

Disorders of cell proliferation (*i.e.,* marked *increase*), particularly of a specific tissue component, probably underlie the neurocutaneous syndromes, outstanding examples of which are as follows:

1. **Neurofibromatosis.** This has as its central feature disordered proliferation of central glia and Schwann cells.* The disturbance of central glia may result in gliomas, particularly of the optic pathway (20%–25% of optic gliomas are in patients with *café-au-lait* spots),[161] less well-organized areas of glial overgrowth within cerebrum,[195] or ependymomas. Meningiomas also occur occasionally in these patients. The peripheral lesions include the several varieties of peripheral neurofibromata and an intracranial Schwann cell tumor, the acoustic neuroma. It is quite possible that these disturbances of cell proliferation have their origin early in development. Manifestations in the neonatal period occur in 43% of cases and include asymmetries of face and skull (which may reflect a more generalized disturbance of cell proliferation and growth); plexiform neurofibromata, particularly around the eye and face; and faint café-au-lait spots.[196] This is an autosomal dominant disorder and a positive family history is present in 50% of cases.[196] The full-blown syndrome usually develops later in infancy and childhood.

2. **Tuberous sclerosis.** The central feature of tuberous sclerosis is disordered proliferation of neurons as well as glia. This results in basically two characteristic lesions within the central nervous system.[132] First, the so-called tubers, hard, pale gyral lesions located in outer layers of cortex, are composed primarily of large collections of abnormal multinucleated, giant astrocytes. In addition, very large neurons of bizarre shapes are found, though in lesser numbers. An abundant proliferation of fibrillary astrocytes results in the firm consistency. A second striking lesion is the subependymal tumor-like structures which may project into the ventricles like "gutterings of a candle," perhaps obstructing the foramen of Monro or aqueduct and causing hydrocepha-

* Neuronal heterotopias deep in cerebral white matter have been described, and it has been suggested that these relate to the intellectual deficits in these patients.[194] The significance and specificity of such findings have been disputed (see discussion below).

lus. These are composed of a proliferation of fibrillary astrocytes, many of which are multinucleated and very large. Abnormal nerve cells may also be located within these lesions. Calcification may occur within the lesions and be visible on x-ray film. These tumors may evolve into glioblastomas.[132] Retinal phakomata appear to have a similar origin. Evidence of a more general disturbance of cell growth is the occurrence of hamartomas of the kidney (80% of cases), rhabdomyomata of the heart and fibroangiomata of the skin (the characteristic adenoma sebaceum). It is interesting that manifestations in the neonatal period are usually very few or none, the triad of mental retardation, seizures, and adenoma sebaceum appearing later in childhood in complete form or in various combinations. However, a good clue that this dominantly inherited disorder is present in the neonatal period is the occurrence of depigmented nevi, white macules with the lance-ovate shape of a mountain-ash leaf.[197,198] Infantile myoclonic spasms with hypsarrhythmia also can occur in very early infancy in this disorder.

3. **Sturge–Weber syndrome** or **encephalofacial angiomatosis.** The central feature of this syndrome is disordered proliferation of endothelial cells, particularly of small veins. The essential neuropathology is venous angiomatosis of the leptomeninges occurring particularly in the parietooccipital region. The lesion is located on the same side as the characteristic facial port-wine stain, which is confined to a pattern similar to that of the branches of the trigeminal nerve, particularly its supraorbital division. The stain is flat, sharply demarcated and present at birth. Associated with the leptomeningeal lesion are atrophic changes in cerebral cortex. These changes are accompanied by iron-calcium depositions both in walls of small vessels and areas of affected cortex, particularly along gyri, thus giving the double curvilinear pattern ("railroad track") seen on x-ray films. The radiologic finding has been noted at birth, although this usually appears after a year or two.[199] The intracranial lesions, certainly the cortical changes, become more severe with age, and the neurologic syndrome of focal seizures, hemiparesis, and mental retardation becomes complete in over 50% of the cases.[199] Occasionally, the hemiparesis is present at birth. In addition to the port-wine stain, the most common and striking

findings at birth are buphthalmos and glaucoma. Several features attest to a more generalized disorder of vascular proliferation; these include angiomas of choroid, mouth, nose, and throat, and various viscera.[199]

Migrational Events

The time period involved is the third to sixth months of gestation. During this period occurs the most remarkable series of events, whereby millions of cells migrate from their sites of origin in the subependymal germinal matrix in the ventricular and subventricular zones to the loci within the nervous system where they will remain for life. Regulation of the timing and direction of these many simultaneous migrations must be highly ordered, but at the present time little is known about these control mechanisms. Nonetheless, it is obvious that these many mechanisms can be altered by inborn genetic errors as well as by exogenous insults.

The major patterns of cell migration have been delineated by the exquisite autoradiographic studies of Sidman and his coworkers and others.[200–204] The critical migratory pattern for formation of the cerebral cortex is from "inside out" (Fig. 39-10). In other words, the neurons of the superficial part of the germinal matrix zone migrate first to the ventricular surface, divide and return to their original position ("to-and-fro" migration), after which they migrate in waves through the intermediate zone into the marginal zone to form the cortical plate. The cells arriving in subsequent waves of migration take more superficial positions. By 16 to 20 weeks, the cortical plate has acquired practically its full complement of neurons by this process of radial migration. The earliest migrating neurons retain some proliferative capacity after arrival and contribute to the final population of the fetal cortex.[63] However, by the end of the sixth fetal month, the cortical plate has its full complement of neurons, mitotic figures are no longer seen, and the six-layered product is grossly very similar to the adult cortex.*

During essentially the same time period as

---

*At approximately this time, at 22 weeks of gestation, Brun's subpial granular layer,[205] cells derived originally from the germinal matrix but arriving in their subpial location by tangential migration from a site in the prepyriform region, reaches its maximal width. These cells migrate inward to the cortex but their contribution to the finished product is still unclear.

that for development of the cerebral cortex, other important radial migrational events are occurring within the nervous system. These events have been well described in the writings of Miale and Sidman, Taber, and Fujita, as well as in the older work of His and Essick.[206–211] Thus, all of the nuclear structures of the basal ganglia, diencephalon, brain stem, cerebellum and spinal cord are formed. Associated with the events within the cerebrum and perhaps the establishment of interhemispheric connections between neurons is the development of the corpus callosum. The earliest crossing fibers of the corpus callosum appear at 11 to 12 weeks, and the structure is complete at 20 weeks.[212] Thus, the frequent concurrence of hypoplastic or absent corpus callosum with the migrational disorders discussed below is understandable.

Disorders. Disorders of neuronal migration obviously will result in severe disturbance of neurologic function. Indeed, although all of the migrational disorders are compatible with life, most are associated with clinical deficits apparent from the first days of life. Nonetheless, the least severe of these disorders is probably present to some degree in all of us. The major disorders,† in order of *decreasing severity,* are

1. *Schizencephaly.* Schizencephaly is the most severe though restricted of these cortical malformations.[215] Here there is believed to be a complete agenesis of the cerebral wall, leaving

---

†Two rare cortical anomalies, migrational disorders in basic nature, are associated with mental retardation as the major neurologic deficit. However, the neurologic syndrome in the neonatal period has not been defined yet, and thus these disorders will be summarized only briefly. The first is the verrucose dysplasia of cerebral cortex, described well by Grcevic and Robert.[213] In this disorder, the dominant feature is the presence of a verrucose malformation of the outer three cortical layers. Most of the verrucose lesions are small and superficial, although some are also intracortical and within areas of microgyric cortex. Despite the presence of polymicrogyria, the distinctive abnormality in this disorder is the verrucose change. The second of these rare cortical dysgeneses is the "driftwood cortex" of Rebeiz, Wolf, and Adams.[214] The major anomaly in this case was the presence of myelinated fiber bundles haphazardly arranged in the outer cortical layers. A number of additional abnormalities were described in this brain, but in view of the ectopic nerve cells in the molecular layer and the severe disarray of superficial cortical layers, the authors suggested that this cortical abnormality was related to a disturbance in the migration of the neurons of Brun's subpial granular layer.[205]

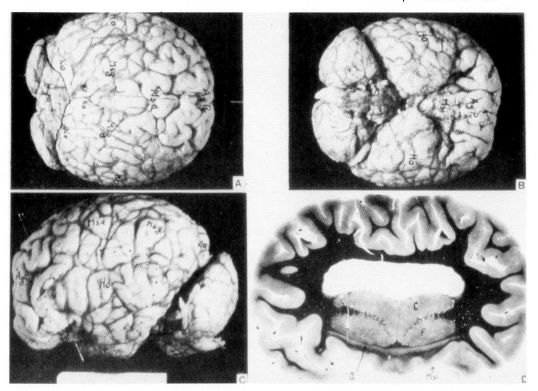

Fig. 39-11. Holotelencephaly. See text for details. In **D.** basal ganglia fused in midline are caudate **(C)**, putamen **(P)**, and claustrum **(C)**. (Courtesy of Dr. Paul Yakovlev)

seams or bilateral clefts in the cerebral walls. In the walls of the clefts, the cortical plate is thick, the density of the nerve cells increased, the normal lamination absent, and the nerve cells arranged in whorls and nests. The lips of the clefts may become widely separated and massive dilatation of the lateral ventricles may occur. Neonates with schizencephaly have distinct neurologic abnormalities, including particularly, increased extensor tone, occasionally with opisthotonus (marked hypotonia may precede the development of hypertonus), markedly decreased spontaneous motility, and seizures. Transillumination will be strikingly increased bilaterally in those cases of separated lips, thus raising the possibility of hydranencephaly secondary to severe vascular or infectious destruction of the brain. Subsequent neurologic development is always severely impaired.

2. *Lissencephaly.* This is a more frequently documented cortical anomaly.[216-220]

Here the brain has few or no gyri. Recent detailed studies of a familial form of lissen-cephaly are of considerable interest.[218-220] The cerebrum was small and had a wall composed of three layers: (1) an outermost, relatively acellular marginal zone; (2) a thick, richly cellular mantle zone; and (3) an innermost thin band of white matter. The pallial wall was said to be very similar to that of the 3-month fetus. These familial cases had a characteristic combination of minor facial anomalies, cloudy corneas, polydactyly, simian creases, congenital heart disease, and other visceral anomalies. They are characteristically severely hypotonic, although most have brisk reflexes and subsequently become spastic. Seizures are frequent and associated with a severely disordered EEG.[220] Neurologic development in lissencephaly is always severely impaired and death in infancy is common.

3. *Pachygyria.* In this condition, the gyri are relatively few, unusually broad, and associated with an abnormally thick cortical plate.[132,221,222] (Fig. 39-11, parasagittal region). Thus, pachygyria is closely related to lissencephaly. The walls of the cerebral hemispheres in pachy-

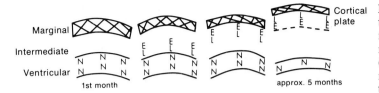

Marginal

Intermediate

Ventricular

1st month

approx. 5 months

Cortical plate

Fig. 39-12. Diagram of basic features of migrational events for formation of cerebral cortex. The germinative cells of the ventricular zone (**N**); earlier migrating cells (**E**); later migrating cells (**L**). See text for details.

gyria are composed of four main layers (Fig. 39-12): (1) the outermost molecular layer which appears normal; (2) a layer of neurons, usually of decreased population and representative of the true cortex, which has not received its full complement of neurons by radial migration; (3) a much thicker layer of neurons, usually poorly organized and arrayed in broad columns, which represent the bulk of heterotopic neurons arrested in their migrations; and (4) a relatively thin layer of white matter, encroached upon by the layer of heterotopic neurons. As in lissencephaly, evidence for other migrational disturbances are apparent in brain stem and cerebellum (*e.g.,* malformed and often aberrantly placed inferior olivary and dentate nuclei), and micrencephaly is the rule. The disturbance of migration resulting in pachygyria originates at a slightly later stage of development than in lissencephaly probably about the fourth month of gestation.

There is as yet no clearly defined neurologic syndrome in the neonatal period associated with pachygyria. Opisthotonus, spasticity, and seizures have been recorded,[221] but others have been described as "normal," only to demonstrate spasticity, seizures, and mental retardation on follow-up.[222]

4. *Polymicrogyria.* This striking disturbance is characterized by a great number of very small plications in the cortical surface, rendering to the external aspect of the cerebrum the appearance of a wrinkled chestnut. The multitude of small gyri are arranged in complicated festoon-like or glandular formations, resulting primarily from failure of separation of their molecular layers (Fig. 39-13, lateral convexity). This abnormality was studied in detail by Bielschowsky and later by Greenfield and Wolfson and by Crome.[223,216,224] The classic cortical structure is four layered.[223,224] The marginal layer is usually sharply demarcated from a richly cellular second layer. The superficial neurons of this layer may be small and round and the deeper ones pyramidal or multipolar[224] The third layer is sparsely cellular and occupied by myelinated fibers. The fourth layer varies in thickness and consists of pyramidal and round cells often in nests and columns. The cerebral white matter is more abundant than in pachygyria. Bielschowsky considered the upper two cortical layers the "true cortex," the third layer arcuate fibers, and the fourth, heterotopic, arrested neurons. The time period of development involved in the generation of polymicrogyria is later than that involved in the generation of pachygyria and is probably approximately the fifth month of gestation. Hallervorden described a case of polymicrogyria in a child whose mother had attempted suicide in the fifth month of pregnancy.[225] The anomaly can probably also occur when migration is affected during this developmental period by infection with cytomegalovirus[226] or by disturbance of vascular supply.[227]

A well-studied example of an inherited (autosomal recessive) disorder of neuromal migration with both polymicrogyria and pachygyria was an instance of *Zellweger cerebrohepatorenal syndrome.*[228] The neuropatholigic disturbance was highly restricted; the migratory abnormality affected posterior hemisphere much more than the anterior, and supralimbic cortex more than limbic. The cortical disturbance involved deeper layers more than superficial ones, suggesting that earlier migrational events were most severely affected and later events relatively spared. These findings in a disease related to presumably a single gene abnormality provide considerable insight into the nature of genetic control of migrational events.

The neurologic syndrome in the patients with Zellweger syndrome is startling and characterized by marked generalized weakness with severe hypotonia and absent deep tendon reflexes, severe recurrent seizures, and absence of any high-level responses to visual, auditory or somesthetic stimuli. Other features of the syndrome include a distinctive craniofacial appearance, hepatomegaly, and multiple renal cortical cysts. The clinical features in the neonatal period of sporadic cases of polymicrogyria are not well-defined, although seizures are recorded most consistently.

5. *Neuronal heterotopias.* The least severe of migrational disturbances is the occurrence of heterotopic collections of nerve cells in subcortical white matter, apparently arrested during radial migration from the periventricular germinal matrix (Fig. 39-14). Such collections are constant accompaniments of the more severe migrational disorders. Whether neuronal heterotopias alone result in significant neurologic disease is not completely clear. Detailed discussion is not appropriate here because they probably never are solely responsible for neurologic manifestations in the neonate. Suffice it to say, neuronal heterotopias have been thought to play a role in the intellectual failure that accompanies neurofibromatosis[194] and myotonic and Duchenne muscular dystrophy[229] The specificity and significance of these latter findings have been disputed by others, particularly by Dubowitz and Crome in a prospective study of 21 cases of Duchenne dystrophy.[230]

Organizational Events

The time period involved begins around the fifth fetal month and continues to at least the end of the second postnatal year. The most significant studies of these events in human brain have been made by Conel.[231] His Golgi–Cox preparations of cerebral cortex from birth to 2 postnatal years demonstrate progressive enrichment of the dendritic and axonal plexus with much smaller increase in size and no proportionate increase in number of individual neurons. Accompanying the elaboration of dendritic and axonal ramifications is the appearance of synaptic connections, development of neurofibrils, and increase in size of Nissl substance in the cytoplasm of cells. These changes have as biochemical correlates increasing cerebral content of RNA and protein relative to DNA.[232] The maturational changes occur relatively more rapidly in rhinic lobe (hippocampus), whereas they occur over a more protracted period in limbic and supralimbic lobes, the latter, of course, of great significance as the locus of the major association areas.

Based on electron microscopic as well as Golgi techniques, more recent studies have amplified these earlier observations.[223-236] Synaptic contacts have been observed in human cerebrum as early as the third month of gestation, and the progression of dendritic development has been defined.

Disorders. With application (albeit limited) of the Golgi technique to the study of human postmortem material, abnormalities of cortical organization have been recently defined.[233,236-241] These abnormalities have escaped attention in the past, because the widely used Nissl method of conventional neuropathology demonstrates only cell bodies, and, thus, even gross aspects of neuronal organization can scarcely be appreciated. Disturbances of the number, length, and spatial arrangements of dendrites and synapses have been demonstrated in infants and children with severe mental retardation and seizures of unknown etiology, Down syndrome, congenital rubella, phenylketonuria, and Rubinstein–Taybi syndrome. Whether the disturbance of cellular organization is the primary neuropathologic abnormality in these disorders remains to be established.

It is of perhaps greatest importance that another critical period of brain development is now defined by these studies. Because its time of rapid developmental progression coincides with the perinatal period, it is most reasonable to ask whether the very frequent insults that affect the human brain in the perinatal period (*e.g.*, hypoxia-ischemia, acidosis, undernutrition, intracranial hemorrhage, and infection) may exert serious consequences on these specific aspects of brain development. It is a clinical truism that many children afflicted with one or more of these perinatal insults may exhibit neurologic sequelae, more severe than might be predicted from the extent of injury recognized by the usual neuropathologic techniques. To what extent such sequelae are related to defects in organizational development is a major topic for future research.

Myelination

The time period involved is very long, beginning around the sixth month of gestation and continuing into adult life. The process of myelination begins with the generation of oligodendrocytes, the cells responsible for myelin

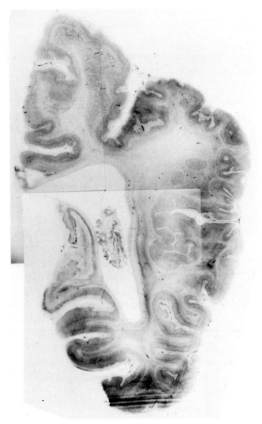

Fig. 39-13. Pachygyria (parasagittal region) and polymicrogyria (lateral convexity) in a case of cerebro-hepato-renal syndrome. Coronal section of left parietal lobe, cresyl violet stain (for Nissl material).

formation in the central nervous system. Using silver techniques, Del Rio–Hortega first clearly implicated the oligodendrocyte in the process of myelination.[242] Since that time, the role of this glial cell in myelination has been clearly defined.[243] The qualitative changes in myelinogenic glial cells in human cerebral white matter during the perinatal period have been described by Mickel and Gilles.[244] However, the *quantitative* aspects of glial development in human brain have not yet been defined. Recent biochemical data indicate that there is a burst of DNA deposition in human brain occurring after 20 to 30 weeks of gestation and thus clearly separate from neuroblast multiplication which is complete by the fifth month (see above).[245] Thus, between 30 weeks and 8 postnatal months, there is an approximately fourfold increase in total brain DNA.[232,245]

Changes in cerebrum, cerebellum and brain stem are roughly coordinate.[246] Despite these informative data, the relative contributions of astrocytes and oligodendrocytes to these changes are unknown.

Unlike the uncertainties surrounding the development of myelin-producing cells, there are excellent descriptions of the process of myelination in the human brain. The most informative of these is the study of Yakovlev and Lecours.[247] Using the Loyez method for staining myelin, these workers defined the development of myelin in 25 areas of the nervous system. A graphical summary of their work is shown in Figure 39-15. Yakovlev summarized this work in part as follows:

In the peripheral nervous system, the ventral roots of the cerebrospinal nerves to the somatic musculature of the body myelinate earliest and rapidly and anticipate myelination of the dorsal root fibers from the recipient surfaces of the visceral and somatic experience. However, in the central nervous system the myelination of fiber-systems mediating sensory input to the thalamus and cerebral cortex generally anticipate myelination of the fiber-systems of correlation and integration of sensory data into movement. Thus, in the brain stem the fiber-systems (*e.g.,* medial longitudinal bundle, lateral lemniscus) mediating vestibular and acoustic modalities of experience myelinate early and rapidly before birth; the fiber-systems mediating the general proprioceptive (muscle sense) and exteroceptive (tactile and pain) somatic experience (*e.g.,* medial lemniscus, outer division of the inferior cerebellar peduncle and brachium conjunctivum) myelinate later and at a slower rate; and the fibers of the middle cerebellar peduncles mediating the integrative activities of the cerebral hemispheres to the cerebellum myelinate only after birth and exhibit a protracted cycle of myelination. Similarly in the forebrain, the specific geniculocalcarine (optic), postcentral (sommesthetic) and precentral (propriokinesthetic) projections from the nuclei of the paramedian thalamus to the cortical ends of the sensory analyzers myelinate rapidly during the first year after birth and, with a singular exception of the geniculotemporal (acoustic) projections the myelination of which is protracted beyond the first postnatal year, anticipate the myelination of the corticofugal systems of motor integration of sensory experience.

Perhaps most important for our purposes is to recognize that myelination of the cerebral hemispheres, particularly those regions involved in higher level associative functions and sensory discriminations, occurs well after

Fig. 39-14. Pachygyric cerebral cortex. Same case as Fig. 39-13. Pial surface is in upper-left hand corner and cerebral white matter in lower right hand corner of photograph. The broad layer of heterotopic neurons contains cells arranged in vertical columns, irregular clumps, and in elliptical and circular configurations.

the neonatal period. It is reasonable to conclude that myelination is not the dominant developmental process in neonatal brain. Present evidence (see above) would indicate that organizational events, the time period for which later overlaps with myelination, are the dominant developmental events in the human neonate.

Disorders. There is no well-defined human example of deficient myelin formation. At least in part, this relates to the inadequacy of standard neuropathologic techniques in quantitating the degree of myelination in the brain. However, a particularly interesting, recently reported series of cases may qualify as the first known disorder of deficient myelination in the human central nervous system (see below). In addition, there are at least five well-defined degenerative diseases of developing myelin, so-called leukodystrophies, which either have been shown to be caused by, or are likely to

be caused by, inborn errors of myelin, glial metabolism, or both (see below).

1. **Cerebral white matter hypoplasia.** Chattha and Richardson described 12 children with severe intellectual and motor deficits, present from the first weeks of life, but nonprogressive in nature.[248] Pregnancy, labor, and delivery were essentially uneventful. Neurologic deficits, including seizures, were present in the neonatal period. The unifying and outstanding neuropathologic feature was a marked deficiency of cerebral white matter. No apparent abnormality of neurons or sign of destructive disease was identifiable. A genetic error was suggested by the fact that the series included several affected families. Biochemical definition of the apparent disorder in myelin formation will be an important topic for future research.

2. **Leukodystrophies.** *Alexander's disease* occasionally begins in the first weeks of life

MYELOGENETIC CYCLES

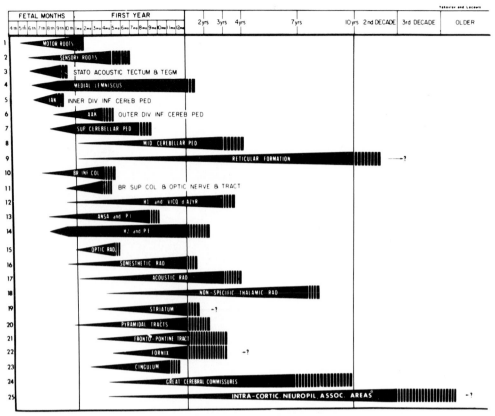

Fig. 39-15. Myelogenetic cycles in the human. The width and length of graphs indicates progression in the intensity of staining and density of myelinated fibers. The vertical strips at the end of graphs indicate approximate age-range of termination of myelination. (Courtesy of Dr. Paul Yakovlev)

with the most frequent initial findings being macrocephaly and failure to attain early motor milestones.[249,252] Progressive spastic quadriparesis and intellectual failure later become prominent and death in infancy of early childhood is most common. The major pathologic features are a severe deficency of myelin and eosinophilic deposits within fibrillary astrocytes, especially in subependymal, subpial, and perivascular locations. These deposits have been shown by electron microscopy to represent an accumulation of disordered glial filaments.[252]

Canavan's disease is an autosomal recessive disorder that also occasionally begins in the first weeks of life, although onset between 3 and 6 months is more common.[253] Signs documented in the first weeks of life have included marked hypotonia, massive spasms, general-

ized seizures, or failure to attain motor milestones. As the disease progresses, hypotonia gives way to spasticity and decorticate posture, intellectual failure, optic atrophy, macrocephaly, and death in the second year. The major pathologic features are strikingly deficient myelin with widespread vacuolization of white matter, especially in subcortical regions. The basic nature of the disease is unknown.

Krabbe's disease is an autosomal recessive disorder that characteristically has its onset between 3 and 6 months of age. The clinical course is that of a white matter degeneration and, therefore, similar in many ways to those just described. Marked spasticity with decerebrate posture and stimulus-sensitive tonic extensor spasms are early prominent features of this disease.[254] The CSF protein is markedly elevated, compatible with the accompanying peripheral neuropathy. The major pathologic features include severe deficiency of myelin and collections of large, multinucleated globoid cells which contain galactocerebroside. A deficiency of beta-galactosidase has been demonstrated in brain.[255]

Pelizalus-Merzbacher disease occasionally begins in the first weeks of life. The early signs are pendular nystagmus with head titubation and hypotonia. The disease is very slowly progressive. Spasticity, optic atrophy and blindness, hearing deficit, and intellectual failure are progressive, but, though bedridden, patients may live many years.[256–258] Most families exhibit X-linked recessive inheritance, but a few females with the disease have been reported.[259] The major pathologic feature is widespread loss of myelin interspersed with islands of preserved myelin. These cases are related to the group of less well-defined "sudanophilic leukodystrophies," a rare case of which may experience a rapid deterioration with death in the neonatal period.[260] The basic nature of these disorders is unknown.

Metachromatic leukodystrophy is an autosomal recessive disorder and does not begin until shortly after 12 months of age. Early signs include hypotonia and ataxia, which progress to spasticity, intellectual failure, and death at 3 to 6 years.[261] Major pathologic features include severe loss of myelin in central and peripheral nervous system with accumulation of metachromatic material in macrophages, central glia, and Schwann cells. The accumulated material is sulfatide,[262] resulting from a deficiency of the degradative enzyme, cerebroside sulfatase.[263]

REFERENCES

1. **Thomas A, Saint-Anne Dargassies S:** Etudes Neurologiques sur le Nouveau-né et le Jeune Nourisson. Masson and Cie, Paris, 1952
2. **Thomas A, Chesni Y, Saint-Anne Dargassies S:** The neurological examination of the infant. Little Club Clin Dev Med 1, 1960
3. **Peiper A:** Cerebral Function in Infancy and Childhood Consultants Bureau, New York, 1963
4. **Prechtl HFR, Bientema D:** The neurological examination of full-term newborn infant. Little Club Clin Dev Med 12, 1964
5. **Saint-Anne Dargassies S:** Neurological maturation of the premature infant of 28-41 weeks' gestational age. In Falkner, F (ed.): Human Development, pp 306–325. WB Saunders, Philadelphia, 1966
6. **Parmelee AH, Schulz HR, Disbrow MA:** Sleep patterns of the newborn. J Pediatr 58:241, 1961
7. **Robinson RJ, Tizard JPM:** The central nervous system in the newborn. Br Med Bull 22: 49, 1966
8. **Robinson RJ:** Assessment of gestational age by neurologic examination. Arch Dis Child 41:437, 1966
9. **Sarnat HB:** Olfactory reflexes in the newborn infant. J Pediatr 92:624, 1978
10. **Amiel-Tison C:** Neurological evaluation of the maturity of newborn infants. Arch Dis Child 43:89, 1968
11. **Paine RS, Brazelton TB, Donovan DE, et al:** Evolution of postural reflexes in normal infants and in the presence of chronic brain syndromes. Neurology 14:1036, 1964
12. **Hogan G, Milligan JE:** The plantar reflex of the newborn. N Eng J Med 285:502, 1971
13. **Moreau T, Birch HD, Turkewitz G:** Ease of habituation to repeated auditory and somesthetic stimulation in the human newborn. J Exp Child Psychol 9:193, 1970
14. **Plum F, Posner JB:** The Diagnosis of Stupor and Coma. FA Davis, Philadelphia, 1966
15. **Patz A:** Comment. In Gellis SS (ed): Yearbook of Pediatrics, p 159. Year Book Medical Publishers, Chicago 1972
16. **Duane A:** Congenital deficiency of abduction, associated with impairment of adduction, retraction movements, contraction of the palpebral fissure and oblique movements of the eye. Arch Ophthalmol 34:133, 1905
17. **Fisher CM:** Ocular bobbing. Arch Neurol 11: 543, 1964
18. **Ellenberger C Jr, Keltner JL, Stroud MH:** Ocular dyskinesia in cerebellar disease: Evidence for the similarity of opsoclonus, ocular dysmetria and flutter-like oscillations. Brain 95:685, 1972
19. **Henderson JL:** The congenital facial diplegia syndrome: clinical features, pathology, and aetiology. Brain 62:381, 1939
20. **Hepner WR:** Some observations on facial paresis in the newborn infant: Etiology and incidence. Pediatrics 8:494, 1951
21. **Millichap JG, Dodge PR:** Diagnosis and treatment of myasthenia gravis in infancy, childhood and adolescence. Neurology 10:1007, 1960
22. **Nelson KB, Eng GD:** Congenital hypoplasia of the depressor anguli oris muscle: differentiation from congenital facial palsy. J Pediatr 81:16, 1972
23. **Pape KE, Pickering D:** Asymmetric crying

facies: An index of other congenital anomalies. J Pediatr 81:21, 1972

24. **Hanson PA, Rowland LP:** Möbius syndrome and facioscapulohumeral muscular dystrophy. Arch Neurol 24:31, 1971

25. **Dodge PR, Gamstorp I, Byers RK, et al:** Myotonic dystrophy in infancy and childhood. Pediatrics 35:3, 1965

26. **Schulman-Galambox C, Galambos R:** Assessment of hearing. In Field TM (ed): Infants Born at Risk. SP, New York, 1979

27. **Brandt S:** Werdnig-Hoffman's Infantile Progressive Muscular Atrophy. Munksgaard, Copenhagen, 1950

28. **Byers RK, Taft LT:** Chronic multiple peripheral neuropathy in childhood. Pediatrics 20:517, 1957

29. **Chambers R, MacDermot V:** Polyneuritis as a cause of "amyotonia congenita". Lancet 1:397, 1957

30. **Foerster, O:** Der atonische astatische Typus der infantilen cerebralen Lähmung. Dtsch Arch Med 98:216, 1910

31. **Drillien CM:** Abnormal neurologic signs in the first year of life in low birthweight infants: possible pronostic significance. Dev Med Child Neurol 14:575, 1972

32. **Alexander E Jr, Davis CH Jr, Kitahata LM:** Hydranencephaly: Observations on transillumination of the heads of infants. Arch Neurol Psychiatr 76:578, 1956

33. **Horner FA, Webb M, Welch K:** Diagnosis of collection of subdural fluid by transillumination. Am J Dis Child 96:594, 1958

34. **Dodge PR, Porter P:** Demonstration of intracranial pathology by transillumination. Arch Neurol 5:594, 1961

35. **Shurtleff DB:** Transillumination of skull in infants and children. Am J Dis Child 107:52, 1964

36. **Sjögren I, Engsner G:** Transillumination of the skull in infants and children. Acta Paediatr Scand 61:426, 1972

37. **Dodge PR:** Personal Communication.

38. **Arey JB, Baird HW:** Hydranencephaly. Am J Pathol Bacteriol 30:645, 1954

39. **McElfresh AE, Arey JB:** Generalized cytomegalic inclusion disease. J Pediatr 51:146, 1957

40. **Altschuler G:** Toxoplasmosis as a cause of hydranencephaly. Am J Dis Child 125:251, 1973

41. **Otila E:** Studies on the cerebrospinal fluid in premature infants. Acta Paediatr 35:8,9, 1948

42. **Arnhold RG, Zetterström R:** Proteins in the cerebrospinal fluid in the newborn. Pediatrics 27(up ps.):279, 1958

43. **Gyllensward A, Malmström S:** The cerebrospinal fluid in immature infants. Acta Paediatr (suppl.) 135:54, 1962

44. **Bauer CH, New MI, Miller JM:** Cerebrospinal fluid protein values of premature infants. J Pediatr 66:1017, 1965

45. **Naidoo BT:** The cerebrospinal fluid in the healthy newborn infant. S Afr Med J 42:933, 1968

46. **Escobedo M, Barton LL, Volpe JJ:** Cerebrospinal fluid studied in an intensive care nursery. J Perinatol 3:204, 1975

47. **Sarff LD, Platt LH, McCracken GH Jr:** Cerebrospinal fluid evaluation in neonates: Comparison of highrisk infants with and without meningitis. J Pediatr 88:473, 1976

48. **Avery ME:** Periodic Breathing. In Kay JL (ed): Physical Diagnosis of the Newly Born p 72. Report of the Forty Sixth Ross Conference on Pediatric Research. Ross Laboratories, Columbus, 1964

49. **Daily WJR, Klaus M, Meyer HBP:** Apnea in premature infants: monitoring, incidence, heart rate changes, and an effect of environmental temperature. Pediatrics 43:510, 1969

50. **Parmelee AH, Stern E, Harris MA:** Maturation of respiration in prematures and young infants. Neuropaediatrie 3:294, 1972

51. **Chernick V, Heldrich F, Avery ME:** Periodic breathing of premature infants. J Pediatr 64:330, 1964

52. **Rigatto H, Brady JP:** Periodic breathing and apnea in preterm infants. Evidence for hypoventilation possibly due to central respiratory depression. (Part I). Pediatrics 50:202, 1972

53. **Rigatto H, Brady JP:** Periodic breathing in preterm infants. Hypoxia as a primary event. (Part II). Pediatrics 50:219, 1972

54. **Deuel RK:** Polygraphic monitoring of apneic spells. Arch Neurol 28:71, 1973 Copyright, A.M.A. 1973

55. **Miller HC, Behrle FC, Smull NW:** Severe apnea and irregular respiratory rhythms among premature infants. Pediatrics 23:676, 1959

56. **Thach BT, Stark AR:** Spontaneous neck flexion and airway obstruction during apneic spells in preterm infants. J Pediatr 94:275, 1979

57. **Plum F, Brown HW:** The effect on respiration of central nervous system disease. Ann NY Acad Sci 109:915, 1963

58. **Wasterlain CG:** Does anoxemia play a role in the effects of neonatal seizures on brain growth? Europ Neurol 18:222, 1979

59. **Caveness WF, Nielsen KC, Yakovlev PI, Adams RD:** Electroencephalographic and clinical studies of epilepsy during the maturation of the monkey. Epilepsia 3:137, 1962

60. **Yakovlev PI:** Maturation of cortical substrata of epileptic events. World Neurol 3:299, 1962

61. **Yakovlev PI, Lecours A-R:** The myelogenetic

cycles of regional maturation of the brain. In Minkowski A (ed): Regional Development of the Brain in Early Life, pp 3–70. FA Davis, Philadelphia, 1967

62. **Conel J:** The Postnatal Development of the Human Cerebral Cortex, Vol I. The Cortex of the Newborn, Harvard University Press, Cambridge, 1941

63. **Yakovlev PI:** Morphological criteria of growth and maturation of the nervous system in man. Ment Retard (Research Publications ARNMD) 39:3, 1962

64. **Purpura DP:** Relationship of seizure susceptibility to morphologic and physiologic properties of normal and abnormal cortex. In Kellaway P, Petersen S (eds): Neurological and Electroencephalographic Correlative Studies in Infancy, pp 117–157 Grune and Stratton, New York, 1964

65. **Purpura DP, Shofer RJ, Housepian, EM, Noback CR:** Comparative ontogenesis of structure—function relations in cerebral and cerebellar cortex. Progr Brain Res 4:187–221, 1964

66. **Purpura DP, Shofer, RJ, Scarff T:** Intracellular study of spike potentials and synaptic activities in immature neocortex. In Minkowski A (ed): Regional Development of the Brain in Early Life, pp 297–325. FA Davis, Philadelphia, 1967

67. **Purpura DP:** Stability and seizure susceptibility of immature brain. In Jasper HH, Ward AA, Pope A (eds): Basic Mechanisms of the Epilepsies, p. 481. Little, Brown, Boston, 1969

68. **Dreyfus-Brisac C, Monod N:** Electroclinical studies of status epilepticus and convulsions in the newborn. In Kellaway P, Petersen S (eds): Neurological and Electroencephalographic Correlative Studies in Infancy, pp 250–272. Grune and Stratton, New York, 1964

69. **Cockburn F, Brown JK, Belton NR, Forfar JO:** Neonatal convulsions associated with primary disturbance of calcium, phosphorus and magnesium metabolism. Arch Dis Child 48:99, 1973

70. **Burke JB:** The prognostic significance of neonatal convulsions. Arch Dis Child 29:342, 1954

71. **Harris R, Tizard JPM:** The electroencephalogram in neonatal convulsions. J Pediatr 57:501, 1960.

72. **Schulte FJ:** Neonatal convulsions and their relation to epilepsy in early childhood. Dev Med Child Neurol 8:381, 1966

73. **McInerny TK, Schubert WK:** Prognosis of neonatal seizures. Am J Dis Child 117:261, 1969

74. **Rose AL, Lombroso CT:** Neonatal seizure states. A study of clinical, pathological and electroencephalographic features in 137 full-term babies with a long-term follow-up. Pediatrics 45:404, 1970

75. **Hopkins IJ:** Seizures in the first week of life. A study of aetiological factors. Med J Aus 2:647, 1972

76. **Volpe JJ:** Neonatal seizures. Clin Perinatol 4:43, 1977

77. **Craig WS:** Convulsive movements in the first ten days of life. Arch Dis Child 35:336, 1960

78. **Koivisto M, Blanco-Sequeiros M, Krause U:** Neonatal symptomatic hypoglycemia: A follow-up study of 151 children. Dev Med Child Neurol 14:603, 1972

79. **Beard A, Cornblath M, Gentz J, et al:** Neonatal hypoglycemia: a discussion. J Pediatr 79:314, 1971

80. **Keen JH:** Significance of hypocalcemia in neonatal convulsions. Arch Dis Child 44:356, 1969

81. **Hogan GR, Dodge PR, Gill SR, et al:** Pathogenesis of seizures occurring during restoration of plasma tonicity in normal animals previously chronically hypernatremic. Pediatrics 43:54, 1969

82. **Scriver CR:** Vitamin B_6-dependency and infantile convulsions. Pediatrics 25:62, 1960

83. **Bejsovec M, Kulenoa Z, Ponca E:** Familial intrauterine convulsions in pyridoxine dependency. Arch Dis Child 42:201, 1967

84. **Herzlinger RA, Kandall SR, Vaughan HG Jr:** Neonatal seizures associated with narcotic withdrawal. J Pediatr 91:638, 1977

85. **Zelson C, Rubir E, Wasserman E:** Neonatal narcotic addiction. Pediatrics 48:178, 1971

86. **Bleyer WA, Marshall RE:** Barbiturate withdrawal syndrome in a passively addicted infant. JAMA 221:185, 1972

87. **Kahn EJ, Neumann LL, Polk G:** The course of the heroin withdrawal syndrome in newborn infants treated with phenobarbital or chlorpromazine. J Pediatr 75:495, 1969

88. **Reddy AM, Harper RG, Stern G:** Observations on heroin and methadone withdrawal in the newborn. Pediatrics 48:353, 1971

89. **Nathenson G, Golden GS, Litt IF:** Diazepam in the management of the neonatal narcotic withdrawal syndrome. Pediatrics 48:523, 1971

90. **Nathenson G, Cohen MI, Litt IF, McNamara H:** The effect of maternal heroin addiction on neonatal jaundice. J Pediatr 81:899, 1972

91. **Nathenson G:** Letter to the Editor. Pediatrics 49:314, 1972

92. **Dodson WE, Hillman RE, Hillman LS:** Brain tissue levels in a fatal case of neonatal mepivicaine (Carbocaine) poisoning. J Pediatr 86:624, 1975

93. **Keith HM:** Convulsions in children under

three years of age: A study of prognosis. Mayo Clin Proc 39:895, 1964

94. **Tibbles JAR, Prichard JS:** The prognostic value of the electroencephalogram in neonatal convulsion. Pediatrics 35:778, 1965

95. **Brown JK, Cockburn F, Forfar JO:** Clinical and chemical correlates in convulsions of the newborn. Lancet 1:135, 1972

96. **Monod N, Dreyfus-Brisac C:** Le tracé paroxystique chez le nouveau-né. Rev Neurol 106:129, 1962

97. **Sarnat HB, Sarnat MS:** Neonatal encephalopathy following fetal distress. Arch Neurol 33:696, 1976

98. **Painter MJ, Pippenger C, et al:** Phenobarbital and diphenylhydantoin levels in neonates with seizures. J Pediatr 92:315, 1978

99. **Prensky AL, Raff MC, Moore MJ, Schwab RS:** Intravenous diazepam in treatment of prolonged seizure activity. N Engl J Med 276:779, 1967

100. **Schiff D, Chan G, Stern L:** Drug combinations and displacement of bilirubin from albumin. Pediatrics 48:139, 1971

101. **McMorris S, McWilliams PKA:** Status epilepticus in infants and young children treated with parenteral diazepam. Arch Dis Child 44:604, 1969

102. **Smith BT, Masotti RE:** Intravenous diazepam in the treatment of prolonged seizure activity in neonates and infants. Dev Med Child Neurol 13:630, 1971

103. **Wallach S, Carter AC:** Metabolic and renal effects of acute hypercalcemia in dogs. Am J Physoil 200:359, 1961

104. **Heaton FW, Fourman P:** Magnesium deficiency and hypocalcemia in intestinal malabsorption. Lancet 2:50, 1965

105. **Austt EG, Ruggia R, Caldeyro-Barcia R:** Effects of intrapartum uterine contractions on the EEG of the human fetus. In Angle CR, Bering EA Jr (eds): Physical Trauma as an Etiologic Agent in Mental Retardation, pp 117–124. U.S. Government Printing Office, Washington, 1970

106. **Aramburu G, Althabe O, Caldeyro-Barcia, R:** Obstetrical factors influencing intrapartum compression of the fetal head and the incidence of dips I in fetal heart rate. In Angle CR, Bering EA Jr (eds): Physical Trauma as an Etiologic Agent in Mental Retardation, pp 125–132. U.S. Government Printing Office, Washington, 1970

107. **Schwarcz RL, Strada-Saenz G, Althabe O, et al:** Compression received by the head of the fetus during labor. In Angle CR, Bering EA Jr (eds): Physical Trauma as an Etiologic Agent in Mental Retardation, pp 133–143. U.S. Government Printing Office, Washington 1970

108. **Mann LI, Prichard J, Symmes D:** EEG and EKG recordings during acute fetal hypoxia. Presented at the American College of Obstetricians and Gynecologists. San Juan, Puerto Rico, 1968

109. **Hon EH:** Observations on "pathologic" fetal bradycardia. Am J Obstet Gynecol 77:1084, 1959

110. **Brady J, James LS:** Heart rate changes in the fetus and newborn infant during labor, delivery and the immediate neonatal period. Am J Obstst Gynecol 84:1, 1962

111. **Kubli FW, Hon EH, Khazin AF, Takemura H:** Observations on heart rate and pH in the human fetus during labor. Am J Obstet Gynecol 104:1190, 1969

112. **Althabe O Jr, Schwarcz RL, Pose SV, et al:** Effects on fetal heart rate and fetal pO_2 of oxygen administration to mother. Am J Obstet Gynecol 98:858, 1967

113. **James LS, Morishima HO, Daniel SS, et al:** Mechanism of late deceleration of the fetal heart rate. Am J Obstet Gynecol 113:578, 1972

114. **Myers R:** Two patterns of perinatal brain damage and their conditions of occurrence. Am J Obstet Gynecol 112:246, 1972

115. **Myers RE:** Atrophic cortical sclerosis associated with status marmoratus in a perinatally damaged monkey. Neurology 19:1177, 1969

116. **Myers R:** Brain pathology following fetal vascular occlusion: An experimental study. Invest Ophthalmol 8:41, 1969

117. **Brann AW Jr, Myers RE, DiGiacomo R:** The effect of halothane induced maternal hypotension in the fetus. Medical Primatology, pp. 637–643. Proc 2nd Conf Exp Med Surg Primates. S. Karger, Basel, 1971

118. **Brann AW, Myers RE:** Chronic fetal compromise and brain damage. Neurology 19:301, 1969

119. **Lou HC, Lassen NH, Friis-Hansen B:** Impaired autoregulation of cerebral blood flow in the distressed newborn. J Pediatr 94:118–121, 1979

120. **Volpe JJ:** Cerebral blood flow in the newborn infant: Relation to hypoxic–ischemic brain injury and periventricular hemorrhage. J Pediatr 94:170–173, 1979

121. **Volpe JJ:** Perinatal hypoxic–ischemic brain injury. Pediatr Clin North Am 23:383–397, 1976

122. **Behrman RE, James LS, Klaus M, et al:** Treatment of the asphyxiated newborn infant. J Pediatr 74:981, 1969

123. **Malamud N:** Trauma and mental retardation. In Angle CR, Bering EA Jr (eds): Physical Trauma as an Etiologic Agent in Mental Retardation, pp 35–51. U.S. Government Printing Office, Washington, 1970

124. **Crothers B, Paine RS:** The Natural History of Cerebral Palsy. Harvard University Press, Cambridge, 1959

125. **McDonald A:** Children of very low birth weight. MEIU Research Monograph No 1, Spastics Society and Heinemann, 1967

126. **Courville CB:** Birth and Brain Damage. MF Courville, Pasadena, 1971

127. **Malamud N, Itabashi H, Castor J, et al:** An etiologic and diagnostic study of cerebral palsy. J Pediatr 65:270, 1964

128. **Banker BQ, Larroche JC:** Periventricular leukomalacia of infancy. Arch Neurol 7:386, 1962

129. **Banker BQ:** The neuropathological effects of anoxia and hypoglycemia in the newborn. Dev Med Child Neurol 9:544, 1967

130. **Towbin A:** Cerebral hypoxic damage in fetus and newborn: Basic patterns and their clinical significance. Arch Neurol 20:35, 1969

131. **Towbin A:** Central nervous system damage in the premature related to the occurrence of mental retardation. In Angle CR, Bering EA Jr (eds): Physical Trauma as an Etiologic Agent in Mental Retardation. U.S. Government Printing Office, Washington, 1970

132. **Norman RM:** Malformations of the nervous system, birth injury and diseases of early life. In Blackwood W, McMenemy WH, Meyer A, et al (eds): Greenfield's Neuropathology, pp 324–440. Williams and Wilkins, Baltimore, 1967

133. **Griffiths AD, Laurence KM:** The effect of hypoxia and hypoglycemia on the brain of the newborn infant. Dev Med Child Neurol 16:308, 1974

134. **Grunnet ML, Curless RG, Bray PF, et al:** Brain changes in newborns from an intensive care unit. Dev Med Child Neurol 16:320, 1974

135. **Schneider H, Ballowitz L, Schachinger H, Hanefeld F, Dröszus J-V:** Anoxic encephalopathy with predominant involvement of basal ganglia, brain stem and spinal cord in perinatal period. Acta Neuropathol (Berlin) 32:287, 1975

136. **Scholz W:** Zur Kenntnis des Status marmoratus (C. & O. Vogt) (Infantile partielle Striatumsklerose). Z Ges Neurol Psychiat 88:304, 1970

137. **Borit A, Herndon RM:** The fine structure of plaques fibromyeliniques in ulegyria and in status marmoratus. Acta Neuropathol 14:304, 1970

138. **Adams RD, Salam MZ:** General aspects of the pathology of cranial trauma in infants and children. In Angle CR, Bering EA Jr (eds): Physical Trauma as an Etiologic Agent in Mental Retardation, pp 53–63. U.S. Government Printing Office, Washington, 1970

139. **Schwartz P:** Birth Injuries of the Newborn; Morphology, Pathogenesis, Clinical Pathology and Prevention. Hafner, New York, 1961

140. **Meyer JE:** Über die lokalisation fruhkindlicher Hirschaden in arteriellen Grenzgebieten. Arch Psychiatr Nervenchr 190:328, 1953

141. **Zulch KJ:** Proceedings of the 2nd International Congress of Neuropathologists 2:613,1955

142. **Brierly JB, Excell BJ:** The effects of profound systemic hypotension upon the brain of *Macacus rhesus.* J Physiol 175:50P, 1964

143. **Norman RM, Urich H, McMenemey WH:** Vascular mechanisms of birth injury. Brain 80:49, 1957

144. **Volpe JM, Pasternak JF:** Parasagittal cerebral injury in neonatal hypoxic–ischemic encephalopathy. Clinical and neuroradiologic features. J Pediatr 91:472, 1977

145. **DeReuck J, Chattha AS, Richardson EP Jr:** Pathogenesis and evolution of periventricular leukomalacia. Arch Neurol 27:229, 1972. Copyright, AMA 1972

146. **Courville CB:** Antenatal and paranatal circulatory disorders as a cause of cerebral damage in early life. J Neuropathol Exp Neurol 18:115, 1959

147. **Malamud N:** Sequelae of perinatal trauma. J Neuropathol Exp Neurol 18:141, 1959

148. **Virchow R:** Zur pathogischen anatomie des yehirns: 1. Congenitale encephalitis und myelitis. Virchow Arch (Pathol Anat) 38:129, 1867

149. **Parrot J:** 1868–1873. In Banker BQ, Larroche JC: Periventricular leukomalacia of infancy. Arch Neurol 7:386, 1962

150. **DeReuck, J:** The human periventricular arterial blood supply and the anatomy of cerebral infarctions. Eu Neurol 5:321, 1971

151. **Vander Eecken H:** Anastomoses Between the Leptomeningeal Arteries of the Brain. Charles C Thomas, Springfield, 1959

152. **Abramowicz A:** The pathogenesis of experimental periventricular cerebral necrosis and its possible relation to the periventricular leukomalacia of birth trauma. J Neurol Neurosurg Psychiatr, 27:85, 1964

153. **Haller ES, Nesbitt RE Jr, Anderson GW:** Clinical and pathological concepts of gross intracranial hemorrhage in perinatal mortality. Obstet Gynecol Surv 11:179, 1956

154. **Craig WS:** Intracranial haemorrhage in the new-born. Arch Dis Child 13:89, 1938

155. **Grontoft O:** Intracranial hemorrhage and blood–brain barrier problems in the newborn, pp 1–114. Acta Pathol Microbiol Scand (Suppl.) Ejnar Munksgaard, C Copenhagen, 1954

156. **Fleming GB, Morton ED:** Meningeal haem-

orrhage in the new-born. Arch Dis Child 5: 361, 1930

157. **Von Reuss, A:** Diseases of the Newborn. MG, London, 1920

158. **Blank NK, Strand R, Gilles FH, et al:** Posterior fossa subdural hematomas in neonates. Arch Neurol 35:108, 1978

159. **Schipke R, Riege D, Scoville W:** Acute subdural hemorrhage at birth. Pediatrics 14:468, 1954

160. **Rabe EF, Flynn RE, Dodge PR:** Subdural collections of fluid in infants and children: Study of 62 patients with special reference to factors influencing prognosis and efficacy of various forms of therapy. Neurology 18: 559, 1968

161. **Matson, D:** Neurosurgery of Infancy and Childhood. Charles C Thomas, Springfield, 1969

162. **Volpe JJ:** Neonatal intracranial hemorrhage. Clin Perinatol 4:77, 1977

163. **Larroche JC:** Hemmorragies cerebrales intra-ventriculaires chez le premature. 1 Partie: anatomie et physiopathologie. Biol Neonate 7:26, 1964

164. **Yakovlev PI, Rosales RK:** Distribution of the terminal hemorrhages in the brain wall in still-born premature and nonviable neonates. In Angle CR, Bering EA Jr (eds): Physical Trauma as an Etiologic Agent in Mental Retardation, U.S. Government Printing Office, Washington, pp. 67–78, 1970

165. **Hambleton, G, Wigglesworth JS:** Origin of intraventricular hemorrhage in the preterm infant. Arch Dis Child 51:651–659, 1976

166. **Larroche JC:** Post-haemorrhagic hydrocephalus in infancy, anatomical study. Biol Neonate 20:287, 1972

167. **Papile L, Burstein J, Burstein R, et al:** Incidence and evolution of subependymal hemorrhage: A study of infants with birth weights less than 1500 gm. J Pediatr 92:529–534, 1978

168. **Ahmann PA, Lazzara A, Dykes FD, Schwartz JF, Brann AW Jr:** Intraventricular hemorrhage: Incidence and outcome. Ann Neurol 4:186, 1978

169. **Harrison VC, Heese H de V, Klein M:** Intracranial hemorrhage associated with hyaline membrane disease. Arch Dis Child 43:116, 1968

170. **Volpe JJ:** Neonatal periventricular hemorrhage: Past, present, and future. J Pediatr 92:693–696, 1978

171. **Ylppö A:** Zum Entstehumgsmechanismus der Blutingen bei Friigeburten und Neugeborenen. Z Kinderhellkid 38:32, 1924

172. **Gilles FH, Price RA, Kevy SV, et al:** Fibrinolytic activity in the ganglionic eminence of the premature human brain. Biol Neonate 18:426–432, 1971

173. **Potter EL, Adair, FL:** Fetal and Neonatal Death. Unversity of Chicago Press, Chicago, 1949

174. **Pape KE, Wigglesworth JS:** Haemorrhage, Ischaemia and the Perinatal Brain. JB Lippincott, Philadelphia, 1979

175. **Lou HC, Lassen NA, Tweed WA, et al:** Pressure passive cerebral blood flow and breakdown of the blood–brain barrier in experimental fetal asphyxia. Acta Paediatr Scand 68:57, 1979

176. **Grunnet ML, Shields WD:** Cerebellar hemorrhage in the premature infant. J Pediatr 88: 605, 1976

177. **Martin R, Roessman U, Fanaroff A:** Massive intracerebellar hemorrhage in low-birth-weight infants. J Pediatr 89:290, 1976

178. **Pape KE, Armstrong DL, Fitzhardinge PM:** Central nervous system pathology associated with mask ventilation in the very low birth-weight infant: A new etiology for intracerebellar hemorrhage. Pediatr 58:473, 1976

179. **Donat JF, Okazaki H, Kleinberg F:** Cerebellar hemorrhage in newborn infants. Am J Dis Child 133:441, 1979

180. **Odeku EL, Adcock KJ:** Neonatal hydrocephalus due to intracerebellar hematoma. Int Surg 51:302, 1969

181. **Schreiber MS:** Posterior fossa (cerebellar) haematoma in the newborn. Med J Austral 2:713, 1963

182. **Lorber J:** Family history of spina bifida cystica. Pediatrics 35:589, 1965

183. **Ingraham FD, Swan H, Hamlin H, et al:** Spina Bifida and Cranium Bifidum. Harvard University Press, Cambridge, 1944

184. **Ingraham FD, Scott HW:** Spina bifida and cranium bifidum. V. The Arnold-Chiari malformation: A study of 20 cases. N Engl J Med 229:108, 1943

185. **List CF:** Neurologic syndromes accompanying developmental anomalies of occipital bone, atlas, and axis. Arch Neurol Psychiatr 45:577, 1941

186. **Russell, DS:** Observations of the Pathology of Hydrocephalus. HM Stationery Office, London, 1949

187. **Lemire RJ, Loeser JD, Leech RW, Alvord EC Jr:** Normal and Abnormal Development of the Human Nervous System. Harper and Row, Hagerstown, 1975

188. **Yakovlev PI:** Pathoarchitectonic studies of cerebral malformations. I Arrhinencephalies (Holotelencephalies). J Neuropathol Exp Neurol 18:22, 1959

189. **DeMyer W, Zeman, W, Palmer CG:** The face predicts the brain: Diagnostic significance of median facial anomalies for holoprosencephaly (arrhinencephaly). Pediatrics 34:256, 1964

190. **Smith DW, Patau K, Therman E, et al:**

The D$_1$ trisomy syndrome. J Pediatr 62:326, 1963

191. **McDermott A, Insley J, Barton ME et al:** Arrhinencephaly associated with a deficiency involving choromsome 18. J Med Genet 5:60, 1968

192. **Bishop K, Connolly JM, Carter C, Carpenter DG:** Holoprosencephaly. A case report with no extracranial abnormalities and normal chromosome count and karyotype. J Pediatr 65:406, 1964

193. **Volpe JJ:** Normal and Abnormal Human Brain Development. Clin Perinatol 4:3, 1977

194. **Rosman NP, Pearce J:** The brain in multiple neurofibromatosis (von Recklinghausen's disease): A suggested neuropathological basis for the associated mental defect. Brain 90:829, 1967

195. **Scharenberg, K, Yanes E:** Diffuse glioma of brain in von Recklinghausen's disease: Study with silver carbonate. Neurology 6:269, 1956

196. **Fienman NL, Yakovac WC:** Neurofibromatosis in childhood. J Pediatr 76:339, 1970

197. **Gold AP, Freeman JM:** Depigmented nevi: The earliest sign of tuberous sclerosis. Pediatrics 36:1003, 1965

198. **Fitzpatrick TB, Szabó G, Hori Y, et al:** White leaf-shaped macules. Arch Dermatol 98:1, 1968

199. **Nelhaus G, Haberland C, Hill BJ:** Sturge–Weber disease with bilateral intracranial calcifications at birth and unusual pathologic findings. Acta Neurol Scand 43:314, 1967

200. **Sidman RL, Miale IL, Feder N:** Cell proliferation and migration in the primitive ependymal zone: An autoradiographic study of histogenesis in the nervous system. Exp Neurol 1:322, 1959

201. **Angevine JB, Sidman RL:** Autoradiographic study of cell migration during histogenesis of cerebral cortex in the mouse. Nature 192:766, 1961

202. **Sidman RL, Angevine JB** Autoradiographic analysis of time of origin of nuclear versus cortical components of mouse telencephalon. Anat Rec 142:326, 1962

203. **Berry M, Rogers AW, Eayrs JR:** Pattern of cell migration during cortical histogenesis. Nature 203:591, 1964

204. **Rakic P, Sidman RL:** Supravital DNA synthesis in the developing human and mouse brain. J Neuropathol Exp Neurol 27:246, 1968

205. **Brun A:** The subpial granular layer of the fetal cerebral cortex in man. Acta Pathol Microbiol Scand (Suppl) 179:3, 1965

206. **Miale IL, Sidman RL:** An autoradiographic analysis of histogenesis in the mouse cerebellum. Exp Neurol 4:277, 1961

207. **Taber E:** Histogenesis of brain stem neurons studied autoradiographically with thymidine-H^3 in the mouse. Anat Rec 145:291, 1963

208. **Fujita S:** Analysis of neuron differentiation in the central nervous system by tritiated thymidine autoradiography. J Comp Neurol 123:311, 1964

209. **Fujita S:** Quantitative analysis of cell proliferation and differentiation in the cortex of the postnatal mouse cerebellum. J Cell Biol 32:277, 1967

210. **His W:** Die Entwicklung des menschlichen Rautenhirns vom Ende des ersten bis zum Beginn des dritten Monats. Herzel, Leipzin 1891

211. **Essick CR:** The development of the nucleus pontis and the nucleus arcuatus in man. Am J Anat 13:25, 1912

212. **Rakic P, Yakovlev PI:** Development of the corpus callosum and cavum septi in man. J Comp Neurol 132:45, 1968

213. **Grcevic N, Robert F:** Verrucose dysplasia of the cerebral cortex. J Neuropathol Exp Neurol 20:399, 1961

214. **Rebeiz JJ, Wolf PA, Adams RD:** Dystopic cortical myelogenesis ("Driftwood Cortex"). Acta Neuropathol 11:237, 1968

215. **Yakovlev PI, Wadsworth RC:** Schizencephalies. A study of congenital clefts in the cerebral mantle. I. Clefts with fused lips. II. Clefts with hydrocephalus and lips separated. J Neuropathol Exp Neurol 5:116, 169, 1946

216. **Greenfield JG, Wolfson JM:** Microcephalia vera. A study of two brains illustrating the agyric form and the complex microgyric form. Arch Neurol Psychiatr 33:1296, 1935

217. **Druckman R, Chao D, Alvord E:** A case of atonic cerebral diplegia with lissencephaly. Neurology 9:806, 1959

218. **Miller JQ:** Lissencephaly in two siblings. Neurology 13:841, 1963

219. **Daube JR, Chou SM:** Lissencephaly: Two cases. Neurology 16:179, 1966

220. **Dieker H, Edwards RH, Zurhein G, et al:** The lissencephaly syndrome. Birth Defects 5:53, 1969

221. **Crome L:** Pachygyria. J Pathol 71:335, 1956

222. **Hanaway J, Lee SI, Netsky M:** Pachygyria: Relation of findings to modern embryologic concepts. Neurology 18:791, 1968

223. **Bielchowsky M, Rose M:** Uber die Pathoarchitectonic ker micro- und pachygyren Rinde und Bezeichnungen zur Morphogenie normaler Rindengebiete. J Psychol Neurol (Lpz) 38:42, 1929

224. **Crome L:** Microgyria J Pathol 64:479, 1952

225. **Hallervorden J:** Allg Z Psychiat 124:289, 1949

226. **Crome L, France NE:** Microgyria and cytomegalic inclusion disease in infancy. J Clin Pathol 12:427, 1959

227. **Bertrand I, Gruner J:** The status verrucosus

of the cerebral cortex. J Neuropathol Exp Neurol 14:331, 1955

228. **Volpe JJ, Adams RD:** Cerebrohepato-renal syndrome of Zellweger: An inherited disorder of neuronal migration. Acta Neuropathol 20:175, 1972

229. **Rosman NP, Kakulas BA:** Mental deficiency associated with muscular dystrophy. A neuropathological study. Brain 89:769, 1966

230. **Dubowitz V, Crome L:** The central nervous system in Duchenne muscular dystrophy. Brain 92:805, 1969

231. **Conel J:** The Postnatal Development of the Human Cerebral Cortex, Vols I–VI. Harvard University Press, Cambridge, 1939–1960

232. **Winick M:** Changes in nucleic acid content and protein content of the human brain during growth. Pediatr Res 2:352, 1968

233. **Huttenlocher PR:** Synaptic and dendritic development and mental defect, pp. 123–140. In Buchwald NA, Brazier MAB: Brain Mechanisms in Mental Retardation. Academic Press, New York, 1975

234. **Marin-Padilla M:** Prenatal and early postnatal ontogenesis of the human motor cortex: A Golgi study. 1. The sequential development of the cortical layers. Brain Res 23:167, 1970

235. **Molliver ME, Kostovic I, Van Der Loos H:** The development of synapses in cerebral cortex of the human fetus. Brain Res 50:403, 1973

236. **Purpura DP:** Normal and aberrant neuronal development in the cerebral cortex of human fetus and young infant, pp 141–170. In Buchwald NA, Brazier MAB: Brain Mechanisms in Mental Retardation. Academic Press, New York, 1975

237. **Bauman ML, Kemper TL:** Curtailed histoanatomic development of the brain in phenylketonuria. J Neuropathol Exp Neurol 30:181, 1974

238. **Kemper TL, Lecours AR, Gates MJ, et al:** Delayed maturation of the brain in congenital rubella encephalopathy. Res Publ Assoc Nerv Ment Dis 51:23, 1972

239. **Marin-Padilla M:** Structural organization of the cerebral cortex in human chromosomal aberrations. A Golgi study. Brain Res 44:625, 1972

240. **Marin-Padilla M:** Structural organization of the cerebral cortex (motor area) in human chromosomal aberrations. A Golgi study. I.D. (13–15) trisomy, Patau syndrome. Brain Res., 66:375, 1970

241. **Pogocar S, Dyckman J, Kemper TL:** Neuropathology of the Rubinstein-Taybi syndrome. J Neuropathol Exp Neurol 34:110, 1975

242. **Del Rio-Hortega P:** Tercera aportacion al conocimiento morfologico et interpretacion funcional de la oligodendroglia. Mem Real Soc Espan Hist Nat 14:5, 1928

243. **Bunge RP:** Glial cells and the central myelin sheath. Physiol Rev 48:197, 1968

244. **Mickel HS, Gilles FH:** Changes in glial cells during human telencephalic myelinogenesis. Brain 93:337, 1970

245. **Dobbing J, Sands J:** Timing of neuroblast multiplication in developing human brain. Nature 226:639, 1970

246. **Winick M, Rosso P, Waterlow J:** Cellular growth of cerebrum, cerebellum, and brain stem in normal and marasmic children. Exp Neurol 26:393, 1970

247. **Yakovlev PI, Lecours AR:** The myelogenetic cycles of regional maturation of the brain. In Minkowski A (ed): Regional Development of the Brain in Early Life, pp. 3–70. FA Davis, Philadelphia, 1967

248. **Chattha AS, Richardson EP:** Cerebral white matter hypoplasia. Arch Neurol 34:137, 1977

249. **Alexander WS:** Progressive fibrinoid degeneration of fibrillary astrocytes associated with mental retardation in a hydrocephalic infant. Brain, 72:373, 1949

250. **Crome L:** Megalencephaly associated with hyaline pan-neuropathy. Brain 76:215, 1953

251. **Wohlwill FJ, Bernstein J, Yakovlev PI:** Dysmyelogenic leukodystrophy. J Neuropathol Exp Neurol 18:359, 1959

252. **Schochet SS, Lampert PW, Earle KM:** Alexander's disease. A case report with electron microscopic observations. Neurology 18:543, 1968

253. **Hogan GR, Richardson EP:** Spongy degeneration of the nervous system (Canavan's disease); report of a case in an Irish-American family. Pediatrics 35:284, 1965

254. **Hagberg B, Kolberg H, Sourand P, Akesson HO:** Infantile globoid cell leukodystrophy (Krabbe's disease). A clinical and genetic study of 32 Swedish cases 1953–1967. Neuropaediatrie 1:74, 1969

255. **Suzuki K, Suzuki Y:** Globoid cell leukodystrophy (Krabbe's disease); deficiency of galactocerebroside betagalactosidase. Proc Natl Acad Sci USA 66:302, 1970

256. **Zeman W, DeMyer W, Falls HF:** Pelizaeus–Merzbacher disease. A study in nosology. J Neuropathol Exp Neurol 23:334, 1964

257. **Norman RM, Tingey AH, Harvey PW, et al:** Pelizaeus–Merzbacher disease: A form of sudanophil leucodystrophy. J Neurol Neurosurg Psychiatr 29:521, 1966

258. **Schneck L, Adachi M, Volk BW:** Congenital failure of myelinization: Pelizaeus–Merzbacher disease. Neurology 21:817, 1971

259. **Rahn EK, Yanoff M, Tucker S:** Neuro-ocular considerations in the Pelizaeus–Merzbacher

syndrome. A clinico-pathologic study. Am J Opthalmol 66:1143, 1968

260. **Sarnat HB, Adelman LS:** Perinatal sudanophilic leukodystrophy. Am J Dis Child 125:281, 1973

261. **Hagberg B:** Clinical symptoms, signs and tests in metachromatic leukodystrophy. In Folch-Pi J, Bauer H (eds): Brain Lipids and Lipoproteins and the Leukodystrophies. Elsevier Publishing, Amsterdam, 1963

262. **Moser HW:** Sulfatide lipidosis (metachromatic leukodystrophy). In Stanbury JB, Wyngaarden JB, Frederickson DS (eds): The Metabolic Basis of Inherited Disease, 3rd ed, pp 688–729, McGraw-Hill, New York, 1971

263. **Jatzkewitz H, Mehl E:** Cerebroside-sulfatase and arylsulfatase A deficiency in metachromatic leukodystrophy. J Neurochem, 16:19, 1969

40

Disorders of Neurosurgical Importance

Thomas H. Milhorat

The surgical treatment of disorders affecting the newborn nervous system has advanced significantly in recent years. Contributing to this advance have been an improved understanding of the developing nervous system, improved methods of neurologic diagnosis, and improvements in surgical technique and supportive management. In some centers, the establishment of specialized units for the care of newborn patients has greatly enhanced the quality of preoperative and postoperative care.

EXCESSIVE CRANIAL ENLARGEMENT

Of the various neurologic disorders requiring surgical attention in the neonatal period, a significant number are associated with increased intracranial pressure. In this age group, owing to the patency of the cranial sutures, the most prominent clinical finding is usually an excessive rate of cranial enlargement. Because expansion of the cranial cavity tends to neutralize a rise in intracranial pressure, this may delay the onset of more obvious signs such as vomiting, papilledema, and cranial nerve palsies. For practical purposes, therefore, the differential diagnosis of an abnormally enlarged head in the neonatal period can be regarded as the differential diagnosis of increased intracranial pressure.

In evaluating patients with excessive cranial enlargement, a systematic approach is desirable. A complete history and physical examination are required, and the diagnosis should be confirmed by plotting the patient's head circumference on a standard chart according to age and sex. More important than any single measurement indicating abnormal enlargement of the head are serial measurements demonstrating an excessive rate of growth. Examination of the head should include percussion, auscultation, and transillumination. Each patient deserves a thorough neurologic examination, and special attention should be given to the following signs of increased intracranial pressure: distention of the scalp veins, palpable separation of the cranial sutures, enlargement and distention of the fontanels, unilateral or bilateral sixth nerve palsies, and a "setting-sun" eye finding. In some cases, it is desirable to obtain routine skull films at the time of the initial evaluation to exclude fractures and to define the pattern of sutural separation.

The diagnostic procedure of choice for evaluating infants with excessive enlargement of the head is cranial computed tomography (CT). This is a noninvasive procedure that can be carried out with little risk to even the smallest infant, and avoids the need for more hazardous tests, such as ventriculography, in most cases.

For screening purposes, a noncontrast scan in the standard axial plane (8 cuts) is usually adequate. The x-ray exposure for this is about the same as for a standard skull series.[1] Contrast scans should be performed in any questionable case and are especially helpful for enhancing vascular lesions such as tumors, subdural hematomas, and arteriovenous malformations.

On the basis of current experience, CT scanning may be regarded as highly reliable in the diagnosis of hydrocephalus, intracranial hemorrhage, and congenital cysts and tumors. The procedure is somewhat less reliable in the assessment of subdural effusions, and will occasionally miss bloody or isodense collections. In the vast majority of neurologic problems of the newborn, the information provided by CT is sufficiently detailed and precise that additional studies are unnecessary, and it is possible to proceed directly on to definitive treatment. It should be emphasized that CT cannot be expected to provide complete or even adequate information in all cases, and that the physician must decide on the basis of available clinical evidence whether or not additional studies are necessary. Overall, CT is best used in conjunction with convential neuroradiologic procedures, and is often helpful in selecting the most appropriate tests for further delineation of the problem.

Benign Enlargements

Benign cranial enlargement may be caused by a number of easily recognizable conditions including cephalohematoma, subgaleal effusion, and edema of the scalp. These disorders are usually the result of birth or neonatal trauma and tend to resolve spontaneously over a matter of days or weeks. Skull films should be obtained to rule out fractures, but surgery is rarely indicated unless the fracture is depressed.

Constitutional macrocephaly is the most important benign condition that can be confused with pathologic enlargement of the head. The diagnosis requires a convincing family history, and, if growth charts, photographs, and skull films of other members of the family are available, these should be examined for comparisons. In patients with true constitutional macrocephaly, the absolute circumference of the head is large, but serial measurements demonstrate a proportional rather than an excessive rate of growth. The neurologic examination is normal and signs of increased intracranial pressure are absent. CT is most reassuring in such cases and reveals normal-sized ventricles without displacement or deformity. If continued follow-up confirms the findings of proportionate head growth and normal development, further diagnostic tests are probably unnecessary.

Pathological Enlargements

Pathologic cranial enlargement may be caused by such neonatal disorders as (1) congenital and acquired hydrocephalus, (2) subdural collections, (3) intracranial hemorrhage, (4) intracranial cysts and tumors, and (5) various disorders causing brain swelling or encephalopathy.

Congenital and Acquired Hydrocephalus. Taken as a group, hydrocephalus constitutes the ranking cause of pathologic cranial enlargement. Congenital and acquired forms are recognized, and examples of the former are more common, in an approximate incidence of 3:1. Table 40-1 indicates the wide spectrum of congenital and acquired lesions that can cause hydrocephalus.

Etiology and Pathology. Etiologic factors responsible for congenital hydrocephalus are for the most part obscure. In a small number of cases, teratogenesis (*e.g.,* exposure to radiation), intrauterine infection (*e.g.,* toxoplasmosis or cytomegalic inclusion disease), maternal malnutrition, and genetic factors (*e.g.,* X-linked hydrocephalus) can be shown to play a role. In patients with acquired neonatal hydrocephalus, the most important etiologic factors include meningitis, trauma, and subarachnoid hemorrhage.

Current knowledge concerning the pathology of hydrocephalus was put on firm ground in 1949 with the publication of *Observations on the Pathology of Hydrocephalus* by Dorothy Russell.[2] One of the most important contributions of this monograph, and one that has been upheld to date, is the observation that in almost every case of hydrocephalus there is a pathologic obstruction at some point along the pathway of cerebrospinal fluid (CSF) circulation. In congenital hydrocephalus, the pathologic obstruction is usually within the ventricular system proximal to the subarachnoid space (noncommunicating hydrocephalus). Lesions of the aqueduct of Sylvius pre-

Table 40-1. Classification of Hydrocephalus.

Noncommunicating hydrocephalus	Communicating hydrocephalus

A. Congenital lesions
  I. Aqueductal obstruction (stenosis)
    1. Gliosis
    2. Forking
    3. True narrowing
    4. Septum
  II. Atresia of the foramina of Luschka and Magendie (Dandy–Walker cyst)
  III. Masses
    1. Benign intracranial cysts
    2. Vascular malformations
    3. Tumors
B. Acquired lesions
  I. Aqueductal stenosis (gliosis)
  II. Ventricular inflammation and scars
  III. Masses
    1. Tumors
    2. Nonneoplastic masses
	A. Congenital lesions
	  I. Arnold–Chiari malformation
	  II. Encephalocele
	  III. Leptomeningeal inflammations
	  IV. Lissencephaly
	  V. Congenital absence of arachnoid granulations
	B. Acquired lesions
	  I. Leptomeningeal inflammations
	    1. Infections
	    2. Hemorrhage
	    3. Particulate matter
	  II. Masses
	    1. Tumors
	    2. Nonneoplastic masses
	  III. Platybasia
	C. Oversecretion of CSF (choroid plexus papilloma)

(Milhorat TH: Pediatric Neurosurgery. Philadelphia, F. A. Davis, 1978)

dominate, and in some cases, there are multiple anomalies of the nervous system. In acquired hydrocephalus, the pathologic obstruction is usually in the subarachnoid space distal to the ventricular system (communicating hydrocephalus). In these cases, chronic inflammation and/or fibrosis of the leptomeninges is the usual histologic finding.

The secondary pathologic effects of prolonged ventricular enlargement have been extensively summarized by Russell and Milhorat.[2,3] The most important findings include diffuse atrophy of the white matter, spongy edema of the brain surrounding the ventricles, and fibrosis of the choroid plexuses. As noted by Penfield and Elvidge,[4] the atrophic process in hydrocephalus involves a sequential destruction of glial cells, myelin, and axonal collaterals.[4] Neurons are selectively spared (Fig. 40-1), and this may explain why the thickness of the cerebral mantle is not a reliable prognostic criterion in patients with neonatal hydrocephalus.[5]

Diagnosis. The diagnosis of congenital hydrocephalus is sometimes obvious at birth on the basis of gross cranial enlargement. In less extreme examples, and in cases of acquired hydrocephalus, the head size at birth is normal and there is gradual cranial enlargement. Whereas early symptoms may be minimal,

anorexia, vomiting, and lethargy and/or hyperirritability are common as the condition advances. The general physical examination may demonstrate any or all the above-mentioned signs of increased intracranial pressure. If there is significant ventricular dilatation, percussion of the head produces a hollow or "cracked-pot" sound over the dilated segments of the ventricular system (Macewen's sign). Transillumination of the head is usually negative unless the cerebral mantle is 1.0 cm or less in thickness. The configuration of the head and the pattern of sutural diastasis may suggest the type of hydrocephalus. In patients with aqueductal stenosis, for example, the cranial vault is expansive and the posterior fossa is small. This is in contrast to patients with communicating hydrocephalus in whom the head is symmetrically enlarged with splitting of all of the major sutures above and below the tentorium. In patients with congenital atresia of the foramina of Luschka and Magendie, there is selective enlargement of the posterior fossa.

Ultimately, the definitive diagnosis of hydrocephalus requires special tests. Without question, the simplest and most reliable of these is CT, and with few exceptions additional studies will be unnecessary (Fig. 40-2). It is generally advisable to obtain both a contrast

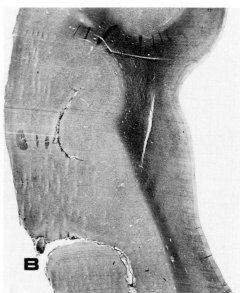
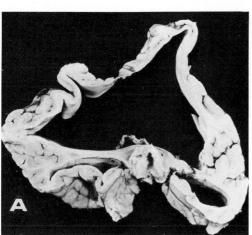

Fig. 40-1. A. Severe hydrocephalus secondary to aqueductal stenosis. The cerebral mantle has been reduced to a thin ribbon and the lateral ventricles resemble a huge monolocular chamber owing to rupture of the septum pellucidum. **B.** Microscopic section (Luxol blue) shows relative sparing of the cortical grey matter and marked atrophy of the white matter (Milhorat TH: Hydrocephalus and the Cerebrospinal Fluid. Baltimore, Williams & Wilkins, 1972)[3]

and noncontrast scan on all new patients with congenital hydrocephalus to rule out unsuspected lesions such as tumors and vascular malformations. In doubtful cases, especially those with a presumed block of the aqueduct of Sylvius, it may be necessary to supplement CT by air or metrizamide ventriculography. The latter studies provide the most complete information concerning ventricular anatomy (Fig. 40-3) and can be performed with relative safety in patients with increased intracranial pressure. In patients who develop abnormal cranial enlargement following meningitis or subarachnoid hemorrhage, pneumoencephalography may be preferable. This procedure, however, is not useful in evaluating most cases of noncommunicating hydrocephalus and is dangerous if the intracranial pressure is significantly elevated. Although cerebral angiography is unnecessary in most cases of congenital hydrocephalus, it is a useful adjunct to CT scanning and is helpful in differentiating arachnoid cysts of the posterior fossa from congenital atresia of the foramina of Luschka and Magendie. Cerebral angiography is also useful in the diagnostic evaluation of acquired hydrocephalus and is essential to rule out

vascular lesions such as aneurysms of the vein of Galen. Under special circumstances, isotope cisternography or ventriculography may be employed to gain added information about cerebrospinal fluid flow and dynamics.

Treatment. Since the introduction of valve-regulated shunts more than 25 years ago, the outlook for patients with neonatal hydrocephalus has improved steadily. As experience has grown, the morbidity and mortality of these operations have been greatly reduced and the 5-year survival rate (unselected series) now approaches 90%.[1] Two operations can be recommended for widespread use (Fig. 40-4): the ventriculoperitoneal shunt and the ventriculoatrial shunt. The former, because it is easier to implant, somewhat easier to revise, and much easier to electively lengthen in growing children, has become the most popular shunting procedure in recent years. It is the preferred shunt for infants and young children, and is probably safer than the ventriculoatrial shunt in patients in whom the CSF has been recently infected.

Unfortunately, for most patients with infantile hydrocephalus, a single operation is rarely curative and multiple revisions are required to

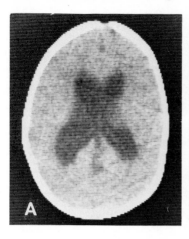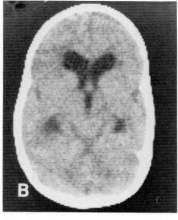

Fig. 40-2. CT scan of infant with congential aqueductal stenosis.

accommodate growth. As a general rule, this means that a shunt inserted during the first 3 months of life will require elective revision between 1 to 2 years, again at 3 to 4 years, and finally between 10 to 15 years of age. If the initial shunt is to a site other than the heart, then a ventriculoatrial shunt can be performed as a definitive procedure once full growth has been reached. The feasibility of an expanding cardiac shunt employing an adult-

length ventriculoatrial catheter coiled in an intrathoracic Silastic pouch has been recently tested and shows promise.[1] Needless to say, only time and experience will determine whether such shunts can be advocated for widespread use. Obstruction and infection are the most common complications of ventriculoperitoneal shunts, and septicemia and thromboembolism are of added concern in patients with ventriculoatrial shunts.

Despite the current popularity of ventricular shunting operations, the treatment of neonatal hydrocephalus is not limited to these procedures. In a small number of cases, direct operations such as the removal of congenital cysts and tumors, suboccipital craniectomy for lesions of the craniospinal junction, and fenestration procedures for Dandy–Walker cysts and septa occluding the aqueduct of Sylvius may be effective in reestablishing the normal flow of cerebrospinal fluid. However, choroid plexectomy has no place in the current treatment of hydrocephalus, and there is no evidence that commercially available drugs such as acetazolamide (Diamox) are of more than temporizing value in the treatment of this disorder.[1,3,6]

Prognosis. The prognosis of patients with neonatal hydrocephalus is uncertain owing to the lack of long-term follow-up. In a most operative series, late complications occur with discouraging frequency, and it is evident that a steady decrease in the survival rate occurs the longer a series is followed.[3] For the purposes of short-term prognosis, it is useful to divide patients in three groups.

1. Patients with progressive hydrocephalus

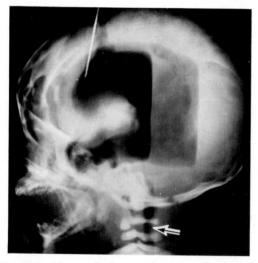

Fig. 40-3. Air ventriculogram demonstrating hydrocephalus secondary to the Arnold–Chiari malformation. The slit-like fourth ventricle extends through the foramen magnum into the upper cervical canal **(arrow).** The ventricular system is well outlined in the brow-up position. (Milhorat TH: Hydrocephalus and the Cerebrospinal Fluid. Baltimore, Williams & Wilkins, 1972[3]

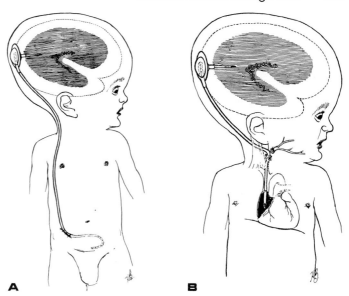

Fig. 40-4. A. Ventriculoperitoneal shunt. **B.** Ventriculoatrial shunt. (Milhorat TH: Hydrocephalus and the Cerebrospinal Fluid. Baltimore, Williams & Wilkins, 1972)[3]

A   **B**

and evidence of irreversible damage of the brain or other major organs (*e.g.,* multiple congenital anomalies, cerebral atrophy secondary to meningitis, and so on). In this group, prognosis is uniformly poor and shunting operations have little to offer.

2. Patients with progressive hydrocephalus and little or no evidence of irreversible brain damage. In this group, prompt treatment is indicated and the prognosis varies according to the severity of hydrocephalus and the success or failure of treatment. Although there is no definite correlation between the thickness of the cerebral mantle and the eventual development of mental and motor skills,[5] a cerebral mantle of 2 cm or more is usually associated with a good prognosis (*i.e.,* the patient is capable of functioning at a competitive level), and a cerebral mantle of 1 cm or less is usually associated with a poor prognosis.[7] To date, the most optimistic results of 5-year follow-up (unselected series) indicate a survival rate of 90%, with approximately two-thirds of the surviving patients having an IQ of 75 or above.[1]

3. Patients with "arrested" hydrocephalus. This diagnosis requires evidence of stable head size (if the head is already enlarged) and continuing psychomotor development with increasing age. If neurologic deficits are present, these remain stable or gradually improve. Patients in this group must be carefully followed

to rule out slowly progressive or "normal pressure" hydrocephalus.[3]

Subdural Collections.   Of the various causes of pathologic cranial enlargement in the neonatal period, the incidence of subdural collections ranks second only to hydrocephalus. Hematoma, hygroma, and effusion are the 3 main pathologic types, and the clinical management of these lesions is sufficiently similar to regard them as a single diagnostic entity.

Etiology and Pathology (See also discussion in Chap. 39). Bleeding into the subdural space is almost always of venous origin and results from the tearing of bridging veins that run from the cerebral surface to the major dural sinuses. Trauma at delivery and postnatal injuries to the head account for the majority of cases. Less commonly, subdural hemorrhage may occur as a consequence of bleeding dyscrasias, immunization reactions, dehydration, and prolonged illnesses associated with cachexia. Hygromatous collections are thought to arise from traumatic laceration of the pia-arachnoid, and subdural effusions are almost always the result of meningeal infection.

In contrast to fluid collections in other parts of the body, accumulations in the subdural space are poorly tolerated. In many instances, the subdural fluid prompts a foreign body response that is characterized by a proliferation of fibroblasts from the dural and pia-arachnoidal surfaces. In time, a thick outer membrane contributed by the dura and a thin inner membrane contributed by the pia-arachnoid may completely envelop the lesion. In cases of acute hematoma, lysis of the clot may produce an osmotic gradient that draws additional fluid into the subdural space, and there is accumulating evidence that an important cause of persistent or enlarging lesions is spontaneous rebleeding from the neovascular membranes.[8] Because subdural hygromas generally have less vascular membranes and contain fluid not unlike CSF, they rarely undergo progressive expansion. In cases of meningitic subdural effusion, the accumulation may spontaneously resolve once the active infection subsides.

Diagnosis. A history of trauma or infection is obtained in most patients with chronic subdural accumulations. In patients with subdural empyema, there is often a history of persistent or recurrent fever following an adequate course of treatment for meningitis. On physical examination, the following findings may be helpful in distinguishing subdural collections from hydrocephalus: (1) the configuration of the head is "squarish" rather than rounded; (2) the transillumination test is positive unless the lesion consists of frank blood or pus; and (3) in cases of acute subdural hematoma, funduscopic examination may reveal subhyaloid hemorrhages as a consequence of blood dissecting through the dural sheaths surrounding the optic nerves.

The diagnostic procedure of choice for screening patients with suspected subdural collections is CT. This usually avoids the need for cerebral angiography and provides much useful information concerning the size and location of the collections, the presence of associated cerebral lesions such as contusions, and the size of the cerebral ventricles. In infants, chronic subdural collections occur bilaterally in approximately 80% to 85% of the cases.[1] CT typically reveals an area of decreased density between the brain and inner table of the skull, although acute clots are invariably dense, and liquifying lesions are often isodense (Fig. 40-5).

X-ray films of the skull are rarely helpful in the diagnostic evaluation of subdural collections, but should be obtained along with films of the long bones in infants who are suspected victims of criminal battering. Isotopic brain scanning is positive in only 40% to 60% of

patients with this lesion,[1] and EEG is abnormal in less than 50% of the cases.

The definitive diagnosis of acute subdural hematoma requires the performing of a burr hole. Negative subdural taps do not exclude this diagnosis because clotted blood may not be recoverable through the needle. In contrast, the definitive diagnosis of chronic subdural collections is made by subdural taps. This is most safely carried out in the hospital rather than in the office or outpatient department, and should be preceded in most cases by a hematocrit to rule out anemia.

Treatment. To date, the surgical treatment of neonatal subdural collections has not been fully standardized. In cases of acute hematoma, the lesion is evacuated through multiple burr holes or a craniotomy. In chronic accumulations, serial taps through the anterior fontanel may be curative and can be repeated on a daily basis for 3 or 4 weeks. If, at the end of this time, there is no evidence that the lesion is resolving, surgical treatment is indicated. Of the many available operations, a subdural shunt to the peritoneal cavity is usually the safest and most effective procedure, unless the lesion is infected or contains more than 500 mg/dl protein. In such cases, external ventricular drainage may be warranted. Subdural peritoneal shunts are usually left in place for 2 to 3 months, at which time they are removed if the CT scan is negative.

Prognosis. The prognosis for patients with chronic subdural collections depends upon (1) the nature and severity of the precipitating illness; (2) the size, location, and duration of the lesion; and (3) the success or failure of treatment. In a small number of cases, communicating hydrocephalus will develop as a late complication. This should be kept in mind in any case in which the expected results of treatment are not achieved.

Intraventricular Hemorrhage of the Newborn (See also Chap. 39). This is a distinctive disorder that occurs in prematures or low-weight, term infants with respiratory distress syndrome, and it is characterized by intraventricular bleeding within the first 24 to 48 hours of life. Although generally referred to as "intraventricular hemorrhage of the newborn," the initial lesion is actually a hemorrhagic infarct of the periventricular white matter that secondarily ruptures into the cerebral ventricles. The bleeding originates from small veins in the

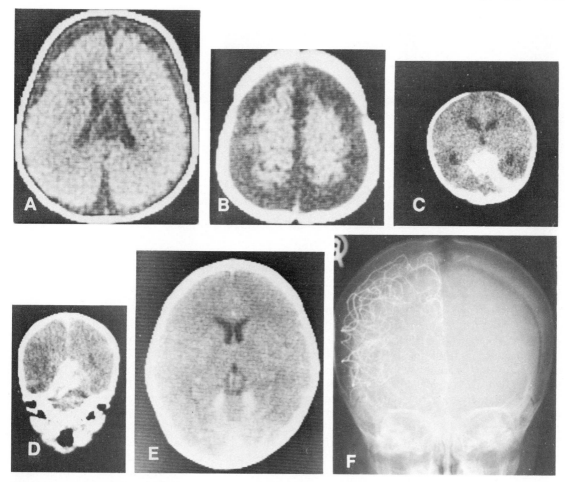

Fig. 40-5. CT scans demonstrating subdural collections of infancy. **A** and **B.** Typical hypodense extra-axial collections indicative of chronic, bilateral subdural collections. **C** and **D.** Acute subdural hematoma appearing as dense clot above and below tentorium in 1-day-old infant following traumatic forceps delivery. **E** and **F.** Isodense subdural hematoma not demonstrated by CT but evident on cerebral angiogram.

subependymal germinal matrix,[9–12] and the hemorrhage frequently extends into the thalamus and white matter of the centrum semiovale, eventually bursting through the ependyma to fill the ventricular system and subarachnoid space (Fig. 40-6). In approximately 40% of the cases, the hemorrhage remains confined to the subependymal white matter and does not enter the ventricular system.

Pathogenesis. The pathogenesis of this condition has not been fully elucidated. Because the strongest association is with events causing hypoxia, it is likely that the combination of increased cerebral venous pressure attendant to respiratory distress, and the vasodilation

that occurs with hypercapnia, results in the rupture of fragile veins surrounding the cerebral ventricles. These vessels reside in a germinal matrix that is almost devoid of supporting connective tissue until term, possibly explaining the almost exclusive occurrence of this condition in premature or low-weight infants.

Clinical Aspects. The diagnosis of intraventricular hemorrhage of the newborn should be considered in any premature or low-weight infant with hyaline membrane disease, pneumonia, or other syndromes of respiratory distress. That the condition is common is suggested by its presence in approximately 70% of infants with hyaline membrane disease com-

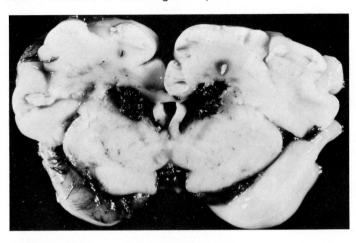

Fig. 40-6. Intraventricular and subarachnoid hemorrhage occurring in hyaline membrane disease.

ing to autopsy,[1] and by the suprisingly high incidence of intraventricular hemorrhage in apparently healthy infants weighing less than 1500 g. In our own institution, CT scans carried out within the first 24 hours of life on infants weighing less than 1500 g have demonstrated periventricular or frank intraventricular hemorrhages in approximately 65% of the cases, regardless of the clinical appearance of the infant. This finding has mandated a policy of routine scans on all premature patients in this weight category.

The clinical findings of intraventricular hemorrhage of the newborn are variable and depend upon the magnitude of bleeding. Small, periventricular hemorrhages frequently produce no clinical signs at all, but massive bleeds are associated with stupor, tonic or generalized convulsions, bulging of the anterior fontanel, and rapidly progressive anemia. If the bleeding is less pronounced, the clinical picture may be characterized by fever, generalized tremulousness, increased muscle tone, and an excessive rate of cranial enlargement.

Before the advent of CT, the diagnosis of intraventricular hemorrhage of the newborn was made by ventricular puncture. This may still be required in some cases, although the finding on CT of an opaque cast that conforms to the outline of the cerebral ventricles is quite characteristic of fresh intraventricular bleeding. For purposes of clinical assessment, four grades of hemorrhage are recognized: (1) petecchial bleeding, which is limited to the subependymal periventricular white matter (grade 1); (2) intraventricular hemorrhage with-out ventriculomegaly (grade 2); (3) intraventricular hemorrhage with ventriculomegaly (grade 3); and (4) intracerebral hematoma with intraventricular hemorrhage and ventriculomegaly (grade 4) (Fig. 40-7).

Treatment and Prognosis. The management of intraventricular hemorrhage of the newborn has been significantly modified by the availability of CT, but it is fair to say that the indications for treatment, as well as the types of treatment, have not yet been fully standardized. It is generally agreed that, unless there are extenuating circumstances, it is unwise to recommend surgical treatment for infants with grade 4 hemorrhages. Bleeding of this magnitude is associated with a mortality rate approaching 90%, and even those infants who are sustained by ventricular drainage and heroic medical management are often severely affected with varying degrees of mental retardation, spastic diplegia, and blindness. In such cases, it is usually advisable to do nothing other than to provide good nursing care and supportive management.

In the less severe examples of intraventricular hemorrhage, CSF drainage may provide life saving decompression and probably reduces the incidence of communicating hydrocephalus in surviving patients. Assisted ventilation is often essential in the early stages of management, and frequent transfusions may be required until hemorrhaging ceases. Anticonvulsants, antibiotics, and parenteral feedings are routinely administered. With grade 3 hemorrhages, external ventricular drainage is preferred to repeated lumbar punctures and can be maintained for days or even weeks

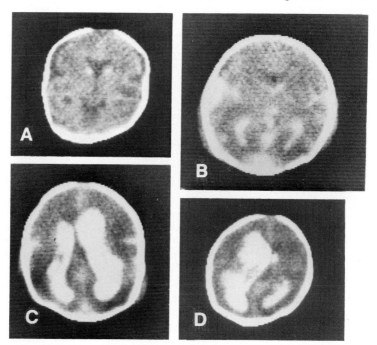

Fig. 40-7. CT scans demonstrating four grades of intraventricular hemorrhage of the newborn. **A.** Grade 1: petecchial hemorrhages in subependymal white matter lateral to frontal horns. **B.** Grade 2: intraventricular hemorrhage without ventriculomegaly. **C.** Grade 3: intraventricular hemorrhage with ventriculomegaly. **D.** Grade 4: intracerebral hematoma, intraventricular hemorrhage, ventriculomegaly.

until the CSF has been cleared of gross blood. CT scans before and after removal of the drain will identify those patients who will eventually need a ventricular shunt, although, in many cases, chronic hydrocephalus seems to be avoided by the early institution of an effective, continuous, external drain.

In patients with grades 1 or 2 hemorrhages, because of the small risk of hydrocephalus, there is a feeling in many institutions that CSF drainage is not indicated. The long-term outcome of such patients has yet to be ascertained, but it is my personal opinion, by no means an established fact, that serial lumbar punctures, carried out until the CSF is clear or only faintly xanthochromic, is probably optimal treatment. This takes advantage of the "lymphatic-like" function of the CSF and helps not only to drain blood out of the ventricles but also to mobilize and remove blood pigments from the periventricular areas of the brain. The long-term benefits of such treatment, with particular reference to mental, motor, and psychological development, will obviously take many years to assess.

Temporal Lobe Hematoma of the Newborn. This is a rare but important complication of birth trauma that results from excessive compression of the temporal or lateral surface of the head during delivery. With few exceptions, the injury is caused by the use of obstetric forceps although it can also result from forceful uterine contractions that crush the head against the pelvic outlet. The clinical picture is characterized by irritability, anemia, hemiparesis, focal or generalized seizures, and episodic apnea. Contusions of the scalp are often evident in the temporal area, but x-ray films of the skull are negative in the majority of the cases. The definitive diagnosis can now be made by CT (Fig. 40-8). Treatment consists of evacuation of the hematoma through a subtemporal craniectomy or osteoplastic craniotomy. The prognosis for survival is good, but seizures, hemiparesis, and mental retardation are common sequelae.

Intracranial Cysts and Tumors. These lesions, though relatively rare, should not be overlooked. Intracranial tumors are exceptional in the neonatal period, but medulloblastoma, teratoma, ependymoma, cerebellar astrocytoma, and craniopharyngioma are all known to occur (Fig. 40-9). Porencephalic cysts may attain sufficient size to produce abnormal cranial enlargement, and arachnoid cysts of the posterior fossa are a relatively common cause of hydrocephalus (Fig. 40-10).

In general, the diagnostic evaluation of pa-

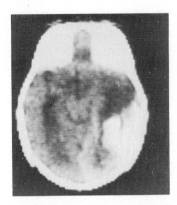

Fig. 40-8. CT scan demonstrating right temporal lobe hematoma in 1-day-old infant following traumatic delivery.

tients with intracranial cysts and tumors is the same as that outlined for hydrocephalus. Treatment is aimed at complete surgical removal, although this is not always possible. In patients with malignant tumors of the brain, radiotherapy, chemotherapy, or both may have something to offer. Ventricular shunting procedures will be required if the lesion produces an obstruction of the CSF pathways which cannot be relieved by direct operation.

Disorders Causing Brain Swelling or Encephalopathy. Encephalopathy is a relatively common cause of pathologic cranial enlargement and is best excluded by a careful history and physical examination. Toxic, metabolic, anoxic, traumatic, and infectious causes are recognized and, of these, lead poisoning is the most important consideration in some regions of the country. Vitamin A deficiency may occur in infants on a milk-substitute diet to which inadequate vitamin supplements have been added. The diagnosis is suggested by the finding of abnormal cranial enlargement in association with xerophthalmia, gynecomastia, and epithelial metaplasia. Hypervitaminosis A may occur after the administration of large amounts of vitamin A (usually 50,000 units per day for several months) and produces signs of increased intracranial pressure in association with cheilosis.

Cranial enlargement of a mild order may occur in the early stages of degenerative brain diseases such as gargoylism, metachromatic leukodystrophy, Tay–Sachs disease, and Canavan's spongy cerebral sclerosis. Such en-

largements are the result of an increased cerebral mass (megalocephaly) and not ventricular dilatation. The history and physical examination are usually sufficient to distinguish these diseases from hydrocephalus and subdural collections.

An unusual rate of cranial enlargement has been reported in otherwise normal infants recovering from severe malnutrition.[13] In extreme examples, there may be roentgenographic evidence of sutural diastasis and other signs of increased intracranial pressure. Although the explanation for this phenomenon is unknown, there is probably a preferential nutrition and growth of the brain during periods of relative deprivation. If adequate nutrition is maintained, the rate of cranial growth and the head-body proportions return to normal in a matter of months.

ABNORMAL CRANIAL CONFIGURATION

An alteration in normal cranial configuration without measurable enlargement of the head is a common clinical problem in the neonatal period. From a diagnostic standpoint, it is important to distinguish examples of benign cranial molding from conditions associated with premature closure of the cranial sutures (craniosynostosis).

Benign Cranial Molding

As a consequence of normal delivery, the fetal head undergoes considerable molding as it passes through the birth canal. The skull, dura, and brain participate in the molding process and compartmental shifts of the CSF probably occur to some extent. At birth, the grossly molded head is lengthened in the occipitofrontal diameter. Flattening of the forehead, narrowing of the biparietal diameter, and protuberance of the occiput are characteristic findings (Fig. 40-11). Examination of the head reveals a palpable patency of the cranial sutures, and this can be confirmed in doubtful cases by obtaining skull films. With few exceptions, the configuration of the molded head improves steadily over a period of days and weeks.

Passive molding of the head may also occur in severely ill or brain-damaged infants on a positional basis. The most common abnormality is bilateral occipital flattening, although asymmetric deformities may occur if the infant

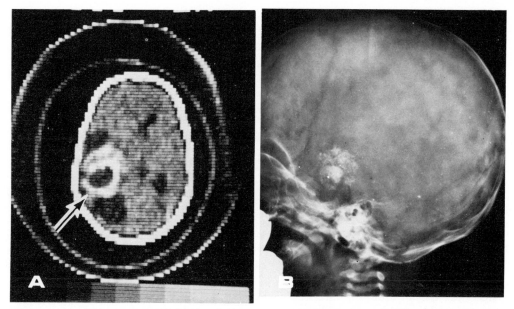

Fig. 40-9. A. CT scan demonstrating a large cystic ependymoma situated within the left lateral ventricle of an infant presenting with cranial enlargement. **B.** Craniopharyngioma in a 1-day-old infant. (Milhorat, TH : Hydrocephalus and the cerebrospinal Fluid. Baltimore, Williams & Wilkins, 1972)[3]

has a preference for lying on one side. X-ray films of the skull should be obtained to rule out premature stenosis of the lambdoid sutures. If the abnormal cranial configuration is of positional origin only, there will be roentgenographic evidence of suture patency.

Craniosynostosis

Craniosynostosis may be regarded as a pathologic condition encompassing a wide spectrum of disorders ranging from premature stenosis of a single cranial suture, to complex syndromes in which there is generalized ste-

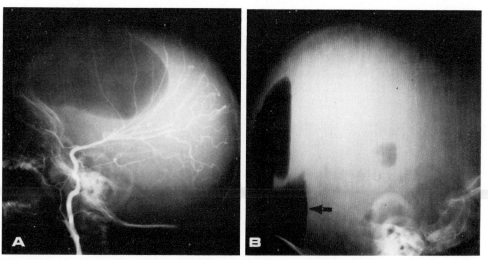

Fig. 40-10. A. A combined air cystogram and cerebral angiogram demonstrates a huge frontal porencephalic cyst. **B.** This air ventriculogram demonstrates an arachnoid cyst of the posterior fossa **(arrow)** causing noncommunicating hydrocephalus.

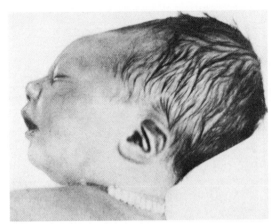

Fig. 40-11. Molded head. (William's Obstetrics, 11th ed. New York, Appleton–Century–Crofts, 1956)

nosis of the cranial vault, midface hypoplasia, and associated systemic anomalies. It is important to distinguish between the primary and secondary types. In primary craniosynostosis, the deformity is present at birth and the premature fusion of the sutures can lead to a restriction of brain growth. In secondary craniosynostosis, the sutures close and the skull fails to grow as a consequence of brain atrophy or agenesis. This is a common occurrence in patients with microcephaly and may develop in patients with treated hydrocephalus if there is marked overlapping of the cranial sutures.

The configuration of the head in patients with craniosynostosis depends upon the suture or sutures involved. In general, the deformity is greatest in the axial direction of the affected suture. In cases of premature closure of the sagittal suture, the lateral growth of the head is limited and the growth of the brain causes the head to expand in the occipitofrontal diameter (scaphocephaly, dolichocephaly, or "boat-shaped" head, Fig. 40-12). In contrast, with premature closure of the coronal sutures, the growth of the head is limited in the occipitofrontal diameter and there marked expansion of the vertex and lateral aspects of the skull (**brachycephaly**; Fig. 40-13). Premature fusion of the metopic suture causes the forehead to assume a bullet-shaped configuration (**trigonocephaly**); and fusion of the squamosal suture, or the squamosal and coronal suture on one side, produces a striking deformity with flattening of the ipsilateral forehead (**plagiocephaly**), and elevation and retraction of the lateral orbital wall (Harlequin eye sign). If there is premature fusion of all the cranial sutures, the skull expands toward the vertex. This is the direction of least resistance and results in a pointed, tower-shaped head (**oxycephaly**).

The etiology of primary craniosynostosis, like that of the other birth defects, is obscure. In occasional patients with coronal synostosis, the disorder will appear in siblings of successive generations, suggesting that genetic factors are important. This is certainly the case when coronal synostosis occurs in association with Apert syndrome, Carpenter syndrome, or Crouzon syndrome, because these conditions follow precise patterns of Mendelian transmission. However, with other types of craniosynostosis (sagittal, metopic, lambdoid), no familial incidence is recognized. There is no evidence that intrauterine infections or disturbances in calcium metabolism are important etiologic factors, but craniosynostosis and accelerated skeletal maturation have been reported in patients with neonatal hyperthy-

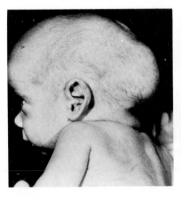
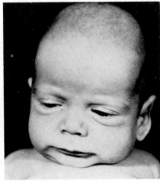

Fig. 40-12. Scaphocephaly secondary to premature stenosis of the sagittal suture.

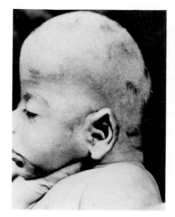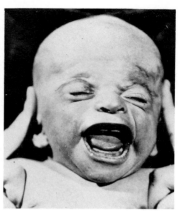

Fig. 40-13. Brachycephaly secondary to premature fusion of both coronal sutures.

roidism.[1] In a few cases of single suture stenosis, there is a history of twin birth, difficult lie, or cephalopelvic disproportion, raising the possibility that compression of the fetal head may play a causal role.

The most common type of craniosynostosis is premature stenosis of the sagittal suture. This accounts for approximately 50% of all cases coming to clinical attention, and is followed in frequency by coronal synostosis, lambdoid synostosis, and metopic synostosis, in that order. Sagittal synostosis occurs about four times as frequently in males as in females, but coronal synostosis exhibits a slight female preponderance.

The clinical features of primary craniosynostosis are related to the cranial deformity, the effects of cerebral compression, and the presence or absence of associated congenital anomalies. In general, when there is premature closure of only one cranial suture, the consequences are mainly cosmetic. When two or more sutures unite before birth, the hazards of restricted brain growth and increased intracranial pressure increase proportionately.

Diagnosis. The diagnostic evaluation of patients with craniosynostosis rarely requires elaborate tests. The configuration of the head usually suggests the diagnosis, and, in most cases, the affected suture can be palpated as an elevated, hyperostotic ridge. Signs of increased intracranial pressure should be sought and a careful funduscopic examination performed to rule out papilledema or optic atrophy.

Three syndromes of craniofacial dysostosis are commonly associated with premature fusion of the coronal sutures. These include Crouzon syndrome, Apert syndrome, and Carpenter's syndrome. In most cases, there is evidence of midface hypoplasia characterized by shallow orbits, exophthalamus, high arched palate, depression of the nasal and malar bones, and choanal atresia (Fig. 40-14). The latter deformity may lead to severe obstruction of the nasopharyngeal airway and is frequently

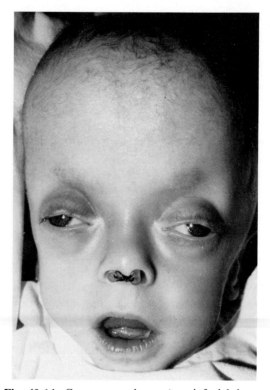

Fig. 40-14. Crouzon syndrome (craniofacial dysostosis) demonstrating exophthalmos and hypoplasia of the facial bones.

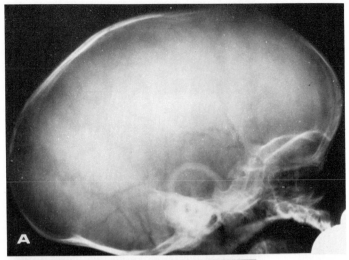

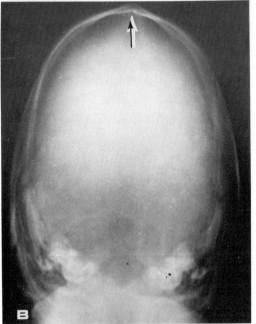

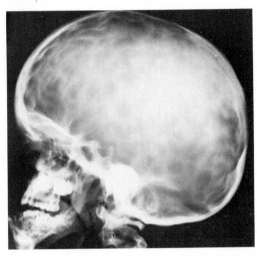

Fig. 40-15. Skull x-ray films demonstrating premature stenosis of the sagittal suture. **A.** Lateral view showing scaphocephaly. **B.** AP view showing hyperostotic sagittal suture.

Fig. 40-16. Skull x-ray films in a 2-year old child with untreated Crouzon's syndrome. Note oxycephaly, increased digital markings, and hypoplasia of facial bones.

a cause of persistent mucoid drainage from the nose and mouth.

The definitive diagnosis of craniosynostosis is made by x-ray examination of the skull. This readily confirms the configuration of the skull and will adequately demonstrate which sutures are fused (Figs. 40-15, 40-16). In patients who exhibit signs of neurologic involvement, EEG and/or CT may be appropriate.

Treatment. There are two principal rationales for operative treatment of primary cran-
iosynostosis: to correct the cranial deformity and to relieve or prevent the effects of cranial or orbital compression. In patients with premature closure of one cranial suture, the considerations are mainly cosmetic. However, when there is involvement of two or more cranial sutures, surgery can be strongly recommended because of the definite risk of progressive visual and neurologic complications. Funduscopic evidence of papilledema or optic atrophy, roentgenographic signs of

increased intracranial pressure, and severe exophthalamos with exposure keratitis are clearcut indications for operative intervention.

There are few indications for operative treatment of secondary craniosynostosis. Surgical procedures should of course be avoided in patients with microcephaly, but in occasional patients with marked overlapping of the cranial sutures following a craniotomy or ventricular shunting procedure, there is evidence of restricted brain growth. In such cases, treatment usually consists of a sizeable cranial decompression followed by a cranioplasty at some later date.

Patients with stenosis of two or more cranial sutures should be operated upon as soon as possible after birth. This is indicated to minimize the effects of cerebral compression during the period of rapid brain growth and is preferable to postponing surgery until symptoms develop. In patients with severe choanal atresia, surgical relief of the airway obstruction is often required before decompression of the cranial vault can be considered.

Operations for stenosis of one cranial suture are performed electively and are best carried out within the first 6 weeks of life. It is advisable not to delay surgery unnecessarily because the rapid growth of the brain during the first 6 months of life is the predominant factor in achieving satisfactory remodeling of the skull and its integuments. Synectectomies performed after 9 months of age usually do not restore normal cranial configuration and after 2 years of age cannot be recommended.

Optimal surgical treatment for primary craniosynostosis consists of completely resecting the affected suture or sutures and lining the bony margins with Silastic film. This is superior to performing parallel craniectomies on either side of the stenotic suture because it recreates the normal anatomy of the skull and removes the hypertrophic ridge which contributes to the cranial deformity. The strip of Silastic film retards bony reunion. In patients with multiple suture synostosis, staged operations, with or without orbital decompression, may be required. The treatment of midface hypoplasia must be postponed until the emergence of secondary dentition (6 to 10 years of age), when a radical craniofacial correction can be carried out. It is important that patients awaiting such cosmetic procedures have adequate

cranial decompressions to prevent neurologic and visual complications.

MENINGOMYELOCELE AND RELATED DISORDERS

Disturbances of fetal development can produce a variety of serious and closely related anomalies. The crucial time for the development of the human nervous system is between the third and fifth weeks of gestation.[15] During this interval, the neural groove closes and the resulting neural tube separates from the overlying ectoderm to become surrounded ventrally, laterally, and dorsally by mesodermal elements (the somites) that later form the vertebral column and supporting soft tissue structures. Any disturbance of this sequence of development, to the extent of the disturbance, can result in incomplete closure of the dorsal midline (dysrhaphism). Less severe developmental errors produce deformities limited to the supporting structures. Of these, the best-known examples are spina bifida, spinal meningocele, cranium bifidum, and cranial meningocele. More severe errors in development produce deformities that include nervous tissue as well as supporting structures (e.g., meningomyelocele and encephalocele). Perhaps the most dramatic example of craniospinal dysrhaphism is anencephaly (Fig. 40-17). In this condition, the brain and spinal cord are exposed, and there is complete failure of the ectodermal and mesodermal layers to close dorsally. In some cases, the exposed nervous tissue contains a persistent neural groove that is mute testimony to the severe and early arrest in development. It is important to emphasize that all of the foregoing dysrhaphic anomalies are closely related and that they differ more in degree than in origin.

Meningomyelocele

This is the most common dysrhaphic disorder referred to the neurosurgeon during the neonatal period. By definition, the lesion contains both meningeal and neural components and is thus distinguished from simple meningocele, which does not contain neural tissue.

Etiology and Pathology. The etiology of meningomyelocele, like that of other congenital anomalies, is poorly understood. The disorder is common and occurs in an approximate

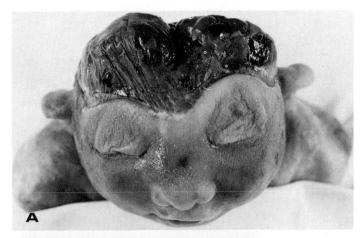

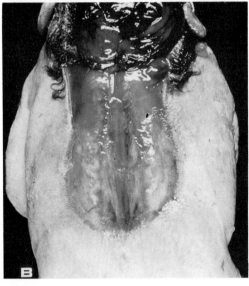

Fig. 40-17. Anencephaly with craniospinal rachischisis and persistent neural groove.

incidence of 1 per 500 live births.[16] Although statistics vary, a familial incidence is recognized, and in families in which one member is affected, the risk that subsequent offspring will be similarly affected approaches 5%.[16] If two ore more members are affected the risk factor increases to 10%.[17] Whereas this pattern of inheritance is too low to indicate direct single gene transmission, it suggests a genetic susceptibility in some families. Meningomyelocele and related disorders occur with greater frequency in whites than in blacks and the sex ratio favors females slightly.[16] In some instances, seasonal outbreaks or "waves" of meningomyelocele appear to correlate with virus epidemics having occurred 8 to 9 months before.[18]

An understanding of the pathology of meningomyelocele is fundamental to correct medical and surgical management. Regardless of the location of the lesion, the spinal cord or nerve roots are displaced dorsally, owing to a lack of posterior supporting structures. Lateral to the lesion, masses of muscle and bone, representing a spina bifida defect, are present. In some cases, the defect is so wide as to accommodate an orange; in other cases, only a dime-sized defect of the posterior elements is present. Overlying the lesion, meninges and skin are present to a variable extent. If the ectodermal covering is complete, the lesion can be confused with a simple meningocele. In most cases, however, the neural elements are incompletely covered and a flattened plaque of nervous tissue (the neuropore) is easily recognizable in the center of the lesion (Fig. 40-18). If the lesion is exposed or if the meninges are ruptured at the time of delivery, the lesion will exude CSF. Meningomyelocele may arise at any point along the vertebral column from C1 to the coccyx but is most common in the lumbar, lumbosacral, and sacral segments.

Associated congenital anomalies are encountered in all but a few cases of meningomyelocele. Except when the lesion is small or sacral in location, an associated Arnold–Chiari malformation (Chiari type II) will be present (see Fig. 40-3). This is a complex hindbrain deformity and is characterized by a small posterior fossa and impaction of the posterior cerebellar vermis through the foramen magnum. Frequently, the cerebellum extends as a tongue-like prolongation to the level of the second to fifth cervical segments. The cisterna magna is obliterated and the fourth ventricle is carried down through the cervical canal as a long slit-like cavity. The herniated cerebellum is usually firmly attached to the back and sides of the cervical canal by arachnoidal adhesions. Frequently, there is an elongation and thinning of the lower pons and upper medulla, and, in severe cases, the lower medulla is dorsally buckled and folded back upon itself at the level of the gracile and cuneate tubercles. The lower cranial nerves are greatly elongated and run upward toward the foramen magnum with the upper cervical nerve roots.

The next most common anomaly associated with meningomyelocele is aqueductal forking. This occurs in approximately 80% of all cases and produces a noncommunicating type of hydrocephalus. Other congenital anomalies that may be associated with meningomyelocele include hydromyelia, syringomyelia, double spinal cord, polymicrogyria, craniolacunia, heterotopias of gray matter, "beak-like" deformity of the quadrigeminal plate, basilar impression, platybasia, Klippel–Feil deformity, congenital heart disease, and intestinal anomalies such as duodenal atresia or pyloric stenosis (Fig. 40-19). Although it has been argued that the Arnold–Chiari malformation may arise as a consequence of traction or "tethering" of the spinal cord, it is likely in view of the multiple associated anomalies that occur in this disorder, that the hindbrain deformity is but one of many closely related maldevelopments.[2,3]

Diagnosis. The diagnosis of meningomyelocele is usually apparent at birth. The head should be carefully examined for signs of hydrocephalus, and serial circumferential measurements are required to rule out an abnormal rate of cranial enlargement. In most cases, CT is performed to determine the size of the ventricular system and to rule out aqueductal stenosis and/or the Arnold–Chiari malformation. EMG may be useful in assessing motor function in the lower extremities and an intravenous pyelogram should be performed to exclude hydronephrosis.

Treatment and Prognosis. Until 1960, the vast majority of infants with meningomyelocele and hydrocephalus were managed conservatively at home. Without surgical treatment, less than 20% survived for as long as 2 years. In patients with large meningomyelo-

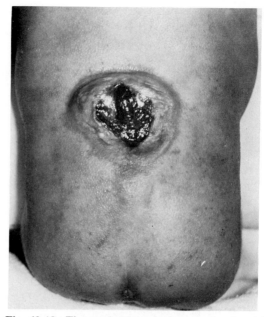

Fig. 40-18. Thoracolumbar meningomyelocele with central neuropore and incomplete covering of meninges and skin.

celes and a severe degree of hydrocephalus, the natural mortality was even higher. In this group, approximately 50% of the patients died within the first month of life and the remainder were dead within 6 months.[19,20]

In 1959, a comprehensive plan of treatment was evolved at the University of Sheffield, England.[21] The "Sheffield plan," as it came to be known, consisted of repairing all meningomyeloceles within the first few hours of life. Hydrocephalus was subsequently treated with a ventriculoatrial shunt and all patients were evaluated and followed by a team of surgeons, physicians, physiotherapists, and social workers. Shunt revisions were performed periodically and many of the patients underwent multiple orthopedic and urologic procedures. This multidisciplinary approach, which was widely adopted, increased the survival rate of all patients with meningomyelocele and hydrocephalus to 60% to 70% at 2 years. However, as experience grew, it became clear that a large number of patients had been sustained who had little or no chance of ever achieving a competitive place in life.[22] Many of the surviving patients had severe handicaps and various degrees of bladder, bowel, and lower extremity paralysis; 30% to 50% were totally

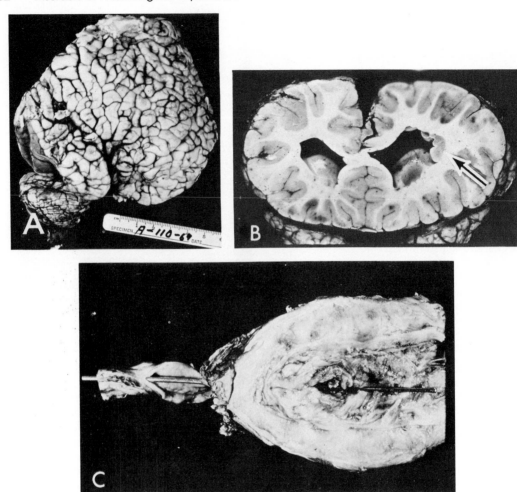

Fig. 40-19. Common anomalies associated with meningomyelocele. **A.** Polymicrogyria. **B.** Heterotopias of gray matter. **C.** Meningomyelocele and hydromyelia. A probe has been passed through the central canal. (Milhorat TH: Hydrocephalus and the Cerebrospinal Fluid. Baltimore, Williams & Wilkins, 1972)[3]

paraplegic, and the average patient required seven orthopedic operations on the lower extremities. It was estimated, furthermore, that only 20% of patients with severe meningomyelocele and hydrocephalus had a normal intellect at 2 to 4 years. These dour statistics, of course, did not include the hardships imposed by multiple operations, the psychological burdens on the patient and his family, or the financial cost of such a comprehensive program.

In view of the foregoing, it is obvious that the management of meningomyelocele is a complicated matter for which there are no easy answers. Arbitrary rules cannot be applied and each case must be judged on an individual basis. After considering all the clinical, prognostic, and ethical factors, however, an attempt should be made to arrive at a clearcut decision. It is rarely possible for parents to evaluate a long list of choices and possibilities objectively, and it is therefore desirable that the physician offer advice and guidance. In many clinics, it is felt that operative procedures on totally paraplegic patients are unjustified.[1,14] Similarly, patients with severe hydrocephalus, multiple anomalies involving the major organ systems, or both, are rarely operated upon. In such cases, conservative management is advised and treatment other than

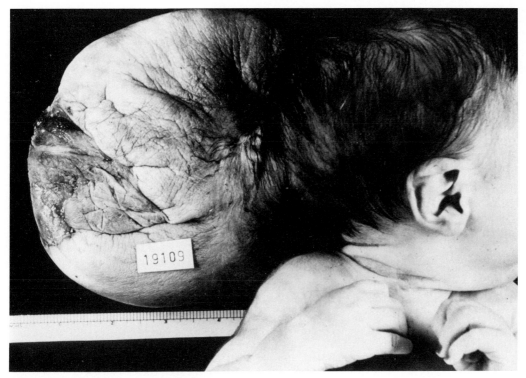

Fig. 40-20. Occipital encephalocele.

that necessary to assure the comfort of the infant is avoided.

In patients who are candidates for surgical treatment, the following plan is appropriate:

1. Whenever possible, the spinal lesion should be closed within the first few hours of life. Prompt surgery cannot be expected to improve neurologic deficits, but is performed to prevent infection and to halt the progressive loss of existing neurologic function. If the lesion is completely epithelialized, elective closure may be performed at some later date. If the lesion is open and the patient is not seen within the first 24 hours of life, surgery should be delayed until superficial contamination of the lesion has been controlled by moist dressings and systemic antibiotics.

2. CT should be performed within the first week of life. Every effort should be made to define the type as well as the severity of hydrocephalus. In patients with minimal ventricular enlargement secondary to the Arnold–Chiari malformation, a suboccipital decompression is sometimes appropriate. More often, a ventricular shunt is performed and

this is required in any patient with aqueductal stenosis. Of the available operations, the ventriculoperitoneal shunt is preferred.

3. Postoperatively, the patient should be fully evaluated to rule out urologic, orthopedic, and general surgical problems.

Encephalocele

Cranium bifidum and encephalocele are much less common than their spinal counterparts. Although these lesions occur in a variety of locations, they are most frequently found in the posterior midline (Fig. 40-20). Occipital and suboccipital encephaloceles show a considerable variation in morbid anatomy. Deformities of the tentorium and hindbrain are common and the external sac may contain a knuckle of occipital lobe, cerebellum, or both. Owing to the distorted anatomy of the posterior fossa in some cases, hydrocephalus may be present or may develop as a delayed complication.[3] Frontal encephaloceles frequently occur in the midline just above the nasion and produce wide lateral displacement of the orbits (hypertelorism). Orbital encephaloceles tend

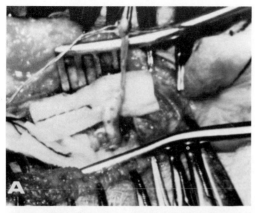

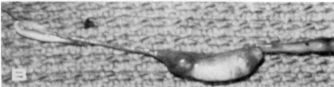

Fig. 40-21. Congenital dermal sinus tract in lumbosacral area. **A.** The operative exposure shows a lesion extending through the dura to end as an intraspinal dermoid tumor. **B.** Surgical specimen.

to present with unilateral exophthalmus, and nasal and nasopharyngeal lesions are occasionally mistaken for nasal polyps.

Although some encephaloceles reach gigantic proportions, the size of the external lesion gives little indication of its contents.[14] It should be emphasized that occipital encephaloceles sometimes communicate with the occipital horn of one or both lateral ventricles, and lesions in the suboccipital area almost invariably communicate with the cisterna magna or upper cervical theca. If the encephalocele is open and draining at birth, it should be repaired immediately. In cases in which the lesion is completely covered by thick skin, it is usually preferable to delay surgery until a complete diagnostic work-up, including skull x-rays, CT scan, and EEG, has been performed. If hydrocephalus is present, a ventricular shunting procedure is usually performed 7 to 10 days after the encephalocele has been repaired.

Cranial and Spinal Meningoceles

These lesions are similar to encephaloceles and meningomyeloceles except that they do not contain nervous tissue. Associated congenital anomalies occur with much less frequency, and, unless the lesions are open and draining at birth, surgical repair can be delayed for several weeks.

Dermal Sinus Tracts

By definition, these lesions consist of a tract of stratified squamous epithelium that extends inward from the skin surface. Like other dysrhaphic disorders, they presumably arise between the third to fifth weeks of gestation as a consequence of imperfect separation of the neuroectoderm and epithelial ectoderm. Dermal sinus tracts, therefore, characteristically occur in the dorsal midline. The most common sites include the sacrum, the lumbar area, and the suboccipital area, in that order. Embryologically, these sites correspond to the location of the posterior neuropore (lumbosacral region) and the anterior neuropore (suboccipital area).

The morbid anatomy of congenital dermal sinus tracts varies considerably. In some cases, the epithelial tube ends blindly just dorsal to the vertebral column or skull. In other instances, the tract extends through a small bony defect to terminate as a large mass (dermoid tumor or lipoma) that may be situated either extradurally or intradurally. In lumbosacral lesions, the intradural component may extend cephalad over many segments (Fig. 40-21). Such lesions are capable of producing an intramedullary mass that is imbedded in the conus medullaris. In suboccipital lesions, the sinus tract may extend through the cerebellar vermis to terminate as a dermoid or teratomatous tumor within the fourth ventricle.

The diagnosis of a congenital dermal sinus tract is occasionally made at birth. It is sufficient to say that any skin dimple or depression overlying the dorsal midline should be carefully examined by the attending physician. X-ray films of the skull or spine may occasionally demonstrate a small bony defect, but the absence of such a finding never excludes this lesion. Unfortunately, in the majority of cases, the disorder comes to attention only after the patient has experienced several bouts of unexplained meningitis. Less commonly, the patient may present with symptoms referable to an expanding intracranial or intraspinal mass.

To fully evaluate the extent of a dermal sinus tract, special diagnostic tests are usually required. Dermal sinography is to be condemned, for it can precipitate or exacerbate a meningeal infection. In patients with sacral or lumbosacral lesions, myelography is usually performed to rule out an intraspinal mass. To evaluate the extent of a sinus tract in the suboccipital area, a CT scan should be obtained.

The surgical treatment of dermal sinus tracts is performed with least risk and fewest complications when there are no signs of active meningeal infection. In patients who present with recurring bouts of meningitis, it is usually best to treat the infection with systemic antibiotics before proceeding with surgery. If persistent fever and meningeal signs suggest the formation of a chronic abscess, however, prolonged medical therapy is unwise. The goal of surgical treatment is to completely remove the sinus tract and its intraspinal or intracranial extensions. This is usually achieved except when past inflammation or infection causes the lesion to adhere intimately to vital structures. In patients who develop hydrocephalus secondary to meningitis, a ventricular shunting procedure may be required.

REFERENCES

1. **Milhorat TH:** Pediatric Neurosurgery. FA Davis, Philadelphia, 1978
2. **Russell DS:** Observations on the Pathology of Hydrocephalus. His Majesty's Stationery Office, London, 1949
3. **Milhorat TH:** Hydrocephalus and the Cerebrospinal Fluid. Williams and Wilkins, Baltimore, 1972
4. **Penfield W, Elvidge AR:** Hydrocephalus and the atropy of cerebral compression. In Penfield W (ed): Cytology and Cellular Pathology of the Nervous System, Vol. 3. Hafner, New York, 1932
5. **Foltz EL, Shurtleff DB:** Five-year comparative study of hydrocephalus in children with and without operation (113 cases). J Neurosurg 20: 1064, 1963
6. **Milhorat TH:** Failure of choroid plexectomy as treatment for hydrocephalus. Surg Gynecol Obstet 139:505, 1974
7. **Paine RS:** Hydrocephalus. Pediatr Clin North Am 14:779, 1967
8. **Rabe EF, Flynn RE, Dodge PR:** Subdural collections of fluid in infants and children. A study of 62 patients with special reference to factors influencing prognosis and the efficacy of various forms of therapy. Neurology 18: 559, 1968
9. **Towbin A:** Cerebral intraventricular hemorrhage and subependymal matrix infarction in the fetus and premature newborn. Amer J Pathol 52:121, 1968
10. **Larroche JC:** Hémorragies cérébrales intraventriculaires chez le prématuré. I. Anatomie et physiopathologie. Biol Neonate 7:26, 1964
11. **Schwartz P:** Birth Injuries of the newborn. Hafner, New York, 1961
12. **Towbin A:** Cerebral hypoxic damage in fetus and newborn: Basic patterns and their clinical significance. Arch Neurol (Chicago) 20:35, 1969
13. **DeLevie M, Nogrady MB:** Rapid brain growth upon restoration of adequate nutrition causing false radiographic evidence of increased intracranial pressure. J Pediatr 76:523, 1970
14. **Matson DD:** Neurosurgery of Infancy and Childhood. Charles C Thomas, Springfield, 1969
15. **Arey LB:** Developmental Anatomy. A Textbook and Laboratory Manual of Embryology, 7th ed, W B Saunders, Philadelphia, 1965
16. **Myrianthopoulous NC, Kurland LT:** Present concepts of the epidemiology and genetics of hydrocephalus. In Fields WS, Desmond MM (eds): Disorders of the Developing Nervous System. Charles C Thomas, Springfield, 1961
17. **Carter CO, Roberts JAF:** The risk of recurrence after 2 affected children with central nervous system malformations. Lancet, 1:306, 1967
18. **Milhorat TH:** Congenital hydrocephalus. In Sano K, Ishii S, LeVay S (eds): Recent Progress in Neurological Surgery. Excerpta Medica Amsterdam, 1974

19. **Laurence KM:** The natural history of spina bifida cystica. Arch Dis Child 39:41, 1964

20. **Rickham PP, Mawdsley T:** The effect of early operation on the survival of spina bifida cystica. Dev Med Child Neurol (Suppl) 11:20, 1966

21. **Sharrard WJ, Zachary RB, Lorber J, Bruce AM:** A controlled trial of immediate and de-layed closure of spina bifida cystica. Arch Dis Child 38:18, 1963

22. **Lorber J:** Results of treatment of meningo-myelocele. An analysis of 524 unselected cases, with special reference to possible selection for treatment. Dev Med Child Neurol 13:279, 1971

41

Neuromuscular Diseases

Gloria D. Eng

The principles of rehabilitation medicine are important in the evaluation and treatment of infants who present with nerve or muscle problems which affect tone, posture, and movement, congenital or traumatic in origin. They include accurate diagnosis, prevention of functional loss, minimizing deformity which exaggerates with growth, training in compensatory movements when function is permanently lost, and effective assistance of infants to reach maximum potential despite permanent disability. The parents are integrally involved and educated in the treatment program which they can apply daily to their infants.

The more common clinical disorders coming under the purview of rehabilitation medicine are herein detailed.

TRAUMATIC PERIPHERAL NERVE PALSIES

Traumatic peripheral palsies in the newborn are usually associated with difficult deliveries. The infant's head and face may be subject to prolonged pressure; the baby may have difficulty slipping his shoulders through the birth canal because of their width; or if he presents in breech position, too much traction may be exerted on his legs. The peripheral nerves lying under the thin skin and subcutaneous tissue are vulnerable to pressure, stretch, or actual avulsion.

Facial Palsy

Frequently following a complicated delivery, facial palsy may occur, particularly where there is extended impingement of the baby's head against the maternal sacrum, prolonged application of forceps, or intracranial bleeding with or without skull fracture. The infant is unable to wrinkle his forehead, close his eye, or suck the nipple without dribbling on the affected side. (Fig. 41-1.) This condition must be differentiated from congenital maldevelopment of the seventh nerve nucleus itself, which is frequently bilateral, and associated with abducens palsy, as seen in the Möbius syndrome. It should not be confused with persistent partial congenital palsies associated with chondrocardiac anomalies (i.e., Klippel–Feil, Sprengel's deformity), phocomelia, and cardiac malformations, or maldevelopment of the visceral arches. Central facial palsy involves the lower portion of the face and is characterized by flattening of the nasolabial fold, a droop of the involved corner of the mouth, and widening of the palpebral fissure. It is usually associated with anoxia at birth. To be distinguished from all the others is a

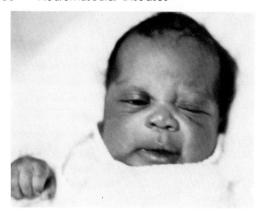

Fig. 41-1. Right facial palsy in a 2-week-old infant.

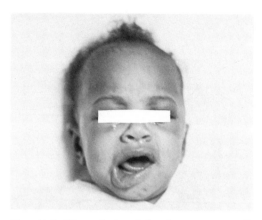

Fig. 41-2. Hypoplasia of the depressor anguli oris muscle in a 2-month-old infant.

benign condition described by Nelson and Eng, of congenital absence or hypoplasia of the depressor anguli oris (triangularis) muscle (Fig. 41-2).[1] In this condition, one corner of the mouth does not move downward and outward with the other when the baby is crying. The rest of the facial muscles are intact allowing the baby to frown, close his eyes, wrinkle his nose, and suck without dribbling because, despite palpable thinning of the lateral portion of the lower lip, the orbicularis oris functions normally.

In birth palsy of the facial nerve, the asymmetry of facial movements may be profound and may not reflect the true integrity of the nerve. Clinical criteria that may predict prognosis—pain about the ear or associated symptoms such as hyperacusis, loss of taste in the homolateral two-thirds of the tongue, and disturbances in lacrimation—cannot be evaluated in an infant. Fortunately, there are simple electrodiagnostic tests that can provide valuable information on the state of the nerve.

1. **Nerve excitability test.** This can be performed 72 hours after onset. The facial nerve is stimulated in front of the ear with surface electrodes, using a square wave pulse of 1 millisecond duration at a rate of 1 per second. The milliamperage is varied until the threshold response of the nerve is reached. The amperage is compared to that required on the unaffected side. If they are the same, then neuropraxia (block of nerve impulse secondary to edema) exists, and recovery should occur in several weeks. Late degeneration of the nerve occurs in 12% to 18% of patients; therefore, repeated testing is necessary at 3- to 5-day

intervals until stabilization or gradual recovery becomes evident.

2. **Nerve conduction latency.** The facial nerve is stimulated in front of the ear, and the impulse is recorded from the frontalis or levator anguli nasi muscles (Fig. 41-3). If the nerve loses all response to electrical stimulation, the prognosis is guarded. This test may be done 7 days after onset.

3. **Chronoxie and strength duration curve.** Electrical stimulus is delivered directly to the facial muscles. The threshold of response rises as the nerve degenerates. These tests may be done 5 days after onset.

4. **Electromyogram (EMG).** This may be done 14 to 21 days after onset. Absence of motor unit activity, presence of fibrillation potentials and sharp waves depict a state of denervation. The study is particularly useful sequentially to evaluate regeneration and gradual improvement.

Because many infants with facial palsy recover spontaneously within several days to 3 weeks following delivery, the pathophysiology in these infants is undoubtedly one of mild neuropraxia. The infants who are referred for consultation are usually more seriously involved, yet their numbers are not large in the total spectrum of facial palsies affecting children. In Manning and Adour's series of 61 children under 14 years of age seen over a 4-year-period, only 5 were the result of birth trauma.[2] We studied 28 patients with facial palsy over a 1-year period.[3] Only 11 were seen in the newborn period; 6 had traumatic palsies, and 5 had congenital palsies associated with other anomalies. Only 1 infant out of the 6

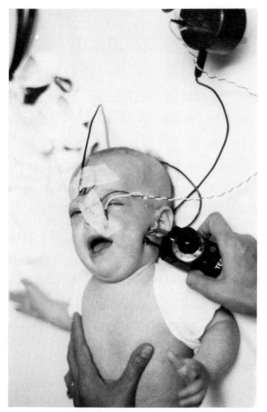

Fig. 41-3. Nerve conduction latency determination in a 6-week-old baby with hypoplasia of the left depressor anguli oris muscle.

traumatic palsies did not recover spontaneously by 5 months of age. If there was evidence of degeneration of the nerve on initial electrodiagnostic studies, then the nerve regenerated at approximately an inch per month. The congenital group did not change on follow-up because, in this group, there was agenesis of a lower branch or the entire lower division of the facial nerve.

General principles of management have been formulated based on our experience with this problem. If the clinical picture and electrodiagnosis suggest mild involvement or neuropraxia, no treatment is required. If partial denervation exists, then physical therapy, including massage, electrical stimulation, and later active exercises, is prescribed. If there is further loss of nerve excitability after 72 hours from onset, surgical decompression may be indicated. In none of our infants was the last consideration necessary. The use of cor-

ticosteroids to suppress edema and inflammation seems to hold no justification in birth palsy. Methylcellulose drops and taping of the involved eye to prevent excoriation of the cornea may be the only treatment indicated.

Brachial Plexus Palsy

The brachial plexus may be injured during delivery when the infant's head has been delivered and his shoulders are trapped in the birth canal. Hyperextension of the head may exert traction on the cervical roots and plexus.

Erb's palsy is paralysis of the muscles of the arm supplied by components of C5 and C6 nerve roots. It is the most common form of paralysis and is clinically obvious in an infant who has a one-side Moro reflex, whose affected arm hangs limply adducted and internally rotated at the shoulder, extended and pronated at the elbow, and with flexed wrist in the typical "waiter's tip" posture (Fig. 41-4).

Klumpke's paralysis affects only the muscles of the hand supplied by C8 to T1 nerve roots. It is rarely seen in infancy as an isolated entity. Total plexus involvement affects all the muscles in the arm because the entire plexus from C5 to T1 has been damaged (Fig. 41-5). The arm lies motionless, usually with absence of sweat and sensation, and the hand is small, dry, and atrophic. The deep tendon reflexes are markedly diminished or regularly absent in the affected arm.

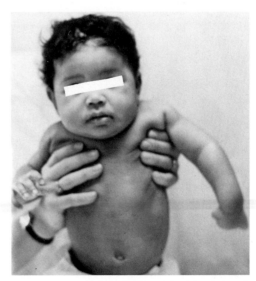

Fig. 41-4. A 2-month-old baby girl with a left Erb's palsy.

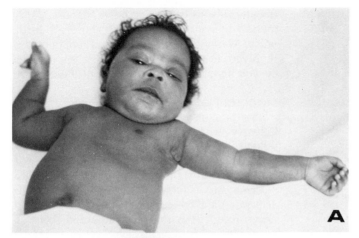

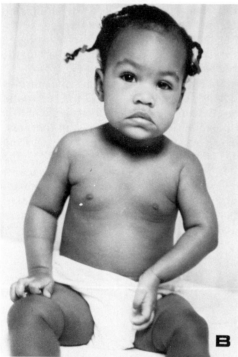

Fig. 41.5. **A.** Newborn baby girl with complete brachial plexus palsy involving the left arm. Note the atrophy of the pectoralis major muscle, also the Horner's syndrome: ptosis of the left lid. **B.** At 1 year of age, she has return of the function of the C5, C6 supplied muscles, but no return of the C7, C8 and T1 muscles. The hand is atrophic and devoid of sensation. Note the persistent Horner's syndrome.

of the cervical spine with evidence of traction injury of the cervical cord; ipsilateral diaphragmatic paralysis; and even periadrenal hemorrhage; all, suggest the traumatic nature of these deliveries. Horner's syndrome associated with complete plexus palsy was seen in eight of our infants.

EMG is extremely useful in accurate anatomic delineation of the extent of pathology in these arms, to determine severity of denervation and estimate prognosis. The first examination can be accomplished 2 to 3 weeks after birth. Serial studies at 6-week intervals will give information on the degree of return. The EMG recovery precedes the clinical return of function by several weeks, and, as in all nerve lesions with the exception of neuropraxia, the regeneration proceeds at approximately an inch per month.

Treatment is critical and includes early and meticulous movement of the joints in the paralyzed extremity. Scapulohumeral winging, limitation of internal and external rotation, abduction of the shoulder, loss of supination of the elbow, flexion deformity of the wrist, and tight adduction of the thumb quickly develop without treatment. Supportive splints to hold the wrist and hand in good alignment may be indicated. Electrical stimulation of the denervated muscle to prevent fibrosis is recommended. To be effective, treatment must be started early, be applied with regularity, and be of sufficient current intensity to cause maximal muscle contraction. As recovery ensues, active exercises to strengthen the proximal shoulder girdle and arm muscles are included.

In our early report and in subsequent study of 135 of those unfortunate infants, the obstetric histories have been complicated.[4,5] Long, difficult labors and the use of general anesthesia were the rule. The babies, with the exception of one, weighed between 3600–7000 g. The incidence of abnormal presentation was high. Associated defects included torticollis; facial palsies; subluxation of the shoulder; fracture of the clavicle and humerus; slippage of the capital head of the radius; subluxation

The infant must be made aware of that extremity as a part of himself.

Sequelae, even in the mildest paralysis, include scapular winging (Fig. 41-6), loss of shoulder abduction, and elbow supination. More serious complications include loss of bone growth (Fig. 41-7), persistent loss of sensation, and total lack of awareness of the arm by the infant even with good neuromotor and sensory recovery.

Lumbosacral Plexus Injury

Such injury is suspect in an infant who presents with paralysis of one leg. The extent of involvement may be determined by clinical examination and substantiated by EMG. The frequency of this injury is undoubtedly low, occurring primarily after frank breech deliveries. In 128 neonatal peripheral palsies studied over a 7-year period, only 3 cases of lumbosacral traction injury have come to our atten-

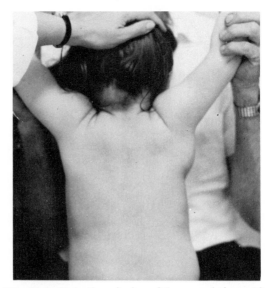

Fig. 41-6. Note the winging of the scapula in an 18-month-old baby girl with a C5, C6, C7 brachial plexus palsy.

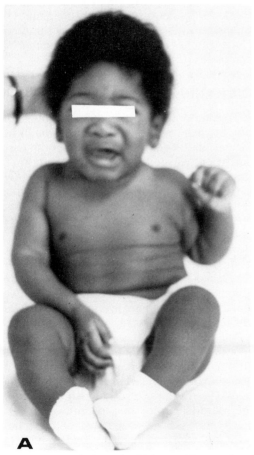 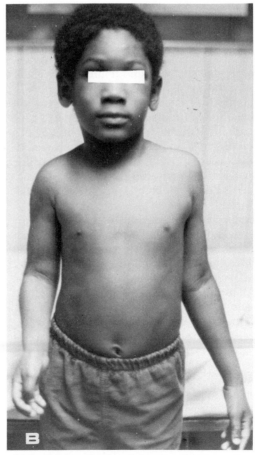

Fig. 41-7. A. A 4-week-old boy with complete brachial plexus palsy involving the right arm. **B.** At 3 years of age. Note the length discrepancy and loss of growth of the right arm. The hand intrinsic muscles are weak and sensation is not intact.

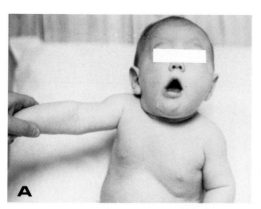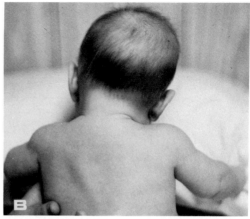

Fig. 41-8. A. Congenital torticollis affecting the right sternocleidomastoid muscle in a 3-month-old baby. **B.** Note the flattening of the left occiput and right head tilt.

tion. Difficulties may arise in the differentiation of this entity from myelomeningocele with asymmetrical involvement, infantile poliomyelitis, flaccid hemiparesis, or trauma from intramuscular injection.

Radiographs of the spine and digital palpation through the rectum would substantiate the presence of a myelomeningocele occulta affecting the lumbosacral plexus. The rectal sphincter may be patulous if the S3 division of the sacral plexus is also involved.

Poliomyelitis causes "spotty" paralysis with sparing of one or more muscles in the extremity, and the affected muscles are not root-related. For example, the tibialis anterior and peroneal longus which are L4, L5, and S1 supplied muscles may be paralyzed; yet, the gluteus maximus, which is also L4, L5, and S1 supplied, may be spared. The rectal sphincter remains unaffected. Stool virus isolation or serologic studies can confirm the diagnosis.

Flaccid hemiparesis affects not only the leg but the arm as well. Careful evaluation of the arm movements will usually distinguish it as abnormal when compared to the unaffected opposite extremity. Deep tendon reflexes are brisk in the involved limbs despite severe flaccidity. The plantar reflex may be persistently extensor on the hemiplegic side.

The most difficult entity to distinguish from lumbosacral plexus injury is trauma to the sciatic nerve in the buttocks by intramuscular injection. In sciatic damage, the muscles supplied by L4, L5, S1, and S2 nerve components are usually paralyzed, whereas in total lum-

bosacral traction injury, the muscles supplied by nerves from L2 and L3 roots are also affected. Furthermore, nerve conduction velocity may be segmentally impaired in sciatic injury. Causalgia (sensitivity to touch and trophic skin changes) was a prominent symptom in two of our infants with traction injury. None of the recoveries in our infants was complete.

CONGENITAL TORTICOLLIS

Torticollis is recognized in an infant who tilts his head persistently to one side, whose face is flattened, with the palpebral fissure narrowed, ear compressed, and the corner of the mouth lowered on the same side, with flattening of the occiput on the opposite side (Fig. 41-8). The affected sternocleidomastoid muscle feels thick and broad and resists stretch of both the clavicular and sternal portions. By the second to the fourth weeks, a hard fusiform mass (the "olive"), is palpable in the belly of the muscle. It may increase in size, then gradually disappear when the infant is between 4 and 7 months of age, leaving a thick, fibrotic noncontractile muscle.

The birth history in an infant with torticollis is remarkable in that it is usually difficult, almost invariably a breech presentation, and occasionally even necessitates a cesarean section. The reason probably lies in the fact that the sternocleidomastoid pathology exists *in utero,* precluding engagement of the infant's head in the birth canal. The concept that there

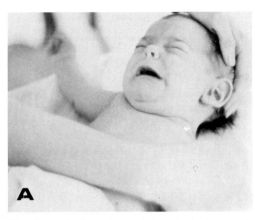
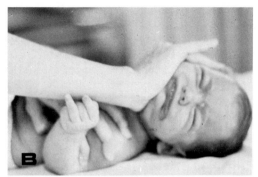

Fig. 41-9. A. Stretching of the clavicular portion of the contracted sternocleidomastoid muscle. **B.** Stretching of the sternal portion of the contracted sternocleidomastoid muscle.

is a hereditary defect in the anlage of the muscle is derived from the discovery of anomalous muscles in relatives or of the association of ipsilateral hip dislocation or clubfoot in the affected infants.[6] Intrauterine denervation or infection have not been substantiated by pathologic dissections of the involved muscle, which usually consists of glistening white fibrous tissue engulfing muscle fibers, without evidence of hemorrhage.[7]

Congenital torticollis must be differentiated from bony anomalies of the cervical spine and shoulder girdle (*i.e.,* Klippel–Feil Syndrome with or without Sprengel's deformity) or acquired wry neck associated with acute trauma, pharyngotonsillitis, adenitis, cerebral irritation secondary to meningitis or posterior fossa tumor, visual and labyrinthine disorders, and postshunting for hydrocephalus. A mass in the neck may represent adenoma, cystic hygroma, dermoid, or rhabdomyoma.

In our experience with over 100 babies with congenital torticollis, only 2 have required surgical tenotomy (both were over a year old when first seen). In a young baby, physical therapy is eminently successful in stretching the contracted muscle. The parents are taught two basic exercises: stretching of the clavicular portion by lateral flexion of the head to the opposite side, and stretching the sternal portion by rotation of the chin to the affected side. (Fig. 41-9**B**). Occasionally, the trapezius must also be stretched, as well as the muscles over the ipsilateral pelvic brim as the baby tends to assume a long C-scoliotic curve. A soft collar can be readily made to hold the head in good alignment (Fig. 41-10). Hanging toy mobiles above the baby's head on the affected side, and placing the crib so that the baby has to turn his head to the affected side to see what is happening in the room, are recommended for active stretching on his part. Later, strengthening exercises will provide balanced flexion of the head. With early treatment, the asymmetry lessens as the skull and facial bones are permitted to remold. At 2 years of

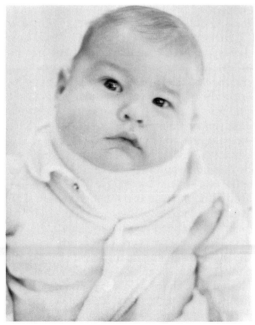

Fig. 41-10. A soft collar is used to keep the head in good alignment in a baby with a left torticollis.

age, the entire contour is appreciably improved.

TONE PROBLEMS

Infants are frequently examined because of problems in tone. In order to separate tonal changes caused by upper motor neuron disorders from peripheral neuromuscular weakness, the concept of tone must be considered.

Tone. Tone is that quality in muscle that resists movement. The French call it "extensibilité" and relate it to slow stretch while moving the muscle through a range of motion.[8] It can also be described as a recoil phenomenon. When the muscle is stretched passively and released, it springs back to its original position. When there is stretch and no rebound, allowing for limpness, this is hypotonia. On the other hand, when there is a constant resistance to stretch associated with a "lead-pipe" delay in relaxation, this is rigidity. Further, if there is stretch with too rapid rebound and too much recoil, this is spasticity.

Mechanism of Tone

Neurophysiologists have attempted to unravel the nervous control of posture and movement for almost a century. It now appears that the gamma nervous system with its muscle spindles, the primary and secondary endings in the spindles, the afferent gamma pathways, the gamma motor neurons in the ventral horn of the spinal cord, and the efferent gamma fibers back to the spindles assume prime roles in the mechanism of tone. The monosynaptic connection between the group Ia gamma afferent fibers and the alpha motor neurons, which send axons to the extrafusal fibers, makes up the important stretch reflex. Supraspinal centers send modifying influences to both the alpha motor and gamma motor neurons (Fig. 41-11).

More specifically, the muscle spindles are sensory structures. They are small and fusiform in shape, lying parallel to skeletal muscle fibers. There are two types of intrafusal fibers in the muscle spindles, a nuclear bag fiber and a nuclear chain fiber. Each nuclear bag and nuclear chain fiber has a sensory ending that unites to form the group Ia sensory afferent nerve. The secondary endings come from nuclear chain fibers and form the group II afferent nerve fibers. Presumably, the primary ending

from the nuclear bag intrafusals is sensitive to the **rate** of change of muscle length in stretch, and the secondary endings are sensitive to change in length. According to Rushworth, group Ia afferent fibers have monosynaptic connections with the alpha motor neurons in the spinal cord not only of the same muscle but also end in motor neurons of the synergistic and antagonistic muscles.[9] The exact function of the secondary endings is not clear, but they conduct more slowly, are polysynaptic, and are thought to facilitate flexor and inhibit extensor alpha motor neurons in the regulation of posture.

In the ventral horn of the spinal cord, the alpha motor neurons send axons back to the extrafusal muscle fibers. Gamma I and gamma II motor neurons in turn send fibers which terminate in the intrafusal muscle fibers as trail endings and plate endings.[10]

The gamma system modulates voluntary movement. According to Matthews, the gamma afferents connect with the alpha motor neuron by way of the spindle loop as a "closed-loop servomechanism" controlling the length of the muscle, while the gamma efferents control the "damping" of this loop and its controlled position.[9]

Rushworth believes that overactivity of the gamma system is the primary disorder of function in spasticity and rigidity.[9] Hypotonia, on the other hand, results from a lack of gamma motor activity. There is withdrawal of cerebellar facilitation that results in flaccid intrafusal fibers and consequent lack of the stretch reflex.

Changes in Tone in the Brain-injured Infant

A cerebrally damaged infant's tone may remain flaccid for days or weeks following delivery. He then progressively assumes abnormal postures and increasing stretch reflex. His tone can be modified by changing his position. Hypotonia in prone may be hypertonia in supine and exaggerated hypertonicity in vertical suspension. The release of descending vestibulospinal impulses from higher cortical control is probably responsible for these shifts in tone. Changing the position of the infant's head will evoke the labyrinthine reflexes that also affect tone. Hyperextension of the head will elicit hyperextension of the trunk and facilitate hypertonicity in the limbs. Flex-

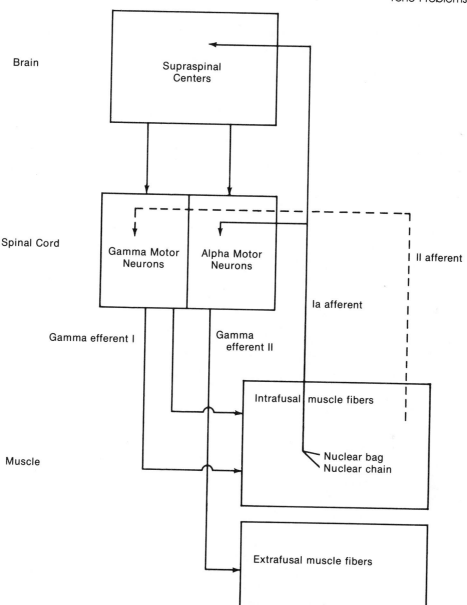

Fig. 41-11. Schematic diagram of the Alpha and Gamma pathways in muscle control.

ion of the head will relieve the hypertonus and relax the limbs. Imposing the tonic neck reflex increases the extensor tone in the limbs on the face side of the infant and the flexor tone on his occipital side. There may exist a discrepancy between hypotonicity affecting neck and trunk muscles and hypertonicity of the limb muscles. Deep tendon reflexes and infantile automatisms, though important in the early assessment of the infant, are frequently un-reliable because they again are subservient to his tone.

The problem in discrimination between brain and peripheral neuromuscular disease lies not in the overtly cerebrally damaged infant with changing tone, but in the infant with persistently depressed tone. It may be hard to determine whether an infant has peripheral neuromuscular disease or brain damage because both conditions have a similar history: varying

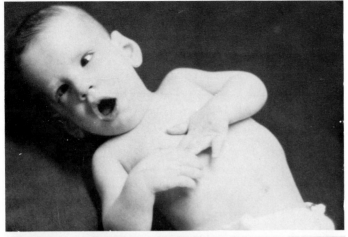

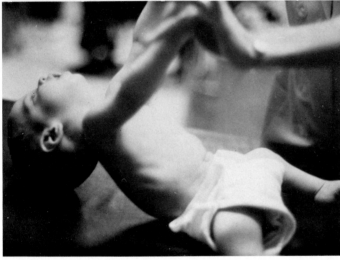

Fig. 41-12. A. Hypotonic 4-month-old infant with myopathic facies. **B.** Extreme head lag on traction of the arms. The diagnosis: myotonic atropthy.

degrees of intrauterine immobility, difficult labor, slow engagement and descent in the birth canal, and a flaccid, immobile, infant with weak cry and a low Apgar score. Prolonged hypotonia may be seen in the kernicteric infant after the initial rigid, opisthotonic state; athetosis may appear at the end of the first year of life. Severe anoxia can produce a depressed baby for several months who then becomes increasingly choreoathetotic. Our experience bears out Paine and Oppe's statement that "persistent and permant hypotonicity of the body as a whole is also occasionally seen with chronic brain syndrome and may include hypo- or arreflexia (and usually severe mental deficiency as well)."[11] In some cases only the laboratory examination or the passage of time may help.

The Hypertonic Infant

On occasion, an infant may present with too much tone. He tends to be stiff in his limbs, his head control is too good, the Landau response shows too much extension of the head and legs. When placed on his feet, he jerks into full vertical extension, rearing into almost an opisthotonic posture. He may show increased jitteriness, regurgitant feeding patterns, brisk jaw jerks and deep tendon reflexes. He usually has a complicated gestational and delivery history, may be premature, or may be a small-for-dates baby. As he grows, the rigidity diminishes and he begins to attain milestones readily, gradually evolving into a perfectly normal baby by 14 to 18 months of age. On the other hand, he may become overtly spastic with delayed development and varying

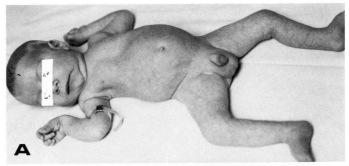

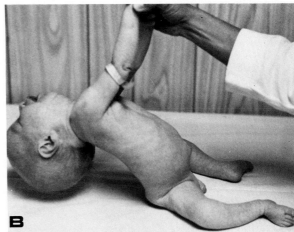

Fig. 41-13. A. A hypotonic 3-month-old infant lying in a typical immobile posture. He appears alert despite profound weakness and paradoxical respirations. The diagnosis: Werdnig-Hoffman disease. **B.** Severe head lag is noted when traction is exerted on the infant's arms.

degrees of psychomotor retardation. Drillien in a prospective study of 300 children of low birth weights, described "transient dystonia" in some of the babies in the first year of life.[12] Mental impairment and hyperactivity were noted in these babies by 2 to 3 years of age as compared to the children who did not show abnormal neurologic signs. The author suggests that those same children will show deficits in language skills, motor perception, behavior, and learning when they attain school age.

The Hypotonic, Peripheral Neuromuscular-diseased Infant

Certain aspects of a hypotonic infant with lower motor neuron involvement may be clinically helpful. He usually assumes a very typical posture without changes in tone when his posture in space is altered. When supine, his arms rest slightly abducted and internally or externally rotated at the shoulder, elbows flexed and pronated, fingers clenched in slight ulnar drift. His hips maintain an abducted

externally rotated position in the so-called pithed-frog posture. The cry is weak, breathing may be paradoxic with asynchronous expansion of the chest cage and the abdomen, and the only spontaneous movements involve small excursions of his fingers and toes. Deep tendon reflexes are depressed and frequently absent. The Moro, tonic neck reflexes, and crossed adductor responses are usually not elicitable. He may have an expressionless facies (Fig. 41-12), but more commonly appears vitally alert despite profound weakness (Fig. 41-13).

The Chronically Ill Infant

Not to be forgotten, also among the hypotonic babies, is the chronically ill infant who has cardiac, renal, adrenal, metabolic, or nutritional problems. He may be severely hypotonic but usually maintains deep tendon reflexes and will move his extremities on stimulus. Moreover, he will look "sick."

Few surveys of populations of infants suffering tonal problems exist. There are deline-

Table 41-1. A Study of Infants with Tone Problems.

331	Infants; newborn to 3 years
230	Cerebral hypotonia
207	Cerebral palsied—diplegia, hemiplegia, quadriplegia, athetosis
23	Psychomotor retardation
18	Rigid babies
7	Normal development
6	Cerebral palsied—spastic
3	Mental retardation and seizures
2	Accelerated motor development
83	Hypotonic infants; studied electrodiagnostically

ations of "amyotonia congenita," or hypotonic infants, where the overtly cerebrally damaged babies have already been segregated. Paine studied 133 floppy babies between the ages of 6 months and 2½ years: 68 had cerebral palsy, 25 had psychomotor retardation, 7 had Werdnig–Hoffmann disease, 1 had congenital myopathy, and 21 had unclassified congenital hypotonia.[13] Because many of the Werdnig–Hoffmann infants are diagnosed under 6 months of age, Paine's survey probably excluded some of these younger infants. Moreover, some of the benign hypotonias could have been rarer muscle disorders not analyzed because of limitation of available techniques.

Results of a Series of Infants with Tone Problems

Over a 3-year-period, we studied 331 infants who presented with problems in tone. Their ages ranged from birth to 3 years (Table 41-1). Of these, 230 were readily categorized as cerebral hypotonic infants who evolved into typical cerebral-palsied children with varying degrees of spastic hemiplegia, diplegia, or quadriplegia, and a lesser number into athetoid cerebral palsy; 10% of the cerebral hypotonic infants did not develop further tonal changes but remained floppy and retarded children; 18 infants presented with hypertonus; 7 of these stiff infants improved and attained normal milestones within the first 14 months of life, 6 became overtly spastic, 2 developed hyp-

sarrhythmia and retardation, 1 deteriorated rapidly with Krabbe's disease, and 2 babies from Africa remained entirely normal, manifesting accelerated muscular development.

A separate category of 83 infants was studied in depth because their clinical picture was not well defined. In this last group, 31 infants were ultimately found to be cerebrally damaged infants (Table 41-2). Thus, only 16% of the total group of hypotonic-hypertonic infants was diagnosed as peripheral neuromuscular disorders.

The most common lower motor neuron disorder in the series was **spinal muscular atrophy (Werdnig–Hoffmann disease).** This is a disorder with a wide spectrum of manifestations. It may occur *in utero,* resulting in diminution of fetal movements. The baby may then be born with arthrogrypotic changes. A baby may appear normal at birth and suddenly develop extreme weakness with severe head-lag, proximal limb girdle muscle paralysis, absent DTRs, and increasing respiratory problems because of bulbar and respiratory muscle involvement. Despite severe flaccidity, the baby's facial muscles are spared and he usually appears alert, wide-eyed, and intelligent. The earlier the onset of the disease, the worse becomes the prognosis. Of our babies who were diagnosed under 5 months of age, 90% were dead before 1 year of age. Some infants with spinal muscular atrophy who are not diagnosed until the end of the first year or during the second year of life have a more benign variant of this disease. They may survive infancy and with good care grow into adulthood. Their disease appears to be nonprogressive and they blend into the adult group of benign limb girdle atrophies.

The inheritance pattern of spinal muscular atrophy is of utmost significance in that it is an autosomal recessive inherited disorder. Although the severity of the disease affecting different siblings in the family may vary, the parents must be counseled on the 25% incidence of transmission to their children. There is no method at this time to detect the carrier state.

Other neuromuscular disorders are much rarer clinical entities and the reader is referred to the many excellent articles and monographs on the subject.[14–20] Except for progressive Duchenne muscular dystrophy, the other dystrophies and rarer myopathies are still ill-de-

Table 41-2. Eighty-three Hypotonic Infants Ages: 4 Days–3 Years.

Brain	Cerebral hypotonia	26
	Degenerating and demyelinating	5
	Tay–Sachs 2	
	Metachromatic leukodystrophy 2	
	Unknown 1	
Cord	Infantile spinal muscular atrophy (Werdnig–Hoffmann)	15
	Juvenile spinal muscular atrophy	4
	Arthrogryposis—secondary to neurogenic atrophy	4
	Traction injury	1
	Infantile poliomyelitis	1
	Multiple anomalies with upper cord lesion	1
	Multiple anomalies with diffuse neurogenic atrophy	1
Roots and Nerves	Polyneuropathy	3
Myoneural Junction	Congenital myasthenia gravis	2
Muscle	Muscular dystrophy	1
	Myopathy—fiber hypotrophy and central nuclei	4
	Inflammatory myopathy	2
	Polymyositis	1
	Myotonic atrophy	5
Metabolic and Chronic Diseases	Hyperthyroidism—myositis	1
	Hypothyroidism—neuropathy	3
	Congenital renal anomaly	1
	Benign congenital hypotonia	2

fined entities, with equivocal modes of inheritance and unknown but relatively benign prognosis.

Suffice it to say, the physician is responsible for prescribing therapy to maintain these infants in as optimal physical condition as possible, regardless of ultimate prognosis. Prevention of contractures, maintenance of good respiratory capacity, and postural drainage in the event of lung complications are standard procedures.

LABORATORY AIDS

The laboratory becomes of inestimable value in the detailed study of infants with hypotonia. Muscle enzymes, EMG, and muscle biopsy are important facets in laboratory confirmation of clinical impression.

Muscle Enzymes

Elevated serum enzyme levels of creatine phosphokinase, aldolase, and transaminases reflect muscle breakdown. They are normal in the cerebral-damaged baby, may be slightly elevated in neurogenic disease, and markedly elevated in some myopathies and dystrophies. Creatinkinase levels are particularly specific for intrinsic muscle disease. However, they may be considerably elevated in normal infants during the first 24 hours of life, gradually tapering to near normal levels by 5 days of age, but may persist in slight elevation throughout the first year of life.[21,22] Cautious interpretation of the enzyme levels is therefore necessary, especially when a baby with possible congenital Duchenne dystrophy is being considered. His values may be lost in the upper limits of normal range during the first few days of life. The enzymes should therefore be drawn after the end of the first week of life. It is also preferable to request enzymes prior to EMG because trauma caused by needle exploration may elevate the creatinkinase for 72 hours. Intramuscular injection will also cause a rise in creatinkinase levels.

Electrodiagnosis

The development of electrodiagnosis in recent years has proved an incomparable adjunct to the neurologic differentiation of hypotonic infants. The electrical studies are well-tolerated by neonates, and give objective evidence of pathology. They include strength-duration curves, study of neuromuscular transmission, nerve conduction velocity determinations, and electromyography. Their application is based on knowledge of maturation of the infant's peripheral nervous system. In this regard, even the gestation age of infants can be estimated by conduction velocities of their peripheral nerves.[23] Term babies' nerve conduction velocities are approximately half those of adults, and mature to adult levels by 3 to 5 years of age. These nerve conduction velocity studies provide information relevant to the integrity of the peripheral nerve, particularly in suspected polyneuropathies.

Neuromuscular transmission likewise improves with maturation and deteriorates when disease states such as myasthenia gravis, or botulism and other poisonous agents intervene.[24] Strength-duration curves are difficult to plot in babies. In paralytic states, there is shift of the motor points, and their localization is made difficult, particularly in the small squirming movements of the baby.

The EMG has proved especially excellent in providing information regarding the state of the muscle. The size and duration of the motor unit potentials, the aggregation of these potentials to form an interference pattern, the tracing when the muscle is at rest—whether it remains silent or shows fibrillation potentials and sharp waves—all reflect the presence or absence of pathology. Irritability of the muscles on needle exploration may signify "sick" muscles. The presence of runs of positive potentials may suggest myotonia. Tolerance to EMG is very good in infants, especially if fine teflon-coated monopolar electrodes are used.

In the EMG studies of normal infants, we have found "minifibrillations" in the muscles from 32-weeks' gestation to 2 months of age, that must be taken into account in interpretation of neuropathic disease in these young infants. These minifibrillations were alluded to by Marinacci[25,26] and von Bernuth.[24] They differ from end-plate potentials in frequency, amplitude (15 to 100 mv), and duration (1 to 2 milliseconds). The physiologic reason for their existence is debated. The muscle membrane excitability may be increased as compared to adults, leading to easy depolarization. They may represent preinnervation fibers discharging spontaneously. Or, because the muscle fiber diameter of infants is relatively small, rapid summation to threshold level of the muscle fiber presumably occurs, causing it to depolarize, upon firing of the end-plate potentials. Whatever the reasons may be, these minifibrillations persist in problems of delayed maturation, in some of the hypotonic infants with metabolic conditions, and even upper motor neuron disease states.

Thus, the interpretation of an EMG as neuropathic merely on the observation of fibrillation potentials alone is invalid in neonates. The amplitude and duration of the motor unit potentials, presence or absence of polyphasic potentials, the interference pattern, and the tracing on muscle rest must all be analytically considered before rendering a conclusion.

Muscle Biopsy

The enzyme and electrodiagnostic data may lead to necessary confirmation of suspected muscle disease by muscle biopsy. The importance of meticulous handling of the biopsy specimen cannot be overemphasized, especially when the possible diagnosis of a rather obscure myopathy is involved. The selection of the biopsy site is important. It should reflect active disease but not so advanced pathologically that all landmarks are destroyed. Avoid a muscle that has been recently studied electromyographically or which has received intramuscular injections. The biopsy then may show inflammatory reaction and frequently identifiable needle tracks. It is preferable not to fix the specimen in formalin because it causes the muscle to shrink and contract. For histochemical techniques, the specimen should be gently anchored in longitudinal alignment on a tongue depressor or deposited on a gauze square soaked in normal saline. It may be transported in ice if the pathologist is in the vicinity, or frozen, for distant mailing.

REFERENCES

1. **Nelson K, Eng G:** Congenital hypoplasia of the depressor anguli oris muscle: differentiation from congenital facial palsy. J Pediatr 1:16, 1972
2. **Manning J, Adour K:** Facial paralysis in children. Pediatrics 1:102, 1972
3. **Eng GD:** The value of electrodiagnosis in facial palsies affecting infants and children. Clin Proc Children's Hospital 10:279, 1971
4. **Eng GD:** Brachial plexus palsy in newborn infants. Pediatrics 48:1:18, 1971
5. **Eng GD, Koch B, Smokvina MD:** Brachial Plexus Palsy in Neonates and Children. Arch Physical Med Rehab 59:458–464, 1978
6. **Hara I, Ikeda T:** On the ipsilateral involvement of congenital muscular torticollis and congenital dislocation of the hip. J Jpn Orthop Assoc 35:1221, 1962
7. **Garceau G:** Congenital muscular torticollis hematoma—fact or myth. Med J Rhode Island 45:401, 1962
8. **Andre-Thomas, Chesni Y, Saint-Anne Daigassis S:** The neurological examination of the infant. Little Club Clinic, No. 1, London, National Spastics Society, 1960
9. **Boyd J, Eyzaguirre C, Matthews P, Rushworth J:** The role of the Gamma system in movement and posture. NY Assoc for the Aid of Crippled Children, 1964
10. **Dubo H, Darling R:** Gamma nervous system and muscle spindles. In Physiological Basis of Rehabilitation Medicine. WB Saunders, Philadelphia, 1971
11. **Paine R, Oppe T:** Neurological examination of children. Clinic in Developmental Medicine 20/21. The Spastics Society in Association with William Heinemann, 1966
12. **Drillien C:** Abnormal neurologic signs in the first year of life in low-birthweight infants: Possible prognostic significance. Develop Med Child Neurol 14:575, 1972
13. **Paine RS:** The future of the "floppy infant;" a follow-up study of 133 patients. Dev Med Child Neurol 5:115, 1963
14. **Campbell E:** Electrodiagnosis of muscular hypotonia in infancy and childhood. In Kiernander B (ed): Physical Medicine in Pediatrics, pp. 155–189. Butterworths, London, 1965.
15. **Walton JN:** The Amyotonia congenital syndrome. Proc R Soc Med 50:301, 1957
16. **Jebson R, Johnson E, Knobloch H, Grant D:** Differential diagnosis of infantile hypotonia: The use of the electromyograph and the developmental and neurological examination as aids. Am J Dis Child 101:8, 1961
17. **Zellweger H, Smith J, Cusminsky M:** Muscular hypotonia in infancy: Diagnosis and differentiation, Rev Can Biol 21:599, 1962
18. **Rabe E:** The hyptonic infant. J Pediatr 62:422, 1964
19. **Dubowitz V:** The floppy infant, clinics in developmental medicine, No. 31, 14. Spastics International Medical Publications, William Heinemann, 1969
20. **Dubowitz V:** Muscle disorders in childhood, Vol. 16. In Series: Major Problems in Clinical Pediatrics. WB Saunders, Philadelphia, 1978
21. **Wharton B, Bassie U, Gough G, Williams A:** Clinical value of plasma creatine kinase and uric acid levels during first week of life. Arch Dis Child 46:356, 1971
22. **Bodensteiner J, Zellweger H:** Creatine phosphokinase in normal neonates and young infants. J Lab Clin Med 77:853, 1971
23. **Thomas J, Lambert E:** Ulnar nerve conduction velocity and H-reflex in infants and children, J Appl Physiol 15:1, 1960
24. **Koeningsberger MR, Patten B, Lovelace R:** Studies of Myoneural Junction in Normal Full-term, Premature and Hypermagesemic Newborn Infants. Presented at the Fourth International Congress of Electromyography, Brussels, 1971
25. **Marinacci AA:** Applied Electromyography. Lee and Febiger, Philadelphia, 1968
26. **von Bernuth CH:** Die neuromuskalore Entwicklung in der abkangigkeit vom Geburtswegwicht und Menstruationsulter. Sonderatdruck ans, Monatsschrift fur Kinderkeilkunde, Band 119, Heft 7, 295, 1971

42

Nutrition

Gordon B. Avery and
Anne B. Fletcher

THE PHYSIOLOGY OF DIGESTION AND ABSORPTION

General Considerations. The gastrointestinal (GI) tract, with its accessory glands, is an organ system with powerful homeostatic capabilities. Diets of widely varying composition and tonicity ordinarily do not upset our internal milieu. There is sufficient reserve in the adult to accomplish almost all absorption of nutrients by the level of the midjejunum. Yet in the neonate, the margin of safety is more narrow. The large energy demands of rapid growth plus the relative diluteness of his milk diet present the infant with a volume load. In addition, his sphincteric and motility control are less mature. The result, in many, is a group of symptoms with which all pediatricians are familiar: regurgitation, distension, air swallowing, flatus, and a wide variation in stool patterns, accompanied all too often by persistent colicky crying. The premature is at even more of a disadvantage. Although able to digest and absorb suitable milk feedings, the small premature is limited by poor sucking and swallowing, a penchant for aspiration, and a small stomach. Initially, he may be able to tolerate only a few milliliters of formula, and thus be forced to endure a period of partial starvation despite minimal caloric reserves.

The intestinal tract of the full-term newborn is about 240 to 300 cm in length. With the exception of pancreatic amylase, the characteristic enzymes and digestive juices are present even in small prematures.[1] Initially sterile, the gut acquires a characteristic flora in the first few days after birth. Amniotic fluid is swallowed during fetal life and contributes to meconium together with intestinal secretions and shed mucosal cells. The newborn, especially the premature, has a relative steatorrhea, excreting 10% to 20% of dietary fat in the stool, compared with a normal of less than 10%. Regional specialization of the intestinal tract is illustrated in Table 42-1, and Figure 42-1 diagrams a typical intestinal unit.

Intestinal motility, gastric acid, and the secretions of the pancreas, bile, and intestinal mucosa wax and wane with the cycle of periodic meals. The complex hormonal mechanisms involved in this coordination are summarized in Table 42-2.[2] In addition, the autonomic nervous system, particularly branches of the vagus nerve, help in the regulation and integration of GI function. Disorders in these regulatory mechanisms, as well as end organ defects, can result in altered digestion and absorption. An example is the hyperacidity and diarrhea resulting in part from decreased secretin and other enteric hor-

Table 42-1. Regional Specialization of the Intestinal Tract.

Mouth

Chewing, moistening, preliminary starch digestion

Stomach

Mixing, liquefaction, formation of acid curd, beginning adjustment of tonicity, preliminary protein digestion, absorption of alcohol, preliminary fat digestion

Duodenum

Chyme rendered isotonic with blood, emulsification of fats, pH raised to neutral, preliminary digestion and absorption of CHO, fat and protein

Jejunum

Final brush border digestion; main absorptive site for CHO, fat and protein; water absorbed passively with nutrients and NaCl; absorption of many vitamins and minerals

Ileum

Na absorbed against gradient; water reabsorption with NaCl; reserve nutrient absorption; absorption of bile salts and vitamin B_{12}; chloride-bicarbonate exchange

Colon

Final salt and water absorption, chloride-bicarbonate exchange, storage prior to evacuation

mones after surgical shortening of the small intestine or bypass of the duodenum.[3]

Motility. The autonomic nervous system plays a prime role in controlling intestinal motility. Reflexes mediated by the vagus nerve stimulate peristalsis throughout the intestinal tract in response to the stimuli involved in feeding. Distension of the stomach triggers contractions of the rectum (gastrocolic reflex). Filling of the rectum initiates motility of both small and large intestine (coloenteric reflex). Although vagotomy causes diarrhea and malabsorption, there is villous atrophy and puddling of barium on x-ray contrast studies.[4] The ganglion cells of the myenteric plexis are evidently necessary for effective peristalsis, and their absence from the lower intestine in Hirschprung's disease results in functional obstruction. Activation of the sympathetic nervous system in general results in decreased intestinal motility.

A number of mechanical and chemical factors are associated with disordered intestinal motility. Partial obstruction, anatomic or functional, may cause stasis and dilation of the proximal segment, and "overflow" diarrhea. Controversy exists over the relative contributions of compromised capillary circulation and bacterial overgrowth to this result. Increased osmotically active material which can-

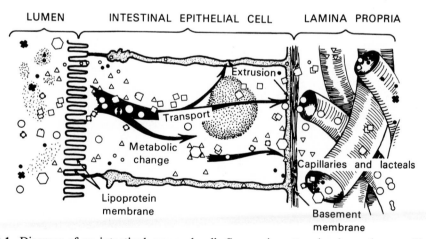

Fig. 42-1. Diagram of an intestinal mucosal cell. Successive steps in absorption are illustrated, including intraluminal digestion, transport across the musocal brush border, metabolic change and transport within the musocal cell, and extrusion into the lamina propria, where food substances are taken up by capillaries and lacteals. (Adapted from Ingelfinger FJ: Nutrition Today, 2:3, 1967)

Table 42-2. Effect of Hormones on the Gastrointestinal System.*

	Gastrin	Chole-cystokinin-pancreozymin	Secretin	Glucagon	Insulin
Number of amino acids	17	33	27	29	51
Source	*Antral Mucosa*	*Mucosa of Upper Intestine*	*Mucosa of Upper Intestine*	*Islets of Langerhans*	*Islets of Langerhans*
Actions					
Stomach					
H+	↑	± ↑	↓	± ↓	↓
Pepsin	± ↑	± ↑	↑	—	?
Motility	↑	↑	↓	↓	↓
Exocrine pancreas					
HCO₃⁻	± ↑	± ↑	↑	↓	?
Enzymes	↑	↑	± ↑	↓	?
Endocrine pancreas					
Insulin	↑	↑	↑	↑	
Glucagon	—	↑		—	
Intestine					
Brunner's gland secretion	↑	↑	↑	↑	?
Motility	↑	↑	↓	↓	?
Gallbladder contraction	± ↑	↑	—	?	?
Hepatic bile HCO₃⁻	± ↑	± ↑	± ↑	± ↑	0

Key: ↑ = increase; ± ↑ = weak increase; — = no effect; ? = unknown; ↓ = decrease; ± ↓ = weak decrease
* (Go VLW, Summerskill WHJ: Am J Clin Nutr 24:160, 1971)[2]

not be absorbed results in rapid intestinal transit. Hypocalcemia may cause increased motility, whereas hypercalcemia or hypokalemia are associated with decreased peristalsis. However, functional obstruction has been observed in some cases of severe tetany. Hyperacidity of the small intestine results in increased motility, perhaps in part through

Table 42-3. Effect of Hormones on Motility.

Increased Motility	Decreased Motility
Gastrin	Secretin
Cholecystokinin-pancreozymin	Glucagon
Thyroid	Adrenal corticosteroids
	Catecholamines (may cause diarrhea by unknown mechanism)
	Parathormone

parasympathetic activation by gastrin. Thyroid, adrenal steroid, catecholamine, parathyroid and gastrointestinal hormones modulate peristalsis, and their disorders may be associated with abnormal motility (Table 42-3).[5]

Clement Smith has summarized x-ray studies of the passage of a barium meal in full-term and premature newborns.[6] In general, the muscular coat of the newborn's intestine is less well developed, rendering him more liable to distension and the puddling of intestinal contents. Contractile activity is more irregular and less predictable in the neonate. Emptying of the stomach is usually nearly complete by 2 hours after a meal, but some residua may be present for as long as 8 hours. Coordination of the peristaltic waves is imperfect, making a "segmentation" pattern not uncommon and leading to confusion with the picture seen in older patients with malabsorption. Compared with the adult, transit is slower in the upper small intestine and more rapid in the ileum and

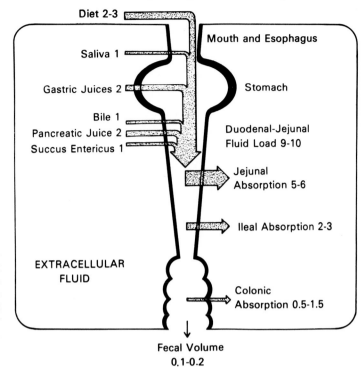

Diet 2-3

Saliva 1

Gastric Juices 2

Bile 1

Pancreatic Juice 2

Succus Entericus 1

Mouth and Esophagus

Stomach

Duodenal-Jejunal
Fluid Load 9-10

Jejunal
Absorption 5-6

Ileal Absorption 2-3

EXTRACELLULAR
FLUID

Colonic
Absorption 0.5-1.5

Fecal Volume
0.1-0.2

Fig. 42-2. Diagram of the adult intestinal tract, illustrating fluid transit at various levels. It will readily be seen that failure of fluid reabsorption in the jejunum, ileum and colon will result in fluid losses from the body greater than total dietary intake. (Adapted from Phillips SF: Hosp Prac 8:138, 1973)

colon. The meal reaches the cecum in 3 to 8 hours, and begins to be evacuated by about 15 hours.

Absorption of Water and Electrolytes. Many similarities have been observed between the function of the intestine and the kidney. In both, a large quantity of fluid is subjected to secretion, differential absorption, and ion exchange, resulting in the final elimination of a vastly reduced volume. In adult man, 10 liters/day are passed through the upper small bowel, comprised of food, drink, saliva, gastric juice, bile, and pancreatic and intestinal secretions. About 1 liter reaches the colon, and only 200 ml comes to the rectum (Fig. 42-2). The infant has a relatively more liquid diet and more rapid water turnover, and hence is especially subject to dehydration should this large fluid volume be lost to the body.

An early step in the process of digestion and absorption is the achieving of isotonicity with blood. In the stomach and upper small intestine, water and sodium chloride diffuse rapidly down osmotic gradients to render the luminal contents isotonic. As absorption proceeds, water is carried back into the blood stream together with osmotically active molecules, notably glucose, amino acids, and electrolytes, which are actively transported across mucosal cells. A sodium pump ejects sodium from the base of mucosal cells into the lamina propria and blood stream, utilizing a specific ATPase. This produces a concentration gradient resulting in sodium reabsorption in the ileum for hypotonic intestinal contents. Potassium is also reabsorbed by active transport, but chloride apparently follows sodium and potassium passively as a consequence of its electronegative charge. In addition to these mechanisms, sodium and chloride are reabsorbed by exchange with hydrogen and bicarbonate ions respectively. Water is absorbed passively along osmotic gradients and there appears to be no such thing as a mucosal "water pump."[7]

Carbohydrate Absorption. Carbohydrate digestion begins with salivary amylase, which acts on polysaccharides, especially starch. In the duodenum, pancreatic amylase is added, with a pH optimum of 5 to 7. Thus, neutralization of strongly acid gastric juice is necessary for optimum carbohydrate digestion. The brush border of the mucosal cells of the small intestine contain four disaccharidases: lactase, sucrase, maltase and isomaltase. These liberate the monosaccharides glucose, galactose, and fructose. Glucose and galactose are actively transported into the mucosal cell, by means of a common energy-dependent kinase which appears to require an adequate intraluminal concentration of sodium. This mechanism is capable of saturation, and shows competitive inhibition between the two sugars. It is specifically inhibited by phlorrhizin. Fructose, on the other hand, is absorbed by facilitated diffusion. The concentration gradient for fructose uptake is maintained by rapid conversion of fructose to glucose in the body. Under ordinary circumstances, most carbohydrate absorption is complete by the level of the midjejunum.

The human newborn is relatively deficient in pancreatic amylase, and this enzyme remains low during the first few months of life. However, lactose is the principle dietary carbohydrate in the milk-fed infant, and is well digested and absorbed by the healthy newborn, including the premature. Unfortunately, lactase is easily diminished by a variety of types of injury to the mucosal brush border, and acquired lactose intolerance is common. The mechanism for glucose absorption is present from the ninth week of gestation, and may be involved in glucose uptake from swallowed amniotic fluid.[1] The presence of bacteria in the duodenum has been associated in infants with diarrhea and carbohydrate intolerance.[8] First lactose intolerance, then generalized disaccharide intolerance, and finally glucose-galactose intolerance were noted with increasing bacterial counts of Klebsiella, *Escherichia coli,* enterococci, and Pseudomonas. Although lactose is the usual dietary sugar for newborns, Andrews and Cook have found no difference in weight gain, distension, or stool patterns whether healthy prematures were fed lactose, glucose, or sucrose.[9]

Protein Absorption. The protein of a milk feeding is coagulated by gastric acid to form a curd. Pepsin and rennin begin digestion in the stomach, and pancreatic proteases are added in the duodenum. These latter have a pH optimum near neutral, and depend for their effectiveness on bicarbonate buffering of the duodenal contents. The pancreatic secretion contains five proenzymes: trypsinogen, chymotrypsinogen, proelastase, and carboxypeptidasogens a and b. Enterokinase from the intestinal mucosa activates trypsin, which in turn activates chymotrypsin, elastase, and the carboxypeptidases. Enterokinase may be rate-limiting for typical activity before 28 weeks gestation.[10] These enzymes are fully capable of protein hydrolysis, but are thought to be quantitatively inadequate without enteric proteases (erepsin) and peptidases (aminopeptidase). The combined effect of these enzymes is to reduce dietary proteins to a mixture of free amino acids and some peptides.

The amino acid mixture in the stomach varies widely with the composition of dietary protein. However, the amino acid composition of the jejunal contents is remarkably constant. Substantial amounts of endogenous protein enters the gut from intestinal secretions, shed mucosal cells, transudates of plasma proteins, and perhaps by diffusion of amino acids from the blood down concentration gradients. It has been estimated that 50% of protein catabolism takes place in this way.[11] The endogenous protein is normally digested and reabsorbed as free amino acids. The buffering effect of this "normal" amino acid mixture may facilitate absorption and may help prevent wide swings in the blood amino acid pattern according to the diet taken. But if, in diarrhea states, this recirculation is prevented, the body experiences protein losses beyond mere fasting.

Transport of amino acids from lumen to blood stream occurs throughout the small intestine but is most prominent in the jejunum. Several mechanisms seem to be involved, but, in general, absorption can occur against a concentration gradient and appears to be energy dependent. The more rapid transfer of L-amino acids compared with their D isomers testifies to the specificity of the process. Several groups of amino acids show competitive inhibition and may share common transport systems. These include the neutral, dibasic, and diacidic groups, and further subgroups probably exist. Radioactive ammonia reaches a maximum in the urine 1 hour after instillation of labeled amino acids into the small intestine. Significant absorption of peptides also occurs, although their metabolic fate is uncertain.[12] In humans, absorption of intact proteins is nutritionally unimportant, but may expose the infant to significant antigens.[1]

Prematures digest and absorb dietary protein comparatively well, and digestive enzymes have been demonstrated in fetuses from midgestation on.[1] Active transport of L-alanine was found in a 10-week fetus. In fact, protein digestion in fetal life may be necessary in order to prevent obstruction of the bowel with inspissated secretions and cellular debris, as apparently occurs in meconium ileus. Postnatal injury to the intestinal mucosa may, however, result in increased absorption of intact protein and antigenic peptides, and be associated with temporary protein intolerance.[13]

Fat Absorption. Fat digestion begins in the stomach under the influence of lingual lipase, a recently described enzyme derived from glands in the tongue with a pH optimum allowing effective activity at gastric pH.[14] This enzyme may be particularly important in the newborn in that it does not depend on bile salts. Further hydrolysis of fats occurs in the duodenum and jejunum under the influence of pancreatic lipase. Bile salts emulsify the fat, rendering it more accessible to lipolysis, and also stabilize the products: free fatty acids (FFA), glycerol, monoglycerides, and some diglycerides. These digestive products are enclosed in a hydrophilic coat of bile salts, forming micelles, and as such are rendered suitable for transport into mucosal cells. The bile salts remain in the lumen and are normally reabsorbed in the ileum and recirculated through the liver. Within the mucosal cell, long-chain (C16–18) fatty acids are resynthesized into triglycerides, enclosed in an envelope of β-lipoprotein, and secreted into the lamina propria, where they enter the blood stream as chylomicrons primarily by way of the lymphatics.

Medium chain triglycerides (C8–10) are handled somewhat differently. Because of their relatively greater water solubility, they are less dependent on bile salts for emulsification and micelle formation. Although readily hydrolysed by pancreatic lipase, there is also direct absorption of medium-chain triglycerides. Within the mucosal cell, resynthesis of triglycerides fails to occur. Rather, medium chain fatty acids are secreted directly into the lamina propria, where they pass to the liver primarily through the portal vein.[15]

Balance studies indicate that the newborn absorbs fat less efficiently than the older child or adult. Pancreatic lipase has been demonstrated in the human fetus by 4 months of gestation.[1] However, it is quantitatively less in prematures than in term infants, and in-

creases during the early weeks of life. Bile salt synthesis and pool size are relatively lower in the newborn when compared to the adult.[16] Human milk fat, having palmitic acid in the 2 position, is better absorbed than butterfat (cow's milk fat). Vegetable fats, notably corn, coconut, and soy oils, are more highly unsaturated and hence better absorbed than butterfat. As a consequence, most commercial formulas are now made with vegetable fats. Foman and coworkers reported fecal excretion of dietary fat in healthy term infants as follows: human milk, 13%; butterfat (cow's milk), 21%; Similac (vegetable), 11.4%; and Prosobee (vegetable), 6.3%.[17] Older estimates suggest that prematures may fail to absorb as much as 30% of cow's milk fat.[18] It seems clear that even small prematures tolerate feedings of human milk or formula, and the relative steatorrhea which they display is not disabling. However, calories may be lost and calcium and fat-soluble vitamins carried out in the stool.

Vitamins. Discussion of the metabolism of individual vitamins, as well as their clinical significance, is found under Specific Nutritional Constituents. In general, the water-soluble vitamins, with the exception of vitamin B_{12}, are readily absorbed, predominantly in the upper small intestine. Storage in the body is more limited than is the case with the fat-soluble group, and excess is excreted in the urine. The fat-soluble vitamins are absorbed in the small intestine, along with other dietary lipids. In general, factors leading to steatorrhea cause malabsorption of fat-soluble vitamins. They are all relatively dependent on bile salts for emulsification, and some utilize additional digestive and absorptive steps in common with neutral fats.[19]

Minerals. The absorption, as well as the metabolism and clinical significance of minerals and trace elements is described under Specific Nutritional Constituents.

Feast-fast Cycle. The ebb and flow of the absorptive tide from the intestinal tract initiates a complex sequence of hormone-modulated biochemical changes resulting in the assimilation and utilization of food substances. The full details of these interactions are not known. Yet it is clear that the metabolic fate of ingested food depends not only on whether it is absorbed, but also on the previous nutritional state of the patient, the combination and balance in which food elements are taken in, the prevailing hormonal and neurohormonal environment, and the activity of several organs, most prominently the liver. Specific adaptive changes occurring in response to starvation are detailed below. Suffice it to say that mere inspection of a bedside intake-output sheet falls far short of explaining whether or not an infant will grow in response to a given allotment of food.

Three hormones, insulin, glucagon, and growth hormone, are the prime regulators of the feast-fast cycle. Insulin is the hormone of energy storage. Under its influence glucose and amino acids are transferred from the plasma into cells. Insulin facilitates glycogen synthesis and blocks glycolysis. Likewise, fat synthesis is aided and plasma FFAs are lowered by insulin's inhibition of hormone-sensitive intracellular lipase while increasing plasma lipoprotein lipase activity. The biologic half-life of insulin is 10 minutes, and falling insulin results almost immediately in a rise in plasma glucose and FFA levels.[20]

Glucagon is, in effect, an antiinsulin, with biologic effects directly opposite to those of insulin. The molar ratio of insulin to glucagon exerts an important effect on the balance between energy storage and energy mobilization: after a carbohydrate meal it is 70:1; after an overnight fast it is 3:1; after a 7-day fast it is less than 1:1.[21] Glucagon increases glycolysis, gluconeogenesis, and probably lipolysis, raising plasma glucose and FFA levels.

Growth hormone has varying effects depending on the availability of calories and accompanying insulin levels. In the presence of calories, amino acids, and high insulin levels, growth hormone facilitates protein synthesis and cell multiplication. In the fasting state, with falling glucose and low insulin levels, growth hormone decreases glucose uptake and stimulates fat mobilization, stabilizing blood glucose and raising plasma FFAs. Growth hormone, like insulin, is labile, with a biologic half-life of 20 to 30 minutes and widely fluctuating levels throughout the day.[22]

Other hormones have important modifying effects on energy metabolism. The catecholamines (epinephrine, norepinephrine) increase glycogenolysis, mobilize FFAs, and inhibit insulin release. Adrenal corticosteroids increase gluconeogenesis, blunt the response to growth hormone, and interfere with cell multiplication. Finally, thyroxine increases respiratory metabolism through action on the flavoenzymes, and appears to be needed for optimal growth hormone effect as well as for normal growth and maturation of the brain and long bones.

Zierlier and Rabinowitz, in a classic study involving serial sampling of the arterial and venous blood perfusing the forearms of adult male volunteers, described the coordination of these metabolic functions after a meal.[23] The essential features of this sequence are detailed in Table 42-4. Phase 1, as absorption begins, is dominated by insulin activity, and is a time of energy storage and movement of nutrients into cells. Phase 2, beginning after about 2 hours, is characterized by the simultaneous availability of insulin, growth hormone, and abundant food elements. This is a time of anabolism and protein synthesis. Phase 3, the postabsorptive phase, demonstrates predominant growth hormone activity with falling insulin. During this time, fat is mobilized and ketones become a major energy fuel, with decreased glucose uptake and stabilized glucose levels.

The general features of the feast-fast cycle are similar in the newborn, but some of the responses are attenuated. Insulin response to a glucose load is more sluggish, although significant levels are reached. Insulin also rises after amino acid loading.[24] Glucose tolerance is somewhat reduced in prematures. Growth hormone responses are normal in newborns after the first few days, and FFAs rise during fasting.[25] There is some evidence for the use of fats (perhaps ketones) for fuel during late fetal life, and the brain may participate in this adaptation.[26] Conceivably, this is why relatively lower blood glucose levels are tolerated by newborns.

The period of relative starvation to which small prematures are frequently subjected gives clinical significance to some of these points. The fasting premature switches rapidly to mobilizing fat for fuel, but has relatively limited fat stores and is prone to metabolic acidosis. The protein-sparing effect of providing basal calories as soon as possible may be particularly important in this situation. It is customary to time oral feedings in prematures primarily around considerations of gastric emptying. However, more study of the effect of very frequent feeding on effective utilization is needed. Clearly, the catecholamine, adrenal

Table 42-4. Metabolic Responses to Assimilation and Starvation.

| | Feast-Fast Cycle | | | Starvation | |
| | Postprandial | | Postabsorptive | | |
	Phase 1 (0–2 hours)	Phase 2 (2–4 hours)	Phase 3 (after 4 hours)	Early (0–7 days)	Late (greater than 7–14 days)
Regulatory hormones	Insulin ↑	Insulin ↑ Growth hormone ↑	Insulin ↓ Growth hormone ↑ ± Catecholamines	Insulin ↓ Growth hormone ↑ ± Catecholamines	Insulin ↓ ↓ Growth hormone ↑ (↓ Basal metabolism)
Carbohydrate	Glucose ↑ Glucose into cells Glycogen synthesis Glucose utilization for energy	Plasma glucose → Glucose uptake →	Stabilized plasma glucose Glucose uptake → Glycogenolysis ↑ Gluconeogenesis ↑	Stabilized plasma glucose Low glucose, utilization (brain, rbc, renal medulla)	Miminal glucose utilization Gluconeogenesis ↓
Fat	FFA ↑ Neutral fats ↑ Intracellular lipase Fat storage in adipose depot	Fat mobilization blocked Plasma FFA→ ↓	↑ Intracellular lipase Plasma FFA and glycerol ↑ Fat mobilization FFA and ketones main energy fuel	Fat mobilization FFA and ketones energy fuel Some use of ketones by brain May have fatty liver	Fat mobilization FFA main muscle fuel Use of ketones by brain ↑
Protein	Plasma amino acids ↑ Transport amino acids into cells	Protein synthesis Nitrogen retention ↓ BUN	Muscle protein breakdown (gluconeogenesis)	Muscle protein breakdown (gluconeogenesis)	Muscle protein breakdown ↓ (↓ gluconeogenesis)

Table 42-5. Body Composition Changes in Starvation.

↓ Cell number (marasmus)
↓ Cell size (kwashiorkor)
↑ Total body water
Hypoproteinemia
Hypomagnesemia
Hypokalemia
Shift of Na and water into cells
Anemia
↓ Fat and muscle mass
Relative increase in visceral cell mass
Variable deficit of Zn^{++}, Cu^{++}, Cr^{+++}
↓ Plasma osmolarity
↓ BUN

cortisteroid, and thyroid responses to stresses, such as chilling, traumatic procedures, and hypoxic episodes, result in a shift toward energy mobilization rather than toward energy storage and growth. Because of the modulation of these latter hormones by the central nervous system, we need to become more aware of the appropriate sensory and psychological environment for these babies. Perhaps psychologically induced marasmus, familiar in the older institutionalized infant, may play more of a role in the poor weight gain of prematures than we realize.

The Biochemistry of Starvation. Some degree of starvation during a time of rapid growth is such a common feature of severe neonatal disease that some attention is given here to the changes accompanying starvation. Certain metabolic adaptations to starvation are illustrated in Table 42-4. Growth hormone is dominant, and fat is mobilized as the main energy source. Glucose is utilized by the brain, red blood cells, and renal medulla, and is supplied primarily by gluconeogenesis from breakdown of muscle protein. The liver synthesizes glucose from lactate and pyruvate returned from the periphery (Cori cycle) and from muscle-derived amino acids, especially alanine. With increased duration of fasting, glucose utilization reaches a minimum and gluconeogenesis decreases. There is adaptation of the brain to the use of ketones (acetoacetate and betahydroxybutyric acid) as fuel.[27] Insulin activity is very low, and insulin response to glucose administration is reduced.[28]

With advanced starvation, profound changes occur in body composition and function. These changes are listed in Tables 42-5 and 42-6. In making up for a significant nutritional deficit, consideration should be given to supplying intracellular ions, especially potassium and magnesium. Caloric allowance should take into consideration the relatively large active cell mass per kg body weight and the large energy requirements of catch-up growth. Relative intolerance to oral feedings is frequent, and diarrhea is a common accompaniment to advanced malnutrition. In addition, temporary deficiencies in renal function, immune competence, and carbohydrate tolerance should be taken into account.

Feeding in Gastrointestinal Development. Oral feeding contributes importantly to the growth and function of the gastrointestinal tract. Widdowsen reported a doubling of intestinal weight in the first 24 hours after birth in piglets suckled by their mother, compared with a decreased weight in controls fed water alone.[33] Heird demonstrated that rats gaining weight on total parenteral nutrition (TPN) exhibited a decrease in intestinal weight and mucosal mass, compared with controls making comparable gains in body weight on oral feedings, whose intestinal mucosal masses increased steadily.[34] Protein/DNA ratios in the mucosa remained constant in the TPN animals, indicating decreased cell number rather than cell size. Activity of brush-border enzymes was preserved per gram of mucosal tissue, but total activity decreased in proportion to the loss of

Table 42-6. Function Changes in Starvation.

↓ Insulin response to glucose
"Diabetic glucose tolerance test
↓ Basal metabolism for ideal weight
↓ Urine flow and osmolarity
↓ Glomerular filtration rate[29]
↓ Tubular function[29]
    Amino aciduria
    Phosphaturia
    ↓ Concentration ability
    Poor excretion of acid load
↓ Immunocompetence[30]
↓ Pancreatic enzymes[31]
↓ Intestinal brush border enzymes
    Delayed regeneration of intestinal lining layer[32]
↓ Wound healing

mucosal mass. Williamson has suggested that mucosal cell proliferation and renewal are reduced, despite adequate systemic nutrition, in the absence of enteric feedings, indicating a direct topical nutritional effect of food on the intestinal lining, which is lacking in TPN.[35] This would be compatible with the observed cephalocaudal gradient of mucosal height, as well as the adaptation of the remaining bowel after partial enterectomy. Enteric stimulation and the hormones secretin and cholecytokinin-pancreatozymin, released by feeding, are important in supporting adequate pancreatic secretion.[36]

The atrophy of the intestinal mucosa, which results from disuse even in the presence of adequate general nutrition, helps to explain the distension, vomiting, diarrhea, and malabsorption noted on refeeding infants who have had prolonged parenteral nutrition. These effects are even more marked when a degree of malnutrition is superimposed. Gradual introduction of feedings of dilute concentration, starting with small volumes, allows for buildup of mucosal bulk, brush-border enzymes, and pancreatic function, before full feedings are reintroduced.

SPECIFIC NUTRITIONAL CONSTITUENTS (SIGNIFICANCE, REQUIREMENTS, DEFICIENCY STATES)

Calories

Underprovision of calories causes tissue breakdown and diverts all food substances into energy production. Thus, it makes no sense to give proteins in expectation of tissue growth when less than basal calories are supplied. Conversely, the provision of even basal calories has a beneficial protein-sparing action in arresting the body's catabolism.

It is particularly important to supply an optimal caloric intake in the newborn period. The minimal fat deposits of the small premature are rapidly exhausted and advanced starvation may occur within a week. A growing literature suggests that severe malnutrition in early infancy, when brain cell multiplication is rapidly approaching completion, may result in a lasting reduction in brain size, cell number, and perhaps intellectual performance.[37,38] (See also Chap. 39.) The contribution of malnutrition to the neurologic sequelae seen in small prematures cannot be accurately evaluated at

this time. On the other hand, overnutrition in infancy may predispose to adult obesity.[39] The juvenile-onset obese (50% of adult obese) have normal birth weights but are significantly overweight by 1 year of age and have an increase in fat cell number which apparently is lifelong.[40]

It is difficult to settle on an ideal caloric allowance for the newborn because of the many variables involved, including the following: fever, cold stress, activity (motility, cardiac, respiratory, muscle tone) cachexia, catch-up growth, and systemic illness. Rose and Mayer, in a study of 4- to 6-month-old infants, reported their 105 cal/kg/day to be apportioned as follows: basal, 57; lost in excreta, 9; specific dynamic action of food, 5; growth, 7; and activity, 29.[41] They found that activity introduced great variability among babies. In the first few days after birth, oxygen consumption was found to rise from 4.8 cc/kg/minute at 2 hours to 6.6 cc/kg/minute at 24 hours, to 7.0 cc/kg/minute at 10 days.[42] However, after the first week of life, basal calories are approximately 50 to 55 cal/kg/day. The figure of 120 cal/kg/day provides a rough rule of thumb that is sufficient for growth in most term newborns and prematures. The factors listed above all tend to increase caloric demand, and some babies will fail to gain on 120 cal/kg/day. Montgomery has shown that basal calories must be exceeded by 60 to 85 cal/kg/day to achieve catch-up growth in a cachexic infant, and requirements may range as high as 160 to 185 cal/kg/day.[43]

Protein

Protein is the basic ingredient of protoplasm, and all net growth depends on an exogenous supply of protein or its constituent amino acids. Kwashiorkor, a state of malnutrition in which protein deficiency predominates, is characterized by edema, growth failure, listlessness, abdominal distension, hypoproteinemia, diarrhea, and skin and hair changes. The body has considerable ability to interconvert amino acids, but nine are considered essential: arginine, lysine, leucine, isoleucine, valine, methionine, phenylalanine, threoine, and tryptophan. In addition, the newborn has a temporary specific requirement for histidine and cystine, and may for a time be unable to convert phenylalanine to tyrosine and methionine to cystine.

Evidence in certain animal species indicates that taurine plays a role in brain and retinal development. A specific deficiency state in humans has not been identified. However, commercial formulas contain less taurine than human milk, and usual parenteral nutrition solutions contain almost none. Low-birth-weight infants on TPN or formula feedings were shown to have lower serum taurine values than others fed human milk in one recent study.[44] Whether these differences are clinically significant remains to be seen.

Protein synthesis is going on with particular rapidity in late fetal and early postnatal life. The data of Fomon and Widdowson indicate that the body increases in protein content from 9.0% at 28 weeks' gestation to 11.4% at term, to 17.5% at 1 year of age.[45,46] Plasma proteins average 1 g/dl lower in term newborns than in adults, and 2 g/dl lower in prematures.

Both human and cow's milk provide protein of good biologic efficiency in terms of favorable amino acid content. Soy protein is relatively deficient in methionine, and certain soy preparations failed to support sustained growth until this problem was realized and methionine supplementation became routine. Breast milk is relatively richer in cystine and cow's milk in methionine. Human milk is lower in electrolytes because of its lower protein content, and Mayer has suggested that the decreased sodium intake may lower the incidence of adult hypertension.[47] Otherwise, formulas have been devised which support adequate growth in infancy based on protein derived from goat's milk, beef, lamb, and casein hydrolysate, as well as soybean and human and cow's milk. Bessman has postulated that a critical internal milieu with respect to amino acid pools is necessary to prevent injury to the developing brain, and that marginal defects in achieving this type of homeostasis may account for some "nonspecific" mental retardation.[48] Much more must certainly be learned about amino acid metabolism in the newborn before we can with impunity attempt feeding with exotic mixtures.

For years, there has been controversy over what protein intake is optimal for prematures. Davidson and coworkers reported most rapid growth of low-birth-weight babies fed 3 to 6 g/kg/day, with decreased gain on 2 g/kg/day and some azotemia on 6 g/kg/day.[49] Kagan, and coworkers found that much of the in-creased weight on high-protein intakes was salt and water retention, and recommended 2.5 to 4.0 g/kg/day of protein.[50] Synderman and coworkers reported different patterns of plasma amino acids in low-birth-weight babies fed 2 versus 9 g/kg/day of protein: the high-protein group showed decreased glycine and increased proline, tyrosine, phenylalanine, methionine, leucine, isolecucine, and valine; whereas the low-protein group had decreased lysine and increased glycine.[51] The results of Goldman and coworkers suggest that excessive protein intake in early infancy may be injurious to the developing nervous system.[52] In a 3-year follow-up study of low-birth-weight infants fed high- and low-protein formulas, an excess of strabismus and mental deficiency was found in the lowest birth-weight groups after high-protein intakes. Unfortunately, virtually all these studies are marred by the use of weight criteria alone, and contain an admixture of true prematures and small-for-dates babies whose protein requirements and tolerances may be quite different.

Räihä and coworkers[53] have reported adequate growth of small prematures fed pooled human milk at 170 ml/kg/day. This amounts to a protein intake of only 1.7 gm/kg/day. However, plasma proteins declined progressively in the study group. Davies reports suboptimal growth of prematures fed human milk for the first month of life.[54] The suitability of human milk to be the sole nutrition of small prematures and the lowest protein intake which will support optimal growth are still in contention.

Until further data are available, it seems reasonable to recommend a relatively modest protein allowance: 3 g/kg/day at birth, 2.2 at 6 months, and 1.6 at 1 year, amounting to about 9% of the total caloric intake.

Carbohydrate. Carbohydrate is one of the body's main energy fuels. Glucose is apparently essential to brain metabolism and normally is oxidized in the periphery to form high-energy phosphates. Thus, there is an **internal** requirement for glucose at all times. Yet there is no specific **dietary** requirement for carbohydrate because glucose can be manufactured in the body from proteins and fats (as well as from many other carbohydrates). Enzymes for these conversions are present in the newborn, and indeed it is possible to concoct a carbohydrate-free diet which will support growth in infancy.[55]

On the other hand, an appropriate intake of carbohydrate is highly desirable. Carbohydrate-free feedings must necessarily have high protein and fat contents, and at the least are very unpalatable. Excess protein may lead to azotemia and acidosis, and excess fat can be associated with ketoacidosis. Too much carbohydrate, however, may cause loose stools, and if supplied as lactose, may exceed the limited capacity of intestinal lactase and result in fermentative diarrhea. The provision of 35% to 50% of calories as carbohydrate seems to be an appropriate compromise and minimizes these difficulties.

Fat. Dietary fat, like carbohydrate, is a major source of energy for biologic reactions. Its inclusion in the diet results in greater palatability and supplies a high density of calories with minimal osmolarity and minimal renal solute load. The biologic oxidation of fat results in 9 (as opposed to 4) cal/g and does not yield nitrogenous wastes or inorganic acids, as does protein. Neither does unabsorbed fat provoke acid diarrhea, as is the case with carbohydrate. Thus, the inclusion of fat in the diet provides what might be called "logistical" advantages. On the other hand, energy needs can be met from other sources, and sustained growth is possible on a fat-free diet provided that essential fatty acid requirements are met. Lipids are part of vital cell structures and neutral fat depots represent the body's main energy stores, but these lipids can be synthesized in the body. Yet some authors challenge the notion that dietary fat is only needed as an energy source and for essential fatty acid supply. Hahn has documented active ketone production by the liver in newborns and postulates ketone-utilization as an important mechanism in the newborn's unexplained resistance to hypoglycemia.[56] He cites evidence in rats that aborting this early ketone utilization by high-carbohydrate feeding was associated with decreased learning in the adult rats. Further work is needed before we can be certain whether provision of 40% to 50% of calories as fat is necessary or merely a convenience.

Two unsaturated fatty acids, linoleic acid and arachidonic acid, must be included in the diet of animals for normal health, and they have been called essential fatty acids. Infants develop poor growth and skin lesions on inadequate linoleic acid intake. Greenberg and Wheeler have suggested that provision of 1.8% of the total calories as linoleic acid satisfies requirements for good health.[57] All diets which they examined appeared to be adequate to maintain plasma arachidonic acid levels. The linoleic acid content of fats varies widely. Fomon lists the percent of linoleic acid in dietary fats as follows: human milk, 8%; cow's milk, 4%; corn oil, 53%; peanut oil, 26%; soybean oil, 51%; and safflower seed oil, 77%.[58] When medium-chain triglycerides are the only source of fatty acids, deficiency of essential fatty acids may potentially develop.

Fatty acid streaking of the arteries begins in infancy, and the question has been raised whether dietary management in early life has any bearing on the ultimate development of coronary artery disease. Cholesterol levels have been reported to be lower in breast milk than in cow's milk.[57] In theory, highly saturated fats such as butterfat should be less desirable than human milk fat, and corn oil should be even better. Unfortunately, tedious and extremely long-term investigations are required to tell whether there is any clinical benefit in adult life to be derived from this sort of nutritional manipulation in infancy.

Vitamins. Vitamin deficiency in infancy is rare for the healthy, term, milk-fed baby without malabsorption. Prematures appear to be somewhat more susceptible to lack of ascorbic acid, folacin, and vitamin E. Vitamin D is inadequate in unfortified milk, and the addition of 400 IU/liter has become standard in both whole milk and prepared infant formulas. Vitamin A may be marginal in the presence of steatorrhea or when skim milk preparations are given. The widespread use of prepared formulas supplemented with multiple vitamins, and the practice of giving preparations containing vitamins A, D, and C to breast-fed infants, have made deficiencies uncommon in this country.

In contrast, developing countries may have infantile malnutrition complicated by severe vitamin lack. Preexisting maternal depletion with reduced neonatal endowment, an early switch from breast milk to carbohydrate gruel, lack of appropriate vitamin supplementation, and intestinal parasites all contribute to this result. Yet even in our own intensive care nurseries, some instances of unexplained growth failure or bizarre symptomatology may be caused by unrecognized deficiency states.

Table 42-7. Vitamin Allowances for the Newborn.

Nutrient	Recommended Daily Intake	Content/liter of milk	
		Cow	*Human*
Vitamin D	400 IU	14 IU	22 IU
Vitamin A	420 μg RE	1025 IU (341 μg RE)	1898 IU (640 μg RE)
Vitamin K	12 μg	60 μg	15 μg
Vitamin E	3 mg TE	0.4 mg	1.8 mg
Ascorbic acid	35 mg	11 mg	43 mg
Thiamin	0.3 mg	440 μg	160 μg
Riboflavin	400 μg	1750 μg	360
Niacin	6 mg NE	(9.2 mg NE)	(18. mg NE)
Pyridoxine	300 μg	640 μg	0 μg
Pantothenic acid	2 mg	3.46 mg	100 mg
Folacin	30 μg	55 μg	1.84 μg
Vitamin B$_{12}$	0.5 μg	4 μg	52 μg
Biotin (μg)	35 μg		0.3

* RE = retinol equivalents
  TE = tocopherol equivalents
  NE = niacin equivalents
(Data of Fomon, Mitchell, and coworkers; RDA)[19,59,60]

The infant with prolonged diarrhea or malabsorption, the child with intestinal or biliary disease, the baby on prolonged synthetic or intravenous feedings, and the very small premature deserve attention in this respect.

Suggested daily vitamin intakes for newborn infants are presented in Table 42-7, together with the vitamin content of unsupplemented human and cow's milk. It should be recognized that these recommended intakes are crude estimates, generally two or three times the minimal daily requirements needed to prevent obvious symptoms. In addition to the imprecision of these estimates, intestinal absorption is inconstant and the vitamin content of natural foods including milk may have considerable variation. Information on the vitamin content of strained baby foods and table foods can found in Fomon's excellent monograph.[61]

Vitamin D is emulsified by bile salts and absorbed in the small intestine, whence it is transported in the lymph as chylomicrons. There is considerable storage in liver, as well as in skin, brain, and bones. Because of initial neonatal stores, rickets is rare in the immediate newborn period. Inactive precursors can be converted into vitamin D in the skin to response to sunlight. Further activitation of 1,25-dihydroxy vitamin D$_3$ occurs in the liver and kidney. Disease of these organs can therefore create a functional vitamin D efficiency. Complex and elegant feedback loops regulate the level of ionized calcium and phosphorus (see Chap. 27). Vitamin D increases intestinal absorption of calcium and phosphorus, renal phosphorus reabsorption, and facilitates both bone mineralization and calcium reabsorption from bone. Deficiency results in clinical tetany or rickets. Excess causes hypercalcemia, anorexia, constipation, and azotemia.

Vitamin A is partly emulsified by bile salts and absorbed directly, and partly hydrolysed by lipase and then reesterified to retinal palmitate in the mucosal cell. Absorption is reduced in the absence of adequate fat. About one-sixth of dietary carotene is converted into active vitamin A, which is stored in the liver and in fat. Vitamin A is a precursor of the photosensitive pigments rhodopsin and iodopsin, and is involved in the synthesis of mucopolysaccharides, the differentiation of mucous membranes, the maintenance of the adrenal cortex, the remodeling of bone, and may play a role in reproduction. Deficiency causes xerophthalmia, poor growth, apathy, mental retardation, keratinization of mucous membranes and night blindness. Excess results in increased intracranial pressure, dry skin, loss of hair, brittle bones, and irritability.

Vitamin K requires emulsification by bile

salts, and absorption is impeded by interfering substances, such as mineral oil, and by prolonged antibiotic therapy. Stores in the liver are relatively modest, and maternal deficiency coupled with the initial absence of intestinal flora predispose to neonatal deficiency of vitamin K, inasmuch as gut bacteria are a substantial source of the vitamin. Several related molecules of the naphthoquinone family have vitamin K activity, although water-soluble preparations of vitamin K_1 are usually selected for therapy. Vitamin K is necessary for manufacture by the liver of several clotting factors, including prothrombin and Factor VII. Deficiency results in hemorrhagic disease of the newborn, and excess may cause hemolytic anemia and interferes with albumin binding of bilirubin.

Vitamin E is poorly absorbed by prematures of less than 32-weeks' gestation, and low levels have been noted despite adequate intake.[62] Furthermore, iron supplementation may interfere with both vitamin E absorption and activity, the latter effect through generation of free radicals which enhance peroxidation of unsaturated fats.[63] Diets high in polyunsaturated fats, such as are commonly given to prematures, increase the vitamin E requirement. Placental transfer of vitamin E is poor, and liver stores may be small. The principle role of vitamin E is to retard oxidation of unsaturated fats, which in turn contributes to the stability of cell membranes. A parallel antioxidant system is provided by glutathione peroxidase, with selenium as a cofactor.[64] The two systems appear to be independent but additive in their protective effects. Thus, peroxidation of fat would be most likely in a premature of less than 32-weeks' gestation, receiving iron but not vitamin E supplementation, who was also fed a diet high in polyunsaturated fats and was selenium deficient. Clinical entities reported to be ameliorated by vitamin E therapy in the premature include hemolytic anemia,[63] retrolental fibroplasia,[65] and bronchopulmonary dysplasia.[66] Several investigators have confirmed the occurrence of lower hemoglobins in vitamin E-deficient prematures. Whether additional studies will support the protection against retrolental fibroplasia and bronchopulmonary dysplasia imparted by parenteral vitamin E prophylaxis is uncertain. In the meantime, it seems prudent to begin vitamin E supplementation soon after birth in the small premature and to continue until a postconception age of 36 to 40 weeks (see below).

Vitamin C (ascorbic acid) is water soluble and is readily absorbed in the upper small intestine. There are no large body stores, and excess is excreted in the urine. Cord levels reflect maternal intake, and deficiency may occur in the immediate newborn period, although symptoms of scurvy are rare before 3 to 4 months of age. The vitamin C content of unfortified cow's milk is marginal, and the vitamin is susceptible to being destroyed by heat during processing. Ascorbic acid participates in many steps in amino acid metabolism, including the hydroxylation of phenylalanine, proline and lysine, the conversion of folic to folinic acid, the synthesis of collagen, and the vitamin is also thought to play a role in the adrenal response to stress. Transient tyrosinemia, which disappears promptly on vitamin C administration, has been reported in prematures immediately after birth, and scurvy in later infancy is not uncommon in unsupplemented milk-fed babies.

Vitamins of the **B-complex** are water soluble and are particularly abundant in yeast. With the exception of vitamin B_{12}, they are all readily absorbed in the upper small intestine. Vitamin B_{12} is absorbed by a specific mechanism involving a carrier molecule, intrinsic factor, and specific binding sites in the ileum where calcium-dependent mucosal cell uptake occurs. Body stores of the B-complex vitamins are minimal, and excess quantities are excreted in the urine. Hence toxic symptoms of overdosage are essentially unknown. Deficiencies in early infancy are rare, the most frequent being folic acid depletion in the premature. Severe deficiencies may occur in later infancy, often associated with advanced general malnutrition. This is seen most commonly in populations where gruel derived from polished rice is substituted for milk after the first few weeks of life.

B-complex vitamins function as coenzymes in many metabolic pathways. **Thiamine** participates in 24 enzyme systems including acetyl CoA, and plays a particularly important role in carbohydrate metabolism. Symptoms of deficiency include anorexia, irritability, fatigue, constipation, and peripheral neuropathy. **Riboflavin** is a component of the flavoenzymes including those active in electron transfer in the Krebs cycle. Deficiency symptoms include cheilosis and photophobia. **Niacin,** the antipellagra vitamin, is part of the NAD–NADP system of the Krebs cycle, and participates in protein and fat synthesis. Dietary tryptophan can substitute for all or part of the niacin requirement, with 60 mg of tryptophan equivalent to 1 mg of niacin. Diarrhea, dermatitis, and central nervous symptoms result from niacin lack. **Pyridoxine** (B_6) is active in transamination, decarboxylation, and desulfation and is needed for protein synthesis. Irritability and convulsions have been reported in infants after accidental pyridoxine destruction during formula processing, and additional deficiency symptoms include weakness, dermatitis, and anemia. **Vitamin B_{12}** is a coenzyme in DNA synthesis, folic acid metabolism, and in the conversion of methylmalonic to succinic acid. Lack of the vitamin causes pernicious anemia and central nervous system damage. **Folacin** (folic acid) is part of five enzyme systems which accomplish 1-carbon transfers in DNA, RNA, methionine, and serine synthesis, and is necessary for histidine utilization. Significant amounts of folacin are supplied by gut bacteria, and hence deficiency is usually associated with malabsorptive states. Folic acid depletion causes megaloblastic anemia, gastrointestinal disturbances, and glossitis. **Pantothenic acid** is part of the coenzyme A system, and participates in energy metabolism as well as in the synthesis of protein, carbohydrate, fat, and porphyrins. Deficiency causes emaciation and loss of hair. **Biotin** is needed for fatty acid synthesis, and may be absorbed from intestinal flora as well as dietary intake. Biotin lack has not been documented in infants, but in adults causes anorexia, malaise, and anemia.

Minerals and Trace Elements

Calcium is absorbed by active transport in the upper small intestine. A calcium-magnesium-dependent ATPase facilitates entry into the mucosal cell, where it is attached to a special calcium-binding protein induced in response to vitamin D.[67] Between 20% and 60% of dietary calcium is absorbed, depending on a variety of factors. Vitamin D, parathormone, and perhaps growth hormone increase calcium uptake.[68] On the other hand, various dietary constituents reduce calcium absorption by forming insoluble complexes in the gut lumen,

notably excess phosphates, fats, phytates, and oxylates. Tsang and coworkers have stated that hypomagnesemia causes refractory hypocalcemia through decreased parathormone production, reduced end organ sensitivity to parathormone, decreased intestinal calcium absorption, and decreased calcium-magnesium exchange at bone surface with consequent reduced calcium release.[69] In the plasma, calcium is partly free and partly bound to protein. The bones represent a large calcium depot, and are the only major site of storage. In addition to bone mineralization, calcium is essential for blood clotting, helps regulate cell membrane permeability, and exerts control over neuromuscular excitability. Deficiency results in tetany and bone demineralization, and excess causes cardiac arrhythmias, paralytic ileus, and ectopic calcifications. Decreased calcium stores, "physiologic" hypoparathyroidism, reduced kidney tubular function, and rapid growth render the premature particularly liable to low calcium states, (see Chap. 27.)

Phosphorus is relatively better absorbed than calcium, about 70% of dietary phosphorus being taken up. Phosphate absorption is increased by vitamin D, which also increases renal phosphate reabsorption. As with calcium, formation of insoluble complexes in the gut lumen may reduce uptake. Phosphate is widely distributed in the body, forming part of the bone mineral as well as being a ubiquitous intracellular anion with important buffering properties. Phosphorus is part of ATP, DNA, RNA, phospholipids, and many other biologically active compunds. Relatively elevated values of plasma phosphorus are normally seen in the first few weeks of life. Clinical rickets is rare in the immediate newborn period, perhaps because of adequate stores of vitamin D and minerals acquired transplacentally. However, a phosphate deficiency state can occur, characterized by listlessness, poor feeding, rapid shallow breathing, muscle weakness, and impaired oxygen release from hemoglobin. This condition is most common in infants on TPN with inadequate phosphorus intake, but also can result from shifts of phosphorus into bone, muscle, and adipose tissue with surges of carbohydrate metabolism resulting from hypertonic glucose administration.

Magnesium and strontium appear to share

some transport mechanisms with calcium, and in general the uptake of these three ions is parallel. Some investigators believe that magnesium absorption at the brush border depends on a common energy-dependent ATPase, although there is disagreement as to whether transport of calcium and magnesium is competitive. The close interdependence of calcium and magnesium metabolism has already been alluded to. Magnesium absorption is increased by vitamin D, parathormone, and probably growth hormone, and is decreased by steatorrhea and dietary phytates. There is significant magnesium deposited in bone mineral, but it is also a prominent intracellular cation which is a cofactor in carbohydrate, protein, and energy metabolism and is necessary for muscle contraction. An early postnatal drop from high fetal values of serum magnesium is commonly observed, and is most prominent in prematures. Magnesium deficiency is associated with weakness, poor feeding, failure to thrive, paralytic ileus, and calcium-resistant tetany.

The electrolytes **sodium, potassium,** and **chloride** share certain features in common. They are readily absorbed from the gastrointestinal tract (see above), are found in water-soluble ionic form in body fluids, and are excreted by the kidney. Sodium and chloride are mainly extracellular and potassium is mainly intracellular, active membrane work being required to maintain this differentiation. Besides providing the ionic milieux in which biologic reactions take place, these ions help to regulate polarization of cell membranes. Values in the newborn period are similar to those in later life, except that serum sodium may be lower and potassium temporarily higher in prematures. The premature below 1250 g is a partial renal salt lose because of immature tubular function. Temporarily, an intake of 4 mmol of sodium per day or more may be required to avoid hyponatremia.

Iron is absorbed by a specific mechanism in the upper small intestine. The proportion of ingested iron which is taken up varies from 5% to 35%, the principal determinant being the degree of saturation of the body with iron. The mucosal cell is a significant storage area for iron, and when replete with iron it effectively shuts off further absorption. The mucosal depot, in turn, is in equilibrium with other body stores such as the liver, spleen, and bone marrow by way of transferrin, a carrier protein in blood. Ferrous iron is better absorbed than ferric, and gastric acidity and reducing agents such as ascorbic acid and vitamin E increase absorption by maintaining iron in the ferrous form. On the other hand, phytates, and certain sulfur-containing compounds form insoluble complexes with iron, trapping it in the gut lumen. Compared with term infants, prematures absorb iron relatively well, perhaps because their stores are less and become more rapidly depleted. Prematures have been reported to take up 32% of the iron in fortified milk. Unsupplemented human and cow's milk contain insufficient iron for growing infants not receiving iron from other sources. Neonatal iron stores, particularly the high initial hemoglobin mass, usually protect against deficiency until 4 to 6 months of age. However, prematurity with rapid dilution by growth, fetal or neonatal hemorrhage, or excess blood sampling may cause earlier iron depletion. Hypochromic, microcytic anemia is the most prominent symptom of iron deficiency, but poor feeding, irritability and listlessness have also been noted. Iron is an integral part of the hemoglobin molecule, as well as muscle myoglobin and the cytochrome enzymes crucial to oxidative metabolism. The relative frequency of iron deficiency in later infancy has led the Committee on Nutrition of the Academy of Pediatrics to recommend routine iron supplementation, beginning at 2 months in prematures and 4 months in term babies.[70,71] The recommended dosage is 1 mg/kg/day for term and 2 mg/kg/day for prematures, up to a maximum of 15 mg/day. The need for iron supplementation in breast-fed infants is controversial because iron content of human milk is low but absorption is good and intestinal blood loss minimal.

Iodine is readily absorbed and transported in the blood as water-soluble iodine. It is concentrated in the thyroid gland, where it becomes a component of the hormones thyroxine and triiodothyronine, and excess is excreted in the urine. Milk of cows or humans may be iodine-deficient in endemic goiter areas where soil is poor in iodine. In addition, soybean formulas may have a low concentration and are customarily fortified with iodine.

Zinc has recently been shown to be a vital trace element in human nutrition.[72] It is part of numerous metalloenzymes including LDH, alkaline phosphatase, carboxypepidase, and carbonic anhydrase. In addition, it is a cofactor of insulin and plays a role in protein synthesis. About one-third of dietary zinc is absorbed by active transport in the distal small intestine. It is interesting to note that iron saturation seems to have a regulatory effect on zinc uptake. Animal zinc is more available than that in plant products because of the formation of insoluble complexes by the latter. It is carried in the blood bound to α_1-globulins, and excretion is through the pancreatic and gastrointestinal secretions. Body stores are apparently limited. Zinc deficiency causes growth failure, retarded bone age, decreased wound healing, hepatosplenomegaly, decreased growth hormone, and adrenal cortical responses, and in older individuals, sexual infantilism. Although zinc levels in cord blood are similar to adult values, they rapidly fall in the first weeks of life, and reach a minimum at 2 to 3 months, rising again by 6 months of age.[73] Both human milk and commercial formulas provide marginal zinc supplies, and parenteral nutrition is often zinc free. Daucey and coworkers report negative zinc balances for the first 60 days of life in preterm infants less than 1500 g fed pooled human milk.[74] Michie and Wirth showed falling zinc levels in infants on TPN.[75] Clinical experience of brisk growth responses after zinc therapy in such infants suggests that monitoring of zinc levels and zinc supplementation in high-risk populations such as prematures and infants on prolonged parenteral nutrition are desirable. Plasma zinc levels below 50 μg/dl might be considered low for newborns until better standards can be developed.

Copper is a component of cytochrome oxidase, tyrosinase, and uricase. In addition, it is necessary for iron utilization in hemoglobin synthesis and participates in nerve myelination and in collagen and elastin formation. Deficiency results in anemia, leukopenia, and brittle bones. Dietary copper is absorbed in the stomach and proximal small intestine by an unknown mechanism. It is transported loosely bound to albumin and stored in liver and muscle, relatively tightly attached to ceruloplasmin. Excretion is through the bile. Newborns ordinarily have good copper stores at birth, but milk is a relatively poor source of the metal. Low serum copper values after birth rise to adult levels by 6 months.[73] Deficiencies have been reported in malabsorptive states such as cystic fibrosis, protein-losing enteropathy, celiac disease, and kwashiorkor.

Manganese is found in mitochondria and apparently participates in carbohydrate metabolism. It is absorbed by an active process in the duodenum, transported bound to a specific β_1-globulin, transmanganin, and excreted in the bile. In animals, deficiency causes growth retardation, bony defects, and abnormal fat metabolism. **Chromium** potentiates the action of insulin in causing glucose uptake into cells. Dietary chromium is poorly absorbed (0.5%–3.0%). In the blood, it is carried by transferrin. Body stores are small, and excretion is through the urine. Diabetic glucose tolerance tests in Jordanian infants with kwashiorkor were corrected by chromium supplementation.[76] **Fluoride** enters the mineral of bones and teeth, resulting in increased hardness. Excess causes mottling of the teeth. Many communities have supplemented fluoride intake by adding 1 part per million to the drinking water. An intake of approximately 1 mg/day is thought to reduce dental caries with minimal danger of fluorosis, including both dietary and drinking water fluoride. Nevertheless, the current recommendation is for no added medicinal fluoride in the first 6 months of life, followed by 0.25 mg/day in breast-fed infants, and in formula-fed infants up to 18 months in areas with drinking water fluoride under 0.2 parts per million.[77] **Molybdenum** is a component of xanthine oxidase, and deficiency causes growth failure and xanthine calculi in chickens. Dietary molybdenum is readily absorbed, and excess is excreted in the urine. There appears to be active placental transfer with cord values higher than maternal. **Selenium** is thought to function as a biologic antioxidant and is a cofactor with 24-glutathione peroxidase. Its deficiency has been associated with liver necrosis in animals. Infants with kwashiorkor in Jamaica and Jordan showed weight gain and reticulocyte responses when given supplemental selenium.[71] It is unclear whether there is a human need for dietary **cobalt** other than as a component of vitamin B_{12}. Because the vitamin cannot be synthesized and must be ingested intact, need for separate cobalt intake may not exist. The body contains trace amounts of aluminum, arsenic, boron, cadmium, and silicon, but biologic roles for these elements have not been defined (see Table 42-8.)

Table 42-8. Minerals and Trace Elements.

Nutrient	Recommended Daily Intake	Content/Liter of Milk	
		Cow	*Human*
Calcium	360.0 mg	1,250.0 mg	340.0 mg
Phosphorus	240.0 mg	960.0 mg	140.0 mg
Sodium	8.0 mmol (184 mg)	25.0 mmol	7.0 mmol
Potassium	8.0 mmol (320 mg)	35.0 mmol	13.0 mmol
Chloride	8.0 mmol (280 mg)	29.0 mmol	11.0 mmol
Iron	10.0 mg	1.0 mg	0.3 mg
Iodine	35.0 μg	47.0 μg	30.0 μg
Magnesium	60.0 mg	120.0 mg	40.0 mg
Zinc	3.0 mg	3.8 mg	1.2 mg
Copper	0.3 mg	0.03 mg	0.03 mg
Manganese	0.8 mg		
Fluoride	0.5 mg		
Chromium	trace		
Cobalt	trace		
Molybdenum	trace		
Selenium	trace		

(Data of Fomon, Mitchell et al; RDA)[19,59,60]

FEEDING THE TERM AND PRETERM INFANT
Feeding the Full-term Infant

Scheduling of Feedings. Because some 2000 feedings occur in the first year of life, it is best that they bring enjoyment to both mother and infant. In general, in the first few days of life, full-term healthy infants will feed at more frequent intervals until the sucking-swallow mechanism is well developed. Thereafter, they usually settle down to a schedule of every 3 to 4 hours with sleep occurring about 60% of the time. To wake an infant for feeding when he is sleepy and will only take small amounts is unnecessary and creates tension for all concerned. Exceptions include the baby who is hypotonic with a poor suck and weak cry, who may require scheduled feedings with careful calculations of intake to insure growth. This latter approach will often alleviate guilt feelings in the parents of a nonthriving baby. Breast-fed infants may feed more frequently, often every 2 to 3 hours. Intake is usually unknown and need only be calculated by weighing before and after feedings when the infant does not thrive. More frequent feedings than every 2 hours should be discouraged.

Where obesity of the infant is seen, the diet should be calculated and restricted in caloric intake. Low caloric-density foods can be sub-stituted (*i.e.,* vegetables substituted for fruits or dinners in place of pure meats). Skim milks should not be used in the first year of life.

As the infant gets older, the number of feedings decrease, so that by 6 months the number of meals should approach 3 to 4 daily.

Breast versus Bottle Feeding. All healthy women should be encouraged, but not forced, to breast feed their full-term infants. No artificial formula has yet been able to fully mimic human milk, whose superiority remains (Table 42-9). With the advent of modified cow's milk formula and sterilization processes, the necessity to breast feed for survival is no longer applicable. This necessity, however, still remains with less-privileged cultures.

The advantages of breast feeding are many. Human milk is always at the correct temperature and requires no sterilization. The protein content is low, but of high quality, gives a small curd, and is easily digestible. The fats are well absorbed. The carbohydrate is relatively high in percentage of lactose but seems to give very few problems. Breast milk imparts a gram-positive intestinal flora, which may play some part in the decreased incidence of diarrhea seen in these infants. Antibodies passed by way of the milk to the infant may help to prevent respiratory infection. The psy-

Table 42-9. Composition of Mature Breast Milk, Cow's Milk, and a Routine Infant Formula.*

Composition/dl	Mature Breast Milk	Cow's Milk	Routine Formula with Iron†
Calories	75.0	69.0	67.0
Protein, g[78]	1.1	3.5	1.5
Lactalbumin %	80	18	
Casein %	20	82	
Water, ml	87.1	87.3	
Fat, g	4.0	3.5	3.7
CHO, g	9.5	4.9	7.0
Ash, g	0.21	0.72	0.34
Minerals			
Na, mg	16.0	50.0	25.0
K, mg	51.0	144.0	74.0
Ca., mg	33.0	118.0	55.0
P, mg	14.0	93.0	43.0
Mg, mg	4.0	12.0	9.0
Fe, mg	0.1	Tr.	1.2
Zn, mg	0.15	0.1	0.42
Vitamins			
A, IU	240.0	140.0	158.6
C, mg	5.0	1.0	5.3
D, IU	2.2	1.4	42.3
E, IU	0.18	0.04	0.83
Thiamin, mg	0.01	0.03	0.04
Riboflavin, mg	0.04	0.17	0.06
Niacin, mg	0.2	0.1	0.7
Curd size	Soft	Firm	Mod. firm
	Flocculent	Large	Mod. large
pH	Alkaline	Acid	Acid
Anti-infective properties	+	±	−
Bacterial content	Sterile	Nonsterile	Sterile
Emptying time	More rapid		

* Composite of a number of sources
† Enfamil

chological benefit to both mother and child is obvious.

In certain instances, breast feeding may not be possible either because of maternal or newborn factors. Cracking of nipples and mastitis are at least temporary reasons to stop. The milk supply may not be adequate because of poor nutrition or psychological factors, and the infant may fail to thrive. Intake of drugs for various reasons may necessitate cessation of feeding because most drugs pass, at least to some extent, into the milk.

Selection of Feedings. A few basic guidelines should be considered when choosing the appropriate feeding for an infant.

1. The diet should contain adequate calories and essential ntrients.
2. The diet should be digestible.
3. Reasonable distribution of calories should be achieved.
4. The diet should be chosen to avoid potential problems suspected from a family history.

Calories and Essential Nutrients. The traditional caloric requirement of 120 cal/kg may be an overestimation. Adequate weight gain of 15 to 30 g/day has been observed with as low as 90 cal/kg, particularly in infants with a decreased daily activity. Fluid requirements in the newborn average 150 ml/kg, but may be as high as 200 ml/kg in the premature. Generally, the full-term infant fed *ad libitum* takes in excess of 150 ml/kg. Both these requirements need only be calculated in the newborn who either gains excessively or poorly. Essential nutrients for weight gain are contained in both human milk and most prepared infant formulas, with the occasional exception of some vitamins.

Digestibility. A digestible diet should contain protein, carbohydrates, and fat in those forms which have a superior nutritive value and allow minimal losses in stools. Breast milk still appears to be the best overall formula. While its protein content is low (1.1%), the excellent lactalbumin:casein ratio (80:20%) makes for small curds and easy digestibility. The presence of a variety of nucleotides enhances protein synthesis in the infant indirectly.[79] Cow's milk or modified cow's milk, as present in most routinely used infant formulas, is also a very adequate source of protein. Although slightly less digestible because of larger curd, reversed lactalbumin:casein ratio, and higher pH, excellent growth is maintained.

Soy protein formulas, while giving adequate growth in term infants, contain only one-third of their available nitrogen as essential or semi-essential amino acids.[80] To obtain optimal growth, approximately 10% more calories are needed in comparison with breast milk or cow protein formulas. In addition, fat losses are increased in the stool as is the loss of various minerals, vitamins, and trace elements because of binding with phytate. Rickets has been seen in low-birth-weight infants consistently fed with these formulas. The predominant use of a soy formula has been in infants with cow's milk allergy or as a supplement to breast feeding. Evidence now suggests that serum antibodies to soy proteins are formed as quickly or even more so, as compared to cow milk protein.[81] Thus, soy formula should not be used without specific therapeutic indications.

Casein hydrolysate is a satisfactory nitrogen source, but a tendency toward acidosis has been observed, particularly in small infants. Routine use is not warranted because of the very high expense.

Most infant formulas contain lactose or sucrose as their major carbohydrate. A few contain glucose and other starch or polysaccharide modifiers. It must be remembered that minor as well as major GI problems can lead to temporary intolerances of any of these, and, when choosing a formula, the carbohydrate source must be kept in mind (Table 42-10).

Table 42-10. Complete Infant Formulas.

Major Protein Source	Major Carbohydrate Source		
	Lactose	*Sucrose*	*Glucose*
Cow's milk protein	Enfamil with or without iron* Evaporated milk† Similac with or without iron* ‡ Similac PM 60/40* ‡ SMA*		Portagen§
Soy	CHO-free*	Isomil* i-Soyalac* Neo-Mull-Soy* Nursoy* Soyalac* CHO-free*	CHO-free* Prosobee*
Hydrosylate		Nutramigen*	Pregestimil§
Other	Human milk	Meat-base	

* Vegetable oils
† Animal fat (butterfat)
‡ Lactalbumin/casein ration = 60/40
§ MCT oil

Table 42-11. High-Protein Milks with Inappropriate Distribution of Calories.

Formula	Normal Dilution (cal/oz)	Protein %	CHO %	Fat %
Probana	20	24.0	47.0	29.0
Skim milk	10	40.0	57.0	3.0
Cow's milk	20	22.0	30.0	48.0
Evaporated milk 1:1	22	19.7	29.0	51.3
2% fat cow's milk	15	20.6	38.4	36.0
Similac advance	17	25.7	47.0	27.3
Meat base	17	20.0	29.0	51.0
Mull-Soy	20	19.0	32.0	49.0
Goat's milk	20	20.0	27.0	53.0

The fat content of several formulas can be seen in Table 42-10. For the most part, infants fed either human milk or formulas with added vegetable oils (corn, coconut, soy, oleo), excrete less than 1 g fat/kg/day. Infants fed whole cow's milk in many instances excrete in excess of 2 g/kg/day, and those fed evaporated milk without additional carbohydrate lose between 1 to 2 g/kg/day.[82] Fat absorption is least good in the first 10 days of life and then increases rapidly. Medium-chain triglyceride oil (MCT) has been shown to have an excellent absorption very early in life.

Distribution of Calories. A distribution of calories appropriate for good infant nutrition is as follows:

Protein	7–16%
Fat	35–55%
Carbohydrate	35–65%

Most infant formulas fall into these ranges and therefore are adequate even when combined with various strained infant foods that are relatively low in fats. Table 42-11 lists those formulas which have abnormal distributions, with a lowering of either fat or carbohydrate and an increase of protein. These milks should be avoided as routine diets for infants and are hazardous when abnormal losses are encountered (diarrhea, vomiting, excessive temperature) because of their high solute load.

With increasing concern over obesity and arteriosclerosis, pediatricians throughout the country have moved toward the use of skim milk and 2% low fat milks in infants after 4 months of age. Fomon has found that infants who consume skim milk have an intake of less than desirable total calories (average = 84 cal/kg) and an abnormal distribution of calories, with high protein and low fat. They also tend to consume an average of 30% more volume, a tendency which may persist beyond infancy.[83] It is therefore recommended that skim milks not be used in the first year of life.

Fortification of Formulas with Iron. Since 1969, it has been recommended by the American Academy of Pediatrics that formulas be fortified with iron. While a full-term infant is born with some reserves of iron, it has been shown that throughout the first year of life, inadequate amounts are ingested in infant foods unless large amounts of commercial dried cereals are given (Table 42-12).[84] The desired intake of iron is in the range of 10 to 12 mg/day. The hesitation to give iron-fortified formulas has been based on poorly documented reports of vomiting, diarrhea, constipation, or poor tolerance, as well as on reports from middle class practices stating a low incidence of iron-deficiency anemia. Because absorption of iron is far superior in breast-fed infants, at least before solid foods are added, it has been suggested that supplemental iron is unnecessary.[85] Oral iron will lead to binding of lactoferrin in the GI tract and as a consequence to an increase in infection.[86] However, breast-fed infants do exhibit low transferrin saturation by 4 months.[87] Thus, we maintain that an infant should have an iron-fortified formula for the first year of life and that breast-fed infants be supplemented by at least 4 months of age.

Infant Formulas and Their Contents. Table 42-10 lists some of the complete proprietary formulas which are available for use in the newborn period and adhere to recommended caloric distribution. They are shown according to major protein and carbohydrate source. Major fats are indicated as footnotes.

The group of formulas with cow's milk protein and lactose are more commonly used for routine feeding. The evaporated milk formula, in order to fit regular caloric distribution, must have added carbohydrate. The usual mixture contains 13 oz milk, 17 oz water and 2 tbsp carbohydrate (Karo).

A true history of milk allergy or primary and secondary lactose intolerance may indicate the long- or short-term use of the next-most commonly used formulas: soy isolates or soy flour protein and sucrose. Because allergy to soy protein is also common, and in light of Barrter's-like syndrome in some infants fed Neo-Mull-Soy, casein hydrolysate preparations may well be preferable despite their additional cost.

Minor Problems—Dietary Manipulation. Frequently, the pediatrician encounters minor problems with "spitting" and changes in stool pattern in the bottle-fed infant. Providing ad-equate growth is maintained, these problems need not require formula changes. Mild constipation can be treated with the addition of Karo syrup to the formula, or by adding prune juice, solid foods, or both to the diet. Severe constipation requiring the constant use of suppositories should be investigated. Loose stools may be helped by elimination of some carbohydrates from the diet. Temporary removal of iron from the diet may help either constipated or loose stools, but it should be reinstituted at a later time to insure adequate iron intake.

Many infants "spit up" small amounts of formula. This can result from overfeeding, and a careful dietary history should be taken. The incidence of chalasia in the newborn population is unknown, but is probably high, and propping after feedings plus thickening of milk with cereal may help. Projectile, bile-stained vomiting, or vomiting with poor weight gain require immediate inquiry.

Feeding the Premature

General Considerations. While advances in knowledge and techniques in management of premature infants have resulted in a lower

Table 42-12. Iron Content of Commercially Prepared Strained and Junior Foods.

Food	Mean Iron (mg/100 g)	Range (mg/100 g)
Dry cereals	71.60–80.1	50.00–100.2
Mixed 1:6 with milk	10.80–11.4	7.10–14.3
Cereal with fruit, strained		
High protein	5.30	—
Rice	0.18	—
Junior cereal with fruit		
Oatmeal	3.91	—
Strained		
Juices	0.46	0.10–0.95
Fruits	0.36	0.10–0.9
Plain vegetables	0.66	0.29–1.32
Creamed vegetables	0.56	0.24–0.88
Meats	1.57	0.70–4.43
Egg yolks	3.12	3.02–3.2
High meat dinners	0.76	0.47–1.71
Soups and dinners	0.51	0.12–2.13
Desserts	0.30	0.10–0.71
*Junior**		
Meat sticks	1.49	0.90–2.00

* Other foods similar to strained.
(Fomon SJ: Infant Nutrition, 2nd ed, Tables 16-1 and 16-2. Philadelphia, WB Saunders, 1974)[84]

mortality rate, feeding the premature infant still requires a very precise nursing and nutritional art because of the special liabilities of the infant. We feel that the aim of feeding should be to approximate intrauterine growth and mineral storage. This, however, is frequently impossible and the ideal growth rate remains unknown in the preterm extrauterine environment.

The problems facing the premature are well known and consist of poor suck and swallowing reflexes, relatively high caloric requirement with a small stomach capacity, poor gag reflexes leading to aspiration, an incompetent esophageal cardiac sphincter, and decreased absorption of essential nutrients.

Whether to feed the premature early or late is no longer a great controversy. All small prematures are now given intravenous feedings, with or without additional protein, until oral intake is adequate. This measure alone has improved survival and alleviated early aspiration. When the infant's condition permits, oral feedings—by gavage, continuous gastric or nasojejunal drip, dropper or nipple, depending on size and gestational age—have been given as early as 3 to 6 hours of age.

Scheduling of Feedings. The first few feedings, as with full-term infants, should consist of either sterile water, ½ normal saline, or 5% dextrose. In experimental animals, sterile water is less injurious to the lung than either milk or 5% dextrose if aspirated.[88] Once the patency of the GI tract is established, milk feedings may begin slowly. Table 42-13 shows suggested intervals and amounts. In infants less than 32-weeks' gestation, skillful gavage may be required until the feeding mechanisms are developed.[89] Because the stomach capacity may differ from one infant to another, gastric residuals should be measured prior to each feeding. If the amount retained in the stomach is equal to the anticipated feeding, no feeding should be given. If there is less, an additional increment to equal the desired amount may be given. Increasing residuals, with or without distension, may be indicative of obstruction or ileus, and further feedings should be given only with great caution.

Special Requirements. The premature infant has only a few requirements that differ from those of the full-term infant.

Protein. A number of studies have shown that protein requirements are greater for the premature than for the full-term infant, for whom 2.0 to 2.5 g/kg/day is adequate;[50,51] 3 to 4 gm/kg of protein is currently recommended for the premature. In the past few years, however, there has been a resurgence of interest in breast milk for feeding prematures. Quality rather than quantity of protein has been explored. Räihä and his group have shown good growth with pooled breast milk, although discharge weight was reached later in the breast-fed group. Higher serum ammonia levels, urea nitrogens, amino acid levels, total proteins, and more late metabolic acidosis were seen in the infants fed high-casein formulas. Cystine, methionine, and taurine levels, those amino acids felt to be essential in late fetal and early neonatal life, were lower in formula-fed infants.[90-93] Though these are studies of considerable importance, they disregard to a great extent, mineral status, lower serum proteins, and the fact that, after 6 weeks of the study, 50% of the breast-fed infants were still hospitalized while only 9% of the formula-fed infants were left in the study. Davies has reported statistically significant decreased increments of weight gain in prematures of less than 32-weeks' gestation fed breast milk during the first month of life despite adequate caloric intake.[94]

Recently, the protein and mineral content of preterm breast milk has been investigated. Compared with milk from term mothers, a higher protein, ranging from 2.015 to 3.26 gm/dl, was shown in the first days of life independent of gestational age. The level fell to a low of 1.46 to 1.79 gm/dl at the end of 28 days.[95,96] Sodium and chloride levels were significantly higher, while calcium, magnesium, and phosphorus remained constant and low.[96] Unfortunately, the number of breast milk samples was small. Until further conclusive studies are performed, infants fed preterm or pooled breast milk should be monitored for adequate nutritional status.

Vitamins. Although most formulas presently contain supplemental vitamins, they are only adequate when a whole formula is taken (usually 26 oz or 780 ml). Of particular importance to the premature are the fat-soluble vitamins A and D, and the water-soluble vitamins B and C. With the addition of polyunsaturated vegetable fats to prepared formulas, absorption of the fat-soluble vitamins may be lessened. Thus Poly-Vi-Sol, 1.0 ml daily is recommended in

Table 42-13. Oral Feeding Schedule for the Low-Birth-Weight Infant.*

Time	Substance	Up to 1000 g		1001–1500 g		1501–2000 g		More than 2000 g	
		Amt.	Freq.	Amt.	Freq.	Amt.	Freq.	Amt.	Freq.
First "drink"	Sterile H$_2$O 0.45% saline 5% glucose	1–2 ml	1 hr	3–4 ml	2 hr	4–5 ml	2–3 hr	10 ml	3 hr
Subsequent feedings 12–72 hr	Formula	Increase 1 ml every other feeding to maximum 5 ml	1 hr	Increase 1 ml every other feeding to maximum 10 ml	2 hr	Increase 2 ml every other feeding to maximum 15 ml	2–3 hr	Increase 5 ml every other feeding to maximum 20 ml	3 hr
Final Feeding Schedule 150 ml/kg	Formula	10–15 ml	2 hr	20–28 ml	2–3 hr	28–37 ml	3 hr	37–50 ml	3–4 hr

* Supplemental IV fluids should be given to fulfill requirements of 140–160 ml/kg (urine specific gravities 1.008–1.010) and caloric requirements of 90–110 ml/kg.

Table 42-14. Commonly Used Premature Formulas.

	Contents per dl (usual dilution)								Osmolality
		CHO		**Protein**			**Fat**		
Formula	*Caloric Content*	*g/dl*	*Type*	*g/dl*	*Whey/casein ratio*	*g/dl*	*Type*		*mosm/kg H₂O*
Enfamil 24 Premature Formula	81	9.1	60% polycose 40% lactose	2.4	60/40	4.1	40% MCT 40% Corn		300
Enfamil 24 w/Iron	81	8.5	lactose	1.8	18/82	4.5	80% Soy		355
Similac Special Care Infant Formula	81	8.6	50% lactose 50% polycose	2.2	60/40	4.4	50% MCT		290
Similac 24 w/Iron	81	8.5	lactose	2.2	18/82	4.3	60% Coconut		360
Similac PM 60/40	68	6.9	lactose	1.6	60/40	3.8	60% Coconut		260
SMA 24	81	4.2	lactose	1.8	60/40	4.2	Oleo, soy coconut		364

addition to the vitamins in prepared formulas. Vitamin K should be given intramuscularly at birth, and thereafter, except in special circumstances, need not be repeated.

Premature infants are born with low serum levels of Vitamin E, and its deficiency has been associated with a hemolytic anemia characteristically seen at 6 to 10 weeks of age.[97] A decreased absorption was reported, particularly in infants of less than 32-weeks' gestation and more so in those supplemented with polyunsaturated fats and large amounts of iron.[98,99] Iron acts as a catalyst in the autooxidation of fatty acids and apparently reduces the absorption of Vitamin E in this manner. With decreased vitamin E, an antiperoxidant, there is red blood cell lysis.

New evidence, however, shows adequate oral absorption of D,L-alpha-tocopherol at 25 units/day in prematures less than 1500 g.[100] Normal plasma levels of >0.05 mg/dl are also maintained when an experimental intramuscular preparation is given in conjunction with iron.[101] It is therefore recommended that oral vitamin E, 25 units/day, be given to prematures until the time of discharge with or without small amounts of iron. These recommendations may change if injectable preparations become available or if its use as protection against oxygen toxicity is proven.

Iron. Iron stores are deficient in prematures at birth. Differences of opinion exist as to when iron supplementation should begin because of its effect on vitamin E and binding with proteins important in bacteriostatic properties (lactoferrin and transferrin). It is recommended that iron supplements of 2 mg/kg up to 15 mg daily be started either after delivery when feeding is allowed, or at least by 2 to 3 months of age, to prevent iron-deficiency anemia. This may be obtained either as medicinal iron (Fer-in-sol) or through supplemented formulas. Additional iron is available in dry cereals with smaller amounts in other strained infant foods (Table 42-12). Beikost is usually not added to the diets of infants until the sixth month of age.

Selection of Feedings for the Premature. The formulas more commonly used for premature infants, with their caloric distributions, may be seen in Table 42-14. All fit well within acceptable caloric distribution. Those with the higher protein concentration will have higher solute loads and ash contents, but have been shown to be within the renal concentration abilities of premature infants. With the addition of the new premature formulas from Mead Johnson and Ross Laboratories, most formulas used in the United States for prematures now contain protein with a 60:40 ratio of lactalbumin to casein, approaching that of breast milk. Calcium and phosphorus ratios are also closer to the 2:1 ratio seen in breast milk. Growth and metabolic studies performed with both the above formulas show better digestibility with improved fat and calcium absorption, a lower osmolality, and an improved weight gain. When beginning an infant on formula, it is suggested that the concentration be started at a 12 cal/oz dilution and increased to 18 to 24 cal/oz over 5 to 7 days.

The use of pooled breast milk or preterm breast milk for even the smallest of infants may have some benefits particularly when beginning feedings. (See previous section on protein requirements.) Its digestibility can not be surpassed and there may be some protection against infection, possibly against necrotizing enterocolitis. It is now becoming more widely used around the country and, in some institutions, it is the only feeding for prematures. Measurements of bone mineral content in premature infants by photon absorptiometry show that the postnatal increase in the first three months of life is considerably less than would be expected *in utero*.[102] The fact remains, that it can not be recommended without qualifications as an adequate feeding because of its low levels of calcium, phosphorus, and magnesium, low sodium content, and marginal protein.

Special Formulas and Their Indications. A variety of special formulas are included in Table 42-10. Specific indications are detailed in Table 42-15 and for the most part, are self-evident. One word of caution is warranted regarding the use of CHO-free. In its undiluted form, the formula contains 22 cal/oz, and on occasion has been given that way without added carbohydrate. This results in an extremely high solute load and danger of hypernatremia. Errors in the addition of carbohydrate have also occurred. Recently, this formula along with Neo-Mullsoy was removed from the market because of an error in the formulation resulting in inadequate chloride content. As a result, failure to thrive with a metabolic alkalosis, and in some cases a

Table 42-15. Therapeutic Indications.

Indications	Diet	Comments
Cow's milk protein intolerance	Soy formula/Nutramigen	Soy protein shown to be as allergenic as cow
Soy protein intolerance	Nutramigen Pregestimil Meat base	
Biliary atresia	Portagen	MCT as main lipid
Hypocalcemia	Similac PM 60/40	Favorable Ca/P ratio
Sodium retention (i.e., congenital heart disease)	Lonalac SMA	Complete formula, low Na (2.5 mg/100 ml), may cause hyponatremia
Convalescent chronic diarrhea	Pregestimil	Start as 5–10 cal/oz increase to 20 cal/oz
Lactose intolerance (primary or secondary)	Sucrose-containing formula (see Table 42-10)	
Sucrose-isomaltose intolerance (primary)	Regular milk (restrict sucrose)	
Glucose-galactose intolerance	CHO-free with fructose or modular formula	Restrict lactose and glucose
Pandisaccharide intolerance (secondary)	Pregestimil	
Congenital chloridorrhea	Similac PM 60/40 SMA	Monitor serum electrolytes, restrict chloride, supplement potassium
Enterokinase deficiency Pancreatic insufficiency Cystic fibrosis	Pancreatic enzyme supplement (Cotazyme, Viokase)	
Celiac disease	Gluten-free diet	
Short bowel	Pregestimil Vitamin supplementation	Injectable B_{12} if ileum is absent
Abetalipoproteinemia	Portagen Pregestimil	MCT as main lipid
Acrodermatitis enteropathica	Breast milk	Zinc supplementation
Aminoacidurias	See Table 42-16 for treatable entities presenting in early infancy	

Bartter-like syndrome, was seen in infants ingesting this formula.[103] The return of these formulas is likely and they are thus included. The episode illustrates well, however, the lack of one element in a diet and the profound effects it may have on a growing infant.

Some aminoacidurias and metabolic diseases presenting in the newborn period are amenable to dietary therapy.[104] Signs and symptoms often overlap with other commonly occurring problems. Persistent vomiting (when GI disturbances are eliminated), jaundice (particularly of the direct variety), lethargy or seizures, and disorders of tone may signify underlying disease (Table 42-16). The management of such patients is difficult and highly specialized and should not be attempted without adequate experience and laboratory back-

Table 42-16. Major Inborn Errors of Metabolism Presenting in the Newborn Period and Amenable to Dietary Therapy.

Name	Clinical Findings	Diet
Aminoacidemias		
Maple syrup urine disease	Hypertonicity, lethargy, maple syrup odor	Restriction of valine, leucine, isoleucine, MSUD diet powder
Hypervalinemia	Feeding difficulty, vomiting	Restriction of valine
Phenylketonuria	No symptoms—picked up by routine screening	Restriction of phenylalanine; Lofenalac formula
Tyrosinemia I	Cirrhosis, renal tubular dysfunction	(Product 3200 AB)
Hyperalanemia	Lethargy, seizures, mental retardation	Vitamin B6—large doses
Organic acidemias		
Isovaleric acidemia	Neurologic dysfunction, "sweaty feet" odor	Restriction of leucine
Propionic acidemia Methylmalonic acidemias	Feeding difficulty, vomiting, lethargy hyperammonemia	Restriction of protein-biotin cyanocobalamin
Urea cycle enzyme deficiencies	Neurologic dysfunction coma, feeding difficulties, hyperammonemia	Restriction of protein
Galactosemia	Vomiting, jaundice, hepatomegaly	Restriction of galactose

Table 42-17. Dietary Supplements.

Substance	Contents	Uses
Casec powder	Casein hydrolysate 88 g protein/100 g powder	May be used as dietary supplement for protein
Dextrimaltose powder	Carbohydrate-cornstarch 97 g/100 g powder	Carbohydrate supplement
MCT oil	Medium chain triglyceride 1 g = 8.3 cal	Calorie supplement, malabsorption
Controlyte	72% carbohydrate cornstarch 24% fat vegetable oil	Calorie supplement, renal failure
Product 80056	CHO, fat, vitamins and minerals	For use in metabolic disorders, where amino acids must be added
Polycose	100% glucose polymers	Carbohydrate supplement liquid (2 cal/ml) powder (4 cal/g)

up. Particular care should be given to the inclusion of iron, calcium and vitamins when low protein diets are necessary.

Dietary supplements are useful for specific conditions. However, they are not complete diets, and care should be given to provide all nutrients required for growth (Table 42-17). MCT oil has been frequently used as a supplement to the diet of prematures. When given, it should be mixed thoroughly with the formula because it has been reported to cause an aspiration lipoid pneumonia when given alone.[105]

SPECIALIZED FEEDING TECHNIQUES IN THE NEWBORN AND PREMATURE INFANT

Gavage Feedings

Feedings by means of the nasogastric or orogastric tube either intermittent or continuous drip, are frequently used in infants who cannot take oral feedings for limited periods of time and whose GI tract is intact. Infants included in this group are those with CNS depression and poor suck reflexes following delivery, or premature infants less than 32-weeks' gestation whose oral intake is initially limited.

A No. 5 or No. 8 French nasogastric tube is inserted through the nose into the stomach prior to each feeding to avoid aspiration. Proper placement of tubing should be checked by aspiration of gastric contents and by injection of air with auscultation for gurgling over the stomach. The formula should run in by gravity and the length of time for feeding should be equal to that allotted to oral feedings of a similar amount. Under no circumstances should a feeding be injected by syringe. Continuous drip is usually done on an hourly basis by pump. The tube is clamped and withdrawn slowly once the feeding is finished to avoid dripping into the esophagus or oropharynx. With each feeding, a fresh tube is placed, although in some centers a No 5 French tube is clamped and left in place.

Hazards of this technique include partial airway obstruction, incompetence of the esophageal-cardiac sphincter when the tube is in place, and, rarely, malplacement into the trachea or perforation of the esophagus. Recent reports of lactobezoars seem more associated with constant drip and the use of high-density formulas, but they have been seen with bolus feeding and low-density formulas as well. If abdominal distention, vomiting or increasing gastric residuals are seen, this complication should be suspected. However, when done carefully, this method has merit and avoids surgical procedures.

Nasojejunal and Nasoduodenal Feedings.

In 1967, the use of nasojejunal feedings as a means of nutritional support for newborns with tetanus was first mentioned.[106] This method has subsequently been refined to include critically ill infants, term and premature, with pneumonia, meningitis, respiratory distress syndrome, congenital heart disease, and other such conditions.[107,108] Nasoduodenal tubes have been used with similar success but with less frequency.[109]

Silicone, silastic, and polyvinyl tubes have all been used. The tube is passed through the infant's nostril into the stomach, allowing for adequate length. The pH is tested at frequent intervals and when one of 5 to 7 is attained, a flat plate of the abdomen is taken to look for placement. Failure to pass the tube into the duodenum or jejunum occurs in approximately 2% of cases. If difficulty occurs, the tube may be guided by fluoroscopy, with its concurrent radiation risks, or, preferably, aided by gastric air insufflation. Ten milliliters of air is placed in the stomach of prematures of less than 1000 g, and increasing amounts are used for larger infants.[110]

Once there is correct positioning, feedings may be started. Glucose water, usually followed by half-strength, then full-strength formula, is given in increasing amounts to ultimately provide the infant's full fluid and caloric needs. This may be achieved by continuous drip or in 10 to 15 ml hourly aliquots. Hypertonic formulas should not be given. Gastric residuals must be checked by way of a nasogastric tube.

Transpyloric tubes, however, have had their ups and downs in frequency of use, complications, and efficacy. While good growth in prematures has been reported, impaired assimilation of fat and potassium and increased bacterial contamination of the jejunum have been documented.[111-113] Duodenal and jejunal perforations, midgut volvulus, and necrotizing enterocolitis have occurred in small numbers.

When either of these techniques is used, it

must be remembered that oral feedings should be instituted as soon as possible and that the infant should be held and fondled to give stimulation if the condition permits.

Gastrostomy. The use of gastrostomy, first suggested in 1837, was successfully carried out in 1876. Enthusiasm for this technique has waxed and waned in the last 100 years, though for surgical patients it is an accepted mode of therapy for decompression, drainage, and feeding. Its use for feeding purposes in the nonsurgical patient is still controversial.

In most instances, the Stamm gastrostomy has been placed using local anesthesia unless accompanied by a major surgical procedure. A size 10 to 12 French mushroom or basket (Pezzery) tube is inserted through a stab wound in the left upper quadrant and sutured to the skin. Special external taping of the tube to the skin has been used to prevent excessive movement of the tip and consequent partial obstruction. The infant is left with nothing by mouth for a variable period according to the initial indication. Feedings, begun with 5% to 10% dextrose, are increased to half-strength and full-strength formula and are dripped in slowly over a 30- to 45-minute period. Residuals are checked prior to the next feeding and the tubing is left open about 10 to 12 cm above the abdominal wall as a "pop-off" valve. Care should be exercised not to elevate the reservoir more than this distance above the stomach.

While accepted for surgical patients, the procedure is not recommended for routine feeding purposes. A number of small uncontrolled series have suggested its use in the small premature and claimed no major complications or increased mortality.[114,115] Vengusamy and coworkers in 1969 reported a controlled study in prematures weighing 750 to 1250 g.[116] Survival was significantly higher in the control group and infection was found more frequently in the gastrostomy group at autopsy. Some have questioned this high incidence of infection because it has not often been seen in other series. More recently, gastrostomy has proved useful for feeding critically ill infants on respirators or with chronic lung disease, but because of uncontrolled studies and limited numbers, its effectiveness in relation to mortality is unknown.[117] Certainly with the use of peripheral intravenous nutrition, the use of gastrostomy has diminished.

Gastrostomy alleviates some of the following problems faced when using either an indwelling or intermittent nasogastric tube:

1. Better decompression can be achieved because of its larger size and posterior position.
2. Obligate nose breathing of infants is protected and competency of the esophageal-cardiac sphincter preserved.
3. Promotes patient comfort over nasogastric tube.

Known major complications of gastrostomy in both surgical and nonsurgical infants amount to 2.5% to 5.8% and include intra-abdominal leaks with peritonitis, leaks around the tube requiring surgical closure, and bleeding. Minor complications, from 4.3% to 10.8%, include leaks not requiring surgery, delayed closure, and displacement of tube. The mortality directly attributed to gastrostomy has been reported from 0.4% to 4.7%.[118,119]

Nutritional Monitoring in Prematures

Feeding the premature by any method is not without its hazards. Thus once the premature begins to feed, it is important to ensure tolerance of milk, prevention of complications, continued growth, and adequate nutritional and laboratory monitoring. In a small retrospective study in our institution, it was shown that by doing systematic nutritional monitoring, premature infants were discharged at the same weight 1 week earlier, with a greater length, and higher albumin levels.[120] Therefore, monitoring was instituted throughout this nursery and nutritional charts with suggestions from the dieticians were placed in the infants' permanent records. Table 42-18 shows what is considered to be adequate monitoring.

Most of the parameters are self-explanatory and, particularly with "tolerance," are intended to look for early signs of necrotizing enterocolitis. Growth may be watched by the usual methods of weight, length, and head circumference. Though normals for skin fold thickness and mean arm circumference are not available in growing premature infants, it is interesting to note whether muscle and fat are being laid down in appropriate proportions.

In measuring plasma zinc, an element essential for growth, it was found that levels at birth are equal to or higher than those of adults, and that they gradually decrease to seemingly deficient levels over a 6- to 8-week

Table 42-18. Nutritional Monitoring in Premature Infants.

Tolerance		Status	
Parameter	*Interval Measured*	*Parameter*	*Interval Measured*
Stools		Anthropometric	
Reducing substances	Each feeding	Weight	Daily
Hematest	Daily	Height	Weekly
Consistency	Each feeding	Head circumference	Weekly
WBCs	As necessary	Mean arm circ	Weekly
Abdominal girth	Daily	Skin fold thickness	Weekly
Gastric residuals	Each feeding	Protein, calorie intake	Daily
Vomiting	Each feeding	Laboratory	
		BUN	7–10 Days
		Albumin	7–10 Days
		Calcium, phosphorus	7–10 Days
		Alkaline phosphatase	7–10 Days
		Zinc (if available)	Biweekly after 4 weeks

period unless supplemented. While symptoms of acrodermatitis enteropathica have been reported in prematures with low plasma zinc levels, this was not seen in our population of infants.[121] Rather, a few infants with plasma levels ranging from 37 to 40 μg/dl were found to have a poor suck, gastric residuals, and poor gastric motility, which responded to supplemental zinc. It is well known that two-thirds of the infant's supply of zinc is transferred across the placenta in the last 10 to 12 weeks of pregnancy and, at least in the small number of balance studies done, prematures remain in negative balance for the first 45 days of life.[122,123] Present ways of feeding these infants do not allow for adequate intake of zinc and other trace elements. What the consequences are in terms of the premature is unknown.

In following alkaline phosphatase levels, 47% of infants of less than 32-weeks' gestation were found to have levels greater than 500 IU, with a few greater than 1000 IU. These were infants supplemented with the recommended amount of vitamin D. Intramuscular vitamin D injections and/or increasing the oral dose to 600 IU daily quickly corrected the abnormality. This may in fact be the earliest sign of chemical rickets because calcium and phosphorus levels were normal and bone radiographs did not show changes. Rickets resulting from inadequate intake of phosphorus, vitamin D, and calcium, as well as the use of soy formulas, has been previously reported.[124–127]

By following serum albumin and blood urea nitrogen values, adequate protein intake has been ensured. Previously we had seen low protein levels and edema in some of these infants.

Parenteral Nutrition in Infants

The concept of *total* parenteral nutrition in infants is relatively new, though the giving of wines and oils by vein dates back to the mid1660s.[128] The first serious attempts to give nutrition by vein, but without positive nitrogen balance, were undertaken by the Japanese in the 1920s with emulsified oils. In 1944, the first intravenous feeding of a complete diet in a 5-month-old patient with Hirschsprung's disease was reported, with maintenance of the infant's weight.[129] Within the last 10 to 12 years, the science of giving total calories and all essential nutrients by vein has progressed to the point

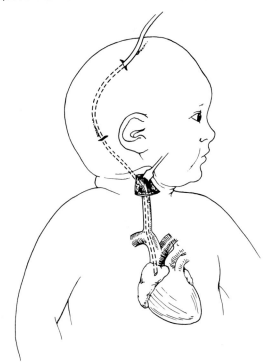

Fig. 42-3. Placing of an internal jugular catheter for total intravenous alimentation is done under strict aseptic conditions. The jugular vein is cut down in the neck and the proximal end threaded into the superior vena cava. The distal end is tunneled subcutaneously to a remote exit point in the scalp. All incisions are closed, and asepsis is carefully observed in dressing and caring for the catheter emergence point.

that sustained weight gain is possible for long periods of time. Total parenteral nutrition has since been the subject of a number of excellent reviews.[130–133]

Technique. In 1968, Dudrick and Wilmore described an aseptic technique for insertion of a silastic catheter into the external or internal jugular vein which is widely used today.[134] Under sterile conditions in the operating room, an incision is made in the neck, and the catheter is advanced into the superior vena cava. The distal end is tunneled subcutaneously to a stab wound on the scalp above the ear and the neck incision is closed (Fig. 42-3). This technique removes the entrance of the catheter into the vein from its exit to the skin and helps prevent contamination. Sterile dressings on the superficial wound should be changed every 2 to 3 days. Through this centrally placed catheter, hypertonic solutions

Table 42-19. Indications for Parenteral Nutrition

Surgical lesions
    Omphalocele
    Gastroschisis
    Complicated anastomoses
    Short gut $\geq$ 18 cm with ileocecal valve
            $\geq$ 40 cm without ileocecal valve
Necrotizing enterocolitis
Intractable nonspecific diarrhea
Premature infants—feedings not tolerated or in conjunction with increasing oral calories

---

may be slowly infused by pump and are rapidly diluted, thus preventing sclerosis of veins and marked changes in blood sugars and serum osmolarities. Placement of catheters through the common facial vein or internal jugular vein into the superior vena cava without ligation of any vessel has decreased the incidence of the superior vena cava syndrome.[135] Subclavian placement has also been successful in infants, as has the use of peripheral lines for partial or total parenteral nutrition. Regardless of route, a 0.22 μ Millipore filter placed in the intravenous line will help prevent infection. Proper placement of the catheter tip *must* be determined by radiography. Neither medications nor blood should be given through the line, and the entire external tubing is changed daily. With strict technique, the catheter can remain in place for periods up to 2 months.

Indications for Use of Total Parenteral Nutrition. There are definite indications for parenteral nutrition in infants (Table 42-19). This technique has reversed the high mortality with omphalocele, gastroschisis, and other severe surgical problems in which oral feedings must be delayed up to 4 to 5 weeks. In 1968, Avery and coworkers reported a 50% mortality in infants with chronic nonspecific diarrhea.[136] Intravenous nutrition has since increased survival significantly. Intensive care of the premature infant has permitted survival of shocky, moribund babies, but among this group an increased incidence of necrotizing enterocolitis has been noted. Oral feedings may not be tolerated for weeks, and total calories by vein have often made the difference between life and death while healing of the bowel takes place.

Parenteral nutrition and prolonged cathe-

terization are hazardous. The technique should be used only where ultimate survival of the child is expected but critical malnutrition may jeopardize recovery. Peripheral intravenous techniques alleviate some of the difficulties now encountered.

Ingredients and Requirements (Tables 42-20 and 42-21)

Although stock solutions for parenteral nutrition are used for infants, children, and adults,[130,160] all solutions should be prepared under careful aseptic conditions, for they readily support the growth of bacteria and fungi.

Protein. Protein lack in humans is known to produce poor growth, delayed wound healing, and generalized weakness. Exact requirements of intravenous protein or amino acids remain unknown. It has been shown that, when infants were given as little as 60 cal/kg/day, including 1% amino acids, weight gain and positive nitrogen balance could be achieved.[137] Dudrick and Wilmore gave 4 g/kg/day with good growth.[134] Perhaps most important to understand is the essentiality of certain amino acids, the ratio of essential to nonessential amino acids, and the nonprotein calories:nitrogen ratio (cal:N) which is most suited for infants. This information is only becoming available. A recent study in surgical infants reports a cal:N ratio of 200 (4 g protein/kg/day) to give good weight gain and a more positive nitrogen balance than a ratio of 400 (2 g protein/kg/day).[138] Suffice it to say that parenteral intakes of protein in the amount of 2.0 to 3.0 g/kg, depending on gestational age, seem to prevent

Table 42-20. Daily Requirements of Total Parenteral Nutrition.

Protein	2–4 g/kg
	(2.5 g/kg for prematures)
Calories	100–120.0 cal/kg
H_2O	125.0 ml/kg or as needed
Na	3–4.0 mmol/kg
K	2–3.0 mmol/kg
Ca	2–2.5 mmol/kg
P	2.5 mmol/day*
Mg	1 mmol/day
Multivitamins (Multivit)	1 ml/day

* Blood levels may be watched at intervals and P as K_2PO_4 given as needed.

Table 42-21. Requirements Given at Intervals.

Vitamin K	1–5 mg	Given weekly or as needed	IM or IV
		Monitored by prothrombin levels	
B$_{12}$	Less than 1 μg/day required	Given weekly	IM or IV
Folic acid	5–50 μg/day	Given daily or weekly	IV
Iron (Imferon)		As needed to maintain Hbg in normal range	IM

excessive complications and give adequate growth.

While Ghademi and Snyderman have each proposed ideal amino acid solutions for infants, there is not yet such a preparation.[139,140] Previously used casein or fibrin hydrolysates have been replaced by solutions of free amino acids. Currently, there are four such products on the market for routine use, which come in various percent solutions (Table 42-22). Only one of the preparations, Aminosyn,* comes with

packets of cysteine HCl which may be added to the parenteral solutions. This amino acid is converted to cystine, which is considered essential in the newborn.

None contain taurine, which may be important in the developing retina, CNS, and cardiac muscle. However, no long-term deficiencies have as yet been reported in infants. Frequently reported complications from the use of the hydrolysates such as acidosis, azotemia, and hyperammonemia have been decreased

Table 42-22. Amino Acid Solution Profile.

Amino Acid mg/dl	Freamine II 8.5%	Travasol* 8.5%	Aminosyn† 7%	Veinamine 8%
Essential				
Isoleucine	590	406	510	347
Leucine	770	526	660	493
Lysine	620	492	510	427
Methionine	450	492	280	427
Phenylalanine	480	526	310	400
Threonine	340	356	370	160
Tryptophan	130	152	120	80
Valine	340	390	560	253
Nonessential				
Alanine	600	1760	900	—
Arginine	310	880	690	749
Histidine	240	372	210	237
Proline	950	356	610	107
Serine	500	—	300	—
Tyrosine	—	34	44	—
Glycine	1700	1760	900	3387
Aspartic Acid	—	—	—	400
Glutamic Acid	—	—	—	426
Total Amino Acid (g/500 ml)	42.50	42.50	35.00	40.00
Total Nitrogen (g/500 ml)	6.25	7.15	5.50	6.65
Essential Amino Acids (%)	48	39	47	35
cal:N	136.10	191.10	154.10	127.10

* Also comes as 5.5% solution
† Also comes as 3.5%, 5%, or 10% solution

with the use of amino acid solutions, providing excessive amounts are not given. Monitoring of their use is still important.

Carbohydrate. Glucose is at present the most common source of carbohydrate used in parenteral solutions. While there are no stated requirements, limited quantities are tolerated by infants. Term and older infants seem to handle up to 14 mg/kg/minute without significant glucosuria, while 100% of premature infants have shown hyperglycemia and glucosuria with this same amount.[141] None of these infants had an osmotic diuresis. Amino acids given with glucose seem to lessen hyperglycemia, perhaps by increasing insulin secretion. However, in view of recent evidence of hyperglycemia worsening asphyxial damage to the CNS, it may be wise to give just that amount of glucose giving normoglycemia or sufficient calories.[142]

Other sources of carbohydrate include fructose, which is infrequently used but does not require or stimulate insulin secretion. However, it is relatively expensive and not as readily available. Galactose in conjunction with glucose has also been used in small numbers of hyperglycemic low-birth-weight infants with subsequent normoglycemia, without signs of toxicity.[143]

Ethyl alcohol, 3 to 5 g/kg/day, has been used as a supplementary caloric source because it provides 7 cal/g metabolized. At this intake, in full-term infants, liver functions have remained essentially normal though elevated alcohol levels have been noted in prematures even with low intake. Alcohol and amino acids are not sufficient for maintenance of positive nitrogen balance unless some other carbohydrate source is also provided.

Fat Emulsions and Essential Fatty Acids. Many oils have been employed with varying success in an attempt to give calories. The first in this country was by L. Emmett Holt and coworkers. In the mid 1950s, Upjohn introduced Lipomul, the first commercially prepared fat emulsion.[128] This preparation was fraught with many problems, including a high percentage of febrile reactions and the "overload syndrome," and was removed from the market. In 1960, the Swedish soybean oil-egg emulsion (Intralipid) was introduced and has been used widely and with great success in Europe, Canada, and the United States.

The syndrome of essential fatty acid deficiency, with decreased growth, dermatitis, and various anatomic, degenerative and pathophysiologic changes in many organs, has been well described. The full syndrome has been rare in infants. However, it has been shown that infants on fat-free parenteral nutrition develop plasma lipid changes and essential fatty acid deficiency quite rapidly within a week.[144,145]

There are presently two 10% fat-emulsion preparations on the market that have been approved for use (Table 42-23). Both came as 20% solutions, but are either not made in this country or not approved in this concentration at present. Most experience, however, resides with the use of Intralipid. Thus, the bulk of this discussion will pertain to this product. With the development of such a stable lipid emulsion, it has become possible to give more balanced intravenous calories and lower concentrations of glucose. All nutrients may now be given by either a central or a peripheral vein.

Generally, term and, to a slightly lesser extent, preterm, appropriate-for-gestational-age infants, tolerate up to 4 g/kg/day of Intralipid. Small-for-gestational-age infants have much more difficulty with fat clearance. Intercurrent illness with any infant may cause hyperlipidemia where previous tolerance had already been established. Fat emulsions are usually added to the glucose-amino acid solutions when acute problems are controlled (*i.e.,* significant hyperbilirubinemia), and when it is apparent that enteral nutrition will be delayed. An initial test dose of 0.1 ml/minute over 10 to 15 minutes is given, watching for acute reactions such as respiratory distress, flushing, or change in temperature. If no untoward reactions occur, the infusion may be given at 1 g/kg initially and increased on successive days to 4 g/kg/day as clearance allows. At no time should more than 60% of calories be given as fat. If only essential fatty acids are needed, there is evidence that as low as 1% of calories, but preferably 4%, given as linoleic acid, will alleviate signs of deficiency.[146]

Intralipid or other fat emulsions should be infused separately from any other IV solution to avoid disturbing the stability of the emulsion, and should be infused over at least 16 hours if not longer to allow time for clearing. It may be run through the same IV near the

Table 42-23. Fat Emulsions (10% Solutions)

Emulsion	Intralipid (Soybean Oil)	Liposyn (Safflower Oil)
Fats:		
Linoleic	54%	77%
Linolenic	8%	—
Oleic	26%	13%
Palmitic	9%	7%
Stearic	—	2.5%
Egg yoke phosphatides	1.2%	1.2%
Glycerol	2.5%	2.5%
pH	7.2–7.9	8.0
Calories	1.1 cal/ml	1.1 cal/ml

infusion site by means of a Y-connector. It should *never* be filtered.

While the use of Intralipid appears to be quite safe for term and premature infants, there are some real and theoretical problems at least to be considered with its use.

1. **Clearance** from the blood stream should be monitored by measuring lipids and triglyceride levels, by nephalometry, and/or by visible clearing from serum. The latter, while widely used, is probably the least reliable.[147]
2. **Displacement of Albumin-Bound Bilirubin by FFA.** This problem is potential rather than actual. Intralipid itself does not compete with bilirubin binding, although it can bind to free sites on the albumin molecule. It is the FFAs that are generated during hydrolysis of Intralipid that may compete for albumin. *In vivo* studies have shown no free bilirubin generated if the molar ratio of FFA to albumin is less than 6.[148] There are also no reports indicating a higher incidence of kernicterus in infants given Intralipid.
3. **Effects on Pulmonary Function.** Fat globules have been noted at autopsy in alveolar macrophages and capillaries.[149] The arterial P_{O_2} has also been shown to fall minimally when 1 g/kg was infused into infants over 4 to 7 hours. Effects on other pulmonary functions were not seen.[150] Until there is further evidence for abnormal function, Intralipid can be used with caution in most infants with lung disease, particularly when the acute stage is over.

4. **Effects on Hepatic Function.** Hyperbilirubinemia has been implicated as a complication of Intralipid infusion. This however was seen with parenteral nutrition solutions alone prior to the use of Intralipid. Fat particles may be seen in the reticuloendothelial system of the liver after emulsion infusion. It seems to have little effect on the infant and at least in rabbits, no effects on endotoxin clearance.[151] It has been recommended for reasons above that Intralipid not be used in infants with marked jaundice.
5. **The Overload Syndrome.** The syndrome, consisting of fever, lethargy, hyperlipemia, liver damage, and disorders of coagulation has never been reported in infants.

In rare instances, an infant may not be able to tolerate intravenous fats, in which case correction of essential fatty acid deficiency has been shown to occur by cutaneous application of sunflower seed oil.[152] However, this procedure cannot be assumed to be uniformly effective and thus absorption must be documented by measurements of essential fatty acids.[153]

Electrolyte, Macro- and Microminerals and Vitamins. Table 42-20 lists approximate estimates of electrolytes that are needed by the premature infants, providing there are no excessive losses for other reasons. Obviously, monitoring of serum electrolytes will help prevent serious deficiencies.

Macrominerals such as calcium, magnesium, and phosphorus are also added to the solution individually. Compatibility tables will help in providing information on how much calcium

Table 42-24. Suggested Daily Intravenous Intake of Essential Trace Elements.

Element	μg/kg/day
Zinc	
Prematures	300
Infants	100
Copper	20
Chromium	0.14–0.2
Manganese	2–10

(Adapted from AMA Department of Foods and Nutrition: JAMA 241:2053, 1979)[158]

and phosphorus may be added in the same solution without precipitating. Some institutions add one element on one day and another the next. Regardless of how this is done, inadequate amounts of these particular elements are often given, resulting in osteoporosis or even rickets if TPN is continued for long periods of time.

We are becoming more knowledgeable about **trace elements.** Until a few years ago, it was felt that twice weekly plasma transfusions were adequate in supplying them. As the technique of TPN has improved, so has the length of time that it may be continued. Both zinc and copper deficiencies have been described and should be avoided.[155–157] Potential deficiencies of chromium, manganese, iodine, or selenium are less well defined.

Some institutions routinely add trace elements to their solutions, but many do not. The AMA Department of Foods and Nutrition has recently made a statement on requirements of some trace elements (Table 42-24).[158] Until monitoring of these elements becomes more adequate, with the exception of zinc which is relatively nontoxic, the rest should be given with caution.

Vitamins. Vitamins play an extremely important basic role in bone metabolism, in development of the eye, in maintenance of the erythrocyte, in coagulation, and in fat, carbohydrate, and protein metabolism. Satisfactory results have been obtained by adding 1 ml of Multivit to present solutions and weekly administration of folic acid, vitamin B_{12} and vitamin K.

Despite these additions, small premature infants are subject to rickets and low vitamin A and E plasma levels. It has also been noted that riboflavin undergoes photodegradation under the bilirubin lights.[159] It is likely that further investigation will call for higher vitamin requirements, particularly in the small prematures.

Management of the Patient

Initially lower concentrations of protein (0.5 g/kg/day) and glucose (10% solution) are begun, rather than starting with the full calculated amounts. This allows the infant to increase his insulin secretion slowly and prevents potential hyperglycemia and osmotic diuresis. Intralipid is usually begun following acute illness and any bilirubin problems, at between 4 to 6 days. A cal:N ratio of 200 to 400:1 seems satisfactory for growth. (6.25 g protein = 1 g nitrogen.)

Table 42-25. Variables to be Monitored in Infants Receiving TPN.

Variable	Frequency
Anthropometric	
Weight	Daily
Length, Head circum.	Weekly
Skin fold thickness	
Mid-arm circumference	Weekly if available
Laboratory	
Electrolytes	Daily until stable Then 3 times weekly
Ca, P, Mg	Initially then weekly
Dextrostix	Daily (glucose as needed)
Albumin	Initially, then weekly
BUN	Initially, then weekly
Bilirubin, SGOT, SGPT	Initially, then weekly or as indicated
Ammonia	As needed
Hemoglobin	2 times weekly
pH, blood gases	As needed
Trace elements (Zn, Cu)	Weekly after 1 month if available
Serum turbidity*	Daily
Urine	
Glucose, specific gravity, protein	At least daily
Detection of Infection	
Clinical observations	Daily
WBC, differential	As needed

* Serum triglycerides and FFAs should be obtained periodically but will not be of help in day-to-day management.

Fastidious attention to detail is necessary in order to minimize complications and to ensure that no essential nutrient is missed. Important parameters to be monitored can be seen in Table 42-25. With each voiding, the urine must be checked for volume, specific gravity, protein and glucose. An increase in urine sugar, once the infant's total parenteral nutrition has been stabilized, suggests that infection may be present. If there is a significant change in activity, a rise in the white blood cell count, a temperature change, or an unexpected bilirubin rise cultures should be taken, antibiotics started, and careful consideration given to removing the catheter. In most cases, once the catheter is removed, the signs of sepsis will disappear. After the catheter has been in place for 30 days or more, the incidence of infection rises regardless of technique or monitoring.

In general, infants requiring parenteral nutrition need it for at least 3 weeks. Thus, the infant with chronic diarrhea or necrotizing enterocolitis is placed on nothing by mouth for this period of time in order to allow healing of the bowel, while the infant with a surgical condition may require even longer before the bowel is functional. The latter can be judged by bowel sounds, the absence of distension, absence of bile-stained gastric aspirates, and the presence of normal stool pattern. While the bowel is at rest, particularly in nonsurgical infants, the passage of small stools may continue throughout the period of parenteral nutrition. This need not be of concern, and is generally the result of intestinal juices and sloughing of cells. If excessive, an additional amount of fluid may be required.

The process of refeeding the infant must progress with caution. Intravenous feeding should overlap the initial period; 5% glucose water is given by mouth for three to four feedings.

Once this is tolerated, one of the following may be introduced: a formula consisting of protein hydrolysate, glucose and MCT oil (Pregestimil); an elemental formula of L-amino acids and glucose (Vivonex); or breast milk. This should be fed at a low concentration of (5 to 7 cal/oz) for the first 2 to 3 days. Then, depending on the indication for parenteral nutrition, progression of feedings may be more rapid or slow (1 to 3 weeks). In general, a good rule is not to increase concentration and volume simultaneously. Occasionally, infants will develop transient diarrhea during refeeding. Dropping back on concentration, decreasing volume or stopping feeding entirely for a short period will usually suffice. Monitoring for tolerance of formula should be performed as previously discussed in this chapter.

Most infants will have loose stools during this period of refeeding, particularly when elemental formulas are used. It has been our policy to continue a non-cow's milk formula for a period of 2 months to allow for good growth. Thereafter changes to more routine formulas can easily be accomplished.

Complications of Parenteral Nutrition

Complications attributed to this form of nutrition have been reported to be as high as 68.5% with a mortality of 8.4%.[133] The success of this technique depends upon the skill and care of the pediatric and surgical team and probably should only be attempted in a center that has adequate experience and laboratory support. With a multidisciplinary approach, morbidity has dropped to less than 10% and mortality is only rarely due to TPN itself. Table 43-26 lists complications according to origin, and in relative decreasing order of frequency.

In general, catheter complications are self-explanatory, and, if good care is given, can be minimized. The metabolic complications are reduced by monitoring, but some may have long-term residua.

One of the most interesting but perplexing complications of TPN is the cholestasis and mild hepatocellular damage that appears after 2 to 3 weeks in up to 50% of infants, and results in an elevated direct and indirect bilirubin, SGOT, SGPT, and occasionally alkaline phosphatase. This appears to happen whether or not Intralipid is used. The cause remains unknown. Lack of oral intake with decreased bile flow,[161] amino acid toxicity,[162] immaturity of bile salt secretion,[163] and sepsis[164] have been postulated. Liver biopsies have shown minimal fibrosis, round cell infiltrates, fatty infiltration,[165,166] and hepatocellular injury without significant inflammatory reaction.[167] All of these seem to disappear when TPN is stopped. As benign as this may sound, progressive liver failure and death has been reported in two infants who needed parenteral nutrition for prolonged periods of time.[168]

Despite the life saving effect of TPN in many

Table 42-26. Known Complications in
Parenteral Nutrition.

Catheter	Metabolic
Central	
Sepsis, bacterial or fungal	Hyperglycemia*
	Glycosuria*
Plugging or dislodgement	Hepatic drainage
	Cholestasis
Local skin infections	Postinfusion
Thrombosis of major vessel or embolism	hypoglycemia*
	Acidosis*
Improper placement	Hypocalcemia*
Hemorrhage	Hypophosphatemia*
Extravasation of fluid	Hypokalemia*
	Essential FA
Peripheral	deficiency* (no
Sloughs	Intralipid)
Local infection	Hyperlipidemia* (with Intralipid)
	Hyperammonemia*
	Radiographic bone changes (Rickets, osteoporosis, Cu deficiency)
	Trace element deficiency* (Zn, Cu)

* Avoided by careful monitoring

infants, it must be remembered that our present solutions fall far short of maintaining completely normal body homeostasis. A small 4- to 7-year follow-up of infants given TPN shows no difference in intellegence quotients between them and controls.[169] More thought and study must be done before all answers are known.

DISORDERS OF NUTRITION

Inadequate Intake

The infant's rhythmic alternation between hunger and satiety, regulated by hypothalamic centers, normally achieves a homeostasis balancing feeding behavior and metabolic needs. Malnutrition caused by inadequate intake is thus the result of disordered feeding behavior, inadequate mothering, the provision of an inappropriate diet, or failure to compensate for increased requirements. **Marasmus** is the deficiency state in which both proteins and calories are proportionately reduced. In **kwashiorkor,** protein deficiency predominates. These conditions are compared in Table 42-27.

Disordered feeding behavior is characteristic of the small premature, the brain-damaged infant, and the infant debilitated by severe or chronic disease. The situation of the small premature, with little disposition to suck and a tendency to regurgitate if his limited stomach capacity is exceeded, is all too familiar. A delay of 2 to 3 weeks before the 1000 g premature regains his birth weight is commonplace; nevertheless, this represents acute starvation at a time of rapid growth with minimal caloric reserves. The infant debilitated by disease may be equally apparent, but it is easy to focus on his primary condition and let considerable time lapse during which inadequate nutrition has compounded the child's problems. The infant with subtle signs of brain damage is easily missed, but his feeding may be poor, and discoordinated sucking and swallowing may result in recurrent aspiration. Some brain-damaged babies will appear to

Table 42-27. Comparison of Two Starvation
Syndromes.

	Marasmus	Kwashiorkor
Growth failure	+ +	+ +
Wasting	+ + + +	+ +
Diarrhea malabsorption	+ +	+ +
Vomiting	+	±
Infections	+ +	+ +
Anemia	+	+ + +
Apathy	+	+ + +
Anorexia	+	+ + +
Edema	−	+ + +
Abdominal distension	+	+ +
Fatty liver	±	+ +
Atrophic skin, exudative lesions	−	+ +
Red or depigmented hair	−	+ +
Hypoproteinemia	+	+ + +
Decreased BUN	±	+ +
Potassium, magnesium deficit	+	+ +
↑ICW, ↓ECW*	+	+ + +
↑ Urine volume, ↓ urine s.g.	+ +	+ +
Ketonuria	+	+

* Increased intracellular water, decreased extracellular water.

suck adequately but will stop before their full caloric needs are met. In all these instances, the physician must monitor growth and insure a sufficient intake.

Inadequate mothering may result from preoccupation with personal problems, psychiatric conditions such as postpartum depression or schizophrenia, life circumstances requiring a chain of poorly motivated baby sitters, and a variety of other conditions. The important subject of mother-infant interaction is discussed in greater detail in Chapter 17. Suffice it to say that the infant is totally dependent for all the aspects of his care, and feeding is the central transaction in this intimate relationship. When maternal deprivation is severe, the baby may retreat into a state of almost catatonic depression, failing to respond to stimuli and even refusing food. Management of this problem requires a team approach. The infant must be coaxed out of his depression; a proper feeding regimen must be initiated and sustained weight gain achieved. The mother must be helped with her problems, coached in the skills of caring for her baby, and allowed to give part of the baby's care in the hospital.

Inappropriate diet may result from unavailability of milk, miscalculation of the baby's needs, misunderstood instructions on how to prepare the formula, or excessive zeal in introducing solid foods. In some parts of the world, the most common cause of infantile malnutrition is the switch from breast milk to inadequate amounts of a carbohydrate gruel. Here, inexperienced mothers may fail to increase feedings to match the baby's growth. Formulas may be overdiluted or may be refused by the infant because of their taste. Finally, the premature introduction of foods suitable for an older infant may result in a diet which is poorly tolerated or is relatively high in protein and carbohydrate and deficient in essential fatty acids.

Increased requirements are seen in babies with hypermetabolism relative to their weight: the severe small-for-dates infant, the cachectic child, the infant with congenital heart disease or chronic pulmonary disease requiring increased work of breathing, the cold-stressed baby, the infant with hyperthyroidism or a catecholamine-secreting tumor, or the spastic or hyperkinetic baby. Under these circumstances, ordinary allowances may underestimate the infant's dietary requirements.

Table 42-28. Causes of Vomiting.

Physiologic "spitting up"
Chalasia
Hiatal hernia
Pyloric stenosis
Intestinal obstruction
   Partial, complete
Protein malabsorption
Infection
Hypoadrenal states
Metabolic
   Ileus—electrolyte imbalance
   Galactosemia
   Amino acidurias
CNS
   Increased intracranial pressure
   CNS hemorrhage
Narcotic withdrawal

Vomiting

The diagnosis and management of surgical lesions which result in vomiting are detailed in Chapter 34. An additional group of miscellaneous causes of vomiting are included in Table 42-28. They should be considered when vomiting sufficient to interfere with weight gain persists, and contrast studies of the intestinal tract fail to reveal a mechanical cause. Diagnosis is reasonably straightforward once the condition is suspected, and all are discussed individually elsewhere in this volume. Management is primarily directed at the underlying disease. The characteristic fluid and electrolyte problems accompanying prolonged vomiting are described in Chapter 29.

Diarrheal States (Malabsorption)

Diarrheal states in infancy are characterized by failure of normal intestinal absorption and usually by loss from the body of substantial amounts of fluid, electrolytes, and even endogenous nutrients such as amino acids. Infantile diarrhea in its milder forms is very common, and after the first few days of life is often caused by viral or bacterial enteric infection. Mild transient diarrhea may result from intolerance to feedings, systemic infections, and so on, and is sometimes unexplained. It is usually brief and self-limiting, and therapy is directed at replacing fluid and electrolyte losses and temporarily putting the bowel at rest by withholding feedings. In a few

Table 42-29. Clinical Classification of Malabsorption Syndromes Based on Type of Stool.*

Watery stools	Fatty stools	Normal stools
Congenital, developmental, and secondary lactase deficiency	Cystic fibrosis	Primary hypomagnesemia
Sucrase-isomaltase deficiency	Pancreatic insufficiency and bone marrow failure	Amino acid malabsorption
Glucose-galactose malabsorption	Celiac sprue	Vitamin B_{12} malabsorption Juvenile pernicious anemia Immerslund's syndrome
Primary immune defects	Short bowel syndrome	Adult type perinicious anemia
Congenital chloridorrhea	Abetalipoproteinemia	Congenital malabsorption of folic acid
Enterokinase deficiency	Intestinal lymphangiectasia	
Cow's milk protein sensitivity	Whipple's disease	
Soy protein sensitivity	Wolman's disease	
Parasites *Giardia lamblia* *Strongyloides sterocoralis* *Capillaria philippinensis* *Coccidia*	Tropical sprue Stasis syndrome Biliary tract obstruction	

* (Adapted from Ament ME: J Pediatr 81:685, 1972)[170]

cases, antibiotic treatment of bacterial enteritis is required. (See Chap. 32 for a discussion of infectious infantile diarrhea.)

In a smaller number of cases, infantile diarrhea may present a serious challenge because of either the severity or the chronicity of the malabsorptive state. In some instances, numerous loose stools call attention to the diarrhea. In other cases, poor weight gain despite adequate intake is the presenting complaint, but on closer examination the baby is found to have bulky, foul-smelling stools that signal malabsorption. The discussion to follow will focus on these more severe diarrheal disorders, and will be divided into three sections: specific malabsorptive states, enterocolitis, and nonspecific intractable diarrhea.

Specific Malabsorptive States. Among infants with intractable diarrhea which fails to respond to ordinary therapy and does not yield a bacterial pathogen, a considerable number are found to have specific malabsorptive states which can be diagnosed by careful work-up. A listing of these conditions according to the characteristic pattern of their stools is found in Table 42-29. A discussion of the individual diagnostic entities is given below.

Considering the size of the differential diagnosis of intractable diarrhea, the number and complexity of the possible diagnostic studies, and the often debilitated condition of the baby, the evaluation must usually proceed in stages. In the extreme case of the severely cachectic premature, all studies may be postponed for a period of several weeks during which bowel rest and intravenous alimentation by a central catheter will allow growth, the replenishment of metabolic reserves, and the interruption of secondary mechanisms of diarrhea caused by starvation itself. The initial studies should be those which are least traumatic and have the highest diagnostic yield. More complex or esoteric tests should follow in evaluating leads turned up by screening procedures, or as forced by the inexorable course of the child's disease. How some of these diagnoses can be approached is given in Table 42-30.

Carbohydrate Intolerance.[170,172] The mechanisms of carbohydrate absorption have been reviewed earlier in this chapter. Whenever substantial amounts of dietary mono- or disaccharides are not absorbed normally, there results a fermentative diarrhea. Bacterial overgrow in the gut lumen and ferment the sugars to organic acids. Water is drawn into the gut by the osmotic activity of the sugars and organic acids, and hence is lost to the body. Intestinal irritation and gas also may be produced.

Carbohydrate intolerance may be divided into congenital and acquired, and may reflect sensitivity to disaccharides (lactose or sucrose and isomaltose) or monosaccharides (glucose and galactose). In general, the congenital form is rare and represents a lifelong enzyme deficiency presumably on a genetic basis. The acquired form is common, particularly lactose intolerance, and it responds to treatment of the primary condition with which it is associated.

Congenital glucose-galactose intolerance is an extremely rare autosomal recessive condition, and probably results from lack of the intestinal kinase enzyme shared by glucose and galactose.[172] Severe diarrhea begins with the earliest feedings and is aggravated even by glucose water. Disaccharides are not tolerated because these in turn must be hydrolysed into glucose or galactose. However, these babies can be made to thrive on special formulas in which fructose is substituted for other carbohydrates. Later management requires severe carbohydrate restriction.

Congenital lactose intolerance is rare in the complete form, although mild lactase deficiency with slight symptoms on exposure to milk, especially beyond infancy, is not uncommon. In the severe form, fermentative diarrhea begins soon after milk feedings are introduced, but monosaccharides are well tolerated. Vomiting and colic may also be symptoms. Management is by using a formula containing sucrose or a monosaccharide, and becomes easier when other foods are introduced because milk is the chief form in which lactose is encountered. Congenital lactose intolerance has been reported in siblings, but the exact mode of inheritance has not been worked out.

Congenital sucrose-isomaltose intolerance is an autosomal recessive condition and is the least rare of the congenital carbohydrate intolerances. Deficient absorption of these two sugars occurs together, and they may well share a common enzyme. The hallmark of this condition is tolerance of milk containing lactose but the onset of diarrhea when sucrose is introduced into the diet. Dietary management consists in the elimination of foods containing sucrose, although with advancing age modest intakes may be tolerated.

Acquired lactose intolerance is common and may follow in the wake of diarrhea of almost any cause. The lactase activity of the intestinal brush border has relatively little reserve capacity and must be constantly regenerated. Injury of the intestinal epithelium from any cause—infection, ischemia, allergy, toxins, and even severe starvation—may be complicated by acquired lactose intolerance which may last for weeks. Fermentative diarrhea is noted on exposure to lactose-containing milks in infants who previously tolerated milk feedings. Usually some precipitating circumstance will be obvious. Management consists in giving lactose-free feedings for 1 to several weeks depending on severity. Complete recovery may take up to 4 months in some cases. The conventional wisdom of temporarily withholding feedings from infants with minor diarrhea probably reflects their mild and transitory intolerance to lactose. Skim milk is obviously contraindicated.

Acquired sucrose-isomaltose intolerance is found in the same circumstances as acquired lactose intolerance, but is less common and less severe. It appears that the enzyme for absorbing these sugars has greater reserve capacity or is less easily destroyed by minor mucosal injury. In more severe cases of secondary lactose intolerance, sucrose and isomaltose may provoke diarrhea as well. In this case a monosaccharide-containing formula may be required.

Acquired glucose-galactose intolerance may occur under the same circumstances as lactose intolerance but requires a more extreme mucosal injury. Once chronic diarrhea has been present for several weeks, it is not uncommon to find that even glucose water exacerbates the condition. Under these circumstances, a period of bowel rest and intravenous alimentation or of carbohydrate-free or fructose-based formula may be required.

Diagnosis in most **carbohydrate intolerances**
(*Text continues on p. 1046.*)

Table 42-30. Diagnostic Studies.*

Condition	First-Step Screening	Second-Step Screening	Specific Diagnostic Studies
ANATOMIC			
Hirschsprung's disease	Abdominal radiograph	Barium enema	Rectal biopsy
Stenosis of the bowel	Abdominal radiograph	Long GI series	Exploratory laparotomy
ALLERGY AND INTOLERANCE			
Dissacharide intolerance	Stool pH; test stool for reducing substances	Tolerance tests for sugars	Enzyme assays
Glucose-galactose malabsorption	Stool pH; test stool for reducing substances	Tolerance tests for sugars	Trial carbohydrate elimination, may use fructose
Milk protein sensitivity	Cow's milk elimination	Rechallenge with cow's milk	Consistent response to cow's milk protein
Celiac disease		Trial of gluten free diet	Intestinal biopsy
INFECTION AND INFESTATION			
Monilial enteritis	Observation of oral thrush	Mycelia on stool smear	Positive culture–monilia
Staphylococcal enteritis	Stool culture		Staphylococcus primary organism
Other enteric infections	Stool culture		Identify pathogen
Enteric infestations	Stool ova and parasites		Identify pathogen
Intra-abdominal infections	Blood and urine cultures	IVP-barium enema	Abdominal exploration

Condition	Clinical clue	Diagnostic test
Pellagra	Look for skin rash and CNS symptoms	Niacin therapy effective
Hypocupremia	Hypochromic anemia	Serum copper and
Hypomagnesemia	Refractory hypocalcemia	magnesium; response to therapy with these ions
ENDOCRINE		
Adrenogenital syndrome	Serum electrolytes	Urinary 17-ketosteroids
Addison's disease	Serum electrolytes	Urinary 17-OH steroids
Neural crest tumors	Urinary cathecolamines	IVP—retroperitoneal air inflation—laparotomy
Thyrotoxicosis	(rare in young children)	$\uparrow$T4 and T_3 $\uparrow$ TSH
MISCELLANEOUS		
Agammaglobulinemia (Swiss type)	Peripheral blood smear ($\downarrow$ lymphocytes)	Biopsy of lymph nodes or thymus; immunoelectrophoresis
Cystic fibrosis	Sweat test	Repeat sweat test; stool trypsin Duodenal drainage
Exudative enteropathy	Serum proteins	Serum proteins RISA or PVP half-life
Ulcerative colitis	Stool guaiac Sigmoidoscopy-barium enema	Rectal biopsy
Achrodermatis enteropathica	Look for skin rash and neurologic signs Serum zinc	Response to zinc Urine zinc excretion
Abetalipoproteinemia	Blood smear $\times$ acanthyocytes Serum cholesterol	Phospholipids-lipoproteins
Congenital chloridorrhea (Darrow–Gamble syndrome)	Serum electrolytes, pH	Stool chloride determinations

* (From Avery GB et al: Pediatrics, 41:718, 1968)[171]

Table 42-31. Tests for Carbohydrate Intolerance.

Test	Procedure	Evaluation
Stool pH	Tes-tape or Combistix, drop of liquid stool	pH less than 5.5 suggestive of fermentative diarrhea
Stool-reducing sugars	Liquid stool mixed 2 parts water, 15 drops reacted Clinitest tablet	Positive result suggestive but not diagnostic of fermentative diarrhea
Oral glucose tolerance (galactose, same procedure except galactose 1 g/kg substituted)	After 2–3 days of adequate caloric intake, 2.5 g/kg glucose as 10–20% solution Blood samples fasting, 30, 60, 120 minutes	Appearance of diarrhea, with flat blood glucose curve, suggestive of intolerance. Prolonged starvation may give flat curve by itself
Oral lactose tolerance test (sucrose same except sucrose 2 g/kg substituted)	After 2–3 days of adequate caloric intake, 2.0 g/kg sucrose given as 10% solution Blood samples fasting 30, 60, 120 minutes	Appearance of diarrhea, with less than 20 mg/dl rise in blood glucose, strongly suggests intolerance
Peroral intestinal biopsy	Biopsy with peroral suction capsule, evaluation of vilae under dissecting microscope Assay of lactase, sucrase on biopsy specimen	Quantitation of brush border enzymes confirms CHO intolerance. May also see sprue-like changes in villae Dangerous in small or cachexic infant

begins with the finding of acid stools which contain reducing sugars. Details of tests for carbohydrate intolerance are given in Table 42-31. The offending sugar may often be identified by the baby's previous response to various feedings, and by a judicious trial of glucose water. Usually the diagnosis is so obvious that further confirmatory tests are unnecessary. In more chronic cases, a lactose intolerance test may be performed. Although lactase assay on a peroral intestinal biopsy specimen is definitive, it is rarely feasible in wasted, debilitated infants whose bowel wall may be paper thin. Except in the congenital sugar intolerances, lactase deficiency is almost always present when the other sugars are not tolerated. Obviously, sucrose and glucose tolerance tests can be performed when indicated.

Immune deficiency states may be associated with chronic diarrhea in infancy.[170] The precise mechanisms are unknown, but overgrowth of flora, deconjugation of bile salts, villous atro-

phy, and bacterial invasion of the bowel wall have been postulated. Immunocytes, which are abundant in the bowel wall, and the production of secretory IgA may normally be important in preventing invasion of the gut by bacteria.

Chronic diarrhea is particularly characteristic of the Wiskott–Aldrich syndrome, thymic alymphoplasia, and certain dysgammaglobulinemias. In the Wiskott–Aldrich syndrome, the presence of thrombocytopenia and eczema, often with bloody stools, is helpful in making the diagnosis. Thymic alymphoplasia is characterized by profound lymphopenia in the peripheral blood, absence of the thymic shadow on chest film, the occurrence of pyogenic infections, and ultimately by global immunoglobulin deficiency. However, the presence of passive maternal gamma globulin may be confusing initially. Numerous and complex patterns of immunoglobulin deficiency are now being described, some of them associated with chronic diarrhea often complicated by giardiasis.[170] In general, specific therapy is not available for diarrhea caused by immune deficiency, although one report suggests that fresh plasma may be of temporary benefit,[173] and nonabsorbable antibodies may sometimes help.

Congenital chloridorrhea or Darrow–Gamble syndrome is a rare inborn error of intestinal chloride reabsorption, resulting in loss of chloride, sodium, and potassium in the stools; osmotic diarrhea; metabolic alkalosis; and contraction of extracellular fluid volume, with secondary increased renin and aldosterone.[174] It is relatively more common in Finland, where extensive metabolic and balance studies have been performed. Onset in infancy is usual, with protracted diarrhea and failure to thrive. However, a therapeutic regimen using a mixture of sodium and potassium chloride supplementation, in the dose of 60 to 216 mmol/m² daily, has been successful in maintaining normal body chemistries and supporting long-term survival. The ratio of sodium to potassium chloride is varied from 3:1 to 1:1, according to electrolyte determinations, and the total supplement is increased to the point where some chloride spill in the urine is noted.

Enterokinase deficiency is an extremely rare lack of the brush-border enzyme responsible for activating pancreatic trypsinogen, chymotrypsinogen, and procarboxypeptidase.[175] The diarrheal stools are watery rather than fatty, probably because of the presence of normal lipase and amylase activity. Low serum proteins may be seen. Absent stool trypsin but normal lipase and amylase support the diagnosis, and a favorable response to exogenous pancreatic enzyme preparations is to be expected.

Sensitivity of exogenous protein is an important if somewhat overdiagnosed cause of chronic diarrhea. It is most common in the infant with an atopic family history, and diarrhea may be accompanied by other manifestations such as vomiting, colicky crying, guaiac-positive stools, eosinophilia, and in later infancy, eczema and iron-deficiency anemia. Symptoms begin shortly after exposure to the offending protein, most commonly cow's milk protein but sometimes soy protein as well. The frequency of sensitivity to ovalbumin is the basis for the usual practice of withholding eggs until after the infant is 6 months of age.

Sensitivity to gluten resulting in celiac disease is a related condition which will be discussed below.

Cow's milk protein sensitivity has been estimated to occur in 3 to 10 per 1000 live births.[172] Milder cases may present insidiously in the latter half of the first year of life. The true incidence of this condition is difficult to establish because of the lack of a satisfactory diagnostic test. In general, Koch's postulates must be fulfilled, that is

1. The symptoms only occur when cow protein is contained in the feedings.
2. Withdrawal of cow protein results in disappearance of the symptoms.
3. Rechallenge with cow protein is accompanied by reappearance of the symptoms.

Although many affected infants have serum antibodies to bovine proteins, the finding is nonspecific and is also found in many nonsensitive infants. Management involves substituting a milk not based on cow protein. A soybean preparation is the usual choice because of ready availability and low cost. However, it should be remembered that many babies are also sensitive to soy protein, and may require a milk in which the protein is hydrolysed. The increased permeability of the gut to intact proteins and large peptides, which is characteristic of newborns, becomes greatly diminished after the first year of life; hence, many babies who are initially sensitive can later accept cow's milk.

Parasitic infestation is an uncommon cause of infantile diarrhea in the United States, but should be considered in certain cases. *Giardia lamblia,* a protozoan, is sometimes associated with watery diarrhea, especially in the presence of immune deficiency. Examination of fresh stool preparations on 3 consecutive days plus examination of fasting duodenal aspirate may serve to make the diagnosis. Treatment is given with metronidazole (Flagyl), 10 mg/day for 10 days. Other parasites should also be considered in tropical areas.

Cystic fibrosis of the pancreas occasionally presents in infancy as chronic, intractable diarrhea, although failure to thrive and steatorrhea are more common. Because of its relative frequency, severity, and the availability of enzyme substitution therapy, tests to rule out cystic fibrosis command a high priority in the evaluation of malabsorptive conditions.

The association of pulmonary infections, unexplained pulmonary hyperaeration, or meconium ileus are, of course, highly suggestive. In some cases, hypoproteinemia and edema may occur. It is not necessary here to deal in detail with cystic fibrosis as a disease entity: lengthy discussions are available elsewhere. The diagnosis is suspected when absent or markedly diminished stool trypsins are encountered, and a sweat test is required to rule out isolated pancreatic insufficiency.

Pancreatic insufficiency and bone marrow failure (Schwachman syndrome) may be a cause of malabsorption in infants who do not have cystic fibrosis.[176] Pancreatic enzymes are markedly reduced, but the sweat test is normal. Neutropenia may be constant or cyclic, and anemia or thrombocytopenia may also sometimes be present. Frequent infections, not confined to the lungs, are observed. Poor growth appears to result from malabsorption, and responds to exogenous pancreatic enzyme therapy. Other occasional associations include metaphyseal dysotosis, Hirschsprung's disease, dwarfism, and mental retardation. The mode of inheritance is likely to be an autosomal recessive trait.

Celiac sprue and tropical sprue are not usually encountered in the newborn period. Although a significant cause of malabsorption in childhood, celiac sprue begins, often insidiously, with the introduction of significant amounts of gluten-containing cereal grains into the diet, and usually is recognized after the patient is 6 months of age. Tropical sprue is poorly understood, but is apparently associated with bacterial overgrowth in the upper intestine.

Short bowel syndrome causes diarrhea because of inadequate absorptive surface. It occurs most commonly in infancy from midgut volvulus associated with malrotation, with infarction of a long segment of small intestine (see Chap. 34). Management often requires a period of intravenous alimentation supplementing poorly absorbed oral feedings during the time that the remaining small intestine hypertrophies and increases its absorptive efficiency. Because of the disuse atrophy which occurs with prolonged withholding of oral feedings, it is best to continue and gradually increase oral intake, even in the face of diarrhea. Some success has been achieved with continuous infusion through a gastric tube of a dilute elemental formula such as Vivonex or Pregestimil. Full enteric adaptation and return to normal stool consistency may require several months.

Several relatively uncommon conditions can result in steatorrhea with malabsorption and fatty stools in infancy.

Abetalipoproteinemia is a defect inherited as an autosomal recessive, and is accompanied by other manifestations such as retinitis pigmentosa, CNS degeneration, acanthocytes on peripheral blood smear, and low serum levels of cholesterol and betalipoprotein.[177] It is the result of intestinal mucosal cells being unable to synthesize β-lipoproteins for secretion into the lymphatics, resulting in accumulation of fat in the mucosal cells and the eventual blockage of absorption.

Intestinal lymphangiectasia may be either congenital or acquired and consists of blockage or abnormal development of the intestinal lymphatics and consequent poor absorption of long-chain fats.[177] Perhaps because of back pressure in the lymphatics, there is a protein-losing enteropathy sometimes accompanied by lymphopenia and increased infection. Low plasma proteins and decreased protein half-life in the absence of liver disease or proteinuria are suggestive. Intestinal biopsy may be needed for definitive diagnosis. Both abetalipoproteinemia and intestinal lymphangiectasia are benefited by feedings of medium-chain triglycerides.

Acrodermatitis enteropathica is a rare, familial autosomal recessive disorder, usually characterized by an exudative rash involving the extremities and mucocutaneous areas, alopecia, neurological signs, growth failure, corneal lesions, and chronic diarrhea.[178] It is accompanied by zinc deficiency and responsive to zinc supplementation at the dosage of 1 to 2 mg/kg/day on a maintenance basis. The pathophysiology is not fully defined, but a defect in intestinal zinc absorption seems likely. Breast milk is usually protective. The diarrhea disappears, skin and corneal lesions heal, and growth resumes upon zinc repletion.

Whipple's disease is thought to be an infectious condition and results in steatorrhea and malabsorption. Characteristic PAS-positive macrophages are seen in the mucosa on intestinal biopsy, and improvement may occur after treatment with antibiotics.

Wolman's disease is a lipidosis, with fatty

infiltration of liver and spleen as well as the intestine.[177] Vomiting, abdominal distension, adrenal calcification, anemia, and vacuolization of peripheral lymphocytes may be seen. No specific therapy is available at this time.

Stasis syndrome is the mechanism by which a variety of anatomic abnormalities of the intestine result in diarrhea (see also Chap. 34). Conditions such as Hirschsprung's disease, malrotation, ileal or jejunal stenosis, scarring from intrauterine peritonitis, and blind loop syndrome are examples of this association. Compromise of the circulation and overgrowth of enteric bacteria play prominent roles. Barium studies of the upper and lower intestinal tract may be useful in diagnosis. Therapy is directed at correcting the underlying anatomic defect, although antibiotics may be of temporary benefit.

Hepatobiliary disease may result in steatorrhea. Faulty emulsification of fats caused by absence of bile salts is the explanation most commonly given. However, portal hypertension and ascites may also interfere with the dynamics of absorption, and result in protein loss. Silverberg and Davidson have stated that infants with biliary atresia absorb only between 20% and 65% of ingested fats, with consequent caloric loss.[179] Deficiencies of the fat soluble vitamins are also common. The diagnosis is usually obvious, with jaundice and an enlarged liver. Provision of extra calories as carbohydrates, substitution of medium-chain triglycerides for part of the fat intake, and supplementation of fat-soluble vitamins at more than the usual dosage are essentials of therapy. The prothrombin time should be monitored, and occasional films taken of the long bones to look for signs of rickets. Intramuscular vitamin D and vitamin K have been necessary in a number of our patients. (See also Chap. 24.)

Malabsorption of specific nutrients without diarrhea may occasionally occur in infants. **Primary hypomagnesemia** resulting from a defect in intestinal absorption has been reported, and is accompanied by hypocalcemia and tetany.[177] Certain of the aminoacidurias are accompanied by specific amino acid absorptive defects.[172] These include phenylketonuria, maple syrup urine disease, Oast-house disease (methionine malabsorption), cystinuria, and blue diaper syndrome. Congenital defects have been reported in the ability to absorb, respectively, folic acid and vitamin B_{12}. The **folic acid deficiency** is manifest by diarrhea, megaloblastic anemia, neurologic deterioration and mouth ulcers, and can be corrected by ordinary doses of folic acid by injection or enormous doses given by mouth.[172] **Congenital vitamin B_{12}** *malabsorption* may result from deficiency of intrinsic factor (pernicious anemia) or from unresponsiveness of the ileum to normal amounts of intrinsic factor (Immerslund's syndrome).[172] In either case, the symptoms are megaloblastic anemia, failure to thrive, and psychomotor retardation. Treatment is vitamin B_{12} by injection, 100 μg per month.

Endocrine states associated with intractable diarrhea include thyrotoxicosis, hypoadrenal states, pheochromocytoma, and other catecholamine-secreting neural crest tumors. In the case of thyrotoxicosis, other manifestations of the disease are usually present and aid in the diagnosis: enlarged thyroid gland, proptosis, tachycardia, sweating, and history of maternal Graves' disease. In newborns, variants of the adrenogenital syndrome are more common than primary hypoadrenalism (Addison's disease). If genital stigmata are absent, presentation may be subtle, and intractable vomiting, diarrhea, or both may be the initial complaints. Catecholamine-secreting tumors are rare, but may present difficult diagnostic problems. Accordingly, when simpler studies fail to reveal the cause of intractable diarrhea, a 24-hour urine should be collected for 17-hydroxy and 17-ketosteroids, and for catecholamines (vanillylmandelic acid). For detailed discussion of these conditions, see Chapter 44.

Enterocolitis

Neonatal necrotizing enterocolitis is a severe and relatively common entity which has been estimated to occur in 2% of all admissions to newborn intensive care units and to account for about 2% of deaths in prematures.[180] Onset is usually within the first week or two of life, and the course is frequently fulminant, with perforation common and death occurring in about 30% of cases.

A definite predisposed group can be identified. The majority of cases occur in prematures. Maternal complications are frequent, especially those associated with fetal distress and neonatal shock and hypoxia. Prolonged rupture of the membranes and maternal infection are also quite common. Low Apgar scores are recorded in many of these babies, and some have severe perinatal illness such as hyaline membrane disease.

Two factors seem paramount in causing neonatal necrotizing enterocolitis: ischemia of the intestine and the action of enteric bacteria. Systemic shock and hypoxia result in powerful responses of the sympathetic nervous system and adrenal medulla, shunting blood to the heart and brain and interrupting flow to the gut and kidney. Analogy has been made to the diving reflex of the seal which conserves oxygen consumption in this way during long dives. However, if intestinal ischemia is too protracted, damage and finally digestion of the mucosa may begin, together with thrombosis of fine vascular channels and local infarction of the bowel. Once shock has been corrected and more normal circulation restored, repair and regeneration can begin. However, the action of enteric bacteria and the onset of feeding may further complicate the situation.

Under these conditions, adynamic ileus and stasis are to be expected. Initial colonization of the gut is followed by overgrowth of enteric bacteria (see above discussion of diarrhea with immune deficiency or intestinal stasis). Invasion of the devitalized bowel wall occurs, and bacteria together with inflammatory cells are seen in the submucosa. Systemic sepsis is a common terminal event.

If the infant is fed at this time, intestinal bacteria are provided with abundant substrate, and further overgrowth occurs in the adynamic upper bowel. Gas is formed in the bowel wall, producing subserosal blebs and sometimes dissecting through the portal system into the liver. Engel and coworkers have shown that the substrate provided by oral feedings is necessary for this intramural gas formation.[181] Large segments of intestine may be involved— sometimes the entire small bowel. Perforation of this thin and friable bowel is common.

A significant association of neonatal enterocolitis with umbilical arterial and venous catheters has been noted. But thrombosis of major mesenteric arteries is rarely seen, and it may be the underlying disease which placed the infant at risk and in turn resulted in both placement of the catheter to facilitate care and critical ischemia of the bowel. Touloukian and coworkers have noted a series of cases associated with exchange transfusion in the absence of many of the usual predisposing perinatal complications.[182] Perhaps, as they suggest, interruption of portal venous flow during the exchange transfusion resulted in vascular compromise of the gut, although this must be a relatively uncommon occurrence.

A peculiar feature of NEC is its tendency to occur in "epidemics." This clustering of cases has been repeatedly observed, but as yet has not been consistently associated with any seasonal or infectious factor, nor has nosocomial spread been proved. The bacteria cultured from affected infants include *E. coli,* Klebsiella, Pseudomonas, Staphylococcus, Enterococcus, and Clostridia. One is tempted to speculate that a virus, an anaerobe, or a toxin (perhaps carried by bacteria as a plasmid) may play a crucial role in pathogenesis. Clostridia enterotoxin has been mentioned in this connection.[183]

Early diagnosis depends upon awareness of the group of infants at risk, and their careful observation for relatively nonspecific signs. Systemic symptoms include temperature instability, lethargy or irritability, apnea, and signs associated with sepsis. GI problems include distension, vomiting, delayed gastric emptying with residua or bile-stained contents, and blood in the stools. Confirmation of the diagnosis can often be made on plain AP and lateral x-ray films of the abdomen demonstrating thickened bowel walls, loops of unequal size, a bubbly appearance of the intestinal contents, and the diagnostic findings of air in the bowel wall, pneumatosis intestinalis. Air in the portal system is a late and ominous sign.

Management consists of withholding oral feedings and placing a tube for gastric drainage, supporting the circulation with blood, plasma, or low-molecular-weight dextran, giving vigorous fluid and electrolyte therapy by vein with as many calories as can be achieved, and administering oral and systemic antibiotics. Because of the frequency of systemic sepsis, we give ampicillin and gentamicin parenterally. A recent report suggests promising results from administration by nasogastric tube of two to three times the systemic dose of gentamicin or kanamycin until 48 hours after subsidence of symptoms.[184] The frequency of perforation requires close following with a pediatric surgeon, with serial evaluation of the abdomen for sudden appearance of tenderness or splinting, and frequent plain films of the abdomen. Although some surgeons favor operating on all cases with pneumatosis intestinalis, it seems advisable to wait for actual or impending perforation, as advised by Stevenson and co-workers.[185] With aggressive management, the mortality from this potentialy devastating condition can be reduced appreciably.

Increased awareness of NEC has caused the diagnosis to be suspected in many high-risk prematures with distension, gastric residua, and hematest positive stools, without waiting for the classic criterion of pneumatosis intestinalis. Therapy instituted at this point will often abort further development of the disease. As with the suspicion of sepsis, however, it is uncertain how often a catastrophic disease process has been interrupted and how often the functionally hypodynamic bowel of the premature has been overdiagnosed as NEC. It certainly seems as though less surgery for perforation has been necessary since early intervention has become usual.

Convalescence from severe NEC may be complicated and prolonged. When enterostomy and intravenous alimentation have been necessary, scarring and stenosis in the distal segment may occur. Diarrhea and malabsorption are common upon refeeding, which must be cautious and gradual. In some cases stenosis, adhesions, or other gross anatomic changes explain the dysfunction. In other instances, it must be the residua of massive necrosis and disruption of the lining layer of the gut, with continuing changes at the microscopic and functional level.

Other Enterocolitis. "Specific" enterocolitis is a term which might be used to denote certain inflammatory intestinal conditions in small infants similar in many ways to the above description of NEC, but sometimes discussed separately in the literature. The predisposed group, the timing of presentation, and the surrounding circumstances may differ, but the pathophysiology is essentially the same. Thus **Hirschsprung's enterocolitis** is probably an instance of stasis syndrome, in which vascular compromise may also occur because of obstruction of capillary flow from increased intraluminal pressure.

Pseudomembranous enterocolitis associated with overgrowth of *Staphylococcus* in the gut is probably a specific instance of an enterotoxic bacterial strain which causes breakdown of mucosal integrity under conditions in which the bowel is already partly compromised. Neo-natal **ulcerative colitis** has been described,[186] but some cases may well be neonatal NEC localized primarily to the colon. In other cases, immune injury to the colon, similar to adult disease, may play a part. We have used the term **nonspecific enterocolitis** to denote a self-perpetuating diarrhea associated with mucosal breakdown which may occur in the wake of many initial diarrheal states (see below).[136] However, once established, many aspects of the pathophysiology and of the bowel histology at autopsy precisely parallel neonatal NEC.

Nonspecific Intractable Diarrhea. In our series, 60% of the intractable cases could be associated with a definite causal factor.[136] Yet a group of babies remains in whom an adequate diagnosis cannot be found, who nevertheless meet the following criteria:

1. Onset of diarrhea in the first 3 months of life
2. Diarrhea continuing more than 2 weeks despite ordinary conservative therapy
3. Three or more negative stool cultures

These cases develop self-perpetuating mechanisms, and form a relatively severe group which we have termed nonspecific enterocolitis. Proctoscopy often reveals colonic inflammation and friability, and examination of the bowel in those who die shows widespread involvement of the small intestine, with loss of mucosa, inflammatory exudate in the submucosa, and invasion of the intestinal wall by bacteria. Systemic sepsis is a frequent complication, although pneumatosis intestinalis and perforation are less common than in postshock neonatal necrotizing enterocolitis.

Diarrhea-perpetuating Mechanisms. The original cause of the diarrhea in these babies is sometimes relatively trivial, and often no cause can be defined. However, once infantile diarrhea has continued for a period of time, secondary changes occur which are the combined result of progressive injury to the gut itself and of acute starvation in an actively growing neonate. Some of these diarrhea-perpetuating mechanisms are listed in Table 42-32. Perhaps the best known is acquired carbohydrate intolerance resulting from loss of mucosal brush border enzymes. In the more severe cases, glucose and galactose, as well as lactose, will exacerbate the diarrhea.

The bowel flora modifies intestinal function and bacterial overgrowth complicates many

Table 43-32. Diarrhea-perpetuating Mechanisms.

Loss of brush-border enzymes
(secondary carbohydrate intolerance)
Sprue-like changes of mucosal villae
(steatorrhea)
Pancreatic insufficiency
(deficient intraluminal digestion)
Abnormal motility
Delayed regeneration of mucosal cells
Specific deficiencies—malnutrition
(Cu, Mg, vitamins, protein)
Deranged bowel flora
Mural invasion of enteric flora
Hyperacidity
Fistula formation
Adjacent infection

diarrheal states. Germ-free animals have long, delicate mucosal villi, with slower cellular turnover rates and higher values of brush border enzymes. Normally, less than 10^3 bacteria/ml are found in the upper small intestine, and bacterial counts of 10^8 or more are associated with diarrhea. Excess bacteria in the upper intestine may deconjugate bile salts to form more irritating acids.

Both starvation and overgrowth of enteric bacteria have been associated with blunting of mucosal villi, similar to the changes in sprue. Intense anabolism is required for the constant regeneration of mucosal cells to replace those sloughed from the villi. This constant renewal appears to be necessary to prevent digestion and breakdown of the intestinal lining layer. It is scarcely surprising that under the catabolic conditions of chronic diarrhea, regeneration is slowed.

Temporary deficiency of the pancreatic digestive enzymes has been reported under conditions of starvation and many interfere with intraluminal digestion. Hyperacidity in the small intestine causes inefficient absorption, and may result both from bacterial fermentation and failure to neutralize gastric acid. The formation of fistulae or walled-off abscesses may result in rapid intestinal transit. Abnormal motility is common, and may take the form of rapid transit or of stasis with accumulation in the lumen of large quantities of fluid and electrolytes. Specific deficiency states, some of them capable of causing diarrhea, are encountered. Thus, recovery may be hampered by lack of protein, vitamins, or ions such as copper or magnesium.

It is easy to construct vicious cycles whereby diarrhea and malnutrition feed upon one another. Once diarrhea is longstanding, malnutrition is inevitable because of severely compromised absorption. Malnutrition, in turn, interferes with the processes of repair and regeneration in the gut. Feedings provoke worse diarrhea, yet the infant has scant caloric reserves to tolerate additional periods of fasting. The integrity of the intestinal mucosa breaks down in the face of chronic injury and requires a period which may last several weeks for complete recovery. The situation is like an

Table 42-33. Organic Causes of Failure to Thrive.

Series	Total No. in Series	CNS	GI (includes CF)	Urinary tract	Cardio-vascular	Respira-tory	Endo-crine	Other
Riley RL, et al 1968[192]	40	10	11	4	2	9		4
Hannaway PJ 1970[191]	49	18	12	5	4	1	5	4
Shaheen E et al 1968*[187]	243	52	43	14	38	16	12	54*
Ambuel and Harris 1963†[189]	68	18	10	4	26	2	5	3
Total	400	98	76	27	70	28	22	65

* Includes all infants and children admitted with weights less than the third percentile. Other causes are congenital anomalies, surgical, blood and tumors, skeletal and miscellaneous
† Includes probable and possible causes of failure to thrive

internal burn, with epithelial breakdown, bacterial invasion, the loss of large volumes of fluid and electrolyte from the damaged surface, and occasional scarring in the recovery process which may result in stenosis or atresia of involved intestine.

Therapy. These above considerations dictate therapy. If conservative management fails and a treatable underlying condition cannot be identified, the bowel should be placed at rest with no oral feedings whatsoever for 2 to 4 weeks. During this period it is essential that nutrition be provided and depleted stores replenished. Hence, support by total intravenous alimentation is necessary. It should be borne in mind that more than ordinary allowances of calories may be required on a per-kilogram basis because the cachectic infant has a large active cell mass for his weight. Great care should be given to maintaining proper fluid and electrolyte homeostasis, repairing deficits of vitamins and specific ions such as magnesium, and detecting and treating systemic sepsis. Some investigators recommend systemic or oral antibiotics even in the absence of an identifiable enteric pathogen. Adequately controlled studies are not yet available. Excellent results have been encountered recently with protracted bowel rest and intravenous alimentation. The latter therapeutic tool has permitted the prognosis in nonspecific enterocolitis to be reversed, so that now survival is usual.

Failure to Thrive

Failure to thrive in infancy is a source of challenge and frustration to clinicians, and has been the subject of several reports.[188-190] Defined as growth failure in an infant with disproportionate lag in weight gain, it identifies a different group from dwarfism, defined by stunted height. Infants with failure to thrive frequently have disorders of nutrition, emotional environment, CNS, heart, kidneys, or GI tract. Many remain unexplained even after exhaustive study.

Approximately one-half of infants who fail to thrive ultimately prove that their condition resulted from inadequate intake or family problems. In one series, Hannaway found that failure to thrive made up approximately 1% of pediatric admissions.[191] Of this group 51% were "nonorganic," predominantly feeding and environmental problems. Of the feeding

problems, 24 of 25 were less than 6 months old; of the organic problems, most were less than 12 months; and the majority of those thought to be deprivation or constitutional were greater than 1 year of age at presentation. The low-birth-weight infant is at greater risk, 20% of this series being less than 2500 g at birth.

Among those who prove to have "organic" lesions, problems of the central nervous system, heart, kidneys and gastrointestinal tract predominate. Individual series vary according to age and criteria for selection, but serve to illustrate the type and variety of lesions represented (Table 42-33).

An exhaustive, stereotyped laboratory evaluation is inadvisable in failure to thrive, because a relatively small number of diagnostic tests actually yield useful information. Most of the conditions which come to light can be suspected from a careful history and physical examination. Many of the initial studies which prove valuable can be performed in an outpatient setting. A list of such general screening procedures includes history, physical examination, evaluation of family, complete blood count, urinalysis including pH and specific gravity, bone age, thyroxine (T_4, TSH), intravenous pyelogram, urine culture, serum urea nitrogen, serum Na, K, Cl, CO_2, sweat test and stool trypsin. Beyond these basic tests, the next step is a period of observation in the hospital to document oral intake and evaluate the response of the child to nurture. Finally, a wide variety of diagnostic possibilities opens up, as partially indicated in Table 42-34. Further studies should be those needed to follow up on particular diagnostic clues.

Individual children vary in the timing of their growth. Many children with failure to thrive resume normal growth despite our inability to supply specific therapy. However, the overall prognosis in failure to thrive must be guarded. In the series of Ambuel and Harris, 69% of the "nonorganic" group achieved normal height and weight, or showed improved growth rates.[189] Yet Bullard and coworkers reported an 8-month to 9-year follow-up of 41 similar patients, of whom only 35% were normal, with one-third still failing to thrive, 15% with IQ below 80, and an equal number with severe emotional disorders.[193] Others have published similar results.[194-196]

Table 42-34. Diagnosis of Failure to Thrive.

Organ System	Specialized Tests	Confirmatory Tests
RENAL		
Urinary infection	24-Hour urine for bicarbonate ti-	Kidney biopsy
Renal tubular acidosis	tratable acid, creatine, Na, K,	Pitressin test for diabetes insipi-
Diabetes insipidus	Ca, PO$_4$	dus
Dysplactic kidney	Cystourethrogram	
Polycystic kidney	Concentration test	
CNS		
Mental retardation	Deveopmental examination	Lumbar puncture
Diencephalic syndrome	Skull films	Ventriculogram, CT scan
	EEG	
GI		
Malabsorptive syndrome	Sweat test	Mucosal biopsy
Cystic fibrosis	Fat balance	Duodenal drainage
Celiac disease	Lactose tolerance	
Pancreatic insufficiency	Xylose tolerance	
Disaccharide intolerance	GI series	
	Barium enema	
CARDIAC		
Large L-R shunts	ECG	Cardiac catheterization
Pulmonary hypertension	Chest film	
Hypoxia	Cardiac series	
ENDOCRINE		
Hypothyroid	Glucose tolerance with insulin	Pneumoencephalogram or CT
Panhypopituitarism	and growth hormone	(only for special indication)
Isolated growth hormone defi-	Insulin and/or arginine stim. of	
ciency	nonresponders	
	Skull films	
GENETIC AND METABOLIC DISEASE		
Idiopathic hypercalcemia	Urine-reducing substances	Amino acid chromatography
Storage diseases	Ferric chloride	Liver biopsy
Errors of metabolism	Urine mucopolysaccharides	Bone marrow
Obscure chromosomal disor-	Nitroprusside	Chromosomal karyotype
ders (Turner)	Dinitrophenylhydrazine	
	Calcium, phosphorus	
	Buccal smear	
INFECTION		
GU infection (see renal)	Chest film	Appropriate cultures
Tuberculosis	Stool culture × 3	Attempted virus isolation
Chronic intrauterine infection	Stool for blood, ova,	
	parasites × 3	
	Skull film	
	Careful funduscopic	
	Specific antibody titers	

REFERENCES

1. **Koldovský O:** Digestion and absorption during development. In Stave U (ed): Physiology of the Perinatal Period. Appleton-Century-Crofts, New York, 1970
2. **Go VLW, Summerskill WHJ:** Digestion, maldigestion, and the gastrointestinal hormones. Am J Clin Nutr 24:160, 1971
3. **Silen W:** Advances in gastric physiology. N Engl J Med 27:864, 1967
4. **Ballinger WF II:** The small intestine following vagotomy. Surg Gynecol Obstet 116:115, 1963
5. **Herbst JJ, Sunshine P, Kretchmer N:** Intestinal malabsorption in infancy and childhood. In Schulman I (ed): Advances in Pediatrics, Vol. 16. Year Book Publishers, Chicago, 1969
6. **Smith CA:** The Physiology of the Newborn Infant, 3rd ed, pp 234–235, 249. Charles C Thomas, Springfield, 1959
7. **Parsons DS:** Salt and water absorption by the intestinal tract. Br Med Bull 23:252, 1967
8. **Coello-Ramirez P, Lifshitz F:** Enteric microflora and carbohydrate intolerance in infants with diarrhea. Pediatrics 49:233, 1972
9. **Andrews BF, Cook LN:** Low birth weight infants fed a new carbohydrate free formula with different sugars. Am J Clin Nutr 22:845, 1969
10. **Grand RL, Watkins JB, Torti FM:** Development of the human gastrointestinal tract. Gastroenterol 70:790–810, 1976
11. **Jeffries GH, Holman HR, Sleisinger MH:** Plasma proteins and the gastrointestinal tract. N Engl J Med 266:652, 1962
12. **Matthews DM:** Intestinal absorption of peptides. Physiol Rev 55:537–608, 1975
13. **Gruskay FL, Cooke RE:** Gastrointestinal absorption of unaltered protein in normal infants and in infants recovering from diarrhea. Pediatrics 16:763, 1955
14. **Hamosh M, Klaeveman RO, Wolf RO, Slow RO:** Pharyngeal lipase and digestion of dietary triglyceride in man. J Clin Invest 55:908–913, 1975
15. **Greenberger NH, Skillman TG:** Medium-chain triglycerides. N Engl J Med 208:1045, 1969
16. **Watkins JB, Ingal D, Scezepanik P, Klein PD, Lester R:** Bile salt metabolism in the newborn. N Engl J Med 288:431, 1973
17. **Fomon SJ, Ziegler EE, Thomas LN, Jensen RL, Filer LJ:** Excretion of fat by normal full-term infants fed various milks and formulas. Am J Clin Nutr 23:1299, 1970
18. **Smith CA:** The Physiology of the Newborn Infant, 3rd ed, pp 285–286. Charles C Thomas, Springfield, 1959
19. **Mitchell HS, Rynbargen HJ, Anderson L, Dibble MV:** Cooper's Nutrition in Health and Disease, 15th ed, JB Lippincott, Philadelphia, 1968
20. **Levine R:** Mechanisms of insulin secretion. N Engl J Med 283:522, 1970
21. **Unger RH:** Glucagon physiology and pathophysiology. N Engl J Med 285:443, 1971
22. **Root A:** Growth hormone. Pediatrics 36:940, 1965
23. **Zierlier KL, Rabinowitz D:** Roles of insulin and growth hormone based on studies of forearm metabolism in man. Medicine 42:385, 1963
24. **Tobin JD, Roux JF, Soeldner JS:** Human fetal insulin response after acute maternal glucose administration during labor. Pediatrics 44:668, 1969
25. **Keele DK, Kay JL:** Plasma free fatty acid and blood sugar levels in newborn infants and their mothers. Pediatrics 37:597, 1966
26. **James EJ, Raye JR, Gresham EL, Makowski EL, Meshia G, Battaglia FC:** Fetal oxygen consumption, carbon dioxide production, and glucose uptake in a chronic sheep preparation. Pediatrics 50:361, 1972
27. **Cahill GF Jr:** Starvation in man. N Engl J Med 282:668, 1970
28. **Parra A, Garza C, Garza Y, Saravia JL, Hazelwood CF, Nichols BL:** Changes in growth hormone, insulin, and thyroxin values, and in energy metabolism of marasmic infants. J Pediatr 82:133, 1973
29. **Alleyne EAO:** The effect of severe protein calorie malnutrition on the renal function of Jamaican children. Pediatrics 39:400, 1967
30. **Chandra RK:** Immunocompetence in undernutrition. J Pediatr 81:1194, 1972
31. **Barbezat EO, Hansen JDL:** The exocrine pancreas and protein–caloric malnutrition. Pediatrics 42:77, 1968
32. **Brunser O, Reid A, Monckeberg F, Maccioni A, Contreas I:** Jejunal biopsies in infant malnutrition: with special reference to mitotic index. Pediatrics 38:605, 1966
33. **Widdowson EM:** The first feed. In Sunshine P, Jeffries JE (eds): Gastrointestinal Development and Neonatal Nutrition, p 16. Ross Laboratories, Columbus, 1977
34. **Heird WC:** Effects of total parenteral alimentation on intestinal function. In Sunshine P, Jeffries JE (eds): Gastrointestinal Function and Neonatal Nutrition, p 68. Ross Laboratories, Columbus, 1977
35. **Williamson RCN:** Intestinal adaptation. N Engl J Med 298:1444–1450, 1978
36. **Walker WA:** Development of gastrointestinal function and selected dysfunctions. In Perinatal Developmental Medicine, Mead Johnson Symposium 11:3–11, 1977
37. **Scrimshaw NW, Gordon JE:** Malnutrition,

Learning, and Behavior. MIT Press, Cambridge, 1968

38. **Winick M:** Cellular growth during early malnutrition. Pediatrics 47:969, 1971

39. **Eid EE:** Follow-up study of the physical growth of children who had excessive weight gain in the first six months of life. Br Med J 2:74, 1970

40. **Heald FP, Hollander RJ:** The relationship between obesity in adolescence and early growth. J Pediatr 67:35, 1968

41. **Rose HE, Mayer J:** Activity, caloric intake, fat storage, and the energy balance of infants. Pediatrics 41:18, 1968

42. **Hill JR, Rahimtulla KA:** Heat balance and the metabolic rate of newborn babies in relation to environmental temperature; and the effect of age and weight on basal metabolic rate. J Physiol 180:239, 1965

43. **Montgomery RO:** Changes in the basal metabolic rate of the malnourished infant and their relation to body composition. J Clin Invest 41:1653, 1962

44. **Rigo J, Senterre J:** Is taurine essential for neonates? Biol Neonate 32:73–76, 1977

45. **Fomon SJ:** Body composition of the infant. In Faulkner F: Human Development, p 245. WB Saunders, Philadelphia, 1966

46. **Widdowson EM:** Growth and composition of the fetus and newborn. In Assali NS: Biology of Gestation, Vol. II, p 23. Academic Press, New York, 1968

47. **Mayer J:** Hypertension, salt intake, and the infant. Postgrad Med 45:229, 1969

48. **Bessman SP:** Genetic failure of amino acid "justification": A common basis for many forms of metabolic, nutritional, and "nonspecific" mental retardation. J Pediatr 81:834, 1972

49. **Davidson M, Levine SZ, Bauer CH, Dann M:** Feeding studies in low-birth-weight infants. I. Relationships of dietary protein, fat, and electrolytes to rates of weight gain, clinical courses, and serum chemical concentrations. J Pediatr 70:695, 1967

50. **Kagan BM et al:** Body composition of premature infants: relation to nutrition. Am J Clin Nutr 25:1153, 1972

51. **Snyderman SE, Holt LE Jr, Norton POM, Phanselkar SV:** Protein requirement of the premature infant. I. Influence of protein intake on free amino acid content of plasma and red blood cells. Am J Clin Nutr 23:890, 1970

52. **Goldman HI, Liebman OB, Freudenthal R, Reuben R:** Effects of early dietary protein intake on low-birth-weight infants: Evaluation at 3 years of age. J Pediatr 78:126, 1971

53. **Raiha NCR, Heinonen K, Rassin DK, Guull**

GE: Milk protein quantity and quality in low-birth weight infants: I. Metabolic responses and effects on growth. Pediatrics 57:659–674, 1976

54. **Davies DP:** Adequacy of expressed breast milk for early growth of pre-term infants. Arch Dis Child 2:296–301, 1977

55. **Schneider HJ, Kinter WB, Stirling CE:** Glucose–galactose malabsorption. N Engl J Med 274:305, 1966

56. **Hahn P:** Lipids. In Stave U: Physiology of the Perinatal Period, Vol. 1, pp 457–492. Appleton-Century-Crofts, New York, 1970

57. **Greenberg LD, Wheeler P:** Influence of fatty acid composition of infant formulas on the development of arteriosclerosis and on the lipid composition of blood and tissues. Nutr Metab 14:100, 1972

58. **Fomon SJ:** Infant Nutrition, 2nd ed, p 212. WB Saunders, Philadelphia, 1974

59. **Fomon SJ:** Infant Nutrition, 2nd ed, pp 362–363. WB Saunders, 1974

60. National Academy of Sciences and National Research Council: Recommended Dietary Allowances, 8th ed. National Academy of Sciences Printing and Publishing Office, Washington, 1973

61. **Fomon SJ:** Infant Nutrition, 2nd ed. WB Saunders, Philadelphia, 1974

62. **Melhorn DK, Gross S:** Vitamin E dependent anemia in the premature infant. II Relationship between gestational age and absorption of vitamin E. J Pediatr 79:581–588, 1971

63. **Williams ML, Schott RJ, O'Neal PL, Oski F:** Role of dietary iron and fat on vitamin E deficiency anemia of infancy. N Engl J Med 292:887–890, 1975

64. **Gross S:** Hemolytic anemia in premature infants: relationship to vitamin E, selenium, glutathione peroxidase, and erythrocyte lipids. Semin Hematol 13:187–199, 1976

65. **Johnson L, Schaffer D, Boggs TL Jr:** The premature infant, vitamin E deficiency and retrolental fibroplasia. Am J Clin Nutr 27:1158–1173, 1974

66. **Ehrenkranz RA, Bonta BW, Ablow RC, Warshaw JB:** Amelioration of bronchopulmonary dysplasia after vitamin E administration. N Engl J Med 299:564–569, 1978

67. **Shafer RB:** Current concepts of calcium absorption. Calif Med 114:91, 1971

68. **Hanna S, Harrison MT, MacIntyre I, Fraser R:** Effects of growth hormone on calcium and magnesium metabolism. Br Med J 2:12, 1961

69. **Tsang RL, Donovan EF, Steichen JJ:** Calcium physiology and pathology in the neonate. Pediatr Clin North Am 23:611–626, 1976

70. Committee on Nutrition, Am Acad Pediatrs:

Iron supplementation for infants. Pediatrics 58:765–768, 1976

71. **Sandstead HH, Burk RF, Booth EH Jr, Darby WJ:** Current concepts on trace minerals. Med Clin North Am 54:1509, 1970

72. **Sandstead HH:** Zinc, a metal to grow on. Nutr Today 3:12, 1968

73. **Henkin RI, Schulman JD, Schulman CB, Bronzert DA:** Changes in total non-diffusible, and diffusible plasma zinc and copper during infancy. J Pediatr 82:831, 1973

74. **Dauncey MJ, Shaw JCL, Urman J:** The absorption and retention of magnesium, zinc, and copper by low-birth weight infants fed pasteurized human breast milk. Pediatr Res 11:991–997, 1977

75. **Michie DD, Wirth FH:** Plasma zinc levels in premature infants receiving parenteral nutrition. J Pediatr 92:798–800, 1978

76. **Mertz W:** Biological role of chromium. Fed Proc 26:186, 1967

77. **Formon SJ, Wei SHY:** Prevention of dental caries. In Formon SJ (ed): Nutritional Disorders of Children, p 90. DHEW Publication No. (HSA) 76-5612, Rockville, 1977

78. **Hambraeus L, Lonnerdal B, Forsum E, Gebre–Medhin M:** Nitrogen and protein components of human milk. Acta Paediatr Scand 67:561, 1978

79. **György P:** Biochemical aspects. Am J Clin Nutr 24:970, 1971

80. **Graham GG, Placko RP, Morales E, Acevedo G, Cordano A:** Dietary protein quality in infants and children. Am J Dis Child 120:419, 1970

81. **Eastham EJ, Lichauco T, Grady MI, Walker WA:** Antigenicity of infant formulas: Role of immature intestine on protein permeability. J Pediatr 93:561, 1978

82. **Fomon SJ, Ziegler EE, Thomas LN, Jensen RL, Filer LJ:** Excretion of fat by normal full-term infants fed various milks and formulas. Am J Clin Nutr 23:1299, 1970

83. **Fomon SJ:** Skim Milk in Infant Feeding. Commentaries on Infant and Child Nutrition. U. S. Department of Health, Education and Welfare, January, 1973

84. **Fomon SJ:** Infant Nutrition, 2nd ed. WB Saunders, Philadelphia, 1974

85. **Saarinen UM, Siimes MA:** Iron absorption from breast milk, cow's milk, and iron-supplemented formula: An opportunistic use of changes in total body iron determined by hemoglobin, ferritin, and body weight in 132 infants. Pediatr Res 13:143, 1979

86. **Bullen JJ, Rogers HJ, Leigh L:** Iron-binding proteins in milk and resistance to *Escherichia coli* infection in infants. Br Med J 1:69, 1972

87. **Woodruff CW, Latham BA, McDavid S:** Iron nutrition in the breast-fed infant. J Pediatr 90:36, 1977

88. **Olson M:** The benign effects on rabbit lungs of the aspiration of water compared with 5% glucose or milk. Pediatrics 46:538, 1970

89. **Gryboski JD:** Suck and swallow in the premature infant. Pediatrics 43:96, 1969

90. **Räihä NCR, Heinonen K, Rassin DK, Gaull GE:** Milk protein quantity and quality in low-birthweight infants: I. Metabolic responses and effects on growth. Pediatrics 57:659, 1976

91. **Rassin DK, Gaull GE, Heinonen K, Räihä NCR:** Milk protein quantity and quality in low-birthweight infants: II. Effects on selected aliphatic amino acids in plasma and urine. Pediatrics 59:407, 1977

92. **Gaull GE, Rassin DK, Räihä NCR, Heinonen K:** Milk protein quantity and quality in low birthweight infants: III. Effects on sulfur amino acids in plasma and urine. J Pediatr 90:348, 1977

93. **Rassin DK, Gaull GE, Räihä NCR, Heinonen K:** Milk protein quantity and quality in low birthweight infants: IV. Effects on tyrosine and phenylalanine in plasma and urine. J Pediatr 90:356, 1977

94. **Davies DP:** Adequacy of expressed breast milk for early growth of perterm infants. Arch Dis Child 52:296, 1977

95. **Atkinson SA, Bryan MH, Anderson GH:** Human milk: Difference in nitrogen concentration in milk from mothers of term and premature infants. J Pediatr 93:67, 1978

96. **Gross SJ, David RJ, Bauman L, Tomarelli RM:** Nutritional composition of human milk in mothers of preterm infants. Pediatr Res 13:400, 1979 (abstr.)

97. **Oski FA, Barnes LA:** Vitamin E deficiency: A previously unrecognized cause of hemolytic anemia in the premature. J Pediatr 70:211, 1967

98. **Melhorn DK, Gross S:** Vitamin E dependent anemia in the premature. I. Effect of large doses of medicinal iron. J Pediatr 79:569, 1971

99. **Melhorn DK, Gross S:** Vitamin E dependent anemia in the premature infant. II. Relationship between gestational age and absorption of Vitamin E. J Pediatr 79:581, 1971

100. **Bell EF, Brown EJ, Milner R et al:** Vitamin E absorption in small premature infants. Pediatrics 63:830, 1979

101. **Graeber JE, Williams ML, Oski FA:** The use of intramuscular vitamin E in the premature infant. J Pediatr 90:1977

102. **Minton SD, Steichen JJ, Tsang RC:** Bone mineral content in term and preterm appro-

priate for gestational age infants. J Pediatr 95:1037, 1979

103. **Garin EH, Geary D, Richard GA:** Soybean formula (Neo-Mull-Soy) metabolic alkalosis in infancy. J Pediatr 95:985, 1979

104. **Burton BK, Nadler HL:** Clinical Diagnosis of the Inborn Errors of Metabolism in the Neonatal Period. Pediatrics 61:398, 1978

105. **Smith RM, Brumley GW, Stannard MW:** Neonatal pneumonia associated with medium-chain triglyceride feeding supplement. J Pediatr 92:801, 1978

106. **Rhea JW, Graham AW Jr, Akhnoukh F, Parthew CT:** Effect of hyperbaric oxygenation on neonatal tetanus. J Pediatr 71:33, 1967

107. **Cheek JA, Staub GF:** Nasojejunal alimentation for premature and full-term newborn infants. J Pediatr 82:955, 1973

108. **Rhea JW, Ghazzawi O, Weidman W:** Nasojejunal feeding: An improved device and intubation technique. J Pediatr 82:951, 1973

109. **van Caillie M, Powell GK:** Nasoduodenal versus nasogastric feeding in the very low birthweight infant. Pediatrics 56:1065, 1975

110. **Schaff–Blass E, Kuhns LR, Wyman ML:** Gastric air insufflation as an aid to placement of oroduodenal tubes. J Pediatr 89:954, 1976

111. **Wells DH, Zachman RD:** Nasojejunal feedings in low-birth-weight infants. J Pediatr 87:276, 1975

112. **Roy RN, Pollnitz RP, Hamilton JR, Chance GW:** Impaired assimilation of nasojejunal feeds in healthy low-birth-weight newborn infants. J Pediatr 90:431, 1977

113. **Challacombe D:** Bacterial microflora in infants receiving nasojejunal tube feeding. J Pediatr 85:113, 1974

114. **Berg RB, Schuster SR, Colodny AH:** The use of gastrostomy in feeding premature infants. Pediatrics 33:287, 1964

115. **Tomsovic EJ, Barringer ML, Gay JH, McBride WP, Nomura FM:** Feeding gastrostomy in small premature infants. Am J Dis Child 112:56, 1966

116. **Vengusamy S, Pildes RS, Raffensperger J, Levine HD, Cornblath M:** A controlled study of feeding gastrostomy in low birth weight infants. Pediatrics 43:815, 1969

117. **Jones PF, Reid DHS:** Gastrostomy in neonatal respiratory failure. Lancet 2:573, 1966

118. **Haws EB, Sieber WK, Kiesewetter WB:** Complications of tube gastrostomy in infants and children. Ann Surg 164:284, 1966

119. **Holder TM:** Gastrostomy: Its uses and dangers in pediatric patients. N Engl J Med 286:1345, 1972

120. **Stave VS, Robbins S, Fletcher AB:** A comparison of growth rates of premature infants

prior to and after close nutritional monitoring. Clin Proc CHNMC 35:171, 1979

121. **Sivasubramanian KN, Henkin RI:** Behavioral and dermatologic changes and low serum zinc and copper concentration in two premature infants after parenteral alimentation. J Pediatr 93:847, 1978

122. **Widdowson EM, Dauncey J, Shaw JCL:** Trace elements in fetal and early postnatal development. Proc Nutr Soc 33:275, 1974

123. **Dauncey MJ, Shaw JCL, Urman J:** The absorption and retention of magnesium, zinc, and copper by low birth weight infants fed pasteurized human breast milk. Pediatr Res 11:991, 1977

124. **Rowe JC, Wood DH, Rowe DW, Raisz IG:** Nutritional hypophosphatemic rickets in a premature infant fed breast milk. N Engl J Med 300:293, 1979

125. **Lewin PK, Reid M, Reilly BJ et al:** Iatrogenic rickets in low birth-weight infants. J Pediatr 78:207, 1971

126. **Kooh SW, Fraser D, Reilly BJ et al:** Rickets due to calcium deficiency. N Engl J Med 297:1264, 1977

127. **Hoff N, Haddad J, Teitelbaum S et al:** Serum concentrations of 25-hydroxyvitamin D in rickets of extremely premature infants. J Pediatr 94:460, 1979

128. **Geyer RP:** Parenteral nutrition. Physiol Rev 40:150, 1960

129. **Helfrick FW, Abelson NM:** Intravenous feeding of a complete diet in a child. J Pediatr 25:400, 1944

130. **Filler RM, Eraklis AJ, Rubin VG, Das JB:** Long term total parenteral nutrition in infants. N Engl J Med 281:589, 1969

131. **Filler RM, Eraklis AJ:** The critically ill child; XII Intravenous alimentation. Pediatrics 46:456, 1970

132. **Shaw JCL:** Parenteral nutrition in the management of sick low birthweight infants. Pediatr Clin North Am 20:333, 1973

133. **Heird WC, Driscoll JM, Schullinger JN, Grebin B, Winters RW:** Intravenous alimentation in pediatric patients. J Pediatr 80:351, 1972

134. **Wilmore DW, Dudrick SJ:** Growth and development of an infant receiving all nutrients exclusively by vein. JAMA 203:860, 1968

135. **Vain NE, Georgeson KE, Cha CC, Swarner OW:** Central parenteral alimentation in newborn infants: A new technique for catheter placement. J Pediatr 93:864, 1978

136. **Avery GB, Villavicencio O, Lilly JR, Randolph JG:** Intractable diarrhea in early infancy. Pediatrics 41:712, 1968

137. **Anderson TL, Muttart ER, Bieber MA, et al:** A controlled trial of glucose vs glucose and

amino acids in premature infants. Pediatrics 94:947, 1979

138. **Endo M, Katsumata K:** Metabolic response to postoperative parenteral nutrition in infants. J Parent Ent Nut 3:360, 1979

139. **Ghademi H:** Newly devised amino acid solutions for intravenous administration, p 393. In Ghodemi H (ed): Total Parenteral Nutrition: Premisis and Promises. John Wiley and Sons, New York, 1975

140. **Snyderman SE:** Recommendations of Dr. SE Snyderman for parental amino acid requirements, p 422. In Winter RW, Hasselmeyer ED (eds): Intravenous Nutrition in the High Risk Infant. John Wiley and Sons, New York, 1975

141. **Cowett RM, Oh W, Pollak A, Schwartz R, Stonestreet BS:** Glucose disposal of low birth weight infants: Steady state hypoglycemia produced by constant intravenous glucose infusion. Pediatrics 63:389, 1979

142. **Myers RE:** Anoxic brain pathology and blood glucose. Neurology (Abstr) 26:345, 1976

143. **Avery GB:** Galactose: Its potential use in the glucose intolerant premature infant, pp 261–65. In Stern L, Oh W, Friis-Hansen B (eds): Intensive Care in the Newborn II. Masson, New York, 1978

144. **White HB, Turner MD, Turner AC, Miller RC:** Blood lipid alterations in infants receiving intravenous fat-free alimentation. J Pediatr 83:305, 1973

145. **Friedman Z, Danon A, Stahlman MT, et al:** Rapid onset of essential fatty acid deficiency in the newborn. Pediatrics 58:640, 1976

146. **Hansen AE, Wiese HF, Boeloche AN, et al:** Rate of linoleic acid in infant nutrition: Clinical and chemical study of 428 infants fed on milk mixtures varying in kind and amount of fat. Pediatrics 31:171, 1963

147. **Schreiner RL, Glick MR, Nordshow CD, Gresham EL:** An evaluation of methods to monitor infants receiving intravenous lipids. J Pediatr 94:197, 1979

148. **Andrew G, Chan G, Schiff D:** Lipid Metabolism in the Neonate II. The effect of Intralipid on bilirubin binding in vitro and in vivo. J Pediatr 88:279, 1976

149. **Freedman Z, Marks KH, Maisels J et al:** Effect of parenteral fat emulsion on the pulmonary and reticuloendothelial systems in the newborn infant. Pediatrics 61:694, 1978

150. **Fox WW, Pereira GR, Schwartz SG:** Effects of Intralipid infusions on arterial blood gases and pulmonary function. Pediatr Res (absr) 12:524, 1978

151. **Tovar JA, Mahour GH, Miller SW, Isaacs H Jr, Smith CN:** Endotoxin clearance after intralipid infusion. J Pediatr Surg 11:23, 1976

152. **Freedman Z, Shochet SJ, Maisels MJ et al:** Correction of essential fatty acid deficiency in newborn infants by cutaneous application of sunflower-seed oil. Pediatrics 58:650, 1976

153. **Hunt CE, Engel RR, Modler S et al:** Essential fatty acid deficiency in Neonates: Inability to reverse deficiency by topical applications of EFA-Rich oil. J Pediatr 92:603, 1978

154. **Kobayshi NH, King JC:** Compatibility of common additives in protein hydrosylate/dextrose solutions. Am J Hosp Pharm 34:589, 1977

155. **Hambidge KM:** Trace elements in pediatric nutrition. Adv Pediatr 24:191, 1977

156. **Sivasubramanian KN, Henkin RI:** Behavorial and dermatologic chances and low serum zinc and copper concentrations in two premature infants after parenteral nutrition. J Pediatr 93:847, 1978

157. **Heller RM, Kirchner SG, O'Neill JA, et al:** Skeletal changes of copper deficiency in infants receiving prolonged total parenteral nutrition. J Pediatr 92:947, 1978

158. Guidelines for Essential Trace Element Preparations for Parenteral Use. A Statement by an expert panel. AMA Department of Foods and Nutrition. JAMA 241:2051, 1979

159. **Tan KL, Chow MT, Karim SMM:** Effect of phototherapy on neonatal riboflavin status. J Pediatr 93:494, 1978

160. **Wilmore DW, Groff DB, Bishop HC, Dudrick SJ:** Total parenteral nutrition in infants with catastrophic gastrointestinal anomalies. J Pediatr Surg 4:181, 1969

161. **Roger R, Finegold MJ:** Cholestasis in immature newborn infants: Is parenteral alimentation responsible? J Pediatr 86:264, 1975

162. **Preisig R, Rennert O:** Biliary Transport and Cholestatic effects of Amino Acids. Gastroenterology (abstr) 73:1240, 1977

163. **Sondheimer JM, Bryan H, Andrews W, Forstner GG:** Cholestatic Tendencies in Premature Infants on and off Parenteral Nutrition. Pediatrics 62:984, 1978

164. **Manginello FP, Javitt NB:** Parenteral nutrition and neonatal cholestasis. J Pediatr 94:296, 1979

165. Presented at a Symposium on Parenteral Nutrition. APS-SPR, Atlantic City, May, 1971

166. **Coran AG:** The long term total intravenous feeding of infants using peripheral veins. J Pediatr Surg 8:801, 1973

167. **Bernstein J, Chang CH, Brough AD, Heidelberger KP:** Conjugated hyperbilirubinemia in infancy associated with parenteral alimentation. J Pediatr 90:361, 1977

168. **Postuma R, Trevenen CL:** Liver disease in

infants receiving total parenteral nutrition. Pediatrics 63:110, 1979

169. **Tejani A, Mahadevan R, Dobias B, et al:** Total parenteral nutrition of the neonate—a long-term follow-up. J Pediatr 94:803, 1979

170. **Ament ME:** Malabsorption syndromes in infancy and childhood, Part I. J Pediatr 81:685, 1972

171. **Avery GB, Villavicencio O, Lilly JR, Randolph JG:** Intractable diarrhea in early infancy. Pediatrics 41:718, 1968

172. **Herbst JJ, Sunshine P, Kretchmer N:** Intestinal malabsorption in infancy and childhood. Pediatrics 16:11, 1969

173. **Binder HJ, Reynolds RD:** Control of diarrhea in secondary hypogammaglobulinemia by fresh plasma infusions. N Engl J Med 277:802, 1967

174. **Holmberg C:** Electrolyte economy and its hormonal regulation in congenital chloride diarrhea. Pediatr Res 12:82–86, 1978

175. **Haworth JC, Gourley B, Hadorn B, Sumida C:** Malabsorption and growth failure due to intestinal enterokinase deficiency. J Pediatr 78:481, 1971

176. **Burke V, Colebatch JH, Anderson CM, Simons MJ:** Association of pancreatic insufficiency and chronic neutropenia in childhood. Arch Dis Child 42:147, 1966

177. **Ament ME:** Malabsorption syndromes in infancy and childhood, Part II. J Pediatr 81:867, 1972

178. **Walravens PA, Hambidge KM, Nelder KH, Silverman A, van Doorninck WJ, Mieran G, Favara B:** Zinc metabolism in acrodermatitis enteropathica. J Pediatr 93:71–73, 1978

179. **Silverberg M, Davidson M:** Nutritional requirements of infants and children with liver disease. Am J Clin Nutr 23:604–613, 1970

180. **Fetterman GH:** Neonatal necrotizing enterocolitis—old pitfalls or new problem. Pediatrics 48:345, 1971

181. **Engel RR, Virnig NL, Hunt CE, Levitt MD:** Origin of mural gas in necrotizing enterocolitis. SPR, San Francisco, May 1972

182. **Touloukian RJ, Kadar A, Spencer RP:** The gastrointestinal complications of neonatal umbilical venous exchange transfusions: a clinical and experimental study. Pediatrics 51:36, 1973

183. **Kliegman RM:** Neonatal necrotizing enterocolitis: Implications for an infectious disease. Pediatr Clin North Am 26:327–344, 1979

184. **Bell MJ, Koslaske AM, Benton C, Martin LW:** Neonatal necrotizing enterocolitis: prevention of perforation. J Pediatr Surg 8:601, 1973

185. **Stevenson JK, Oliver TK Jr, Graham CB, Bell RS, Gould VE:** Aggressive treatment of neonatal necrotizing enterocolitis: 38 patients with 25 survivors. J Pediatr Surg 6:28, 1971

186. **Enger NB, Hijonamo JC:** Ulcerative colitis beginning in infancy. J Pediatr 63:437, 1963

187. **Shaheen E, Alexander D, Truskowsky M, Barbero GJ:** Failure to thrive: A retrospective profile. Clin Pediatr 7:255, 1968

188. **Root AW, Bongiovanni AM, Eberlein WR:** Diagnosis and management of growth retardation with special reference to the problems of hypopituitarism. J Pediatr 78:737, 1972

189. **Ambuel JP, Harris B:** Failure to thrive: A study of failure to grow in height or weight. Ohio State Med J 59:997, 1963

190. **Luzzuti L:** Failure to thrive. A diagnostic approach. Postgrad Med 35:270, 1964

191. **Hannaway PJ:** Failure to thrive: A study of 100 infants and children. Clin Pediatr 9:96, 1970

192. **Riley RL, et al:** Failure to thrive: An analysis of 83 cases. Calif Med 108:32, 1968

193. **Bullard DM, Glaser HH, Heagarty MC, Pivchik EC:** Failure to thrive in the "neglected" child. Am J Orthopsychiatr 37:680, 1967

194. **Chase HP, Martin HP:** Undernutrition and child development. N Engl J Med, 282:933, 1970

195. **Glaser HH:** Physical and psychological development of children with early failure to thrive. J Pediatr 73:690, 1968

196. **Elmer E:** Late results of the failure to thrive syndrome. Clin Pediatr 8:584, 1969

43

Dermatologic Conditions

Andrew M. Margileth

Careful assessment of skin in the sick newborn frequently provides clues for a presumptive diagnosis of a primary cutaneous, a systemic disease, or both. During the initial examination, an exact dermatologic diagnosis is often difficult to make. However, the diagnosis evolves by analysis of the descriptive morphology, configuration, and distribution of the skin lesions. Close observation with a bright light and small magnifying glass identifies the type of primary and secondary cutaneous lesions (Tables 43-1 and 43-2). Configuration refers to patterning of lesions (*e.g.,* annular, circinate, serpiginous or gyrate, linear, iris, zosteriform, along lines of cleavage, marbled, and multiform). Distribution refers to the body area, sites of predilection, and whether symmetrical, localized or circumscribed, scattered, generalized, single or multiple, and discrete or confluent. With a good history, including that of family and prior medication, presence or absence of pruritus, and a descriptive analysis of the lesions, common dermatologic entities are quickly identified or ruled out. Finally, if the diagnosis is not clear after a short period of observation with a few selected tests, dermatologic consultation is indicated.[1-4]

The cutaneous disorders to be discussed were chosen because of their frequency, including the important skin lesions seen in premature, full-term and young infants, and those distinguishing cutaneous manifestations noted in systemic neonatal diseases. Lesions have been further classified according to origin—traumatic, neoplastic, or infectious—metabolic importance, and include common skin disorders of unknown etiology peculiar to neonates.

Skin consists of epidermis, a relatively impermeable membrane, and dermis which constitutes the main bulk of skin. Dermis consists of minimally cellular fibrous tissue containing collagen and elastin fibers. The epidermis is an avascular, cellular structure composed chiefly of keratinocytes (keratin-forming cells) stratified into five layers.[1-3] Prenatal and postnatal epidermal changes are discussed in detail by Solomon and Esterly and include a review of the functional components of skin (pH, sebum, bacterial flora, epidermal permeability, vasomotor tone, sweating.)[3]

PHYSIOLOGIC AND GENETIC VARIATIONS

The appearance of newborn skin primarily depends upon maturation (premature, full-term, dysmature), state of nutrition, racial

Table 43-1 Primary Cutaneous Lesions.

Lesions < 1 cm in Size		Lesions > 1 cm in Size		Lesions of Varying Size	
Macule	Nodule	Patch	Tumor	Pustule	Burrow
Papule	Vesicle	Plaque	Bulla	Wheal	Telangiectasia
Comedo					

origin, and amount of vernix caseosa. Activity, distribution and amount of fat, hemoglobin and bilirubin level, and the type and intensity of available light produce variations in the skin. The premature has thin, taut skin, while in dysmature infants the skin is loose and wrinkled.

Keratinization. The degree of desquamation, part of the keratinization process, varies with maturity, nutritional state and presence of cutaneous disease. Normally, term infants show little or no desquamation until 1 or 2 days of age, and peeling is usually complete within a few days. Desquamation does not occur in prematures until the second or third week after birth. At birth, desquamation is abnormal, and occurs frequently in the dysmature or full-term infant with acute intrauterine anoxia. No treatment is necessary. Although collodion-like skin may be seen in the dysmature infant, desquamation at birth is rarely a result of congenital ichthyosiform dermatosis.

Macular Hemangiomas. Macular hemangiomas of the nape, eyelids, and glabella are found in 50% of newborns. These salmon patches have diffuse borders and become pinker when the infant cries; most eyelid lesions fade by 1 year of age. The nuchal and glabellar lesions persist longer and may appear transiently when anger occurs in the child or adult. Unna's nevus is a persistent nuchal salmon patch. No therapy is indicated.

Cutis Marmorata. Cutis marmorata is a physiologic generalized marbling effect in infants who become chilled. The mottling resembles a net-like pattern caused by dilatation of the capillaries and venules. Marbling usually dis-

appears with rewarming and is uncommon after several months of age unless prolonged exposure to low environmental temperatures occurs. Persistent cutis marmorata is frequent in trisomy 18 and 21 and De Lange syndrome.[5] Localized marbling or reticulation which becomes intense with crying or change in temperature is called **cutis marmorata telangiectatica congenita.** This vascular ectasia involves both capillaries and veins, and its usual course is one of steady improvement.[3]

Harlequin Color Change. Harlequin color change is a very rare phenomenon observed only in neonates, especially low-birth-weight (LBW) infants. A sharply demarcated deep red color develops in the dependent half of the body when lying on that side compared to the pale superior half. The color change lasts from 1 to 20 minutes and reverses sides if the infant is rotated to the opposite side. The harlequin sign, observed in well and sick infants, is of no pathologic significance.[3]

Milia. Epidermal inclusion cysts or milia are multiple yellow or white 1-mm papules noted over the cheeks, nasal bridge, forehead, nasolabial folds, palate, and alveolar ridges (Epstein's pearls). Epstein's pearls, seen in 85% of newborns, usually rupture soon after birth. Milia, observed in 40% of full-term infants as grouped, noninflamed papules, invariably disappear within a few weeks.

Sebaceous Gland Hyperplasia. In contrast to milia, many full-term infants have innumerable tiny (<0.5 mm) white or yellow spots involving the pilosebaceous follicles of the nose, upper lip and malar areas. These hyperplastic sebaceous glands, rare in preterm infants, spontaneously become smaller and disappear by 2 to 3 weeks of age.

Acne Neonatorum. This disorder, seen more often in boys, occasionally develops during the first or second postnatal months, (Figure 43-1). Characteristically, erythematous comodones and papules are seen; pustules, nodules, and cystic lesions are rare. Lesions occur over

Table 43-2 Secondary Skin Lesions.

Atrophy	Excoriation	Scar
Crusts	Fissure	Scale
Erosion	Pigmentation	Ulcer

the cheeks primarily, but also on the chin and forehead. Most lesions disappear by one or two years of age; rarely, they may persist to puberty. Most patients require no therapy; daily cleansing with a mild soap (Dove) and water is sufficient. Petrolatum, baby oils, and lotions should be avoided. Keratolytic agents or benzoyl peroxide preparations may be needed for more severe cases.[2,4]

Miliaria. Retention of sweat as a result of edema of the stratum corneum blocking eccrine pores results in 4 types of miliaria (m.): m. rubrum (prickly heat), m. crystallina (sudamina), m. pustulosa, and m. profunda.[2-4] The latter two conditions are rarely seen in temperate climates. M. rubra (small-grouped erythematous papules) is commonly observed in infants but rarely during the early neonatal period, unless environmental temperature is excessive with high humidity. M. crystallina, clear, 1- to 2-mm, superficial vesicles without inflammation, are commonly observed over the forehead, neck, intertriginous areas, and occasionally in the diaper area (Fig. 43-2). Their distribution and grouping of vesicles that contain no eosinophils help to differentiate them from erythema toxicum. These infants are usually well and removal to a cooler environment effects rapid clearing. Recurrence may be expected in an excessively warm, humid situation. M. pustulosa, resulting from leukocytic infiltration of the vesicles, is rare. Aspiration and culture of a pustule is necessary to rule out staphylococcal impetigo.[7] Rapid resolution of the eruption by keeping the infant cool and dry helps to differentiate m. pustulosa from a pyoderma.

Erythema Toxicum. This benign, self-limiting, perifollicular eruption is usually seen at birth or shortly thereafter. Its peak incidence is at 24 to 48 hours of life; but it may appear up until 1 or 2 weeks of age. The lesion, observed in 30% to 70% of full-term infants, is a firm, 1- to 3-mm white or pale yellow papule or pustule with an erythematous base (Fig. 43-3). Occasionally, only erythematous macules (up to 3 cm) are seen. These may become confluent, especially over the trunk, but any body area may be involved except the palms and soles. The infant is invariably well, and the lesions usually fade spontaneously in a few hours or days. Diagnosis can be confirmed if a smear of an aspirated pustule shows numerous eosinophils (Wright's stain) and no

bacteria are cultured. Etiology is unknown and treatment is unnecessary.

Transient Neonatal Pustular Melanosis. Newly described, transient vesicopustular melanosis occurs more often in the healthy newborn than is generally appreciated.[2,6] Three stages of lesions may be observed: (1) noninflammatory pustules, (2) ruptured vesicopustules with a collarette of scale usually surrounding a central hyperpigmented macule (Fig. 43-4), and (3) hyperpigmented macules which may persist for up to 3 months of age. Cultures are sterile; aspirated pus shows a few inflammatory scales and debris. The pustules last 1 to 3 days or so, and may not be observed because a few newborns have demonstrated only hyperpigmented macules at birth. This dermatosis is benign, self-limited, and requires no treatment. Differential diagnosis of vesicopustules is discussed later.[2]

Pigmentary Lesions. **Mongolian spot,** the most common pigmented lesion seen at birth, is present in 90% of Black, Indian, and Oriental infants. It occurs in 1% to 5% of Caucasian infants. These large (2- to 10-cm) macular, slate blue or gray lesions, usually seen over the lumbosacral area, may also be observed over buttocks, flanks or shoulders. Lesions may be single or multiple and are caused by infiltration of melanocytes deep in the dermis. The spots usually fade during late infancy but may persist into adulthood.

Café au lait spots (tan or brown macules), seen occasionally in newborns, may develop during infancy. Single lesions under 3 cm in length are found in 19% of normal children.[3] An infant with five or less café au lait spots (<1.5 cm), and a negative family history for Recklinghausen's disease, is probably normal. Subsequently, if six or more spots (>1.5 cm) develop, a diagnosis of cutaneous neurofibromatosis should be considered and the patient followed closely.[2,5]

Melanocytic nevi (flat, junctional nevi) are noted in 1% of newborns; pigmented lesions occur in 4%.[8] These nevi are brown or black; their size varies from one to several centimeters and usually very few lesions are present at birth. Subsequently, the number increases with age. They may be associated with neurofibromatosis, tuberous sclerosis, bathing trunk nevi, lentiginosis, or xeroderma pigmentosum.[3] Therapy is rarely necessary, however, lesions larger than 3 cm should be removed.[2]

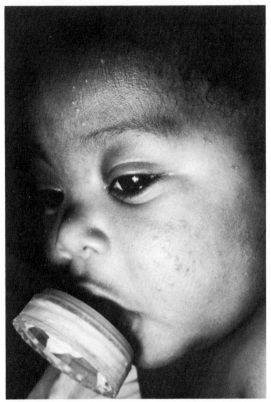

Fig. 43-1. Acne neonatorum of cheeks in a 4-month-old male; comedones developed at age 4 weeks. Note miliaria pustulosa (× 6 lesions) on forehead. There was much improvement in 1 month after vaseline was discontinued.

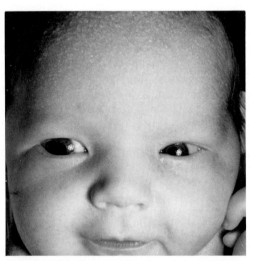

Fig. 43-2. Miliaria crystallina in a 5-day-old infant. Cooling resulted in disappearance of the lesions overnight.

Diffuse hyperpigmentation in the newborn is unusual. The degree and location of hyperpigmentation must be considered in view of the infant's racial and genetic background. Diffuse hyperpigmentation may be caused by congenital Addison's disease, nutritional disorders (pellagra, sprue), hepatitis or biliary atresia, hereditary disorders (lentiginosis, melanism),[2,3] metabolic disease (Hartnup, porphyria) or to unknown causes such as bronze discoloration in Niemann–Pick disease. Androgens may produce hyperpigmentation of the labial folds with clitoral hypertrophy as a result of transplacental passage during pregnancy. Therapy depends upon the basic disorder. We observed a newborn male with slate gray melanosis at birth secondary to maternal malignant melanoma with placental metastases. The mother died 6 weeks postpartum; however, the infant survived without treatment and was well at 10 years of age. Although his

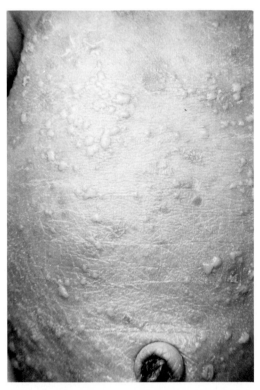

Fig. 43-3. Erythema toxicum in a 12-hour-old full-term infant. At birth many pustules were present and continued to form. Wright's stain of aspirate showed numerous eosinophils. The skin cleared spontaneously in 1 week.

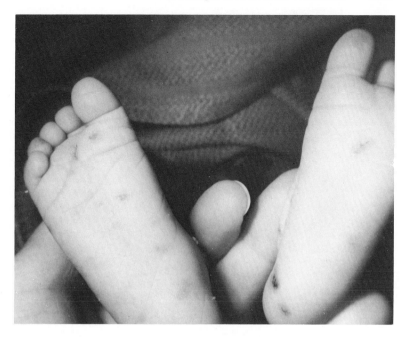

Fig. 43-4. Transient neonatal pustular melanosis in a 6-day-old black infant. Vesicles noted over the entire body, extremities, palms, and soles at birth began scaling at 24 hours. A few vesicopustules developed. Note collarette of scales surrounding the hyperpigmented macules which were very prominent by age 1 month. TORCHES studies were negative.

deciduous teeth were brown, his permanent teeth were normal.

Hypopigmentation, a diffuse or localized loss of pigment in the neonate, may be the result of genetic (piebaldism, vitiligo, tuberous sclerosis, albinism), metabolic (phenylketonuria), endocrine (Addison's), traumatic or postinflammatory causes.[2] The melanocytes may be sparse or absent.

Hypomelanosis of Ito, a neurocutaneous syndrome, may be associated with seizures, delayed development, and ocular and musculoskeletal anomalies. The skin lesions resemble those of incontinentia pigmenti as a negative image.[9]

Albinism, an autosomal recessive disorder, occurs in all races. The infant shows markedly reduced pigmentation, yellow or white hair, pink pupils, grey irides, and photophobia with photosensitivity. Nystagmus with reduced vision is common. Small stature, mental retardation, and deafness may occur. Protection from ultraviolet light is necessary to prevent actinic keratoses and squamous cell carcinomas.[2]

Piebaldism or partial albinism, an autosomal dominant disorder, present at birth, is easily detected in the dark-skinned infant. Usually amelanotic (off-white) macules involve the scalp, widow's peak, and forehead with ex-

tension to the base of the nose, chin, trunk, and extremities. Because an isolated white forelock may be the only manifestation, and deafness may develop much later, Klein–Waardenburg syndrome must be considered.[3] Other diagnoses in the newborn are vitiligo, nevus anemicus, Addison's disease, and white macules of tuberous sclerosis. Most of these entities may be excluded by the characteristic distribution of the hypomelanotic areas in piebaldism which contain normal pigmented islands (1- to 5-cm macules). Vitiligo (pure white macules) usually develop after 6 months of age at sites of repeated trauma.[1,2] When illuminated with a Wood's light, these amelanotic areas exhibit a brilliant whiteness.

Nevus achromicus or depigmentosus, present at birth, appears as irregularly shaped, long, linear streaks of hypomelanosis which are very small or may cover half the body (Fig. 43-5). The area of hypopigmentation is uniform in color and usually unilateral. Rubbing the lesion produces a normal vasodilation response in contrast to nevus anemicus which is unresponsive and remains pale compared to normal adjacent vasodilated skin. Therapy is not necessary for either lesion because each usually occurs in covered areas.[2]

White macules (leukoderma, white spots) detected in 90% of infants with tuberous scle-

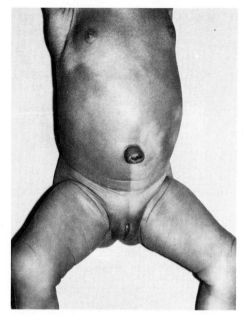

Fig. 43-5. Nevus achromicus of the right chest, left abdomen, and leg in a healthy 3-week-old premature. Hypopigmentation was noted at 10 days of age. A normal flare response developed after rubbing. Family history was negative for hypopigmented lesions. (Courtesy Dr. M. Renfield and Dr. F. Bowen)

rosis (epiloia) may be present at birth. One patient was detected in 1000 newborns.[10] These spots may be missed in lightskinned infants unless a Wood's lamp is used. The macules are about the size of a thumbprint or mountain ash leaf,[2] vary in number (4 to 100), are usually seen over the trunk or buttocks, and have a normal physiologic response to stroking. All infants with seizures should be carefully examined with a Wood's lamp. Not all white spots are caused by epiloia. Four infants out of 1000 showed depigmented nevi that may have been caused by nevus anemicus, a developing hemangioma, or macules associated with neurofibromatosis.[10] Because other cutaneous features[11] (angiofibromata, shagreen patch and periungual fibroma) of epiloia take years to develop, careful follow-up is essential.[2]

TRAUMA

Caput Succedaneum. A diffuse edematous, occasionally hemorrhagic, swelling of the presenting part, occurs secondary to compression of local vessels associated with prolonged labor. The scalp, scrotum, labia majora or an extremity (Fig. 43-6) may be involved. Edema recedes in a week or so; ecchymoses, if present, clear in several weeks. No therapy is needed and sequelae are not reported.

Sucking Blisters. Occasionally, a few intact or ruptured bullae (1 cm) may be noted on the thumb, index finger or lip in a healthy newborn. The blisters contain sterile, serous fluid, resolve rapidly without treatment, and are presumably a result of vigorous sucking *in utero*.

Skin Trauma. Ocassionally, abrasions, ulcerations, ecchymoses, or areas of pressure necrosis of the presenting part are seen following prolonged labor or possibly after forceps application. Subconjunctival hemorrhage and petechiae may be seen. These lesions are usually inconsequential and spontaneously disappear in a week or two. Ulcerated areas should be kept clean and dry, especially if a deep ulcer develops from pressure necrosis.[3] If serous drainage occurs, application of tap water or normal saline dressings (changed every 4 hours) for 1 or 2 days will effectively minimize exudate formation and infection. A povidone-iodine (Betadine) surgical scrub, four times daily, followed by application of 0.1% gentamicin cream, will be effective for a secondary superficial infection that rarely occurs.

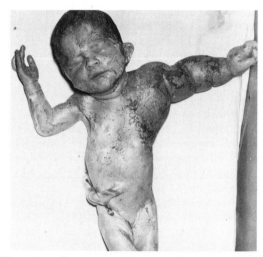

Fig. 43-6. Caput succedaneum edema and ecchymoses of the presenting part in a 1-day-old premature. Labor was prolonged; a cesarean section was necessary. Swelling disappeared spontaneously in 1 week; the arm functioned normally.

Fat necrosis, an uncommon, sharply circumscribed, indurated subcutaneous nodule or plaque appearing on the extremities, trunk or buttocks during the first weeks of life, has been attributed to trauma, shock, cold, and asphyxia. The lesion is nonpitting, hard, and may have a deep reddish or purplish discoloration. The disease occurs in well infants and resolves spontaneously over weeks to months. Residual atrophy or scarring are unusual.

Sclerema neonatorum more commonly affects the preterm or debilitated infant. It may have the same etiology and adipose tissue abnormality in the subcutaneous tissues as noted in fat necrosis.[3] The British have shown that low environmental temperature alone can produce the injury. A diffuse hardening of subcutaneous tissue develops with cold, stony hard, nonpitting skin. The extremities may be involved at first, but generalized involvement occurs within 3 to 4 days. Most infants are severely ill. If survival occurs, the sclerematous changes rarely persist beyond 2 weeks. Differential diagnosis includes edema neonatorum, Milroy's and Turner's syndrome, and panniculitis.[3] Therapy is based upon the underlying systemic disease, restoration of body temperature, and adequate nutrition.

DIAPER DERMATITIS

Napkin or diaper dermatitis is a common, transient, erythematous eruption localized to the diaper area. Maceration and scaling are common; eventually nodular ulcerations develop after improper care. Neonatal skin is more permeable and susceptible to irritation. Predisposing factors are inheritance of a reactive skin with a seborrheic or atopic diathesis; systemic disease such as syphilis, acrodermatitis enterophatica, or Letterer–Siwe disease; activating factors such as occlusive moist heat or retention of sweat; secondary infection caused by pyogenic invaders, viruses or yeasts; mechanical irritation; contact factors (retained urine and stool); and maternal factors such as overcleansing or inability to carry out proper skin care or therapeutic directions.[2,12]

Contact Diaper Dermatitis. Primary irritant or contact dermatitis, a common problem, is often caused by direct application of harsh soaps, detergents, lanolin, sensitizers (neomycin, nystatin, parabens, ethylenediamine,

sulfur)[13] or secondary to recurrent diarrhea, especially with alkaline stools. Petrolatum or mineral oil, tolerated in older infants or young Black infants, may cause maceration with sweat retention in Caucasian infants. When the intertriginous areas are clear and the eruption involves the mons pubis, scrotum, penis, medial thighs, and buttocks, then a clinical diagnosis of contact dermatitis is likely (Fig. 43-8).

Therapy consists of frequent diaper changes, keeping the area clean, dry and cool, and elimination of the offending irritant after it is determined by a careful history. Impermeable plastic pants foster heat and sweat retention and are to be avoided, especially if diaper dermatitis is present. In the acute stage, rapid healing will occur if no diapers are used for 24 to 48 hours. Irritation will be diminished especially at night by application of Lassar's paste or a dusting powder containing equal parts of zinc oxide and talc, and use of four cotton diapers that have been rinsed thoroughly. A final rinse with addition of ½ to 1 cup of white vinegar may be necessary. Nonmedicated neutral soap should be used for cleansing. Aveeno or starch baths are soothing. Disposable paper diapers should be tried in resistant cases. However, some products are perfumed, which may cause mild irritation.

Intertrigo, a symmetrical moist eruption in skin folds and creases, is secondary to excessive sweating and close approximation of opposing gluteal or inguinal surfaces. It is managed in the same way as contact diaper dermatitis. Ointments must be avoided. Because secondary yeast or bacterial infection occurs, cultures or smears should be considered in each patient.

Primary Irritant Diaper Dermatitis. Ammonia dermatitis may be caused by urea-splitting bacteria or nonalkaline irritants produced by putrefactive enzymes. Dry erythematous skin resembling a scald is found on the convex surfaces.[12] A pungent ammonia odor is invariably present when the first morning diaper is changed. Frequent changing of diapers, maintenance of dry, clean skin and feeding of D,L-methionine, 0.2 g bid for 7 to 10 days, will clear the rash in 5 to 10 days. Recurrences are unusual. Secondary monilia infection may be present.

Monilial Diaper Dermatitis. Diaper dermatitis is occasionally caused by or associated with

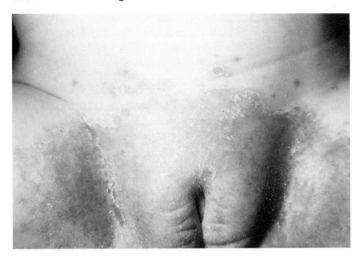

Fig. 43-7. Monilial diaper rash persisted for 3 weeks in a 6-week-old infant. There was no response to nystatin ointment. However, gentian violet, 1% aqueous, applied t.i.d. for 3 days was effective. Note the satellite lesions.

monilia. Over several days, a vesicular eruption becomes confluent to form a moist, bright red macerated rash. Diagnosis is suspected by the presence of many, 0.5- to 1-cm, superficial satellite erosions or moist patches, and pustules outside the diaper rash (Fig. 43-7) or perianal eruption. *Candida albicans* can be cultured or quickly identified by gram stain of scrapings. Oral thursh with white plaques over the tongue and soft and hard palates, is usually seen during the second week of life while cutaneous lesions may occur at any age. Untreated infants may develop a generalized rash, especially if an endocrinopathy or immunologic deficiency exists. Prolonged antibiotic therapy, diabetes mellitus, and excessive sweating are predisposing factors. Simple candidial diaper dermatitis is treated with Burrow's solution (1:20) soaks followed by nystatin (Mycostatin) powder or cream (100,000 units/g) applied tid for 7 to 10 days. Because of cost and occasional failure of nystatin (Fig. 43-7), 1% aqueous gentian violet, applied tid for 3 days, is recommended for monilial dermatitis and oral thrush. A second 3-day course of therapy is occasionally necessary after 3-day's lapse following the initial treatment. It is essential that the diaper area remain clean and dry to effectively eradicate the infection. Generalized cutaneous and systemic candidial infections are quite rate in infants.[2]

Seborrheic Diaper Dermatitis. Seborrhea of the diaper area, rarely seen in the absence of scalp or truncal involvement (discussed later

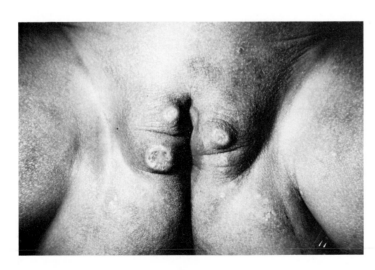

Fig. 43-8. Chronic ulceronodular contact diaper dermatitis and secondary staphylococcal infection in a month-old infant. The rolled edges of the ulcers are characteristic. Note the absence of skin involvement in the thigh folds.

in this chapter), is characterized by patchy redness, fissuring, scaling, and occasional weeping, especially in intertriginous (gluteal) folds. The scalp and postauricular regions should be examined carefully for an oily, scaly, minimally erythematous eruption. Diagnosis is suspected if, by scraping the scales and rubbing them between one's fingers a soapy sensation is produced. The eruption, rarely seen during the first week of life, may become widespread (truncal) by 1 or 2 months of age. Spontaneous healing may occur 6 to 8 weeks later. Therapy consists of 0.5% hydrocortisone cream tid for 7 to 14 days or 3% vioform in 0.5% hydrocortisone cream tid for 10 days. Recurrence is uncommon after 6 months of age.[14]

Secondary Diaper Dermatitis—Subacute and Chronic. Diaper rash may occur in association with cutaneous or systemic bacterial, viral, or fungal infections; diarrhea; or atopic eczema.[12] Secondary staphylococcal infection superimposed upon eczematous diaper dermatitis can produce an erosive nodular eruption (Fig. 43-8) that can be resistant to local therapy.[3] Elimination of the primary irritant, allergic and physical agents (cold, heat), and use of a systemic antibiotic (penicillin G or a semisynthetic penicillinase-resistant penicillin), will clear the infection. Hydrocortisone, 0.5% cream alone or 1% hydrocortisone in zinc oxide ointment or in 3% vioform cream will provide excellent antiinflammatory action and protection from irritants in infants with atopic dermatitis. Coal tar baths,[1,13] for 15 minutes tid using 1 to 2 tsp of Zetar or Balnetar, or 1 oz of liquor carbonis detergens, are very effective for pruritus and also cleansing. Alkali soaps must be avoided. Basis or Lowila soap or Cetaphil lotion are excellent substitutes. Dry heat using a 75- or 100-watt light bulb positioned about 18 inches from the uncovered diaper area is effective. Education of the mother is essential to avoid recurrence.[14]

MISCELLANEOUS SKIN LESIONS

Redundant Skin. Loose skin folds are observed over the neck posteriorly in Turner, Down, and trisomy 13 syndromes. Redundant skin in a more generalized distribution is seen in infants with trisomy 18 and combined immunodeficiency syndrome with dwarfism and alopecia. Dermatomegaly or cutis laxa and

cutis hyperelastica (Ehlers–Danlos syndrome), although rare, must be differentiated. Their diagnostic features[3] may not be fully developed in the neonatal period.[15]

Congenital Fistulas. Auricular, branchiogenic and thyroglossal fistulas and cysts are relatively common and easily detected in the ear, or anterolateral neck. Most fistulae may be noted in the neonatal period; cysts develop in later infancy or childhood, particularly, when secondary infection develops. Surgical excision is definitive.

Umbilical Anomalies. After the cord has separated, a small (3 to 7 mm) dull red, dry, velvety granuloma may slowly develop. Purulent exudate caused by secondary infection may occur. Daily application of a silver nitrate stick will effectively cauterize the granuloma and cause it to recede, whereas the rare umbilical polyp (persistent remnant of the omphalomesenteric duct or urachus) will not. The latter lesions require surgical excision.

Aplasia Cutis Congenita. Congenital absence of skin, not uncommon, may present as a localized midline posterior scalp defect, or several small, or one large defect involving upper or lower extremities and occasionally the trunk. The typical scalp lesion is a 2- to 3-cm, circular, sharply marginated area (Fig. 43-9). At birth, the lesion is usually covered by a smooth membrane that often desquamates, leaving a dry ulcer. These lesions heal slowly over several months by reepithelialization, leaving a hypertropic (Fig. 43-10) or atrophic scar. Infection is rare. Other malformations, cleft lip and palate, defects of hands and feet, and trisomy 13 may be associated.[3,16]

Extensive congenital defects of the skin present at birth (Fig. 43-11**A**) are usually multiple and heal spontaneously by epithelial growth from the borders. The end result is an acceptable thin scar (Fig. 43-11**B**). Histologically, these areas show an absence of epidermis, few appendageal structures, and decreased dermal elastic tissue. Infection should be prevented by reverse isolation, local cleansing (Betadine or surgical soap), and application of bacitracin ointment or 0.1% gentamicin cream 2 to 4 times daily. Extensive aplasia cutis may be associated with epidermolysis bullosa.[3] In either case, skin grafting should be avoided because in our experience surgical trauma may result in severe secondary infection.

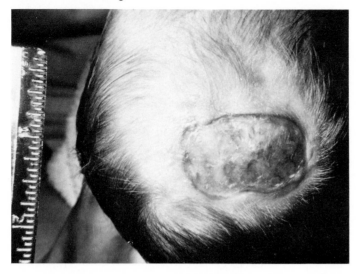

Fig. 43-9. Cutis aplasia of the scalp in a 1-month-old with trisomy 13. Healing was spontaneous by 4 months of age.

Hypoplasias. Focal dermal hypoplasia (Goltz's syndrome) is characterized by linear areas of thinning or absence of dermis with herniation of fat through surrounding skin.[5] The areas resemble red or yellow-brown deflated balloons. Atrophic scars, aplasia cutis, telangiectasias, intense whealing after stroking and red papillomas (peri- and intraoral, perianal, vulvar) may be found. Additional skin (alopecia, nail), skeletal, eye, dental, hearing, and mental defects may be present.[3] Therapy is symptomatic and based upon the major findings.

NAIL, SWEAT, AND HAIR DEFECTS

Nail Disorders. Total absence (anonychia), partial absence or dysplasia of nails occurs in 25 known disorders.[3,5] Well-known entities include anhidrotic ectodermal dysplasia, Apert's, Ellis–Van Creveld, trisomy, and nail-patella syndromes. Many of these conditions will be apparent in the neonatal period; a large number are familial (Fig. 43-12). In general, etiology and pathogenesis are poorly understood; therapy is not available or needed. Beau's lines, single transverse depressions

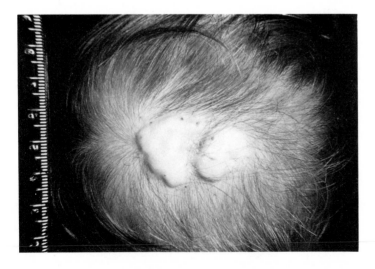

Fig. 43-10. Keloid of the scalp of a normal 1-year-old who had an isolated posterior scalp defect at birth. A hypertrophic scar developed spontaneously during the first 3 months of life.

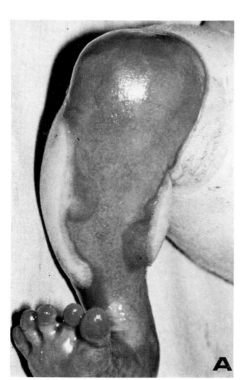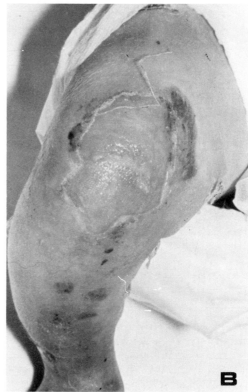

Fig. 43-11. Cutis aplasia and epidermolysis bullosa simplex in a 4-day-old with **(A)** absent epidermis of the leg. Note bullae on the toes. **B.** The same patient with spontaneous healing at 6 weeks of age. (Courtesy K. A. Gill, Jr., M.D.)

occurring in one or more nails, are seen frequently after infectious diseases or other systemic disorders. These gradually disappear with nail growth.

Hypertrophic nails, rarely observed in the neonate, may occur as familial onychogryposis, congenital onychauxis, or associated with congenital hemihypertrophy or the pachyonychia congenita syndrome.[3] Treatment is relatively ineffective; amputation may be necessary to restore function.

Sweat Disorders. **Anhidrotic** (hypohidrotic), absent, or decreased sweating occurs in several disorders.[5] Anhidrotic ectodermal dysplasia with hypotrichosis and defective dentition is the most striking disorder and may be recognized during early infancy. Facies are distinctive with frontal bossing, flattened nasal bridge, depressed central face, and absent eyebrows. Alopecia occurs later. The skin is thin, dry, hypopigmented, and vessels are prominent. Absence of sweat can be detected

early by the sweat chloride plate. Hyperpyrexia with fever of undetermined origin, caused by marked heat intolerance, is often the first major clue that brings the infant to the physician's attention. Therapy consists of cool environmental temperatures, with application of wet towels or clothing for the older infant during warm weather. Deficient lacrimation can be palliated by regular use of artificial tears; a wig will conceal severe alopecia. Genetic counseling is indicated because the disease is inherited in an X-linked dominant fashion. Congenital ectodermal dysplasia of the face with localized absence of sweating must be considered.[3]

Hair Abnormalities. Hair disorders rarely present as isolated defects.[5] Hypertrichosis, hypotrichosis and abnormal morphology (twisted, ringed, beaded, node-like hair) are usually not appreciated until after the neonatal period. Exceptions are hypertrichosis of the De Lange syndrome, with gingival fibroma-

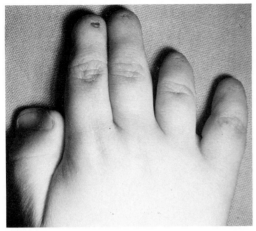

Fig. 43-12. Anonychia and hypoplasia of the nails in an infant who was otherwise normal. Similar nail defects with broad thumbs were present in five siblings and family members for five generations.

tosis, and localized hairiness seen in congenital hemihypertrophy and diastematomyelia. Alopecia totalis congenita may occur alone or with hidrotic ectodermal dysplasia. Changes in hair color, caliber, and fragility may suggest a specific diagnosis. The best test is to perform dissecting microscopic examination of the hair shaft. Therapy is based upon the specific diagnosis because many systemic disorders are associated with hair disorders.[3,5,17]

NEVI AND TUMORS

Many nevi and cutaneous tumors are not present at birth but develop during the early months of life. A nevus is a localized, highly differentiated, proliferative malformation aris-

Table 43-3. Epidermal Nevi.

Keratinocytic Nevi
  Nevus unius lateris
  Small verrucoid nevi
  Systematized verrucoid nevi
  Epidermal nevus syndrome
Appendageal (Organoid) Nevi
  Sebaceous nevi
  Hair follicle nevi
  Apocrine duct nevi
Melanocytic Nevi
  Junction (flat melanocytic) nevi

Table 43-4. Dermal Nevi.

Melanocytic
  Blue nevi; dermal melanocytoma
  Intradermal nevi
  Compound nevi
  Giant hairy nevus
Vascular Nevi
Connective Tissue Nevi
  Juvenile fibromatosis
  Osteoma cutis
Nervous Tissue Nevi
Mixed Nevi

ing from keratinocytes, melanocytes, or appendageal (organoid), or vascular structures. A partial list of epidermal and dermal nevi found in young infants is noted in Table 43-3 and Table 43-4. The type of nevus is best described by its origin or location, hence the terms melanocytic nevus, sebaceous nevus, or systematized nevus. Rare types have been discussed recently.[2,3]

Malignant skin tumors are rarely observed in the newborn period (Table 43-5). Congenital melanoma has been described in one infant; sarcomas and parotid gland adenocarcinomas are rare.[2,3]

Because of undue concern about cutaneous nevi in a newborn, active therapy is requested and initiated at times. A basic principle of management of nevi is to avoid overzealous treatment so that tragic cosmetic results do not occur. After obtaining a detailed history, the lesion should be examined carefully using a magnifying lens; it should be palpated and measured accurately. In cosmetically objectionable lesions a photograph is invaluable for subsequent reference. Repeat visits help the physician to decide whether active therapy is needed. In each patient, the individual circumstances (appearance, location, and rate of growth) provide the best guidelines for continued observation or need for histopathologic

Table 43-5. Congenital Skin Tumors.

Dermoids
Lipomas
Neuroblastomas
Sarcomas
Teratomas

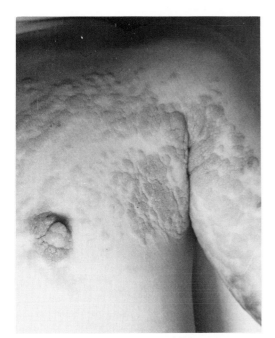

Fig. 43-13. Epidermal nevus syndrome. The left chest of a 5-month-old with a large epidermal nevus covering the left scalp, forehead, face, and upper chest at birth. Infantile spasms, and severe mental retardation occurred at 2 months of age.

examination or complete removal of the lesion. Dermatologic consultation resolves most problems.

Epidermal Nevi. Verrucoid nevi commonly seen in the neonate are local or systematized nevi and nevus unius lateralis. The latter lesion initially consists of long, unilateral, barely palpable streaks that become verrucous and pigmented with age. They are usually found over the neck, trunk or an extremity at a single site or occasionally at multiple sites. Pruritus and inflammation may occur. Rarely, one-half of the body is involved and appears identical to congenital ichthyosiform erythroderma. Widespread linear verrucous lesions (systematized) may involve the oral mucosa, ocular conjunctiva, or scalp.[3] Recently, 23 patients with epidermal nevi, skeletal defects, vascular anomalies and severe mental retardation and/ or convulsions (Fig. 43-13) were studied by Solomon, and designated as the epidermal nevus syndrome.[3] Therapy should be withheld for several years to allow full growth of the lesion.[18] Keratolytic creams (3% salicylic acid) will keep lesions soft. Subsequently, plastic repair or electrodesiccation will improve the cosmetic appearance.

Nevus Sebaceous. This lesion, commonly observed in the newborn over the scalp (Fig. 43-14) or forehead, is a discrete, yellowish, cobblestoned, oval, hairless plaque. It occasionally occurs on the face, ears or neck. Untreated, these lesions change little, if at all, for years. A few eventually transform into basal cell epitheliomas; therefore, simple excision during late childhood is advised. Juvenile xanthogranuloma and syringocystadenoma papilliferum[2] must be considered differentially in the young infant. Rarely, a variation of the epidermal nevus syndrome, called the linear sebaceous syndrome, is seen.[19]

Melanocytic Nevi. **Junctional, compound, and intradermal** nevi are rarely encountered at birth. They are classified histologically as follows: in junctional nevi, all melanocytes are above the basement membrane; in compound nevi, all melanocytes are in the epidermis and dermis; and in intradermal nevi, all melano-

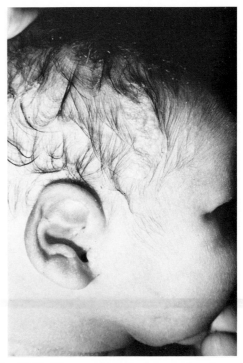

Fig. 43-14. Nevus sebaceous in a newborn's scalp. The cobblestone yellowish lesion remained unchanged over several years.

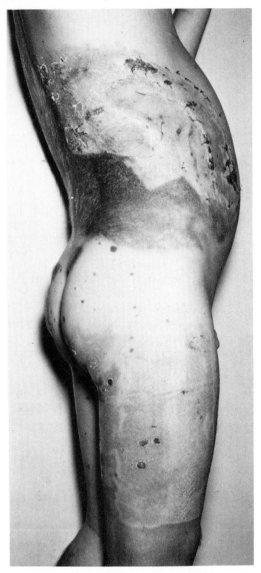

Fig. 43-15. Giant hairy nevus in a 5-year-old boy. First-stage resection and skin grafting were necessary because of local radiation keratoses that developed several years after x-ray therapy.[2]

cytes are in the dermis. Pigmented nevi occur in 2.4% of newborn Caucasian infants, are few in number, and are found on any part of the body.[20] The majority require no therapy unless a sudden change occurs in growth, color, or bleeding, or unless ulceration develops. Removal by simple excision or shave excision (Walton) will suffice for cosmetic reasons or for functional or anatomic reasons: irritation, trauma, and infection.[18] Whatever method is used for removal, pathologic examination is mandatory.

Blue nevi in newborns present in two forms. The common Mongolian spot (cellular dermal melanocytoma) has been discussed. The **dermal melanocytoma** (blue nevus) appears rarely at birth as a grayish or steel blue papule or nodule (1 to 3 cm), which grows slowly. Found on the buttocks and upper body, these nevi may be difficult to differentiate clinically from vascular lesions. If diagnosed clinically, routine follow-up is sufficient, otherwise simple complete elliptical excision with histologic diagnosis is curative.

Giant hairy nevus (nevus pigmentosus et pilosus, bathing trunk nevus) present at birth may be found anywhere on the body. The more extensive lesions involving the lower part of the trunk are commonly known as "bathing trunk" nevi. Less commonly found lesions on the neck and scalp may be associated with leptomeningeal melanocytosis. Epilepsy or signs of focal neurologic abnormalities may be present. Complete excision (Fig. 43-15) with plastic reconstruction should be performed if possible before puberty because the lesions are associated with an incidence of malignant melanoma of 10% in adults.[1-3] Depilation alone of associated small, hairy, intradermal nevi may produce a cosmetically acceptable result. Shave excision and electrodesiccation of hairy nevi in special areas (*e.g.,* eyebrow) may be more desirable than total excision with skin grafting.[18]

Nervous Tissue Nevi. Nevi of neural origin, found in neurofibromatosis, are rarely observed in the newborn. Occasionally, these nevi may be part of a mixed cutaneous malformation with osseous defects (Fig. 43-16A). These congenital lesions may consist of hemangioma or lymphangioma tissue, nevus pigmentosus et pilosus, and plexiform neuromas. Localized hypertrophy with or without elephantiasis of tissues is usually seen; rarely, atrophy of the affected part is observed (Fig. 43-16B). In selected cases, surgical resection will improve function and appearance (Fig. 43-17). Fortunately, these lesions change very slowly over many years.

Congenital Tumors (Table 43-5). **Dermoids** (epidermal inclusion cysts), present at birth or

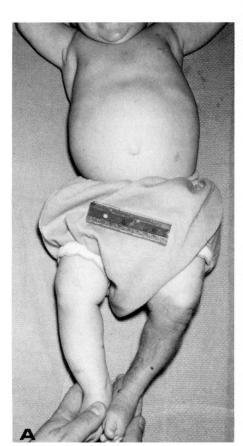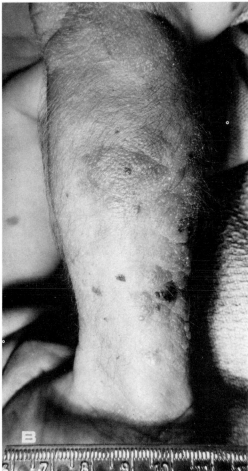

Fig. 43-16. A. Mixed nevus with atrophy of the leg in a 3-month-old. Over six café au lait spots (>1.5 cm) were present. **B.** Elements of lymphangioma circumscriptum (angioma cystica), hairy pigmentation, ''shagreen'' plaques are seen.

soon thereafter, are round or ovoid subcutaneous tumors (1 to 10 cm) of soft or rubbery consistency. They are encapsulated and contain sebaceous material and hair, and are often located at the outer ends of eyebrows, or on the neck, sternum, scrotum, perineal raphe, or the sacrum. They were observed in 7% of 110 dermal lesions.[11] Simple surgical excision is effective.

Neuroblastoma, the most common cutaneous cancer at birth, is detected in one-third of affected infants by the presence of 5 to 30 small (3 to 6 mm), bluish, or pale blue nontender nodules (Fig. 43-18). Hepatomegaly and a retroperitoneal primary neuroblastoma are frequently present. Prognosis in this age group

is excellent (90%) with surgery and chemotherapy.[2]

Teratomas present as neck, intraoral, or sacrococcygeal tumors. They are large (3 to 10 cm), firm, nontender, and fixed to underlying tissue. Multiple calcifications are often seen on x-ray films. Epignathi (intraoral teratomas) contain structures resembling fetal parts (Fig. 43-19). Prompt surgical excision is necessary for functional and cosmetic reasons. After the patient is 5 months of age, these tumors tend to reveal embryonal carcinomatous elements. Recurrences, if they appear, will do so within 2 years after removal. Epulis, a fibrous tumor of the gums, tends to resolve spontaneously.[21]

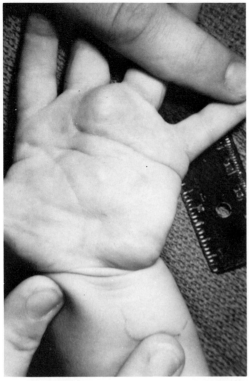

Fig. 43-17. Neurofibroma of the left wrist and hand in an infant. The larger left hand and swelling was noted at 9 months of age. A painful plexiform neuroma of the palmar area was resected at 2 and 6 years of age with improved function.

DEVELOPMENTAL VASCULAR ABNORMALITIES

Angiomas or vascular "nevi" are very common cutaneous congenital malformations seen during early infancy. Classification (Table 43-6) and description of these vascular tumors have been reported.[11] Two major groups seen in children are the involuting and noninvoluting vascular lesions, which may be flat (telangiectatic) or raised (hemangiomatous).

Studies of the common involuting types (erythema nuchae, salmon patch, spider nevi or teliangiectases, strawberry, cavernous, mixed strawberry-cavernous) have shown that no active therapy is necessary. A program of planned, intelligent neglect is essential in order to avoid disfiguring scars. Management consists of a detailed history, close scrutiny of the lesions with three-dimensional measurements, and evaluation of the growth pattern of the hemangioma. The natural pattern for the strawberry or cavernous hemangioma is rapid growth (to double or triple in size) within several weeks or months during early infancy. At birth the skin usually appears normal or shows a macular lesion which has a pink flush or off-white color.[10] Occasionally, a tumor will be present at birth (Fig. 43-20**A** and **B**). By 2 months of age, the strawberry lesion is bright red, or blue if a cavernous type, in about 90% of infants. When maximal size is attained, usually between 9 and 12 months of age, the color becomes a dark red.

At this time the hemangioma remains quiescent; its growth rate is the same as that of the infant. By 12 to 18 months, often earlier, spontaneous involution begins. The color gradually fades to a grayish pink; a gray-white hue appears in the center of the lesion and spreads until the whole area becomes white or pink. There is a decrease in tenseness as involution progresses. Although the bulk of the lesion

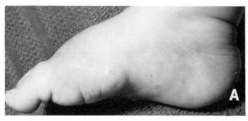
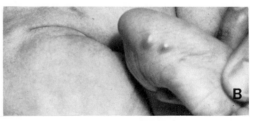

Fig. 43-18. A. Neuroblastoma. Cutaneous nodules (×30) and hepatosplenomegaly in a 1-month-old. The nodules regressed following surgical removal of a retroperitoneal neuroblastoma and cyclophosphamide therapy for 1 year. The patient was well at 4 years of age. (Courtesy Dr. S. Leikin) **B.** A 2-month-old with 13 violaceous nodules; excision of 8 revealed neuroblastoma. No primary tumor was found; no treatment was given. The nodules involuted by 6 months of age; the patient well at 3 years of age. (Courtesy Dr. J. L. Kennedy, Jr.)

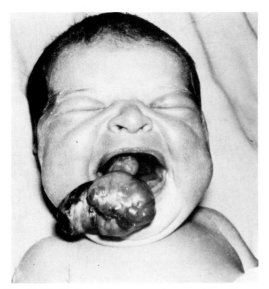

Fig. 43-19. Epignathi in a newborn arising from a hard palate. Surgical removal was done at 1 day of age; no recurrence was seen at 1 year of age. (Courtesy Dr. W. Bason and Dr. M. Museles)

diminishes, the area of discoloration decreases very slowly over several years.

Telangiectatic Nevi (Flat Lesions). **Involuting nevi,** the salmon patch (erythema nuchae) and cutis marmorata congenita or livedo reticularis have been discussed previously.

Noninvoluting nevi, seen less commonly in the newborn, are the port-wine nevus or stain, and rarely, the pyogenic granuloma. Granuloma pyogenicum is a rapidly growing, solitary, small (3–10 mm), dull red, papular lesion that easily bleeds. It is composed of granulation tissue with many capillaries and usually develops after minor skin trauma. Simple exision is best to avoid recurrence. Histologic examination is recommended to detect the rare benign juvenile melanoma.

The **port-wine** (nevus flammeus) nevi present at birth, is a capillary angioma consisting of mature capillaries, dilated and congested, directly beneath the epidermis. It is flat, sharply delineated, does not grow in area or size, and blanches minimally. The lesion may be very small (a few millimeters in diameter) or cover almost one-half of the body. In Black infants, they appear jet black. The characteristic red or red-purple color intensifies with the infant's crying. Unfortunately, facial lesions are common and may follow the distribution of a cutaneous nerve, such as the fifth cranial nerve. The presence of convulsions, mental retardation, hemiplegia (contralateral), and/or intracortical calcification suggests the Sturge–Weber syndrome.[3] Most port-wine nevi occur as isolated defects. They may occur in trisomy 13, Rubinstein–Tabyi, Wiedemann–Beckwith and pseudothalidomide syndromes.[3,5] In a few children the lesions may become lighter with age; however, they rarely disappear. A water-repellent cosmetic cream (Covermark, Retouch) will effectively conceal

Table 43-6. Developmental Cutaneous Vascular Abnormalities in Early Infancy.

Telangiectatic Nevi (Capillary Nevi)
Involuting
  Salmon patch, erythema nuchae; infantile
    hemangioma
  Cutis marmorata congenita (livedo reticularis)
Noninvoluting
  Port-wine nevus (nevus flammeus)
  Pyogenic granuloma (granuloma
    telangiectaticum)
Angiomatous Nevi (Involuting)
  Strawberry (capillary-endothelial nevus)
  Cavernous-superficial, subcutaneous types
  Mixed capillary-cavernous (combined type)
  Hemangioendothelioma
  Giant hemangioma with thrombocytopenia
    (Kasabach–Merritt)
Cutaneous Nevi with Systemic Hemangiomatosis
  Congenital multiple hemangiomatosis
Phacomatoses
  Sturge–Weber, tuberous sclerosis
  Blue rubber bleb nevus
Vascular Nevi and Cutaneous Vascular Tumors
  Phlebectasia (venous cavernous angiectasia)
  Hemangiectatic (angiectatic) hypertrophy
    (Klippel–Trenaunay–Weber)
Angiokeratoma
  Circumscriptum; Mibelli
  Racemose hemangiomata (cirsoid arterial or
    venous aneurysm)
Lymphangiomas (Vasoformative, Noninvoluting) and Lymphedema
  Simple lymphangioma
  Lymphangioma circumscriptum
  Cystic lymphangioma or hygroma
  Diffusive cavernous lymphangiomas
  Lymphedema, congenital, hereditary

(Margileth A: Pediatr Clin North Am 18:774, 1971)

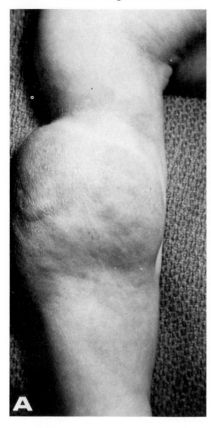
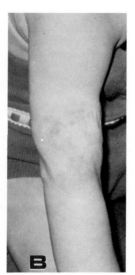

Fig. 43-20. A. A cavernous hemangioma of the arm in 6-day-old infant. The mass (6 × 10 cm × 1 cm elevated) was compressible (50%), blanched, and felt like a bag of worms. **B.** The same patient at 15 months of age; no therapy was used. (Courtesy Dr. E. Kraybill)

the mark. Tattooing can not be recommended because of possible scar formation, and inability to properly match the color of the normal skin. Plastic surgical repair may be necessary in the older child, because of the development of a verrucous, thickened nodular surface. Laser beam therapy appears to be effective cosmetically in the older child.[22]

Angiomatous Involuting Nevi(Raised Lesions). **Strawberry hemangioma** or hemangioma simplex is a capillary hemangioma, usually bright red or purplish red with well-defined margins. Rarely present at birth, it usually appears within a few days or weeks as a pink or red macule, resulting from myriads of tiny capillaries. The lesion enlarges during the first 5 to 6 months. The strawberry nevus blanches incompletely with pressure, and on palpation is a firm rubbery mass that compresses minimally. It is found on any part of the cutis and rarely involves mucous membranes. One or two are common; rarely, 20 or 30 lesions may be observed in an infant (Fig. 43-21**A** and **B**).

The **cavernous hemangioma** arises deeper in the dermis usually with poorly defined borders (Fig. 43-22**A**); but may be well circumscribed and elevated (Fig. 43-22**B**). The tumor, composed primarily of large venous channels and vascular lakes lined by mature endothelial cells, usually imparts a red-blue discoloration to the overlying normal skin. On palpation, these lesions are often cystic and feel like a bag of worms. The swelling usually compresses to half the original size and quickly resumes its usual size upon release of pressure. When the infant strains and cries, the tumor often becomes larger and darker blue. The **mixed (combined) hemangioma** consists of a cavernous lesion with an overlying strawberry component (Fig. 43-23**A** and **B**).

Natural Course of Hemangioma. The natural growth pattern of the strawberry, cavernous and mixed hemangioma is a noticeable increase in size during the first 3 to 6 months of life, a stationary period of several months, during which the hemangioma grows at the

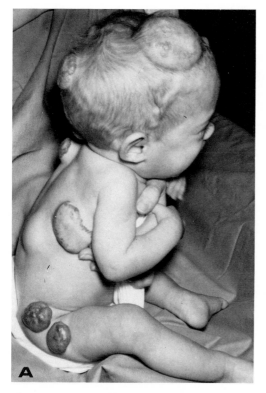
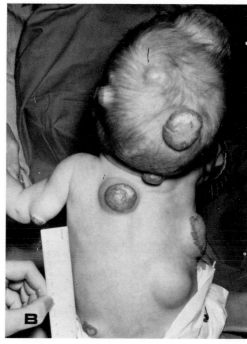

Fig. 43-21. A 7-month-old infant with 21 hemangiomas (strawberry, cavernous, and mixed types). No lesions were seen until 1 month of age. Between 7 and 8 months 1 new lesion developed. **A.** Lateral—9 hemangiomas visible over the scalp, back, and thigh. **B.** Posterior—11 lesions visible over the scalp, back, and left upper arm.

same rate as the patient, and then spontaneous involution occurs. Based upon the size of the hemangioma at 1 to 3 months, 80% of 420 hemangiomas we observed in 308 children, grew less than double in size during the first 1 to 2 years of observation.[11] About 5% tripled and 2% quadrupled their size. Six lesions continued to show minimal growth during the second year of observation. Because hemangiomas are benign and diagnosis is made easily by careful evaluation and repeated observation, a biopsy is not indicated.[3] In our series extending over 20 years, the strawberry, cavernous, and mixed hemangiomas regressed spontaneously and at similar rates during an 8- to 10-year period. By 5 years of age, one-half of these had involuted spontaneously. One infant we observed had 33 hemangiomas that involuted spontaneously by 3 years of age.

Treatment of Vascular Nevi. Those vascular nevi located in exposed areas often cause great parental concern because of the cosmetic ef-

fect. Parental anxiety increases as the hemangioma grows and causes deformity of tissue especially in the breast, lip, ear or eye. Additional concern develops when ulceration or bleeding occurs from trauma, maceration, or infection. Such situations often disturb the physician and create a feeling of urgency to do something. Nonetheless, the basic principle *primum nil nocere* should be followed.

The most important factor to evaluate is the parents' and, often, the grandparents' or friends' reactions. Preconceived notions about birth defects and advice by previous physicians must be reviewed before effective counseling. Search for a family history of hemangioma (10% of our series) was useful because most of the birthmarks of relatives had regressed spontaneously.

Complications following therapy were significant and occurred in 12 of 20 (60%) of our patients treated elsewhere.[11] Radiation and injection therapy caused greater morbidity and

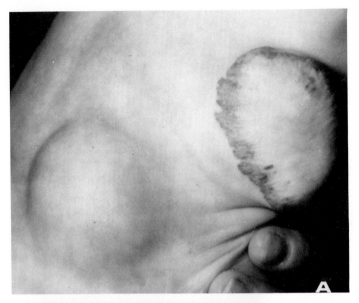

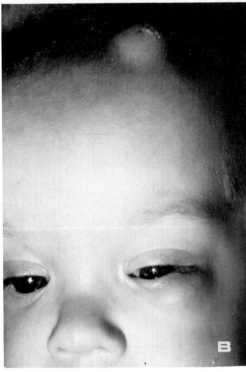

Fig. 43-22. The same patient (Fig. 43-21) at 8½ months of age before prednisone. **A.** Right chest and back—(upper) combined hemangioma with involuting strawberry component; (lower) subdermal cavernous, hemangioma. All lesions softened after 8 weeks of oral prednisone therapy. **B.** Face—a dermal cavernous hemangioma noted in the lower eyelid, and a combined lesion over the left forehead. By 6 years of age only three involuting lesions remained.

resulted in more extensive scarring than did surgery or dry ice. Seven of 19 hemangiomas showed subsequent growth within a few months after therapy. All of these have involuted spontaneously.

By contrast, complications during spontaneous involution are infrequent. In decreasing frequency these were ulceration, bleeding, and infection. Therapy consisted of local saline or tap water compresses, cleansing measures and a bacitracin ointment when indicated. Bleeding and secondary infection appeared to be natural processes which were beneficial and hastened spontaneous involution. Residual scarring af-

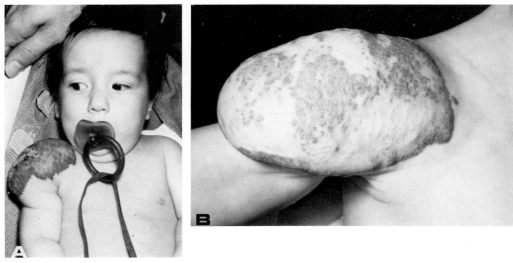

Fig. 43-23. A. A combined hemangioma in a 4-month-old was noted at 1 month of age. Rapid growth occurred until 2½ months of age. Ulceration developed at 3 months. The volume was 284 cm³. **B.** The same lesion at 17 months; the volume was then 180 cm³, a spontaneous reduction of 37%. By 5 years of age the lesion had involuted 90%.

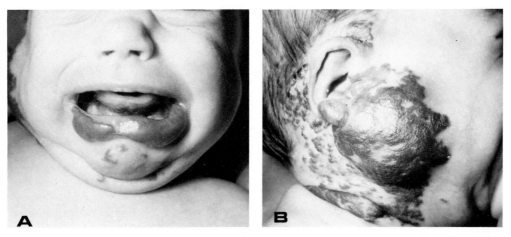

Fig. 43-24. A. A strawberry hemangiomata of the lip and chin. **B.** A combined dermal and right parotid hemangioma in a 6-week-old. The lesions were first noted at 5 days of age and are still enlarging with new strawberry hemangioma appearing on the neck and chin.

ter complete involution was uncommon and rarely unsightly. Minimal bleeding was observed in about 5% of 375 children; it was stopped by direct local pressure.

Active treatment is rarely needed and must be determined individually. Color photographs (35 mm) should be taken of lesions on exposed areas. Reassuring parents of the probability of spontaneous involution using serial photographs of similar cases has been most effective.

Observation of the child for several years is usually necessary to continue reassurance. In rare instances in which the diagnosis is uncertain (atypical growth pattern or no evidence for a vascular lesion), excisional biopsy may be necessary. In a patient in whom a hemangioma enlarges rapidly (within a few weeks) and vital structures are compromised (Fig. 43-24A and B) tissue destruction results, prednisone should be considered. If symptomatic

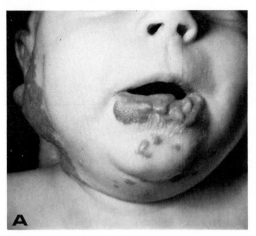 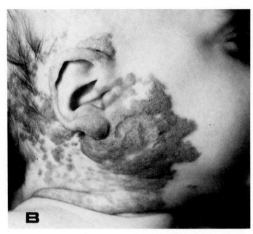

Fig. 43-25. The same patient (Fig. 43-24) at 3 months of age after 20 days of oral prednisone (10 mg/day). **A.** Note the ulceration of the lip. **B.** There was less redness and swelling of the parotid mass which was occluding the right external auditory canal.

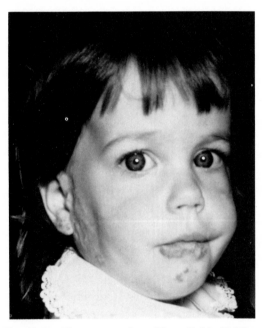

Fig. 43-26. The same patient (Figs. 43-24, 43-25) at 18 months of age. There was no recurrence after a 3-month course of prednisone: 10 mg on alternate days during the last 6 weeks.

thrombocytopenia occurs, prednisone may be effective also. Prednisone, 2 mg/kg/day in 2 or 3 divided doses orally for 3 to 4 weeks, has been beneficial in 24 of our 28 patients with hemangiomas obstructing the nares, auditory canal, or vision.[11] If signs of involution (Fig. 43-25A and B) occur after several weeks of daily prednisone, therapy should be continued 4 more weeks on alternate days in the same or double the dose. After 8 weeks, prednisone should be discontinued and the lesion watched carefully for recurrence of swelling, redness, or both. Regrowth may occur; it was not noted in 26 of our 28 patients (Fig. 43-26). A second course of prednisone has been effective in one series in which 20 to 40 mg of prednisone were given orally on alternate days for 1 to 3 months with 4 to 6 weeks between successive courses.[23] Plastic surgery may be necessary for redundant tissue persisting after spontaneous regression, or in a 5- or 6-year-old child whose lesion has not regressed. Compression treatment of large hemangiomas may be very effective.[24]

Giant Hemangioma with Thrombocytopenia (Kasabach–Merritt Syndrome). Over 72 patients with hemangioma and thrombopenia have been seen during early infancy in 30 years.[3,25] The hemangioma may be large (over 5 to 6 cm) or consist of small, multiple hemangiomas involving dermal and/or internal organs. These hemangiomas are usually cavernous, the majority occurring during the first few months of life. Thrombocytopenia with or without hemorrhagic manifestations may be found shortly after birth or appear only after several weeks or months. Sequestration of platelets in the hemangioma has been demonstrated by infusion of Cr^{51}-tagged platelets and by biopsy studies. The hemangioma itself may suddenly enlarge because of bleeding.

Anemia, splenomegaly, and purpura (with or without thrombopenia) are frequently observed. Spontaneous resolution has been reported in a significant number of patients who were treated conservatively or who did not respond to x-ray therapy or splenectomy.[11] Prednisone (2 mg/kg orally 2 or 3 times daily) for 1 or 2 months appears to be the treatment of choice. Compression of the tumor by a tight dressing and surgery, if feasible, have also been effective.[24] Although x-ray therapy may be effective,[26] the long-term effects are potentially serious.[11] Death may occur from infection or hemorrhage.

Cutaneous Nevi with Systemic Hemangiomatosis. Diffuse neonatal hemangiomatosis, an extremely rare condition, results in an early death in infants resulting from cardiac failure, gastrointestinal hemorrhage, infection, or hydrocephalus from aqueductal compression by hemangioma. Criterion for diagnosis is the recognition of nonmalignant visceral hemangiomas in three or more organ systems; cutaneous hemangiomas in varying numbers (1 to over 100) are found concomitantly.[27]

Therapy is supportive. Perhaps oral prednisone in large doses (4 to 10 mg/kg daily) should be tried initially in these seriously ill infants whose mean survival time is 71 days. Diffuse neonatal hemangiomatosis should be differentiated from the hamartomatous, Riley's, and blue rubber bleb nevus syndromes.[1–3,11]

Other Vascular Nevi and Cutaneous Vascular Tumors. **Phlebectasia** or venous ectasia, a rare vascular lesion consisting of dilated mature vessels in the dermis and subcutaneous tissues, presents in two forms in the newborn or young infant. Single or multiple tumors resembling cavernous hemangiomas grow slowly and may be associated with hypertrophy of the extremity.[11] We observed three children with neck varicosities and four with unilateral leg or forearm lesions. The other form, cutis marmorata telangiectatica with generalized phlebectasia, is apparent at birth and may have underdevelopment of subcutaneous and osseous tissues. In both types, therapy is rarely necessary because steady improvement occurs with growth.[3]

Hemangiectatic hypertrophy (Klippel–Trenaunay–Weber syndrome) of a limb associated with an extensive cutaneous nevus and a developmental hypertrophy of underlying bone and soft structures (osteohypertrophic varicose nevus) is a rare congenital abnormality. It is seen more frequently in males. The three major clinical features—hypertrophy of an extremity, vascular nevus, and venous varicosity—are not necessarily proportionate in extent and severity.[2] The nevus may be unilateral and the hypertrophy bilateral; minimal hypertrophy may be associated with an extensive nevus. Varicosity of the superficial veins with deep subcutaneous involvement may be a conspicuous feature noted at birth (Fig. 43-27A). The nevus may be capillary or cavernous with thickening and deformity of subcutaneous tissues. Occasionally, atrophy of bone, muscle, and soft tissue develop and, in fact, did occur in 1 of our 3 patients. Selective amputation of a grossly malformed digit and orthopedic measures to prevent limb hypertrophy will improve appearance and function. (Fig. 43-27B). Surgical extirpation of a giant lymphangiohemangioma was very effective in one of our patients.

Racemose hemangiomas usually found on the scalp, trunk or limbs at birth are usually 2 to 5 cm, elevated, warm, bluish, and occasionally pulsating vascular tumors. A central artery feeds the partially compressible tumor which has prominent peripheral radiating veins. The venous racemose aneurysm is more compressible and nonpulsating. The venous racemose aneurysm usually may involute spontaneously[11] while the arterial type may require selective artery ligation of associated arteriovenous fistulae or surgical excision. These lesions may arise from multiple glomus tumors.[3]

Lymphangiomas. Tumors of lymphatic origin are less common than hemangiomas and are hamartomatuous malformations consisting of dilated lymph channels of various sizes lined by normal lymph endothelium. Of four major types observed, each may be present at birth or develop during infancy or childhood.[25] Generally tumors are slow growing or may not grow at all.

Simple lymphangioma is the least common, and presents as a solitary, well-defined, skin-colored dermal or subcutaneous tumor on the face or neck. Mucous membranes are rarely involved. Simple surgical excision is usually satisfactory.

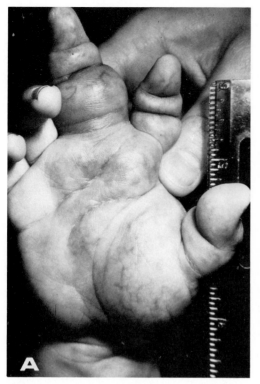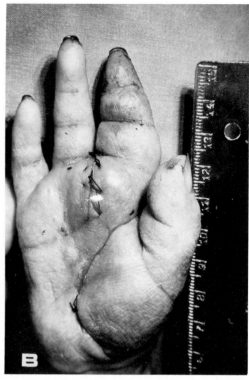

Fig. 43-27. A. Hemangiectatic venous hypertrophy of the hand, arm, and shoulder of a 3-year-old. The lesion was present at birth and enlarged slowly during the first 6 months of life. There was no growth in the past 2 years but the hand functioned poorly. **B.** The same patient at 3½ years of age, 7 days postamputation of the middle finger. Subsequently, useful function of the hand returned.

Lymphangioma circumscriptum, observed most commonly, consists of small, thick-walled vesicles in the skin resembling frog spawn (Fig. 43-28B). Sites commonly involved are axillary folds, neck, shoulder, proximal limbs (Fig. 43-28A), perineum, tongue, and buccal mucous membrane. Usually localized, such lesions may be extensive. Often a hemangiomatous component is present including blood-filled vesicles (Fig. 43-28B). Rarely, after several years of observation during which the lesion remains unchanged, the tumor will enlarge suddenly because of spontaneous bleeding or trauma.[11] Spontaneous involution is uncommon (one of nine patients in our series). Satisfactory results will follow complete surgical excision which is necessary to avoid recurrence.[25]

Cystic lymphangioma or **hygroma** occurs most often in the neck (hygroma colli) and axilla, but may occur in inguinal, popliteal and retroperitoneal regions and as mesenteric cysts. These are large unilocular cysts but may also be multilocular, especially in the neck. Transillumination will be present unless bleeding occurs. Because these lesions may grow rapidly with infiltration of vessels and nerves, surgical excision should be considered, but surgical results are often unsatisfactory.[28] Spontaneous regression may occur.

Diffuse or cavernous lymphangiomas are diffuse, ill-defined cystic dilatations, involving the skin, muscles and mucous membranes, and large areas of the face, trunk, and limbs (elephantiasis lymphangiectatica). Macroglossia and macrocheila[11] may occur because of involvement of the tongue and lips. Recurrent local infections (pre- and postoperative) are common and will usually respond to specific antibiotic therapy. Surgical excision will effectively remove small lesions, although recurrences are common. Surgical extirpation of

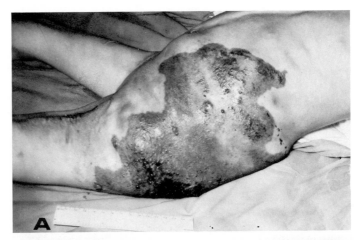

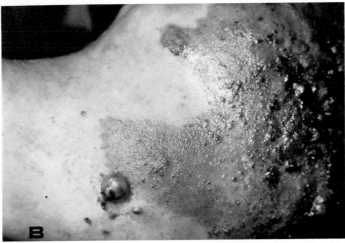

Fig. 43-28. A giant hemolymphangioma involving the upper thigh, flank, and retroperitoneal areas has been present since birth. Radical extirpation was necessary to drain a staphylococcal abscess within the mass. **B.** Lymphangioma circumscriptum in the same patient, showing thick-walled vesicles (frog spawn) overlying the tumor.

more diffuse lesions using multiple procedures is often unsatisfactory.[28,29]

Lymphedema. Congenital lymphedema occurs in two forms: as primary lymphedema, especially in females, mainly involving the lower extremities; and as Milroy's disease (hereditary lymphedema), almost always confined to the legs and feet. In Milroy's disease the edema is firm, easily pitted, and the temperature of overlying skin is elevated. Its pathogenesis is unclear; treatment during infancy is unnecessary. In both conditions upper extremities and genitalia may be involved.[3]

Infants with congenital lymphedema rarely may develop chylothorax and chylous ascites. The edema is brawny, and at first will partially respond to diuretics, pressure dressings, and elevation of the part. Edema becomes permanent as progressive fibrosis of tissue occurs.

Antibiotics are effective for secondary streptococcal or staphylococcal infections. Reconstructive surgery may be helpful during childhood. Chronic recurrent obstructive jaundice with associated cutaneous hemangiomas, lymphatic anomalies, and lymphedema has been reported in several families.[30] Similar therapy is effective.

INFECTIONS OF THE SKIN

Blistering disorders in the neonate frequently result from infection of bacterial, fungal, or viral origin (Table 43-7). Blistering has not been reported in congenital rubella, toxoplasmosis, or cytomegalovirus (CMV) infections. Maculopapular eruptions, usually without purpura, occur in the neonate (Table 43-8) as a result of fungal, parasitic, and viral infec-

Table 43-7. Vesicobullous Eruptions.

Infectious

BACTERIAL
Bullous-impetigo of newborn
Listeriosis
Mima and Herellea
Phagedenic ulcer
Toxic epidermal necrolysis (Ritter–Lyell)

FUNGAL
Cutaneous candidiasis
Oral candidiasis (thrush)
Mucocutaneous candidiasis

SPIROCHETAL
Congenital syphilis

VIRAL
Varicella
Variolovaccinia
Herpes simplex
Herpes zoster

Table 43-8. Maculopapular Eruptions.

NONPURPURIC
Aspergillosis
Coccidioidomycosis
Congenital syphilis*
Molluscum contagiosum
Toxoplasmosis*
Warts

PURPURIC OR PETECHIAL
Cytomegalovirus disease
Hematologic disorders
Histiocytosis X
Listeriosis
Rubella syndrome
Septicemia: streptococci, gram-negative bacilli

* Purpura may occur

tions. When purpura or petechial maculopapular eruptions are seen (Table 43-8), the clinician must look for bacterial sepsis, hematologic disorders, histiocytosis X, or viral (CID, rubella) infections. Noninfectious disorders (Table 43-9) producing vesicobullous eruptions will be discussed in the next subsection.

With a detailed history and a description of the morphologic characteristics of the cutaneous lesion (*e.g.*, maculopapular with or without purpura or vesicobullous) it is easy to think of the differential diagnosis of a specific eruption (Tables 43-7 and 43-8). Although a skin biopsy is simple and clearly delineates the cutaneous level of blister formation[3] or histologic nature of the eruption, we rarely request a biopsy. Routine in-office cultures, special cultures (fungal, viral), stained smears, scrapings using 10% KOH solution, and/or antibody titers, coupled with the history and morphologic findings, will provide a diagnosis in most infants.[1–3,31,32]

Vesicobullous Eruptions. **Bullous impetigo** of the newborn, a superficial vesiculopurulent pyoderma involving the stratum corneum, commonly occurs in the neonate and infant and is usually caused by staphylococci. The blisters vary from small vesicles to large, flaccid bullae filled with clear or straw-colored fluid. These rupture quickly and leave a red, moist denuded area (Fig. 43-29). Lesions may be widely dispersed and vary from a few single ones to large denuded areas. Because of thick stratum corneum, blisters over the palms and soles are less likely to rupture. Regional lymphadenopathy is rare unless secondary infection occurs with insect bites, eczema, scabies, herpetic lesions, or varicella.

Coagulase-positive *Staphylococcus aureus* frequently are cultured upon aspiration of bullae. Rarely, beta-hemolytic streptococcus will be isolated. Group A streptococci usually produce omphalitis, paronychia, erysipelas, perianal cellulitis, or sepsis.[1–3,31] Although very rarely, skin abscesses or umbilical lesions occur as a result of group B streptococci.[33] Coagulase determination of staphylococci isolated and antibiotic sensitivity tests are necessary only when the patient has had recurrent

Table 43-9. Vesicobullous Eruptions.

NONINFECTIOUS
Acrodermatitis enteropathica
Arthropod-induced blisters
Bullous ichthyosiform erythroderma
Epidermolysis bullosa
Erythropoietic porphyria
Incontinentia pigmenti
Juvenile dermatitis herpetiformis
Urticaria pigmentosa (mastocytosis)

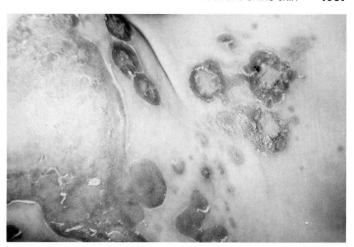

Fig. 43-29. Bullous impetigo in a young infant of 48-hours' duration. *Staphylococcus aureus,* penicillin sensitive, was cultured from a pustule.

or severe skin infections or during nursery epidemics. Blood cultures should be done if sepsis is suspected. Aseptic technique is essential for prevention in the premature nursery. Infected infants should always be isolated.

Topical therapy consists of cleansing of the lesions with povidone-iodine (Betadine) surgical scrub three to four times daily for 5 to 7 days until no new lesions appear. Concomitantly, a bacitracin ointment, 500 units/g, should be applied locally. A systemic antibiotic is indicated in newborns. Penicillin G, 25,000 to 50,000 U/kg/24 hours in two divided doses for 5 to 7 days will be effective unless the *S. aureus* is penicillin resistant. Oxacillin, 50 mg/kg/24 hours in two divided doses, or another penicillinase-resistant, semisynthetic penicillin may be the drug of choice depending upon the percent of resitant *S. aureus* strains in a particular hospital. If group A beta-hemolytic streptococci are recovered, a full 10-day course of penicillin is necessary. For patients with penicillin sensitivity, oral erythromycin, 40 mg/kg/24 hours in four divided doses or cephalexin, 25 mg/kg/24 hours given in four divided doses every 6 hours may be substituted.[33]

Toxic epidermal necrolysis (Ritter-Lyell syndrome) begins with an acute painful generalized erythema, followed rapidly by spreading bullous eruption and intraepidermal peeling, which closely resembles scalded skin. The skin is shed in sheets with minimal trauma (Nikolsky sign). In our series of 46 children with the staphylococcal skin syndrome, five infants less than 6 months of age were ob-

served; three had Ritter–Lyell's disease, two had bullous impetigo.[7] Characteristically, the skin was often tender, edema was noted about the mouth and eyes; low-grade fever (101° F) occurred in 56% of 35 children with toxic epidermal necrolysis (TEN). Within 24 hours of onset, vesicobullae were filled with clear sterile fluid. Conjunctivitis, often purulent, developed with prominent perioral wrinkling of the skin (Fig. 43-30). Within 1 to 2 days most bullae ruptured spontaneously with large, red, moist denuded areas which became dry and tan or bronze colored. Within 48 hours of onset, the infants were less toxic and exfoliation with large sheets of epidermis was widespread. Within 3 to 5 days, desquamation involved most of the erythematous areas, and by the sixth to twelfth days desquamation was complete. Cultures were positive for *S. aureus,* coagulase positive, in all five of the infants.

This syndrome in children includes Ritter's and Lyell's diseases, scarletiniform eruption, staphylococcal scarlet fever, and bullous impetigo of infancy. The first three disorders have generalized cutaneous involvement; bullous impetigo is usually localized. In each disorder, beta-hemolytic *S. aureus* can usually be isolated from the nose, throat, conjunctivae, or skin. Bullae are usually sterile because they result from an exfoliative exotoxin produced by *S. aureus.* The staphylococci are usually phage type 71, group II, and often penicillin resistant. In our series 50% of *S. aureus* were resistant to penicillin.[7]

Differential diagnoses may include syphilis, listeriosis, epidermolysis bullosa, and bullous

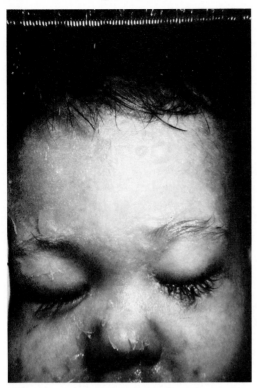

Fig. 43-30. Ritter–Lyell disease (TEN) in a 14-month-old. The second day there were associated sterile bullae on the forehead, trunk, and extremities. Note the positive Nikolsky sign (upper forehead) and purulent conjunctivitis due to *S. aureus*.

erythema multiforme (Table 43-7 and 43-9). Erythema multiforme, extremely rare in young infants, is easily recognized by the typical target or iris lesions. Cultures and smears or dark-field examination would exclude bacterial or spirochetal infection. Family history and close observation over several days should exclude epidermolysis bullosa.

Management in mild cases, especially the older infant or child at home, consists of thorough washing of lesions using a surgical soap (Betadine), two or three times daily, followed by 0.1% gentamicin cream or bacitracin ointment, 500 units/g for 3 to 5 days and close observation by parents and physician. For moderate or severe cases, especially in young infants, hospitalization is mandatory. Infants should be placed in reverse isolation and given IM penicillin or oral dicloxacillin, 25 to 50 mg/kg/24 hours orally in four divided doses, administered for 7 to 10 afebrile days.

After appropriate cultures are taken, fluids, electrolytes, and temperature should be monitored carefully. Lesions should be washed three times daily. Steroids are contraindicated. If denudation is extensive compresses of sterile water or normal saline, to which 0.1% silver nitrate has been added, are effective. Tepid baths twice daily followed by application of cold cream U.S.P. XVIII are effective for dry skin in the healing phase. Sulfacetamide sodium solution, Bleph-10 or Bleph-30, 100 to 300 mg/ml, or ointment, 100 mg/g, applied qid is effective for conjunctivitis. Recovery in most cases is complete in 9 or 10 days or less. Prognosis is excellent under 5 years of age; death has been reported in 0% to 7% of cases. One death occurred in 46 of our children.[7]

Phagedenic ulcers (ecthyma-like) are small, circumscribed ulcers with black necrotic centers and erythematous areolas complicating preexisting lesions (*e.g.,* varicella or puncture wounds). Severe debilitating disease, dysgammaglobulinemia, leukemia, or prematurity may be predisposing factors. The umbilicus may serve as a portal of entry. Initially, the lesions appear as grouped erythematous opalescent vesicles which rapidly become green and/or pustular and hemorrhagic at times. *Pseudomonas aeruginosa* is usually cultured; rarely, *S. aureus* may be isolated. Septicemia may be associated. Because tissue is destroyed beyond the epithelium, ecthyma is usually followed by scars. Treatment should be prompt and vigorous. Systemic antibiotics, gentamicin and carbenicillin, should be administered, especially if the lesions are extensive or sepsis is suspected. Gentamicin dose is 5 mg/kg/24 hours IM in three doses. Carbenicillin dose is 300 to 400 mg/kg/24 hours IV in six divided doses for 10 to 14 days. For local lesions polymyxin B, 0.1% solution in 1% acetic acid, may be useful. Silver nitrate, 0.5%, soaks are also effective. Soaks are applied locally for 1 to 2 hours 2 or 3 times daily for 7 to 10 days.

Listeriosis caused by *Listeria monocytogenes,* may produce severe infection (sepsis, meningitis) or disseminated miliary granulomatosis in the neonate.[3] A small percentage of infants show gray papules or papulopustules that resemble miliary abscesses at times. These may be widespread or localized to the back, oropharynx, or conjunctiva where they appear as small white foci. Occasionally, generalized erythema, maculopapular, or petechial-purpuric eruptions (Table 43-8) have been reported. The organism may be isolated from the pustule, blood, or spinal fluid. It is a gram-positive bacillus that produces hemolysis on blood agar. Infants should recover if intravenous penicillin or ampicillin is given promptly. Penicillin G dose is 50,000 to 100,000 units/kg/24 hours in two divided doses; ampicillin is 100 to 200 mg/kg/24 hours in four to six divided doses. Fatality rate with therapy varies from 30% to 55%.[34,35]

Mima polymorpha and *Herellea vaginicola,* normal residents of skin, vagina, and conjunctiva, may produce skin pustules, septicemia, meningitis, endocarditis and urinary tract infections. The cutaneous lesions are sharply demarcated with an elevated red base surmounted by a cluster of 1 to 3 mm pustules. When isolated from sick infants these gram-negative rods, resembling Neisseria on blood agar, should be regarded as pathogens. The primary skin lesions tend to be indolent[3] unless treated with gentamicin or the appropriate antibiotic as indicated by sensitivity studies.

Fungal infection of skin in the newborn is extremely uncommon except for candidial vesicopustular diaper rash and thrush (discussed previously). **Paronychial** infections occasionally seen in young infants are most often secondary to thumbsucking or local injury. Continuous wetness and sucking results in maceration and secondary mixed infection caused by Candida and *S. aureus* or *P. aeruginosa.*[34] Red, swollen skin at the nail base with purulent discharge suggests a bacterial infection. Exudate is rarely seen with Candida infection. After cultures are taken, wet soaks for 2 to 3 hours, three to four times daily, will effect purulent drainage. Systemic antibiotics will eradicate bacterial infection. Candidial paronychia usually responds to topical application of nystatin cream with a cotton applicator to fill the gap between the nail plate and posterior nail fold. The finger must be kept perfectly dry, since Candida thrives in a moist environment. A course of oral nystatin (Mycostatin) suspension, 1 to 2 ml, four times daily is occasionally helpful in recalcitrant infections.

Congenital syphilis, if untreated, will produce a maculopapular or bullous skin eruption in about 90% of infants between 2 and 6 weeks of life.[36] Bullae are occasionally seen at birth on the palms and soles; these infants tend to have a more severe disease. These blisters are of irregular size, and contain a cloudy fluid teeming with spirochetes that can be seen by darkfield examination. When the lesions rupture, the denuded area usually dries and crusts or macerates if moisture is present. The most common eruption consists of erythematous or copper-colored maculopapular ovoid lesions of the palms and soles which may spread over the entire body. Mucocutaneous lesions about the mouth, anus, and genitalia, and snuffles with a highly infectious nasal discharge may be the first clinical manifestations of the disease. Fissures may develop in these moist areas which upon healing result in fine periorificial scars (rhagades). Raised, flat, moist lesions, condylomata lata, may appear at angles of the mouth, nares, or anogenital region. Mucous patches may be seen on the lips, tongue, and palate. If untreated, the skin lesions regress spontaneously in 1 to 3 months leaving residual hyper- or hypopigmentation.

The routine VDRL on the mother is invariably positive. If the infant is infected, the serology will be positive in 85% of infants at 1 month of age, 95% at 2 months of age, and 100% by 3 months of age. An infant's serologic titer higher than the maternal titer is diagnostic. Other clinical features are reviewed elsewhere (see Chap. 32).[3] Therapy consists of IM aqueous procaine penicillin, 50,000 units/kg/24 hours given twice daily over 10 days.[35] Therapy should continue with the infant having a monthly quantitative titer for 6 months, then every 3 months for a year to insure adequate therapeutic response. Serologic reversal is usually expected in one year. An examination of CSF is recommended 12 to 24 months after therapy.[36] All physicians should be alert for this disease because of its increased incidence in the past decade.

Viral epidermal lesions usually present in the neonate or young infant with a characteristic morphologic picture. Vesicles are seen in varicella, variolovaccinia, herpes simplex, and herpes zoster; the virus may be isolated from early lesions. Multinucleated ''balloon'' cells and eosinophilic mononuclear cells may be seen on a Giemsa-stained smear from scrapings of the base of a fresh vesicle in the herpes group (simplex, varicella-zoster).[32] Rarely, they are detected in the pox group (variola, vaccinia). Petechial-purpuric lesions occur in cytomegalovirus inclusion disease and con-

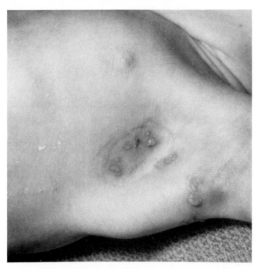

Fig. 43-31. Herpes simplex vesicles in axilla of a 12-day-old with severe herpes, type 2, encephalitis of 3 days' duration. The lesions cleared in 12 days. Severe mental retardation developed.

genital rubella. Papular eruptions are characteristic of molluscum contagiosum and warts (Table 43-8).

Herpesvirus hominis (simplex) infection, one of the most potentially serious viral diseases in young infants, should be differentiated from other vesiculobullous eruptions (Table 43-7). Cutaneous lesions may be noted at birth or during the neonatal period in most of the affected infants. Lesions vary from a few scattered depressed scars or a local boggy swelling to one (Fig. 43-31) or many discrete groups of vesicles. A zosteriform distribution may occur.[32] Vesicles may coalesce and become erosive. In a group of 11 infants, seven survivors continued to exhibit recurring crops of vesicles for months, until two years of age. Each recurrence was less severe with fewer vesicles and shorter duration of each episode. Concomitantly, erythema multiforme occurred in some infants. Antiviral therapy should be considered (see Chap. 33) because the prognosis is guarded.[37] Two-thirds of infants developing encephalitis either die or live with mental retardation or hemiparesis.

Varicella-zoster, a rare transplacental infection, is one of the least-threatening infections to the fetus and newborn. Varicella occurring in the first 10 days of life has probably been acquired in utero because the incubation period is 10 to 21 days. The vesicular eruption, lesions, and course of disease are identical to varicella at any age. Although a mortality of 20% has been reported, the course of neonatal varicella has been mild in most patients. In two of our patients, depressed white scars were observed at birth; each mother had varicella during the first trimester. Scars in a zosteriform distribution have been seen.[3] No therapy is needed unless secondary infection develops.

Vaccinia virus and **variola** infections are rarely seen in the neonate. Abortion or stillbirth may occur if the mother is vaccinated or maternal variola occurs.[3] Congenital vaccinia may be associated with cutaneous scars, ocular damage, and hypoplastic bony defects.

Petechial, Purpuric, and Maculopapular Eruptions with Infection (Table 36-8). **Cytomegalovirus inclusion disease** (CID) is usually recognized in a small-for-dates infant with jaundice, lethargy, pallor, petechiae, and/or purpura with hepatosplenomegaly and chorioretinitis. Thrombocytopenia accounts for the purpuric lesions. In a few infants, generalized dark-blue, magenta papules or nodules occur as a result of collections of extramedullary dermal erythropoiesis. These regress in 2 to 3 weeks leaving dark red to pale gray macules. Differential diagnosis includes sepsis, toxoplasmosis, rubella, syphilis, and herpes simplex infections. Isolation of CMV virus from urine or liver biopsy with a rising complement fixation titer will confirm the diagnosis. No satisfactory treatment is available.

Rubella infection in the neonate produced purpura in 35% of 200 infants. Petechiae and purpura are often seen at birth; new lesions rarely develop after several days of age unless thrombocytopenia is severe. Most lesions have faded by the second week and are gone by 4 to 6 weeks of age. The most unusual cutaneous finding is the "blueberry muffin" lesion noted at birth in severely affected infants. These firm, bluish-red papules, 2 to 8 mm in diameter, occur over the head, trunk, and extremities. They are caused by dermal erythropoiesis and resolve spontaneously in 2 to 3 weeks, unless death occurs. Cutis marmorata, slate-blue discoloration of dependent extremities and capillary flushing, are reported.[3] Isolation of these infants from susceptible personnel is mandatory because the virus is excreted for months. Septicemia caused by streptococci or gram-negative bacilli, toxoplasmosis, CMV, and syphilis should be considered in the differential diagnosis. Therapy is supportive.

Molluscum contagiosum, very rarely seen in neonates, is caused by a pox virus. The benign lesions are characterized by discrete, waxy papules with a pink, tan, or ivory hue and central umbilication. Size varies from 1 mm to 1 cm, and lesions are found anywhere. The lesions are self-limiting after 6 to 9 months. Treatment is not necessary unless new lesions develop by autoinoculation. Treatment consists of removal by curettage, or by blistering with either a light application of liquid nitrogen or 0.7% cantharidin in colloidin, used in minute quantities under an occlusive plastic tape for 12 hours to enhance blister formation. Examination of a curetted plug after clearing debris with 10% KOH will reveal the typical molluscum bodies.[32]

Warts, extremely uncommon in the newborn or young infant, are caused by a virus of the papova group. Mucous membrane warts (condylomata acuminata) are occasionally seen in older infants on moist mucosa of the anus, genitalia, or mouth. A VDRL should always be done. The treatment of choice is 15% podophyllin in compound tincture of benzoin, applied carefully to the lesion for 3 hours and then washed off. Applications are repeated weekly for several weeks. Suggestion therapy for common warts is discussed elsewhere.[34]

Toxoplasmosis, relatively uncommon in neonates, is caused by an intracellular parasite, *Toxoplasma gondii.* It is a transplacental infection with features simulating those found in erythroblastosis fetalis, rubella syndrome, CMV, or bacterial sepsis. A generalized maculopapular rash has been seen in 25% of infants with hepatosplenomegaly, jaundice, fever, and anemia. The rash tends to spare the scalp, palms and soles, and rarely persists longer than 2 weeks. Desquamation and hyperpigmentation have followed severe eruptions. Diagnosis is made by noting rising titers measured by the Sabin–Feldman dye test. Specific therapy is discussed by Remington.[34]

Both **coccidioidomycosis** and **aspergillosis,** exceedingly rare in the neonate, may produce maculopapular nonspecific eruptions. Vesicopustules have been reported in aspergillosis,

and vesicles have occurred in the former disease. Erythema nodosum has not been reported in very young infants. Clinical features and therapy are discussed elsewhere.[38]

BLISTERING DISEASES: NONINFECTIOUS

Acrodermatitis Enteropathica. The classic tetrad of diarrhea, periorificial vesiculobullous dermatitis, alopecia, and apathy is diagnostic of this rare disorder. Acrodermatitis enteropathica usually presents during the first year of life and is characterized by remissions and exacerbations. Symmetrical vesicopustules which usually evolve into erythematous eczematous patches may be seen over the trunk and extremities. Zinc therapy, 50 mg orally tid, for years, is very effective.[12]

Arthropod-induced Blisters. Bites and stings, although uncommon in the young infant, may produce erythema, blisters, wheals, and rarely a gangrenous slough. Lesions tend to be localized or in a linear arrangement. Spiders (brown recluse) or scorpions can produce severe reactions locally and systemically.[2] Intense erythema rapidly progresses through a blister, sometimes hemorrhagic, to sloughing of skin. The blister beetle may produce a subepidermal blister. Papular urticaria, caused by flea, fly, mosquitoe, bedbug, moth, wasp, or bee stings, characteristically develops on the distal extremities in a symmetrical pattern. Lesions may become purpuric and occasionally develop over the trunk and face if repeated bites occur. Pruritus with secondary excoriations are often seen in the infant. Local therapy consists of cool tap water compresses or baths, diphenhydramine (Benadryl), 4 to 6 mg/kg/24 hours, and 3% vioform in 0.5% hydrocortisone cream applied tid. Oral steroids are rarely necessary.[2]

Mite infestations (scabies) may be considered, especially if the parent, sibling, or family pet has a pruritic rash.[2,3] The gray- or flesh-colored burrows vary in length up to 1.5 cm, and commonly occur on the palms, soles, scalp, face, and neck. Vesicles often appear at the end of the burrow. Because of intense pruritus excoriations, eczematous changes and secondary infection are common. Diagnosis is confirmed by presence of ova or mites seen microscopically from scrapings of burrows. Ten percent KOH should be used to clear

Table 43-10. Epidermolysis Bullosa.

Nonscarring Types

Epidermolysis bullosa simplex	Autosomal dominant
Epidermolysis bullosa letalis (junctional bullous)	Autosomal recessive

Scarring: Dermolytic Bullous Dermatosis

Dominant dystrophic	Autosomal dominant
Recessive (polydysplastic) dystrophic	Autosomal recessive

debris. Larva of Diptera may be similarly identified.[1-3] A very effective treatment for the entire family with scabies is gamma hexabenzene (Kwell ointment) or 10% crotamiton (Eurax) which is preferred for infants due to potential toxicity of Kwell, applied twice daily for 2 days followed by bathing. In 5 to 7 days, a second course may be given. Bacitracin ointment applied tid will be effective for secondary infection.

Epidermolysis Bullosa. Pearson has classified this rare hereditary mechanobullous disease into two major subgroups: nonscarring and scarring epidermolysis bullosa (EB). Four of the subtypes (Table 43-10) may occur at birth or in early infancy.[2,3,39] The disorder is further identified by location of blister formation in the intra-epidermal or subepidermal layers produced as a result of minor trauma.[2]

Nonscarring *EB* presents in 2 forms: epidermolysis bullosa letalis (EBL), which is extremely rare; and epidermolysis bullosa simplex (EBS), which is commonly seen by comparison. Characteristically, in EBS the legs, feet, and scalp show erosions which heal slowly without scars. Blisters can be produced within a few hours by gentle rubbing, as in most forms of EB. Bullae may contain blood (Fig. 43-32). Pyogenic infection may be prevented by proper skin care and aseptic technique. Protection from minor trauma is essential. Clean, soft cotton dressings may be helpful over pressure points. Bacitracin ointment should be used after surgical soap cleansing two or three times daily for secondary infection. Maceration must be avoided. Emollients (Nivea or Aquaphor cream) will avoid dry skin. Prognosis for EBS is good with a tendency to improve by puberty.

Sheets of epidermis loosen (dermal-epidermal separation) with minimal trauma in EBL. The resulting moist erosions become infected, ulcerate, and develop vegetating granulomas. Septicemia, growth retardation, and anemia are common. The prognosis is poor when frequent, large, denuded areas continually develop. In some children, lesions heal spontaneously and completely. Treatment is protective, palliative and supportive. Iron and steroid therapy is often helpful during critical periods. Heat should be avoided; cool water compresses to traumatized skin and air conditioning are helpful. Local and systemic antibiotics are indicated for secondary infection[2,3]

Dominant dystrophic EB (dermolytic bullous dermatosis), seen uncommonly in the new-

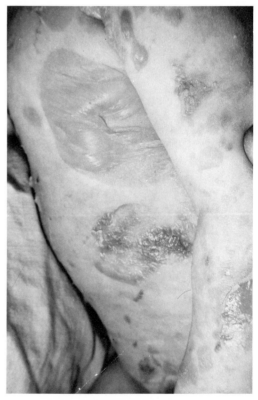

Fig. 43-32. Nonscarring epidermolysis bullosa (EB) in 4-month-old whose sister died in infancy of EB letalis. The vesiculobullae noted at birth recurred often until the patient was 2 years of age when improvement began. The patient is much improved at 17 years of age.

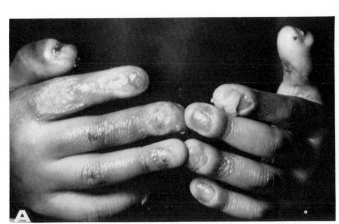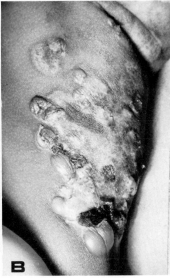

Fig. 43-33. Dystrophic scarring epidermolysis bullosa in a 3½-year-old boy with finger and toenails absent at birth. At 1 week of age, recurrent clear and hemorrhagic blisters developed after minor trauma. **A.** Atrophic scarring of fingertips. **B.** The thigh at 18 months of age with blisters and dystrophic scars.

born, is less severe than the recesive type of scarring EB (Table 43-10). Lesions usually appear well after birth on the hands, feet, and sacrum secondary to minimal trauma. Nails may be lost but deforming scars and contractures are not frequent. Mucous membrane lesions occur but are mild. Hypo- and hyperpigmentation with soft, wrinkled scars are observed with healing. Therapy is the same as noted previously for EB simplex. Paper tape should be used for diapers instead of pins; adhesive tape should never be used on the skin.

Recessive scarring EB (polydysplastic and dystrophic) initially appears benign in the neonate. Eventually after many months, the toe and finger blisters heal with pseudofusion of the digits and loss of nails (Fig. 43-33A). Finally, over several years, the hands and arms become fixed in a flexed position and contractures ensue. A positive family history helps to differentiate this type from EB simplex and dominant scarring EB. Consanguinity has been reported. During early infancy, a skin biopsy to localize blister formation (Fig. 43-33B) may be helpful to differentiate the severe scarring and nonscarring types,[2,3] and to rule out bullous congenital ichthyosiform erythroderma. Therapy is similar as above. Vitamin E, 200 to 3200 I.U. daily has been beneficial in some patients.[1]

Erythropoietic Porphyria Congenita. This very rare hereditary disease, caused by a defect in heme synthesis, may be seen in the newborn. Because of severe photosensitivity, burning, pruritus, erythema, and vesicobullous eruptions develop upon sun exposure. Ulcerations and secondary infection are common. Scarring and loss of nails, digits and cartilage (ears, nose) develop later. The urine may be pink; when teeth erupt they are stained pink-brown and have a red fluorescence under ultraviolet illumination. Systemic and cutaneous manifestations are progressive with a decreased life expectancy. Excess uroporphyrin-1 and orange-red fluorescence of erythrocytes are diagnostic. Therapy is symptomatic and includes protection from light with application of sunscreen creams, and appropriate management of hemolytic anemia and infection.[2] Oral administration of beta-carotene, (Solatene), 60 to 180 mg daily coupled with topical UV-A, sunscreen increases tolerance to sun exposure at least three times.[1]

Incontinentia Pigmenti. Nevus continuous reticularis et pigmentosus or incontinentia pigmenti is an uncommon hereditary (X-linked dominant) disorder affecting skin primarily.

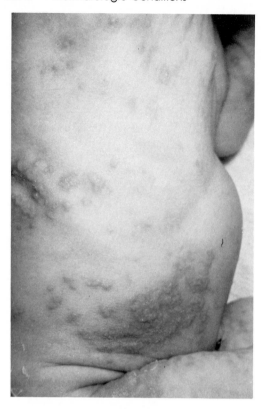

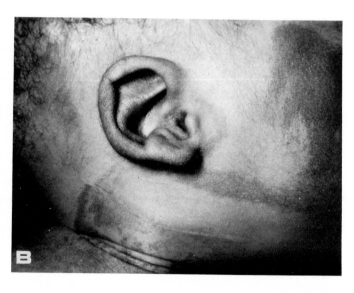

Fig. 43-34. Incontinentia pigmenti in a week-old infant. Erythematous vesicles and papules developed at 4 days of age and progressed to pigmented whorls by 6 months of age. No other defects were present. The mother had similar pigmented linear macules on the thigh.

Extracutaneous defects of the eyes, CNS, teeth, heart, and bones, are often seen after neonatal period. The female to male ratio is 9: 1 or greater. At birth or shortly thereafter, inflammatory vesicobullae and papules (Fig. 43-34) erupt in crops over the trunk or limbs. After several months pigmented hypertrophic or verrucous lesions appear that gradually resolve and form macular pigmented whorls and brush-stroke lines (Fig. 43-35A and B). These bizarre brown or slate-gray macules are diagnostic and should alert the physician to watch for retarded development, microcephally, seizures, ocular pseudotumors, pegged teeth, and cardiac defects. Eosinophilia (50%) is present during the vesicular stage; the subcorneal vesicles are filled with eosinophils. No therapy is required for the skin. Genetic counseling is advisable.[2,3]

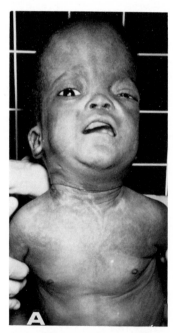

Fig. 43-35. A. Bloch–Sulzberger syndrome in a 6-month-old: incontinentia pigmenti, ocular pseudogliomas, mental retardation, hydrocephalus, heart disease. **B.** Note the typical pigmented brown brush strokes on the face.

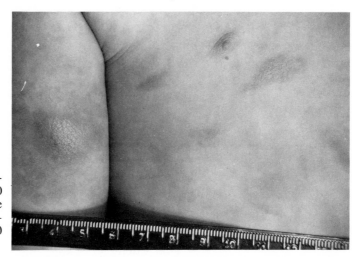

Fig. 43-36. Urticaria pigmentosa (mastocytosis) in a healthy infant with 30 maculopapular truncal lesions. Note the positive Darier sign on the arm produced after stroking a similar lesion 10 times.

Juvenile Dermatitis Herpetiformis. This chronic, pruritic, vesiculbullous dermatitis is extremely uncommon in young infants. Crops of small, clear, tense blisters are seen on the buttocks, face, genitalia, and limbs in an otherwise well infant. The lesions are sterile, thus excluding impetigo. Recurrent bouts of vesicles or bullae occur over many months or years, when spontaneous resolution occurs. Treatment with dapsone (diaminodiphenylsulfone) or sulfapyridine should be individualized to avoid side effects and should be used only during acute phases. Topical therapy is usually unnecessary. Diphenhydramine (Benadry), 5 mg/kg/24 hours, or cyproheptadine (Periactin), 0.25 to 0.5 mg/kg/24 hours, may alleviate pruritus.

Urticaria Pigmentosa. **Cutaneous mastocytosis** (mast cell disease) rarely observed in the newborn, is not uncommon during infancy. In young infants the lesions may be single or multiple bullae (sterile), appearing primarily on the trunk, limbs, or scalp. A single mastocytoma (2 to 6 cm) may be seen. In older infants, disseminated maculopapular or nodular eruptions occur. As many as 20 to 40 tan to light-brown lesions may gradually develop. Minimal rubbing may produce urtication (Darier sign; Fig. 43-36) within minutes to 1 hour or so in some patients. This reaction is diagnostic. Spontaneous resolution of lesions occurs over several years, but a few many persist through puberty with residual hyperpigmentation.[1,2]

Systemic mastocytosis is rare in infants. Dif-

fuse mast cell proliferation occurs in the skin, bone, liver, nodes, spleen, and bone marrow. In addition to presenting with multiple blisters (Fig. 43-37), these infants manifest episodes of flushing, irritability, tachycardia, respiratory distress, hypotension, pruritus, diarrhea, and abdominal pain. Eosinophilia and elevated urine histamine levels occur. Therapy, rarely necessary for cutaneous lesions, is difficult in infants with extensive lesions. Cyproheptadine

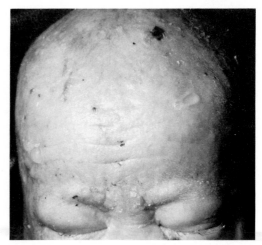

Fig. 43-37. Systemic mastocytosis in a 2-month-old. At 2 days of age, bright red macules were noted which urticated and vesiculated with trauma. Episodes of flushing and severe diarrhea occurred. Hepatosplenomegaly, pulmonary infiltrates, and anemia were present. (Courtesy N. Movassaghi, M.D.)

Table 43-11. Types of Ichthyosis in Young Infants.

Condition	Age of Onset/Inheritance	Clinical Features	Associated Features
Ichthyosis vulgaris (ichthyosis simplex)	Usually after 3 months of life Autosomal dominant	Scales: fine, branny, white Forehead, cheeks involved Back more affected than abdomen Flexures spared Increased palmar and plantar markings	Localized shiny hyperkeratosis of knees and elbows Atopic dermatitis common Family history positive for atopy Keratosis pilaris common
Sex-linked ichthyosis	Birth to one year X-linked; female to male transmission	Scales: thick, dark brown, large Lateral face, neck and scalp most severely affected Abdomen more than back Limbs: total involvement common Flexures variably affected Palms and soles normal	"Dirty" appearance of scales Only males affected Occasionally have collodin membrane at birth Deep corneal dystrophy by slit lamp Normal cellular kinetics
Nonbullous congenital ichthyosiform erythroderma (Lamellar ichthyosis)	Birth Autosomal recessive	Scales: flat, dark, large, coarse Upper face more than lower Uniform generalized hyperkeratosis of trunk Limbs generalized involvement Flexures always affected (dry) Palms and soles thickened	Background erythroderma Prematurity common May have collodin membrane Harlequin fetus, the most rare and severe Ectropion present and progressive Increased epidermal motitic rate
Bullous congenital ichthyosiform erythroderma (Epidermolytic hyperkeratosis) (Ichthyosis hystrix)	Birth to 6 months Autosomal dominant	Scales: coarse, verrucous, small Lower face more than upper Limbs, trunk variably affected Flexures always affected (moist) Palms and soles usually affected	Background erythroderma Bullae during infancy and childhood Increased epidermal mitotic rate

HC1 (Periactin), not to exceed 0.5 mg/kg/24 hours in four divided doses, or diphenhydramine (Benadryl), 5 mg/kg/24 hours in three or four doses orally, will alleviate pruritis and irritability. Rubbing of skin and hot water must be avoided. Aspirin, codeine and procaine are contraindicated, because severe reactions may occur after histamine release from mast cell granules.[1-3] Prognosis is good for cutaneous mastocytosis but poor for systemic mastocytosis.

SCALING DISORDERS

Desquamation of skin occurs in 75% of newborns. It is commonly observed in infants of 40- to 42-weeks' gestation and rarely, if ever, in those less than 35-weeks' gestation. Maximum shedding is observed by the end of the first week of life. Differential diagnosis of the scaly infant includes physiologic desquamation, dysmaturity and the rare ichthyosiform dermatoses. Three of the four major types of ichthyosis (Table 43-11) may be present at birth. These are sex-linked ichthyosis, nonbullous congenital ichthyosiform erythroderma, and bullous congenital ichthyosiform erythroderma. Ichthyosis vulgaris, the most common and benign form, is rarely observed before the third month. Well-known terms, "harlequin fetus" and "collodion baby" are descriptive only, and not separate types of ichthyosis (Table 43-11). Extremely rare types, ichthyosis linearis circumflexa and erythrokeratoderma variabilis will not be discussed. Nor will very rare syndromes (Netherton, Sjögren–Larsson, Rud, Conradi, Refsum, Tay) with scaling dermatosis, since they have been reviewed recently.[1-3,5,39]

X-Linked Ichthyosis. This relatively mild disorder occurs in males only; however, in female heterozygotes scaling of the arms and lower legs may be present. In males, the entire body is involved except palms and soles, midface, and flexural areas. Scales are large, yellow to dark brown and thick. (Fig. 43-38). At birth, the infant may present as a collodion baby or simply as a scaly infant. In one series, 36% were affected at birth; only 6% were unaffected by 3 months of age. Prognosis is good and therapy (discussed later) is simple.

Nonbullous Congenital Ichthyosiform Erythroderma (Lamellar Ichthyosis). At birth, this autosomal recessive disorder may present in

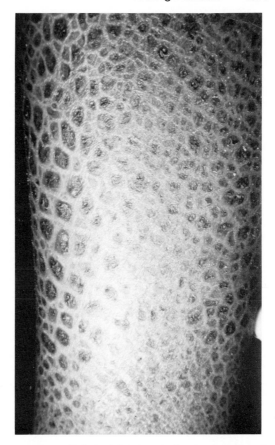

Fig. 43-38. X-linked ichthyosis in the leg of a 5-year-old boy. Five other males in the family were affected. Note the large, thick, and dark scales.

a healthy infant with generalized brilliant erythema or as the rare collodion baby (Fig. 43-39A and B). Desquamation is universal and with drying the skin assumes a parchment-like appearance. In general, these infants do well with gradual fading of the erythroderma. After the neonatal period, scales develop that vary from a yellow to brown-black color, and eventually form warty excrescences or thick horny plates covering large body areas in childhood. Secondary infection may occur if the skin becomes macerated, especially in intertriginous areas. Prognosis is generally good except for the extremely rare Harlequin fetus for whom therapy is ineffective; death usually occurs from sepsis during the neonatal period (Fig. 43-40).[1,3,39]

Bullous Congenital Ichthyosiform Erythroderma (CIE). Infants born with this disorder

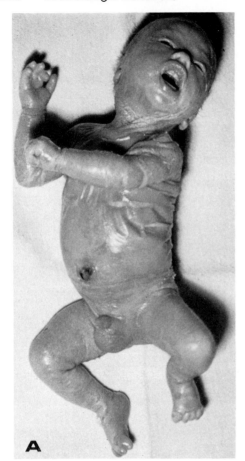 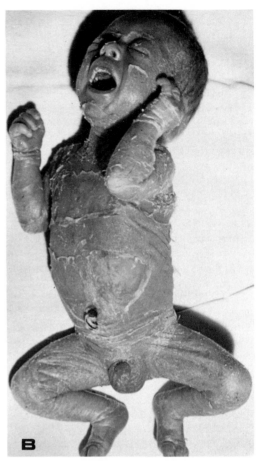

Fig. 43-39. A collodion baby. **A.** Shortly after birth. **B.** At 3 days of age. The yellow collodion membrane peeled and shed in sheets leaving large, coarse, lamellar scales. The older sister had dry minimally scaly hyperkeratotic skin and a similar appearance at birth.

have widespread bullae (0.5–20 cm), erythema, and dry, peeling skin. The blisters commonly appearing in crops during childhood differentiate this disease from nonbullous CIE. In the newborn, extensive denudation with secondary infection and sepsis occur often because of beta-hemolytic streptococci or staphylococci. In older infants, hyperkeratosis may remain generalized or localized to flexural areas. Scales are small, hard, and coarse and shed in large quantitites. Normal bacteria in the thickened horny layers produce a putrid odor as in lamellar ichthyosis. Bacterial population may be decreased with antiseptic baths. It is common to find several affected family members because this is an autosomal dominant disorder.

Management of ichthyosis is primarily the continued use of topical preparations. Daily hydration and lubrication of the skin are essential. One or two baths are given daily, containing a water dispersable bath oil (Alphakeri), followed by application of an ointment or cream (Aquaphor)[22] several times daily. In severely affected localized areas, use of a keratolytic ointment (salicylic acid, 3% to 10%) or 10% urea in an ointment base, is an effective alternative.[1,4] It is most important to avoid detergents and soaps that are drying and irritating. Basis soap, Lowila bar, are excellent but pHisoderm or Dermolate are excellent substitutes. Dry indoor heat should be avoided. Topical steroid creams or ointments used for short periods are effective for primary irritant dermatitis. Oral prednisone (1 mg/kg/ 24 hours) may be necessary for children with

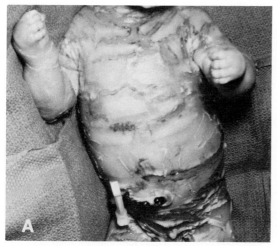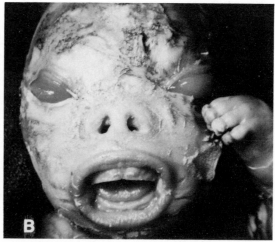

Fig. 43-40 A, B. Nonbullous ichthyosiform erythroderma. Harlequin fetus, age 1 day, with severe ectropion, eclabion and fissures, scaling, and deformity of hands, feet and ears. Death resulted from sepsis and extensive bacterial abscesses at 1 month of age. Patient was the first baby and family history was negative. (Courtesy A. Fletcher, M.D., CHNMC)

widespread bullous CIE. Diphenhydramine (Benadryl) is effective for pruritus. Dramatic improvement has been reported in patients with ichthyosis vulgaris and X-linked ichthyosis using diluted (40%–60%) propylene glycol with an occlusive plastic overnight.[40] Topical vitamin A acid (0.1%) with an occlusive plastic wrap for 24 to 48 hours has also been effective.

In our experience and that of others, oral 13-cis-retinoic acid in limited trials has been beneficial to older children with lamellar ichthyosis and epidermolytic hyperkeratosis.[41] Genetic counseling is essential for these patients and their families.

ECZEMA IN THE NEWBORN

Eczema, "to boil over," a common problem in the infant over 2 months of age, is much less common in the newborn. Nevertheless, it is such a difficult problem for the infant, mother, and physician and its causes are so varied (Table 43-12) that two of the common conditions will be discussed. Several have been reviewed here and elsewhere.[1–3,5,14] The four phases of eczema are usually seen simultaneously in the same patient. Pruritus, the major symptom, occurs in all phases. Initially, acute **erythema** proceeds rapidly to microvesicles with **weeping.** A burst of epidermal mitotic activity leads to **scaling,** and finally to **lichen-ification** (thickened skin with prominent normal markings). Hypo- or hyperpigmentation eventually develops. Exogenous types of eczema observed during early infancy are noted in Table 43-12. Primary irritant diaper dermatitis, and infectious eczema, including physical agents, were discussed earlier. Allergic contact or drug dermatitis is extremely rare.[3] Some of the endogenous types of eczema (Table 43-12) have been discussed previously or are so rare as to be dismissed.[2,3,12,14]

Atopic Dermatitis. **Atopic or infantile eczema,** the most common type of eczematous eruption after 2 months of age, is a difficult management problem of unknown etiology.[14,42] Diagnostic features are a healthy child with a highly pruritic erythematous, oozing symmetrical eruption of the cheeks, extensor surfaces of limbs and diaper area, and patchy lesions of the scalp and trunk; family history of allergy; rapid response to topical therapy and environmental measures; and recurrent exacerbations with a chronic (1- to 3-year) course. Elimination of possible exogenous causes and continued consideration of other systemic disorders (Table 43-12) that may be excluded by time, course of the patient's disease and a few specific tests (*i.e.,* 10% $FeCl_3$ test of fresh urine for phenylketonuria) make atopic dermatitis the likely diagnosis. Rarely, histologic examination of skin may be necessary to exclude a diagnosis of nonbullous CIE.

Table 43-12. Causes of Eczema in the Newborn.

Exogenous
  Contact primary irritant dermatitis
  Allergic, contact or drug dermatitis
  Infectious eczematoid dermatitis
  Physical-light, cold, heat dermatitis
Endogenous
  Atopic infantile dermatitis
  Congenital ichthyosiform erythroderma
  Seborrheic dermatitis
  Systemic diseases
    Acrodermatitis enteropathica
    Histidinemia
    Anhidrotic ectodermal dysplasia
    Histiocytosis X
    Leiner's disease—C_5 dysfunction
    Phenylketonuria
    Wiskott-Aldrich syndrome
  Psoriasis

(Adapted from Solomon and Esterly)[3]

Seborrheic dermatitis is the most difficult entity to differentiate from atopic dermatitis. In seborrheic dermatitis the eruption usually begins on the scalp and is most often found behind the ears, in skin folds of the neck, axillae and inguinal regions. Diaper area involvement is common. If the eruption becomes generalized it is known as exfoliative erythroderma or Leiner's disease. The scales are greasy and with drying develop into the "potato chip" scale. Patchy redness with weeping and fissuring may develop. Pruritus is minimal or absent in contrast to atopic dermatitis. At times, it is nearly impossible on clinical and morphologic grounds to determine which of the two entities is present. Rarely, they may occur simultaneously in the same patient. In most infants several visits with careful observation and assessment of the therapeutic response will decide the proper diagnosis. This occurred in one of our infants who at 2 months of age developed typical seborrheic dermatitis which responded to therapy. At 6 months of age, after a severe exacerbation, a diagnosis of atopic erythroderma was made and a therapeutic response was effected with remission by 11 months of age. At 2 years psoriasis developed.[3,12,14]

Cradle cap and seborrheic dermatitis may be treated with Sebulex shampoo or 10%
sodium sulfacetamide (Sebizon) cream rubbed in nightly followed by a neutral shampoo (Johnsons) in the morning. Five or six courses may be necessary, and then once or twice weekly thereafter. This disorder is usually self-limiting, lasting only a few months; recurrences are rare.

Management of the eczematous dermatoses must be individualized. Detailed written instructions for each infant must be given to nurses or parents to avoid confusion and each step must be carried out properly. Rapport is essential between the physician and parents. Environmental factors, clothing, hygiene, and socioeconomic and emotional aspects must be reviewed during each visit. The details of management are reviewed elsewhere and include parental reassurance, elimination of pruritus, topical medications, baths, avoidance of dry heat and skin irritants, treatment of secondary infections and avoidance of complications of therapy.[2,4,12,14,42]

IDIOPATHIC DERMATOSES

Histiocytosis X. Only the Letterer–Siwe variant of the nonlipid reticuloendothelioses has been seen during the neonatal period. The cutaneous features that may precede systemic signs (fever, hepatosplenomegaly, lymphadenopathy, anemia) are valuable clues to the diagnosis. In our experience, initial lesions are usually papular, scaly, and become petechial with or without purpura. An eczematous, seborrheic eruption is also common; however, maculopapules, pustules, and widespread erythema have been observed. The eruption usually occurs over the neck, groin, axillae, and scalp. Skin biopsy will reveal histiocytic infiltration and establish the diagnosis. Topical therapy is limited to emollients, steroid cream, or both for eczematous lesions. Systemic steroids, alkylating agents, or vinblastine are effective for the basic disease.[34]

Connective Tissue Diseases. **Scleroderma,** "hard skin," rarely seen in the neonatal period, may develop as local lesions during early infancy. Localized scleroderma occurs in 2 forms: morphea and linear scleroderma. Morphea develops insidiously as purplish indurated areas of shiny skin or nodules. Lesions may be multiple and are found on the face, trunk, and limbs. Spontaneous resolution occurs in 3 to 5 years and leaves a brown

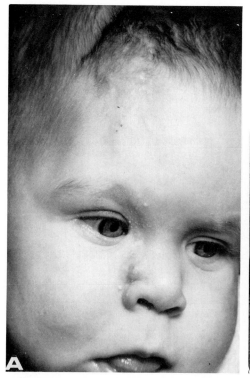
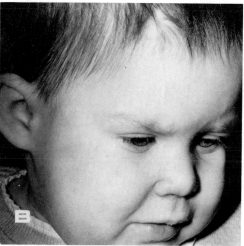

Fig. 43-41. A. Scleroderma, localized with "en coup de sabre" defect, noted at birth. Note the areas of calcinosis cutis. **B.** Good postoperative (resection and plastic graft) result was seen at 18 months of age.

pigmentation.[1] Linear scleroderma usually involves the scalp, face or limbs and often coexists with morphea. A particular type of linear scleroderma, the *"en coup de sabre,"* was so named because of its resemblance to a saber cut (Fig. 43-41A). This type shows a linear depressed groove in the frontoparietal region that may extend into the scalp and down to the chin and neck. Progressive atrophy of underlying structures including the skull may occur. Plastic surgical excision is beneficial (Fig. 43-41B). One report of good results in 14 patients treated with Pencillamine is encouraging.[43]

Disseminated lupus erythematosus has been reported in newborns of both affected and unaffected mothers. These infants are usually ill with petechial and purpuric lesions secondary to thrombocytopenia. Very rarely, discoid lupus erythematosus (DLE) without systemic involvement has been reported in newborns. Family history has been positive for collagen disease. Skin lesions in DLE are erythema-

tous, sharply demarcated areas of variable size located over the scalp and face, but rarely extending into the neck or upper back. Skin within these lesions is atrophic, telangiectatic, and scaly. Alopecia is often present and may be permanent with healing. Biopsy of an active lesion is often diagnostic.[3] If not, a portion of the tissue may provide additional information by doing immunofluorescent studies that demonstrate deposition of IgG in the basement membrane zone in 90% of patients with lupus erythematosus.

Therapy consists of avoiding sunlight and physical trauma to the skin, and use of sunscreen creams. Topical use of fluorinated steroid creams is effective for the skin lesions.[1,2]

Juvenile Xanthogranuloma. This benign, self-limiting disorder is often seen at birth or shortly thereafter. The typical lesion often restricted to the head, neck, and upper trunk, is a firm, nontender, yellow-brown, or reddish nodule. Size varies from 0.3 to 3 cm in diameter (Fig. 43-42), and numbers from a few to nu-

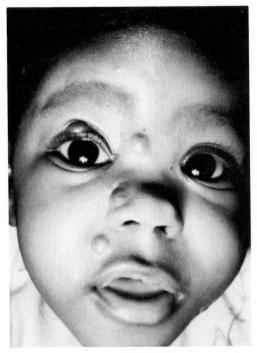

Fig. 43-42. Juvenile xanthogranuloma noted at birth. The nodules slowly grew in size and increased in number to a total of 22. At 16 months of age, most lesions were involuting.

merous, widely scattered or closely grouped lesions. Biopsy is diagnostic, showing a dense infiltrate of histiocytic cells throughout the dermis in early lesions, and Touton giant cells in mature lesions. Spontaneous regression usually occurs within 6 months to 2 years.

Of major importance is that ocular, lung, testicular, and pericardial lesions may occur. The ocular infiltrates may involve the iris, ciliary body, or orbit. Before ocular surgery is done, an infant should be examined thoroughly for skin tumors. Thus a major ophthalmologic procedure may be avoided. Eye involvement may predate the onset of skin nodules.[2,3]

REFERENCES

1. Stewart WD, Danto JL, Maddin S: Dermatology, Diagnosis and Treatment of Cutaneous Disorders, 4th ed CV Mosby, St. Louis, 1978

ACKNOWLEDGMENT

The author is grateful to Miss Ellee Margileth for secretarial assistance, and to Doctors Mervyn Elgart and John Kenney for their critical review and comments.

2. **Weinberg S, Hoekelman RA:** Pediatric Dermatology for the Primary Care Practitioner. McGraw Hill, New York, 1978
3. **Solomon LM, Esterly NB:** Neonatal Dermatology. WB Saunders, Philadelphia, 1973
4. **Arndt KA:** Manual of Dermatologic Therapeutics, 2nd ed Little Brown, Boston, 1978
5. **Smith DW:** Recognizable Patterns of Human Malformation, 2nd ed WB Saunders, Philadelphia, 1976
6. **Ramamurthy RS, Reveri MR, Esterly NB, et al:** Transient neonatal pustular melanosis. J Pediatr 88:831, 1976
7. **Margileth AM:** Scalded skin syndrome: Diagnosis, differential diagnosis and management of 42 children. South Med J 68:447, 1975
8. **Walton RG, Jacobs AH, Cox AJ:** Pigmented lesions in newborn infants. Br J Dermatol 95: 389, 1976
9. **Schwartz MF Jr, Esterly NB, Fretzin DF, Pergament E, Rozenfeld IH:** Hypomelanosis of ito (incontinentia pigmenti achromians) neurocutaneous syndrome. J Pediatr 90:236, 1977
10. **Kennedy JL, Kalish GH:** Incidence of depigmented nevi in 1,000 healthy newborns. Mod Probl Pediatr 17:211, 1975
11. **Margileth AM:** Developmental vascular abnormalities. Pediatr Clin North Am 18:713, 1971
12. **Jacobs AH:** Eruptions in the diaper area. Pediatr Clin North Am 25:209, 1978
13. **Schmidt LM:** Topical dermatologic therapy for the Pediatrician. Pediatr Clin North Am 25: 191, 1978
14. **Margileth AM:** Allergic dermatoses. Ann Pediatr 8:50, 1979
15. **Agha A, Sakati NO, Higginbottom MC, Jones KL, Bay C, Nyhan WL:** Two forms of cutis laxa presenting in the newborn period. Acta Paediatr Scand 67:775, 1978
16. **Mannino FL, Jones KL, Benirschke K:** Congenital skin defects and fetus papyraceus. J Pediatr 91:559, 1977
17. **Price VH:** Disorders of the hair in children. Pediatr Clin North Am 25:305, 1978
18. **Walton RG:** Pigmented nevi. Pediatr Clin North Am 18:897, 1971
19. **Mollica F, Pavone L, Guiseppe N:** Linear sebaceous nevus syndrome. Am J Dis Child 128: 868, 1974
20. **Jacobs AH, Walton RG:** The birthmarks in the neonate. Pediatrics 58:218, 1976
21. **O'Brien FV, Pielou WD:** Congenital epulis: Its natural history. Arch Dis Child 46:559, 1971
22. **Apfelberg DB, Maser MR, Lash H:** Argon laser treatment of cutaneous vascular abnormalities. Am Plast Surg 1:14, 1977
23. **Brown SH Jr, Neerhout RC, Fonkalsrud EW:** Prednisone therapy in the management of large

hemangiomas in infants and children. Surgery 71:168, 1972

24. **Miller SH, Smith RL, Skochat SJ:** Compression treatment of hemangiomas. Plast Reconstr Surg 58:573, 1976

25. **Margileth AM:** Cutaneous vascular tumors. Mod Probl Paediatr 17:101, 1975

26. **Pyesmany A, Ebert H, Williams K, Hittle R:** Intravascular coagulation secondary to cavernous hemangioma in infancy: response to radiotherapy. Can Med Assoc J 100:1053, 1969

27. **Kellar L, Bluhm JF III:** Diffuse neonatal hemangiomatosis. A case with heart failure and thrombocytopenia. Cutis 23(3):295–7, 1979

28. **Barand KG, Freeman NV:** Massive infiltrating cystic hygoma of the neck in infancy. Arch Dis Child 48:523–531, 1973

29. **Saijo M, Munro IR, Mancer K:** Lymphangioma: Longterm follow-up study. Plast Reconstr Surg 56:642, 1975

30. **Sharp H, Kruit W:** Hereditary lymphedema and obstructive jaundice. J Pediatr, 78:491, 1971

31. **Koblenzer PJ:** Common bacterial infections of the skin in children. Pediatr Clin North Am 25:321, 1978

32. **Jarrett M:** Viral infections of the skin. Pediatr Clin North Am 25:339, 1978

33. **Breese BB, Hall CB:** Beta Hemolytic Streptococcal Diseases. Houghton Mifflin, Boston, 1978

34. **Gellis SS, Kagan BM:** Current Pediatric Therapy, 8th ed WB Saunders, Philadelphia, 1978

35. **McCracken GH Jr, Nelson JD:** Antimicrobial therapy for newborns. Grune and Stratton, New York, 1977

36. **Margileth AM:** What is your diagnosis? Clin Proc Child Hosp Nat Med Center 29:77, 1973

37. **Blough HA, Giuntoli RL:** Successful treatment of human genital and herpes infections with 2-deoxy-glucose. JAMA 241:2798, 1979

38. **Jacobs PH:** Fungal Infections in childhood. Pediatr Clin North Am 25:357, 1978

39. **Watson W:** Selected genodermatoses. Pediatr Clin North Am 25:263, 1978

40. **Goldsmith LA, Baden HP:** Propylene glycol with occlusion for treatment of ichthyosis. JAMA 220:579, 1972

41. **Peck GL, Yoder FW, Olsen TC, et al:** Treatment of Darier's disease, lamellar ichthyosis, pityriasis rubra pilaris, cystic acne, and basal cell carcinoma with oral 13-cis-retinoic acid. Dermatologica 157:11, 1978

42. **Moss EM:** Atopic dermatitis. Pediatr Clin North Am 25:225, 1978

43. **Moynahan EJ:** Penacillamine in treatment of morphea and keloid in children. Postgrad Med J (suppl) 50:39, 1974

44. **South DA, Jacobs AH:** Cutis marmorata teliangiectatica congenita. J Pediatr 93:944–949, 1978

45. **Kopf AW, Bart RS, Hennessey P:** Congenital nevocytic nevi and malignant melanomas. J Am Acad Dermatol 1:123–130, 1979

44

Endocrine Disorders in the Newborn

*Alfred M. Bongiovanni and
Thomas Moshang, Jr.*

Almost from the moment of conception, endocrine physiologic processes are actively involved in the growth and development of the human fetus. Disturbances of the interplay of these complex hormonal processes can cause somatic or biochemical alterations in the fetus or newborn infant. Therefore, the clinical disorders of endocrine function in the newborn are reflections of altered physiologic function, in either the fetus or the mother, during intrauterine life. Moreover, these disturbances of endocrine physiologic function can occur during different stages of fetal development, resulting in different clincal situations. Knowledge concerning the physiologic fetomaternal hormonal processes and the ontogeny of the fetal endocrine glands make the clinical disorders of endocrine function in the newborn more readily understandable.

SEXUAL AMBIGUITY AND GONADAL DISORDERS

Normal Sexual Differentiation

A schematic representation of the controls of sexual development is depicted in Figure 44-1. The gonadal anlagen are recognized as genital ridges by the fifth or sixth fetal week. These primitive gonads are bipotential, consisting of cortical (ovarian) and medullary (testicular) components. The differentiation of the gonadal anlage into either a testis or an ovary is generally believed to be directed by the genetic information contained within the sex chromosomes. However, a recent report of a family with XX males in 2 generations suggests that an autosomal gene for maleness is also necessary for direction of the bipotential gonad to become a testis.[1]

The differentiated gonads in turn play a critical role in directing the differentiation of the internal genital ducts as well as the external genitalia. The classic experiments by Alfred Jost clearly demonstrate the active role of the fetal testis.[2] The fetal testis secretes two hormones, a large molecular weight hormone, probably a polypeptide,[3] which inhibits the müllerian duct, and an androgen, probably testosterone, which stimulates the wolffian duct to proliferate into the vas deferens, seminal vesicle, epididymis, ejaculatory ducts, and promotes growth of the genital tubercle and fusion of the urogenital slit. The fetal ovary, on the other hand, is passive in terms of sexual differentiation, and persistence of the müllerian duct, regression of the wolffian duct, and development of female external genitalia do not depend upon hormone action or on the presence of functioning gonads.

NORMAL SEXUAL DIFFERENTIATION

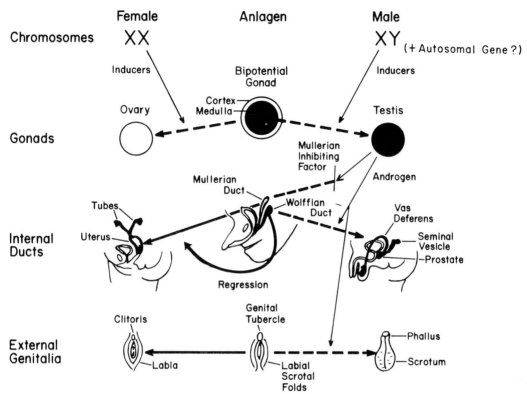

Fig. 44-1. Various inducers (*thin arrows*) are necessary for differentiation of the gonads and masculine development (*broken heavy arrows*). In the absence of these inducers, the differentiation is female (*solid heavy arrows*).

Sex Chromosome Abnormalities

The normal complement of sex chromosomes directs the bipotential gonad to differentiate into either ovary or testicle. Many varieties of sex chromosome aberrations have been reported. Some of these are lethal to the fetus (*e.g.*, YO) and some probably cause very little somatic or biochemical abnormalities in terms of sexual differentiation (*e.g.*, XXX). It is clear that the type and degree of sex chromosome aberration influences the gonadal differentiation. Studies of natural chromosomal disorders indicate that at least two X chromosomes are required for complete ovarian development. Although more than two X chromosomes do not interfere with gonadal differentiation, a percentage of the reported patients with X polyploidy developed early menopause.[4,5] It is generally true that a Y chromosome is necessary for testicular development. However, case reports of true hermaphrodites and normal male phenotypes with only XX chromosomes are well documented.[1,6,7] The presence of testicular tissue in the absence of a Y chromosome is difficult to explain except for the possibility of undetected mosaicism. It is now possible to recognize the presence of Y chromosome material in cells by detection of the H-Y surface antigen, presumably a determinant of the male sex chromosome. In a true hermaphrodite with ovotestes and an apparent 46 XX genotype, the H-Y antigen was found in the testicular elements of the ambiguous gonad. This discovery has wide application in the understanding of ambiguous sexual development or discordant clinical conditions, as in the genotypic XX male.

The classic sex chromosomal aberrations occur relatively frequently as determined by newborn screening. In the New Haven study, XXY occurred once in 545 males, XYY occurred once in 728 males, XXX occurred once in 727 females, with only one case of 45 XO in 2,181 female newborns.[8] However, the diagnosis of Turner's syndrome is made with much more frequency than the other sex chromosomal aberrations because of the associated somatic abnormalities. Various combinations and deletions of sex chromosomal material have been reported, causing various gonadal and sexual differentiation. The interested reader is referred to the discussion by Morishima and Grumbach concerning the interrelationship of various sex chromosome aberrations and phenotype.[9]

Turner Syndrome (Bonnevie–Ullrich Syndrome, Gonadal Dysgenesis). The term Turner syndrome is used in preference to other eponymic or descriptive terms because of the linking of this eponym with the association of the somatic characteristics with the 45 XO chromosomal karyotype. The terms gonadal dysgenesis or ovarian dysgenesis can be confused with those embryologic situations designated as "pure gonadal dysgenesis" (discussed below). The classic chromosomal abnormality is loss of a total X chromosome. However, other chromosomal abnormalities have been reported, such as mosaicism of cells with an XO cell line with normal 46 XX cells, or deletion of part of an X chromsome (such as 46 X isochromosome X). The loss of some of the genetic information in the X chromosomes results in varying degrees of the somatic abnormalities of Turner syndrome. The presence of a 46 XX cell line in mosaicism does not modify the short stature or somatic abnormalities to a great degree, but does seem to influence gonadal development. In the study by Goldberg and associates, spontaneous female sexual development occurred in 3 of 25 patients with mosaic karyotypes but in none of the XO group.[10]

Ullrich described in 1930[11] and Bonnevie in 1934[12] a syndrome in three female neonates in which lymphedema of the hands and feet was found in association with pterygium colli. Most endocrinologists believe that this syndrome (Bonnevie–Ullrich) is a description of Turner syndrome in the neonate. The pterygium colli is most often seen as redundant folds about the posterior neck. The lymphedema involves the dorsa of the hands and feet. A host of associated somatic defects have been described in this syndrome,[13] most of which

become more readily identifiable with age and growth of the child. The most common defects include triangular facies with low-set ears, high-arched palate, low hairline, shield-like chest with widespread and hypoplastic areolae, and cubitus valgus. Coarctation of the aorta is a common cardiovascular abnormality, as are hemangiomata. Other skin manifestations include cutis laxa, pigmented nevi, dysplastic nails, and tendency to keloid formation. Skeletal abnormalities such as "beaking" of the medial tibial condyle, drumstick-shaped distal phalanges, and vertebral anomalies have been described.[14] Palmar simian creases, distal axial triradius, and increased number of digital ulnar whorls are documented as dermatoglyphic abnormalities. The most consistent characteristics are seen in the older child and these are short stature and sexual infantilism.

The diagnosis should be suspected in female neonates of low birth weight with lymphedema, pterygium colli, or coarctation of the aorta. The confirmatory finding would be a chromatin-negative buccal smear or definitive chromosomal analyses. The sex assignment is almost invariably female except in the mixed gonadal dysgenesis conditions (see below). There is no specific therapy for this syndrome unless the developmental anomalies create a clinical problem, such as coarctation of the aorta. These children have a high incidence of recurrent otitis media, chronic lymphocytic thyroiditis, and idiopathic hypertension. There is an increased incidence of mental retardation, but there are certainly many intellectually bright children with Turner syndrome. Hormonal therapy at the appropriate age is indicated for the treatment of sexual infantilism. There have been efforts to increase the final height in these patients with the use of growth hormone or androgens. Androgen therapy seems to be the most beneficial regimen at present.[15] The use of pharmacologic doses of growth hormone, when a synthetic growth hormone or the growth-promoting fragment of growth hormone becomes available, may be even more efficacious.[16]

In Turner syndrome with XO/XY or XX/XY mosaicism (or variations), the gonadal elements will frequently contain testicular components. In these situations, the presence of both medullary and cortical elements in gonadal remnants is referred to as mixed gonadal dysgenesis.

Various genital phenotypes in this variant of Turner syndrome have been documented, including normal female, normal male, intersex, female with clitoromegaly, and male with hypospadias and unilateral cryptorchidism. The most frequent phenotypes, however, are usually female, occasionally with clitoromegaly. In nine cases of XO/XY chromosome mosaicism described by Morishima and Grumbach, only one had male genital development.[9] These patients may have many of the somatic abnormalities typical of classic XO Turner syndrome. However, in mixed gonadal dysgenesis, especially in the presence of a Y chromosome, the likelihood for malignant degeneration of the gonadal tissues is markedly increased. Because any gonadal hormonal function in this disorder is more likely to be androgenic in nature and inappropriate for the usual phenotype, early gonadectomy is recommended for this specific variant of Turner syndrome.[17]

Other Sex Chromosome Aberrations. The other common sex chromosome abnormalities (XXY, XXX, and XYY) do not present with problems during the neonatal period.

Klinefelter's Syndrome. XXY is the most frequent sex chromosomal abnormality as determined by newborn screening studies. The most characteristic finding is small and firm testes. The classic histologic finding in the testis is hyalinization of the seminiferous tubules, which is seen only after puberty.

Superfemale Syndromes. In the superfemale syndrome, or polyploidy X syndromes, the one consistent finding is mental retardation. Ovarian differentiation and postpubertal function do not appear to be impaired by the presence of extra X chromosomes, although a number of these patients have early menopause.[4,5]

XYY Syndrome. The concern of the XYY syndrome involves not sexual assignment or physical abnormalities but socially deviant behavior. In an excellent review of this syndrome, Hook concludes that there is a definite association between XYY state and presence in mental and penal institutions.[18] However, because there are many socially normal XYY individuals, the nature and degree of risk of this association is not clear. This creates a dilemma for the pediatrician concerning informing the parents when this genotype is found in the young. This problem is further compounded by the knowledge that even in those children with documented socially deviant behavior there is no information yet as to what forms of environmental or psychiatric manipulations can be recommended as beneficial.

Gonadal Abnormalities

A number of conditions have been documented in which there is gonadal failure of one degree or another. The etiologies of these disorders may include sex chromosome aberrations, but in many reported conditions, no chromosome aberrations have been noted. Certainly various teratogens including irradiation, viruses, and drugs might cause *in utero* gonaditis and damage to the developing gonad. The degree and timing of the damage to the developing testis will cause varying levels of failure of development of the internal ducts and external genitalia.

Pure Gonadal Dysgenesis. Complete dysgenesis of the genital ridges results in normal phenotypic females. These girls tend to be tall and eunuchoid with primary amenorrhea and sexual infantilism. The chromosomal karyotype may be either 46 XY or 46 XX. It is suspected that teratogenic factors are the cause of the dysgenesis of the gonads in this condition. A high incidence of neoplasia has been reported in pure gonadal dysgenesis.

Partial Gonadal Dysgenesis. Teratogenic factors which damage the new testis at later stages of fetal development cause varying clinical situations. Dysgenesis of the testis late during pregnancy may cause complete anorchia in a perfectly well-formed male. Lesser damage early in gestation may cause hypospadias and cryptorchidism.

True Hermaphroditism refers to that state in which both cortical and medullary gonadal elements are present. This may be comprised of an ovary on one side and a testis on the contralateral side, or an ovary or a testis and an ovotestis contralaterally, or 2 ovotestes. Therefore, this also includes those patients with mixed gonadal dysgenesis associated with sex chromosome aberrations, discussed above. In those patients without chromosome aberrations, two-thirds have a 46 XX karyotype with one-third having a 46 XY karyotype. The development of medullary tissue in the XX karyotype has been postulated to be a result of Y chromosome elements.[1]

The development and differentiation of the internal duct structures and external genitalia depend on the degree of functioning medullary tissue. The sex differentiation of the gonaduct corresponds to the gonad on the same side. As for external genitalia, the majority of the true hermaphrodites have ambiguous genitalia.

Gonaducts and External Genital Derangements

Derangements of the gonaducts and external genitalia can occur in the presence of normal gonads and sex chromosomes. Such derangements may be secondary to teratogens causing defective embryogenesis or to inappropriate hormonal changes. Teratogenic factors are believed to be the explanation for an anatomic derangement such as agenesis of the müllerian ducts in otherwise normal females.

Derangements of the external genitalia may create a state of pseudohermaphroditism. In pseudohermaphroditism, the gonads are generally normal and appropriate for the genotype, but the external genitalia are either ambiguous or totally inappropriate for the genotype. Therefore, by this definition, a disorder such as cryptorchidism with severe third-degree hypospadias is a form of male pseudohermaphroditism.

Female Pseudohermaphroditism. Masculinization of the female fetus is usually caused by androgens either formed by the fetus or transmitted by the mother. The formation of a urogenital sinus with fusion of the labia is a result of the effects of androgens before the twelfth week of fetal life. Enlargement of the clitoris, on the other hand, can develop at any time of life prenatally or postnatally.

The Adrenogenital Syndrome. The adrenogenital syndrome is the most common cause of virilization in the female. The more common inherited enzymatic deficiencies of adrenal biosynthesis, namely, the 21-hydroxylase, the 11-hydroxylase, and the 3-β-hydroxysteroid dehydrogenase defects, all cause virilization of the female. The gonaducts remain normal with persistence and development of the müllerian ducts. This is as expected because these patients are true females without testes and therefore do not have the testicular polypeptide factor which suppresses müllerian duct development. The adrenal androgens however cause fusion of the labia, creation of a urogenital sinus, and clitoral enlargement. In those

disorders of adrenal steroid biosynthesis associated with virilization, the urinary excretion of 17-ketosteroids are elevated, and, without therapy, increase with age. The various enzymatic defects of this disorder, the method of diagnosis and treatment are more fully discussed in the section below dealing with adrenal disorders.

Drug-induced Female Pseudohermaphroditism. A number of female newborns have been virilized by progestational agents or androgens used during the first trimester of pregnancy. The incidence of drug-induced female pseudohermaphroditism has decreased in recent years because, with recognition of this iatrogenic cause of virilization of the fetus, there has been a decreased use of the incriminated drugs. Such drugs are most commonly used during the first trimester of gestation in order to prevent spontaneous abortion or to maintain pregnancy in patients with habitual abortion. When these drugs are used during the first trimester of gestation, the anatomic changes are similar to those found in the adrenogenital syndrome. These will be fusion of the labioscrotal folds with formation of a urogenital sinus and clitoromegaly. Rarely, virilization can be so extreme as to cause complete external masculinization. When used after the first trimester, these drugs will cause only phallic enlargement without fusion of the labioscrotal folds. The bone age is often advanced at birth. However, there is no progressive virilization, nor progressive acceleration of growth, bone age, or sexual development postnatally. The 17-ketosteroids are not elevated. These children will feminize normally at puberty and are quite capable of bearing children. The only therapy necessary is surgical correction of the labioscrotal fusion and clitoromegaly when these findings are present.

The drugs that have been incriminated include testosterone, 17-methyltestosterone, 17α-ethinyl-19-nortestosterone (Norlutin), 17α-ethyl-19-nortestosterone (Nilevar), 17α-ethinyltestosterone (Pranone, Lutocylol, Progesteral), progesterone, diethylstilbestrol, 17α-hydroxyprogesterone, 17-methylandrostenediol and the combination of ethinyl estradiol 3-methylester and 17α-ethinyl-19-nortestosterone (OrthoNovum).

Virilizing Disorders in the Mother. The virilization of a female fetus as the result of an androgen-producing tumor of the mother is a relatively rare condition. These tumors are almost always caused by an ovarian lesion, although in one report the lesion was a benign adrenal adenoma.[19] The reported tumors have included arrhenoblastomas, Krukenberg tumors, luteomas, a lipoid tumor of the ovary, and a stromal cell tumor. Haymond and Weldon reviewed the reported cases and noted that maternal virilization has been characterized by clitoromegaly, acne, deepening of the voice, decreased lactation, hirsutism, and elevated excretion of urinary 17-ketosteroids.[20] The offspring tend to have a low birth weight as well as virilization. The degree of virilization of the fetus is variable.

Idiopathic Female Pseudohermaphroditism. There are two forms of idiopathic female pseudohermaphroditism. There is a small group of genotypically normal females in whom virilization of the external genitalia is seen in association with congenital anomalies of the gastrointestinal and urinary tracts. The reported anomalies include imperforate anus, renal agenesis, urinary tract obstructions, urethrovaginal fistulas, and defective formation of müllerian ducts. The masculinization of these infants cannot be explained on the basis of androgens and is thought to be caused by nonhormonal factors. There is another group of female pseudohermaphrodites in whom there are no associated anomalies and no history of maternal exposure to androgens. It is possible that in this latter form there is an as yet unknown disturbance of steroid metabolism either in the mother or the placenta.

Male Pseudohermaphroditism. Incomplete masculinization of the male fetus may be secondary to an enzymatic deficiency of testosterone synthesis, unresponsiveness to testosterone action or teratogenic damage to either the gonad or the genital anlagen. Damage to the fetal testis may lead to states in which the testis may be completely absent (anorchia or pure gonadal dysgenesis) or to partial deficiencies of testicular tissue. The degree of incomplete masculinization of the external genitalia depends not only upon the amount of damage to the fetal testis but upon the timing during gestation as well. Anorchia represents dysgenesis of the fetal testes after formation of the male external genitalia have been completed. Hypospadias can be caused by either gonadal damage early during the first trimester

of pregnancy or damage to the external genital anlagen directly.

The Adrenogenital Syndrome. The adrenogenital syndrome can cause incomplete masculinization of the male fetus when the enzyme deficient in the adrenal is also deficient in the testes and necessary for testosterone synthesis. Deficiency of the 3β-hydroxysteroid dehydrogenase enzyme causes a block early in the biosynthetic pathway of cortisol synthesis, resulting in a severe salt-losing syndrome.[21] The inability of the testis to form testosterone, indicating that the enzymatic defect also affects testicular steroid biosynthesis,[22] causes hypospadias in the male to a varying degree. The testes are usually within the scrotum. Other defects of adrenal steroid biosynthesis affecting testicular synthesis of testosterone include the deficiencies of 17α-hydroxylase, and the 20,22 desmolase enzymes.

The Syndrome of Testicular Feminization. This disorder has complete and partial varieties. These patients are XY male pseudohermaphrodites with fairly normal testes, differentiated male internal genital structures, and absence of müllerian duct structures. The external genitalia are normal female in the complete form and ambiguous in the partial (or incomplete) form of this disorder. Both variants are inherited disorders and the degree of ambiguity is consistent with siblings. The inheritance of this syndrome is compatible with either an X-linked disorder or an autosomal recessive disorder that is limited to males.

The testes may occasionally be detected as masses located above the symphysis pubis or labia. When the diagnosis is made during childhood, it is usually because of these testicular masses or when testicular tissue is found during a herniorrhaphy. Internally, there are well-formed vas deferens and epididymes. There are usually no müllerian duct structures, although a rare patient with rudimentary müllerian elements has been described. The lower third of the vagina is present but ends in a blind pouch. At puberty, feminization occurs with good breast development and estrogenization of the labia minora and the vagina. However, the majority of the affected patients have very little pubic hair and approximately one-third have total absence of sexual hair. In all other respects, including height, habitus, voice, and breast development, these individuals are completely feminine. They frequently marry and can have normal sexual relations. Because of the lack of formation of a uterus, these patients will also present because of primary amenorrhea.

All of the accumulated data suggest that this disorder is caused by an inherited defect of end-organ unresponsiveness to testosterone. There has been no abnormality of testosterone biosynthesis demonstrated. The testes are histologically similar to those described for cryptorchid males, although the Leydig cells after puberty tend to be hyperplastic and in clumps. Testosterone levels in both plasma and urine are in the normal male range after puberty. Wilkins showed that large amounts of methyltestosterone administered orally caused no growth of sexual hair or clitoral enlargement in a patient with this disorder.[23] Recent studies indicate that the biologic action of testosterone may be mediated through an enzymatic conversion of testosterone to 5α-androstan-3-one-17β-ol (5α-dihydrotestosterone), a more potent androgen in certain bioassays. Wilson and Walker demonstrated that perineal skin from patients with testicular feminization converts testosterone to 5α-dihydrotestosterone at a lower rate than normal male perineal skin *in vitro*.[24] However, Strickland and French demonstrated that the administration of 5α-dihydrotestosterone did not increase urinary excretion of nitrogen, phosphorus, or citric acid in a patient with this syndrome.[25] This study and evidence from several animal models indicate that the defect is not caused by a deficiency of an enzyme necessary for the conversion of testosterone to 5α-dihydrotestosterone. The intracellular defect of testosterone metabolism in this syndrome still remains to be elucidated.

Evaluation of Sexual Ambiguity

It is imperative that the evaluation of a newborn with ambiguous genitalia be carried out immediately after delivery if the baby's condition permits. Table 44-1 outlines a schema for the evaluation of the newborn with ambiguous genitalia, with the diagnostic studies divided into three levels. Certainly all studies at level I can be performed and gender assignment made within the first 72 hours, even in the most ill infant. The urgency for making as correct a diagnosis and gender assignment as soon as possible cannot be overemphasized. It has been shown that genotype, gonads, or sex hormones contribute very little to final psychosexual inclinations and behavior, and that psychosexual differentiation is influenced mainly by sex assignment and environmental conditions of rearing. The classic studies by Money and the Hampsons emphasize that adult psychosexual orientation is most closely correlated with the sex of rearing and that the firm ascertainment of the gender role is established during early infancy and can rarely be reversed.[26–28] Parents must not be left in doubt or confused about the infant's gender. It has been our policy to recommend that parents remain in seclusion and not notify relatives or friends, if possible, of the birth of the child until a gender has been assigned.

Level I Studies. The buccal smear for determination of sex chromatin pattern should be carried out immediately. Although it has been documented that the percentage of positive chromatin bodies in a buccal smear of a normal 46 XX female may be diminished during the immediate newborn period, there are usually a respectable number of Barr bodies. A child with a positive buccal smear should be considered to have the adrenogenital syndrome until all studies are complete. The adrenogenital syndrome is the most common disorder causing virilization of the female. Moreover, one must be alert for the possibility of salt-losing adrenal crisis within the first several weeks of life.

The determination of 17-ketosteroid and pregnanetriol excretion can be performed within the first 72 hours. Although the level of 17-ketosteroid excretion in 24 hours may be as high as 2.5 mg in the normal newborn, there is an inclination for this level to decline and serial determinations may establish the diagnosis. Moreover, pregnanetriol excretion is elevated, as determined by gas liquid chromatography, in the newborn with the 21-hydroxylase defect.[29] The infant with 3β-hydroxysteroid dehydrogenase deficiency will have markedly elevated 17-ketosteroid excretion as well as high Δ^5 steroids, such as dehydroepiandrosterone.

The search for a possible drug or teratogen must be detailed. It is not enough to query about known androgens or progestational

Table 44-1. Evaluation of Ambiguous Genitalia.

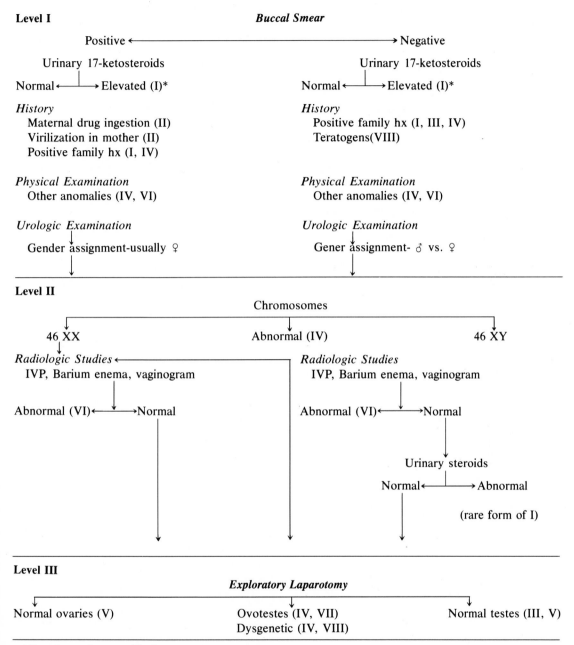

Level I

Buccal Smear

Positive ← → Negative

Urinary 17-ketosteroids

Normal ←⊥→ Elevated (I)*

History
  Maternal drug ingestion (II)
  Virilization in mother (II)
  Positive family hx (I, IV)

Physical Examination
  Other anomalies (IV, VI)

Urologic Examination
  Gender assignment-usually ♀

Urinary 17-ketosteroids

Normal ←⊥→ Elevated (I)*

History
  Positive family hx (I, III, IV)
  Teratogens(VIII)

Physical Examination
  Other anomalies (IV, VI)

Urologic Examination
  Gener assignment- ♂ vs. ♀

Level II

Chromosomes

46 XX   Abnormal (IV)   46 XY

Radiologic Studies ←
  IVP, Barium enema, vaginogram

Abnormal (VI)←→Normal

Radiologic Studies
  IVP, Barium enema, vaginogram

Abnormal (VI)←→Normal

Urinary steroids

Normal←⊥→Abnormal

(rare form of I)

Level III

Exploratory Laparotomy

Normal ovaries (V)   Ovotestes (IV, VII)   Normal testes (III, V)
                            Dysgenetic (IV, VIII)

* Parentheses refer to possible diagnoses:

I. Adrenogenital syndrome. II. Maternal virilization of fetus. III. Testicular feminization syndrome. IV. Chromosomal aberrations. V. Idiopathic. VI. Idiopathic associated with multiple anomalies. VII. True hermaphroditism. VIII. Gonadal dysgenesis.

drugs, but every drug, including tradenames, every illness or unusual dietary habit must be elicited. Vitamins with the addition of anabolic compounds can be a source of androgens. Severe viral illnesses may be a cause of gonadal damage.

The physical examination must include a urologic surgeon's opinion. In the chromating-positive child, the gender assignment will almost always be female. However, in the infant with a negative buccal smear, the sex assignment must be made on the basis of potential future sexual function. Those males with complete or almost complete female external genitalia should be raised as females. Substitution therapy with estrogens after puberty will cause feminization and plastic surgical correction of an inadquate vagina will provide satisfactory sexual function.

In those patients not diagnosed as having the adrenogenital syndrome, further studies are in order. However, the above studies should have provided enough information to assign a gender to the infant and further studies can be pursued more leisurely.

Levels II and III Studies. In order to establish a diagnosis, it may be necessary to perform a careful exploratory laparotomy with gonadal biopsies. However, before resorting to laparotomy, as much information as possible should be obtained through ancillary studies. A female infant virilized by a known drug associated with virilization of the fetus, with a normal karyotype, may be spared an exploratory laparotomy. Similarly, an infant with ambiguous genitalia, normal chromosome analysis, and multiple congenital anomalies, such as unilateral renal agenesis as determined by IVP, might be spared further surgical procedures. Further urinary steroid studies are indicated in a male with incomplete masculinization in order to look for the more unusual forms of the adrenogenital syndrome, such as elevation of desoxycorticosterone and corticosterone found in the 17α-hydroxylase defect. In an infant with sex chromosomal aberrations and the possibility of mixed gonadal dysgenesis, exploratory laparotomy and gonadal biopsy should be carried out at a later age. If the gonads are grossly dysgenetic, it is recommended that castration be carried out because of the increased incidence of malignancy.[16]

DISORDERS OF THE ADRENAL GLAND
Development and Function of the Adrenal Gland

The adrenal gland is in reality two separate glands, the adrenal cortex and the adrenal medulla. The fetal adrenal cortex is of mesodermal origin, whereas the chromaffin cells of the adrenal medulla are probably of neuroectodermal origin. The classes of hormones secreted by these 2 glands differ and are fairly independent of each other, although Wurtman and Axelrod have suggested that the intraadrenal level of glucocorticoids may influence the level of the enzyme, phenylethanolamine-N-methyl transferase, necessary for the conversion of norepinephrine to epinephrine.[30] It is certainly possible that the influence of these two glands upon each other may be greater than appreciated by present knowledge. Inasmuch as the knowledge concerning the development and function of the fetal adrenal medulla is scanty, and that diseases of the adrenal medulla during the neonatal period are extremely rare, this section will focus on the adrenal cortex.

The anlage of the adrenal cortex arises as two large masses on either side of the aorta at about the level of the first thoracic nerve. Immediately adjacent are the medullary cells which have migrated from the neural crest. Fetal adrenal cortical cells can be identified by the fourth week of gestation. By 7 weeks of gestation, the medullary cells begin to migrate to the interior of the adrenal cortex. These original adrenal cortical cells make up the fetal zone of the adrenal cortex. There is a second downgrowth of coelomic epithelium which envelops the original cortical cells and remains as an outer shell. The fetal adrenal gland is extremely large during gestation but involutes during the last half of pregnancy and especially after birth. The adult adrenal cortex slowly develops from the outer shell with involution of the fetal zone. The fetal zone is extremely active in steroid metabolism and the rapid involution after birth suggests a role in the maintenance of pregnancy.

The trophic hormonal control of the fetal adrenal is not clear. In anencephalic fetuses, the fetal adrenal appears to be normal during the first 12 weeks of gestation with subsequent involution of the gland. It has been suggested that some other trophic hormone (perhaps human chorionic gonadotropin; HCG) stimulates adrenal growth during the first trimester and subsequently a hypothalamic-pituitary hormone (ACTH) maintains the adrenal gland during the last half of pregnancy.[31] However, in patients with enzymatic defcts of cortisol biosynthesis, the excessive androgen production in association with hyperplasia of the adrenal glands during the first 12 weeks of gestation suggests that ACTH must play some role during that time.

The adrenal cortex secretes three main groups of steroid hormones. The glucocorticoids and mineralocorticoids have 21 carbon atoms, whereas the androgens have 19 carbon atoms. The glucocorticoids, of which cortisol (hydrocortisone) is the most important, exert their major physiologic effects on carbohydrate, protein, and fat metabolism. The mineralocorticoids, desoxycorticosterone and aldosterone, maintain salt and water balance by promoting sodium retention in exchange for hydrogen and potassium in the distal convoluted tubules of the kidney. The adrenal androgens, dehydroepiandosterone, Δ^4-androstenedione, and 11β-hydroxyandrostenedione, are protein anabolic and responsible for the development of sexual hair in females at puberty. Adrenal androgens are not secreted in appreciable amounts until puberty, except during the neonatal period. The slightly higher levels of adrenal androgens during the neonatal period may be secondary to the relative deficiency of 3β-hydroxysteroid dehydrogenase in the fetal zone of the fetal adrenal cortex.

The tissue concentration of adrenocortical steroids is controlled by means of a hypothalamic-pituitary-adrenal homeostatic mechanism. The hypothalamus contains an ACTH-releasing factor, corticotrophin-releasing hormone, which provokes release of ACTH from the pituitary gland. The hypothalamic center is sensitive to both tissue levels of cortisol and to stress. ACTH in turn stimulates adrenocortical steroid biosynthesis, mainly cortisol. Increased levels of cortisol inhibit the production of ACTH (a "negative feedback" control), probably acting at the level of the hypothalamus or pituitary.

The regulation of aldosterone, on the other hand, is influenced by many factors. It is generally believed that the main regulatory homeostatic mechanism controlling aldosterone secretion is the reninangiotensin system. Acute changes in pressure receptors, perhaps in the renal afferent arterioles, control the release of renin from the juxtaglomerular cells of the kidney. Increased levels of circulating renin in turn increase angiotensin II. Angiotensin II acts on the zona glomerulosa of the adrenal to increase aldosterone secretion as well as directly causing vascular contractility. Increased pressure within the arterial receptors secondary to the contracted vessels and increased blood volume produced by elevated aldosterone operate a negative feedback inhibition of the renin-angiotensin system.

Other mechanisms are involved in a secondary fashion in the control of aldosterone secretion. A low-sodium or high-potassium intake will increase aldosterone excretion. It has been demonstrated that the sodium or potassium concentration in the blood perfusing the adrenals has a direct effect on aldosterone secretion.[32] ACTH will also cause a transient, albeit unsustained, increase in aldosterone excretion,[33] and aldosterone secretion will be diminished in the absence of ACTH.[34] Finally, cortisol itself may have a permissive role in aldosterone action at the tissue level.[35]

Adrenal Insufficiency

The disorders of the adrenal cortex during the neonatal period consist almost entirely of those conditions which cause adrenal insufficiency. The inborn errors of steroid biosynthesis (adrenogenital syndrome) can cause excessive production of various steroids, but Cushing's syndrome or cortisol excess rarely occurs during the neonatal period. Adrenal insufficiency can result from lack of trophic hormone stimulation, damage to fetal adrenal gland, inherited degenerative disorders or inborn errors of steroid biosynthesis.

ACTH Insufficiency. There have been a number of neonatal deaths following shock and peripheral vascular collapse associated with severe hyponatremia and hyperkalemia in which the adrenal glands were noted to be hypoplastic at autopsy. Some of these cases of failure of development of the adrenal cortex after involution of the fetal zone have been reported in infants with anencephaly and in patients with partial or total pituitary aplasia. The probable basis of the developmental failure in these cases is the lack of ACTH.

However, the possibility that the lack of another central nervous system factor might also be involved in these cases is suggested by the patients with congenital hypopituitary dwarfism. In the latter group of patients, the adrenal insufficiency is limited to decreased cortisol production but normal mineralocorticoid function.[36] Such patients have a tendency toward hypoglycemia, poor feeding, and failure to thrive. These patients can, however, maintain water and electrolyte balance and can respond to sodium deprivation with increase in aldosterone excretion. The limitation of the developmental failure to only the zona fasciculata and reticularis with ACTH deficiency can be explained by the fact that the trophic hormone for zona glomerulosa function is angiotensin II and not ACTH.

ACTH Unresponsiveness. Migeon and associates have postulated that the dichotomy of control of the various zones of the adrenal cortex may be the explanation for a familial syndrome of isolated glucocorticoid deficiency. This syndrome was initially reported by Shepard and associates in 1959.[37] It presents in early childhood with hyperpigmentation, hypoglycemia, failure to thrive, and poor feeding. These patients have cortisol insufficiency and can not increase 17-hydroxysteroid excretion in response to ACTH stimulation. These patients can, however, respond to sodium deprivation with increased aldosterone excretion and decreased sodium excretion. Migeon and associates, based on in vitro experiments, have suggested that this syndrome is the result of an inherited defect in the ACTH receptor system.[38] This syndrome has since been referred to as "the syndrome of ACTH unresponsiveness." However, we have reported a family with this syndrome in whom the pathogenesis of the disorder appears to be more compatible with a degenerative process (see below).[39] It is probable that this familial syndrome is caused by a variety of defects including ACTH unresponsiveness.

Damage to the Adrenals. Adrenal insufficiency can occur during the newborn period as a result of damage to the relatively large and hyperemic adrenal glands. Trauma in association with a difficult delivery, hemorrhagic diseases, or infectious processes can damage the adrenal glands. Minor hemorrhage or unilateral damage may not cause adrenal insuffi-

ciency and may present, subsequently as calcification of the adrenal glands.

It is extremely difficult to diagnose acute adrenal insufficiency in the newborn. The characteristic clinical findings are nonspecific (see below).

Degenerative Disorders of the Adrenal. The most common cause of chronic adrenal insufficiency is idiopathic atrophy or degeneration of the adrenal glands. However, chronic adrenal insufficiency (Addison's disease) is extremely uncommon in childhood and unheard of during the newborn period if one excludes the cases of congenital hypoplasia of the adrenal glands. It is possible that some of the cases of congenital hypoplasia of the adrenals are caused by a degenerative process, especially when the central nervous system, including the pituitary gland, is intact.

Familial isolated glucocorticoid insufficiency can occur during the neonatal period. These infants present during the neonatal period with shock, hyperpigmentation, and hypoglycemia. Some of the families with this syndrome probably have a defect in ACTH responsiveness. However, there are a substantial number of case histories with a clinical course suggestive of an inherited degenerative process.

We have studied a family of which five siblings had hyperpigmentation, hypoglycemia, convulsions, and deficient glucocorticoid production.[39] Mineralocorticoid function was normal. Of these five children, two were studied during early infancy, and glucocorticoid function was normal initially. The development of deficient glucocorticoid production at a later age in these two patients suggests an inherited degenerative process of the adrenal glands as the pathogenetic basis for this syndrome in this family.

The adrenogenital syndrome is a genetic disorder involving deficiency of one of several enzymatic systems required for normal steroid biosynthesis. It is suggested that the generic terminology "congenital virilizing adrenocortical hyperplasia" be discarded because there are now several recognized enzymatic defects in steroid biosynthesis that do not cause virilization, and in fact may cause deficient masculine embryogenesis. The various clinical manifestations of this syndrome can be correlated with the different defects of cortisol

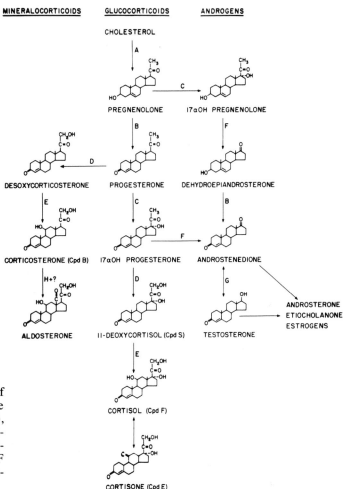

MINERALOCORTICOIDS   GLUCOCORTICOIDS   ANDROGENS

CHOLESTEROL

PREGNENOLONE   17αOH PREGNENOLONE

DESOXYCORTICOSTERONE   PROGESTERONE   DEHYDROEPIANDROSTERONE

CORTICOSTERONE (Cpd B)   17αOH PROGESTERONE   ANDROSTENEDIONE

ALDOSTERONE   11-DEOXYCORTISOL (Cpd S)   TESTOSTERONE

ANDROSTERONE
ETIOCHOLANONE
ESTROGENS

CORTISOL (Cpd F)

CORTISONE (Cpd E)

Fig. 44-2. The biosynthetic pathways of adrenal steroid biosynthesis. The enzyme systems include A (the 20,22 desmolase), B (the 3β-hydroxysteroid dehydrogenase), C (the 17-hydroxylase), D (the 21-hydroxylase), E (the 11-hydroxylase), F (the 17,20 desmolase), G (the 17 reductase) and H (the 18-hyroxylase).

synthesis. The biochemical basis of this syndrome has recently been extensively reviewed.[40] The principal biochemical reactions in the conversion of cholesterol into active adrenocortical steroids require a series of hydroxylations (Fig. 44-2). The 3 synthetic pathways lead to (1) mineralocorticoids with the final production of aldosterone, (2) glucocorticoids leading to cortisol, and (3) androgens which can be converted to testosterone, which in turn can be converted to estrogens. Both steroidogenesis and adrenocortical growth are stimulated by the trophic influence of ACTH. Deficient cortisol synthesis secondary to an enzymatic deficiency causes increased ACTH production. Increased ACTH production in turn causes a compensatory hypertrophy of the adrenal cortex and in this manner the block

in the biosynthetic pathway may be partially overcome. However, this increased production of ACTH also leads to an increased production and accumulation of precursor steroids. The clinical findings as well as the urinary steroidal patterns of the individual defects are summarized in Table 44-2.

Virilization of the female is secondary to the elevation of adrenal androgens caused by those enzymatic defects subsequent to 17-hydroxylation. In most cases there is some fusion of the labioscrotal folds with clitoral enlargement, which may be bound down by chordee. Occasionally, virilization may be so severe that phallic urethra becomes developed. Virilization of the male is not noted during the neonatal period and, in the nonsalt-losing forms of this disorder, the male will be often undetected

Table 44-2. Diagnosis of the Adrenogenital Syndrome.

Deficiency	Clinical Viriliz-ation (♀)	Incomplete Masculin-ization (♂)	Salt Loss	Other	Biochemical Dominant Steroid-Secreted	Urinary 17-Keto-steroids	Urinary 17 OH-steroids	Primary Abnormal Urinary Steroid
Desmolase	0	+ + + +	Usually	Lipid-filled adrenals	? Cholesterol	Low	Low	Virtually absent
3β-Hydroxy-steroid de-hydrogenase	+	+ + +	Usually		Δ^5-3β-OH compounds	Elevated	Low	Pregnene-triol
11-Hydroxylase	+ + + +	0	No	BP↑	S+DOC	Elevated	Elevated	Tetrahydro-S Tetrahydro-DOC
17-Hydroxylase	0	+ +	No	BP↑	B+DOC	Low	Low	Tetrahydro-DOC
21-Hydroxylase	+ + + +	0	Often		17-Hydroxy-progesterone	Elevated	Low or normal	Pregnanetriol

until age 5 or 6 years, at which time he is noted to be large for his age, muscular, and demonstrating secondary sexual changes. The classic virilizing form of the adrenogenital syndrome is the result of a deficiency of the 21-hydroxylase enzyme. This defect is also the most common, accounting for almost 90% of the cases currently recognized.

Incomplete Masculinization. Failure of complete masculine development occurs in those forms in which synthesis of testosterone is blocked (20,22-desmolase, the 3β-hydroxysteroid dehydrogenase, and the 17α-hydroxylase defects). The incomplete masculinization in the male, which is under fetal testicular control,[2] suggests that the enzymatic deficiency in these defects occurs in both the adrenal and the testis. It has been possible to demonstrate that the lack of the enzyme 3β-hydroxysteroid dehydrogenase occurs in both the adrenal and the testis.[21] In the 3β-hydroxysteroid dehydrogenase defect, the block results in secretion of steroids that consists almost entirely of compounds with Δ^5-3β-OH configuration. Its lack in the fetal testis,[22] interfering with testosterone synthesis, causes incomplete masculinization in the male. The marked elevation of Δ^5-3βOH adrenal androgens, especially dehydroepiandrosterone, on the other hand, accounts for the virilization of the female infant. The cases of genetic males with the 20,22-desmolase defect and the 17α-hydroxylase defect reported bear out the hypothesis that the adrenal and testicular enzymatic mechanisms for testosterone biosynthesis share common genetic controls.

Hypertension has been associated with enzymatic blocks resulting in excessive secretion of mineralocorticoids. A deficiency of 11-hydroxylase causes an accumulation of desoxycorticosterone (DOC), a potent mineralocorticoid, as well as 11-deoxycortisol.[41] The 17α-hydroxylase defect blocks 17-hydroxylation of progesterone, interfering with cortisol and androgen biosynthesis, and the mineralocorticoid excess again results in hypertension.[42-44] However, hypertension in these forms of the adrenogenital syndrome is an inconstant feature. Whether the hypertension is related to the duration of excessive secretion of mineralocorticoid, the degree of the defect, or variations in sodium intake is not clear. It is not known whether hypertension occurs during the newborn period in the infants with these forms of the adrenogenital syndrome.

Salt Loss. The salt-losing form of the 21-hydroxylase defect, the 3β-hydroxysteroid dehydrogenase defect, and the 20,22-desmolase defect block steroid synthesis early in the biosynthetic pathway, resulting in mineralocorticoid insufficiency, and causing severe sodium loss. The electrolytes are initially normal but, within a week of life, serum sodium concentration will slowly decrease with a concomitant increase in serum potassium concentration. These infants may develop acute adrenal crisis with shock, peripheral collapse and dehydration by the tenth to fourteenth day of life.

The underlying metabolic defects for two varieties of the 21-hydroxylase enzyme defect are still not clearly understood. Bongiovanni and Eberlein postulated that both varieties are the result of the same hydroxylase deficiency.[45] In the salt-loser, there is almost complete 21-hydroxylase deficiency, whereas in the compensated patient there is sufficient 21-hydroxylase to permit aldosterone synthesis. Childs and associates and Prader found one form or the other (salt-loser or non-salt-loser) consistent within individual families and proposed separate genotypes.[46,47] On the other hand, Rosenbloom and Smith described salt-losers and non-salt-losers within the same siblings.[48] Bartter has favored the thesis of two 21-hydroxylases and that the compensated form is caused by a genetic error in which only the 21-hydroxylase specific for 17-hydroxyprogesterone is deficient, whereas the salt-losing form is the result of a second 21-hydroxylase specific for progesterone as well. Aldosterone hypersecretion in the compensated form has been reported by Bartter and associates.[49] However, his very high values for aldosterone secretion have not been generally confirmed, although there are reports of modest elevations.

Another factor which must be included is the possibility of a sodium-losing hormone. No such steroid or other adrenal hormone has yet been clearly identified.

Two important developments make prenatal diagnosis of the 21-hydroxylase deficiency feasible. The amniotic fluid shows elevated levels of 17-hydroxyprogesterone.[50] Better standards and more experience are needed. However, the serum levels of this steroid are elevated in the affected newborn. Normal newborn levels are 37.8 ± 12 ng/dl, whereas affected infants have shown 67 to 360 ng/dl, and this may serve as a screening device as well.[51] In addition, HL-A typing may prove useful since the locus for this enzyme is on chromosome 6 and closely linked to this system,[52] but there is no single HL-A type characteristic of this disorder, and the value lies in intrafamily recognition and prenatal diagnosis.

A few instances of aldosterone deficiency because of a specific defect of 18-dehydrogenase (the last enzymatic transaction toward aldosterone) have been described.[53,54] There is salt and water loss without the other clinical consequences of congenital adrenal hyperplasia. It is possible that some of the infants described by Jaudon to have transient adrenal insufficiency of the newborn had the same defect.[55]

Diagnosis and Treatment of Acute Adrenal Insufficiency

Diagnosis. It is difficult to make the diagnosis of acute adrenal insufficiency in the newborn. There must be a high index of suspicion in any acutely ill infant with shock, peripheral collapse, and a rapid and weak pulse, or in an infant with poor feeding, or failure to thrive, or intermittent pyrexia, or even hypoglycemia and convulsions. Decreased serum sodium and chloride and increased serum potassium levels are suggestive of mineralocorticoid deficiency. Certainly, ambiguous external genitalia at birth should always suggest the possibility of the adrenogenital syndrome.

The 24-hour output of 17-hydroxycorticosteroids is low in acute adrenal insufficiency. The use of ACTH to determine adrenal responsiveness is not indicated in the acutely ill infant in adrenal crisis; ACTH will often aggravate the clinical situation. The ACTH stimulation test, in the older child, may differentiate between primary adrenocortical insufficiency and cortisol insufficiency secondary to absence of ACTH. However, in the infant with congenital ACTH deficiency there may be complete hypoplasia of the adrenal gland. In the adrenogenital syndrome, it is occasionally necessary to use ACTH to increase the concentration of the abnormal urinary steroid metabolites in order to more clearly establish a diagnosis in the partial enzyme deficiency states.

The diagnosis of the specific enzyme defect in the adrenogenital syndrome can be established by the urinary steroidal pattern. Generally the total 17-ketosteroids will be elevated (except in the more rare forms) and the 17-hydroxysteroids will be low (except in the 11-hydroxylase form). The typical urinary steroidal patterns in the various forms are summarized in Table 44-2. It is important to note that although the measurement of 17-hydroxycorticosteroids is generally an index of the amount of cortisol or its metabolites in the urine, the Porter-Silber reaction will also measure other steroids, such as tetrahydro-S. It is for this reason that the level of urinary excretion of 17-hydroxycorticosteroids is elevated in the 11-hydroxylase defect. The urinary "ketogenic steroids" are used by some laboratories as an index of cortisol excretion and are even less specific and will be elevated in most forms of the adrenogenital syndrome, including the most common form, a deficiency of 21-hydroxylase.

Treatment. The immediate need of the critically ill infant in adrenal crisis is for cortisol. If possible, one should withhold cortisol until the diagnosis can be established by the appropriate urinary steroid studies. On the other hand, if a newborn infant is in shock and in extremis, one may be justified in the use of glucocorticoids as a life-saving measure, whatever the diagnosis. In the usual situation, salt and water alone will relieve the clinical crisis. Intravenous isotonic saline in 5% glucose water should be infused at a rate of 100 to 120 ml/kg during the first 24 hours. If the infant is in severe shock, the use of plasma 5 ml/kg might be necessary as well as cortisol. Hydrocortisone hemisuccinate or phosphate, 1.5 to 2.0 mg/kg should be given intravenously immediately. Hydrocortisone (or cortisone acetate) 2 mg/kg is to be given intramuscularly simultaneously and to be repeated daily for several days. In order to aid restoration of electrolyte balance, desoxycorticosterone acetate is often employed intramuscularly in a dose of 2 mg on the first day and 1 mg each day thereafter. The infant with severe shock may at times require a vasopressor. It is important to note that in severe adrenal cortical insufficiency, vasopressor drugs may be without effect until after the administration of hydrocortisone.

In the adrenogenital syndrome, the treatment of the acute crisis, especially in an undiagnosed male, is the same as discussed above. We have often found it possible to use fluids and desoxycorticosterone acetate alone in order to treat the patients with the salt-losing forms of the adrenogenital syndrome. This regimen permits the collection of urine in an effort to establish the diagnosis. Certainly, in the newborn female with ambiguous genitalia, it is possible to treat the patient expectantly and collect the necessary urine because acute adrenal crisis is not likely to occur until several days after birth.

Hydrocortisone (or cortisone acetate) in the dose of 15 to 25 mg/m²/day is the mainstay for long-term treatment of patients with adrenal insufficiency. The newer steroid analogues, especially in the patient with mineralocorticoid deficiency, should be avoided. Many of these analogues were synthesized with the express aim of eliminating the sodium-retaining property of hydrocortisone. In fact, some of these drugs, such as dexamethasone, promote sodium excretion. Cortisone acetate can also be given intramuscularly every 3 days for long-term replacement therapy, but this regimen is seldom necessary. During severe stress, such as pernicious vomiting or surgery, cortisone acetate (25 mg/m²) should be given parenterally on a daily basis.

9α-Fluorohydrocortisone (Florinef) in the dose of 0.05 to 0.1 mg/day orally is at times a necessary adjunct for chronic therapy. This oral mineralocorticoid has generally supplanted the use of desoxycorticosterone acetate (DOCA) for chronic therapy except in unusual circumstances because DOCA can be given only parenterally or as a pellet implanted subcutaneously. Furthermore, DOCA has been implicated as a cause of hypertension as a consequence of excessive dosage, and, in the case of the pellet, adrenal crisis has been known to occur with unexpected loss of potency of the drug.

DISORDERS OF THE THYROID

Development and Function of the Thyroid Gland

The fetal thyroid begins as a thickening of epithelium at the base of the tongue. The thyroid anlage subsequently migrates down the trachea, leaving the thyroglossal duct as an embryonic remnant. During its caudal mi-

gration, the thyroid anlage assumes a more bilobate shape. Thyroid function is apparent by 12 weeks of gestation, the ability to accumulate and concentrate iodide then being present. Organification of iodine with synthesis of thyroxine and triiodothyronine occurs by 14 weeks of gestation. The fetal hypothalamic-pituitary feedback mechanisms are operative by the latter part of gestation and the fetal thyroid is responsive to thyrotropin (TSH). There is no placental transfer of maternal or fetal TSH, although long-acting thyroid stimulating hormone (LATS), a 7S gamma globulin, will cross the placenta. Free thyroxine and, more so, triiodothyronine are capable, to a small degree, of crossing the placenta in either direction.[56,57]

The biosynthesis of thyroid hormones is illustrated in Figure 44-3. Circulating plasma iodide is concentrated by the thyroid gland. The concentrated iodide is then oxidized by a thyroid peroxidase and bound to tyrosine to form monoiodotyrosine and diiodotyrosine. The iodotyrosines are held in peptide linkage to thyroglobulin. These iodotyrosines are then coupled to form thyroxine and triiodothyronine, still linked to thyroglobulin. The thyroid hormones are cleaved from thyroglobulin by thyroid proteases and thyroxine and triiodothyronine secreted into the circulatory system. Intrathyroidal iodotyrosines and iodothyronines are deiodinated by the dehalogenase enzymes and remain within the intrathyroidal iodide pool to be reused. The thyroid gland secretes both thyroxine and triiodothyronine. However, a large percentage of the circulating triiodothyronine is secondary to diiodination of thyroxine by the peripheral tissues.[58] The iodide released from the peripheral metabolism of iodothyronines enters the circulatory system to be reconcentrated by the thyroid gland or excreted by the kidneys. The iodothyronines are transported in the plasma by proteins. Thyroxine-binding globulin (TBG), an alpha globulin, is the major carrier of thyroxine. TBG will bind triiodothyronine to a lesser extent. Thyroxine is also bound by thyroxine-binding prealbumin and by albumin. At the cell level, the free thyroxine and triiodothyronine are active. Disorders, either genetic or acquired, that quantitatively change the concentration of TBG will alter the level of total thyroxine in serum without altering biological thyroid status.

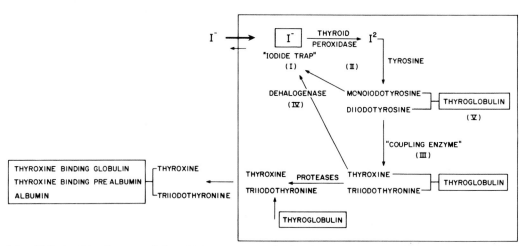

Fig. 44-3. In this diagram of thyroid hormone synthesis, the roman numerals represent described enyzmatic defects of thyroxine synthesis.

The secretion of the thyroid hormones is under hypothalamic pituitary control. The hypothalamus secretes a tripeptide, thyrotropin-releasing hormone (TRH), which provokes release of TSH from pituitary.[59,60] TSH in turn stimulates the production of thyroid hormones. Every step of thyroid hormone biosynthesis and release from iodide accumulation to proteolysis of thyroglobulin, is under TSH stimulation. The thyroid hormones in turn exercise negative feedback control of TSH response to TRH at the pituitary level.

Thyroid Function Tests

Thyroid function tests in the newborn are elevated in comparison to values obtained for older children. The total T_4 ranges from 7.3 to 20.9 μg/dl during the first month of life, with a mean value greater than 10 μg/dl (Table 44-3).

Congenital Hypothyroidism

The causes of congenital hypothyroidism are many and include disorganized embryogenesis, genetic disorders including errors of

Table 44-3. Range of Values and Means for Thyroid Hormones and TSH During Neonatal Period.[61-64]

	T_4 μg/dl	T_3 ng/dl	rT_3 ng/dl	TBG mg/dl	TSH μU/dl
Newborn	11.0 ± 2.0	50 ± 18	136 ± 29	5.4 ± 2.1	9.5 (2.4–20.0)
30 min					86.0 (13–149)
1 hour	12.5				68 (43–94)
24 hours	16.2	419		5.4	17.1 (8.6–33)
48 hours	14.5	191			12.8 (5–23)
2 weeks	10.3 (7.8–12.7)				

Means are shown with either ±1 SD, or range in parentheses. T_4 = thyroxine; T_3 = triiodothyronine; rT_3 = reverse T_3; TBG = thyrosine binding globulin; TSH = thyrotropin.

thyroxine biosynthesis, and environmental factors.

Clinical Diagnosis. It is useful to classify congenital hypothyroidism into the following subgroups.

1. Agenesis of the thyroid gland (athyrotic cretinism) or dysgenesis of the thyroid gland (thyroid hypoplasia, thyroid ectopia)
2. Endemic goitrous hypothyroidism
3. Inborn errors of thyroxine synthesis (familial goitrous cretinism)
4. Drug-induced hypothyroidism
5. End-organ unresponsiveness to thyroid hormone.
6. Thyroid unresponsiveness to thyrotropin.

Agenesis or Dysgenesis of the Thyroid Gland. Disorganization of embryogenesis of the thyroid gland is the most frequent cause of congenital hypothyroidism in the United States. Although congenital endemic goitrous hypothyroidism may have been more prevalent throughout the world at one time, the frequency of this disorder has declined over recent years with the introduction of iodine into endemic areas.

• Etiology: At this time, little is known of the causes of defective fetal thyroid development. There may be genetic factors. Athyrotic congenital hypothyroidism has been documented in siblings[65,66] and in identical twins.[67] Nonetheless, athyrosis is generally a sporadic disorder. Thyroid antibodies have been detected in greater incidence among mothers of children with hypothyroidism.[68] However, most mothers with thyroid antibodies have normal children and, conversely, most mothers who deliver children with congenital hypothyroidism do not have thyroid antibodies. Thyroid hypoplasia has been reported in children with congenital toxoplasmosis but *in utero* infectious disorders have not been commonly implicated as a cause of thyroid dysgenesis.

• Central Nervous System: There is considerable evidence for the essential role of the thyroid hormones in the growth and development of the central nervous system.[69] The final outcome of mental development in children with congenital hypothyroidism depends on the severity, the time of onset (*in utero*) and duration of thyroid insufficiency.

• Symptoms: Symptoms of agenesis of the thyroid gland are detectable by 6 weeks of age. However, a number will have clinical manifestations at birth or during the immediate neonatal period. The signs during the early neonatal period are subtle and include prolonged neonatal jaundice, poor suck, poor feeding, lethargy ("the quiet baby"), respiratory difficulties, and intermittent cyanosis. Later, the more classic symptoms of cretinism appear. The progressive myxedema causes coarsening of the facies with puffy eyelids, flattened nasal bridge, and enlarged tongue. The cry is hoarse secondary to myxedema of the larynx and epiglottis. The infant is extremely lethargic and hypotonic. Constipation, poor feeding, poor weight gain, dry hair, umbilical hernia, and pallor become more notable with time.

Infants with ectopic or residual thyroid tissue ("dysgenetic cretinism") will often produce enough thyroid hormone to delay the onset of clinical symptoms. Although the signs and symptoms are similar to the athyrotic cretin, the outlook for mental prognosis is greatly improved.

• Diagnosis: The diagnosis can be confirmed by a serum thyroxine level, and low normal values should be viewed suspiciously in light of the relatively elevated values in normal newborns. Radiographic skeletel age is often helpful, in that half of the infants with congenital hypothyroidism will not have the osseous centers normally present at birth. A thyroidal radioactive iodine uptake is useful in detecting the presence of residual or ectopic tissue.

The incidence of congenital hypothyroidism has been estimated to be 1/6000 births. In view of the desirability of early diagnosis and treatment, screening programs of newborn infants employing filter paper "spots" as with PKU has been undertaken, using radioimmunoassay. Some 34% of low T_4 values by this method will *not* be the result of true hypothyroidism and often represent diminished thyroxine binding globulin (TBG). If the initial T_4 is more than 2.4 SD below the mean for a given set of tests, a TSH is determined on the same sample, and if this is greater than 1.0 μU per spot (= $40\mu1$) the infant is recalled for further study. Some methods use a smaller paper spot. If the T_4 is between -2.3 and -2.6 SD and the TSH is low, the result is regarded as normal. If the T4 is -4 SD of the mean, the infant is recalled at once. When the initial results are doubtful, a repeat filter paper specimen is obtained. If this last reveals a T_4 more than -2.6 SD, a serum sample is obtained and studied in detail to rule out secondary, tertiary hypothyroidism, or TBG deficiency. If the T_4 is greater than 7 μg/dl, it is regarded as normal.[70] Note the need to avoid using specimens in the early hours following birth because of the normal surge of TSH (Table 44-3).

Endemic Goitrous Hypothyroidism. Although endemic goiter still remains one of the most widespread nutritional diseases in the world, the introduction of iodine into various foods, including infant formulas, has markedly decreased the incidence of endemic goitrous hypothyroidism. The dietary requirements for iodine vary, but 40 to 100 μg/day is sufficient for most children. In areas of endemic goiters, it is probable that factors other than iodine, such as enzymatic defects, other genetic factors, and other dietary factors (such as goitrogens) may contribute to goiter formation. The contributory factors are suggested by the evidence that females are more commonly afflicted than males, many of the population within the endemic area may not be afflicted, and the incidence of endemic cretinism varies in different areas. In the Alps, deaf-mutism is a common finding in association with endemic cretinism, suggesting possibly an associated enzymatic defect of organification of iodide. When cretinism occurs in conjunction with an endemic goiter, the signs and symptoms are similar to the dysgenetic form of cretinism except for the presence of a goiter and an elevated radioactive iodine uptake.

Inborn Errors of Thyroxine Synthesis. The inherited disorders of thyroxine synthesis involve deficiencies in one or more of the enzymes necessary for hormonogenesis or release of thyroid hormones resulting in hypothyroidism. A compensatory increase in TSH production produces hyperplasia and enlargement of the thyroid gland, creating the clinical picture of "familial goitrous cretinism." These defects of thyroxine biosynthesis have recently been reviewed.[76]

• Iodide Trap Defect: The thyroid gland has the ability to concentrate iodide so that the intrathyroidal iodide concentration may be 40-fold greater than the serum concentration. In this rare inherited defect of thyroxine synthesis, this ability is lost. As would be anticipated, the 24-hour radioactive iodine uptake is negligible. Several other organs, including the salivary glands, share the ability to concentrate iodide and this defect can be distinguished from athyrosis because the salivary iodide concentration is also low and there is usually a goiter. The serum T_4 and PBI are also low in this defect. In a manner of speaking, this defect represents iodine deficiency and high dosages of iodide can overcome this defect to some degree.

• Organification Defect (Peroxidase Defect): A defect in the organification of iodide is one of the more frequent defects of thyroxine synthesis. In this defect, the thyroid has an increased uptake for iodide but is unable to oxidize it and cannot combine it with tyrosine. This leads to the accumulation of free iodide in the gland, and the administration of anions such as perchlorate or thiocyanate will cause a discharge or release of the unbound iodide. Iodine that is bound to tyrosine or thyronines cannot be discharged. These findings have led to a simple test for the organification defect. The patient is given a tracer amount of radioactive iodine and the radioactivity over the thyroid gland is noted. In a patient with the organification defect, the radioactive iodine is rapidly concentrated into the gland. When the radioactivity over the gland has plateaued, a dose of potassium perchlorate (or thiocyanate) given orally (0.5–1.0 g) will displace the unorganified iodine, causing a rapid discharge of the radioactive iodine from the thyroid gland. The measurements of T_4, PBI, and BEI are usually low.

A variant of this form of familial goiter secondary to a defect in organification is associated with deaf-mutism (Pendred's syndrome). The clinical pattern differs slightly from the full organification defect in that the Pendred group often has only small goiters and the perchlorate discharge is not as complete. The hearing loss in this variant is neurosensory. Intelligence is usually normal.

• Coupling Defect: The failure of coupling of monoiodotyrosine (MIT) and diiodotyrosine (DIT) into thyroxine and triiodothyronine has been identified as a cause of goitrous hypothyroidism. The coupling of the iodotyrosines into the final product of the thyroid hormones is probably a complex intermediate step involving many processes, and the block should not be thought of as a defined enzymatic deficiency. The inability of the thyroid gland to couple MIT and DIT into thyroxine and triiodothyronine leads to the accumulation of large amounts of MIT and DIT in the gland, with the small amounts of T_4 and T_3 synthesized being immediately released into the circulation. Thus, when extracts of the thyroid gland are subjected to chromatographic analysis after radioactive iodine labeling, large amounts of MIT and DIT are detected with only trace quantities of T_4 and T_3. The PBI is usually low. The radioactive iodine uptake by the thyroid gland is rapid and high. Definitive diagnosis requires thyroidectomy and chromatographic analysis of the iodotyrosines and iodothyronines.

• Dehalogenase Defect: The deiodination of the iodotyrosines and iodothyronines occurs intrathyroidally as well as in the liver, kidney, and other organs. The inherited inability of the thyroid to deiodinate MIT and DIT causes leakage of these precursors from the gland and depletion of iodide stores. This loss of iodide causes decreased hormone synthesis, resulting in compensatory TSH release, thyroid hyperplasia, increased synthesis of MIT, DIT, and the iodothyronines. The loss of iodide is compounded by further intermediate formation and their increased loss. The goitrous hypothyroidism in this defect is not caused by a biosynthetic block but, in a sense, by iodine deficiency. Radioactive iodine is rapidly accumulated and turned over. Large amounts of iodine can permit adequate hormone synthesis. The increased circulating levels of MIT and DIT may cause the PBI determination to be normal, whereas the BEI and T_4 determinations will be low. Because this defect is extrathyroidal as well as intrathyroidal, administered radioactive MIT or DIT appears unchanged in the urine.

• Abnormal Thyroglobulin: Thyroglobulin is synthesized exclusively within the thyroid. The iodination of the tyrosyl residues within the thyroglobulin complex lead to formation of MIT and DIT and coupling of these iodinated tyrosyl residues lead to formation of T_4 and T_3. A "defect" of thyroglobulin formation actually incorporates a group of disorders. Errors of thyroglobulin synthesis resulting in an abnormal thyroglobulin as well as decreased synthesis are possible. Deficient protease activity for thyroglobulin degradation has also been postulated to result in deficiency of thyroid hormone release.[72]

These disorders are characterized by ab-normal, nonbutanol extractable iodoproteins in the thyroid and the serum. These peptides have sometimes been described as albumin-like and have been identified by Savoie and associates as an iodoalbumin (thyroalbumin) in which the major iodinated compounds appear to be monoiodohistadines and diiodo-histadines.[73,74] These investigators conclude that the abnormality of thyroglobulin causes iodination of inappropriate proteins, mainly albumin with subsequently a low yield of thyroxine. A compensatory increase in TSH secretion causes thyroid hyperplasia and a rapid turnover of thyroxine-poor albumin. Proteolysis of the iodohistadine-thyroalbumin results in a high secretion of iodohistadine which can be detected in the urine.

Drug-induced Neonatal Goiter. Many drugs such as paraaminosalicylic acid, cobalt, iodides, and the thiourea drugs, as well as foods (cabbage, turnips, rutabaga) have been demonstrated to be goitrogenic. In the newborn infant, the most commonly implicated drugs are iodides and thiourea derivatives used for treatment of maternal thyrotoxicosis. The use of these drugs has caused not only goiter in the newborn but also has been associated with scattered reports of hypothyroidism.[75] Although the correlation between the dose of the drug and the occurrence of goiter is poor, prolonged administration of thiourea drugs to the mother increases the risk of fetal goiter. Herbst and Selenkow suggest lowering the dose of thiourea drugs during the last trimester and the use of thyroid hormone as well when treating a thyrotoxic pregnant female.[76] In these infants, it is necessary to distinguish the drug-induced goiter and the LATS-induced goiter. A low T_4 suggests that the goiter is secondary to the drug, whereas a high T_4 is more compatible with a LATS-induced goiter and possible neonatal hyperthyroidism. Treatment is usually not necessary for the infant with a drug-induced goiter unless the goiter is asphyxiating or, more rarely, if the infant is hypothyroid. Thyroid hormone will cause the goiter to subside. However, if the goiter is suffocating, subtotal thyroidectomy may be necessary.[77]

Unresponsiveness to Thyroid Hormones. Refetoff and associates reported a family with deaf-mutism, stippled epiphyses, delayed bone age, goiter, and an elevated serum T_4.[78] The children appeared to be euthyroid. The serum thyroid hormone-binding proteins as well as hormone biosynthesis appeared to be normal. This family has been postulated to represent tissue unresponsiveness to thyroid hormone.

Partial target organ resistance has been postulated by Bode and associates as an explanation for a clinically euthyroid 8-year-old male with goiter and elevated thyroid function tests.[79] Thyroxine-binding proteins were normal. Despite the elevated levels of thyroid hormones, TSH determinations were normal. TSH levels increased with the use of methimazole. TRH caused a brisk increase in TSH, unlike thyrotoxicosis. Glucocorticoids and triido-L-thyronine caused a blunting of the TSH responses to TRH. These latter TSH findings are consistent with a euthyroid state. This patient, unlike the family reported by Refetoff and associates, had no defect in auditory function or skeletal processes. Lamberg reported a 25-year-old female with similar findings.[80]

Unresponsiveness to TSH. Stanbury and associates reported a severely retarded 8-year-old male with a normal thyroid gland, a low PBI, normal radioactive iodine uptake, and high endogenous levels of biologically active TSH.[81] Exogenous TSH did not stimulate the thyroid gland *in vivo* nor increase glucose metabolism by thyroid slices *in vitro*. TSH unresponsiveness of the thyroid gland was postulated by these investigators as an explanation for this clinical syndrome.

Treatment and Prognosis of Congenital Hypothyroidism

It is possible to treat some of the forms of inborn errors of thyroxine synthesis with iodide, but substitution therapy with thyroid hormone is inexpensive and effective for all of the disorders causing congenital hypothyroidism. The synthetic thyroid hormones rather than desiccated thyroid are preferred. Desiccated thyroid is generally effective but variations in thyroxine content is common and low thyroxine content has been reported.[82] The U.S.P. standardization for desiccated thyroid is based on iodide content and not hormonal content. The cost of L-thyroxine is now low.

The dose of thyroid hormone prescribed should be adequate and increased rapidly to assure high euthyroid levels of serum T_4. The dosages of 15 to 30 mg of desiccated thyroid commonly used as initial doses are too low.

These low initiating doses are not necessary because the symptoms of myxedema cardiac failure or headache, commonly seen in adults with hypothyroidism with rapid increase in thyroid replacement therapy, are not seen in infants. L-thyroxine at 0.05 mg/day orally should be initiated once the diagnosis is established. The dosage may be increased to 0.1 mg rapidly and the infant maintained on this dose.

The prognosis for mental development has been correlated with onset of therapy. Several series have indicated that the prognosis is best if therapy has been initiated before 6 months of age.[83,84] Klein and associates studied 31 patients and, in 9 treated before the age of 3 months, the mean IQ was significantly greater than all the children treated after 3 months of age, including the group between 3 and 6 months of age.[85] However, in the individual child the prognosis must be guarded despite the statistics.

Congenital Thyrotoxicosis

Thyrotoxicosis occurring in the neonatal period is extremely rare, slightly more than 40 cases having been reported. These infants are almost always born of mothers with either active thyrotoxicosis or past histories of thyrotoxicosis. It appears that the etiologic factor for neonatal thyrotoxicosis is the placental transfer of maternal LATS. LATS has been demonstrated in both mother and infant in over 90% of studied cases.

Neonatal thyrotoxicosis is manifested by poor weight gain or excessive weight loss, goiter, irritability, tachycardia, flushing, and exophthalmos. A number of these infants have tended to be small for gestational age. In an infant of a thyrotoxic mother, a high normal T_4 should be viewed with suspicion and the child followed closely. Onset usually occurs within the first week of life but may be delayed until the second week. Arrhythmias, such as paroxysmal atrial tachycardia,[86] cardiac failure, and death may occur if thyrotoxicity is especially severe. However, the prognosis is generally good because the thyrotoxic state is transient. In several reported cases, there has been a rapid advance in skeletal maturation with advanced bone age and premature closure of the cranial sutures.[87,88]

The therapeutic concerns in neonatal thyrotoxicosis are tracheal obstruction secondary to goitrous encroachment or cardiac failure. Subtotal thyroidectomy may be necessary with tracheal obstruction. Iodide is usually reserved for preoperative management of thyrotoxicosis because the duration of its therapeutic effects is limited. However, because neonatal thyrotoxicosis is a self-limiting disorder, iodide is the drug of choice, for it not only interferes with thyroxine synthesis but also release of thyroid hormones. In the most severe cases, digitalis, sedation, or a β-adrenergic blocking agent such as propanolol hydrochloride, may be necessary.

REFERENCES

1. **Winters SJ, Wachtel SS, White BJ, Kov GC, Javadpour N, Loriaux L, Sherins RJ:** H-Y antigen mosaicism in the gonad of a 46, XX true hermaphrodite.
2. **Jost A:** Embryonic sexual differentiation: Morphology, physiology, abnormalities. In Jones HH, Scott WW (eds): Hermaphroditism, Genital Anomalies and Related Disorders, p. 16. Williams and Wilkins, Baltimore, 1971.
3. **Josso N:** Permeability of membranes to the mullerian-inhibiting substance synthesized by the human fetal testis in vitro: A clue to its biochemical nature. J. Clin Endocrinol Metab 34:265, 1972.
4. **Jacobs PA, et al:** Evidence for the existence of the human "super-female," Lancet 2:423, 1959.
5. **Johnston AW, Ferguson-Smith MA, Handmaker SD Jr, Jones HW, Jones GS:** The triple-X syndrome. Clinical, pathological, and chromosomal studies in three mentally retarded cases. Br Med J 2:1047, 1961.
6. **Shah PN, Naik SN, Manajan PK, Dave MJ, Paymasters JC:** A new variant of human intersex with discussion on the developmental aspects. Br Med J 2:474, 1961.
7. **Therkelsen AJ:** Sterile male with the chromosome constitution 46 XX. Cytogenetics 3:207, 1964.
8. **Lubs HA, Rudd FH:** Chromosomal abnormalities in the human population: estimation of rates based on New Haven Newborn Study. Science 169:496, 1970
9. **Morishima A, Grumbach M:** The interrelationship of sex chromosome constitution and phenotype in the syndrome of gonadal dysgenesis and its variants. Ann NY Acad Sci 155:695, 1968
10. **Goldberg MB, Scully AL, Solomon IL, Steinbach HL:** Gonadal dysgenesis in phenotypic female subjects. Am J Med 45:529, 1968

11. **Ullrich O:** Über typische kombinations bilder multipler abartunigen. Zschr Kinderh 49:271, 1930
12. **Bonnevie K:** Embroyological analysis of gene manifestation in Little and Bagg's abnormal mouse tribe. J Exp Zool 67:443, 1934
13. **Haddad HM, Wilkins L:** Congenital anomalies associated with gonadal aplasia. Pediatrics 23:885, 1959
14. **Preger L, Steinbach HL, Moskowitz P:** Roentgenographic abnormalities in phenotypic females with gonadal dysgenesis. Am J Roentgenol 104:899, 1968
15. **Johanson AJ, Brasel JA, Blizzard RM:** Growth in patients with gonadal dysgenesis receiving fluoxymesterone. J Pediatr 75:1015, 1969
16. **Tsagonnis M:** Response to long term administration of human growth hormone in Turner's syndrome. JAMA 210:2373, 1969
17. **Moshang T, Vallet HL, Cintron C, et al:** Gonadal function in XO/XY or XX/XY Turner's syndrome. J Pediatr 80:460, 1972
18. **Hook EB:** Behavioral implications of the human XYY genotype. Science 179:139, 1973
19. **Mürset G, et al:** Male external genitalia of a girl caused by virilizing adrenal tumor in the mother. Acta Endocrinol 54:181, 1967
20. **Haymond MW, Weldon VV:** Female pseudohermaphroditism secondary to a maternal virilizing tumor. J Pediatr 82:682, 1973
21. **Bongiovanni AM:** Adrenogenital syndrome with deficiency of 3β-hydroxysteroid dehydrogenase. J Clin Invest 41:2086, 1962
22. **Bongiovanni AM, Eberlein WR, Goldman AS, New M:** Disorders of adrenal steroid biogenesis. Recent Progr Horm Res 23:375, 1967
23. **Wilkins LW:** The Diagnosis and Treatment of Endocrine Disorders. In Childhood and Adolescence, p 321, Charles C Thomas, Springfield, 1965
24. **Wilson JD, Walker JD:** The conversion of testosterone to 5α-Androstan-17β-ol-3-one (Dihydrotestosterone) by skin slices of man. J Clin Invest 48:371, 1969
25. **Strickland AL, French FS:** Absence of response to dihydrotestosterone in the syndrome of testicular feminization. J Clin Endocrinol Metab 29:1284, 1969
26. **Money J, Hampson JG, Hampson JL:** Hermaphroditism: Recommendations concerning assignment of sex, change of sex and psychologic management. Bull Johns Hopkins Hosp 96:253, 1955
27. **Hampson JG, Money J, Hampson JL:** Hermaphroditism: Recommendations concerning case management. J Clin Endocrinol 16:547, 1956
28. **Money J:** Hermaphroditism, gender and precocity in hyperadrenocorticism: Phsyicologic

findings. Bull Johns Hopkins Hosp 96:253, 1955

29. **Bongiovanni AM, Eberlein WR, Moshang T Jr:** Urinary excretion of pregnanetriol and Δ5-Pregnenetriol in two forms of congenital adrenal hyperplasia. J Clin Invest 50:2751, 1971

30. **Wurtman RJ, Axelrod J:** Adrenaline synthesis. Control by the pituitary gland and adrenal glucocorticoids. Science 150:1464, 1956

31. **Gardner LI, Walton RL:** Plasma 17-ketosteroids in the human fetus: Demonstration of concentration gradient between cord and maternal circulation. Helvet Paediatr Acta 9:311, 1954

32. **Denton DA, Goding JR, Wright RD:** Control of adrenal secretion of electrolyte-active steroids. Adrenal stimulation by cross-circulation experiments in conscious sheep. Br Med J 2: 522, 1959

33. **Newton MA, Laragh JH:** Effect of corticotropin on aldosterone excretion and plasma renin in normal subjects, in essential hypertension and in primary aldosteronism. J Clin Endocrinol Metab 28:1006, 1968

34. **Davis JO, Yankopoulos NA, Lieberman F, et al:** Role of the anterior pituitary in the control of aldosterone secretion in experimental secondary hyperaldosteronism. J Clin Invest 39: 765, 1960

35. **Eberlein WR, Bongiovanni AM:** Steroid metabolism in the "salt-losing" form of congenital adrenal hyperplasia. J Clin Invest 37:889, 1958

36. **Peters JP, German WI, Man EB, Welt LG:** Functions of gonads, thyroid and adrenals in hypopituitarism. Metabolism 3:118, 1954

37. **Shepard TH, Landing BH, Mason DG:** Familial Addison's disease. Am J Dis Child 97:154, 1959

38. **Migeon CJ, Kenny EM, Kowarski A, et al:** The syndrome of congenital adrenocortical unresponsiveness to ACTH. Pediatr Res 2:501, 1968

39. **Moshang T, et al:** Familial glucocorticoid insufficiency. J Pediatr 82:821, 1973

40. **Bongiovanni AM:** Disorders of adrenocortical steroid biogenesis. In Stanbury JB, Wyngaarden JB, Fredrickson DS (eds): The Metabolic Basis of Inherited Disease, p 857. McGraw-Hill, New York, 1972

41. **Eberlein WR, Bongiovanni AM:** Plasma and urinary corticosteroids in hypertensive form of congenital adrenal hyperplasia. J Biol Chem 223:85, 1956

42. **Biglieri EG, Herron MA, Brust N:** 17-Hydroxylation deficiency in man. J Clin Invest 45: 1946, 1966

43. **Goldsmith O, Solomon DH, Horton R:** Hypogonadism and minealocorticoid excess: The 17-hydroxylase deficiency syndrome. N Engl J Med 277:673, 1967

44. **Mallin SR:** Congenital adrenal hyperplasia secondary to 17-hydroxylase deficiency. Ann Intern Med 70:69, 1969

45. **Eberlein WR, Bongiovanni AM:** Defective steroidal biogenesis in congenital adrenal hyperplasia. Pediatrics 21:661, 1958

46. **Childs B, Grumbach MM, Van Wyk JJ:** Virilizing adrenal hyperplasia: A genetic and hormonal study. J Clin Invest 35:213, 1956

47. **Prader A:** Die Hanfigkeit des Kongenitalen Adrenogenitalen syndromes. Helv Paediatr Acta 13:426, 1958

48. **Rosenbloom AL, Smith DW:** Varying expression for salt losing in related patients with congenital adrenal hyperplasia. Pediatrics 38: 215, 1966

49. **Bartter FC, Henkin RI, Bryan GT:** Aldosterone hypersecretion in "non-salt-losing" congenital adrenal hyperplasia. J Clin Invest 47:1747, 1968

50. **Fraser SD, Thorneycroft IH, Weiss BA, Horton R:** Elevated amniotic fluid levels of 17-hydroxyprogesterone in congenital adrenal hyperplasia. J Pediatr 86:310, 1975

51. **Pang S, Hotchkiss J, Drash AL, Levine LS, New MI:** Microfilter paper method for 17-hydroxyprogesterone RIA: Screen for congenital adrenal hyperplasia. J Clin Endocrinol Metab 45:1003, 1977

52. **Dupont B, Oberfield SE, Smithwick EM, Levine LS:** Close genetic linkage between HLA and congenital adrenal hyperplasia (21-hydroxylase deficiency). Lancet ii:1309, 1977

53. **Ulick S, Gautier E, Vetterik K, et al:** An aldosterone biosynthetic defect in a salt-losing disorder. J Clin Endocrinol Metab 24:669, 1964

54. **Visser HK, Cost WS:** A new hereditary defect in the biosynthesis of aldosterone: Urinary C 21-cortico-steroid pattern in three related patients with a salt-losing syndrome, suggesting an 18-oxidation defect. Acta Endocrinol 47: 589, 1964

55. **Jaudon JC:** Addison's disease in children. Pediatrics 28:737, 1946

56. **Fisher DA, Hobel CJ, Garza R, Pierce CA:** Thyroid function in the pre term fetus. Pediatrics 46:208, 1970

57. **Dussault J, Row VV, Lickrish G, Volpe R:** Studies of serum triiodothyronine concentration in maternal and cord blood: Transfer of triiodothyronine across the human placenta. J Clin Endocrinol Metab 29:595, 1969

58. **Pittman CS, Chambers JB, Jr, Read VH:** The extrathyroidal conversion rate of thyroxine to triiodothyronine in normal man. J Clin Invest 50:1187, 1971

59. **Burgus R, et al:** Characterization of ovine hy-

pothalamic hypophysiotropic TSH-releasing factor. Nature 226:321, 1970

60. **Nair RMG, Barrett JF, Bowers CX, Schally AV:** Structure of porcine thyrotropin releasing hormone. Biochem 9:1103, 1970

61. **Erenberg A, Phelps DL, Oh W, Fisher DA:** Total and free thyroxine and triiodothyronine in the newborn period. Pediatrics 53:211, 1974

62. **Fisher DA, Odell WD:** Acute release of thyrotopin in the newborn. J Clin Invest 48:1670, 1969

63. **Abuid J, Stimson DA, Larson PR:** Total and free triiodothyronine and thyroxine in early infancy. J Clin Endocrinol Metab 39:263, 1974

64. **Aruskin TW:** Measurements of free and total serum T4 and T3 in pregnant subjects and neonates. Am J Med Sci 271:309, 1976

65. **Lowrey GH, et al:** Early diagnostic criteria of congenital hypothyroidism. Am J Dis Child 96:131, 1958

66. **Childs B, Gardner LI:** Etiologic factors in sporadic cretinism. Ann Hum Genet 19:90, 1954

67. **Greig WR, Henderson AS, Boyle JA, McGirr EM, Hutchison JH:** Thyroid dysgenesis in two parts of monozygotic twins and in a mother and child. J Clin Endocrinol Metab 26:1309, 1966

68. **Blizzard RM, et al:** Maternal autoimmunization to thyroid as a probable cause of athyrotic cretinism. N Engl J Med 263:327, 1960

69. **French FS, Van Wyk JJ:** Fetal hypothyroidism. I. Effects of thyroxine on neural development. II. Fetal versus maternal contributions to fetal thyroxine requirements. III. Clinical implications. J Pediatr 64:589, 1964

70. **Committee on Genetics, American Acad Pediatr:** screening for congenital deficiency of thyroid hormone. Pediatrics 60:389–404, 1977

71. **Stanbury JB:** Familial goiter. In Stanbury JB, Wyngaarden JB, Fredrickson DS (eds): The Metabolic Basis of Inherited Disease, p 223. McGraw-Hill, New York, 1972

72. **Reinwein D:** Hormonsynthese und enzymspektrum bei erkrankungen der menschlichen schilddruse. Acta Endocrinol (Kbh.): (Suppl) 47 94:1, 1964

73. **Savoie JC, Thompoulos P, Savoie F:** Studies on mono and diiodohistidine. I. The identification of histadines from thyroidal iodoproteins and their peripheral metabolism in the normal man and rat. J Clin Invest 52:106, 1973

74. **Savoie JC, Massin JP, Savoie F:** II. Congenital goitrous hypothyroidism with thyroglobulin defect and iodohistidine-rich iodoalbumin production. J Clin Invest 52:116, 1973

75. **Burrow GN:** Neonatal goiter after maternal popylthiouracil therapy. J Clin Endocrinol Metab 25:403, 1965

76. **Herbst AL, Selenkow JA:** Hyperthyroidism during pregnancy. N Engl J Med 273:627, 1965

77. **Bongiovanni AM, Eberlein WR, Jones IT:** Sporadic goiter of the newborn infant. Dallas Med J 43:167, 1957

78. **Refetoff S, DeWind LT, De Groot LJ:** Familial syndrome combining deaf-mutism, stippled epiphyses, goiter, and abnormally high PBI: Possible target organ refractoriness to thyroid hormone. J Clin Endocrinol Metab 27:279, 1967

79. **Bode HH, et al:** Partial target organ resistance to thyroid hormone. J Clin Invest 52:776, 1973

80. **Lamberg BA:** Congenital euthyroid goiter and partial peripheral resistance to thyroid hormones. Lancet 1:854, 1973

81. **Stanbury JB, Rocmans P, Butler UK, Ochi Y:** Congenital hypothyroidism with impaired thyroid response to thyrotropin. N Engl J Med 279:1132, 1968

82. **Mangieri CN, Lund MH:** Potency of United States Pharmacopeia desiccated thyroid tablets as determined by the antigoitrogenic assay in rats. J Clin Endocrinol Metab 30:102, 1970

83. **Smith DW, Blizzard RM, Wilkins L:** Mental attainments of hypothyroid children. Review of 128 cases. Am J Dis Child 81:233, 1951

84. **Man EB, Mermann AC, Cooke RE:** The development of children with congenital hypothyroidism. J Pediatr 63:926, 1963

85. **Klein AH, Meltzer S, Kenny FM:** Improved prognosis in congenital hypothyroidism treated before age 3 months. J Pediatr 81:912, 1972

86. **Riopel DA, Mullins CE:** Congenital thyrotoxicosis with paroxysmal atrial tachycardia. Pediatrics 50:140, 1972

87. **Farrehi C:** Accelerated maturity in fetal thyrotoxicosis. Clin Pediatr 7:134, 1968

88. **Hollingsworth DR, Mabry CC, Eckard JM:** Hereditary aspects of Graves' disease in infancy and childhood. J Pediatr 81:446, 1972

45

Eye Disorders in Neonates

David S. Friendly

A thorough discussion of the multitudinous ocular abnormalities that appear during the first 4 weeks of life is beyond the scope and purpose of this chapter. Rather, the author has elected to concentrate on those disorders that have particular importance because of high incidence, impairment of vision, and bearing on general health.

HISTORY AND EXAMINATION TECHNIQUES

The **history** obtained from parents may be of considerable importance when confronted with an infant with eye abnormalities. The existence of hereditary ocular disease should be explored in depth and, when indicated, should include examination of the parents and siblings. A prenatal history of maternal drug ingestion and of rubella or other illnesses may be highly significant. Whenever relevant, questions should be asked concerning the possibility of parental veneral disease. The birth history should include specifics pertaining to the likelihood of perinatal anoxia. The Apgar score should be noted as well as details concerning the administration of supplemental oxygen. The birth weight and gestational age of the patient may provide evidence of prematurity.

Helpful information regarding visual behav-ior often can be obtained from attendants in the nursery. The training, experience, and relative objectivity of nurses generally make their observations more reliable than those of family members.

The general medical findings may be essential in arriving at a specific and comprehensive diagnosis. Particular attention should be directed to the central nervous system. Because the optic vesicle and cup develop from the embryologic forebrain, malformations of the globe are associated with developmental defects of the brain.

Examination of the eyes of newborns may be conveniently divided into structural and functional components. Structural aspects of importance include the size of the eye, the size and clarity of the cornea, the transparency of the lens, and abnormalities of the uveal tract (iris, ciliary body, and choroid), vitreous, retina, and optic disc.

The size of the eye can be grossly estimated by inspection or by inspection coupled with palpation. There is a tendency to equate corneal diameter and eyeball diameter. This tendency should be consciously resisted because, while these two determinations generally correlate, they do not always have the same significance. Eyeball diameter may be precisely, simply, and safely measured with ultrasound equipment. Ultrasound is also a useful modality for exploring the interior of the eye in the presence of corneal and lenticular opacities as well as other conditions that interfere with visualization of the posterior segment of the eye.

Corneal diameter is generally measured with ruled calipers. The axial diameter of the human eye at term is about 17 mm; the corneal diameter is usually between 9.5 and 10.5 mm.

Functional ophthalmologic aspects of importance which can be tested during the newborn period include pupillary light responses, induced eye movements, ocular fixation, and tracking or following eye movements.

Pupillary responses to light are normally present even in premature infants. They should be elicited prior to mydriasis. A strong light— preferably that of the indirect ophthalmoscope—should be used, although a conventional flashlight is usually adequate. Pocket flashlights are generally not sufficiently powerful. Pupillary responses should be demonstrated several times to differentiate conclusively reflex responses to light from random changes in pupillary size. The presence of pupillary responses to light demonstrates intactness of pupillary afferent and efferent pathways, and, by inference, intactness of subcortical visual pathways. Blink responses to light in newborns are likewise indicative of subcortical visual function. Supranuclearly-induced horizontal ocular rotations can be stimulated by manual rotation of the head about the longitudinal axis of the body, or by rotational stimulation with the infant held facing the examiner. The former will produce doll's-head movements while the latter will produce deviation of the eyes toward the direction of rotation. Such simple maneuvers are helpful in identifying paretic ocular muscles early in life.

Ocular fixation of stationary objects and eye tracking of moving objects are present in some term newborns but are not generally well developed until 4 to 6 weeks. The absence of fixation or following at birth need not cause concern but their presence is reassuring. Using sophisticated optokinetic stimulation and electrooculographic recordings, visual acuities of 20/150 have been demonstrated during the first few days of life. For clinical purposes, a bright light or a human face are optimal test objects for eliciting fixation and following movements.

Examination of the lens, vitreous, and fundus is best deferred until after pupillary mydriasis has been obtained. Optimal mydriasis requires both anticholinergic and sympathetic drugs. Recommended agents are 0.5% cyclopentolate (Cyclogyl) and 2.5% phenylephrine (Neo-Synephrine). One drop of each should be instilled in each eye. Because the conjunctival recesses of the newborn can accommodate far less than a single drop of fluid, most of the medication will flow out of the eye. Excess fluid should be absorbed with tissues. If pupillary dilation is inadequate after 45 minutes, the above medications may be repeated. Bauer and coworkers report paralytic ileus and necrotizing enterocolitis following topical instillation of 6 drops of cyclopentolate in the eyes of newborns.[1] One death occurred. The authors recommend not using more than a total of 4 drops (2 drops in each eye) of the 0.5% solution. Darkly pigmented irides (such as those of most Blacks) require a second instillation of drops. Caution should be observed in repeating anticholinergic drops in lightly pigmented individuals because such patients are more likely to develop erythema, hyperthermia, and tachycardia. Ten percent phenylephrine should not be instilled in the eyes of premature infants. Its use in such infants has been reported to produce transient systemic hypertension.[2] The possibility of inducing angle closure glaucoma in infants is so remote as not to constitute a realistic danger. Atropine drops or ointment should never be used in infants for routine diagnostic purposes because of possible adverse reactions.

Opacities of the lens are best visualized by slit-lamp examination. Hand-held slit lamps which can readily be brought to the patient are presently commercially available. A bright light and plus lens magnification—such as is obtained with the indirect ophthalmoscope without the hand-held condensing lens—is a convenient although less precise diagnostic instrument. Another useful technique is to retroilluminate lenticular opacities by means of a retinoscope. The latter instrument is a readily available, diagnostic device generally used for objective estimation of refractive error.

Much information regarding the anterior segment of the eye may be obtained by simple inspection. There are four important principles to consider. First, in order to obtain maximum magnification, the examiner should reduce the

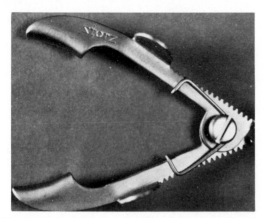

Fig. 45-1. Spring action, self-retaining infant eyelid speculum.

distance between his eyes and the eyes of the patient as much as possible. If the examiner is presbyopic, reading glasses should be worn. Second, the object must be well illuminated. A conventional type flashlight such as is used for transillumination of the head is adequate. Third, the object must be well exposed. This can be accomplished best by means of a small self-retaining speculum (Fig. 45-1), specifically designed to separate the eyelids of infants. A topical anesthetic such as 0.5% proparacaine hydrochloride (Ophthaine) should be instilled to anesthetize the cornea and dull conjuctival sensitivity prior to insertion of the speculum. If a speculum is employed, normal saline should be dropped on the cornea from time to time to maintain corneal transparency. If a speculum is not available, an assistant should be asked to separate the lids. A tissue placed between the fingers and the lid surfaces will ensure dryness and reduce slippage. In order to obtain maximal exposure, the lids should be grasped as close as possible to their margins. The assistant's fingers should actually touch the cilia of both the upper and lower lids. Gentle pressure must be applied to the globe in order to obtain adequate exposure. This pressure may blanch the optic disc by interfering with its circulation. The unwary may misinterpret this induced blanching as optic atrophy. Slight pallor of the discs is a normal finding in about one-third of newborns.[3] Fourth, the patient's eye must be centered and more or less immobile. Correct positioning may at times be difficult to attain particularly

in the presence of an active Bell's phenomenon (*i.e.,* the tendency of the anterior portion of the eye to roll upward toward the brow as the lids are forcibly separated against the contracting orbicularis oculi). It is frequently helpful to feed the baby during this and other portions of the examination or to place a pacifier in the baby's mouth.

The fundi are best visualized after mydriasis by indirect ophthalmoscopy (Fig. 45-2). Familiarity with the indirect ophthalmoscope is unfortunately not widespread outside the specialty of ophthalmology. The instrument has the disadvantage of producing an inverted as well as reversed image. For screening purposes, however, this inconvenient feature is of little importance. The instrument is far superior to the conventional direct ophthalmoscope because it provides a panoramic stereoscopic view. Opacities of the media do not significantly interfere with fundus visualization unless they are dense and extensive. As with handling any other unfamiliar instrument, a certain amount of practice is required until

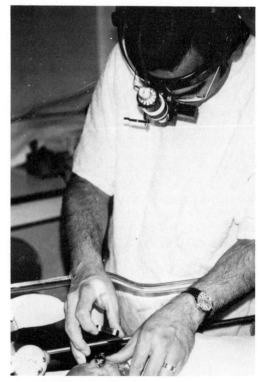

Fig. 45-2. Indirect ophthalmoscopy in the nursery.

proficiency is obtained. The effort is well worth making.

The infant's eyes are closed much of the time after birth. When open, a moderate divergence is generally noted. The eyes do not move together in a smooth, well-coordinated (conjugate) manner immediately after birth. In this sense, all newborns may be thought of as having strabismus during the first several weeks of life.[4] Definitive diagnosis of nonparalytic (concomitant) strabismus is rarely possible before the third month. For this reason, this subject has little importance in neonatal pediatric ophthalmology.

OPHTHALMIA NEONATORUM (CONJUNCTIVITIS) (See also Chap. 32)

Conjunctivitis is one of the most frequently encountered problems in the newborn. Although a vast number of microorganisms are capable of producing such infections, for practical purposes the list of most likely causes can be narrowed to silver nitrate drops, staphylococci, inclusion conjunctivitis agents, and gonococci. Although gonorrheal ophthalmia is far less prevalent than the other types, it alone is capable of producing damage sufficient to interfere with vision. In the United States and elsewhere, an epidemic of gonorrhea is being experienced. Indeed, it has been said to be the most common contagious disease next to the common cold. An upsurge in the incidence of gonorrheal ophthalmia neonatorum is therefore to be expected and actually appears to be occurring.[5]

Antibiotics have radically altered the prognosis in the presence of established disease. From 1906 to 1911, 24% of children admitted to American schools for the blind had visual disability secondary to ophthalmia neonatorum. During 1958 to 1959, only 0.3% of these children were sightless because of this disease. The rarity of serious complications in proven cases of gonococcal conjunctivitis in newborn infants has been documented.[6] However, in view of rising incidence rates of the venereal form of the disease and the development of penicillin resistance, complacency toward this potentially blinding disease must not be allowed to develop.

At the present time, all 50 of the United States require some form of prophylaxis; 22 of them specify that silver nitrate alone must be used. There is little question that silver nitrate prophylaxis is imperfect. Yet there is good evidence that its use has materially reduced the incidence of gonorrheal ophthalmia neonatorum. Until a well-controlled, parallel double-blind study is reported, there seems little to be gained by abandoning silver nitrate in favor of other chemotherapeutic agents or antibiotics with possibly superior or possibly inferior therapeutic indices.

Although there is no lack of papers extolling the relative virtues of particular prophylactic agents, very little has been written recently about techniques of instillation. It must be emphasized that no topically applied drug, however potent, will have the slightest effect unless it comes into contact with the pathogenic organisms. Faulty technique is undoubtedly widespread and probably accounts for at least as many cases of gonorrheal ophthalmia neonatorum as does drug failure.

Laboratory procedures are essential for etiologic diagnosis of conjunctivitis. With the exception of silver nitrate conjunctivitis, which invariably begins within 24 hours after prophylaxis, incubation periods are of little practical use in differential diagnosis. The clinical appearance of the eye (Fig. 45-3) and the discharge from the eye are likewise nonspecific.

A gram stain of the discharge is sufficient to make a presumptive diagnosis of staphylococcal or gonococcal infection. Giemsa stains of scrapings from the conjunctiva of the lower lid may be used to demonstrate the basophilic paranuclear cytoplasmic inclusions characteristic of inclusion conjunctivitis. Specific fluorescein antibody techniques are presently available for demonstrating the etiologic agents of both inclusion conjunctivitis and gonorrheal conjunctivitis. However, immunofluorescent staining and interpretation are technically difficult.

If the initial gram stain fails to demonstrate gram-negative diplococci, 30% sulfacetamide drops may be prescribed for 2 or 3 weeks on the assumption that the infection is the result of inclusion conjunctivitis agents or to bacterial organisms other than the gonococcus. If symptoms continue or become more pronounced while on this regimen, bacteriologic cultures should be repeated.

If the initial gram stain demonstrates gram-negative diplococci, cultures should be obtained on the selective medium of Thayer–

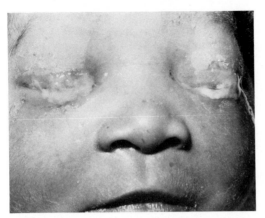

Fig. 45-3. Gonorrheal ophthalmia neonatorum.

Martin, as well as on conventional media. The patient should be admitted to the isolation unit of the hospital for a 2- or 3-day course of treatment with systemic aqueous penicillin G. A dose of 30,000 units/kg should be given every 12 hours. The eyes should be periodically irrigated with normal saline solution and if the cornea is involved, atropine 0.5% drops should be instilled once or twice a day. Ophthalmologic consultation is recommended. A serologic test for syphilis is advisable. The case should be reported to the local public health authority for biostatistical purposes and for assistance in bringing the parents to treatment.

A response of gonorrheal ophthalmia neonatorum to treatment with systemic aqueous penicillin G should be evident within 24 to 48 hours. If, after 2 days of therapy, the erythema, edema, and discharge have not subsided, additional cultures and conjunctival scrapings should be obtained.

Obstructed tear ducts may cause discharging eyes during the first month of life. Because the obstruction is usually at the distal end of the nasolacrimal duct, where it empties into the nose at the inferior meatus, digital pressure on the nasolacrimal sac usually produces a reflux of purulent material through the lacrimal puncta which are located on the upper and lower lid margins near the inner canthus. Infants with obstructed nasolacrimal excretory passages have recurrent episodes of conjunctivitis and constant tearing; usually, only one eye is involved. Occasionally, a tear sac will become obstructed superiorly as well as inferiorly. This will lead to distention (Fig. 45-4)

and possibly to spontaneous rupture of the sac. At other times an obstructed nasolacrimal sac will become distended by clear fluid, forming a mucocele.

Patients with purulent dacryocystitis or mucoceles should be seen by ophthalmologists without delay. Infants without gross infection or distention of the lacrimal sac may be treated conservatively with topical antibiotics and massage of the sac. The duct frequently opens spontaneously in such cases. If symptoms persist beyond 6 to 9 months, a probing of the nasolacrimal outflow passages by a qualified specialist is indicated. This is best performed under general anesthesia and is successful in about 80% of cases.

CATARACTS

The causes of cataracts in infants and children are legion. A tabulation in 1969 listed 50 known causes and associations.[7] A survey of 386 cases reported finding ''etiologic factors'' in about two-thirds of all cases.[8] Details are given in Table 45-1. It is significant that the birth weight was below 2500 g in 52% of the patients with CNS damage and in 22% of the cases for which a cause could not be established. The mechanisms whereby perinatal hypoxia and low birth weight contribute to the incidence of infantile cataracts is unknown. Hypoglycemia may play a role in some cases. It is of interest that cataracts associated with neurologic abnormalities and prematurity, as well as rubella cataracts, may develop postnatally.

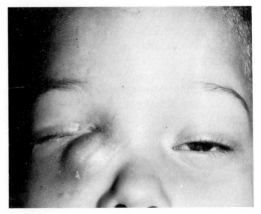

Fig. 45-4. Acute dacryocystitis with enlargement of the right nasolacrimal sac.

Table 45-1. Etiology of Infantile Cataracts (386 Cases).

	Number	**Percent**
Hereditary	32	8.3
(Other family members affected)		
Congenital rubella syndrome	74	19.1
Systemic disease	46	11.9
(Down syndrome, multiple congenital malformations, Lowe syndrome, galactosemia, and so on)		
Other ocular disease	23	6.0
(Excluding microphthalmus)		
Central nervous system disorders	88	22.8
(Mental retardation, convulsions, paraplegia, hemiplegia and cerebral palsy)		
Unknown	123	31.9

(Based on Table 1 of Merin S, Crawford JS: Can J Ophthalmol 6:178, 1971)[8]

In galactosemia, cataracts may appear as early as 7 days after birth. The most characteristic type of lens opacity resembles an oil droplet. These cataracts are always bilateral and are observed in approximately 75% of affected patients. The classic disease is caused by deficiency of the transferase enzyme which, in the presence of uridine diphosphoglucose, converts galactose-1-phosphate to glucose-1-phosphate. Cataracts of a similar type may occur within 5 months of birth in galactokinase deficiency. Galactokinase deficiency results in an inability to phosphorylate galactose. This disorder, like galactose transferase deficiency, is inherited as an autosomal recessive trait. Urinary reducing substances by Clinitest but not with glucose-oxidase testing strips are present in both disorders. Systemic abnormalities are present in transferase deficiency but—with the possible exception of mental retardation—not in galactokinase deficiency. Prompt diagnosis is of the utmost importance, because in both disorders early dietary restriction of galactose (the major source of which is the lactose of milk) can prevent cataracts from developing and can also cause regression of established cataracts.

Transient bilateral cataracts of obscure etiology have recently been described in premature infants.[9] Of 513 prematures examined for possible retrolental fibroplasia, transient cataracts were noted in 19.[10] These cataracts were clearly related only to gestational age and birth weight. The cataracts were not invariably present at the time of initial examination. Symmetrical fluid vacuoles were noted in the region of the posterior lens sutures. At times, these cataracts were sufficiently dense to obscure fundus details. Complete spontaneous clearing invariably occurred over a periods of several weeks.

The principal difficulty in rehabilitating eyes with severe congenital monocular cataracts is the presence of a particularly pernicious form of amblyopia. Experimental work in monocularly deprived kittens suggests that irreversible anatomic changes at the level of the lateral geniculate body and neurophysiologic alterations in striate cortical synapses occur very early in life and are responsible for the poor postreatment prognoses of individuals with congenital monocular cataracts.[11,12] Patients with congenital bilateral symmetrical cataracts may fare better, presumably because of less severe or absent competitive interaction between the neural pathways from the two eyes, resulting in less severe amblyopia.

INFANTILE GLAUCOMA

Glaucoma in infants may be primary or secondary. The primary or idiopathic variety has generally been thought to be caused by autosomal recessive inheritance with incom-

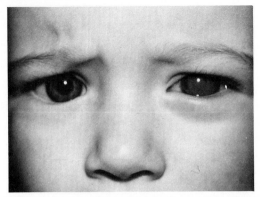

Fig. 45-5. Unilateral congenital glaucoma in an 11-months-old infant. Note the enlargement and the cloudiness of the left cornea.

plete penetrance. This time-honored concept has recently been challenged.[13] and a multi-factorial genetic basis has been proposed. The secondary forms of infantile glaucoma are associated with other anomalies or disorders of the eye and of the body generally and, with a single exception, will not be considered in this discussion.

The incidence of primary infantile (or less accurately, congenital) glaucoma is said to be approximately 1 in 12,500 births. The low incidence of the disease, combined with the high incidence of obstructed nasolacrimal ducts in the same age group, make for a high proportion of misdiagnoses and late referrals. In both conditions, tearing may be the chief complaint. Neonates with glaucoma, however, have light sensitivity and blepharospasm in addition to tearing. All infants with tearing should have careful corneal examinations. The hallmark of infantile glaucoma is corneal cloudiness (Fig. 45-5), occurring as a result of the passage of intraocular fluid, which is under abnormally high pressure, into the corneal stroma. Breaks in Descemet's membrane occur as the cornea stretches and increases in size in response to the raised intraocular pressure. The entire eye may eventually share in the enlargement, producing buphthalmos.

Approximately 70% of the optic discs of normal newborns show some degree of cupping.[3] This is nearly always symmetrical. Assymetric and extensive cupping of the optic discs is a relatively early sign of infantile glaucoma. Such findings should suggest the possibility of this diagnosis.

There is a slight but definite tendency for the disorder to occur preferentially in males. For reasons equally obscure, approximately 25% of cases are monocular.

Immediate recognition and early referral are critically important. In late cases, irreversible damage to the angle region (where aqueous humor egresses from the eye) makes control of pressure difficult. Corneal scarring and retinal and optic nerve damage are largely preventable by prompt surgery.

The prognosis is related to the patient's age at the onset of corneal opacification. The earlier the corneal edema becomes apparent, the poorer the prognosis is for vision.

The treatment of infantile glaucoma is surgical. Attempts at long-term control by medications are inadvisable, except in instances in which surgery cannot be performed or is only partially successful. Although new operations are presently being introduced (such as trabeculotomy), goniotomy is still generally recognized as the operation of choice. The raised intraocular pressure can be brought under control by this procedure in approximately 80% of cases. The success rate in terms of vision, however, is not nearly as favorable, primarily because of unrecognized or treatment-resistant amblyopia secondary to unequal refractive errors. Poor vision can also result from corneal scarring and irregular astigmatism.[14]

The glaucoma which is occasionally seen in infants with the rubella syndrome is an exact phenocopy of primary infantile glaucoma. The diagnosis may be made on the basis of associated findings and serologic tests. Only very rarely do patients with the rubella syndrome have both cataracts and glaucoma.

Megalocornea is an inherited binocular condition largely confined to males. Affected eyes are asymptomatic and are normal except for an enlarged anterior segment. The corneas, although enlarged, are clear and do not have breaks in Descemet's membrane.

Prolonged labor, anatomic crowding during delivery and, in particular, the application of obstetric forceps to an eye during birth may cause ruptures of Descemet's membrane and corneal edema. The intraocular pressure of such traumatized eyes is low and there is no corneal enlargement. Patients with perinatal corneal injuries may develop myopia, amblyopia, and strabismus. Some of these patients develop bullous keratopathy in adult life.[15]

RETROLENTAL FIBROPLASIA

The term **retrolental fibroplasia** (RLF) was introduced in 1942 by Terry who first described the condition.[16] He believed that the essential disturbance was an overgrowth of embryonic connective tissue behind the lens. Heath in 1951 introduced the term **retinopathy of prematurity.**[17] This term more accurately identifies the site of the initial pathologic processes but has not achieved widespread acceptance.

Historical Aspects and Incidence

In the early 1950s a number of investigators suggested that excess oxygen was causally associated with RLF. Three controlled nursery studies published in 1951, 1954, and 1955 convincingly demonstrated the toxic effects of excess oxygen on the retinal vessels of premature infants.[18-20] Production of the condition in experimental newborn animals raised with supplemental oxygen provided further confirmation of the detrimental effect of hyperoxia on growing retinal vessels.

The "epidemic" of RLF which occurred in the 1940s and early 1950s in association with the unrestricted use of oxygen was followed by a period of low incidence during which supplemented oxygen was markedly curtailed. More recent studies have shown that the restricted use of oxygen resulted in an increase in mortality[21] and in cerebral palsy.[22] As a result, oxygen is now being used more liberally; but unlike the period following World War II, it is being used more selectively. An upsurge in the incidence of RLF may nevertheless occur as a result of this most recent swing of the therapeutic pendulum.

The incidence of RLF is inversely proportional to birth weight. In one study, retinal vessel changes in premature infants receiving oxygen occurred in 6 of 17 infants (35%) below 1500 g, while such changes occurred in only 10 of 58 infants (17%) over 1500 g.[23] In a retrospective survey, Silverman found that 82% of all cases of RLF occurred in infants under 1500 g birth weight.[24] For reasons unknown, infants of multiple births are more likely to develop cicatricial RLF than are singleton infants of the same gestational age and weight.[20]

In 1970, Tasman found the overall incidence of cicatricial RLF to be 0.9% in 995 live births.[25] This investigator showed, by citing his own experience as well as the recorded experience of others, that very few cases of RLF develop in infants over 5 pounds (2268 g) at birth but that

all gradations of severity . . . may be found no matter what the premature weighs at birth and no matter what the gestational age.

The history of oxygen therapy and retrolental fibroplasia has been recently reviewed.[26]

Pathophysiology

In a series of animal experiments, Ashton and coworkers have shown that excess oxygen produces a vasoconstriction of immature retinal vessels.[27-30] This vasoconstriction, which is reversible in its early stages, occurs first in the terminal arterioles and in the arteriolar side of the capillary tree. It is followed by an irreversible vasoobliteration, at which stage the vessel walls are adherent and show degenerative changes. Cytopathic effects are first noted in the endothelium of immature retinal capillaries. Vasoproliferation typically occurs following normalization of oxygen tension. The severity of the vasoobliteration is directly proportional to the duration and concentration of excess oxygen and to the degree of immaturity of the retinal vascular system. The toxic effects of oxygen can be prevented in kittens by intermittent air breathing. Thus, kittens alternately receiving 1-hour periods of 80% to 90% ambient oxygen and normal air showed no evidence of vaso-obliteration.

Completely vascularized retinas of animals and humans are immune to the toxic effects of oxygen. The occasional case of RLF in a full-term infant is probably best explained by the fact that the human retina is incompletely vascularized at term.[31] Intrauterine hypoxia may be the basis for the rare development of RLF in infants who do not receive supplemental oxygen. It is hypothesized that, in such infants, the abnormally great postnatal increase in blood oxygen tension is sufficient to produce vasoobliteration. This theory is, however, entirely speculative and it should be

Table 45-2. Classification of Retrolental Fibroplasia.

Stage	Active Phase Fundus changes
O	Severe constriction of retinal vessels
I	Dilation and tortuosity of retinal vessels with peripheral neovascularization
II	Neovascularization with retinal hemorrhages; increased vitreous haziness
III	Proliferation into vitreous; localized peripheral retinal detachment
IV	One half retina detached
V	Entire retina detached

Grade	Cicatrical Phase Fundus changes
I	Small areas of retinal pigment irregularities; small scars in retinal periphery
II	Disc distortion
III	Retinal fold
IV	Incomplete retrolental mass; partial retinal detachment
V	Complete retrolental mass; total retinal detachment

(Classification of Reese, Owens, and King, modified by Patz)[33,34]

recognized that there are important unknown factors in the development of proliferative retinopathy in newborns.[32]

The disorder usually makes its appearance between 10 days and 1 month after birth. Bilateral involvement is nearly invariable but pathologic changes are frequently asymmetrical. The active phase generally subsides in a few months and in mild cases is frequently followed by spontaneous regression. The completeness of the regression varies directly with the severity of the morphologic derangement during the active stages.

The Reese, Owens, and King classification of RLF as modified by Patz is given in Table 45-2.[33,34] Patz introduced the concept of pre-retrolental dibroplasia or stage O to describe the stage during hyperoxygenation when retinal vessels show severe constriction. Stages I through V describe the events that may take place following removal from excess oxygen.

Flynn and coworkers have identified, by means of fluorescein angiography, a function-

ing arteriovenous shunt located between avascular and vascularized retina.[35] The shunt is virtually always present in the temporal fundus but, in severe cases, may extend circumferentially. Neovascularization develops from vessels posterior to the shunt. In mild cases of RLF, vasoproliferation occurs only in the retinal periphery, but in severe cases, the entire retina will undergo neovascularization. Early changes occur predominantly in the temporal periphery, presumably because this area is the last to become vascularized.

Newly formed vessels are strikingly abnormal. They tend to leak blood and plasma. Organization of hemorrhages and exudates leads to the formation of retinal and vitreous membranes and retinal detachments. Cicatricial changes start to develop at approximately 6 months after birth. Temporal traction of the vessels as they leave the disc is commonly noted (Fig. 45-6). The proliferation of retrolental fibrous tissue produces leukokoria (abnormal pupillary reflex; (Fig. 45-7) and visible ciliary processes that become elongated by traction.

In more severe cases, peripheral anterior synechiae and angle closure by forward movement of the lens iris diaphragm result in glaucoma. Such eyes are usually blind but may be preserved by lens aspiration and iridectomy. The most severely affected eyes become microphthalmic, soft, atrophic, and eventually phthisical.

Long-term Effects

Myopia is present in a great preponderance of eyes with cicatrical RLF. At times corrected central acuity may be poor because of foveal damage that may not always be readily apparent on ophthalmoscopy. Temporal displacement of the macula in cicatricial RLF may give the false impression of exotropia (pseudoexotropia).

All eyes with cicatrical RLF are susceptible to late retinal detachment. Detachments are most frequently discovered in the first and second decades of life but may occur at any age. There is a direct relationship between the degree of myopia and the incidence of retinal detachment.

Detection and Prevention

Although vasoconstriction is the earliest adverse effect of oxygen on developing retinal

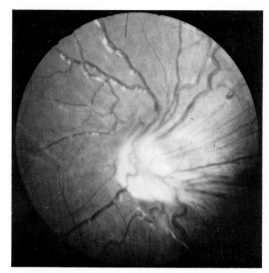

Fig. 45-6. Temporal traction of vessels from the optic disc in the left eye of an 8-month-old infant with grade II cicatricial retrolental fibroplasia.

vessels, attempts to detect this narrowing ophthalmoscopically have been unrewarding.[36] The presence of vitreous haziness in low-birth-weight infants may interfere with visualization of the retinal vessels even when the indirect ophthalmoscope is used. Persistence of the hyaloid system and the tunica vasculosa lentis may be the cause of this vitreous haze. The degree of opacification varies inversely with the birth weight. There is also a poor correlation between arterial P_{O_2} levels and retinal vessel caliber. Therefore, daily monitoring of the fundi would seem to have little practical value in assessing the oxygen tension of arterial blood.

RLF is quite rare although not unknown in the presence of cyanosis.[37] However, the risk cannot be estimated by inspection alone once the skin color has become pink. At normal hemoglobin levels, cyanosis is observed when hemoglobin is between 75% and 85% saturated with oxygen, which for fetal hemoglobin corresponds to oxygen tensions of 32 to 42 torr. This does not mean that supplemental oxygen should be withheld until cyanosis appears. The respiratory distress syndrome is by far the most common condition for which supplemental oxygen is given to newborns. It is highly desirable to monitor the arterial P_{O_2} levels of such infants. This is particularly important after the infant's cardiopulmonary system has

begun to improve. It is after recovery from the respiratory distress syndrome that arterial P_{O_2} levels are likely to reach retinotoxic levels if supplemental oxygen is not curtailed.

The safe upper level of retinal artery P_{O_2} is unknown. However, when possible, it is desirable to keep umbilical artery P_{O_2} levels below 100 torr. Unfortunately, maintenance below this level will not invariably prevent development of RLF. Susceptibility to oxygen is known to depend on multiplicity of birth, degree of immaturity, duration of oxygen exposure, and the level of arterial oxygen tension.

Newborns receiving oxygen should be ophthalmologically examined prior to discharge from the nursery. Indirect ophthalmoscopy with maximum pupillary mydriasis is mandatory. Attention should be primarily directed to the temporal retinal periphery. If no abnormalities are noted, it is wise to repeat the examination in the office at 5 or 6 months of age. A satisfactory negative examination at this age practically eliminates the presence of the disease or the possibility of its future development. If abnormalities are noted at any age, subsequent ophthalmologic examinations must be planned according to the extent and severity of the changes and the rate of progression.

Treatment

Indications for treatment during the active stages are not definitely established. In the presence of progressive vasoproliferation and

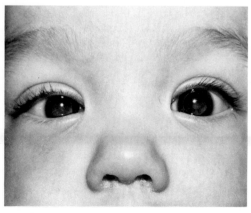

Fig. 45-7. Grade V retrolental fibroplasia in both eyes of a 7-month-old infant.

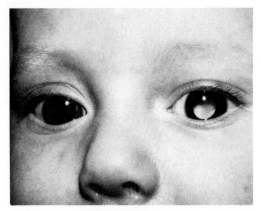

Fig. 45-8. This 2-month-old infant presented with leukokoria caused by retinoblastoma of the left eye but had bilateral disease. The left eye was more severely involved and was enucleated. The right eye was successfully treated with radiation.

vitreous hemorrhages,[38] argon laser photocoagulation, or cryotherapy should be considered. While treatment in carefully selected cases appears at times to be effective, the long-term sequelae of intervention during the active stages remain unknown.

It is essential that patients with significant cicatricial disease receive periodic fundus evaluations by ophthalmologists because of the possibility of late retinal detachment. This recommendation is particularly important in view of the favorable results of surgery for late retinal detachments associated with RLF.

RETINOBLASTOMA

The incidence of retinoblastoma is presently approximately 1 in 20,000 births and appears to be increasing. The diagnosis is only rarely made in the neonatal period except when examining siblings and progeny of affected individuals. The condition generally becomes manifest during infancy and is most frequently recognized between 17 and 18 months of life.[39] The mortality in the United States is approximately 25%. If untreated, the mortality is nearly 100%.

The presenting signs are leukokoria (abnormal pupillary reflex) in about 60% (Fig. 45-8) and strabismus in about 20 percent of cases. Approximately one-third of patients have bilateral involvement.

The disease occurs in both familial and sporadic forms. The familial form (defined as such whenever there is at least one other affected family member) is only one-tenth as common as the sporadic form. The familial form is dominantly inherited and is more likely to be bilateral.

According to Knudson, retinoblastoma requires two mutational events (two-hit theory).[40] In the dominantly inherited form, one mutation is inherited (prezygotic), while the second occurs in the somatic cells (postzygotic). In the sporadic form of the disease, both events occur postzygotically. Tumors arising from multiple origins (*e.g.*, bilateral disease) signify the presence of the hereditary form.

In a relatively small proportion of retinoblastoma patients, a deletion on the long arm of chromosome 13 has been found.[41] Clinical findings in these 13q− patients have included mental retardation, microcephaly, hypertelorism, absence or hypoplasia of the thumb, short fingers, pelvic girdle anomalies, and anogenital malformations. Eye findings have included microphthalmos and colobomata.

Patients with the hereditary form of the disease (including all bilaterally affected patients) have a tendency to develop other malignancies later in life,[42] the most common of which is osteogenic sarcoma.

Because cure rates vary according to the size and multiplicity of the tumors, it is vital that all patients with a history or physical findings indicating an abnormal pupillary reflex (cat's-eye reflex) be referred to competent specialists as early in life as possible. In favorable cases, cure rates approach 100%. X-ray therapy and chemotherapy are the mainstays of conservative management. In unilateral cases, enucleation is generally performed.

Because progeny and siblings of retinoblastoma patients may be affected, it is most important to examine thoroughly the retinas of all such persons shortly after birth. Thorough examination of suspected and high-risk cases requires indirect ophthalmoscopy with careful visualization of the entire retina of both eyes. Such examinations can be satisfactorily performed only under general anesthesia.

ANIRIDIA

In 1964, Miller and associates found in a retrospective study that of 440 children with

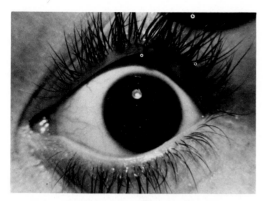

Fig. 45-9. Aniridia in the left eye of a child. Note that iris tissue is only visible in the superior nasal quadrant.

Wilms' tumor, 6 had aniridia (Fig. 45-9).[43] This rate of 1 in 73 is much higher than the expected rate of aniridia in the general population, which is about 1 in 50,000 births. Mental retardation, hypospadias, undescended testicles, and congenital hemihypertrophy were also found to have a higher than expected incidence in patients with Wilms' tumor. In 1968, Fraumeni and Glass found seven cases of Wilms' tumor among 28 children hospitalized with aniridia.[44] In several patients with the triad of aniridia, ambiguous genitalia, and mental retardation, an interstitial deletion of the short arm of chromosome 11 has been reported.[45] Hence, patients with aniridia and other congenital abnormalities should receive high-quality chromosomal banding analysis.

Aniridia occurs in both familial and sporadic forms. The familial form is somewhat more common. With a single possible exception, all patients with both Wilms' tumor and aniridia reported to date have been sporadic.

The implication of the association of Wilm's tumor with aniridia is obvious. All infants with rudimentary or apparently absent irides without a positive family history of aniridia should be followed with periodic physical examinations, urinalyses, renal scans, and ultrasonograms until at least 3 years of age.

TOXOPLASMOSIS

Human toxoplasmosis is primarily acquired by the handling and consumption of raw and undercooked meat and by contact with feces from infected cats. Desmonts found that of infants born to mothers who acquired the disease during pregnancy, only 11% were overtly affected.[46]

The clinical manifestations of congenital toxoplasmosis vary widely. In severely affected infants, chorioretinitis, microphthalmos, hydrocephalus, jaundice, hepatosplenomegaly, anemia, fever, and failure to thrive may be observed. As in other congenital infections, low birth weight and prematurity are common. Occasionally, microcephaly, meningoencephalitis, convulsions, and a maculopapular rash are present. In some cases, only the retinas are affected. Retinal lesions may not appear, however, for days or even weeks after birth.

The most constant feature is a chorioretinitis or more properly a retinochoroiditis because the organisms lodge in the retina, producing a primary necrotizing retinitis with secondary choroidal involvement. The foveas are a favored location. There may be one or multiple foci in each fundus. The retinal lesions, when first observed, are usually bilateral and sharply outlined. They are generally quiescent, consisting of flat scars with pigmented borders (Fig. 45-10). The vitreous is usually clear. X-rays may reveal diffuse intracranial calcifications. Specific hemagglutination antibody titers and Sabin and Feldman dye titers will be raised in both mother and infant. Elevated assays for immunoglobin M (IgM) antibodies

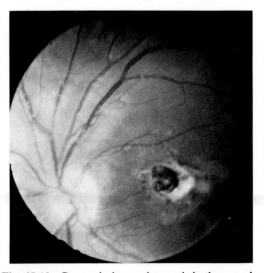

Fig. 45-10. Congenital toxoplasmosis in the macular region of the left eye of a child.

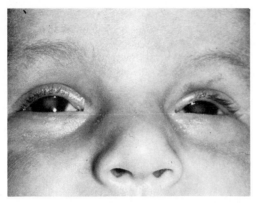

Fig. 45-11. Rubella cataracts in a 7-week-old infant.

in the infant are particularly significant because maternal IgM does not cross the normal placenta.

Treatment of active toxoplasmosis is not very satisfactory. Administration of pyrimethamine (Daraprim), sulfadiazine, steroids, and folinic acid does not result in dramatic improvement. Furthermore, steroids to a moderate extent and pyrimethamine to a marked extent are dangerous drugs with serious side effects (see Chap. 33).

Reactivation of congenital lesions may occur at any time throughout life. Late rupture of cysts situated at the pigmented margins of the retinal scars liberates viable organisms that produce characteristic satellite lesions. It is probable that the majority of adult cases of ocular toxoplasmosis infection represents relapses of congenital disease.

CYTOMEGALOVIRUS DISEASE (CMV)

Transplacental infection of the fetus with CMV virus results in clinical manifestations that vary from death to asymptomatic involvement. Hepatosplenomegaly is the most common physical finding. The lung, hematopoetic system, and the brain may be affected producing pneumonitis, thrombocytopenia, and encephalitis with calcifications that are characteristically but not invariably periventricular in distribution. Approximately 25% of infants with severe neonatal CMV have retinochoroiditis.[47,48] Most infected infants are asymptomatic.[49]

The retinal lesions are usually described as similar to those of toxoplasmosis but tend to

be less pigmented and more peripheral in location. They may not become manifest until some time after birth.

Diagnosis can be made on the basis of serologic tests including elevated IgM levels, virus culture and the finding of enlarged cells with intranuclear and, less frequently, intracytoplasmic inclusions in freshly prepared urinary sediment.

At the time of writing, there is no effective treatment for the disease (see Chap. 33).

RUBELLA SYNDROME

Sir Norman Gregg in 1941 first described the rubella syndrome.[50] The virus was not isolated, however, until 1962. Today, congenital rubella is recognized as a major cause of serious eye malformations including retinopathy, glaucoma, cataract, microphthalmos, and anterior uveitis.

The classic syndrome, as originally described, consists of the triad of eye, ear, and heart defects. Involvement of other organ systems is now recognized. Microcephaly, encephalitis, hepatosplenomegaly, jaundice, anemia, thrombocytopenia, skin, and bone abnormalities are not uncommon manifestations of congenital infection. Infants with the syndrome tend to have low birth weights, fail to thrive, and have a high incidence of mental retardation (see Chap. 33).

An atypical retinitis pigmentosa-like retinopathy is frequently noted. Diffuse or localized pigment epithelium hypertrophy and atrophy are present giving rise to a "salt-and-pepper" configuration. The retinopathy is not progressive and is not associated with significant visual loss. It may be either unilateral or bilateral.

The glaucoma which occurs in the rubella syndrome has been previously discussed.

Cataracts, the most common clinical ocular finding in the rubella syndrome, are usually (but not invariably) bilateral and have a characteristic morphology. A dense white opaque nucleus is seen centrally with gradually decreasing opacification toward the periphery of the lens (Fig. 45-11). Involved eyes are usually microphthalmic and have an anterior uveitis which results in variable degrees of iris atrophy and poor pupillary dilation with topical medications.

Treatment of rubella cataracts is similar to

treatment of other types of congenital cataracts. Surgical discission and aspiration of the lens is the procedure of choice. An iridectomy should be done at the time of cataract surgery to prevent postoperative glaucoma from pupillary blockage of aqueous humor flow. It is important to obtain and retain pupillary dilation for several months after surgery by means of topical medications. Surgery for rubella cataracts can be safely performed in early infancy.[51] Delay for ocular reasons beyond 6 months is unnecessary according to most authorities despite the fact that virus has been isolated from lenses of congenital rubella patients up to 35 months old. In order to obtain functional visual results, it is necessary for surgery be performed as promptly as possible and that contact lenses be fitted early in the postoperative period.

RETINAL DANGERS ASSOCIATED WITH PHOTOTHERAPY FOR HYPERBILIRUBINEMIA

Phototherapy for hyperbilirubinemia has become increasingly popular since it was introduced in England in 1958 by Cremer and coworkers.[52] Light, obtained from ordinary fluorescent bulbs, is used to photooxidize bilirubin in the skin and subcutaneous tissues, thereby reducing the required number of exchange transfusions.

Noell in 1966 and Kuwabara in 1968 exposed rats to 750 foot-candles of illumination from ordinary fluorescent lights for periods of time ranging from one hour to several weeks.[53,54] Damage to the outer retinal layers was observed. Sisson in 1970 exposed newborn piglets to 300 foot-candles of illumination for periods of time ranging from 12 to 72 hours.[55] Irreversible changes in the outer retinal layers were demonstrated.

Commercial phototherapy units for hyperbilirubinemia produce approximately 300 foot-candles of illumination in the incubator.[56] In view of the above-cited animal experiments, it would appear to be necessary to shield the eyes of infants receiving phototherapy. This may be accomplished by an opaque mask secured by an elastic strap or by eye pads held in place by adhesive tape. Both eyes should be completely occluded. Incomplete occlusion of one eye is undesirable not only because of the retinotoxic effects of intense light but also for reasons related to animal experiments.

Hubel and Wiesel have shown in kittens that monocular occlusion for merely a few days during the fourth or fifth weeks of life (period of maximum sensitivity to unilateral occlusion in kittens) results in permanent amblyopia.[57]

The effects of monocular occlusion observed in kittens is also potentially applicable to newborns with unilateral cataracts, ptosis, or lid tumors which are sufficiently severe to occlude the pupillary aperture. Strenuous efforts should be made to eliminate the monocular occlusion at a very early age in such cases.

REFERENCES

1. **Bauer CR, Trottier MC, Stern L:** Systemic cyclopentolate (Cyclogyl) toxicity in the newborn infant. J Pediatr 82:501, 1973
2. **Borromeo-McGrail V, Bordiuk JM, Keitel H:** Systemic hypertension following ocular administration of 10% Phenylephrine in the neonate. Pediatrics 51:1032, 1973
3. **Khodadoust AA, Ziai M, Briggs SI:** Optic disc in normal newborns. Am J Ophthalmol 66:502, 1968
4. **Dayton GO, Jones MH, Aiu P, Rawson RA, Steele B, Rose M:** Developmental study of coordinated eye movement in the human infant. Arch Ophthalmol 71:865, 1964
5. **Snowe RJ, Wilfer CM:** Epidemic reappearance of gonococcal ophthalmia neonatorum. Pediatrics 51:110, 1973
6. **Friendly, DS:** Gonorrheal ophthalmia, reappearance of an old problem. Trans Am Acad Ophthalmol Otolaryngol 74:975, 1970
7. **Scheie HG, Albert DM:** Adler's Textbook of Ophthalmology, 8th ed, p 123. Philadelphia, W.B. Saunders, 1969
8. **Merin S, Crawford JS:** The etiology of congenital cataracts. Can J Ophthalmol 6:178, 1971
9. **McCormick AQ:** Transient cataracts in premature infants. A new clinical entity. Can J Ophthalmol 3:202, 1968
10. **Alden ER, Kalina RE, Hodson A:** Transient cataracts in low-birth-weight infants. J Pediatr 82:314, 1973
11. **Wiesel TN, Hubel DH:** Effects of visual deprivation on morphology and physiology of cells in the cat's lateral geniculate body. J Neurophysiol 26:978, 1963
12. **Wiesel TM, Hubel DH:** Single-cell responses in striate cortex of kittens deprived of vision in one eye. J Neurophysiol 26:1003, 1963
13. **Merin S, Morin D:** Heredity of congenital glaucoma. Br J Ophthalmol 56:414, 1972
14. **Shaffer RN, Weiss DI:** Congenital and pediatric glaucomas. CV Mosby, St. Louis, 1970

15. **Sugar HS, Airala MA:** Birth injuries of the cornea. J Pediatr Ophthalmol 8:26, 1971

16. **Terry TL:** Extreme prematurity and fibroblastic overgrowth of persistent vascular sheath behind each crystalline lens. I. Preliminary report. Am J Ophthalmol 25:203, 1942

17. **Heath P:** Pathology of the retinopathy of prematurity; retrolental fibroplasia. Am J Ophthalmol 34:1249, 1951

18. **Patz A, Hoeck LE, DeLaCruz E:** Studies on the effect of high oxygen administration in retrolental fibroplasia. I. Nursery observations. Am J Ophthalmol 35:1248, 1952

19. **Lanman JT, Guy LP, Dancis J:** Retrolental fibroplasia and oxygen therapy. JAMA 155:223, 1954

20. **Kinsey VE, Hemphill FM:** Etiology of retrolental fibroplasia, and preliminary report of a cooperative study of retrolental fibroplasia. Trans Am Acad Ophthalmol Otolaryngol 59:15, 1955

21. **Avery ME, Oppenheimer EH:** Recent increase in mortality from hyaline membrane disease. J Pediatr 57:553, 1960

22. **McDonald AD:** Cerebral palsy in children of very low birth weight. Arch Dis Child 38:579, 1963

23. **Aranda JV, Saheb N, Stern L, Avery ME:** Arterial oxygen tension and retinal vasoconstriction in newborn infants. Am J Dis Child 122:189, 1971

24. **Silverman WA:** Prematurity and retrolental fibroplasia. Sight Sav Rev 39:42, 1969

25. **Tasman W:** Vitreoretinal changes in cicatricial retrolental fibroplasia. Trans Am Ophthalmol Soc 68:548, 1970

26. **James LS, Lanman JT:** History of Oxygen Therapy and Retrolental Fibroplasia. Pediatrics (Suppl) 57:591–642, 1976

27. **Ashton N, Ward B, Serpel G:** Role of oxygen in the genesis of retrolental fibroplasia: Preliminary report. Br J Ophthalmol 37:513, 1953

28. **Ashton N, Ward B, Serpell G:** Effect of oxygen on developing retinal vessels with particular reference to the problem of retrolental fibroplasia. Br J Ophthalmol 38:397, 1954

29. **Ashton N, Pedler C:** Studies on developing retinal vessels. IX. Reaction of endothelial cells to oxygen. Br J Ophthalmol 46:257, 1962

30. **Ashton N, Garner A, Knight G:** Intermittent oxygen in retrolental fibroplasia. Am J Ophthalmol 71:153, 1971

31. **Cogan D:** Development and senescence of the human retinal vasculature. Trans Ophthalmol Soc UK 83:465, 1963

32. **Karlsberg RC, Green R, Patz A:** Congenital retrolental fibroplasia. Arch Ophthalmol 89:122, 1973

33. **Reese AB, Owens WG, King M:** Classification of retrolental fibroplasia. Am J Ophthalmol 36:1333, 1953

34. **Patz A:** Retrolental fibroplasia. Surv Ophthalmol 14:1, 1969

35. **Flynn JT, O'Grady GF, Herrera J, et al:** Retrolental Fibroplasia: 1. Clinical Observations. Arch Ophthalmol 95:217–223, 1977

36. **Cantolino SJ, O'Grady GE, Herrera JA, Israel C, Justice J, Flynn JT:** Ophthalmoscopic monitoring of oxygen therapy in premature infants. Am J Ophthalmol 72:322, 1971

37. **Kalina R, Hodson WA, Morgan BC:** Retrolental fibroplasia in a cyanotic infant. Pediatrics 50:765, 1972

38. **Payne JW, Patz A:** Treatment of acute proliferative retrolental fibroplasia. Trans Am Acad Ophthalmol Otolaryngol 75:1234, 1971

39. **Ellsworth R:** Tumors of the retina. In Tasman W (ed): Retinal Diseases of Children. Harper and Row, New York, 1971

40. **Knudson AG, Hethcote HW, Brown BW:** Mutation and childhood cancer: A probabilistic model for the incidence of retinoblastoma. Proc Nat Acad Sc: 72:5116–5120, 1975

41. **Knudson AG, Meadows AT, Nichols WW, Hill R:** Chromosomal deletion and retinoblastoma. N Engl J Med 295:1120–1123, 1976

42. **Abramson DH, Ellsworth RM, Zimmerman LE:** Nonocular cancer in retinoblastoma survivors. Trans Am Acad Ophthalmol Otolaryngol 81:454–457, 1976

43. **Miller RW, Fraumeni JF Jr, Manning MD:** Association of Wilms' tumor and aniridia, hemihypertrophy and other congenital malformations. N Engl J Med 270:922, 1964

44. **Fraumeni JF Jr, Glass AG:** Wilms' tumor and congenital aniridia. JAMA 206:825, 1968

45. **Riccardi VM, Sujansky E, Smith AC, Francke U:** Chromosomal imbalance in the Aniridia-Wilms' tumor association: 11p interstitial deletion. Pediatrics 61:604–610, 1978

46. **Desmonts G, Couvreur J:** Congenital toxoplasmosis. A prospective study of 378 pregnancies. New Eng J Med 290:1110–1116, 1974

47. **Eichenwald HF, Shinefeld HR:** Viral infections of the fetus and of the premature and newborn infant. Adv Pediatr 12:249, 1962

48. **Weller TH, Hanshaw JB:** Virologic and clinical observations on cytomegalic inclusion disease. N Engl J Med 266:1233, 1962

49. **Lonn LI:** Neonatal cytomegalic inclusion disease chorioretinitis. Arch Ophthalmol 88:434, 1972

50. **Gregg NM:** Congenital cataract following German measles in the mother. Trans Ophthalmol Soc Austr 3:35, 1941

51. **Boniuk V, Boniuk M:** The incidence of phthisis bulbi as a complication of cataract surgery in the congenital rubella syndrome. In Boniuk

(ed): Rubella and Other Intraocular Viral Diseases in Infancy Vol 12. Int Ophthalmol Clinics. Boston, Little Brown, 1972

52. **Cremer RJ, Perryman PW, Richards DH:** Influence of light on the hyperbilirubinemia of infants. Lancet 1:1094, 1958
53. **Noell WK, Walker VS, Kang BS, et al:** Retinal damage by light in rats. Invest Ophthalmol 5: 450, 1966
54. **Kuwabara T, Gorn RA:** Retinal damage by visible light, an electron microscopic study. Arch Ophthalmol 79:69, 1968
55. **Sisson TRC, Glauser SC, Glauser EM, Tasman W, Kuwabara T:** Retinal changes produced by phototherapy. J Pediatr 77:221, 1970
56. **Kalina RE, Forrest GL:** Ocular hazards of phototherapy for hyperbilirubinemia. J Pediatr Ophthalmol 8:116, 1971
57. **Hubel DH, Wiesel TN:** The period of susceptibility to the physiological effects of unilateral eye closure in kittens. J Physiol 206:419, 1970

46

Drugs and the Perinatal Patient

George P. Giacoia and
Sumner J. Yaffe

INTRODUCTION

A number of iatrogenic therapeutic mishaps affecting the human fetus and neonate have been reported in recent years. These have aroused concern over the pharmacologic pollution of the intrauterine environment and have prompted many medical practitioners to condemn the use of drugs during the pregnant state. Implicit in this type of therapeutic nihilism was the frustration of the practitioner over the lack of information concerning the ability of the fetus to defend itself from the intrusion of foreign compounds. The situation of the neonate was not very different. For years, therapeutic regimens for him were based on miniaturization of adult dosages without regard for the biologic peculiarities of this period of human development.

Fortunately, basic scientific disciplines and allied clinical specialties today are focusing their attention upon the biologically immature and developing organism. This interdisciplinary partnership is already bearing fruit. The functional limitations of the fetus and newborn, characteristics of their biochemical milieus and alteration by pharmacologically active molecules are beginning to be known, albeit in a rudimentary fashion. Eventually this type of knowledge will permit the use of drugs based on fundamental pharmacologic princi-

ples rather than on empirical formulations or on extrapolation from knowledge gathered in adult patients. It can be anticipated that drugs will be given to the mother not only to treat maternal disorders, but specifically, for the benefit of the fetus. This goal can be achieved only when the pharmacokinetics of the different drugs in the maternal-placental-fetal unit is precisely characterized. A new dimension has been recently added with the observation that drug exposure of the father may influence the outcome of pregnancy.[1]

General Considerations

The intensity and duration of drug effects depend on a number of variables: absorption, distribution, metabolism, excretion, and intrinsic interaction between drug and specific tissue receptors. The rate of absorption varies with the route of administration. The major factors determining the rate of absorption by the oral route are: rate of drug dissolution, water solubility and degree of ionization of the drug, gastric and intestinal pH, gastric emptying time, composition of intestinal contents, intestinal motility and mesenteric blood flow. Water solubility, degree of ionization, physicochemical composition and blood flow are determinant factors in drug absorption by intramuscular, subcutaneous, or peridural routes. After absorption, drugs are distributed in the body according to their lipid solubility, degree of ionization and binding properties to plasma and tissue proteins. All of these factors determine their "volume of distribution." This is a useful though theoretical parameter that permits one to relate the amount of drug in the blood at a given time to the different tissues and elimination sites. From the pharmacologic standpoint, a drug can be eliminated either by renal or biliary excretion or by metabolic degradation into pharmacologically inactive metabolites.

PHARMACOLOGY OF PREGNANCY

Distribution. The changes in oncotic pressure, total amount and distribution of body water, together with hemodynamic alterations which occur during pregnancy can affect the distribution of drugs. The reduction in oncotic pressure during the last trimester averages 20%. This decrease is caused by the lowering in the concentration of albumin by about 1 g/dl. This relative hypoalbuminemia is mainly responsible for the diminished binding capacity for sulfisoxazole and congo red found in pregnant women at term compared to nonpregnant controls.[2]

Excretion. The profound changes in renal function during pregnancy may be expected to influence the renal excretion of drugs. Glomerular filtration rate (GFR) increases during pregnancy. This increase is sometimes accompanied by comparable changes in tubular reabsorptive capacity (*e.g.,* sodium). For other substances, a glomerular tubular imbalance favors excretion when the increased filtered load exceeds the tubular capacity for reabsorption (glucose). During late pregnancy, renal elimination of drugs may be markedly influenced by changes in body position. Urine volume and clearances of inulin and PAH decrease markedly in the supine position.

Metabolism. Metabolic disposition of drugs may be altered in pregnancy. Glucuronic conjugation of endogenous and foreign compounds is inhibited during late pregnancy and some of the oxidative biotransformation systems are also affected. Glucuronidation has also been found deficient in pregnant women who receive salicylamide.[3] The demethylation of pethidine occurs less readily in pregnancy.[4] The high tissue levels of progesterone and pregnanediol

which are found in pregnancy may be responsible for the inhibition of glucuronyl transference activity.

In vitro studies of drug metabolism performed in pregnant rats in our laboratories uncovered a more complex picture. While oxidative reductive pathways have been found inhibited, sulfation actually increased. Present knowledge in this area is quite limited and further research is urgently needed. In order to make a valid assessment of the metabolic limitations of pregnancy in relation to drug disposition, the contributions of maternal, placental, and fetal tissues to drug metabolism must be evaluated at different stages of pregnancy. It is likely that the alterations in drug metabolism in the maternal organism are modulated by hormonal changes. The results of *in vitro* studies in experimental animals cannot be extrapolated to the situation in human pregnancy without considering the profound physiologic differences among species.

It must also be emphasized that *in vitro* studies need to be related to the intact subject. For example, alterations in liver blood flow may substantially modify the metabolic inactivation of drugs. Total blood volume and cardiac output increases during the last trimester of human pregnancy, while hepatic blood flow remains practically unchanged. Consequently, a smaller proportion of the cardiac output irrigates the liver in pregnancy. Contrary to the situation in experimental animals, no increase in the size of the liver occurs in human pregnancy. Therefore, despite changes in the proportion of total blood flow that perfuses the liver, blood flow per unit of hepatic mass varies very little in normal pregnancy.

Complications of Pregnancy. In toxemia of pregnancy, there is an increase in the amount of body water, mainly in the extracellular space; consequently, changes in drug distribution are likely to occur. The decrease in the filtration fraction and the frequency of abnormal "liver tests" in toxemia accentuate the need to study the pharmacokinetics of drugs commonly used in pregnancy. Of interest are reports of tetracycline toxicity in pregnant women who were treated for acute pyelonephritis. A number of patients had prolonged half-lives of the antibiotic as a consequence of depressed GFR. In addition, it has been postualted that there is a special hepatic tissue sensitivity to tetracycline during pregnancy. It should be kept in mind that pyelonephritis and other infections are known to produce alterations in liver function.

The Role of the Placenta. The transfer of drugs across the placenta is influenced by

1. physicochemical characteristics of the drug.
2. physiologic properties of the placental tissue.
3. maternal and fetal blood flow through the placenta.

Physicochemical characteristics of the drug. The molecular size of any given substance plays an important role in the transfer rate across the placenta. Drugs with molecular weight of less than 400 cross the placenta rather easily. With increasing molecular size, other factors, such as lipid solubility, degree of ionization, molecular configuration, and protein-binding properties become increasingly important.

Recent work attests to the fact that studies of drug transfer utilizing other semipermeable membranes (*e.g.,* gastrointestinal tract) do not apply to the placental membrane. When drugs are listed according to their lipid solubility, degree of ionization, and molecular weight, marked differences have been found between the transfer rates of the placenta and other biologic model systems.

Substances cross the placenta by different transfer mechanisms: simple diffusion, facilitated diffusion, activated transport, and pinocytosis. Most drugs cross the placenta by simple diffusion from regions of higher to lower concentration. Only rarely do drugs cross by facilitated diffusion or active transport. Sometimes, a drug has a structural molecular configuration similar to an endogenous material that normally uses either one of the latter mechanisms. Because of the similarity between endogenous pyrimidines and **5-fluorouracil,** it is likely that transfer of the latter may be facilitated. It is also possible that drugs containing amino acids with chemical configurations similar to those of essential amino acids may utilize common transport-carrier systems. These drugs may achieve higher concentrations in the fetus, as seems to be the case with **alpha methyldopa.**

Because most drugs reach the fetal side of the placenta by simple diffusion, it is not surprising that highly ionized drugs with poor lipid solubility, such as **tubocurarine,** fail to achieve significant concentrations in fetal blood. Placental impermeability to specific compounds is always relative because it would be unlikely for a drug not to cross to the fetal side of the placenta when it is present in very high concentrations on the maternal side. The important factors, however, are the rate of transfer and the ability of the placental tissue to modify or be modified by the drug in question.

The structural characteristics of the placenta change substantially during the course of pregnancy. The concomitant decrease in thickness and increase in surface area that occurs with advancing placental age is not always associated with an increase in permeability to drugs. Unfortunately, little is known about the effect of degenerative changes such as villous edema, on drug transfer.

Physiologic Properties of the Placental Tissue. The realization that the placenta is an extremely competent metabolic organ has stimulated interest in its drug biotransformation capabilities. The interpretation of studies of drug biotransformation reactions *in vitro* using cell-free preparations of placenta, is plagued with difficulties. This heterogenous mixture of all components from different types of cells may contain substances that can markedly alter the pattern of drug metabolic reactions. In addition, contamination of the preparation with erythrocytes, plasma, or both may vitiate the results obtained. Several enzyme systems present in red cells or plasma may act as catalysts in some types of drug biotransformation reactions.

In vitro studies of drug metabolism in human placental homogenates have demonstrated the presence of oxidation reactions for prototype compounds such as **aniline** and **benzpyrene.** Placental homogenates are known to contain catalysts for the reduction of a number of foreign substances. However, those catalysts seem to be of a nonenzymatic nature. No glucuronidation reactions have been found in placental tissue preparations. The importance of the placenta as an organ of drug biotransformation cannot be assessed on the basis of the fragmentary evidence provided by *in vitro* studies.

Future studies should concentrate on the following aspects: (1) characterization, isolation, and purification of enzymes or catalysts involved in drug biotransformation reactions; (2) study of possible interaction between drugs and endogenous compounds in relation to the different drug biotransformation systems; (3) characterization of metabolites generated in drug metabolic reactions and their effects on the developing fetus; (4) application of pharmacokinetic techniques to *in vitro* studies to calculate transfer rates of different substances from mother to fetus and vice versa. *In situ* perfusion studies, using an experimental model that closely resembles the human placenta, can provide valuable help in unraveling the complexities of drug transfer across the placenta.

Maternal and Fetal Blood Flow through the Placenta. The rate of drug transfer across the placenta is markedly influenced by the maternal and fetal placental blood flow. Despite the difficulties of obtaining adequate measurements of uterine blood flow, different studies have shown an increase in mean uterine blood flow per kilogram of total tissue (uterus, placenta, fetus) toward term. However, when the rate of uterine blood flow is expressed per kilogram of fetus, it decreases at the end of pregnancy. In diabetes, preeclampsia, and chronic hypertension, uterine blood flow is decreased. It is not known to what extent this diminished uterine blood flow affects the transfer of drugs across the placenta. During labor, the decrease in uterine blood flow which occurs with uterine contraction may protect the fetus from receiving large amounts of anesthetics and analgesic drugs, especially if given intravenously during the last minutes of labor. It is also conceivable that this mechanism may be, on occasion, detrimental to the fetus because drugs may be "trapped" in the fetus and be unable to equilibrate with a lower maternal concentration during the drug distribution phase.

Uterine blood flow may be decreased by drugs such as **methoxamine** or **epinephrine,** and thus, potentiate the pharmacologic effect in the fetus of **analgesics** or **anesthetics** previously given to the mother. The uptake of drugs by the fetus depends on the blood flow through the umbilical circulation. Under hypoxic conditions, the umbilical flow is increased because most hypoxic conditions in the fetus are generated by hemodynamic alterations in the uterine blood flow. The net effect may be a decrease in the transfer rate of drugs given during the hypoxic episode. The effect of drugs on the fetal circulation has not been adequately studied. Alterations in fetal hemodynamics induced by certain pharmacologic agents (anesthetics, CNS depressant) may affect the placental transfer of other drugs given concomitantly.

Fetal Pharmacology

Once a drug reaches the fetal side of the placenta, its likelihood of producing adverse effects in the fetus depends upon a myriad of factors: the type of drug, amount of drug actually transferred, rate of elimination from the fetus, distribution in fetal tissues, length of gestation, and state of the specific receptor function in the fetus. The effects of drugs given chronically during gestation need to be distinguished from those occurring after the acute administration of a drug during labor and delivery. In the first case, the drug may accumulate in the fetus and produce long-term effects. Drugs given during the first trimester may have teratogenic effects. They were reviewed in Chapter 37. Unfavorable effects of drugs administered acutely during parturition are usually shortlived, but may affect the neonatal adaptation to extrauterine life. (Table 46-1).

Drug Distribution in the Fetus. Body composition and drug disposition. During normal fetal growth and development, there are considerable changes in body composition. Total body water content decreases from about 94% of total body weight at 16-weeks gestation to about 76% at term. A marked decrease in the amount of extracellular water is largely responsible for this decrease. The expanded extracellular fluid volume, characteristic of the fetal period, affords some protection to the fetus by enlarging the volume of distribution of drugs that are mostly dissolved in water. Fat is virtually absent in fetuses of less than 1000 g. Most fetal fat deposition occurs during the last trimester of pregnancy. The amount and distribution of fat determines the distribution in fetal tissues of such lipid-soluble drugs as **thiopental, glutethimide,** and **diazepam.** The changes in composition of individual organs are particularly important if they are the primary site of pharmacologic action of specific drugs. For example, the relatively high water content of the fetal brain, but its low myelization, limits the distribution of lipo-

Table 46-1. Drugs and the Fetus.

Maternal or Paternal (?)	
Exposure Prior to Conception	
Mutagenesis	
Maternal Therapy	
During Pregnancy	
Preimplantation	Acute
First trimester	or
Late gestation	Chronic
Throughout pregnancy	
During delivery	
Fetal Therapy	
Maternal route	
Amniotic route	
Peritoneal route	

phylic drugs. Lipid solubility may cause some drugs to distribute into tissues pharmacologically inert, away from their primary sites of action. A good illustration of this process is the distribution of **diphenylhydantoin.** Fetal adrenal cortex, myocardium, and corpora lutea contain amounts of the drug that greatly exceed the amount present in the central nervous system.[5] The ability of drugs to combine with pharmacologic receptors depends on specific factors of drug distribution in the tissues.

In vitro binding studies comparing adult versus neonatal plasma have generally shown an increase in the proportion of unbound drug in neonatal plasma. Because most drugs are bound to albumin, the lower concentration of plasma proteins in the newborn explains many of the observed results. Recent studies have shown that for certain drugs there are also qualitative differences in the binding properties of neonatal plasma. The different binding capacity of neonatal plasma may also be because of drug binding to other plasma proteins, intrinsic changes in the binding sites or competition for binding sites by endogenous substances.

Contrary to the situation in the adult, α_1-globulin has a higher binding affinity than albumin does to bind **nafcillin.** The interaction between endogenous compounds (hormones, free fatty acids, and so on) and neonatal plasma proteins has not been adequately assessed. The evidence for differences in binding sites or alterations in the basic structure of neonatal plasma proteins is largely inferential.

Regardless of the mechanism involved an increase in the amount of free drug changes the pattern of drug distribution, this being largely responsible for toxic effects of drugs in the fetus and newborn. The few studies of drug binding by fetal and newborn plasma proteins indicate that the fetus is less able to bind drugs than the newborn. Furthermore, drug binding to maternal plasma proteins may be decreased during pregnancy, with obvious consequences upon maternal-fetal drug distribution.

Role of the Fetal Circulation in Drug Distribution. After crossing the placenta, drugs enter the umbilical vein. Although most of the blood flow through the umbilical vein (60%–80%) perfuses the liver by way of the portal vein, a sizable proportion of the umbilical blood flow (20%–40%) is shunted to the inferior vena cava by way of the ductus venosus. Consequently, a rather large proportion of the drug transfer across the placenta can reach the heart and brain without being diluted by the portal vein circulation. In addition, if the drug is inactivated to any extent in the fetal liver, a relatively large amount would escape degradation. These effects are somewhat minimized by the dilutional effect of blood flowing through the superior vena cava. It should be emphasized, however, that the fetal brain receives a larger share of cardiac output than in any other period in life.

During hypoxic conditions, the circulation through the brain may be increased in association with low Pa_{O_2} and high Pa_{CO_2}. The composition of fetal blood is also important in determining drug distribution. For example, fetal blood can take up more **trichloroethylene** than can maternal blood. This is related to the greater total mass of fetal red cells, because trichloroethylene is bound to red cell lipids. Because a great number of drugs are transported in plasma bound to plasma proteins, the study of the protein-binding characteristics of fetal blood has considerable pharmacologic significance.

Receptor Function. The pharmacologic effects of drugs depend on the functional integrity of specific receptor sites. There is a dearth of information concerning the pattern of development of those receptors during fetal life. This information is not only of theoretical but also of practical importance. Most theories of drug addiction explain withdrawal reactions as a result of hyperactivity or lack of inhibition of certain neural pathways. The concentration of specific neurotransmitters is altered by the interaction of drugs (especially **narcotics**) and pharmacologic receptors. Changes in the turnover rate of neurotransmitters become evident as signs of autonomic dysfunction once the addictive drug is withdrawn. In the case of fetal narcotic addiction, it is not known when the specific receptors become functionally active. It is likely that during a considerable period of gestation, the fetus may be incapable of developing physical dependence on narcotics, and these drugs may be abruptly discontinued without fearing a fetal withdrawal syndrome. Looking at the functional development of individual organs in the fetus, it can be inferred that maturation of pharmacologic receptors is likely to proceed at varying rates in different organs. Studies of autonomic receptors in the isolated ileum from human fetuses (12–24 weeks) have shown that while beta-receptors increased their functional response during this interval in gestation, alpha-receptors were inactive.[6]

Drug Metabolism. In general, fetal tissues have little or no enzymatic activity for a number of biotransformation reactions. One of the major metabolic activities of the liver is to transform nonpolar compounds into water-soluble substances that can be easily excreted into the urine (for example, glucuronidation). Because the placenta is the major excretory organ for waste products in the fetus and lipid solubility is an important factor in determining drug transfer across the placenta, it is not surprising to note that on teleologic grounds that enzymes that mediate the conversion of endogenous compounds or drugs to polarized metabolites are not fully developed during fetal life. The most significant pathways of drug biotransformation are oxidative reactions.

The drug oxidizing enzymes located in the microsomal fraction of hepatocytes not only oxidize drugs, but more important, play a major role in the metabolism of steroids and fatty acids. The different components of the oxidizing system constitute what has been termed the electron-transport chain. Cytochrome P-450, the last component in the chain, catalyzes the incorporation of oxygen into the substance being oxidized. It has been demonstrated that the amount of cytochrome P-450 per gram of tissue present in liver micro-

somal preparations from human fetuses (14–25 weeks) is similar to that found in adults. Furthermore, the other components of the electron-transport chain (NADPH—specific cytochrome c reductase and NADPH cytochrome P-450 reductase) were present in concentrations necessary for drug hydroxylation reactions. These findings were somewhat surprising in view of the inability of several investigators to detect cytochrome P-450 or cytochrome P-450-dependent hydroxylation reactions in liver microsomes from fetuses of several animal species (rodent, rabbit, guinea pig) even at very late stages of gestation. The existence of such striking species differences has great significance for evaluation of the safety and efficacy of drugs administered during pregnancy.

Despite the presence of adequate amounts of cytochrome P-450, no detectable oxidizing enzyme activity was found with several drug substrates in *in vitro* studies. In contrast to exogenous compounds, testosterone and fatty acids have been reported to be hydroxylated at significant rates by human fetal liver microsomes. It is likely that endogenous substances have a much higher affinity for the terminal oxidase in the microsomal system than do xenobiotics. Positive results were obtained later for the oxidative N-demethylation of **demethylimipramine** and **ethyl morphine** and p-hydroxylation of **aniline** in human fetal liver preparations *in vitro*.[7,8]

Although the liver is the center of drug-metabolizing activity in the adult subject, this may not be the case in the fetus. The human fetal adrenal gland performs extremely important biochemical functions, and is particularly active with respect to steroid biotransformation. It would not be unexpected that significant biotransformation of exogenous substrates could take place in the organ. Indeed, recent studies have shown that the specific activities of several drug-metabolizing enzymes are higher in the human fetal adrenal gland than in the fetal liver and that the concentration of cytochrome P-450 was exceptionally high. Such studies have considerable potential significance because of the large size of the fetal adrenal and the key role that adrenal-mediated steroid biosynthesis plays in fetal development.

Experimental evidence accumulated during the last decade points to the fact that most other drug-metabolizing enzymes are inactive during fetal life. However, a major discovery of recent years has been that enzyme activity can be dramatically increased by certain pharmacologic substances (drug induction). This finding has stimulated research into the possible clinical application of altering the timetable of enzyme maturation. Recently, it has been reported that even in early pregnancy, the activity of liver microsomal enzymes may be induced *in vitro*.

Drug Excretion in the Fetus. Renal. Although the placenta serves as the major excretory organ for the fetus, other routes of drug excretion need to be considered. Unless significant transfer across fetal membranes is demonstrated, secondary excretory routes may prolong the disappearance rates of drugs. Some drugs may be excreted by the fetal kidneys. It is generally agreed that during the last trimester of pregnancy, fetal urination is a major contributor to the production of amniotic fluid. By extrapolating from figures derived from the primate fetus, it has been estimated that the rate of urine production at term would be about 15 to 20 ml/hour. The composition of fetal urine differs markedly from that of the amniotic fluid; it contains two to five times more urea, creatinine, and uric acid than does amniotic fluid, but has no protein or glucose. The presence of drug metabolites in fetal urine cannot be taken as evidence of fetal drug metabolism, because the placenta is permeable not only to drugs but also to many of their metabolites. For example, the urine of newborns whose mothers were treated with **chlorpromazine** was compared with urine from newborns treated with chlorpromazine after birth. The study demonstrated a number of conjugated metabolites in the former group not present in the latter. It was concluded that the extra metabolites were of maternal origin.[9]

Intestinal. The fate of compounds gaining access to the amniotic fluid depends on their chemical characteristics. The main route of disposal for proteins appears to be fetal swallowing. It has been demonstrated that maternal albumin can find its way into the amniotic fluid; after being swallowed by the fetus, it is digested in the fetal intestinal tract. It is possible that drugs bound to amniotic fluid proteins may be reabsorbed by the fetal intestine. Because fetal swallowing constitutes a bulk

disposal mechanism (all constituents disappearing simultaneously), the amount of free drug cleared from the amniotic fluid will be limited only by the volume of fluid swallowed by the fetus. In late pregnancy, it has been estimated that the fetus can swallow 5 to 70 ml/hour.

The early maturation of the enzyme β-glucuronidase in the intestinal mucosa may allow conjugated compounds excreted by the fetal kidney to be reabsorbed by the fetal intestine. It is possible, therefore, that certain drugs may be recirculated before leaving the fetus. The net effect of this process would be prolonged fetal exposure, and increased risk of fetal toxic effects.

Skin. The fetal skin has been found to be permeable to water and other substances including drugs. Its significance in distribution and elimination of drugs has not been investigated. It seems likely that the distribution and excretion of drugs in the fetus are part of a complex process, and that at least for certain substances, their pharmacokinetic behavior can be explained only on the basis of a multicomparmental system with different transfer-rate constants.

NEONATAL PHARMACOLOGY

During pregnancy, the fetus has at his disposal the metabolic and excretory capabilities of the maternal organism. During the first few days of life, the newborn must adjust to the realities of a different environment, while trying to achieve the homeostatic flexibility and safety that he enjoyed during fetal life.

Absorption

This process determines the rate of appearance of drugs into the blood stream as well as the absolute amount reaching the circulation. The route of administration influences the intensity and duration of therapeutic effects.

Gastrointestinal (GI) Absorption

The general principles governing the transfer of drugs across biologic membranes have been discussed (see above). The type of pharmaceutical preparation can markedly influence the bioavailabiility of drugs. Newborns receive only solutions or suspensions because of their inability to handle solid dosage forms. This facilitates absorption because it bypasses the dissolution phase of tablets, which is a rate-limiting step.

Although absorption can occur along the whole length of the GI tract, the chemical characteristic of each drug will determine its site and degree of absorption. As with other biologic membranes, drugs with small molecular weight, low degree of ionization, and high lipid:water partition ratio tend to be rapidly absorbed, usually by the process of passive diffusion.

The peculiar characteristics of absorptive processes in newborn infants may substantially modify the bioavailability of drugs given orally. Absorption of different compounds depends on the surface area available for absorption. The GI tract represents a larger portion of the body in the newborn than in later life. In addition, studies in neonatal animals from different species indicate that the permeability of the intestinal tract is increased during the neonatal period. The transfer of intact protein molecules through the gastrointestinal tract mucosa has been studied in detail because of its immunologic implications, and has been shown to take place. The existence of intact protein transfer depends on two factors: gastric digestion and the functional characteristics of the mucosa of the small intestine. Because drug molecules are much smaller, the effect of increased permeability upon drug absorption is probably of little consequence.

It is of interest that the hypoglycemic effect of orally administered **insulin** to newborn infants was observed only during the first 20 minutes of life. The decrease in gastric pH occurring during this period of time has been correlated with the hydrolysis of insulin in the gastrointestinal lumen.[10] This change in gastric pH in early life may markedly alter the absorption of ionizable drugs.

The slower transit rate through the GI tract during the neonatal period may result in prolonged absorption of orally administered medications. This factor may be responsible for the prolonged absorption of orally administered **riboflavin.**[11]

No systematic studies of the absorption of different drugs in newborn infants has been published. The available data deal mainly with the GI absorption of chemotherapeutic agents. Long-acting **sulfonamides** have been found to be well absorbed in newborn infants. A new antimycotic agent, **chlortrimazole,** has been found to be well-absorbed in neonates, including premature infants. Satisfactory serum levels for systemic *Candida* infections have been found after the oral administration of this new antimycotic agent.[12]

The study of the blood serum levels of **potassium** and **procaine penicillin G** following their oral administration to newborn infants demonstrated higher levels in this age than in older infants.[13] It is possible that the lower gastric pH in the younger group may be in part responsible for the observed difference. The study of the gastrointestinal absorption of other antibiotics (**nafcillin, ampicillin, cephalexin, erythromycin, tetracycline**) has shown that while therapeutic blood levels may be reached, they are always significantly below those obtained following the parenteral administration of a similar dose.[14]

Comparison of the serum levels of anhydrous ampicillin, sodium nafcillin, and cephalexin attained after oral administration to newborn infants and adults revealed a slower disappearance rate in the newborn because of the decreased rate of renal excretion. Peak serum concentration of these antibiotics occurred later in newborn infants, indicating a slower absorption rate.[15,16] During the neonatal period, a less efficient mechanism for the oral absorption of **phenobarbital, nalidixic acid,** and **phenytoin** has been reported.[17,18] In contrast, **digoxin** and **diazepam** are more efficiently absorbed.[19,20]

It must be emphasized that the above-mentioned studies have been performed in normal newborns. The situation may be quite different in critically ill newborns. For example, changes in GI blood flow associated with many neonatal conditions may substantially modify the power of absorption of these infants. It is important to emphasize that the rapidly changing physiology and biochemistry of the GI tract during early postnatal life mandates systematic investigation of the absorption of drugs by this route. Studies from older age groups cannot be relied upon for dosage recommendations in the neonate.

Absorption of Drugs from Parenteral Routes

Experiments with newborns and adult animals have demonstrated that the rate of absorption of morphine after intramuscular administration was similar in both age groups.

The major determinant of drug absorption from intramuscular and subcutaneous sites is local blood flow. Under hypoxic conditions, newborns may selectively curtail circulation in muscles and skin, thus hindering absorption of drugs given intramuscularly or subcutaneously. Because, under those circumstances, kidney function may also be compromised, drug concentration in blood after repetitive dosage may not be significantly lowered.

Distribution

The changes in body composition occurring in late fetal life continue in the newly born infant. Prematurely born infants have a larger extracellular fluid volume and total body water than full-term infants. The decrease in extracellular fluid volume during the first month may be modified by the type of feeding they receive. Milk with high-ash content prevents the decrease in extracellular fluid volume with age. On the other hand, milk with a high potassium-protein ratio may increase the amount of intracellular water.

Consequent with the changes in body composition, premature infants have a larger volume of distribution of **bromsulphalein** than full-term infants. The degree of plasma protein binding can substantially modify the volume of distribution of drugs. The unbound fraction can freely cross membranes and is the one exerting pharmacologic action.

Depending on the relative affinity for the receptor sites in the protein molecule, endogenous compounds can displace or be displaced by foreign compounds. The increased levels of bilirubin in the early neonatal period, especially in premature infants, can significantly alter the disposition of drugs. For example, *in vitro* studies have shown that bilirubin appears to compete with **diphenylhydantoin** for binding to plasma albumin. The amount of unbound diphenylhydantoin can be doubled by increasing bilirubin concentrations to more than 20 mg/dl. Recently, it has been demonstrated that **sodium benzoate** can cause displacement of bilirubin from its binding to albumin. This substance is used as a preservative in commercial preparations of **caffeine** and **diazepam.** *In vitro* studies have shown that administration of diazepam to the mother does not substantially affect the binding of bilirubin to albumin. The decrease in the binding capacity of albumin may contribute to the exquisite sensitivity

of the newborn to various drugs. The permeability of the neonatal blood-brain barrier during the first few days of life is greater than later on in life. As a consequence, certain unbound drugs can penetrate the newborn brain and reach higher brain concentration per unit dose than in the adult brain. Such drugs must be used at smaller doses to prevent toxic symptoms.

Drug Metabolism

The picture emerging from newborn, human and animal studies is one of a limited ability of the newborn patient to effect biotransformation of drugs. The deficiency of conjugation reactions is somewhat compensated for by the adequacy of sulfation reactions. This is especially important for the metabolism of endogenous steroids.

The evaluation of the conjugating capacity of the liver by *in vitro* studies is hampered by the existence of factors that are unrelated to the intrinsic enzymatic activity of the reaction in question. Decreased hepatic uptake, low concentrations of intracellular carrier proteins, and a decrease in the rate of bile production may act synergistically with a deficient conjugating ability. This may explain the long half-life of **sulfobromophthalein** in premature infants. Beside limited ability to form glucuronides, other conjugation mechanisms are incompletely developed in early neonatal life. Administration of **sodium benzoate** results in delayed formation and excretion of hippuric acid.

The metabolism of **paraaminobenzoic acid** is altered, resulting in the formation of a different pattern of metabolites. Conjugation with glycine is delayed, and there is a preponderance of acetylated metabolites. This is at variance with the limited ability of newborns to acetylate **sulphonamides.** Although after birth there are rather drastic changes in oxidoreduction reactions, experimental evidence points to a deficiency in both oxidizing and reduction ability during the neonatal period. It has been shown that the newborn has an impaired capacity to hydroxylate **diphenylhydantoin** and oxidize **tolbutamide.**

The possibility of inducing new enzyme formation or activity has found clinical application in the treatment of neonatal hyperbilirubinemia. Although several compounds have been found to possess induction capabilities,

phenobarbital has been the drug of choice for this purpose. Retrospective studies have shown that infants born to mothers who received inducing agents (*e.g.,* **phenobarbital, heroin**) had a lower incidence of hyperbilirubinemia. This induced stimulation of neonatal metabolism occurs within 4 to 5 days and at doses of phenobarbital that do not appear to affect the infant's well-being as judged by his clinical status and the time he took to regain birth weight. Induction as implied above also may be produced by prenatal administration of the inducer shortly before term. It is important to recognize that induction is a nonspecific phenomenon and that other endogenous substrates, such as steroid hormones, will have an accelerated catabolism, as well as bilirubin and drugs. The significance of induction and any long-term effects upon growth and development have not been assessed. Until such has occurred, induction should be regarded as potentially hazardous.

Excretion

From the pharmacologic standpoint, a drug is eliminated whenever it is excreted or metabolized into inactive metabolites. Because most drugs are poorly metabolized, excretion constitutes the most important factor in the termination of drug action. Although some excretion of drugs may occur through the bile, it is of subordinate importance. The bulk of drug excretion is accomplished by the kidney.

The renal excretory mechanisms (GFR and renal secretion) are imperfectly developed at birth. GFR is usually measured using a substance that, after it is filtered at the glomeruli, is neither reabsorbed nor secreted in the tubules. The polymeric carbohydrate **inulin** has been widely used in the adult for this purpose. The evidence that inulin in the newborn is a purely glomerular substance is mostly indirect. Endogenous creatinine has also been used as a glomerular marker. In adults, the results obtained with both substances have been quite similar. In newborns, endogenous creatinine clearance and inulin clearance can be markedly different under conditions of osmotic diuresis. The increase in creatinine clearance observed under those circumstances suggests tubular secretion of creatinine.

Inulin clearance in newborns has been compared in a hydropenic state and under conditions of osmotic diuresis. The rise in inulin observed under conditions of osmotic diuresis may be caused by changes in GFR, but the results obtained may also be intereperted by postulating tubular reabsorption of inulin under hydropenic conditions. Another problem is selection of the parameter to be used as the basis of comparison with results obtained in adults. However, regardless of the parameter used, it is evident that GFR is low at birth and does not significantly increase until the end of the first week of life. This change in glomerular filtration is reflected by a marked increase in the half-lives of those antibiotics excreted solely by glomerular filtration (*e.g.,* **aminoglycosides**).

Studies of kidney function during the neonatal period have demonstrated that renal tubular secretory mechanisms are incompletely developed at birth. Their inefficiency is particularly prominent in premature infants.

The effects of the inefficiency of this renal excretory pathway depend on the conditions of drug intake. A rapidly absorbed drug will be slowly eliminated. This situation is not detrimental to the newborn, if, with subsequent doses, the dose interval is increased. Indeed, in the case of **penicillins,** the duration of action of a single dose is prolonged, permitting a decrease in the frequency of administration. With drugs that are slowly absorbed, the potential for toxic reaction is increased. Under those circumstances, both rate of absorption and of elimination must be taken into account when formulating a therapeutic program. The limited ability of the perinatal kidney to acidify the urine may hinder the excretion of weak bases. Whenever kidney function is significantly decreased by pathologic conditions, both magnitude and spacing of doses must be tailored to the degree of kidney failure. The use of formulas derived for the adult (*e.g.,* relation of dose interval to creatinine level) in the newborn, is ill-advised. Drugs known to produce toxic effects (*e.g.,* **digoxin**) should be monitored by frequent measurements of drug concentration in plasma, and the dosage regimen should be adjusted accordingly.

Receptor Function

The functional status of pharmacologic receptors at birth has not been adequately characterized. The reactivity of the iris in premature and full-term infants to different sympathomimetic amines has been recently studied. Mydriasis followed instillation of **phenylephrine.** This response has been taken as evidence of the functional activity of alpha-adrenergic receptors. The mydriatic effect of **tyramine** and **hydroxyamphetamine,** which depends on the release of norepinephrine, was observed only in the more mature babies. This suggests a limited ability to produce and/or release neurotransmitters. The knowledge of the state of maturity of adrenergic receptors in pathologic circumstances may have important therapeutic applications. For example, a shock-like state occurs in a number of neonatal conditions and may be an important factor contributing to neonatal mortality. Plasma expanders are usually used to combat the marked hypotension accompanying this state. If sympathetic reflexes are absent, it may be possible to treat this cardiovascular disturbance effectively with synthetic sympathomimetic amines, provided receptors are present and functional.

SPECIFIC DRUGS: CLINICAL CONSIDERATIONS

Compared with the adult patient, the therapeutic armamentarium used to treat neonatal conditions is rather limited and will not be discussed here. On the other hand, the newborn is the unwanted recipient of a wide variety of drugs given for the benefit of the mother.

In this section, different groups of drugs will be considered in relation to their pharmacologic and toxic effects in the perinatal patient. No attempt has been made to include all drugs known to exert adverse effects upon the neonate. Rather, drugs have been selected for discussion based upon frequency of use and availability of some data. It is obvious that there are wide gaps in our knowledge. These must be closed if we are to use agents for either the mother or fetus (or both) with maximal effect upon the intended recipient and minimal harm to the symbiotic partner.

Drugs Given During Labor and Delivery

Regional anesthesia has been used in obstetrics since the beginning of the 20th century. This form of anesthesia includes subarachnoid, lumbar, peridural, caudal, and paracervical block. The drugs used for this purpose are water-soluble salts of lipid-soluble alkaloids

and may be divided according to their chemical structure into two groups: esters and amides. The esters (*e.g.,* **procaine**) have a slow onset of action, short duration of pharmacologic effect, and penetrate poorly into tissues. They are metabolized by hepatic and plasma esterases. The amides (*e.g.,* **bupivacaine, lignocaine, mepivacaine,** and **prilocaine**) are the group most commonly used in conduction anesthesia because of their rapid onset of action and prolonged duration of pharmacologic effect. These drugs are inactivated by hepatic amidases. Because they are weak bases, urinary excretion depends on the urine pH. However, even with an acid pH, urinary excretion of the unchanged drug is not important in the overall elimination of amides. Both amides and esters cross the placenta; the amides are poorly metabolized by the fetus. For example, in the adult only about 5 to 10 percent of mepivacaine is excreted unchanged in the urine. Newborns whose mothers have received mepivacaine (epidural block) eventually excrete mostly unchanged mepivacaine in their urine.

Plasma pseudocholinesterase hydrolyzes procaine and other local anesthetics. The rate of procaine hydrolysis is low at birth. Consequently, the half-life of procaine in newborn infants is prolonged (1.4 minutes versus 0.66 minutes in adults).[21] For this reason, pharmaceutical preparations of **penicillin-containing procaine** are not recommended during the neonatal period.

The fetus may be affected by the direct action of the drug, or indirectly by the changes that the anesthetic produces in the maternal organism.

Spinal anesthesia, *per se,* has no direct effect on the fetus. The amount of anesthetic used is too small to achieve toxic levels in the fetus. The neonatal depression that complicates spinal anesthesia is usually secondary to maternal hypotension. The hypotensive effect of spinal anesthesia is probably the result of the elimination of the increased vasoconstrictor tone prevailing in pregnancy. Presumably, this increase in neurogenically controlled vasoconstrictor tone compensates for the augmented venous pooling in the legs produced by the pregnant uterus. When this compensatory mechanism is blocked by spinal anesthesia, both the venous and arterial systems collapse. A decrease in venous return, a drop in cardiac output, and a fall in arterial blood pressure are the consequences of this vascular collapse.

The effect of maternal hypotension on the fetus and newborn depends on a number of factors: stage of labor, duration and severity of maternal hypotension, presence of other obstetrical complications, and concomitant use of fetal-depressant drugs. Treatment of spinal hypotension with vasopressors (**methoxamine**) may decrease uterine blood flow and further compromise the fetus. Drugs with minimal vasoconstrictor action must be used. **Ephedrine** and **mephentermine,** for example, raise arterial pressure primarily by increasing cardiac output. Hypotension may also complicate caudal block when large doses of local anesthetics are used. Under these circumstances, significant amounts of anesthetics may reach the fetus. A rare complication of caudal block was reported several years ago. **Mepivacaine** was accidentally injected into the fetal scalp: four newborn infants were affected and two of them died. To avoid this complication, it is recommended that caudal block not be performed when the fetal head has advanced low into the pelvis.

Lumbar peridural block has a number of advantages over subarachnoid block, including a decreased incidence of maternal hypotension, but requires six to ten times the amount of drug used for subarachnoid block. Studies have shown that pregnant women at term require less drug (40%–50%), because during the last trimester there is an engorgement of the internal vertebral plexus that reduces the capacity of the peridural space. The absorption of local anesthetics from the peridural space and their appearance in fetal blood has been the object of several studies.[22] **Lidocaine** has been found in maternal blood 2 to 3 minutes after a peridural injection reaching a peak level in 15 to 30 minutes. The drug was still detected several hours after the injection. Lidocaine concentration in umbilical vein blood has been found to be about 50% to 60% of that present in the maternal arterial blood. Similar studies with other local anesthetics (**bupivacaine, mepivacaine, prilocaine**) have shown the same pattern of distribution.

The concomitant use of **epinephrine** reduces the rate of absorption of local anesthetics from the peridural space. Maternal arterial blood levels of local anesthetics have been reduced by 40% with the addition of epinephrine 1:200,000. However, it appears that the reduction in maternal and fetal blood levels produced by epinephrine occurs only during the initial 30 minutes after the peridural injection. As maternal arterial concentrations peak during this period, epinephrine is a welcome addition to the technique of peridural block. Toxic effects stemming from the use of epinephrine are not likely to occur with total doses of less than 100 mg. The effects of epinephrine on the placental vasculature and the metabolic activity of the organ may militate against its use in regional anesthesia. Absorption from the peridural space is not always predictable. Occasionally, infants are born depressed and their cord blood contains high levels of local anesthetic. This situation has been reported with lidocaine and mepivacaine.

Fetal bradycardia and acidosis have frequently complicated paracervical block. The evidence on hand suggests that the bradycardia is caused by rapid absorption of the local anesthetic into the blood vessels perfusing the placenta with immediate transfer into the fetal circulation.

The amide group of local anesthetics at toxic levels have a quinidine-like effect on the myocardium, which is responsible for the alterations in heart rate. It is of practical importance to differentiate between drug-induced bradycardia and that resulting from fetal asphyxia. The latter may be an indication for immediate obstetrical intervention while drug-induced bradycardia should be treated by delaying delivery until fetal blood concentration has fallen to nontoxic levels.

The amide group of local anesthetics have a selective depressant effect on the CNS; twitching, convulsions, apnea, and death have been found in intoxicated newborns. It should be stressed that with equal amounts of drug taken into the body, the fetus is better able to recover from toxic doses because of elimination across the placenta. After birth, the newborn is unable to metabolize amides.

Although **prilocaine** has been mentioned among the local anesthetics, it is not being used at present because it can produce methemoglobinemia in the newborn. (Actually, it is not the drug itself, but a toluidine derivative which causes the methemoglobinemia.)

General Anesthetics. Gaseous anesthetics, especially those with high lipid solubility, are rapidly transferred into the fetus. For example, within 90 seconds of maternal administration, **cyclopropane** has been found in cord blood.[23,24] **Methoxyfluorane,** which dissociates poorly and is highly lipid, is also transferred early. Within 2 minutes of maternal administration, umbilical vein levels of methoxyfluorane were 65% of the concentration present in maternal blood.[25] The intermittent administration of general anesthetics may permit the metabolism of the drug by the mother while levels in the fetus remain elevated. In a study which compared the levels of **trichloroethylene** found in maternal and fetal blood at the time of delivery, trichloroethylene was given by intermittent inhalation of the anesthetic. In four out of ten patients, the fetal concentration was higher than the maternal concentration. It must be emphasized that the fetus is deficient in "halogenotransferase" which appears to play an important role in the metabolism of aliphatic chlorinated substances.[26] Studies on the placental transmission of **nitrous oxide** have shown that the average concentration in cord blood approaches 50% of the maternal drug concentration.[27] When nitrous oxide is given to produce anesthesia rather than analgesia, a concentration of 75% in the inspired gas is required. At this concentration, a number of infants are born depressed. However when nitrous oxide is given in a mixture containing 40% to 60% of the gas to provide moderate analgesia, no significant neonatal asphyxia is observed. **Cyclopropane** in concentrations of 3% to 5% does not produce ill-effects in the fetus.[28]

Barbiturates are weak acids occurring as undissociated molecules at physiologic pH. Although they are largely fat soluble, lipid solubility is not the only factor to be considered in assessing the effect on the fetus of barbiturates given to the mother. An experimental study on the distribution of ^{14}C labeled **thiopental** has demonstrated that transfer to the fetus proceeded at a much slower rate than to the maternal brain. Despite a different rate of transfer between maternal brain and fetus, it is widely accepted that most barbiturates cross the placenta rapidly.

Secobarbital, a short-acting barbiturate, has been found in the newborn cord blood 1 minute after the intravenous administration to the mother. When equilibrium was established (3–5 minutes), cord blood contained 70% of the maternal blood concentration.[29] Although it has been found that secobarbital does not produce neonatal depression when given to the mother before the last 25 minutes prior to delivery, it may affect the sucking behavior of the newborn for several days after delivery.[30] The type of delivery may affect the amount of short-acting barbiturates transferred to the fetus. This seems to be the case with thiopental. A study compared the neonatal outcome between vaginal delivery and caesarean section when thiopental was used to produce anesthesia. Significant neonatal depression was found in those newborns delivered by caesarean section.[31] Hemodynamic changes in the uteroplacental unit during vaginal delivery may have protected the newborns from receiving depressing amounts of thiopental. The slow rate of oxidation of short- and ultrashort-acting barbiturates in the newborn explains the prolonged depression observed in some infants. The role of other factors affecting the transfer of barbiturates to the fetal brain has not been elucidated, and the distribution of barbiturates in fetal tissues has not been studied. An animal study compared the distribution of two barbiturates, **barbital** and **pentobarbital**, into amniotic fluid after maternal administration.[32] Both drugs appear in amniotic fluid in concentrations much lower than that found in maternal and fetal blood. However, a greater proportion of the dose of sodium barbital, which is more water soluble, was found in the amniotic fluid.

One important factor in the distribution of barbiturates is plasma protein binding. As much as 60% to 70% of thiopental is bound to plasma proteins. The thiopental protein binding by neonatal and adult plasma has been studied by equilibrium dialysis. At a concentration of 2×10^{-4}M, the unbound fraction was 7.2% in adult plasma and 13% in neonatal plasma.[33] If a marked decrease in protein binding occurs at the concentrations found at birth following maternal administration, the concomitant increase in the unbound fraction will facilitate barbiturate uptake by the infant's brain. Barbiturates penetrate more readily into the unmyelinated white matter of the neonatal brain than into its gray matter. The increased rate of transfer of barbiturates into the neonatal brain produces a greater pharmacologic effect.

Sleeping times in neonatal animals, a measure of this pharmacologic effect, is much longer than in adult animals given a similar dose per unit of body weight.

Chronic ingestion of barbiturates may produce fetal addiction, which is manifested by barbiturate withdrawal symptoms after birth. Very rarely, a convulsive state at birth has been attributed to barbiturate withdrawal.

Systemic Analgesics. Almost all the potent analgesics that have been used to relieve the pain and discomfort of labor produce some degree of neonatal depression. **Morphine**, the oldest of this group of analgesics, is known to rapidly cross the placenta and produce significant respiratory depression in the newborn. Because of this, morphine is used very infrequently in present obstetric practice. Diacetylmorphine (**heroin**) has been banned from the United States since the year 1915. Its importance in producing neonatal addiction will be considered later (see narcotic withdrawal syndrome). **Meperidine** is widely used as an analgesic in obstetrics. Meperidine is hydrolyzed in the liver to meperidinic acid, which is in turn partially conjugated. The most important metabolic pathway of meperidine in humans is its N demethylation to normeperidine, which is further hydrolyzed to normeperidinic acid. In the adult, excretion of unchanged meperidine is not important in limiting the pharmacologic effects of the drug, because meperidine is transformed to metabolites that are rapidly excreted. While nonpregnant adults excrete mostly normeperidine, newborns and pregnant patients excrete significant amounts of unchanged meperidine in the urine.[34] Meperidine crosses the placenta with ease. After an intravenous injection (50 mg) to the mother, meperidine has been found within 2 minutes in fetal blood.[35] The peak cord blood concentration after intramuscular injection to the mother ranges between 80% to 130% of the maternal levels.

The timing of the intramuscular administration of meperidine is important in determining the presence or absence of respiratory depression of infants at birth. If given within 1 hour of delivery, no interference with the initiation of breathing has been observed; however, if the drug is given between 1 and 3 hours before delivery, a significant increase in the number of depressed babies is seen.

A recent work has implicated maternal meperidine metabolites as being responsible for the infant respiratory depression when greater than 60 minutes has elapsed since the administration of meperidine. The study of meperidine and its metabolites in maternal serum has shown a marked increase in meperidine me-

tabolites 60 minutes after the intravenous administration of the drug. It has been proposed that meperidine meabolites are more toxic to the fetus than is the parent drug.[36]

Chloral hydrate owes its sedative properties to one of its metabolites, trichloroethanol. Both drugs and metabolites are excreted in the urine. Chloral hydrate and its metabolites, trichloroacetic acid and trichloroethanol, have been detected in fetal blood for more than 8 hours after rectal and oral administration to the mother. **Paraldehyde** passes the placenta and the cord blood levels parallel the maternal blood levels.

Drugs Given to Stop Premature Labor. Many factors have been invoked to explain the initiation of human parturition. Pharmacologic approaches to the inhibition of premature labor require a better understanding of the triggers of premature labor. The lack of uniform success with any of the many available drugs illustrates the lack of specificity of the available therapy. Ethyl alcohol has been used to suppress premature labor. Intravenous alcohol seems to inhibit labor by suppressing oxytocin release. Although this therapy has been termed successful by the proponents of the method, recent studies cast some doubt on its effectiveness.

Studies on the transfer of alcohol to the fetus have shown that the placenta does not significantly slow down the rate of transfer of the drug. During the first 30 minutes of an alcohol infusion, there is delay in transfer, judging by the slower rate of increase of fetal blood alcohol concentration, when compared to the changes occurring in maternal blood.[37] Thereafter, cord blood concentrations are not significantly different from maternal blood concentrations. The rate of disappearance of alcohol from the infant's blood after birth is much slower than that in the mother.

The higher water content of the tissues in the newborn may increase the volume of distribution of alcohol precluding its rapid elimination from the body. The only rate-limiting factor for ethanol oxidation is the activity of the liver alcohol dehydrogenase, which has been found to be decreased in the fetus and newborn. This limited capacity to metabolize alcohol is more important in determining its slow elimination from the body than are distributional changes.

No significant CNS depression has been found in premature infants who were born with a significant concentration of alcohol in the blood. The concomitant use of other drugs may potentiate the depressing effects of alcohol. Experimentally, a marked decrease of oxygen transfer to the fetus occurred when ethanol was infused to pregnant animals under pentobarbital anesthesia. In contrast, a similar ethanol infusion when the animals were under spinal anesthesia resulted in an increase in oxygen transfer across the placenta. Ethanol can produce hypoglycemia in fasting subjects by a decrease in hepatic glucose output. Because the susceptibility to alcohol-induced hypoglycemia seems to be inversely related to the size of hepatic glycogen stores, the fasting newborn infant (especially if prematurely born) may be at risk of suffering this complication. The metabolic effect of alcohol has been studied in a group of full-term infants born to mothers who received alcohol infusion in amounts similar to those used to prevent premature delivery. No significant alterations in glucose or insulin levels could be demonstrated. In another study, alcohol was given intravenously to premature infants 31 to 53 hours of age. No significant hypoglycemia was found.[38] Because of the limited caloric intake during the first few days of life, premature infants born from alcohol-treated mothers should have their blood sugar monitored during the first 24 hours.

In addition to alcohol, a number of other drugs have been tried in threatened premature labor. Beta-adrenergic receptor stimulants have been tested, but their cardiovascular effects (*i.e.*, maternal hypotension and tachycardia) have limited their clinical application. The ideal beta-adrenergic agonist should primarily influence the beta-receptors of the uterus and have a minimal effect on the beta-receptors of the heart and blood vessels. Drugs with relative specificity for the beta-receptors of the uterus include **ritodrine, terbutaline, buphenin, hexoprenaline,** and **salbutamol.** The first beta-adrenergic drug was **isoxuprine.** Maternal hypotension limits its usefulness. Ritodrine does not produce hypotension and the increased maternal heart rate and pulse pressure seems to indicate an increase in cardiac output during therapy. The accelerated fetal growth observed during prolonged ritodrine treatment could be explained by an increase in placental perfusion. Salbutamol, a recently developed beta-adrenergic stimulant, has been praised by some obstetricians because the presence of ruptured membranes does not appear to influence the outcome of the treatment. There is no evidence of direct effect of salbutamol in the fetus other than fetal tachycardia accompanying maternal tachycardia. Clinical evidence suggests inhibition of premature labor by **indomethacin.** Considerable concern exists however, as to the possibility of fetal closure of the ductus arteriosus caused by this prostaglandin inhibitor.

Despite advances in the understanding of labor, its pharmacologic control has not been achieved. A single compound that is effective, safe, and devoid of undesirable effects is not yet available. A multitarget approach that acts concomitantly on different target organs, regulatory mechanisms, or both may prove to be more effective than relying on a single treatment.

Drugs Given to Induce Labor. For years, **oxytocin** has been the drug of choice to induce labor. The quantitative transfer of oxytocin across the placenta has not been determined. The physicochemical similarities between oxytocin and insulin make it likely that insignificant amounts of oxytocin would reach the fetus. In addition, the presence of oxytocinase in the placenta is apt to destroy the small amounts of oxytocin transferred. The recent demonstration that, during spontaneous labor, oxytocin is produced by the fetal membranes and found in the maternal circulation raises the possibility that transport in the opposite direction may occur.[39] There is considerable epidemiologic evidence of an association between maternal administration of oxytocin and neonatal jaundice. No satisfactory theory has been advanced to explain this correlation.[40] Recently, **prostaglandins** have been used successfuly for this purpose. Our present knowledge on the fate of prostaglandins in the fetus is quite rudimentary. Prostaglandins, which are C20 unsaturated fatty acids, have not been found in the fetal and maternal blood at term and in the first void urine of the newborn. Prostaglandins have been found in amniotic fluid and umbilical cord vessels. It has been demonstrated that, physiologically, the prostaglandins in the amniotic fluid originate in decidual cells.

The fetal distribution of therapeutic doses of prostaglandins given to the mother has not been studied. Endogenously produced prostaglandins are involved in the mechanism producing middle trimester abortion induced by hypertonic saline.[41] Because pharmacologically active prostaglandins are rapidly inactivated by metabolic processes, it is possible that their metabolites may reach the fetus in higher concentration than the parent compound.

Drugs Given During Pregnancy

Antimicrobial Drugs. The present interest in the transmission of antibiotics from mother to fetus is directed toward their possible therapeutic and toxic effects. The possibility of treating intrauterine infections has attracted the interests of obstetricians for many years. Unfortunately, the lack of an effective therapeutic program is responsible for the widespread practice of early delivery in premature rupture of membranes and amnionitis. Most antibiotics have molecular weights of 500 or less and are believed to cross the placenta by a process of passive diffusion. The degree of antibiotic binding to plasma proteins can markedly influence the amount transferred to the fetus. **Dicloxacillin** is highly bound (96%) to serum albumin at therapeutic levels. Consequently, only the small, free, diffusible fraction crosses the placenta, resulting in low cord blood levels and insignificant amniotic fluid levels. In contrast, **methicillin**, which is 40% bound to albumin, crosses the placenta barrier rather easily, achieving significant fetal and amniotic fluid concentrations. The rate of transfer of antibiotics given to the mother is important in the prevention of infections acquired by the ascending route. Studies on normal amniotic fluid have demonstrated the presence of several factors with antibacterial properties. However, these natural defenses are unable to eradicate a large inoculum of microorganisms. The knowledge of the antibacterial properties of the amniotic fluid is also important in the interpretation of antibiotic concentrations measured by bioassay techniques. If antibacterial factors are not destroyed (for example, by heating) spuriously elevated levels of antibiotics may be found.

Ampicillin, and to a lesser degree, **penicillin**, appear to reach significant concentrations in amniotic fluid. The transfer of ampicillin to the amniotic fluid, after the intravenous administration of the drug to pregnant patients near term, has been studied by placing a catheter in the amniotic cavity and obtaining simultaneously maternal blood and amniotic fluid samples. Cord blood samples were also taken at birth. Analysis of the data revealed that ampicillin reached the amniotic fluid after some delay. This lag period was more prolonged in cases of fetal death.[42] It is generally accepted that ampicillin reaches the amniotic fluid through the fetal urine. The concentration of ampicillin in amniotic fluid allows recirculation of the drug in the fetus.

Studies of the ampicillin concentration of amniotic fluid after oral administration of drugs to the mother have shown inconsistent results, probably because of factors that influence gastrointestinal absorption in late pregnancy. When ampicillin has been injected into the amniotic fluid, there is a slow transfer into the maternal circulation.[43] Under those circumstances, very high levels of ampicillin in fetal blood have been found at birth.

The study of the placental transmission of **colistimethate** is of interest in view of its high molecular weight (1200). After a single 150 mg dose administered intravenously to the mother, fetal blood levels greater than 2 μg/ml were reached within minutes and remained above 1 nm/ml for 8 hours. No colistimethate was found in the amniotic fluid 3 hours after the administration to the mother. When colistimethate was injected into the amniotic fluid, 20% to 30% of the amount injected was still present 18 hours postinjection. The transfer between amniotic fluid and maternal blood is very slow and occurs only when a high concentration of the drug is introduced into the amniotic sac. **Streptomycin, chloramphenicol, tetracycline,** and **chlortetracycline** resemble colistimethate in not achieving appreciable levels in amniotic fluid after maternal administration of therapeutic doses.

Some antibiotics can produce toxic manifestations even if present in small amounts in fetal tissues and must not be used to treat maternal infections. Tetracycline, when given to the mother during late pregnancy, accumulates in the fetal skeleton. The administration of tetracycline to premature infants during the neonatal period resulted in a decrease in skeletal growth. Similar findings have been reported in experimental animals exposed to tetracycline during intrauterine life. Discoloration of teeth occurs when the drug is given during the second trimester of pregnancy, and can be associated with enamel hypoplasia. Streptomycin can reach the fetus from early pregnancy. Although its administration to pregnant women with tuberculosis has resulted in only a handful of reported cases of congenital deafness, it is very likely that minor degrees of acoustic nerve damage may be common. **Nitrofuradantoin** and **sulfonamides,** when given during pregnancy, have produced hemolysis at birth in G-6-PD-deficient newborns. **Isoniazid** may reach higher levels in fetal blood than in maternal blood, suggesting an active placental transfer of this compound.

Antiprotozoal drugs (**quinine, primaquine, pentaquine,** and **metronidazole**) are transferred across the placenta. Quinine has been considered contraindicated in obstetrics because of its reputation as an abortifacient. Analysis of the literature reveals that, in therapeutic doses, quinine poses less of a danger to the fetus than is commonly stated in standard textbooks. Some of the antiprotozoal drugs are likely to produce hemolysis in G-6-PD-deficient newborns.

Antidiabetic Drugs. Although **insulin** crosses the placenta at term, the amount transferred is too small to be of clinical importance. It can affect the fetus indirectly by producing maternal hypoglycemia. **Sulfonylureas** constitute a group of hypoglycemic agents that have achieved widespread popularity for the treatment of adult-onset diabetes. Although they have been occassionally used in pregnant patients, they are presently not recommended for this purpose because of their potential toxic effects in the fetus.

The sulfonylureas have a beta-cytotrophic effect which facilitates the release of insulin. It is known that **tolbutamide, chlorpropamide,** and **acetohexamide** cross the placenta and can produce beta-cell hyperplasia in the fetal pancreas. Because of the slow metabolism of the drugs by the liver, their pharmacologic effects may persist for several days after birth. A marked prolongation of tolbutamide half-life has been demonstrated in full-term infants. Although similar studies for chlorpropamide have not been performed, several cases of prolonged intoxication in offspring of treated mothers have been reported. The protracted symptomatic hypoglycemia seen in intoxicated infants has responded to prolonged intravenous glucose administration in some cases, while others necessitated exchange transfu-

sions to remove the offending drug from the body. The addition of fructose and the elimination of leucine from the diet have been other forms of therapy used to diminish the stimulation of insulin release.

Iodides and Thyroid Preparations. For years, the maternal ingestion of **iodides** has been implicated in the production of congenital goiter. The minimal maternal intake of elemental iodide needed to cause fetal goiter is not known with certainty. In one study, the calculated maternal intake ranged between 12 to 1650 mg of elemental iodide.[44] Only a small number of patients who take iodides develop a goiter. It has been suggested that fetuses who develop congenital iodide goiters have an abnormal pituitary-thyroid feedback mechanism resulting in an excess of thyroid-stimulating hormone. Infants with congenital iodide-induced goiters may present signs of hypothyroidism at birth. On occasion, deaths have resulted from mechanical obstruction of the trachea by massive goiters. Congenital iodide-induced goiters usually disappear with or without therapy. **Thiouracil** administered to the mother may also produce congenital goiter. Some infants develop hypothyroidism associated with the goiter. In most cases, however, the thyroid enlargement disappears spontaneously without medication. The placental transfer of **carbimazole** is largely unknown, although clinical studies have failed to demonstrate any alteration in neonatal thyroid function.

Cardiovascular Drugs. The transplacental transfer of digitalis glucosides has not been adequately studied. Both **digoxin** and **digitoxin** cross the placenta. Digitoxin has been implicated in the death of a newborn whose mother took a toxic dose of the drug.[45] Both maternal and infant ECGs showed evidences of digitalis toxicity. Unfortunately, the cord blood concentration of digitoxin at birth was not measured.

A recent study provides suggestive evidence that digitalis glucosides may be handled differently in the pregnant state. A group of pregnant women with rheumatic heart disease who received an oral maintenance dose of digoxin have been studied before and after delivery. The digitoxin levels during the last trimester of pregnancy almost doubled one month after delivery.[46] The reason for this striking difference is not known, but changes in absorption and/or distribution of the drug occurring during pregnancy may be responsible for the lowering of serum digitoxin concentrations. In the same study, maternal serum and umbilical cord blood digitoxin concentrations were compared. No significant difference was found, suggesting passive transfer as the mechanism of transport across the placenta. The quantitative aspects of digoxin disposition in the maternofetal-placental unit has been recently studied in the pregnant ewe. Digoxin accumulated in the amniotic fluid where it exceeded the concentrations found in fetal plasma.

The injection of **adrenaline** and **noradrenaline** into the fetal circulation of experimental animals has yielded conflicting results. A new technique for studying the effects of cardioactive drugs in cultured fetal hearts has been described.[47] By employing this technique, it may be possible to determine the potential toxicity of new compounds and the chronic effects of presently used cardioactive drugs on the performance of human fetal hearts at different periods of fetal development. The injection of sympathetic amines into the maternal circulation appears to affect the fetus not directly but by vasoconstrictor effects upon the uterine vessels. However, direct passage of labeled catecholamine has been demonstrated following the injection of ^{14}C epinephrine in pregnant women of anencephalic or hydrocephalic fetuses.[48]

Diuretics. **Thiazides** cross the placenta and have been reported to produce thrombocytopenia in the newborn. This toxic effect of thiazides has been recently disputed.[49,50] The true incidence of this complication is not known at present. Chronic thiazide administration during pregnancy can cause electrolyte imbalance in the fetus. Marked hyponatremia and extrarenal azotemia have been found at birth. Present knowledge on the transfer, distribution, and pharmacologic effects of diuretics on the fetal renal tubule is rudimentary. The realization that diuretics have been overprescribed during pregnancy in recent years has stimulated obstetricians to reassess the therapeutic value of this group of drugs in the treatment of preeclampsia. Hopefully, this will be followed by decreased usage and thus fewer adverse effects in the fetus and newborn.

Anticoagulants. The treatment of thromboembolic disorders in the pregnant woman has raised the question of the safety of anticoagulant therapy with regard to the fetus. **Heparin,** being of relatively large molecular size, and with an electronegative charge, crosses the placenta with difficulty and when given in therapeutic doses, does not affect the fetus. There is convincing evidence that **coumarin** drug therapy during pregnancy can lead to hemorrhagic manifestations and death in the newborn. When both maternal and fetal blood prothrombin levels have been measured a greater reduction has been found in the fetus. Nevertheless, neonatal hemorrhagic death is not common when maternal oral anticoagulant therapy is rigidly controlled. This fact has stirred a controversy among obstetricians on the advisability of using coumarin derivatives during pregnancy. Those favoring its use claim that coumarin can be safely used, provided these two requirements are met:

1. The dose must be adjusted and kept within the therapeutic range.
2. Therapy must be discontinued long before delivery in order to allow the fetal prothrombin concentration to return to normal or near normal levels for age.[51]

The pregnant patient with cardiac valve replacement poses a special problem. In addition to the risks of fetal hemorrhage the potential teratogenic effects of **warfarin** needs to be carefully considered because anticoagulant therapy is given during the organogenic period.[52] Indeed, a fetal warfarin syndrome has been described in infants whose mothers had prosthetic mitral valves and received the anticoagulant during pregnancy.[53] The syndrome includes an abnormal facies (hypoplastic nose and low nasal bridge) stippled epiphisis, and vertebral and CNS dysfunction, including mental deficiency.

Anticonvulsant Medications. Because convulsive disorders are frequently exacerbated after conception, anticonvulsant drugs are frequently used during pregnancy. Chronic administration of **diphenylhydantoin** results in similar maternal and fetal blood concentrations. After birth, diphenylhydantoin half-life is significantly prolonged when compared to the average adult half-life. Plasma levels and clearance rates of diphenylhydantoin in newborns whose mothers received phenobarbital in addition to diphenylhydantoin did not differ from those of mothers treated with diphenylhydantoin alone. Chronic administration of **phenobarbital** during pregnancy can produce a withdrawal syndrome virtually identical to that seen in newborns born of opiate-addicted mothers. The onset of barbiturate withdrawal symptoms, however, occurs at a later age (up to 2 weeks after birth). Although suspected for a long time, epidemiologic evidence linking the use of anticonvulsants during pregnancy and congenital anomalies has only recently been presented.[54] The existence of a fetal hydantoin syndrome seems well established.[55] Newborns born to epileptic mothers receiving anticonvulsive medications have a greater risk of hemorrhage caused by depletion of vitamin K-dependent factors.

Cholinesterase Inhibitors. Only fragmentary information is available on the transfer of these compounds. The chemical structure of **neostigmine, edrophonium,** and **pyridostigmine** is such that ready transfer across the placenta is not likely. However, even the amount of drug transferred can perhaps affect the fetus. This is illustrated by the report of a newborn who developed myasthenia gravis from the administration of **pyridostigmine** to the mother.[56]

Neuromuscular Blocking Agents. **Succinylcholine** crosses the placenta in insignificant amounts. **Tubocurarine,** on the other hand, can reach significant concentrations in fetal blood and is, therefore, not recommended for use in obstetrics. The newborn infant is resistant to the action of succinylcholine. A fourfold increase in dosage is necessary in the newborn, compared with the adult dosage, to maintain apnea.[57] Theoretically, this resistance to succinylcholine may be because of an increased rate of inactivation, a larger volume of distribution of the drug, or an increased number of motor end plates. The decreased levels of plasma pseudocholinesterase rule out an increased metabolic degradation of succinylcholine. The familiar resistance of the newborn to **decamethonium,** a depolarizing muscle relaxant, suggests a common mechanism. Both drugs are highly ionized and it is likely that their distribution in the enlarged extracellular volume of the newborn may explain the decrease in pharmacologic effect.

Another type of muscle relaxant, tubocurarine, does not exhibit any difference in pharmacologic effect in newborns and adults when given in equivalent doses. Marked binding of tubocurarine to plasma albumin limits the distribution of the drug to the extracellular water compartment.[58]

Antihypertensive Medication. Various drugs have been used to treat the hypertensive syndromes occurring in or that are exacerbated by pregnancy. **Reserpine** has been known to produce respiratory depression at birth in addition to a stuffy nose and lethargy. Prolonged treatment with reserpine can produce depletion of catecholamine stores. Because the response to cold is mediated by catecholamines, the possibility that reserpine may block the neonatal adaptation to cold has been investigated in experimental animals. Despite depletion of both epinephrine and norepinephrine, the ability of newborn piglets to increase oxygen consumption in response to cold was not impaired.[59]

Magnesium sulfate has been widely used in the past for the treatment of preeclampsia and eclampsia. In addition, clinical studies have shown that magnesium sulfate can stop spontaneous labor, but additional controlled studies are needed to establish its usefulness to inhibit preterm labor. Frequent administration of the drug to the mother may result in high levels of magnesium in the fetus, which has been associated with neonatal respiratory depression. In addition to central depression, the magnesium ion has a curare-like action at the neuromuscular motor end plate. A decrease in serum calcium has been observed in newborns born with high serum magnesium levels.[60]

Diazoxide, a benzothiadiazine with hypotensive and hyperglycemic properties occasionally has been used to treat severe preeclamptic toxemia. Diazoxide crosses the placenta and reaches the amniotic fluid through fetal kidney excretion. Despite urinary excretion, fetal levels remain stable during the first 24 hours of life and can be demonstrated in the urine up to the first week of life. Hypertrichosis lanuginosa, a common complication of diazoxide treatment in children, has been reported in a newborn born of a mother treated with the drug. Alopecia has also been noticed in three other infants born to women treated with oral diazoxide during pregnancy.[61]

Psychopharmacologic drugs are widely used as sedatives and for the treatment of neurotic conditions. On occasion, chronic administration of these compounds during pregnancy is necessary for the management of psychotic disorders.

Phenothiazines have been known to produce extrapyramidal signs in infants of treated mothers. These signs, including opisthotonus, hypertonia, tremors, and hand posturing, have persisted in some infants for several months after birth.

Chlorpromazine has been implicated as a cause of fetal retinopathy. The existence of such retinopathy has been recently questioned. Some psychopharmacologic agents (*e.g.*, chlorpromazine) may interfere with the central regulation of temperature, resulting in hypothermia during the first days of life.

Lithium carbonate is currently used for the treatment of manic depressive psychosis. Although this drug has been used in pregnancy without demonstrable toxic effects in the fetus, a recent report described lithium intoxication in the newborn of a treated mother. The infant manifested cyanosis and a marked hypotonia.[63]

Self-administered Medications. Although suspected for some time, the surprisingly high rate of fetal exposure to medications not prescribed by the physician has been recently documented in several studies.

The teratogenic effects of chronic maternal **alcohol** ingestion has recently been recognized and the resulting dysmorphic and behavioral abnormalities have been termed fetal alcohol syndrome.[62] The salient features of the syndrome include CNS system dysfunction (including mental retardation), growth deficiencies, a characteristic facial appearance, and variable association with other major and minor congenital anomalies. The facial appearance is characteristic. Key features are short palpebral fissures, absent or diminished philtrum, and thin upper lip. Prospective epidemiologic studies uncovered a great variability of phenotypic expression. A crude dose-response relationship has been established but the lowest safe level of ethanol consumption has yet to be determined. Drinking behavior in the month preceding the recognition of pregnancy strongly correlates with fetal outcome. Mental retardation, a common problem associated with ethanol teratogenicity, seems to be the result of prenatal exposure to alcohol rather than postnatal environmental circumstances. While the pervasive effect of prenatal exposure to alcohol is no longer in doubt, the mechanism(s) by which alcohol or its breakdown products produce their effect during organogenesis remains to be elucidated. The

"dosing" of alcohol consumption (*e.g.*, steady consumption versus binge drinking) and the possibility of potentiation effects by other drugs used frequently by alcoholics (*e.g.*, nicotine, tranquilizers, coffee) needs to be determined.

Smoking may be considered a form of self-administered medication. **Nicotine** and other active components of smoke are likely to affect the fetus. Indeed, a reduction in birth weight has been amply demonstrated in offspring of smoking mothers.

The decrease in birth weight may be related to nutritional deficiencies of smoking mothers or to the toxic effects of specific componenents of cigarette smoke. Although there is animal data lending support to the nutritional theory, this possibility has not been investigated in human pregnancy. The toxicologically active components of cigarette smoke (nicotine, **carbon monoxide**) have been implicated in the birth-weight reduction observed in mothers who smoked continuously during pregnancy.

The pharmacologic effects of nicotine upon the fetus have been studied in experimental animals. Nicotine resembles acetylcholine in its action on the CNS, skeletal muscle, and upper sympathetic and parasympathetic ganglia: initially, it produces stimulation followed by depression. The multiple sites and mechanisms of action of nicotine make the evaluation of its pharmacologic effects exceedingly difficult. It has been found that mature fetuses are more sensitive to the effects of nicotine than are immature fetuses. The developmental pattern of specific receptors probably explains the relative insensitivity of the young fetus.

Nicotine may produce vasoconstriction of uterine circulation with consequent reduction in placental exchange. The amount of nicotine inhaled in average smoking may reach concentrations in the maternal organisms high enough to interfere with the supply line to the fetus. Similarly, the combination of inhaled carbon monoxide with hemoglobin, producing carboxyhemoglobin, is likely to reduce the oxygen-carrying capacity of maternal and fetal blood. It is not known whether these factors acting alone or in combination are responsible for the decrease in birth weight.

Another aspect of cigarette smoking that deserves consideration is the effect of smoking on drug disposition by the maternofetal-placental unit. There is evidence that cigarette smokers metabolize certain drugs (**phenacetin, pentazocine**) more rapidly than do nonsmokers.[64,65] The effect of smoking on drug metabolism during the pregnant state and in fetal life has not been investigated. Cigarette smokers have greater activity of benzpyrene hydroxylase in the placenta.

Antepartum Glucocorticoids and Prevention of Hyaline Membrane Disease. Much evidence has accumulated to support the concept that glucocorticoids are effective in accelerating fetal lung maturation[66] and preventing hyaline membrane disease. Exogenous steroids influence fetal lung development during a critical period of gestation (less than 34 weeks) and require delayed parturition for 48 hours for maximal therapeutic yield. Betamethasone, at a dose of 12 mg given twice, reaches levels in fetal blood which mimic a physiologic stress response and saturate the fetal corticosteroid lung receptors, giving an optimal response.[67] This effect is short lived and disappear's after 7 days. If delivery does not occur, repeat treatment may be needed at weekly intervals until a gestational age of 32 to 34 weeks is reached. Recent evidence seems to indicate that response to antenatal steroids is sex related. When both sexes are matched for gestational age, males are less likely to respond to prophylactic use of steroids. Although risk associated with this type of prophylactic therapy seems low and potential long-term effects remain hypothetical, there is little doubt that many enzymes and body systems are affected by glucocorticoid exposure in late fetal life. Future research is needed to unravel the precise mechanism(s) by which steroids exert their effect. With this knowledge it may then be possible to identify a compound which promotes fetal lung development specifically.

Drug Addiction. The dramatic increase in drug addiction in recent years has not spared women of child-bearing age. Although the gamut of drugs used is impressive, **narcotic** addiction has remained the most serious problem facing the fetus. Other drugs (for example, **phenobarbital** and **alcohol**) are known to produce withdrawal symptoms soon after birth; but the low frequency and mild nature of such symptoms have minimized their importance.

The pathophysiologic consequences of sustained exposure to narcotics *in utero* are poorly understood. Several theories have been advanced to explain the increased autonomic reactivity characteristic of the narcotic withdrawal syndrome. So far, no theory has solid experimental evidence to support its postulation. It is of interest that under the influence of narcotics, infants of low birth weight achieve a state of functional readiness far advanced for their gestational age. Acceleration in lung maturation, induction of liver glucuronidation reactions, and lowering of the pharmacologic threshold for sweating are recently discovered evidences of such alterations in functional development. It is not known at present whether the acceleration in the pattern of development in different tissues is associated with long-term implications. There is evidence in adult narcotic addicts on methadone that their hypothalamic pituitary nycterohemeral periodicity is altered. Similarly, animal studies indicate that narcotics may affect the hypothalamic-adrenal axis. The possibility that long-term fetal exposure to narcotics may influence the hypothalamic-pituitary-adrenal axis has not been investigated.

Fetal and Neonatal Intoxication. It is not possible to set forth in any detail all currently known facts regarding accidental intoxication of the fetus and newborn; however, a few examples will be given.

Fetal poisoning has been the result of attempted suicide in the mother, mistaken medications, or ingestion of toxins unknown to the mother. The fetus has been affected directly by the transplacental passage of the toxic agent or indirectly as a result of hypoxia. On occasion, the toxic agent has been a gas: **carbon monoxide.** The fate of the fetus depends on the time of exposure and ranges from fetal death to severe mental retardation.

Pollution of the environment with industrial waste products has resulted in prenatal poisoning by contamination of food. Congenital Minamata disease has been the result of ingestion by the mother of fish contaminated with **methylmercury.** Fetal death or crippling neurologic disease occurred as a consequence of intrauterine exposure to this toxic agent.

Contamination of cooking oil with **tetrachlorobiphenyl** in Japan has produced a disorder known as ''Yusho'' or rice-oil disease. Nine pregnant women and their fetuses have been affected by this type of intoxication. Two fetuses were stillborn. All nine infants presented at delivery with a dark-brown discoloration of the skin, for which these infants

of oral diphenylhydantoin and the alkalinity of parenteral diphenylhydantoin makes both the oral and intramuscular routes undesirable for the neonate.

Digoxin

Controversy surrounds the use of digoxin in newborns. Recently, it has been doubted whether digitalis glycosides are needed to treat certain types of congestive heart failure (e.g., that associated with patent ductus arteriosus). The use of loop diuretics alone, such as furosemide, may lessen the need for digoxin, which has the lowest therapeutic index (effective:toxic dose ratio) of any drug commonly used in newborns. Small preterm infants are especially susceptible to the toxic effects of this drug. In sick preterm infants, the problem is compounded by the frequent association in these patients of factors which increase the sensitivity of the myocardium (e.g., electrolyte imbalance, hypoxia).

The time honored regimen of digitalization has recently been challenged. It has been argued that, because digoxin is rapidly and selectively bound to the myocardium with immediate onset of action, subjecting small infants to potentially toxic levels is not warranted. By giving the maintenance dose (0.01 mg/kg) from the beginning, the steady state level can be reached in approximately 1 week. Another approach recently reported consists of giving a loading dose calculated to saturate body stores, followed by a maintenance dose.[84] For full-term neonates, the loading dose is 0.025 mg/kg and the maintenance dose is 0.010 mg/kg. Regardless of the therapeutic scheme used, dose requirements differ in preterm and full-term infants. The premature infant, because of limited renal excretory capacity, requires a lower dose. In contrast, full-term infants *tolerate* serum levels of digoxin higher than those that are tolerated by older children and adults. Setting aside the pharmacodynamic explanation for this phenomenon, the key issue to be resolved is not tolerance, but the minimal dosage necessary to achieve optimal pharmacologic response.

CONCLUSION

The first 10 months of existence from conception until the end of the first month of life seem small in comparison with the number of years which comprise the human life span. Yet, there is no other 10-month period in life so rich in contrasting physiologic and biochemical events. During intrauterine existence, the symbiotic relationship between mother and fetus imposes physiologic patterns on them that will vanish when both partners assume independent statuses. During this entire period the infant is peculiarly vulnerable to exogenous substances. (Table 46-2).

Table 46-2. Drugs Reported to Affect the Fetus.

Drug	Effect		
	Morphologic	*Functional*	*Delayed*
Analgesics			
Narcotics		Withdrawal syndrome	?
		↓ Hyperbilirubinemia	
Salicylates	↑ Minor anomalies	Platelet dysfunction	
		↓ Factor XII	
Anesthetics			
General		Depression	
Local		Depression	
		Bradycardia	
		Acidosis	
		Methemoglobinemia	
Antimicrobials			
Sulfonamides		Kernicterus	
Nitrofurantoin		Hemolysis	

(Table continues on following page.)

Table 46-2. Drugs Reported to Affect the Fetus (continued).

Drug	Effect		
	Morphologic	*Functional*	*Delayed*
Antimicrobials (continued)			
Tetracyclines	Teeth staining Enamel hypoplasia		
Streptomycin		8th nerve damage	Deafness
Isoniazide		Encephalopathy	
Anticonvulsants			
Diphenylhydantoin	Cleft lip and palate	Coagulation defects	?
Phenobarbital		Coagulation defects Enzymes induction	?
Barbiturates		Addiction Enzymes induction ↓ Sucking	
Anticoagulants			
Coumarin		↓ Prothrombin time Hemorrhages	
Diuretics			
Thiazides		Thrombocytopenia Hyponatremia ? Electrolyte imbalance	? ?
Antihypertensive Drugs			
Reserpine		Nasal stuffiness	
Cancer Chemotherapeutic drugs			
Aminopertin	Bone defects Intrauterine growth retardation		Retarded growth
Methotrexate	Malformation of head		
Chlorambucil	Unilateral absence of kidney and ureter		
Immunosuppressants			
Azathioprine	?	?	?
Psychopharmacologic Drugs			
Phenothiazine		?	Behavioral changes
Chlorpromazine	? (Eyes)	Extrapyramidal dysfunction	
Imipramine	? Limb defects		
Lithium	?	Toxicity	
Diazepam	?	? Temperature	
Antithyroid			
Potassium iodide	Goiter		
Thiouracil	Goiter	↓ Thyroxine syntheses	
I_{131}		Hypothyroidism	? Malignant changes

Table 46-2. Drugs Reported to Affect the Fetus (continued).

Drug	Effect		
	Morphologic	*Functional*	*Delayed*
Antidiabetic Agents			
Tolbutamide	Anomalies	Thrombocytopenia	?
Chlorpropanide	Anomalies	Severe hypoglycemia	?
Cyclamates		?	?
Saccharin		?	?
Hormones			
Cortisone	Cleft palate ?	? Hemorrhages ? Hypoglycemia Normal adrenal activity	
Prednisolone	Anecephaly ? Low birth weight ?	? Hemorrhages ? Hypoglycemia Normal adrenal activity	
Androgens	Masculinization female	Tomboyish behavior	
Progestins	Masculinization female	Tomboyish behavior	
Diethylstilbestrol	Clitoris hypertrophy		Adenocarcinoma vagina (adolescence)
Smoking	Low birth weight ↑Stillborn		Smaller at 1 year of age
Alcohol			
Chronic intake	Intrauterine growth failure	Fetal alcohol syndrome	Developmental delay
Acute administration		Withdrawal symptoms	?
Pollutants and Pesticides			
Mercury		Severe neurologic defects	Severe handicaps Mental retardation
Lead	Low birth weight	↑ Abortions Anemia	
DDT and metabolites		Enzyme induction	
Parathion	? Teratogen		
Fungicides	?	?	
Herbicides	?	?	
Miscellaneous			
Atropine		Tachycardia	
Hexamethonium		Ileus	
Tubocurarine	? Arthrogryposis Multiplex Congenita	Muscular paralysis	
LSD	? Minor limb deformities		?
Cloroquine		Deafness	

The awakening of enzymatic activities in the fetus follows a timetable which will determine its metabolic capabilities at different stages of gestation. It is over this constantly changing background that drugs will exert their pharmacologic or toxic effects.

From the point of view of the obstetrician treating the mother, the fetus could be considered little more than a nuisance. Despite continuous efforts to identify adverse effects, the lack of precision of clinical evaluation for detecting biochemical and behavioral lesions imposes restrictions on the use of drugs during pregnancy. Hopefully, present day empiricisms will be replaced by a sophisticated type of fetal pharmacology. Information must be gathered on the amounts of each drug transferred to the fetus, as well as the distribution, excretion, biochemical actions, and long-term effects of these drugs on growth and development.

The natural consequence of the acquisition of this type of knowledge will be consideration of the fetus as a treatable patient and a rational approach to neonatal therapeutics.

A concentrated effort also must be made to uncover the adverse effects of environmental pollutants on the fetus and newborn and to find ways to eliminate them.

In summary, many gaps in perinatal pharmacology must be filled, but this task is not unsurmountable and it can be predicted that future years will witness an extraordinary growth in this relatively new discipline.

REFERENCES

1. **Joffe JM:** Influence of drug exposure of the father on perinatal outcome. Clin Perinatol 6: 21, 1979
2. **Csogor SJ, Custak J, Pressler A:** Modifications of albumin transport capacity in pregnant women and newborn infants. Biol Neonate 13: 311, 1968
3. **Rauramo LM, Pulkiven M, Hartiala K:** Glucuronide formation in parturients. Ann Med Exp Biol Fenn 41:32, 1963
4. **Crawford JS, Rudofsky S:** Some alterations in the pattern of drug metabolism associated with pregnancy, oral contraceptives, and the newly born. Br J Anaesth 38:446, 1966
5. **Mirkin BL:** Diphenylhydantoin placental transport, fetal localization, neonatal metabolism and possible teratogenic effects. J Pediatr 78:329, 1971
6. **Boreus LO:** Pharmacology of the human fetus dose effect relationships for acetylcholine during ontogenesis. Biol Neonate 11:328, 1967
7. **Rane A, Sjogvist F, Orrenius S:** Drugs and fetal metabolism. Clin Pharmacol Ther 14:666, 1973
8. **Rane A, Ackermann E:** Metabolism of ethylmorphine and aniline in human fetal liver. Clin Pharmacol Ther 13:663, 1972
9. **O'Donoghue SEF:** Distribution of pethidine and chlorpromazine in maternal, fetal, and neonatal biological fluids. Nature 229:124, 1971
10. **Znamenacek K, Pribylova H:** Glucose and insulin application or glycaemic curves in newborn infants. Cesk Pediatr 18:104, 1963
11. **Jersko WJ, Khanna N, Levy G, Stern L, Yaffe SJ:** Riboflavin absorption and excretion in the neonate. Pediatrics 45:945, 1970
12. **Weingaertrier L, Sitka V, et al:** Studies on the activity of a new antimycotic agent (Bay b 5097) in children. Int J Clin Pharmacol 6:358, 1972
13. **Huang NN, High RH:** Comparison of serum levels following the administration of oral and parenteral preparations of penicillin to infants and children of various age groups. Pediatrics 42:657, 1953
14. **Boothman R, Kerr MM, et al:** Absorption and excretion of cephalexin by the newborn infant. Arch Dis Child 48:147, 1973
15. **Salverio J, Poole JW:** Serum concentrations of ampicillin in newborn infants after oral administration. Pediatrics 51:578, 1973
16. **Grossman M, Ticknor W:** Serum levels of ampicillin, cephalathium, cloxadthium, and nafcillin in the newborn infant. Antimicrob Agents Chemother 5:214, 1965
17. **Wallin A, Jalling B, Boreous LO:** Plasma concentrations of phenobarbital in the neonate during prophylaxis for neonatal hyperbilirubinemia. J Pediatr 85:392, 1974
18. **Rohwedder HJ, Simon C, Kubler W, Hohfnauer M:** Untersuchungen Uber Die Pharmakokinetik Von Nalidixinsaure GEl Kinder Verschiedenen Alters. Z Kinderheilkd 109:124, 1970
19. **Morselli PL, Assael BM, Gomeni R, Mandelli M, Marini A, Reali E, Visconti U:** Digoxin pharmacokinetics during human development. In Morselli PL, Garattini S, Sereni F (eds): Basic and Therapeutic Aspect of the Perinatal Pharmacology, pp 377—392. New York, Raven Press, 1975
20. **Morselli PL, Principi N, Tognoni G, Reali E, Belvedere G, Standen SM, Sereni F:** Diazepam elimination in premature and full term infants and children. J Perinat Med 1:133, 1973
21. **Reidenberg MM, James M, Dring LG:** The rate of procaine hydrolysis in the serum of normal subjects and diseased patients. Clin Pharmacol Ther 13:279, 1972

22. **Shnider SM, Way EL:** Plasma levels of lidocaine in mother and newborn following obstetrical conduction anesthesia. Clin Applicat Anesth 29:951, 1968

23. **Moya F, Smith BE:** Uptake, distribution, and placental transport of drugs and anesthetics. Anesthesiology 26:465, 1965

24. **Joelsson I, Adamson K:** The effects of pharmacologic agents upon the fetus and newborn. Am J Obstet Gynecol 96:437, 1966

25. **Siker ES, Wolfson B, Stewart WD, et al:** Placental transfer of methoxyflurane. Br J Anaesth 40: 588, 1968

26. **Laham S:** Studies on placental transfer of trichloroethylene. Industr Med Surg 39:46, 1970

27. **Smith CA:** The effect of obstetrical anesthesia upon the oxygenation of maternal and fetal blood with particular reference to cyclopropane. Surg Gynecol Obstet 69:584, 1939

28. **Stenger VG, Andersen T, Eitzmen D, et al:** Cyclopropane anesthesia. Am J Obstet Gynecol 96:201, 1966

29. **Root B, Eichner E, Sunshine I:** Blood secobarbital levels and their clinical correlation in mothers and newborn infants. Am J Obstet Gynecol 81:948, 1961

30. **Kron RE, Stein M, Goddard KE:** Newborn sucking behavior affected by obstetric sedation. Pediatrics 37:1072, 1966

31. **Finster M, Mark LC, Morishima HO, et al:** Plasma thiopental concentrations in the newborn following delivery under thiopental nitrous oxide anesthesia. Am J Obstet Gynecol 95:621, 1966

32. **Carrier G, Hume A, et al:** Disposition of barbiturates in maternal blood, fetal blood, and amniotic fluid. Am J Obstet Gynecol 105: 1069, 1969

33. **Ganshorn A, Kurz H:** Unterschiede zwischen der proteinbindung neugeborener und ihre bedeutung fur die pharmakologische wirkung. Arch Pharmakol Exp Pathol 260 (2/3)117:118, 1968

34. **Crawford JS, Rudolfsky S:** The placental transmission of pethidine. Br J Anaesth 37:929, 1965

35. **Shnider SM, Way EL, Lord MJ:** Rate of appearance and disappearance of meperidine in fetal blood after administration of the narcotic to the mother. Anesthesiology 27:227, 1966

36. **Morrison JC, Wiser SI, et al:** Metabolites of meperidine related to fetal depression. Am J Obstet Gynecol 115:1132, 1973

37. **Idanpaan-Heikkila J, Jouppila P, Akerblom HK, et al:** Elimination and metabolic effects of ethanol in mother, fetus, and newborn infant. Am J Obstet Gynecol 112:387, 1972

38. **Wagner L, Wagner G, Guerrero J:** Effect of alcohol on premature infants. Am J Obstet Gynecol 108:308, 1970

39. **Dawood MY, Wang CF, Gupta R, et al:** Fetal contribution to oxytocin in human labor. Obstet Gynecol 52:205, 1978

40. **Davis DP, Gomersall R, Robertson R, Gray OP, Turnbull AC:** Neonatal jaundice and maternal oxytocin infusion. Br Med J 3:476, 1973

41. **Puri CP, Baliga N, Aggarival N, Hingoram V, Jaumus KR:** Prostaglandin F2L disappearance and concentration in amniotic fluid and blood of women undergoing abortion with intra-amniotic hypertonic saline. Prostaglandins 12: 679, 1975

42. **Bray RE, Boe RW, Johnson WL:** Transfer of ampicillin into fetus and amniotic fluid from maternal plasma in late pregnancy. Am J Obstet Gynecol 96:938, 1966

43. **MacAuley Abou Sabe M, Charles D:** Placental transfer of ampicillin. Am J Obstet Gynecol 96:943, 1966

44. **Hutchinson JH, Carswell F, et al:** Congenital goitre and hypothyroidism produced by maternal ingestion of iodines. Lancet 1:1241, 1970

45. **Sherman JL, Locke RV:** Transplacental neonatal digitalis intoxication. Cardiology 6:834, 1960

46. **Rogers MC, Willerson JT, et al:** Serum digoxin concentration in the human fetus, neonate, and infant. N Engl J Med 287:1010, 1972

47. **Armstrong SR, Longmore DBL:** The effects of cardioactive drugs on the performance of cultured fetal hearts. Nature 243:350, 1973

48. **Sandler M, Ruthren CR, Constractor SF, Wood C, et al:** Transmission of noradrenaline across the human placenta. Nature (London) 197:598, 1963

49. **Rodriguez SV, Leikin SL, Miller MC:** Neonatal thrombocytopenia associated with antepartum administration of thiazide drugs. N Engl J Med 270:881, 1964

50. **Merenstein, GB, et al:** Effect of maternal thiazides on platelet counts of newborn infants. J Pediatr 76:766, 1970

51. **Bloomfield DK:** Fetal deaths and malformations associated with the use of coumarin derivatives in pregnancy. Am J Obstet Gynecol 107:883, 1970

52. **Fillmore SJ, McDevitt E:** Effects of coumarin compounds on the fetus. Ann Intern Med 73: 731, 1970

53. **Shaul WL, Emery H, Hall JG:** Chondrodysplasia punctata and maternal Warfarin use during pregnancy. Am J Dis Child 129:360, 1975

54. **Monson RR, Rosenberg L, Hartz SC:** Diphenylhydantoin and selected congenital malformations. N Engl J Med 289, 1049, 1973

55. **Hanson JW, Myrianthopoulos NC, Harvey MAS, Smith DW:** Risks to the offspring of

women treated with hydantoin anticonvulsants with emphasis on the fetal hydantoin syndrome. J Pediatr 89:662, 1976

56. **Blackhall MI, Buckley GA, Roberts DV, et al:** Drug-induced neonatal myasthenia. J Obstet Gynaecol Br Commonw 76:157, 1969

57. **Nightingale DA, Glass AG, Bachmann L:** Neuromuscular blockade by succinylcholine in children. Anesthesiology 27:736, 1966

58. **Cohen EN, Cobascio A, Fleischli G:** The distribution and fate of d-tubocurarine. J Pharmacol Exp Ther 147:120, 1965

59. **Towell ME, Hyman AI, Stanley L, et al:** Reserpine administration during pregnancy. Am J Obstet Gynecol 92:711, 1965

60. **Savory J, Monif GRG:** Serum calcium levels in cord sera of the progeny of mothers treated with magnesium sulfate for toxemia of pregnancy. Am J Ostet Gynecol 110:556, 1971

61. **Milner RDG, Chourkrey SK:** Effects of fetal exposure to diazoxide in man. Arch Dis Child 47:537, 1972

62. **Clarren SK, Smith DW:** The fetal alcohol syndrome. N Engl J Med 298:1063, 1978

63. **Woody JN, London WL, Wilbanks GD:** Lithium toxicity in a newborn. Pediatrics 47:94, 1971

64. **Pantuck EJ, Kuntzman R, Conney AH:** Decreased concentration of phenacetin in plasma of cigarette smokers. Science 175:1248, 1972

65. **Keeri-Szanto M, Ronieray JR:** Atmospheric pollution and pentazocine metabolism. Lancet 1:947, 1971

66. **Liggins GC:** The prevention of RDS by maternal betamethasone administration. In Stern L (ed): Lung Maturation and the Prevention of Hyaline Membrane Disease. pp 189–198. Ross Lab, Columbus, 1975

67. **Ballard P, Benson B, Breliner A:** Glucocorticoid effects in the fetal lung. Ann Rev Resp Dis (Suppl) 115:29, 1977

68. **Miller RW:** Cola-colored babies chlorobiphenyl poisoning in Japan. Teratology 4:211, 1971

69. **Herbst AL, Poskanzer DC, Robboy SJ, Friedlander L, Scully RE:** Prenatal exposure to stilbestrol. N Engl J Med 292:334, 1975

70. **Brown BW:** Fatal phenol poisoning from improperly laundered diapers. Am J Public Health 60:901, 1970

71. **McGrail VB, Bordiuk JM, Keitel H:** Systemic hypertension following ocular administration of phenylephrine to the neonate. Am J Pediatr Res 6:144, 1972

72. **Bauer CR, Trottier MCT, Stern L:** Cyclogyl toxicity in the neonate. J Pediatr 82:501, 1973

73. **Aldridge AB, Aranda JV, Neims AH:** Caffeine metabolism in the newborn. Clin Pharmacol Ther 25:447, 1979

74. **Aranda JV, Turmen T:** Methylxanthines in apnea of prematurity. Clin Perinatol 6:87, 1979

75. **Evans M, Bhat R, Vadepalli M, Fisher E, Hastreiter A, Vidyasagar D:** Disposition of indomethacin in premature infants. Pediatr Res 12:404, 1978

76. **Freidman Z, Whitman V, Maisels MJ, Berman W, Marks KH, Vesell ES:** Indomethacin disposition in indomethacin induced-platelet dysfunction in premature infants. J Clin Pharmacol 18:272–279, 1978

77. **Bell EF, Brown EJ, Sinclair JC, Zipursky A:** Vitamin E absorption in small premature infants. Pediatrics 63:830, 1979

78. **Ehrenkranz RA, Bonta BW, Ablow RC, Warshaw JB:** Amelioration of bronchopulmonary dysplasia after vitamin E administration. N Engl J Med 299:564, 1978

79. **Phelps D, Rosenbaum AL:** The role of tocopherol in oxygen induced retinopathy: Kitten model. Pediatrics 59:998, 1977

80. **Johnson L, Schaffer D, Boggs TR Jr:** The premature infant, vitamin E deficiency and retrolental fibroplasia. Am J Clin Nutr 27:1158, 1974

81. **Aranda JV, Perez J, Sotar DS et al:** Pharmacokinetic disposition and protein binding of furosemide in newborn infants. J Pediatr 93:507, 1978

82. **Pitlick W, Painter M, Pippenger C:** Phenobarbital pharmacokinetics in neonates. Clin Pharmacol Ther 23:346, 1978

83. **Painter MJ, Pippenger C, MacDonald H, Pitlick W:** Phenobarbital and diphenylhydantoin levels in neonates with seizures. J Pediatr 92:315, 1978

84. **Nyberg L, Wettrell G:** Digoxin dosage schedules for neonates and infants based on pharmacokinetic considerations. Clin Pharmacokinet 3:453–461, 1978

Appendices*

Contents

* The editor wishes to thank the following persons for their help in preparing the Appendix tables: Roger Boeckx, Ph.D., Naomi Luban, M.D., Sandra Robbins, R.D., Mhairi MacDonald, M.D., Douglas Smith, Ph.D., Steven Shapiro, M.D., Samuel Shelburne, M.D., Edward J. Ruley, M.D., Peter Holbrook, M.D., and William Rodriguez, M.D.

A

Laboratory Values

1. BLOOD CHEMISTRIES

Appendix A-1**A**. Normal Blood Chemistry Values, Term Infants.

Determination	Sample Source	Cord	1–12 hr	12–24 hr	24–48 hr	48–72 hr
Sodium, mmol/l	Capillary	147 (126–166)	143 (124–156)	145 (132–159)	148 (134–160)	149 (139–162)
Potassium, mmol/l		7.8 (5.6–12)	6.4 (5.3–7.3)	6.3 (5.3–8.9)	6.0 (5.2–7.3)	5.9 (5.0–7.7)
Chloride, mmol/l		103 (98–110)	100.7 (90–111)	103 (87–114)	102 (92–114)	103 (93–112)
Calcium, mg/dl		9.3 (8.2–11.1)	8.4 (7.3–9.2)	7.8 (6.9–9.4)	8.0 (6.1–9.9)	7.9 (5.9–9.7)
Phosphorus, mg/dl		5.6 (3.7–8.1)	6.1 (3.5–8.6)	5.7 (2.9–8.1)	5.9 (3.0–8.7)	5.8 (2.8–7.6)
Blood urea, mg/dl		29 (21–40)	27 (8–34)	33 (9–63)	32 (13–77)	31 (13–68)
Total protein, g/dl		6.1 (4.8–7.3)	6.6 (5.6–8.5)	6.6 (5.8–8.2)	6.9 (5.9–8.2)	7.2 (6.0–8.5)
Glucose, mg/dl		73 (45–96)	63 (40–97)	63 (42–104)	56 (30–91)	59 (40–90)
Lactic acid, mg/dl		19.5 (11–30)	14.6 (11–24)	14.0 (10–23)	14.3 (9–22)	13.5 (7–21)
Lactate, mmol/l†		2.0–3.0	2.0			

(* Acharya PT, Payne WW: Arch Dis Child 40:430, 1965
† Daniel SS, Adamsons K Jr, James LS: Pediatrics 37:942, 1966, Copyright © American Academy of Pediatrics, 1966)

Appendix A-1**B**. Normal Blood Chemistry Values, Low-Birth-Weight Infants, Capillary Blood, First Day.

Determination	<1000	1001–1500	1501–2000	2001–2500
Sodium, mmol/l	138	133	135	134
Potassium, mmol/l	6.4	6.0	5.4	5.6
Chloride, mmol/l	100	101	105	104
Total CO_2, mmol/l	19	20	20	20
Urea, mg/dl	22	21	16	16
Total protein g/dl	4.8	4.8	5.2	5.3

(Pincus JB et al: Pediatrics, 18:39, 1956; Copyright © American Academy of Pediatrics, 1956)

1175

Appendix A-1**C**. Blood Chemistry Values in Premature Infants During the First 7 Weeks of Life (Birth Weight 1500–1750 g).

Constituent	Age 1 Week			Age 3 Weeks			Age 5 Weeks			Age 7 Weeks		
	Mean	SD	Range	Mean	SD	Range	Mean	SD	Range	Mean	SD	Range
Na (mmol/l)	139.6	±3.2	133–146	136.3	±2.9	129–142	136.8	±2.5	133–148	137.2	±1.8	133–142
K (mmol/l)	5.6	±0.5	4.6–6.7	5.8	±0.6	4.5–7.1	5.5	±0.6	4.5–6.6	5.7	±0.5	4.6–7.1
Cl (mmol/l)	108.2	±3.7	100–117	108.3	±3.9	102–116	107.0	±3.5	100–115	107.0	±3.3	101–115
CO_2 (mmol/l)	20.3	±2.8	13.8–27.1	18.4	±3.5	12.4–26.2	20.4	±3.4	12.5–26.1	20.6	±3.1	13.7–26.9
Ca (mg/dl)	9.2	±1.1	6.1–11.6	9.6	±0.5	8.1–11.0	9.4	±0.5	8.6–10.5	9.5	±0.7	8.6–10.8
P (mg/dl)	7.6	±1.1	5.4–10.9	7.5	±0.7	6.2–8.7	7.0	±0.6	5.6–7.9	6.8	±0.8	4.2–8.2
BUN (mg/dl)	9.3	±5.2	3.1–25.5	13.3	±7.8	2.1–31.4	13.3	±7.1	2.0–26.5	13.4	±6.7	2.5–30.5
Total protein (g/dl)	5.49	±0.42	4.40–6.26	5.38	±0.48	4.28–6.70	4.98	±0.50	4.14–6.90	4.93	±0.61	4.02–5.86
Albumin (g/dl)	3.85	±0.30	3.28–4.50	3.92	±0.42	3.16–5.26	3.73	±0.34	3.20–4.34	3.89	±0.53	3.40–4.60
Globulin (g/dl)	1.58	±0.33	0.88–2.20	1.44	±0.63	0.62–2.90	1.17	±0.49	0.48–1.48	1.12	±0.33	0.5–2.60
Hb (g/dl)	17.8	±2.7	11.4–24.8	14.7	±2.1	9.0–19.4	11.5	±2.0	7.2–18.6	10.0	±1.3	7.5–13.9

(Adapted from Thomas J, Reichelderfer T: Clin Chem 14:272, 1968)

38

Appendix A-1**D**. Other Serum Values.

Ammonia nitrogen (μg/dl) newborn	Up to 150
Carotene (μg/dl)	
Birth	70 (0–400)
1 year	340 (300–1800)
Cholesterol (mg/dl)	
Premature, cord	67 (47–98)
Full-term, cord	67 (45–98)
Full-term, newborn	85 (45–167)
3 days–1 year	130 (69–174)
2–14 years	188 (138–242)
Copper (μg/dl)	
0–6 months	<70
6 months–5 years	27–153
Serum enzymes*	
Leucine amino peptidase (units/l)	29–59
CPK (IU/l)	
Premature	0–210
Full-term 0–3 weeks	22–367
3 weeks–3 months	15–134
3 months–9 months	7–97
9 months–1 year	0–47
SGOT, newborn (IU/l)*	Up to 54
Free fatty acids (μmol/l)	[Depends on fasting interval]
Newborn	435–1375
Child (after 14-hour fast)	500–898
Magnesium (mmol/l)	0.75–1.25
Osmolarity (mosm/l)	270–290
Phenylalanine (mg/dl)	
Newborn	Up to 4.0
Older child	0.8–1.8
Zinc (μg/dl)	77–137

* Normal values depend on method used
(Data from Normal Values for Pediatric Clinical Chemistry, Special Committee on Pediatric Clinical Chemistry, American Association of Clinical Chemists, August, 1974)

Appendix A-1E. Serum Amino Acids (μmol/dl).

Amino Acid	1st Day	16 Day–4 Mo	9 Mo–2 Yr	3 Yr–10 Yr	11 Yr+	Adult
Taurine	10.5–25.5		1.4–9.1	5.7–11.5	3.3–16.5	2.7–16.8
OH-Proline	0–8.0			2.5		0
Aspartic acid	0–2.0	1.7–2.1	0–0.9	0.4–2.0	0.08–5.4	0–2.4
Threonine	15.5–27.5	14.1–21.3	3.3–12.8	4.2–9.5	7.9–19.0	7.9–24.6
Serine	19.5–34.5	10.4–15.8	2.4–17.2	7.9–11.2	6.5–19.3	6.7–19.3
Asp + Glu	65.5–115.5		4.6–29.0	5.7–46.7		41.3–69.0
Proline	15.5–30.5	14.1–24.5	5.1–18.5	6.8–14.8	11.1–44.7	10.0–44.2
Glutamic acid	3.0–10.0			2.3–25.0	1.1–10.5	1.4–19.2
Glycine	18.5–73.5	17.8–24.8	5.6–30.8	11.7–22.3	14.4–48.8	12.0–55.3
Alanine	32.5–42.5	23.9–34.5	9.9–31.3	13.7–30.5	21.0–50.2	20.9–65.9
Valine	8.0–18.0	12.3–19.9	5.7–26.2	12.8–28.3	11.6–31.7	11.6–31.5
Cystine	5.5–7.5	3.3–5.1		4.5–7.7	3.7–14.0	4.8–14.1
Methionine	3.0–4.0	1.5–2.1	0.3–2.9	1.1–1.6	1.4–3.6	0.6–3.9
Isoleucine	2.0–6.0	3.1–4.7	2.6–9.4	2.8–8.4	3.5–9.8	3.5–9.7
Leucine	4.5–9.5	5.6–9.8	4.5–15.5	5.6–17.8	7.1–17.5	7.1–17.5
Tyrosine	2.0–22.0	3.3–7.5	1.1–12.2	3.1–7.1	3.6–8.7	2.1–8.7
Phenylalanine	7.0–11.0	4.5–6.5	2.3–6.9	2.6–6.1	3.8–11.6	3.7–11.5
Ornithine	7.0–11.0	3.7–6.1	1.0–10.7	2.7–8.6	2.6–10.6	2.9–12.5
Lysine	13.0–25.0	11.7–16.3	4.5–14.4	7.1–15.1	11.5–27.0	8.2–23.6
Histidine	3.0–7.0	6.4–9.2	2.4–11.2	2.4–8.5	3.7–11.7	3.1–10.6
Arginine	3.0–7.0	5.3–7.1	1.1–6.5	2.3–8.6	4.1–15.7	2.1–13.7
Tryptophan	1.5–4.5				0–7.3	
Citrulline					0–5.5	
Ethanolamine					0–1.2	
Alpha-amino- n-butyric acid					0.83–2.9	
Methylhistidine					0–0.96	(1 methyl)
					0.18–0.58	(3 methyl)

(Dickinson JC, Rosenblum H, Hamilton PB: Pediatrics 36:7, 1965; Copyright © American Academy of Pediatrics; Scriver CR, Lamm P, Clow CL: Am J Clin Nutr 24:876, 1971; Bio-Cal automatic amino acid analyzer)

2. URINE

Appendix A-2**A**. Urinary Values. (See also Chap. 30.)

	17-Ketosteroids	17-Hydroxycorticoids	Pregnanetriol
Adrenal Steroids (*mg/day*)			
Newborn–1 wk	2.0–2.5	0.05–0.3	0.01
1 wk–3 mo	0.5	0.05–0.5	0.01
3 mo–1 yr	0.5	0.1–0.5	0.01
Electrolytes (*depend on intake*)			
Sodium (mmol/l urine)	18–60		
Potassium (mmol/l urine)	10–40		
Chloride (mmol/kg/day)	1.7–8.5		
Bicarbonate (mmol/l)	1.5–2.0		
Calcium (mmol/kg/day)	<2.0		
Other Urinary Values			
Ammonia (μmol/min/m^2)			
infants 2–11.5 mo	4.0–40		
older children	5.9–16.5		
Creatinine (mg/kg/day)			
premature 2–12 wks	8.3–19.9		
full-term 1–7 wks	10.0–15.5		
child 2–3 yrs	6.4–21.9		
Glucose (mg/l)	50		
Osmolarity (infant) (mosm/l)	50–600		
VMA-infant (μg/mg creatinine)	5–19	(<1 mg/24h)	
HVA (μg/mg creatinine)	3–16		
Protein	Trace		
Urea nitrogen (mg/l)	300–3,000		
(depends on intake)			
Titratable acidity (μmol/min/m^2)	[minus bicarbonate]		
Premature	0–12		
Term	0–11		

(Data from Normal Values for Pediatric Clinical Chemistry, Special Committee on Pediatric Clinical Chemistry, American Association of Clinical Chemists, August, 1974)

Appendix A-2**B**. Average Values for Clearance in Infants, Children, and Adults. (Collected from the literature by Weil)

	Premature	Newborn	3 mo	6 mo	12 mo	24 mo	Adult
Clearance (ml/min/1.73 m^2)							
Urea	25	30	45	50	60	70	70
Endog. Creatinine		40–65*		75	100		100
Mannitol	45	50	70	105	120	125	125
Inulin	45	40	70				125
Diodrast		70					650
PAH	150	200	300	500	550	650	650
Phosphate		7		13		15	17
Tm (mg/min/1.73 m^2)							
PAH	13	25	40	65	70	75	75
Glucose		60	170				350

* Normal Values for Pediatric Clinical Chemistry
(Adapted from Smith CA: Physiology of the Newborn. p. 327. Springfield, (Ill.), Charles C Thomas, 1959)

3. CEREBROSPINAL FLUID

Appendix A-3. Cerebrospinal Fluid Values in
Healthy Newborns.

	Range	Mean	2 SD
Red blood cells	0–1070	9	0–884
Polymorphs	0–70	3	0–27
Lymphocytes	0–20	2	0–24
Proteins (mg/dl)	32–240	63	27–144
Glucose (mg/dl)	32–78	51	35–64

CSF protein* (mg/dl)	
premature	50–130 mg/dl
full-term	40–120 mg/dl
older child	15–40 mg/dl
LDH* (IU/l)	
Infant, 2½ hr–10 day	2.3–84
Infant >10 day	6.3–30

* Normal Values for Pediatric Clinical Chemistry
(Naidoo T: South Afr Med J 42:933, 1968)

4. THYROID FUNCTION TESTS

Appendix A-4. Range of Values for PBI, BEI, Total T_4, and the T_3 Resin Uptake During the Neonatal
Period.

Age	PBI Range (mean) μg/dl	BEI Range (mean) μg/dl	T_4 Range (mean) μg/dl	T_3RU Range (mean) % standard
Cord	4.3–9.5 (5.9)	3.6–7.4 (5.5)	7.3–15.3 (11.3)	64–100 (84)
1–3 Days	7.2–16.8 (12.0)	5.7–14.1 (9.9)	10.1–20.9 (15.5)	90–140 (115)
1–2 Weeks	{3.8–11.0 (7.4)}	3.5–7.9 (5.1)	9.8–16.6 (13.2)	74–114 (94)
2–5 Weeks			8.2–16.6 (12.3)	66–114 (90)

PBI = Protein-bound iodine
BEI = Butanol-extractable iodine
T_4 = Total thyroxine (determined by competitive binding assays)
T_3RU = Triiodothyronine resin uptake

B
Hematologic Values

1. HEMOGLOBIN

Appendix B-1. Normal Hematologic Values During the First 12 Weeks of Life in the Term Infant as Determined by an Electronic Cell Counter.

Age	No. of Cases	Hb g/dl ± SD	RBC × 10^6 ± SD	Hct % ± SD	MCV μ^3 ± SD	MCHC % ± SD	Retic % ± SD
Days							
1	19	19.0±2.2	5.14±0.7	61±7.4	119±9.4	31.6±1.9	3.2±1.4
2	19	19.0±1.9	5.15±0.8	60±6.4	115±7.0	31.6±1.4	3.2±1.3
3	19	18.7±3.4	5.11±0.7	62±9.3	116±5.3	31.1±2.8	2.8±1.7
4	10	18.6±2.1	5.00±0.6	57±8.1	114±7.5	32.6±1.5	1.8±1.1
5	12	17.6±1.1	4.97±0.4	57±7.3	114±8.9	30.9±2.2	1.2±0.2
6	15	17.4±2.2	5.00±0.7	54±7.2	113±10.0	32.2±1.6	0.6±0.2
7	12	17.9±2.5	4.86±0.6	56±9.4	118±11.2	32.0±1.6	0.5±0.4
Weeks							
1–2	32	17.3±2.3	4.80±0.8	54±8.3	112±19.0	32.1±2.9	0.5±0.3
2–3	11	15.6±2.6	4.20±0.6	46±7.3	111±8.2	33.9±1.9	0.8±0.6
3–4	17	14.2±2.1	4.00±0.6	43±5.7	105±7.5	33.5±1.6	0.6±0.3
4–5	15	12.7±1.6	3.60±0.4	36±4.8	101±8.1	34.9±1.6	0.9±0.8
5–6	10	11.9±1.5	3.55±0.2	36±6.2	102±10.2	34.1±2.9	1.0±0.7
6–7	10	12.0±1.5	3.40±0.4	36±4.8	105±12.0	33.8±2.3	1.2±0.7
7–8	17	11.1±1.1	3.40±0.4	33±3.7	100±13.0	33.7±2.6	1.5±0.7
8–9	13	10.7±0.9	3.40±0.5	31±2.5	93±12.0	34.1±2.2	1.8±1.0
9–10	12	11.2±0.9	3.60±0.3	32±2.7	91±9.3	34.3±2.9	1.2±0.6
10–11	11	11.4±0.9	3.70±0.4	34±2.1	91±7.7	33.2±2.4	1.2±0.7
11–12	13	11.3±0.9	3.70±0.3	33±3.3	88±7.9	34.8±2.2	0.7±0.3

(Matoth Y et al: Acta Paediatr Scand 60:317, 1971)

2. WHITE BLOOD CELLS

Appendix B-2. The White-Blood-Cell Count and the Differential Count During the First 2 Weeks of Life.

Age	Leukocytes	Neutrophils			Eosinophils	Baso-phils	Lymphocytes	Monocytes
		Total	*Seg*	*Band*				
Birth								
Mean	18,100	11,000	9400	1600	400	100	5500	1050
Range	9.0–30.0	6.0–26			20–850	0–640	2.0–11.0	0.4–3.1
Mean %	—	61	52	9	2.2	0.6	31	5.8
7 Days								
Mean	12,200	5500	4700	830	500	50	5000	1100
Range	5.0–21.0	1.5–10.0			70–1100	0–250	2.0–17.0	0.3–2.7
Mean %	—	45	39	6	4.1	0.4	41	9.1
14 Days								
Mean	11,400	4500	3900	630	350	50	5500	1000
Range	5.0–20.0	1.0–9.5			70–1000	0–230	2.0–17.0	0.2–2.4
Mean %	—	40	34	5.5	3.1	0.4	48	8.8

3. PLATELETS

Appendix B-3**A**. Venous Platelet Counts* in Normal Low-Birth-Weight Infants.

Day	No. of Infants	Mean (mm³)	Range (1,000's)
0	60	203,000	80–356
3	47	207,000	61–335
5	14	233,000	100–502
7	52	319,000	124–678
10	40	399,000	172–680
14	50	386,000	147–670
21	47	388,000	201–720
28	40	384,000	212–625

* Manual method
(Appleyard WJ, Bunton WA: Biol Neonate 17:30, 1971)

Appendix B-3**B**. Platelet Counts in Full-Term Infants.

Day	Mean	Range
Cord	200,000	100,000–280,000
1	192,000	100,000–260,000
3	213,000	80,000–320,000
7	248,000	100,000–300,000
14	252,000	

(Behrman R (ed): Neonatology: Diseases of the Fetus and Infant. St. Louis, CV Mosby, 1973)

4. BONE MARROW

Appendix B-4. The Bone Marrow Differential During the First Week of Life.

	0–24 hours (%)	7 days (%)	Adult (%)
Myeloblasts	0–2	0–3	0.3–50
Promyelocytes	0.5–6.0	0.5–7.0	1.0–8.0
Myelocytes	1.0–9.0	1.0–11.0	5.5–22.5
Metamyelocytes	4.5–25.0	7.0–35.0	13.0–32.0
Band forms	10.0–40.0	11.0–45.0	—
Erythroblasts	0–1.0	0–0.5	1.0–8.0
Proerythroblasts	0.5–9.0	0–0.5	2.0–10.0
Normoblasts	18.0–41.0	0–15.0	7.0–32.0
Myeloid:erythroid ratio	1.5:1.0	6.5:1.0	3.5:1.0

(Oski FA, Naiman JL: Hematologic Problems in the Newborn, 2nd ed. Philadelphia, WB Saunders, 1972; Adapted from Shapiro, Bassen, 1941; and Gardner D et al: Arch Dis Child 27:214, 1952)

5. SERUM IRON, IRON-BINDING CAPACITY

Appendix B-5. Serum Iron and Iron-binding Capacity in the Newborn and Mother.

Serum iron (μg/dl)		Total iron binding capacity (μg/dl)		
Infant	*Mother*	*Infant*	*Mother*	**Author**
173	98	259	470	Hagberg (1953)
147	80	226	446	Laurell (1947)
193	—	240	—	Sturgeon (1954)
(145–240)		(147–468)		
159	—	—	—	Vahlquist and others (1941)
(106–227)				

(Oski FA, Naiman JL: Hematologic Problems in the Newborn, 2nd ed. Philadelphia, WB Saunders, 1972)

Appendix B-6. Coagulation Factor Activity Levels for Preterm and Term Infants.

Subject	I (mg/100 ml)	II	V	VII-X	VIII	IX	XI	XII	XIII	Plasminogen	Antithrombin III	Prekallikrein (Fletcher Factor)	HMW Kininogen
					Coagulation Factor—Percent Activity								
Normal adult	315±60†	100	100	100	100	100	100	100	100	61–125	98±9	100	100
Preterm infant 24–31 wks	282†	31†	73†	39†	87†	22†	20†	20†	—	—	27†	27†	28†
Preterm infant 27–31 wks	256±70‡	30±8‡	91±30‡	38±14‡	90†	27†	—	27†	—	24±8†	29±3‡	—	—
Preterm infant 32–35 wks	260±80‡	33±11‡	90±12‡	42±20‡	120†	34±14‡	—	33†	—	330±10†	44±10‡	—	—
Preterm infant 36–39 wks	230±50‡	52±20†	85±15†	43±20†	125†	43±13‡	—	—	—	35±11†	51±10‡	—	—
Term infant	215±35†	54±15*	114(56–200)* 99(40–150)†	56±16*	97(50–180) 168†	28*(15–42)	31*	47±18*	50†	43±16†	60±16†	33±6*	56±12.5*
Older infant	340±70‡ (21 days)	97±4† (45–60 days)	100‡ (21 days)	92±10‡ (21 days)	—	72±15‡ (21–45 days)	—	100† (14 days)	100† (1 mo)	61† (6 mo)	82† (6 mo)	—	—

Values represent smoothed means ± 1 standard deviation or (ranges) from cord,* venous,* or capillary‡ samples in the first 24 hours of life. Other values are given for older infants at age when values approximate adult levels. All data taken from material referenced in the text.
(Hathaway WE, Bonnar J: Perinatal Coagulation. New York, Grune & Stratton, 1978)

C
Physiologic Values

1. BLOOD PRESSURE

Appendix C-1. Average Systolic, Diastolic, and Mean Blood Pressures During the First 12 Hours of Life in Normal Newborn Infants Grouped According to Birth Weight.

Birth Weight	Hour	1	2	3	4	5	6	7	8	9	10	11	12
1001 to 2000 g	Systolic	49	49	51	52	53	52	52	52	51	51	49	50
	Diastolic	26	27	28	29	31	31	31	31	31	30	29	38
	Mean	35	36	37	39	40	40	39	39	38	37	37	38
2001 to 3000 g	Systolic	59	57	60	60	61	58	64	60	63	61	60	59
	Diastolic	32	32	32	32	33	34	37	34	38	35	35	35
	Mean	43	41	43	43	44	43	45	43	44	44	43	42
Over 3000 g	Systolic	70	67	65	65	66	66	67	67	68	70	66	66
	Diastolic	44	41	39	41	40	41	41	41	44	43	41	41
	Mean	53	51	50	50	51	50	50	51	53	54	51	50

(Kitterman JA, Phibbs RH, Tooley WH: Pediatrics, 44:959, 1969; Copyright © American Academy of Pediatrics, 1969)

2. BLOOD PRESSURE BY BIRTH WEIGHT

Appendix C-2. Parabolic Regression (**middle line**) and 95% Confidence Limits (**top** and **bottom** lines) of Mean Aortic Blood Pressure on Birth Weight in Normal Newborn Infants During Hours 2 to 12 of Life.

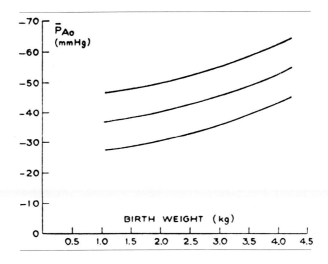

(Kitterman JA, Phibbs RH, Tooley WH, Pediatrics 44:959, 1969; Copyright © American Academy of Pediatrics, 1969)

3. ACID-BASE STATUS

Appendix C-3. Acid-base Status.

Determination	Vigorous Term Infants, Vaginal Delivery	Birth	1st hr	3rd hr	24 hr	2 Days	3 Days
pH	Umbilical artery	7.26					
	Umbilical vein	7.29					
pCO_2 torr	Arterial	54.5	38.8	38.3	33.6	34	35
	Venous	42.8					
O_2 sat.	Arterial	19.8	93.8	94.7	93.2		
	Venous	47.6					
pH	Left atrial		7.30	7.34	7.41	7.39 (temp. artery)	7.38 (temp. artery)
CO_2 content, mmol/l			20.6	21.9	21.4		

	Prematures						
	Capillary						
pH	<1250 g				7.36	7.35	7.35
pCO_2 torr					38	44	37
pH	>1250 g				7.39	7.39	7.38
pCO_2 torr					38	39	38

(Data of Weisbort LM et al: J Pediatr 52:395, 1958; Bucci E et al: Biol Neonate, 8:81, 1965)

4. SIGGAARD-ANDERSEN NOMOGRAM

Appendix C-4. Siggaard—Andersen Nomogram.

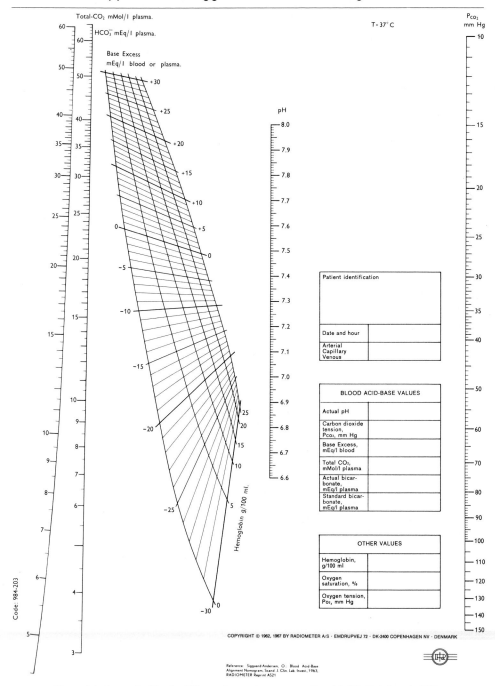

(Siggaard-Andersen O: Blood acid-base alignment nomogram, Scand J Clin Lab Invest, 1963, RADIOMETER Reprint AS21)

5. RIGHT-LEFT SHUNT CURVES

Appendix C-5. Right-Left Shunt Curves. (Arterial oxygen tensions at different right-to-left shunts, breathing 40%, 70%, and 100% oxygen. Calculations assumed hemoglobin 16 g/dl, arterial pH 7.4, temperature 37°C, constant arterial-venous saturation difference 13.8%, and no change in cardiac output or oxygen consumption.)

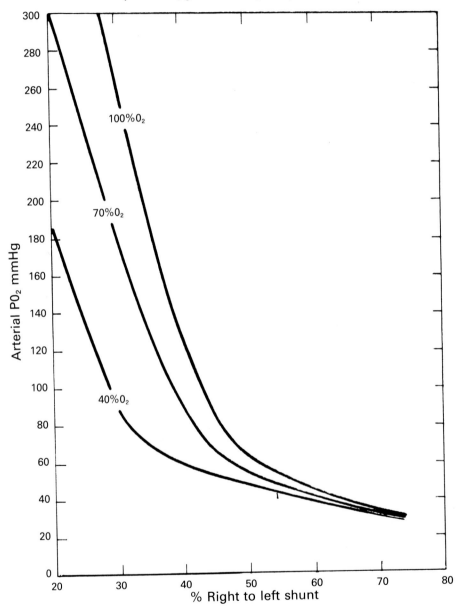

(Barnett H (ed): Pediatrics, 15th ed. Englewood Cliffs, NJ, Appleton-Century-Crofts, 1972)

6. HEMOGLOBIN-OXYGEN DISSOCIATION CURVES

Appendix C-6. Oxygen Dissociation Curves of Fetal and Adult
Hemoglobins at a pH of 7.4, Temperature 37° C.
(Cyanosis is observed at 5g unsaturated
hemoglobin, which corresponds to different arterial
tensions in the adult and the infant.)

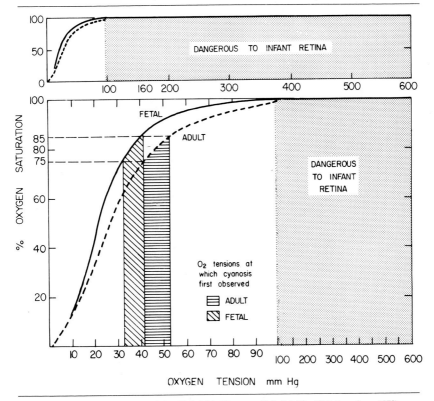

(Klaus MH, Fanaroff AA: Care of the High Risk Neonate. Philadelphia, WB Saunders, 1973)

D

Growth Parameters

1. GESTATIONAL AGE ASSESSMENT

Appendix D-1A. Clinical Estimation of Gestational Age. An Approximation Based on Published Data. Confirmatory Neurologic Examination to Be Done After 24 Hours. (See Figs. 12-5 and 12-6.)

Examination First Hours

WEEKS GESTATION (20–48)

PHYSICAL FINDINGS		Findings across gestational weeks
Vernix		Appears (~21) · Covers body, thick layer (24–33) · Scant, in creases (~39–40) · No vernix (~43)
Breast tissue and areola		Areola and nipple barely visible, no palpable breast tissue (~23–26) · Areola raised (~34) · 1–2 mm nodule (~36) · 3–5 mm (~38) · 5–6 mm (~40) · 7–10 mm (~41) · ?12 mm (~44)
Ear	Form	Flat, shapeless (~27) · Beginning incurving superior (~33) · Incurving upper 2/3 pinnae (~36) · Well-defined incurving to lobe (~39)
	Cartilage	Pinna soft, stays folded (~28) · Cartilage scant, returns slowly from folding (~32) · Thin cartilage, springs back from folding (~37) · Pinna firm, remains erect from head (~42)
Sole creases		Smooth soles without creases (22–32) · 1–2 anterior creases (~33) · 2–3 anterior creases (~35) · Creases anterior 2/3 sole (~37) · Creases involving heel (~39–40) · Deeper creases over entire sole (~43)
Skin	Thickness & appearance	Thin, translucent skin, plethoric, venules over abdomen, edema (27–32) · Smooth, thicker, no edema (~34) · Pink (~36) · Few vessels (~39) · Some desquamation, pale pink (~40) · Thick, pale, desquamation over entire body (~43)
	Nail plates	Appear (~22) · Nails to finger tips (~34) · Nails extend well beyond finger tips (~45)
Hair		Appears on head (~23) · Eye brows and lashes (~25) · Fine, woolly, bunches out from head (~30) · Silky, single strands, lays flat (~37) · ?Receding hairline or loss of baby hair, short, fine underneath (~45)
Lanugo		Appears (~21) · Covers entire body (24–25) · Vanishes from face (~35) · Present on shoulders (~38) · No lanugo (~44)
Genitalia	Testes	Testes palpable in inguinal canal (~30) · In upper scrotum (~37) · In lower scrotum (~41)
	Scrotum	Few rugae (~29) · Rugae, anterior portion (~37) · Rugae cover (~40) · Pendulous (~43)
	Labia & clitoris	Prominent clitoris, labia majora small, widely separated (31–32) · Labia majora larger, nearly cover clitoris (~37) · Labia minora and clitoris covered (~42)
Skull firmness		Bones are soft (~25) · Soft to 1″ from anterior fontanelle (~30) · Spongy at edges of fontanelle, center firm (~36) · Bones hard, sutures easily displaced (~39) · Bones hard, cannot be displaced (~43)
Posture	Resting	Hypotonic, lateral decubitus (22–24) · Hypotonic (~27) · Beginning flexion, thigh (~30) · Stronger hip flexion (~33) · Frog-like (~35) · Flexion, all limbs (~37) · Hypertonic (~39) · Very hypertonic (~44)
	Recoil - leg	No recoil (~21) · Partial recoil (~33) · Prompt recoil (~40)
	Recoil - arm	No recoil (21–28) · Begin flexion, no recoil (~35) · Prompt recoil, may be inhibited (38–40) · Prompt recoil after 30″ inhibition (~42)

Appendix D-1B. Examination: First Hours.

Confirmatory Neurologic Examination To Be Done After 24 Hours

Weeks Gestation: 20 21 22 23 24 25 26 27 28 29 30 31 32 33 34 35 36 37 38 39 40 41 42 43 44 45 46 47 48

Tone

Physical Findings	Progression across weeks of gestation
Heel to ear	No resistance (≈25–28); Some resistance (≈30–32); Impossible (≈36–38)
Scarf sign	No resistance (≈21); Elbow passes midline (≈30–33); Elbow at midline (≈37); Elbow does not reach midline (≈43)
Neck flexors (head lag)	Absent (≈21); Head in plane of body (≈39–40); Holds head (≈43)
Neck extensors	Head begins to right itself from flexed position (≈33); Good righting cannot hold it (≈36); Holds head few seconds (≈39); Keeps head in line with trunk > 40″ (≈41–42); Turns head from side to side (≈44)
Body extensors	Straightening of legs (≈33); Straightening of trunk (≈37); Straightening of head and trunk together (≈43)
Vertical positions	When held under arms, body slips through hands (≈29); Arms hold baby, legs extended? (≈34); Legs flexed, good support with arms (≈38); Head above back (≈43)
Horizontal positions	Hypotonic, arms and legs straight (≈28); Arms and legs flexed (≈37); Head and back even, flexed extremities (≈40)

Flexion angles

Physical Findings	Progression across weeks of gestation
Popliteal	No resistance (≈22); $150°$ (≈29); $110°$ (≈33); $100°$ (≈35); $90°$ (≈39); $80°$ (≈41)
Ankle	$45°$ (≈33); $20°$ (≈37); 0 (≈41); A pre-term who has reached 40 weeks still has a $40°$ angle
Wrist (square window)	$90°$ (≈28); $60°$ (≈33); $45°$ (≈37); $30°$ (≈39); 0 (≈41)

Reflexes

Physical Findings	Progression across weeks of gestation
Sucking	Weak, not synchronized with swallowing (≈26); Stronger, synchronized (≈32); Perfect (≈35); Perfect, hand to mouth (≈39); Perfect (≈43)
Rooting	Long latency period slow, imperfect (≈27); Hand to mouth (≈31); Brisk, complete, durable (≈35); Complete (≈43)
Grasp	Finger grasp is good, strength is poor (≈28); Stronger (≈33); Can lift baby off bed, involves arms (≈40); Hands open (≈45)
Moro	Barely apparent (≈22); Weak, not elicited every time (≈28); Complete with arm extension, open fingers, cry (≈35); Arm adduction added (≈40); ?Begins to lose Moro (≈45)
Crossed extension	Flexion and extension in a random, purposeless pattern (≈27); Extension, no adduction (≈33); Still incomplete (≈36); Extension, adduction, fanning of toes (≈39); Complete (≈43)
Automatic walk	Minimal (≈31); Begins tiptoeing, good support on sole (≈33); Begins tiptoeing (≈35); Fast tiptoeing (≈37); Heel-toe progression, whole sole of foot (≈39); A pre-term who has reached 40 weeks walks on toes (≈43); ?Begins to lose automatic walk (≈47)
Pupillary reflex	Absent (≈21); Appears (≈29)
Glabellar tap	Absent (≈21); Appears (≈32)
Tonic neck reflex	Absent (≈21); Appears (≈29)
Neck-righting	Absent (≈21); Appears (≈35); Present after 37 weeks

(Kempe CH, Silver HK, O'Brien D: Current Pediatric Diagnosis and Treatment, 3rd ed. Los Altos, California, Lange, 1974)

2. INTRAUTERINE GROWTH CURVES

Appendix D-2. The Colorado Intrauterine Growth Charts. (The Colorado curves give percentiles of intrauterine growth for weight, length and head circumference.)

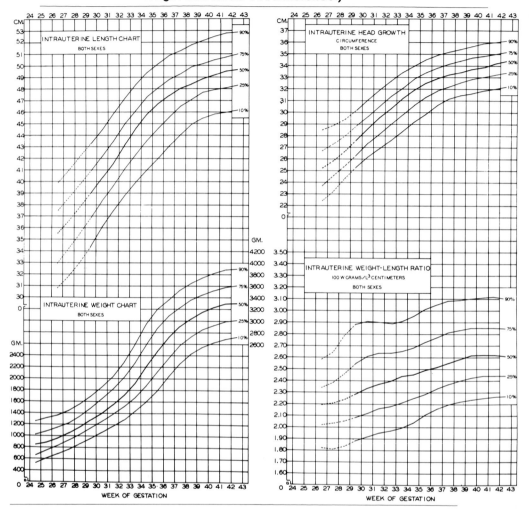

(Lubchenco LO, Hansman C, Boyd E: Pediatrics 37:403, 1966; Copyright © American Academy of Pediatrics, 1966)

3. TWINS—INTRAUTERINE GROWTH

Appendix D-3 **A.** Monochorionic Twins. **B.** Dichorionic Twins. Intrauterine Growth Charts for Both Sexes. (The weights of liveborn monochorionic twins at gestational ages from 24 to 42 weeks are graphed as percentages.)

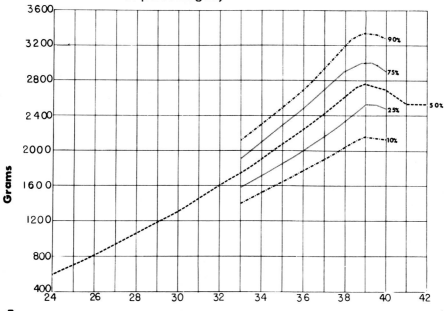

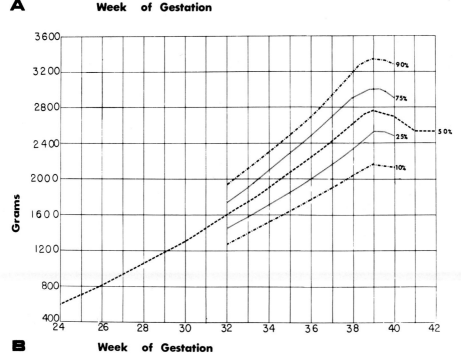

(Naeye R, Bernirschke K, Hagstrom J et al: Pediatrics 37:409, 1966; Copyright © American Academy of Pediatrics, 1966)

4. POSTNATAL GROWTH CURVES, TERM

Appendix D-4 **A.** Postnatal Growth Curves, Boys.

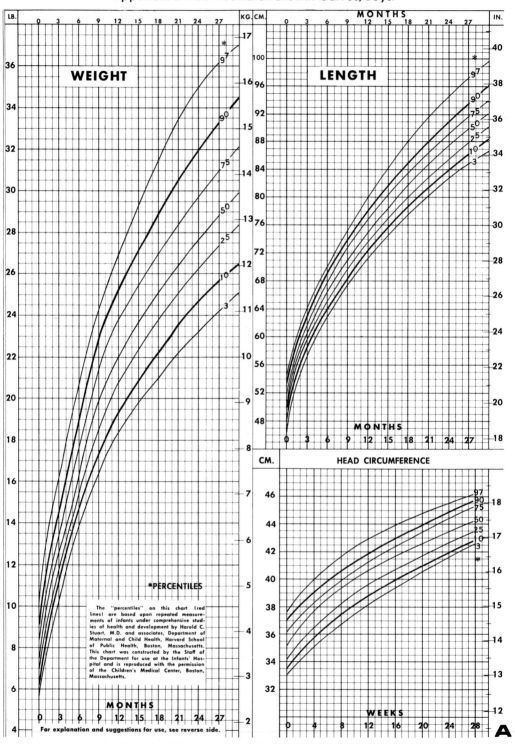

For explanation and suggestions for use, see reverse side.

(The Children's Medical Center, Boston, Massachusetts)

Appendix D-4. **B.** Girls.

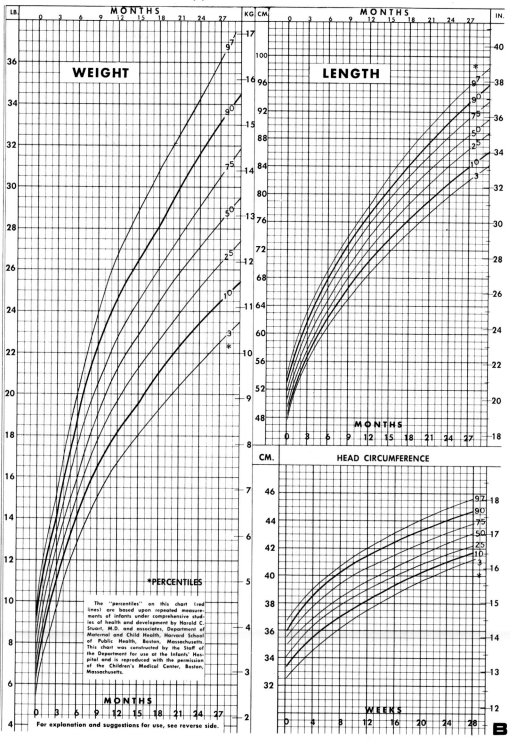

WEIGHT

LENGTH

HEAD CIRCUMFERENCE

*PERCENTILES

The "percentiles" on this chart (red lines) are based upon repeated measurements of infants under comprehensive studies of health and development by Harold C. Stuart, M.D. and associates, Department of Maternal and Child Health, Harvard School of Public Health, Boston, Massachusetts. This chart was constructed by the Staff of the Department for use at the Infants' Hospital and is reproduced with the permission of the Children's Medical Center, Boston, Massachusetts.

For explanation and suggestions for use, see reverse side.

B

5. HEAD CIRCUMFERENCE

Appendix D-5 **A.** Head Circumference Chart, Boys.

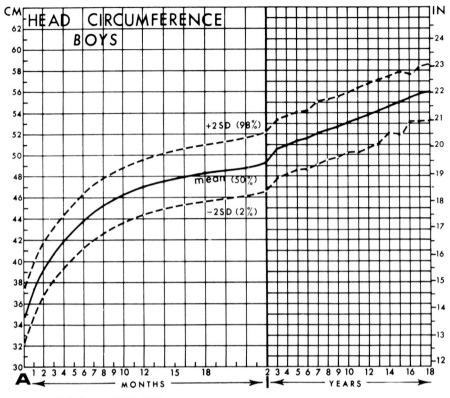

(Nellhaus G: Pediatrics 41:106, 1968)

Appendix D-5 **B.** Head Circumference Chart, Girls.

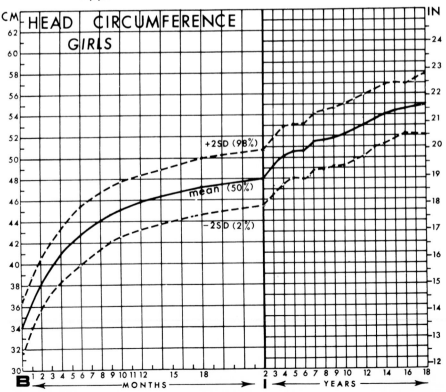

6. CONVERSION, POUNDS TO GRAMS

Appendix D-6. Conversion of Pounds and Ounces to Grams.

POUNDS	OUNCES 0	1	2	3	4	5	6	7	8	9	10	11	12	13	14	OUNCES 15
0	—	28	57	85	113	142	170	198	227	255	283	312	340	369	397	425
1	454	482	510	539	567	595	624	652	680	709	737	765	794	822	850	879
2	907	936	964	992	1021	1049	1077	1106	1134	1162	1191	1219	1247	1276	1304	1332
3	1361	1389	1417	1446	1474	1503	1531	1559	1588	1616	1644	1673	1701	1729	1758	1786
4	1814	1843	1871	1899	1928	1956	1984	2013	2041	2070	2098	2126	2155	2183	2211	2240
5	2268	2296	2325	2353	2381	2410	2438	2466	2495	2523	2551	2580	2608	2637	2665	2693
6	2722	2750	2778	2807	2835	2863	2892	2920	2948	2977	3005	3033	3062	3090	3118	3147
7	3175	3203	3232	3260	3289	3317	3345	3374	3402	3430	3459	3487	3515	3544	3572	3600
8	3629	3657	3685	3714	3742	3770	3799	3827	3856	3884	3912	3941	3969	3997	4026	4054
9	4082	4111	4139	4167	4196	4224	4252	4281	4309	4337	4366	4394	4423	4451	4479	4508
10	4536	4564	4593	4621	4649	4678	4706	4734	4763	4791	4819	4848	4876	4904	4933	4961
11	4990	5018	5046	5075	5103	5131	5160	5188	5216	5245	5273	5301	5330	5358	5386	5415
12	5443	5471	5500	5528	5557	5585	5613	5642	5670	5698	5727	5755	5783	5812	5840	5868
13	5897	5925	5953	5982	6010	6038	6067	6095	6123	6152	6180	6209	6237	6265	6294	6322
14	6350	6379	6407	6435	6464	6492	6520	6549	6577	6605	6634	6662	6690	6719	6747	6776
15	6804	6832	6860	6889	6917	6945	6973	7002	7030	7059	7087	7115	7144	7172	7201	7228
16	7257	7286	7313	7342	7371	7399	7427	7456	7484	7512	7541	7569	7597	7626	7654	7682
17	7711	7739	7768	7796	7824	7853	7881	7909	7938	7966	7994	8023	8051	8079	8108	8136
18	8165	8192	8221	8249	8278	8306	8335	8363	8391	8420	8448	8476	8504	8533	8561	8590
19	8618	8646	8675	8703	8731	8760	8788	8816	8845	8873	8902	8930	8958	8987	9015	9043
20	9072	9100	9128	9157	9185	9213	9242	9270	9298	9327	9355	9383	9412	9440	9469	9497
21	9525	9554	9582	9610	9639	9667	9695	9724	9752	9780	9809	9837	9865	9894	9922	9950
22	9979	10007	10036	10064	10092	10120	10149	10177	10206	10234	10262	10291	10319	10347	10376	10404

E
Nutritional Values

1. BASIC REQUIREMENTS

Appendix E-1. Food and Nutrition Board, National Academy of Sciences—National Research Council Recommended Daily Dietary Allowances, Revised 1980.*
(Designed for the maintenance of good nutrition of practically all healthy people in the U.S.A.)

	Age (years)	Weight (kg)	Weight (lb)	Height (cm)	Height (in)	Protein (g)	Fat-Soluble Vitamins A (µg RE)†	D (µg)‡	E (mg α-TE)§	Water-Soluble Vitamins C (mg)	Thiamin (mg)	Riboflavin (mg)	Niacin (mg NE)||	B-6 (mg)	Folacin (µg)#	B-12 (µg)	Minerals Ca (mg)	P (mg)	Mg (mg)	Fe (mg)	Zn (mg)	I (µg)
Infants	0.0–0.5	6	13	60	24	kg × 2.2	420	10	3	35	0.3	0.4	6	0.3	30	0.5**	360	240	50	10	3	40
	0.5–1.0	9	20	71	28	kg × 2.0	400	10	4	35	0.5	0.6	8	0.6	45	1.5	540	360	70	15	5	50
Children	1–3	13	29	90	35	23	400	10	5	45	0.7	0.8	9	0.9	100	2.0	800	800	150	15	10	70
	4–6	20	44	112	44	30	500	10	6	45	0.9	1.0	11	1.3	200	2.5	800	800	200	10	10	90
	7–10	28	62	132	52	34	700	10	7	45	1.2	1.4	16	1.6	300	3.0	800	800	250	10	10	120

| | | Weight | | Height | | Protein | Fat-Soluble Vitamins | | | | Water-Soluble Vitamins | | | | | | | Minerals | | | | | |
	Age (years)	(kg)	(lb)	(cm)	(in)	(g)	A (μg RE)†	D (μg)‡	E (mg α-TE)§	C (mg)	Thia-min (mg)	Ribo-flavin (mg)	Niacin (mg NE)‖	B-6 (mg)	Fola-cin# (μg)	B-12 (μg)	Ca (mg)	P (mg)	Mg (mg)	Fe (mg)	Zn (mg)	I (μg)
Males	11–14	45	99	157	62	45	1000	10	8	50	1.4	1.6	18	1.8	400	3.0	1200	1200	350	18	15	150
	15–18	66	145	176	69	56	1000	10	10	60	1.4	1.7	18	2.0	400	3.0	1200	1200	400	18	15	150
	19–22	70	154	177	70	56	1000	7.5	10	60	1.5	1.7	19	2.2	400	3.0	800	800	350	10	15	150
	23–50	70	154	178	70	56	1000	5	10	60	1.4	1.6	18	2.2	400	3.0	800	800	350	10	15	150
	51+	70	154	178	70	56	1000	5	10	60	1.2	1.4	16	2.2	400	3.0	800	800	350	10	15	150
Females	11–14	46	101	157	62	46	800	10	8	50	1.1	1.3	15	1.8	400	3.0	1200	1200	300	18	15	150
	15–18	55	120	163	64	46	800	10	8	60	1.1	1.3	14	2.0	400	3.0	1200	1200	300	18	15	150
	19–22	55	120	163	64	44	800	7.5	8	60	1.1	1.3	14	2.0	400	3.0	800	800	300	18	15	150
	23–50	55	120	163	64	44	800	5	8	60	1.0	1.2	13	2.0	400	3.0	800	800	300	18	15	150
	51+	55	120	163	64	44	800	5	8	60	1.0	1.2	13	2.0	400	3.0	800	800	300	10	15	150
Pregnant						+30	+200	+5	+2	+20	+0.4	+0.3	+2	+0.6	+400	+1.0	+400	+400	+150	††	+5	+25
Lactating						+20	+400	+5	+3	+40	+0.5	+0.5	+5	+0.5	+100	+1.0	+400	+400	+150	††	+10	+50

* The allowances are intended to provide for individual variations among most normal persons as they live in the United States under usual environmental stresses. Diets should be based on a variety of common foods in order to provide other nutrients for which human requirements have been less well defined. See text for detailed discussion of allowances and of nutrients not tabulated. See Table E-3 for suggested average energy intakes.

† Retinol equivalents. 1 retinol equivalent = 1 μg retinol or 6 μg β carotene. See text for calculation of vitamin A activity of diets as retinol equivalents.

‡ As cholecalciferol, 10 μg cholecalciferol = 400 IU of vitamin D.

§ α-tocopherol equivalents. 1 mg d-α tocopherol = 1 α-TE. See text for variation in allowances and calculation of vitamin E activity of the diet as α-tocopherol equivalents.

‖ 1 NE (niacin equivalent) is equal to 1 mg of niacin or 60 mg of dietary tryptophan.

The folacin allowances refer to dietary sources as determined by Lactobacillus casei assay after treatment with enzymes (conjugases) to make polyglutamyl forms of the vitamin available to the test organism.

** The recommended dietary allowance for vitamin B-12 in infants is based on average concentration of the vitamin in human milk. The allowances after weaning are based on energy intake (as recommended by the American Academy of Pediatrics) and consideration of other factors, such as intestinal absorption; see text.

†† The increased requirement during pregnancy cannot be met by the iron content of habitual American diets nor by the existing iron stores of many women; therefore the use of 30–60 mg of supplemental iron is recommended. Iron needs during lactation are not substantially different from those of nonpregnant women, but continued supplementation of the mother for 2–3 months after parturition is advisable in order to replenish stores depleted by pregnancy.

2. SELECTED VITAMINS AND MINERALS

Appendix E-2. Estimated Safe and Adequate Daily Dietary Intakes of Selected Vitamins and Minerals*

	Age (years)	Vitamins		
		Vitamin K (μg)	Biotin (μg)	Pantothenic Acid (mg)
Infants	0–0.5	12	35	2
	0.5–1	10–20	50	3
Children and Adolescents	1–3	15–30	65	3
	4–6	20–40	85	3–4
	7–10	30–60	120	4–5
	11+	50–100	100–200	4–7
Adults		70–140	100–200	4–7

	Age (years)	Trace Elements†					
		Copper (mg)	Manganese (mg)	Fluoride (mg)	Chromium (mg)	Selenium (mg)	Molybdenum (mg)
Infants	0–0.5	0.5–0.7	0.5–0.7	0.1–0.5	0.01–0.04	0.01–0.04	0.03–0.06
	0.5–1	0.7–1.0	0.7–0.1	0.2–1.0	0.02–0.06	0.02–0.06	0.04–0.08
Children and Adolescents	1–3	1.0–1.5	1.0–1.5	0.5–1.5	0.02–0.08	0.02–0.08	0.05–0.1
	4–6	1.5–2.0	1.5–2.0	1.0–2.5	0.03–0.12	0.03–0.12	0.06–0.15
	7–10	2.0–2.5	2.0–3.0	1.5–2.5	0.05–0.2	0.05–0.2	0.10–0.3
	11+	2.0–3.0	2.5–5.0	1.5–2.5	0.05–0.2	0.05–0.2	0.15–0.5
Adults		2.0–3.0	2.5–5.0	1.5–4.0	0.05–0.2	0.05–0.2	0.15–0.5

	Age (years)	Electrolytes		
		Sodium (mg)	Potassium (mg)	Chloride (mg)
Infants	0–0.5	115–350	350–925	275–700
	0.5–1	250–750	425–1275	400–1200
Children and Adolescents	1–3	325–975	550–1650	500–1500
	4–6	450–1350	775–2325	700–2100
	7–10	600–1800	1000–3000	925–2775
	11+	900–2700	1525–4575	1400–4200
Adults		1100–3300	1875–5625	1700–5100

* Because there is less information on which to base allowances, these figures are not given in the main table of RDA and are provided here in the form of ranges of recommended intakes.

† Because the toxic levels for many trace elements may be only several times usual intakes, the upper levels for the trace elements given in this table should not be habitually exceeded.

(Food and Nutrition Board, National Academy of Sciences—National Research Council)

3. ENERGY

Appendix E-3. Mean Heights and Weights and Recommended Energy Intake.*

Category	Age (years)	Weight (kg)	Weight (lb)	Height (cm)	Height (in)	Energy Needs (with range) (kcal)		Energy Needs (with range) (MJ)
Infants	0.0–0.5	6	13	60	24	kg × 115	(95–145)	kg × 0.48
	0.5–1.0	9	20	71	28	kg × 105	(80–135)	kg × 0.44
Children	1–3	13	29	90	35	1300	(900–1800)	5.5
	4–6	20	44	112	44	1700	(1300–2300)	7.1
	7–10	28	62	132	52	2400	(1650–3300)	10.1
Males	11–14	45	99	157	62	2700	(2000–3700)	11.3
	15–18	66	145	176	69	2800	(2100–3900)	11.8
	19–22	70	154	177	70	2900	(2500–3300)	12.2
	23–50	70	154	178	70	2700	(2300–3100)	11.3
	51–75	70	154	178	70	2400	(2000–2800)	10.1
	76+	70	154	178	70	2050	(1650–2450)	8.6
Females	11–14	46	101	157	62	2200	(1500–3000)	9.2
	15–18	55	120	163	64	2100	(1200–3000)	8.8
	19–22	55	120	163	64	2100	(1700–2500)	8.8
	23–50	55	120	163	64	2000	(1600–2400)	8.4
	51–75	55	120	163	64	1800	(1400–2200)	7.6
	76+	55	120	163	64	1600	(1200–2000)	6.7
Pregnancy						+300		
Lactation						+500		

* The data in this table have been assembled from the observed median heights and weights of children, together with desirable weights for adults for the mean heights of men (70 in) and women (64 in) between the ages of 18 and 34 years as surveyed in the U.S. population (HEW/NCHS data).

Energy allowances for children through age 18 are based on median energy intakes of children of these ages followed in longitudinal growth studies. The values in parentheses are 10th and 90th percentiles of energy intake, to indicate the range of energy consumption among children of these ages.

(Food and Nutrition Board, National Academy of Sciences—National Research Council)

4. COMPOSITION OF FREQUENTLY USED FORMULAS

Appendix E-4. Composition of Frequently Used Formulas.

| Formula | Cal/dl | Percentage Composition | | | | mmol/dl | | mg/dl | | Type of Carbohydrate | Type of Protein | Remarks |
		Pro	Fat	CHO	Na	K	Ca	P			
Advance	54	2.0	2.7	5.5	1.3	2.2	51	39	Corn syrup, lactose	Cow, soy	16 cal/oz
Cow milk	67	3.5	3.7	4.9	2.2	3.5	117	92	Lactose	Cow	
Enfamil	67	1.5	3.7	7.0	1.2	1.8	55	46	Lactose	Cow	
Enfamil with Iron	67	1.5	3.7	7.0	1.2	1.8	55	46	Lactose	Cow	
Enfamil Premature Formula	81	2.4	4.1	8.9	1.4	2.3	95	48	Corn syrup solids, lactose	Whey from cow, cow	Fat = 40% MCT; Whey: Casein = 60:40
Goats milk	67	3.2	4.0	4.6	1.5	4.5	129	106	Lactose	Goat	Insufficient folate
Human milk	74	1.1	4.5	6.8	0.7	1.3	34	121	Lactose	Human	
Isomil	67	2.0	3.6	6.8	1.3	1.8	70	50	Corn syrup, sucrose, corn starch	Soy, methionine	
Soyalac	67	2.1	3.8	6.7	1.4	1.9	63	52	Sucrose, tapioca	Soy, methionine	
Lofenalac	67	2.2	2.7	8.8	1.4	1.7	63	47	Corn syrup solids, tapioca	Specially processed casein, hydrolysate	Designed for PKU
Meat base	67	2.8	3.3	6.3	0.8	1.0	99	66	Sucrose, tapioca	Beef	High protein, low sodium, free of branched chain amino acids, designed for maple syrup urine disease
MSUD	67	1.1	2.6	8.2	1.3	1.1	66	36			

Formula	Cal/dl	Percentage Composition			mmol/dl		mg/dl		Type of Carbohydrate	Type of Protein	Remarks
		Pro	Fat	CHO	Na	K	Ca	P			
Nursoy	67	2.3	3.6	6.8	0.9	1.9	64	44	Sucrose	Soy, methionine	
Nutramigen	67	2.2	2.6	8.8	1.4	1.7	63	47	Sucrose, tapioca	Casein hydrolysate	
Pregestamil	67	1.9	2.7	9.1	1.4	1.8	63	42	Corn syrup solids, tapioca	Casein hydrolysate, cystine, tyrosine, and tryptophan	Fat = 40% MCT
Portagen	67	2.4	3.2	7.8	1.4	2.1	63	47	Corn syrup solids Sucrose	Na caseinate	Fat = 88% MCT
Probana	67	4.2	2.2	7.9	2.7	3.1	116	89	Dextrose, banana, lactose	Cow, banana, casein hydrolysate	High protein
ProSobee	67	2.5	3.4	6.8	1.8	1.9	79	53	Corn syrup solids	Soy, methionine	
Similac	67	1.6	3.6	7.2	1.1*	2.0*	51	39	Lactose	Cow	
Similac with Iron	67	1.6	3.6	7.2	1.1*	2.0*	51	39	Lactose	Cow	
Similac Special Care Infant Formula	81	2.2	4.4	8.6	1.5	2.5	144	72	Lactose, 50% polycose	Cow	Fat = 50% MCT
Similac PM 60/40	67	1.6	3.5	7.6	0.7	1.5	40	20	Lactose	Casein, whey	60/40 lactalbumin:casein
Soyalac	69	2.2	3.8	6.6	1.5	2.0	63	52	Dextrose, maltose, sucrose	Soy, methionine	
SMA	67	1.5	3.6	7.2	0.6	1.4	44	33	Lactose	Whey from cow, cow	60/40 lactalbumin:casein
Vivonex	67	1.4	0.1	15.4	2.4	2.0	37	37	Glucose, glucose oligosaccharides	Amino acids	Low fat, low Ca

* Slightly higher if made from powder

(Ross Laboratories Product Handbook, Jan, 1979; Infant Formula Products Nutrition Information, Mead Johnson, October, 1979; Children's Hospital National Medical Center, Diet Manual, 1979)

5. STRAINED BABY FOODS

Appendix E-5. Proximate Mineral and Vitamin Composition of Commercially Prepared Strained and Junior Baby Food (Constituents/100 g).

A. Strained Foods.

Category	Number of Products	Energy (kcal)	Water	Protein	Fat	Carbohydrate Total	Fiber	Ash
Juices*	32	65 (45–98)*	83.6 (75.7–88.4)	0.3 (0.0–0.7)	0.2 (0.0–0.4)	15.6 (10.9–22.8)	0.0 (0.0–0.1)	0.3 (0.1–0.4)
Fruits*	33	85 (69–125)	78.2 (68.4–81.4)	0.4 (0.1–1.9)	0.2 (0.1–0.7)	20.4 (16.4–29.7)	0.5 (0.1–1.5)	0.3 (0.1–0.4)
Vegetables								
Plain	24	45 (27–78)	87.7 (80.5–91.8)	1.5 (0.7–4.3)	0.3 (0.1–1.3)	9.0 (5.0–15.5)	0.7 (0.4–1.2)	0.8 (0.5–1.1)
Creamed	6	63 (42–94)	84.0 (76.5–88.8)	1.8 (0.9–2.7)	0.8 (0.2–1.8)	12.2 (6.0–20.4)	0.3 (0.2–0.5)	0.9 (0.5–1.3)
Meats	25	106 (80–194)	79.2 (71.6–82.1)	13.6 (9.9–16.4)	5.6 (2.8–17.1)	0.4 (0.0–2.2)	0.1 (0.0–0.2)	1.1 (0.8–1.4)
Egg yolks	4	192 (184–199)	70.8 (70.3–71.2)	10.0 (9.6–10.7)	16.1 (14.1–17.8)	1.7 (0.0–3.5)	0.1 (0.0–0.1)	1.3 (1.2–1.5)
High-meat dinners	15	84 (62–106)	82.8 (80.6–85.1)	6.0 (5.3–6.6)	4.0 (1.4–6.6)	6.0 (4.4–8.3)	0.2 (0.1–0.3)	1.0 (0.7–1.4)
Soups and dinners	42	58 (39–94)	86.9 (79.8–89.5)	2.2 (1.1–4.4)	2.0 (0.1–5.7)	7.8 (5.8–11.4)	0.2 (0.1–0.4)	0.9 (0.4–1.4)
Desserts	37	96 (70–136)	76.6 (70.0–81.7)	1.0 (0.1–6.2)	0.8 (0.0–4.7)	21.1 (16.9–28.6)	0.2 (0.0–0.9)	0.4 (0.1–0.9)

| | | | | | | Proximate Analysis (g) | | |

* Calories in some products currently are lower as a result of decreased added sugar.

B. Junior Foods.

Category	Number of Products	Energy (kcal)	Water	Protein	Fat	Carbohydrate Total	Carbohydrate Fiber	Ash
Fruits*	30	85 (69–116)	78.1 (70.2–81.5)	0.4 (0.1–2.2)	0.2 (0.0–0.5)	20.4 (16.5–28.3)	0.6 (0.1–1.3)	0.3 (0.1–1.1)
Vegetables								
Plain	16	46 (27–71)	87.5 (81.2–91.8)	1.3 (0.7–3.6)	0.4 (0.1–1.2)	9.3 (5.3–15.7)	0.6 (0.3–1.3)	0.8 (0.5–1.3)
Creamed	5	64 (45–72)	84.5 (81.7–88.1)	1.9 (0.9–2.7)	1.2 (0.2–2.8)	11.2 (6.2–16.1)	0.3 (0.2–0.5)	0.9 (0.3–1.5)
Meats	17	103 (88–135)	79.4 (75.6–81.6)	14.3 (13.0–15.7)	4.9 (3.7–8.3)	0.3 (0.0–1.1)	0.1 (0.0–0.2)	1.1 (0.9–1.4)
Meat sticks	6	168 (112–204)	71.3 (67.0–78.6)	13.5 (9.8–15.9)	12.0 (6.5–15.6)	1.5 (0.4–3.4)	0.2 (0.1–0.2)	1.5 (1.2–1.7)
High-meat dinners	15	85 (64–110)	82.6 (77.7–85.1)	6.2 (5.1–7.1)	4.1 (1.2–6.4)	5.9 (3.9–9.3)	0.2 (0.1–0.3)	1.0 (0.6–1.4)
Soups and dinners	45	61 (39–100)	86.2 (78.7–89.9)	2.2 (1.1–4.4)	2.0 (0.1–5.8)	8.4 (6.6–12.5)	0.2 (0.1–0.5)	0.9 (0.4–1.6)
Desserts	32	93 (73–112)	77.0 (72.1–81.4)	0.8 (0.1–3.1)	0.7 (0.0–2.7)	21.0 (16.3–26.8)	0.2 (0.0–0.6)	0.3 (0.1–0.7)

*Calories in some products are currently lower as a result of decreased added sugar.

(Anderson TA, Fomon SJ. In Fomon SJ (ed): Infant Nutrition, 2nd ed, pp 412–415. Philadelphia, WB Saunders, 1974)

1205

6. INTRAVENOUS ALIMENTATION

Appendix E-6. Daily Requirements of Total Parenteral Nutrition.

Protein (5% amino acid mixtures)	2–4 g/kg (Recommended 3 g/kg/24 hours)
Calories	100–120 cal/kg
H_2O	125 ml/kg
Na	3–4 mmol/kg
K	2–3 mmol/kg
Ca	2–2.5 mmol/kg
P	2.5 mmol/day
Mg	1 mmol/day
Multivitamins (Multivit)	1 ml/day

7. SERUM FOLIC ACID

Appendix E-7. Serum Folic Acid ng/ml.

Age	Range	Mean ± SD
NORMAL PREMATURE INFANTS		
1–4 days	7.17–52.00	29.54 ± 0.98
2–3 wk.	4.12–15.62	8.61 ± 0.55
1–2 mo.	2.81–11.25	5.84 ± 0.35
2–3 mo.	3.56–11.82	6.95 ± 0.50
3–5 mo.	3.83–16.50	8.92 ± 0.86
5–7 mo.	6.00–12.25	9.02 ± 0.74
NORMAL CHILDREN		
1–6 yr.	4.12–21.25	11.37 ± 0.82
NORMAL ADULTS		
20–45 yr.	4.50–28.00	10.29 ± 1.14

(Klaus MH, Fanaroff AA: Care of the High Risk Neonate. Philadelphia, WB Saunders, 1973; Adapted from Shojania A, Gross S: J Pediatr 64:323, 1964)

8. SERUM VITAMIN E

Appendix E-8. Serum Vitamin E (mg/dl)—Mean ± (1 SD).

Weeks	1	2	3	4	5	6	7	8	9	10
<1500 g	0.40	0.30	0.25	0.25	0.25	0.25	0.25	0.25	0.35	0.45
28–32 weeks	[0.05]	[0.04]	[0.03]	[0.03]	[0.03]	[0.03]	[0.03]	[0.03]	[0.04]	[0.05]
1500–2000 g	0.45	0.40	0.40	0.45	0.45	0.45	0.50	0.50	0.60	0.70
32–36 weeks	[0.05]	[0.05]	[0.05]	[0.05]	[0.05]	[0.05]	[0.05]	[0.05]	[0.06]	[0.06]
2000–2500 g	0.50	0.45	0.50	0.60	0.70	0.75	0.75	0.75	0.75	0.80
36–40 weeks	[0.05]	[0.05]	[0.05]	[0.06]	[0.06]	[0.06]	[0.60]	[0.60]	[0.60]	[0.70]
>2500 g	0.55	0.55	0.55	0.60	0.75	0.80	0.85	0.85	0.85	0.85
Term	[0.60]	[0.60]	[0.60]	[0.60]	[0.70]	[0.70]	[0.80]	[0.80]	[0.80]	[0.80]

(Klaus MH, Fanaroff AA: Care of the High Risk Neonate. Philadelphia, WB Saunders, 1973)

F

Technical Procedures

1. LOCATION OF ABDOMINAL AORTIC BRANCHES

Appendix F-1. Distribution of the Major Aortic Branches Found in 15 Infants. (**Filled symbols** represent infants with, and **open symbols** without cardiac and/or renal anomalies.)

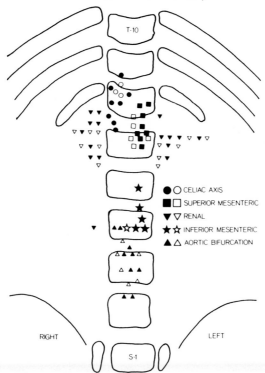

(Phelps DL, Lachman RS, Leake RD, Oh W: J Pediatr 81:337, 1972)

2. PLACEMENT OF UMBILICAL CATHETERS

Appendix F-2A. The Relation Between the Length of Catheter Inserted into the Umbilical Artery in Order to Reach the Bifurcation of the Aorta, the "Diaphragm," or the Aortic Valves, and the Total Body Length of an Infant.

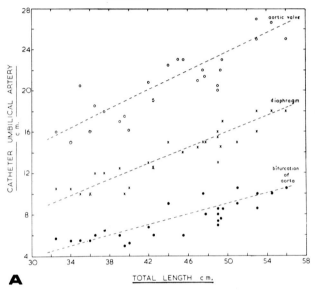

A

Appendix F-2B. The Relation Between the Length of Catheter Inserted into the Umbilical Vein in Order to Reach the "Diaphragm" (**x**) and the "Left Atrium" (**o**), and the Shoulder-umbilicus Length of an Infant.

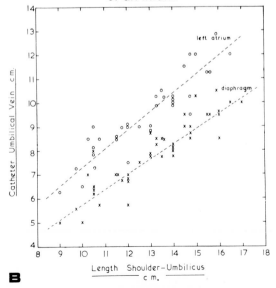

B

(Dunn PM: Arch Dis Child 41:71, 1966)

3. ENDOTRACHEAL TUBE SIZE

Appendix F-3. Endotracheal Tube Size.

Infant weight (g)	ET Tube Diameter	
	(*Inside*)	(*Outside*)
Less than 1000	2.5 mm	12 Fr.
1000–1500	3.0 mm	14 Fr.
1500–2200	3.5 mm	16 Fr.
2200 and over	4.0 mm	18 Fr.

4. INSERTION DISTANCE, ENDOTRACHEAL TUBE

Appendix F-4. Insertion Distance, Endotracheal Tube.

Infant Weight (g)	Cord-carina Distance (cm)	Insertion Past Cords (cm)
1000–1500	4.0	1.5–2.0
1500–2500	4.5	2.0
2500–3500	5.0	2.2
3500–4000	5.5	2.5

G

Miscellaneous

1. PREGNANCY OUTCOME, WEIGHT AND GESTATION

Appendix G-1. Neonatal Mortality by Small-for-gestational-age Blocks.

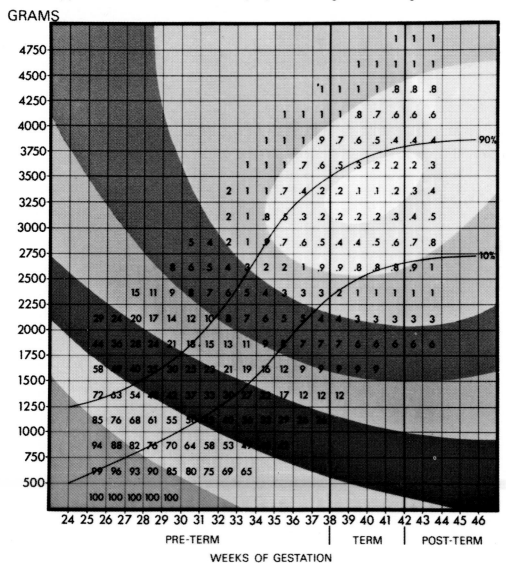

(Lubchenco LO: J Pediatr 81:814, 1972)

2. COMPOSITION, FETUS AND NEWBORN

Appendix G-2. Chemical Composition of Human Fetuses and Infants.

Sex	Body Wt. (g)*	Water (g)*	Nitrogen (g)*	Fat (g)*	Potassium (mmol)†	Calcium (g)†	Phosphorus (g)†	Nitrogen (g)†	Water (g)†	Reference
M	105	932	9.8	5.1						1
	115	887	11.8	7.0	43.0	3.2	2.2	11.9	895	2
F	157	907	9.6	5.4						1
	179	877	12.5	24.2	43.8	4.5	3.1	12.8	899	3
	192	885	11.9	20.8	43.1	4.1	2.9	12.1	904	3
	198	875	17.7	5.0	44.0	4.6	3.2	17.8	880	4
M	225	870	16.3	6.0	44.0	4.2	3.1	16.4	875	4
M	236	898	10.3	5.7				10.4	902	1
M	244	910	11.4	2.8				11.5	915	1
M	259	873	13.4	8.0	45.0	4.9	3.5	13.5	880	2
F	264	889	12.3	5.2				12.4	892	1
	271	880	13.3	5.0	46.0	3.0	2.3	13.4	885	4
M	286	893	12.9	5.0	38.0	4.7	3.5	13.0	895	4
F	299	893	11.7	6.0				11.9	909	1
	314	882	13.1	5.0	39.0	4.6	3.2	13.2	885	4
	335	877	12.7	7.0	35.7	4.7	3.3	12.8	882	2
F	346	862	14.6	24.0	45.0	5.1	3.2	14.9	883	3
M	362	892	10.7	7.2				10.8	900	1
F	400	879	14.9	6.0	47.0	4.3	3.1	15.0	880	4
M	478	889	13.5	5.0	45.0	4.4	3.0	13.6	890	4

F	490	876	12.5	7.0	37.0	6.7	4.1	12.6	881	2
	493	837	17.4	27.5	46.7	6.6	3.9	17.9	861	3
	570	855	14.9	13.0	30.8	5.7	3.9	15.1	865	2
F	575	864	12.5	10.6				12.6	872	1
	590	855	14.9	12.0	40.0	6.4	4.2	15.1	865	2
F	652	848	15.4	32.2	46.5	5.5	3.4	15.9	876	3
M	673	876	13.6	15.0	42.0	5.7	3.6	13.8	890	4
F	687	828	19.2	18.1	36.9	9.9	5.2	19.6	843	3
M	771	838	14.2	19.8				14.5	855	1
M	787	875	14.5	9.0	41.0	6.1	3.7	14.6	880	4
M	832	835	18.2	27.0				18.6	854	1
F	836	839	17.8	22.1				18.2	856	1
F	910	826	18.9	34.7				19.6	855	1
M	911	887	12.3	12.0	45.0	5.7	3.5	12.5	900	4
M	928	829	16.7	24.4				17.1	850	1
	960	831	17.1	22.0	38.0	7.2	4.3	17.5	850	2
F	1000	828	15.1	49.3	45.9	6.7	3.9	16.0	871	3
	1010	855	14.4	22.0	39.6	5.1	3.5	14.9	880	2
M	1117	848	14.6	23.6				14.9	868	1
	1205	825	15.4	35.0	48.5	5.8	3.9	16.0	855	2

* Expressed per kg. whole body weight.
† Expressed per kg. fat free body weight.
([1] Fehling, 1877; [2] Iob and Swanson, 1934; [3] Fee and Weil, 1963; [4] Widdowson and McCance, 1964; [5] Camerer, 1900 and 1902)
(Owen GM and Brožek J. In Faulkner F (ed): Human Development, p 236. Philadelphia, WB Saunders, 1966)

(Continued)

Appendix G-2. Chemical Composition of Human Fetuses and Infants. (continued)

Sex	Body Wt. (g)*	Water (g)*	Nitrogen (g)*	Fat (g)*	Potassium (mmol)†	Calcium (g)†	Phosphorus (g)†	Nitrogen (g)†	Water (g)†	Reference
F	1479	801	17.4	60.1	42.5	8.3	4.8	18.7	852	3
M	1496	739	28.6	51.1				30.2	779	1
F	1536	774	19.2	71.9	43.8	10.8	5.5	20.7	834	1
	1545	822	16.4	34.0	45.0	6.0	4.1	17.0	853	2
	1555	796	17.1	48.0	45.2	6.3	4.2	18.0	837	2
	1615	810	17.4	39.0	46.3	6.2	4.2	18.1	841	2
M	1761	747	20.2	87.0				22.1	816	1
M	1866	800	16.7	68.1	38.8	7.9	4.2	17.9	859	3
M	1966	813	18.6	42.0	41.0	7.9	4.4	19.4	850	4
M	2057	779	17.3	84.5	39.6	8.8	4.9	19.0	851	3
F	2295	778	18.9	75.0	47.0	7.8	4.8	20.4	840	4
F	2476	730	19.8	109.0	41.0	8.5	5.8	22.2	820	5
F	2616	718	17.9	143.0	46.0	5.9	3.5	20.9	830	5
M	2652	797	17.6	67.0	41.0	8.1	4.1	18.8	850	4
M	2683	728	21.8	102.0	50.0	7.4	5.0	24.2	810	5
M	2755	692	18.3	161.0	46.0	7.8	5.6	21.8	825	5
M	2915	755	19.7	67.0	46.2	8.9	5.5	21.1	808	2
F	3048	720	19.7	120.0	49.0	8.7	5.0	22.4	820	5
F	3050	726	19.1	125.0	53.0	8.8	5.3	21.8	830	4
F	3090	699	18.8	155.0	55.0	9.7	5.2	22.2	825	4
M	3105	721	22.1	110.0	53.0	9.4	5.8	24.9	810	4
M	3294	741	18.9	91.0				20.8	815	1
M	3348	722	21.0	113.0	48.0	8.4	4.9	23.6	815	5
F	3767	697	19.7	152.0	50.0	8.8	5.5	23.2	820	4
M	3994	722	17.4	139.0	48.0	10.3	5.7	20.3	840	4
M	4373	585	16.9	283.0	55.0	10.3	6.0	23.5	820	4

* Expressed per kg. whole body weight.
† Expressed per kg. fat free body weight.
(¹ Fehling, 1877; ² Iob and Swanson, 1934; ³ Fee and Weil, 1963; ⁴ Widdowson and McCance, 1964; ⁵ Camerer, 1900 and 1902)
(Owen GM and Brožek J. In Faulkner F (ed): Human Development, p 236. Philadelphia, WB Saunders, 1966)

3. DENVER DEVELOPMENTAL SCREENING TEST

Appendix G-3. Denver Developmental Screening Test.

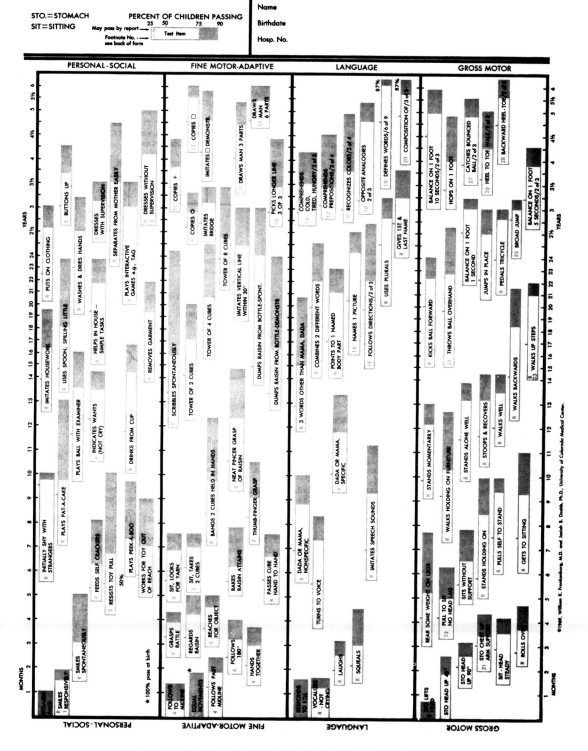

(Frankenburg WK, Dodds JB, University of Colorado Medical Center)

H

Drugs

1. DRUGS IN BREAST MILK

Appendix H-1. Drugs in Breast Milk*

Drug or Agent	Contra-indicated	R$_x$ With Caution	No Apparent Harm	Insufficient Information	Comment
Analgesics					
Acetaminophen			x		
Aspirin			x		
Propoxyphene (Darvon)			x		
Anticoagulants					
Ethyl biscoumacetate	x				Bleeding infant
Phenindione	x				Bleeding infant
Heparin			x		No passage into milk
Warfarin Na (Coumadin)			x		
Bishydroxycoumarin (Dicumarol)		x			
Anticonvulsants					
Phenobarbital			x		Low levels in infant
Primadone (Mysoline)			x		? Drowsiness
Carbamazepine				x	Significant infant levels; no reported effects
Diphenylhydatoin (Phenytoin, Dilantin)			x		Low levels in infant, methemoglobin, one case
Antihistamines					
Diphenhydramine (Benadryl)			x		Small amounts excreted
Trimeprazine (Temaril)			x		Small amounts excreted
Tripelennamine (Pyrabenzamine)			x		Small amounts excreted
Anti-infective Agents					
Aminoglycosides (Kanamycin, gentamicin)			x		Significant excretion in milk; not absorbed

* (Data derived from Anderson PO: Drugs and breast-feeding. Semin Perinatol 3:271–278, 1979; Yaffee SJ, Waletzky L (eds): DHEW Publication No. (HSA) 79-5107, 1979, p 77; Hervada AR, Feit E, Sagraves R: Drugs in breast milk. Perinatal Care 2:19–25, 1978).

Appendix H-1. Drugs in Breast Milk (continued)

Drug or Agent	Contra-indicated	R_x With Caution	No Apparent Harm	Insufficient Information	Comment
Anti-infective Agents					
Chloramphenicol	x				Bone marrow depression; GI and behavioral effects
Penicillins			x		Possible sensitization
Sulfonamides		x			Hemolysis, G-6-PD deficiency, bilirubin displacement
Tetracyclines			x		Limited absorption by infant
Nalidixic acid		x			Hemolysis
Nitrofurantoin		x			Possible G-6-PD hemolysis
Metronidazole (Flagyl)		x			Low absorption but potentially toxic
Isoniazid		x			High levels in milk, possible toxicity
Pyramethamine	x				Vomiting, marrow suppression, convulsions
Chloraquine			x		Not excreted
Quinine		x			Thrombocytopenia
Anti-inflammatory					
Aspirin			x		
Indomethacin		x			Seizures, one case
Phenylbutazone		x			Low levels, ? blood dyscrasia
Gold	x				Found in baby; nephritis, hepatitis, hematologic changes
Steroids				x	Low levels with prednisone and prednisolone
Antineoplastic					
Cyclophosphamide	x				Neutropenia
Methotrexate	x				Very small excretion
Antithyroid					
Radioactive iodine	x				Thyroid suppression
Propylthiouracil	x				Thyroid suppression
Bronchodilators					
Aminophylline			x		Irritability, one case
Iodides	x				Thyroid suppression
Sympathomimetics				x	Inhalers probably safe
Cardiovascular Agents					
Digoxin			x		Insignificant levels
Propanolol			x		Insigificant levels
Reserpine	x				Nasal stuffiness, lethargy
Guanethidine (Ismelin)			x		Insigificant levels

(Continued)

Appendix H-1. Drugs in Breast Milk (continued)

Drug or Agent	Contra-indicated	R$_x$ With Caution	No Apparent Harm	Insufficient Information	Comment
Cardiovascular Agents					
Methyldopa (Aldomet)				x	
Cathartics					
Anthroquinones (Cascara, danthron)	x				Diarrhea, cramps
Aloe, senna		x			Safe in moderate dosage
Bulk agents, softeners			x		
Contraceptives, Oral†					
Diethylstilbestrol	x				Possible vaginal cancer
Depo-provera		x			May affect lactation
Noresthisterone		x			May affect lactation
Ethinyl estradiol		x			May affect lactation
Diuretics					
Chlorthalidone				x	Low levels, but may accumulate
Thiazides		x			May affect lactation; low levels in milk
Spironolactone			x		Insignificant levels
Ergot Alkaloids					
Bromcriptine	x				Lactation suppressed
Ergot	x				Vomiting, diarrhea, seizures
Ergotamine				x	
Ergonovine	x				Brief postpartum course may be safe
Methylergonovine	x				Brief postpartum course may be safe
Hormones					
Corticosteroids				x	Low levels with short-term prednisone or prednisolone
Sex hormones (see above oral contraceptives)					
Thyroid (T$_3$ or T$_4$)			x		Excreted in milk; may mask hypothyroid infant
Insulin			x		Not absorbed
ACTH			x		Not absorbed
Epinephrine			x		Not absorbed
Narcotics					
Codeine			x		In usual doses
Meperedine (Demerol)				x	
Morphine			x		Low infant levels on usual dosage

† Controversy in literature; long-term effects uncertain; one case of gynecomastia

Appendix H-1. Drugs in Breast Milk (continued)

Drug or Agent	Contra-indicated	R$_x$ With Caution	No Apparent Harm	Insufficient Information	Comment
Narcotics					
Heroin	x				Addiction, withdrawal in infants
Methadone		x			Minimal levels
Psychotherapeutic Drugs					
Lithium	x				High levels in milk
Phenothiazines		x			Drowsiness; chronic effects uncertain
Tricyclic antidepressants				x	Low levels; effects uncertain
Diazepam (Valium)	x				Lethargy, wt. loss, EEG changes
Meprobamate (Equamil)	x				High levels in milk
Chlordiazepoxide (Librium)			x		Low levels in milk
Radiopharmaceuticals					
^{131}I	x				72 hr, no breast feeding
Technetium (99M Tc)	x				48 hr, no breast feeding
^{131}I albumin	x				10 days, no breast feeding
Sedatives-hypnotics					
Barbiturates		x			Short-acting less depressant
Chloral hydrate		x			Drowsiness
Bromides	x				Depression, rash
Diazepam (Valium)	x				Depression, wt. loss
Flurazepam (Dalmane)				x	Chemically related to diazepam
Nitrazepam				x	
Social-recreational Drugs					
Alcohol			x		Milk levels equal plasma, moderate consumption apparently safe, high levels inhibit lactation
Caffeine			x		Jitteriness with very high intakes
Nicotine			x		Low levels in milk
Marijuana			x		Minimal passage in milk
Miscellaneous					
Atropine		x			May cause constipation or inhibit lactation
Dihydrotachysterol		x			Renal calcification in animals

2. NEONATAL PHARMACOPOEIA

Appendix H-2. Neonatal Drug Dosages

(Note: Dosages in this table are single dose per kilogram. Frequency is suggested in next column, but may vary with maturity and rate of metabolism.)

Drug	Dose/kg	Route and Frequency	Comments
Acetazolamide (Diamox)	Diuretic, 5 mg Glaucoma, 5 mg	PO or IV q24h PO q6–8h	May cause acidosis, K depletion
ACTH (aqueous)	1 mg (1 unit)	IM q6h	Steroid complications
Adrenalin (epinephrine)	0.1–0.5 ml 1:10,000 aqueous solution (prepare dilution from 1:1000)	Repeat in 2–4h prn SC, IV, or intracardiac. Drip 0.5 μg/kg/min	Higher dosage is for cardiac resuscitation
Albumin (5%)	1.0 g (20 ml)	IV, slowly	Avoid circulatory overload
Amikacin	Loading 10 mg Maintenance 7.5 mg	IM, IV q12h	Nephro-, ototoxicity
Aminophylline	Loading 3–5 mg Maintenance 2 mg	IV, PO Maintenance q8–12h	Monitor blood levels (10–15 μg/ml) tachycardia, distention GI hemorrhage, seizures
Amoxicillin	7–10 mg	PO q8h	Like ampicillin
Amphotericin B	0.25–1.0 mg test dose 0.1 mg	IV by slow drip daily; dilute 1 mg/10 ml	Flushing, febrile reactions; nephrotoxic, hypokalemia ?CNS in high dose
Ampicillin	Sepsis 50 mg Meningitis 100–150 mg	IM or IV First week q12h thereafter q8h First wk q12h thereafter q8h	
Atropine sulfate dilute to 0.1 mg/ml	0.01–0.02 mg	SC q2h prn; resusc.-IV or endotracheal	May cause hyperthermia, urinary retention, tachycardia
Bacitracin	500 units	IM or IV q12h	Nephrotoxic, resistant organisms only
Belladonna tincture	0.1 ml (0.03 mg atropine)	PO q4h	Hyperthermia, flushing, dry secretions
Bicarbonate dilute to 0.5 mmol/ml	1–2 meq Maximum 7 mmol/24 hr	Increase cautiously to flushing push < 1 mmol/min	Transient hyperosmolarity; alkalosis. Must hyperventilate ($CO_2\uparrow$)

Drug	Dose/kg	Route and Frequency	Comments
Caffeine citrate	Loading 20 mg Maintenance 5 mg	Daily maintenance begins after 48h, IV or PO	Monitor blood levels, tachycardia, abdominal distention, seizures.
Calcium gluconate solution (9% calcium)	Therapeutic 125–250 mg	IV q6h PO q6h	Bradycardia, slough if infiltrated, gastric irritation, potentiates digitalis (slow IV infusion only)
Calcium lactate solution (13% calcium)	125 mg	PO q6h	Gastric irritation, potentiates digitalis
Calcium chloride solution (10% calcium)	75 mg Resuscitation 20 mg	PO q6h Slow IV push	Gastric irritation, potentiates digitalis
Carbenicillin	First week 75 mg, thereafter 100 mg	IM or IV; prematures first week q8h; all others q6h	Slough with infiltrate; hypernatremia
Cephalothin Na (Keflin)	25 mg	IV q6h	Nephrotoxicity, neutropenia, allergic rash, false pos. Coombs, poor passage blood-brain barrier
Chloral hydrate	Sedative 25 mg hypnotic 50 mg	PO or PR	Gastric infiltration, paradoxical excitement
Chloramphenicol (Chloromycetin)	25 mg	IV or PO <1.5 kg or < 6 wks qd >1.5 kg or > 6 wks q12h > 3.0 kg or > 8 wks q6h	High blood levels with poor excretion may cause "gray syndrome" Monitor blood levels (10–20 μg/ml) Potentiates Dilantin
Chlorpromazine (see Thorazine)			
Chlorthiazide (Diuril)	10–15 mg	PO q12h	K depletion, hyperglycemia
Cholestyramine (Questran)	1 g (total, not per kg)	PO q4–6h with feedings	Steatorrhea, GI dysfunction, malabsorption fat soluble vitamins, binds other drugs, Metabolic acidosis
Clindamycin (Cleocin)	5–10 mg	IM or IV q6h	GI toxicity if given PO (*Continued*)

Appendix H-2. Neonatal Drug Dosages. (continued)

Drug	Dose/kg	Route and Frequency	Comments
Colistin (Colistimethate)	2.5 mg	IM q12h first week, q8h there-after	Nephrotoxic
Cortisone	Replacement: 0.25 mg Pharmacologic: 2.5 mg	PO q6h	Infection; hypertension; salt retention; adrenal suppression
Desoxycorticosterone acetate (DOCA)	1 mg	IM q24h	Dose adjusted according to serum electrolyte determination
Dexamethasone (Decadron)	0.1 mg	PO or IV q6–8h loading dose 0.2–0.5 mg)	Infection; hypertension; salt retention; adrenal suppression
Dextran (low molecular wt) (10% solution)	Up to 2 g	IV q24h	Avoid circulatory overload
Diazepam (Valium)	Status seizures 0.1–0.3 mg	IV by slow push not above 2 mg/24h	Na benzoate vehicle displaces bilirubin from albumin
Diazoxide (Hyperstat)	5 mg	IV push, repeat q4–8h or prn	Na and water retention; hypotension; hyperglycemia
Dicloxacillin	4–8 mg	PO q6h	Penicillin sensitivity
Digoxin (Elixir, 0.05 mg/ml; Injection, 1 ml ampule, 0.1 mg/ml)	Oral digitalizing: preterm 0.03–0.04 mg term 0.05 mg maintenance 0.005 mg IV or IM digitalizing: preterm 0.02–0.03 mg term 0.04 mg maintenance 0.004	Initial digitalizing: ½ dose stat ¼ dose in 6h ¼ dose in 12h prn Maintenance dose q12h	Toxicity: bradycardia, PVCs, vomiting, poor feeding, arrhythmias; Check ECG trace during digitalization and periodically
Dopamine	10 μg/min (5–20 according to effect)	IV drip	Monitor blood pressure and pulse pressure; pulmonary hypertension
Edrophonium (see Tensilon)			
Epinephrine racemic (see also Adrenalin)	1:100 aqueous solution 0.25 ml total dose in 3 ml distilled H_2O	Inhaled by nebulizer q4h prn	Overdose: tachycardia, arrhythmia
Erythromycin	5 mg	IV or PO q6h	IV solution unstable; antagonist with clindamycin; may potentiate theophylline

Drug	Dose/kg	Route and Frequency	Comments
Ethacrynic acid (Edecrin)	1 mg	PO or IV over 5–10 min; repeat q8h prn	Na, K depletion; may be oto-toxic with aminoglycosides
Fibrinogen	50 mg	IV; repeat prn	
Furosemide (Lasix)	1–3 mg	PO, IM, or IV over 3 min; repeat q8h prn	Na, K depletion; dehydration, oxotoxicity with aminogly-cosides
Gentamicin	2.5 mg	IM first wk q12h, thereafter q8h	Renal and 8th nerve toxicity in adults
Gentian violet	1% solution	Topically q12h	Messy
Glucagon	50–100 μg	IM q6–12h prn	Rebound hypoglycemia
Heparin	100 units	IV q4h prn	Follow clotting time
Hydralazine (Apresoline)	0.5 mg	PO, IM, or IV q4–6h	Tachycardia, hypotension
Hydrocortisone (Solu-cortef)	2.5 mg	PO, IM, or IV q6h	Infection; hypertension, salt retention, adrenal suppres-sion
	Shock: 25 mg	IV stat	
Indomethacin (Indocin)	0.2 mg	IV or PO may repeat q12h × 3	Renal toxicity, liver, ↓ platelet aggregation
Insulin	Diabetic acidosis: 1 unit	SC q4h prn (taper with im-provement)	Hypoglycemia; follow blood sugar closely
	Massive glycosuria with IV alimentation: ¼ unit	SC q6h prn (titrate blood sugar)	
	Hyperkalemia: ¼ unit		
Isoniazid	10 mg	PO q24h	With IV glucose 1–2 g
			B₆ depletion; liver damage
Isoproterenol (Isuprel)	0.05–0.1 μg/min	IV, slow infusion of dilute so-lution (1–5 μg/ml)	Follow heart rate; arrhythmia with overdose; hypotension
Kanamycin	7.5 mg	IM < 7d, q12h; > 7d, q8h	Renal and 8th nerve toxicity
Kayexalate	1 g (as 25% solution)	PO or PR repeat q6h prn	Follow serum electrolytes
Lidocaine	1–2 mg	IV over 5 min	Hypotension
Magnesium sulfate	0.2 ml of 50% solution	IM q12h to max. 3 doses	Hypotension; depression
Mannitol	0.25–0.5 g (as 15–20% solu-tion)	IV in 30–60 min repeat 8–12h prn	Rebound edema; circulatory overload
Meperedine (Demerol)	1 mg	PO or IM q4h prn	CNS depression
Methicillin (Staphcillin)	Under 2 wks: 50 mg	IV, IM q12h	Penicillin allergy
	Over 2 wks: 50–75 mg	IV, IM q6h	*(Continued)*

Appendix H-2. Neonatal Drug Dosages. (continued)

Drug	Dose/kg	Route and Frequency	Comments
Methyldopa (Aldomet)	2.5–5 mg	PO or IV q8h Increase gradually prn	Hemolytic anemia, positive Coombs, liver damage, hypotension
Methylene blue (1% solution)	1–2 mg	IV slowly	Reducing agent: may ↓ hemoglobin O_2 capacity
Morphine sulfate	0.1 mg	SC q4–6h prn	Depression antidote: naloxone HCl (Narcan) 0.005 mg/kg
Mycostatin	100,000–200,000 units total dose	PO q6h	
Naloxone HCl (Narcan)	0.005–0.01 mg	IM or IV stat, repeat prn	
Neomycin	12.5–25 mg	PO q6h	Nephrotoxic if absorbed
Neostigmine	Myasthenia test: 0.04 mg	IM stat	Cardiac arrhythmia (atropine antidote)
Nitroprusside	Maintenance: 0.5 mg 1–8 μg/min	PO q6h IV drip	Hypotension; cyanide toxicity (hemoglobin binding); tachyphylaxis; photodegradation of drug
Oxacillin (Prostaphlin)	Under 2 wks: 50 mg Over 2 wks: 50–75 mg	IV, IM q12h IV, IM q6h	Penicillin sensitivity
Pancuronium Br (Pavulon)	0–7d, 40 μg 7–21d, 60 μg >21d, 90 μg	IV, repeat prn	Voluntary muscle paralysis; short half-life
Paraldehyde	0.15 ml	PO, PR, IM q4–6h prn IV, 4% solution (titrate drip rate)	Depression with overdose; use fresh q24h; avoid plastic containers; photodecomposition
Penicillin (aqueous)	First wk: 50,000 units After first week: 50,000 units Group B Strep 100,000 units Meningitis 150,000 units	IV or IM q12h IV or IM q6–8h q6h q6h	
Phenobarbital	Status: 15–20 mg Maintenance 1–2 mg	IM or IV stat IM, PO q8h	Depression with overdose; blood levels (20–40 μg/ml)

Drug	Dose/kg	Route and Frequency	Comments
Phenytoin (Diphenylhydantoin) (Dilantin)	Load: 15 mg Maintenance: 1–3 mg	IV stat PO or IV q8h	Blood levels (5–20 μg/ml) bone marrow depression
Pitressin (aqueous 20 units/ml)	0.3–1.0 ml total dose	SC q8h	Fluid overload, electrolyte imbalance
Polymyxin B	1.0 mg Intrathecal 1 mg total dose	IM, IV q8h Intrathecal q24h × 3–5	Nephrotoxic; neurotoxic
Potassium (Potassium Triplex 3 mmol/ml)	0.7 mmol	PO q8h	
Prednisone	0.5 mg	PO q6h	Infection; hypertension; salt retention; adrenal suppression
Propanolol	0.05–0.15 mg	½ IV stat, repeat prn in 2 min	Atropine for excess bradycardia
Protamine sulfate	Maintenance 0.2–0.5 mg 1 mg/mg heparin in past 4 h	PO q6h IV stat	
Pyrimethamine (Daraprim)	0.5–1.0 mg	IV q24h	Folic acid deficiency; bone marrow depression
Pyridoxine (vitamin B$_6$)	Therapeutic: 2–5 mg total	PO q24h	
	Dependency: 50 mg (total)	IV stat PO maintenance	
Quinidine	4–10 mg	PO q6h	Discontinue if QRS interval > 0.10 sec
Spironolactone (Aldactone)	0.5–1.0 mg	PO q8h	Avoid in hyperkalemia Contraindicated in renal failure
Sulfadiazine	25 mg	PO q6h	Contraindicated first 3 weeks or in presence of jaundice
	15 mg	IV q6h	Contraindicated first 3 weeks or in presence of jaundice
Sulfisoxazole (Gantrisin)	25 mg	PO q6h	
	75 mg	SC q12h	
Tensilon (Edrophonium)	Test for myasthenia: 0.5 mg (See Chap. 29)	SC or IM stat	
THAM (tris-hydroxy-methylamino methane) (0.3M soln)	Equivalent acid buffering to equal mmol of NaHCO$_3$)	IV over several minutes, central vessel	Hypoglycemia; apnea; hyperkalemia; sclerosing
Thorazine (Chlorpromazine)	0.5 mg	IV, IM, PO q6-8h	hypotension hypothermia
Thyroxine	(See Chap. 44)		
Thyroid extract	(See Chap. 44)		

(Continued)

Appendix H-2. Neonatal Drug Dosages. (continued)

Drug	Dose/kg	Route and Frequency	Comments
Ticarcillin	Loading: 100 mg First wk: 75 mg Thereafter: 100 mg	IV stat IM q6–8h IM q4–6h	Hypernatremia Bleeding problems
Tobramycin	2.0 mg	First week: IM q12h Thereafter: IM q8h	Renal and ototoxicity
Tolazoline (Priscoline)	Test dose: 1 mg Maintenance: 1–2 mg/hr	IV (10 min) IV drip	Hypotension; GI hemorrhage; may have paradoxical further hypotension with dopamine (R$_x$ Ephedrine drip, 2 μg/kg/min)
Tubocurarine Cl (Curare)	0.3–0.6 mg	IV push, repeat prn	Hypotension; histamine-like effect Voluntary muscle paralysis
Vitamin K$_1$ oxide	Prevention: total dose 0.5–1.0 mg Therapy: 2.5–5.0 mg	Single dose IM Repeat q6–12h prn	Follow prothrombin time

Index